SIXTH EDITION

ESSENTIALS
OF MANAGED
HEALTH CARE

Peter R. Kongstvedt, MD, FACP

Senior Health Policy Faculty
Department of Health Administration and Policy
George Mason University
Fairfax, VA

Principal, P.R. Kongstvedt Company, LLC
McLean, VA

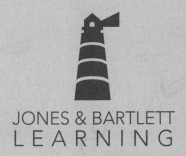

JONES & BARTLETT
LEARNING

World Headquarters
Jones & Bartlett Learning
5 Wall Street
Burlington, MA 01803
978-443-5000
info@jblearning.com
www.jblearning.com

Jones & Bartlett Learning books and products are available through most bookstores and online booksellers. To contact Jones & Bartlett Learning directly, call 800-832-0034, fax 978-443-8000, or visit our website, www.jblearning.com.

Substantial discounts on bulk quantities of Jones & Bartlett Learning publications are available to corporations, professional associations, and other qualified organizations. For details and specific discount information, contact the special sales department at Jones & Bartlett Learning via the above contact information or send an email to specialsales@jblearning.com.

Production Credits
Publisher: Michael Brown
Managing Editor: Maro Gartside
Editorial Assistant: Kayla Dos Santos
Editorial Assistant: Chloe Falivene
Production Assistant: Rebekah Linga
Senior Marketing Manager: Sophie Fleck Teague
Manufacturing and Inventory Control Supervisor: Amy Bacus
Composition: Laserwords Private Limited, Chennai, India
Cover Design: Kristin E. Parker
Cover Image: © Barauskaite/ShutterStock, Inc.
Printing and Binding: Courier Kendallville
Cover Printing: Courier Kendallville

To order this product, use ISBN: 978-1-4496-5331-6

Library of Congress Cataloging-in-Publication Data
Essentials of managed health care / [edited by] Peter R. Kongstvedt.—6th ed.
p. ; cm.
  Rev. ed. of: Essentials of managed health care / edited by Peter R. Kongstvedt. 5th ed. c2007.
Includes bibliographical references and index.
  ISBN-13: 978-1-4496-0464-6 (pbk.)
  ISBN-10: 1-4496-0464-1 (pbk.)
  I. Kongstvedt, Peter R. (Peter Reid) II. Essentials of managed health care.
  [DNLM: 1. Managed Care Programs—organization & administration—United States. 2. Delivery of Health Care—economics—United States. W 130 AA1]
  362.1´04258—dc23

2011044614

6048

Printed in the United States of America
16 15 14 13 12   10 9 8 7 6 5 4 3 2

Contents

Introduction

The sixth edition of *Essentials of Managed Health Care* is the most significant structural overhaul since the second edition morphed into the third back in 1996. And while it is a hefty volume at just under a half a million words, it remains svelte in comparison to the fourth and, as of 2001 the last edition of its antecedent, *The Managed Health Care Handbook*, which was three times the size. This does not reflect a shrinking healthcare sector nor a movement from complexity to simplicity, since neither is the case. It does reflect the commitment of the book's contributors to providing a broad and sufficiently detailed overview of the key elements of health insurance and managed health care to meet the needs of one or more of its types of readers. At the same time, it means that some things are left out. As the editor, I bear full responsibility for any decisions about what to include and what to exclude, as well as any errors that may be contained in this text.

■ WHO BENEFITS FROM THIS BOOK

This book is much like the original Swiss Army Knife® designed by Karl Elsener in 1891, which had a cutting blade, a screwdriver, a can opener, and a reamer (or awl).[1] That tool served four different purposes depending on the needs of the user, and this book also serves four different purposes, depending on the needs of the reader. Unlike the knife, however, there is considerable overlap in how those purposes are served. The four primary users of this book also overlap in many ways, and are loosely categorized next.

Teaching and Academics

This represents the largest number of users, but there are differences in how it might be used in a graduate program. Some topics will be of considerable use for classroom teaching, such as the chapters on history, the types of payers and integrated health systems, network structure, payment, care management, and so forth. But even the operational chapters can be useful since even now it is easier to think we know how these things are done and why, when in fact what we "know" are assumptions, not reality.

Day-to-Day Payer Operations and Administration

Those who work in the payer industry or in other industries that provide services to payers benefit the most from those chapters that focus on operations. As becomes quickly apparent, all operations are interconnected and what affects one part of a payer organization often ripples out to exert an effect on other parts. For example, errors in eligibility affect claims payment, provider services, consumer services, and financial management. Beyond the "tab A goes into slot B" descriptions of operational business processes, knowing as well the background about why operations are carried out as they are will go a long way in understanding the business as a whole. This is especially the case for those in management, where understanding the whole is a requirement for assuming greater responsibilities.

Health Policy

Certain sections of the book are right in the middle of the world of health policy, and overlap with those most useful in academics and teaching. But the book provides something else, something often missing in health policy resources, and that's a picture of what this sector actually looks like *as a whole*. Policy and theory are valuable and critical for our future, but policy that ignores the incredibly messy and complex reality of the sector, or that is built upon assumptions that are "widely understood" but are in fact thoroughly misunderstood, will produce elegant but ultimately useless results—much like a hand-carved, solid walnut SCUBA tank. The systems and operational processes we have today were not found under a loose board; they all came about in direct or indirect response to policy decisions, including policy omissions, whether intended or not.

Health Administration

Those who are preparing to enter the world of health administration or are already working in it, regardless of type of provider, public health or private, and whose organization in any meaningful way interacts with commercial payers will benefit from knowing how payers actually operate, why they do what they do, and under what circumstances. Just as there is great heterogeneity in types of providers and provider organizations, even when they fall under the same descriptive type, there is equal heterogeneity not only between payers but between the different business units within any payer organization. By understanding the payer environment better, and knowing at least the basics of certain operations, legal requirements, and constraints, the business-to-business relationship has a better chance of working at least a little better.

There is another reason for those in health administration to know more about the payer sector, and that is the continually evolving sector itself. At the height of the managed healthcare boom in the late 1980s through the late 1990s, providers sought to take on more risk, and even to "cut out the middle man." Many did not survive that decision, although some did quite well. Those times are not likely to be repeated, but recently we've seen a stronger push to make providers more accountable for costs, and costs are related to risk.

Health systems, especially those with regional market strength and those that now employ a large number of physicians, have been able to negotiate higher prices and not worry much about cost control. That is ultimately an unsustainable model, though, and with Medicare leading the charge, the flow of money will over time be affected more and more by overall performance (which is not the same as pay for performance, discussed in Chapter 5). And it is managed healthcare methodologies that will be used to do it, even if they are referred to under a kinder and gentler name.

Others Who May Benefit

The book has been useful beyond the four primary constituencies noted previously. The legal profession has often turned to it to be better informed both in matters involving litigation or arbitration, and in constructing legal agreements that encompass specific operational aspects between a payer and other parties. Regulators have also used the book, particularly when looking at regulations with a potential impact beyond the intended target. Journalists and nonacademic writers may turn to it to gain a better understanding of some aspect of the industry that is the subject of an article or story. It is fair to say that the book has been used by individuals in all parts of the health sector, not just those noted here. It has also been used in a number of other nations around the globe as they look to addressing issues similar to our own, even if their overall system differs.

■ HOW THIS BOOK IS STRUCTURED

The book has 30 chapters, divided into six parts.

Part I: Introduction to Health Insurance and Managed Health Care

The three chapters that open the book provide a broad overview of the historical roots of health insurance and managed health care in the United States; the different types of insurers, managed care organizations, and integrated delivery systems; and their basic governance and management structure. They are all updates of prior versions, but the updates found in the first two of these are considerable.

Part II: Network Contracting and Provider Payment

Part II underwent a major structural overhaul for this edition, and is composed of three long chapters that describe in some detail how payer networks are structured; the astonishing array of provider payment methodologies and payment modifiers, and how different providers respond to them; and the core structural elements of a contract between a payer and a provider that support all of those elements. These topics no longer completely separate facilities, professionals, and ancillary services, but look at common elements first, and those specific to type of provider second. It also separates payment from all the other aspects of network development, structure, and management in order to keep the focus on each. The content within each chapter has been updated as appropriate, and expanded considerably to address new elements and new dynamics because when it comes to payment, we are all endlessly inventive. Finally, the chapters may address these topics from a payer point of view, but in our currently evolving system, much of what they cover may migrate to new types of organizations, including provider organizations.

Part III: Management of Utilization and Quality

Along with Part II, Part III makes up what is generally considered to be managed health care. It addresses basic utilization management (UM), a topic that has been significantly restructured and expanded in order to illuminate the varied elements of UM that are interconnected, but often treated as though they are not. Part III also addresses the more advanced and specialized forms of UM, including those focused on specific types of utilization such as behavioral health and the prescription drug benefit.

Part III also sees a new contributor addressing a topic that last appeared in the fourth edition, which is changing physician behavior, something that has taken on renewed relevance as physicians are employed increasingly by health systems and payers. It concludes with a chapter focusing on quality management (QM) in payer organizations and on accreditation of health plans and related services, something that is tied deeply to QM.

As in Part II, the topics are addressed from a payer point of view, but they all are relevant to providers and others as our system evolves and greater accountability—and financial performance—are diffused out into the health sector.

Part IV: Sales, Finance, and Administration

The eight chapters of Part IV are the most operationally oriented chapters in the book, describing the nuts and bolts of nonclinical administration. It also includes two entirely new topics never before addressed in this book: enrollment and billing, and fraud and abuse. The chapter on information technology has been completely rewritten and expanded in scope to better cover multiple elements of what can only be described as the backbone of any payer organization. The material covered in this section may not make up the bulk of the book, but these chapters describe what makes up the bulk of all payer operations.

Part V: Special Markets

Where the book overall looks at the why and how of managed care, Part V looks at four specific and unique market segments for payers, which are health plans and Medicare, managed Medicaid, military managed health care, and managed health care in a global setting. Of particular importance, the chapters on health plans and Medicare and Medicaid managed health care have been completely rewritten by new authors, and both are expansive in scope to address all of the most important elements of managed health care in those programs.

Part VI: Laws and Regulations

The three chapters here have been entirely rewritten by a new author, and provide a succinct review of the state and federal legal and regulatory underpinnings affecting health insurance and managed health care, including the Patient Protection and Affordable Care Act (ACA), a law passed but not yet fully implemented at the time this is being written. At nearly 1,000 pages, the ACA affects all health sectors, but its impact on health insurers and health benefits plans is far greater than its impact on any other sector, so that chapter is confined to just those portions of the ACA.

■ WHERE TO FIND CURRENT INFORMATION

Before this book is even printed, something in it will be outdated. The topic at greatest risk for this is the ACA, but it can and does occur for other topics as well. Even when the basic information does not change, metrics and other data do. Rather than attempt to provide individual sources for updated information, data, and analyses here, they are all available through a page on my website devoted to useful links, where you can find a brief description of each useful website as well as an active link. If you find any of those links to be dead or now redirected, please contact me at the e-mail address provided on that page.

The Useful Links page may be accessed at www.kongstvedt.com/useful_urls.html.

■ ACKNOWLEDGMENTS

My appreciation and thanks go first to Dr. P.J. Maddox, Chair, Department of Health Administration and Policy, College of Health and Human Services, George Mason University here in northern Virginia for her support of my efforts with the book and within the department overall.

I also want to acknowledge Tracy Immel, my graduate research assistant at George Mason University, for working to add to the store of information used to update my own chapters, as well as helping to pull together many of the varied structural elements needed for the book as a whole.

I also wish to thank the following individuals who provided their insights or otherwise supported the creation of this edition: Sorin Davis; Jeff Emerson; Richard Frye; Joe Gifford, MD; Paul Marchetti; Julie Mascari; Lawrence R. Muroff, MD; Joshua Raskin; Andy Reynolds; and Miranda Woolston.

It is no hyperbole to express my deepest thanks and appreciation to my wife Emily and my stepsons Aaron and Benjamin for not only resisting the justifiable and well-deserved urge to regularly beat me with sticks, but to actually support me in a hundred different ways. It is one thing to read *Dr. Jekyll and Mr. Hyde*, it is quite another to live with Mr. Hyde for the 6 months in which Dr. Jekyll vanished without a trace. Fortunately, he's back, albeit with his arm in a sling, a glazed look in his eyes, and a noticeable limp.

Finally, thank you. If you were not reading this book, or at least those parts of it that you find valuable enough to take the time to read, there would be no reason to write this Introduction and write or edit the half a million words that now follow. Thanks again, and don't be a stranger.

Peter R. Kongstvedt

Endnote

1. www.victorinox.com/us/content/history_page. Accessed October 18, 2011.

Preface

Is Health Insurance?

PETER R. KONGSTVEDT

The easy answer is mostly no. For one thing, as discussed in Chapter 2, the majority of individuals covered under commercial health benefits plans are in employer self-funded plans, not in fully insured benefits plans. But that is a technical distinction, and while it is important for several reasons that are addressed in the book, it is not the reason to ask the question, "Is health insurance?" The reason to ask it is to illuminate the underlying dynamics in health insurance in order to better make sense of it. Because on its surface it looks like chaos—which it is*—but it is also a very rational system, although not always rational in a good way.

For half a century, the cost of health insurance has stubbornly increased faster than the general rate of inflation. There are myriad reasons why this occurs, many of which are addressed in Parts II and III of the book as well as extensively in published articles.[1] But there are also attributes intrinsic to health insurance itself that contribute to cost inflation. But it is not profits. As shown in Chapter 5, margins for health insurers and hospitals are nearly the same, and well below other health sector industries. One can argue about health insurer profit motives, but it is now moot. As discussed in Chapters 21 and 30, the Patient Protection and Affordable Care Act (ACA) singled out the health insurance industry to control profits indirectly through minimum medical loss ratio requirements, allowing only a narrow margin for administration, marketing, and profits.

These intrinsic attributes are directly related to its being treated as insurance in the first place. All insurers face these attributes all the time, regardless of type of insurance such as property/casualty, life, annuity, and health insurance. All have developed methods to reduce their impact on cost increases, although health insurers have been more limited than other types of insurers and will be markedly limited under the ACA.

Going under the semantically misleading terms "moral hazard" and "inherent vice," these interrelated principles are not difficult to understand in isolation, though regrettably they are often approached that way. But they do not exist in isolation; they exist as a set of related but differing expressions. Moral hazard and inherent vice are not totally ignored in the ACA, but there is considerable variation in what and how effectively they are addressed.

In his landmark 1963 paper, economist and Nobel laureate Kenneth Arrow addressed moral hazard and its application to health insurance, including the pooling of unequal risks, asymmetric knowledge, and issues of trust and delegation.[2] Writing before the passage of Medicare and Medicaid, Arrow argued that the lack of a truly competitive market for health insurance (i.e., no market to insure sick older adults and poor people) means society must fill the void. Two years later, economist Mark Pauly argued that the existence of health insurance must lead to an increase in demand as the direct cost to an individual of an episode of care goes down, and that some things are simply not insurable.[3]

Since then, moral hazard has traditionally been the domain of economists, and they have written extensively on the topic, including further excellent detailed discussions specifically about health insurance.[4] But it is important for noneconomists to understand the concepts as well, particularly for those involved in health policy. The goal of this preface therefore is to illustrate the core concepts of moral hazard and inherent vice as applied to health insurance now and under the ACA, and to do so using plain English, without the use of such terms as price elasticity, welfare losses, marginal utility, or redistributive policy. And there will be no math.

■ MORAL HAZARD

Moral hazard is not a synonym for Las Vegas or the wages of sin. It is usually thought of that way when discussed in the popular press,[5] but it actually has nothing to do with morals as we commonly use the term. It's uncertain when it first came into use, although several researchers found publications from the 19th century associating it with good and bad behavior, such as a person who deliberately burns down an insured building.[6] Others also placed it in

---

*In the sense that the entire health sector conforms to complexly adapting systems theory, also known as chaos theory, which is why pundits must continually rewrite speeches about what the future will hold for the healthcare sector.

the 19th century, but only through recognition that having insurance can itself create a motive to behave differently.[7]

Still others, including this author, believe it appeared earlier, perhaps as early as the 18th century, with the word "moral" referring only to a state of mind.[8] This is similar to one aspect of its current definition in the *Oxford English Dictionary* as "...psychological rather than physical or practical: *moral support.*"[9] The word "hazard" may have referred to the familiar definition of "...a danger or risk," but it's more likely it referred to a popular form of gambling, a dice game called "hazard" that is a forerunner of today's craps.[10] This is further supported by the origin of the word "hazard" from the "...old French *hasard*, from Persian or Turkish, 'dice'."[11] In other words, moral hazard means the outcome is influenced more by the insured's state of mind than by the random chance of a roll of the dice.

In simplest terms, moral hazard means that the presence of insurance changes the behavior of the insured party in a way that increases an insurer's risk because the insured party no longer bears the full cost. For example, a shipping company that is fully insured may be more willing to order its ships to sail through pirate-infested waters because quicker arrival means more profit, but losses to pirates are covered by the insurer, at least until such time as the insurer wises up and boosts the premium.

Beyond this general concept, the expression of moral hazard is seen in four interrelated ways. While each is an expression of a single principal, it is highly instructive to examine all four separately, since addressing one does not equate to addressing them all, and ameliorating one does not ameliorate the others. They are:

- The pooling of unequal risks,
- Asymmetric knowledge and purchasing behavior,
- Induced demand (which has two expressions), and
- The agent–principal problem.

Inherent vice is similar in concept and related to moral hazard, but it refers to physical properties rather than direct behaviors, so it is discussed separately.

The Pooling of Unequal Risks

In an ideal insurance market, all who are insured in a single risk pool have an equal risk of incurring losses. While a perfect market does not exist for any type of insurance, insurers typically identify substantial risk differences and place customers into risk-similar pools; for example, individuals with poor driving records are in a higher risk pool and pay more for their auto insurance, or a malpractice carrier will place all neurosurgeons in a state into a different risk pool than it will place family physicians. In this way, the cost of insurance is related to the level of risk. If significantly unequal risks are pooled, premium costs go up for lower-risk individuals or groups, and they are more likely to exit the risk pool altogether.

Insurers also avoid pooling unequal risks by simply refusing to insure high-risk individuals or organizations. For example, a life insurance company typically will not insure the life of somebody with widespread cancer, or a property/casualty insurer will not insure a coastal home built on a sandbar jutting into the Atlantic.

In health insurance, unequal risk may be separated through age-banding (younger people are in a different risk pool than older people) or categories of products (e.g., a very costly high-risk pool for individuals with high health needs). Experience rating is another way of separating unequal risks, in which employer groups with high costs also have higher premiums. Medical underwriting is another way health insurers avoid pooling unequal risk by not insuring high-risk individuals.

Beginning in 2014, the ACA requires complete pooling of unequal risks in the small group and individual markets, and insurers must charge the same premium rates to individuals or to small employer groups whether they purchase through an exchange or a broker or through direct sales.* Many states have required community rating for small groups for many years, so that is not different. Risk pools for individuals and small groups are not comingled, however, unless a state chooses to do so. Any insurer's risk pool may be sicker or healthier on average, but the exchange will be able to offset this through risk adjusters to premiums. The ACA also creates temporary risk corridors for insurers in an exchange, giving them a few years to address disparities.

The ACA does allow some age-banding for individuals, but limits it to a threefold difference, not eight or tenfold differences found today. This will necessarily increase the premium cost to younger and healthier individuals. The ACA recognizes this by allowing for a less expensive high-deductible "catastrophic" plan with preventive benefits and a small number of office visits for individuals under the age of 30.

The real impact of the ACA on the pooling of unequal risk is guaranteed issue, meaning an insurer must sell coverage to any individual or group that wants it, meaning the least insurable individuals or groups will now be able to have coverage, and for individuals and small groups at least, pay the same price as everyone else. This is a laudable goal, but it also means higher premium costs, which in turn affects purchasing behavior, discussed next.

Asymmetric Knowledge and Purchasing Behavior

Asymmetric knowledge means that one party, the insured, knows something that the other party, the insurer, does not know. The first place this occurs is the decision to purchase insurance. Because the decision to purchase occurs before coverage is in effect, this type of moral hazard is sometimes

---

* All of the elements in the ACA discussed in this Preface are described in detail in Chapter 30 as well as throughout the book.

referred to as "ex ante," meaning "before the event." The other three expressions of moral hazard are referred to as "ex post," meaning after the event.

To illustrate this, imagine an 18th century shipping company learns of an increased density of Jolly Rogers in the Caribbean. The company buys insurance but does not tell the insurer about seeing the pirates and thus obtains a favorable rate because the insurer is unaware of the recent increase in risk. This concept is equally applicable to chronically heightened risk such as driving a truck load of unstable nitroglycerin across rough terrain, or to a single event such as wrecking your car yesterday or a recent diagnosis of cancer.

All insurers address this in several ways. Underwriters require prospective customers to submit all relevant information to allow them to determine risk or even decline coverage. Policies are written to negate coverage if the insured failed to disclose relevant information. An insurer may also directly obtain it; for example, by inspecting ship's logs, obtaining medical records as part of a life insurance evaluation, or requiring an applicant to undergo a physical examination. And coverage is almost never provided for anything occurring prior to applying for it; for example, no auto insurer is required to cover you for yesterday's car wreck. Health insurers accomplished this through medical underwriting by evaluating a group's prior claims or an individual's medical history.

The ACA will not prohibit medical underwriting for experience rating in large groups, but does prohibit rescissions and exclusions for preexisting conditions and, as already discussed, requires guaranteed issue regardless of medical condition. In other words, in 2014 health insurers lose all ability to reduce the impact of asymmetric knowledge except for calculating rates in large insured groups.

Combined with community premium rating requirements in the individual and small group markets, meaning no variations in rates, those facing high medical expenses will be able to buy health insurance for less than the cost of care. This is justifiably the most socially important aspect of the ACA, and has also been the most contentious. But as is now widely understood, if the only individuals or groups who purchase coverage are the sickest, their added high costs will accelerate premium cost inflation since more money goes out than comes in.

Worse, healthy individuals could afford to go without insurance until such time as they needed it, knowing they couldn't be turned down. Barely sustainable right now, the costs for the newly aggregated risk pool would rise so dramatically that it would rapidly become unsustainable, a dynamic that insurers refer to as a "death spiral."

To offset it, the ACA contains requirements on employers to offer coverage or face fines, with exemptions and subsidies for some. The ACA also has an individual "mandate," which, as a result of political compromise, is actually a structured series of modest and slowly increasing fines

for not having coverage. Some people would be exempt from these fines, and low-income individuals will receive subsidies.*

Purchasing behavior needn't be confined to an up-front decision by someone who is currently uninsured. The ACA will allow individuals (or employers) to opt in and back out of the insurance pool with no penalty beyond the fines. If there is no mechanism to prevent opting in and out at will, it sharply increases the impact of moral hazard on purchasing behavior. But the ACA allows each state to determine when an individual or small group may apply for and obtain guaranteed coverage, referring to special-enrollment periods as defined under the Employee Retirement Income Security Act (ERISA) as well as a general open-enrollment period. Should states use the strictest approach, meaning allowing purchase only after a qualifying event such as losing group coverage or getting married, and otherwise limit open enrollment to 1 month per year, this would offset this problem, but only for 11 months or less. A state allowing continuous open enrollment would actually encourage this form of moral hazard.

Professor Paul Starr of Princeton University suggested an alternative to an individual mandate, allowing individual adults to opt out without facing a fine, but doing so would subject them to exclusions on preexisting conditions for 5 years.[12] This may have mitigated the risk of this form of moral hazard more effectively than the relatively modest fines defined in the Act, although it is difficult to know how the two compare. Nevertheless, this or a similar concept may yet come into play.

Induced Demand

Induced demand means that having insurance actually encourages its use. The amount of induced demand varies widely, and most types of insurance have natural limits on induced demand. For example, moral hazard may lead a shipping company to be more willing to sail vessels through risky waters if they are insured, but not to the point of losing half their fleet. And absent felony fraud, the existence of homeowner's insurance does not induce people to burn their houses down. And generally speaking, induced demand in insurance is typically confined to a single or a few events.

Health insurance is exactly the opposite. Having health insurance may not induce you to break your leg, but it does result in increasing the amount of healthcare services received, and the less one pays out of pocket the more healthcare services are used.[13] This is not necessarily a bad thing since the uninsured do not get the care they need and suffer poorer outcomes. Also at some point, increasing

---

* At the time of publication, the individual "mandate" was the subject of conflicting judicial rulings, and the U.S. Supreme Court had not yet heard the case, so it may or may not be a moot point by the time you are reading this.

usage drives up costs while providing diminishing returns. But the heart of induced demand is this: you are supposed to use health insurance to pay for medical services on an ongoing basis, not just when you break your leg.

There are two distinct pathways for induced demand: demand induced by consumers and demand induced by providers. Consumer-induced demand is described here. Provider-induced demand, which is more important, is discussed in combination with the next form of moral hazard, called the agent–principal problem.

While there is no question that the existence of health insurance leads to an increase in consumers' demand for healthcare services, it is unclear how important that is. For example, consumer-induced demand is the precise focus of direct-to-consumer (DTC) advertising by pharmaceutical manufacturers. While there is evidence that DTC increases consumer demand,[14,15,16] it may be offset by physicians' advice.[17,18] Furthermore, as has been argued in the popular press,[19] except for a small number of troubled individuals, nobody really wants to go to the doctor to have a colonoscopy or get stuck with a needle. On the other hand, in today's medicalized society it is not uncommon for a patient to begin an office visit with a request for a diagnostic procedure. In the end, it is difficult to really gauge the impact of consumer-induced demand since a desire to avoid an unpleasant medical intervention must compete with a desire to be healthy.

One way insurers address induced demand is through cost-sharing via deductibles. Losses that are less than the deductible do not result in a claim, and a loss that is only slightly higher than the deductible is unlikely to generate a claim either. For example, if there was no deductible on an auto policy, car owners would have every scratch and ding removed.*

Health insurers do the same via copayments, coinsurance, and deductibles. This reaches its peak in high-deductible health plans (HDHPs), including consumer-directed health plans (CDHPs) with associated pretax funds, as described in Chapter 2. The new standardized benefits plans required under the ACA and described in Chapters 16 and 30 allow for the same significant level of cost-sharing as a typical CDHP, so little changes there.

Health insurers can also use a reduction in cost-sharing to deliberately induce demand, as does the ACA by removing cost-sharing for wellness and preventive care, with the deliberate goal of increasing consumer demand for prevention. Similar approaches to selectively increasing consumer demand have been used recently by insurers as well, using value-based insurance benefits design to lower economic barriers for preventive services, and sometimes for certain drugs and interventions in order to increase compliance in chronically ill individuals.[20]

_____
* They would also pay very high premiums!

The Agent–Principal Problem

This fourth major expression of moral hazard occurs when the financial interests of a principal's agent are not aligned with those of the principal and as a result, the agent's behavior may increase the principal's costs. Non–health insurers address this by requiring certain functions to be done by their own employees or an agent with aligned incentives. For example, a disability insurer might pay a private detective 10% of a recovered fraudulent payout, or an auto insurer will employ a damage assessor to determine exactly what repairs will be covered rather than having the body shop make that determination.

In health care, we typically think of physicians acting as their patients' agent, looking out for their patients' best interest. And that is certainly true, using the broad concept of an agent. In insurance, and in moral hazard in particular, the physician is also the *health insurer's* agent because the physician (or other professional, really) makes decisions that use the insurer's money. This is the result of the third-party payment system in which there is no alignment at all between the insurer's (the principal's) financial interests and those of the physician (the agent). It is made far worse by the fee-for-service (FFS) system that rewards providers for doing and charging more, at little perceived cost to themselves or their patients. It is also a primary reason physicians have turned away from relatively low-paid primary care and toward more highly paid procedure-based specialties.

The impact can be exacerbated by provider-induced demand. Not only does FFS reward providers for doing more, it rewards them for inducing demand that might not otherwise have existed. As discussed extensively in Chapters 5 and 7 for example, physician ownership of costly devices (e.g., cardiac imaging) is associated with significantly higher levels of utilization when compared to physicians with no ownership interest.

In health care, as prepayment to providers in early 20th century models gave way to insured products, alternate payment models such as capitation were designed to align incentives, but as HMOs declined in popularity, so did capitation. Prospective payment methods such as diagnosis-related groups (DRGs) were also designed to better align incentives, but as discussed in Chapter 5, charge-based outlier payment diminished its impact. Recent approaches such as shared savings and value-based payment for accountable care organizations (ACOs) are another example of attempts to realign incentives between the agent and the principal.

Health insurers, and HMOs in particular, also address the agent–principal problem through utilization management for the most costly types of clinical services. The use of clinical algorithms for precertification of coverage for elective procedures or high-cost drugs are examples, as is the capitated primary care gatekeeper model found in most HMOs, as discussed in Chapters 2 and 7. And on a broader basis, most large insurers use their claims database to look for patterns of regular overutilization, irregular billing, or other expressions of the agent–principal problem.

The ACA essentially ignores the agent–principal problem, except for a few provisions applicable to Medicare and Medicaid. It calls for the collection of hospital charge data, although it is not clear how that would differ from chargemaster data currently collected by Medicare, and the relationship between cost and charges in the chargemaster is loose, at best.[21] More encouraging is the creation of an Independent Advisory Board to provide recommendations to Congress on pricing, and which go into effect unless Congress passes legislation for an alternative with equivalent savings. But how such a board will operate is yet to be defined, and it is confined to Medicare, so will have little impact on commercial insurance except to further increase cost-shifting to private payers, as described in Chapter 5.

■ INHERENT VICE

Inherent vice is more than the title of Thomas Pynchon's fine 2009 novel.[22] Inherent vice is an insurance term used most often, but not exclusively, in marine insurance. It refers to an inherent physical property that may cause deterioration or damage, for example, rotting fruit, a truck full of unstable nitroglycerine, or 3 tons of metallic sodium on a leaky ship. Even if discovered after the policy has been issued, a marine insurer will not pay for losses incurred as a result of undisclosed or undetected inherent vice. Inherent vice is simply the other side of the moral hazard coin—where moral hazard refers to a willful behavior, inherent vice refers to a physical state (i.e., structure rather than process).

If it were confined to that, it would not be worth discussing. But inherent vice is a broader concept because life itself is ultimately a fatal condition. As we age, we accumulate more clinical events and conditions, even if we were perfectly healthy when we were first insured. At some point that risk passes from a commercial insurer to Medicare, but the underlying dynamics do not change.

Health insurers address inherent vice through several mechanisms. For reasons discussed earlier, all-or-none approaches such as medical underwriting, exclusions of pre-existing conditions, and rescissions may be used. Experience rating of groups at least partially reflects actual and predicted costs, but it doesn't work for individuals. The individual market therefore typically uses age-banding as a proxy for actual inherent vice, but this will be limited under the ACA.

Inherent vice also increases risk through real vice, for example, smoking, obesity, alcohol and drug abuse, reckless driving, and so forth. To its credit, the added risk caused by unhealthy behavior is recognized in the ACA, and a strong emphasis has been put on wellness and prevention, including in the benefits designs and funding for prevention programs. The ACA even addresses it in a way that is stronger than what is currently permitted by allowing for significant "incentives" for participation in preventive services. These incentives may take the form of premium contribution, in effect allowing for differences of up to 30% (or even 50% if allowed by the Secretary). Furthermore, premium rate adjustments of up to 1.5 for individuals and small groups will be allowed based on tobacco usage.

These measures will certainly improve health, but will not offset the increased risks created by removal of the more traditional approaches of medical underwriting and coverage limitations. In counterpoint, a recent analysis of prevention concluded that "less than 20 percent of the preventive options (and a similar percentage for treatment) fall in the cost-saving category—80 percent add more to medical costs than they save."[23] In this way, the effect of inherent vice on costs will actually be amplified. Prevention is important and the right thing to do, but not because it will lower costs.

■ INSURANCE VERSUS FINANCING

Moral hazard and inherent vice are insurance terms, and broadly speaking, insurance means indemnifying a person or company against unanticipated or unlikely financial losses from a one-time or rare event or cost, for example, a house fire, a sinking ship, or hurricane damage. It can also refer to premature loss or damage when the risks are highly predictable in large populations, for example, life, disability, and long-term care insurance.

Conversely, services that are used repeatedly are often financed, even if their use varies by individual. In some cases, this is through taxation, for example, property taxes to pay for public schools or income tax to pay for police and fire departments. In other cases, it is done through private subscription, for example, monthly payments for telephone service, cable television, or Internet access. Most individuals do not see a doctor as often as they watch television or use online social media each day, but they do see a doctor far more often than they wreck their car or lose a ship to pirates. In this way, health care more closely resembles goods and services that are financed, not insured.

As described in some detail in Chapter 1, the origin of health insurance and managed health care in the United States was also through financing, not through insurance. The earliest forms of coverage were all prepaid plans, including prepaid group practice plans similar to modern group model health maintenance organizations, and prepaid service plans that were the forerunners of today's Blue Cross and Blue Shield plans. That financing of health services became an insurance product is at least in part due to its inclusion as an employee benefit under the 1942 Stabilization Act that imposed wage and price controls on businesses.

Many nations finance health care by using a combination of taxation and fees. In most cases of financed services, the entities collecting the taxes or subscription fees also provide the service directly or strictly control its delivery.

For example, the school district owns the building and hires the teacher; or the cable company owns the copper, fiber, and descrambler box, and sells only prepackaged bundles of cable channels. The same often applies in other nations, where the state owns the hospitals and employs hospital-based specialists. In this way, they are less subject to cost and revenue fluctuations because those facilities operate under a budget, distribution of high-cost services is centrally planned, and governments are better positioned to demand favorable pricing on devices and drugs.

Governments that finance health benefits and in which at least some healthcare services are provided by private providers also usually attempt to offset at least some of the impact of moral hazard through price controls on providers, blunting the capacity for price inflation. Medicare does this in the United States, and a recent analysis of Maryland's all-payer hospital rate setting system concluded that for the commercial sector it was an "enduring and successful cost containment program."[24] Government can also blunt the impact of moral hazard through cost-sharing or other means, since anything in finite supply may be considered in economic terms; for example, time is in limited supply, so queuing is a form of cost-sharing.

Other nations are far from immune to increasing healthcare cost pressures, of course. They face the same issues of new technology, aging populations, new procedures, and so forth. As a result, while other nations spend far less per capita than the United States does for healthcare services, they too face inflation rates above their general rates of inflation. The response by other nations is a combination of greater spending and greater queuing, while spending increases are the primary response in the United States.

It would be misleading, though, to simply conclude that the answer to "Is health insurance?" to be "It is health financing." Financing is applied more easily to regular services for most individuals. It is more easily budgeted and resources may be more fairly allocated. But as discussed in Chapter 7, a small percentage of unfortunate individuals experience medical problems that generate catastrophic levels of cost, and in those cases it is the insurance aspect that protects them from losses. By eliminating annual* and lifetime benefit maximums, the ACA will finally reduce or end the serious medical debt and bankruptcies we have today,[25] although it increases the insurance aspect of protection that indemnifies individuals from catastrophic financial exposure.† In any event, as demonstrated during the rancorous debate culminating in passage of the ACA, our society is not ready to embrace approaches used by other industrialized nations to finance their healthcare systems.‡ That being the case, the insurance elements will continue to exert significant influence.

■ CONCLUSION

So the answer to "Is health insurance?" is "Sometimes it is, most of the time it is not." As necessary as reform is, focusing only on health insurance *as insurance* will have the unintended effect of increasing the impact of moral hazard, potentially accelerating cost inflation in the commercial sector. Having a healthier population and reducing human suffering is important, humane, and long overdue. But the cost of doing so will increase under the provisions in the ACA due to perfectly rational economic behaviors of patients and providers that are in no way "immoral." But health insurance reform is insurance reform, not health reform, which is yet to come.

Endnotes

1. See, for example, the entire September/October 2009 issue of *Health Affairs* (Vol. 28); or McKinsey & Company's December 2008 report, "Accounting for the Cost of U.S. Health Care: A New Look at Why Americans Spend More."
2. Arrow K. Uncertainty and the Welfare Economics of Medical Care. *American Economic Review*. December 1963; 53:941–973; updated 1968.
3. Pauly MV. The Economics of Moral Hazard: Comment. *American Economic Review*. 1968;58:531–537.
4. In addition to Arrow and Pauly, see, for example, Glied SA, Remler DK. What Every Public Finance Economist Needs to Know about Health Economics: Recent Advances and Unresolved Questions. *National Tax Journal*. December 1, 2002.
5. See, for example, Gladwell M. The Moral-Hazard Myth. *New Yorker*. August 29, 2005.
6. See, for example, the Suburban Emergency Management Project report, "What is Moral Hazard?" *Biot Report* #415, April 4, 2007. Available at: www.semp.us/publications/biot_reader.php?BiotID = 415. Accessed April 7, 2010.
7. See, for example, Baker T. *Insuring Morality*. University of Connecticut Law School; 2000. Available at: http://lsr.nellco.org/cgi/viewcontent.cgi?article = 1001&context = uconn_wps. Accessed April 7, 2010.

---

* Though gradually for "grandfathered" plans, as discussed in Chapter 30.
† Of course, it is possible to separate the two elements; for example, the government providing reinsurance (presumably through Medicare or Medicaid) while the private sector undertakes the financing for routine health care, as proposed by Senator John Kerry in his 2004 presidential bid.

---

‡ I am well aware that many nations finance their systems through "insurance premiums," including two that come closest now to what will exist in the United States after 2014 (Switzerland and the Netherlands), but reject the notion that generally speaking, "health insurance" in a European nation is the equivalent of health insurance in the United States.

8. See, for example, White MC. What is a Moral Hazard? The Big Money. *Slate Magazine*, Sept. 19, 2008. Available at: www.thebigmoney.com/articles/moral-hazard/2008/09/19/what-moral-hazard?page = full. Accessed April 7, 2010; or Winston M. What Ever Happened to Moral Hazard? *Open Salon*. August 24, 2009. Available at: http://open.salon.com/blog/tun/2009/08/24/what_ever_happened_to_moral_hazard. Accessed April 7, 2010.

9. Oxford English Dictionaries. Available at: www.askoxford.com/concise_oed/moral?view = uk. Accessed April 3, 2010.

10. Jay, Ricky, Dice: Deception, Fate & Rotten Luck. New York: The Quantuck Lane Press; 2003.

11. Oxford English Dictionaries. Available at: www.askoxford.com/concise_oed/hazard?view = uk. Accessed April 3, 2010.

12. Starr P. Averting a Health-Care Backlash. *The American Prospect*. December 8, 2009. Available at: http://www.prospect.org/cs/articles?article = averting_a_health_care_backlash. Accessed Jan. 8, 2010; and The Opt-Out Compromise. *The American Prospect*. March 9, 2010. Available at: www.prospect.org/cs/articles?article = the_opt_out_compromise. Accessed March 23, 2010.

13. Manning WG, et al. Health Insurance and the Demand for Medical Care: Evidence from a Randomized Experiment. *American Economic Review*. June 1987;77:251–277; RAND. *The Health Insurance Experiment*. Santa Monica, CA: RAND Corporation; 2006. Available at: www.rand.org; Newhouse JP. RAND *Health Insurance Experiment [in Metropolitan and Non-Metropolitan Areas of the United States], 1974–1982*. Ann Arbor, MI: Inter-university Consortium for Political and Social Research; 1999.

14. Bradford WD, Kleit AN, Nietert PJ, et al. How Direct-to-Consumer Television Advertising for Osteoarthritis Drugs Affects Physicians' Prescribing Behavior. *Health Affairs*. 2006;25:1371–1377.

15. Weissman JS, Blumenthal D, Silk AJ, et al. Physicians Report on Patient Encounters Involving Direct-to-Consumer Advertising. *Health Affairs*. Web Exclusive. 2004;W4:219–233; doi:10.1377/hlthaff.w4.219. Accessed April 12, 2010.

16. Wikes MS, Bell RA, Kravitx RL. Prescription Drug Advertising: Trends, Impact and Implications. *Health Affairs*. 2000;19:110–128.

17. Bradford. Op. Cit.

18. Weissman. Op. Cit.

19. See, for example, Noah T. Health Reform and Moral Hazard: Would Health Reform Boost Frivolous Doctor Visits? *Slate Magazine*, posted Feb. 3, 2010. Available at: www.slate.com/id/2243560/pagenum/all/#p2. Accessed April 7, 2010.

20. See, for example, Braithwaite RS, Omokaro C, Justice AC, Nucifora K, Roberts MS. Can Broader Diffusion of Value-Based Insurance Design Increase Benefits from US Health Care without Increasing Costs? Evidence from a Computer Simulation Model. *PLoS Med*. 2010;7: e1000234. doi:10.1371/journal.pmed.1000234.

21. The Lewin Group for MedPAC. A Study of Hospital Charge Setting Practices. December 2005, No. 05-4.

22. Pynchon T. *Inherent Vice*. New York: Penguin; 2009.

23. Russell LB. Preventing Chronic Disease: An Important Investment, But Don't Count on Cost Savings. *Health Affairs*. 2009;28:42–45.

24. Murray R. Setting Hospital Rates to Control Costs and Boost Quality: The Maryland Experience. *Health Affairs*. 2009;28:1395–1405.

25. Seifert RW, Rukavina M. Bankruptcy is the Tip of a Medical-Debt Iceberg. *Health Affairs*. 2006;25:w89–w92. doi: 0.1377/hlthaff.25.w89.

About the Author

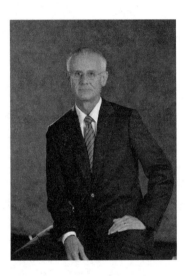

Dr. Peter R. Kongstvedt is an independent strategic advisor and a Senior Health Policy Faculty member in the Department of Health Administration and Policy at George Mason University. With over 30 years of industry experience as both a senior-level executive and with global consulting firms, he is a well-known national authority on the healthcare industry, with particular expertise in health insurance and managed health care. Dr. Kongstvedt is also the author of *Managed Care, What it Is and How it Works*, and recently created an online multimedia training program on health insurance and managed care. Prior to passage of health reform, he consulted with and made several appearances on *The CBS Evening News* and also appeared on NBC's *Today Show*.

He is principal of the P.R. Kongstvedt Company, LLC, and Kongstvedt Learning Solutions, LLC, in McLean, Virginia, and may be reached through his website at www.kongstvedt.com.

Contributors

Emily Adrion, MSc
PhD Candidate, Department of Health Policy and Management
Johns Hopkins Bloomberg School of Public Health
Baltimore, Maryland

Joann Albright, PhD
SVP QI Outcomes and Research
Magellan Health Services
Columbia, Maryland

Catherine K. Anderson, MPA
National Vice President, Complex Care Products
United Healthcare Community and State, a United Health
    Group Company
Driggs, Idaho

Rodney C. Armstead, MD, FACP
President, Northeast Region
United Healthcare Community and State, a United Health
    Group Company
Clinical Associate Professor of Medicine
University of Arizona College of Medicine, Phoenix Campus
Phoenix, Arizona

Kelli D. Back
Law Offices of Mark S. Joffe
Washington, DC

Stephen J. Balcerzak, MSW, MBA
Executive Vice President
Gorman Health Group, LLC
Washington, DC

Richard Birhanzel
Senior Executive, Accenture
Minneapolis, Minnesota

Wendy K. Burger
President
Write on the Dot, LLC
Mount Airy, Maryland

Christopher R. Campbell
CFO Small Group and Individual, Aetna Inc.
Hartford, Connecticut

Dale F. Cook
Vice President, Head of Small Group, Aetna
Hartford, Connecticut

M. Nicholas Coppola, MHA, MS, PhD, FACHE
Lieutenant Colonel (Ret.), U.S. Army
Founding Director, Army-Baylor MHA/MBA Program 2005–
    2008
Director and Associate Professor, Texas Tech University Health
    Sciences Center
Lubbock, Texas

Joanna Case Famadas, PhD, MBA
Senior Decision Support Specialist
UMass Memorial Health Care
Worcester, Massachusetts

Troy M. Filipek, FSA, MAAA
Principal & Consulting, Milliman
Brookfield, Wisconsin

Donald L. Fowler, Jr.
Vice President, Operations Services and Support
Blue Cross Blue Shield of North Carolina
Durham, North Carolina

Peter D. Fox, PhD
Independent Consultant
Denver, Colorado

Lawrence Fulton, PhD, MHA, MSStat
Lieutenant Colonel (Ret.), U.S. Army
CSciCStatPStat(R) CQE CSSBB FACHE
CIS and QM Department, McCoy School of Business, Texas
    State University
San Marcos, Texas

Nancy Garrett, PhD
Director, Health Economics and Reimbursement
Boston Scientific
St. Paul, Minnesota

Djordje Gikic, MD, MPH
Country Director Rwanda
Clinton Health Access Initiative—CHAI
Kigali, Rwanda

John K. Gorman
Chairman
Gorman Health Group, LLC
Washington, DC

Rusty Hailey, PharmD, DPh, MBA, FAMCP
President, Pharmaceutical Operations
Senior Vice President
Health Spring, Inc.
Nashville, Tennessee

Jeffrey P. Harrison, PhD, MBA, MHA, FACHE
Lieutenant Commander (Ret.), U.S. Navy,
Vice President, UNF Faculty Association
  and Chair, Department of Public Health
Associate Professor Brooks College of Health,
University of North Florida
Jacksonville, Florida

Deborah Heggie, PhD
Corporate Chief Clinical Officer
Magellan Health Services
Columbia, Maryland

Amy Huang
Student
Oberlin College
Westlake, Ohio

Ronald P. Hudak, JD, PhD, FACHE
Colonel (Ret.), U.S. Army Office of Strategy Management
Office of the Assistant Secretary of Defense (Health Affairs)
Washington, DC

Mark S. Joffe
Law Offices of Mark S. Joffe
Washington, DC

Bernard J. Kerr, Jr., EdD, FACHE
Professor, Health Administration Division, School of Health
  Sciences
The Herbert H. and Grace A. Dow College of Health
  Professions
Central Michigan University
Mt. Pleasant, Michigan

Forest S. Kim, PhD, MHA, MBA, MA, FACHE
Major, U.S. Army
Assistant Professor and Chair of Research Committee
Army-Baylor Graduate Program in Health & Business
  Administration
San Antonio, Texas

Kevin Knarr
Vice President, Enterprise Operations
United Health Group
Washington, DC

Anthony M. Kotin, MD
Chief Medical Officer
Magellan Health Services
Avon, Connecticut

Karl V. Kovacs, ACSW, MBA
Holt, Michigan

Jean D. LeMasurier
Senior Vice President for Public Policy
Gorman Health Group, LLC
Washington, DC

William A. MacBain
Senior Vice President
Gorman Health Group, LLC
Washington, DC

Marc Manley, MD, MPH
Vice President and Chief Prevention Officer
Blue Cross and Blue Shield of Minnesota
Eagan, Minnesota

Scott McDaniel
Director, Analytics
MEDSOLUTIONS
Franklin, Tennessee

Christie A. Moon, JD, CHC
Chief Compliance Officer, Rady Children's Hospital and
  Health Center
San Diego, California

Elizabeth Cabot Nash
Vice President, Health Exchanges
United Healthcare Community and State, a United Health
  Group Company
Washington, DC

Robert P. Navarro, PharmD
Clinical Professor
Department of Pharmaceutical Outcomes and Policy, University of Florida College of Pharmacy
President, Navarro Pharma, LLC
Gainesville, Florida

Margaret E. O'Kane
President, National Committee for Quality Assurance (NCQA)
Washington, DC

Elizabeth A. Pascuzzi, EdD
Principal Consultant, Managed Care Learning
Bradford Woods, Pennsylvania

Dave W. Plocher, MD
Affordability Solutions, LLC
Stillwater, Minnesota

Connie Salgy
Director, Product Development and Innovation
Magellan Health Solutions
Avon, Connecticut

Pamela B. Siren, RN, MPH
Vice President, Quality and Compliance
Neighborhood Health Plan, Inc.
Boston, Massachusetts

James S. Slubowski
Senior Vice President, Healthcare
High Point Solutions, LLC
East Norriton, Pennsylvania

Craig S. Stern, PharmD, MBA
President
Pro Pharma Pharmaceutical Consultants, Inc.
Northridge, California

Michael G. Sturm
Principal and Consultant, Milliman
Brookfield, Wisconsin

Wanda Sullivan, MPH
Director, Product Innovation
Magellan Health Services
Avon, Connecticut

Eric R. Wagner
Executive Vice President for External Affairs and Diversified Operations
MedStar Health
Columbia, Maryland

Jay Want, MD
Principal, Want Healthcare LLC
Denver, Colorado

Hugh R. Waters
Deputy Director, Health Care Outcomes and Quality Program
RTI International
Research Triangle Park, North Carolina

Frederick R. Waxenberg, PhD
Chief Clinical Officer, Nonmedical
Magellan Health Services
Merrick, New York

Jonathan P. Weiner, DrPH
Professor, Department of Health Policy and Management
Johns Hopkins Bloomberg School of Public Health
Baltimore, Maryland

Tom Wilder
Senior Counsel, America's Health Insurance Plans
Washington, DC

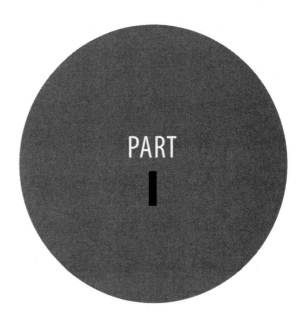

PART

I

Introduction to Health Insurance and Managed Health Care

"You know more than you think you do."

Benjamin Spock, MD
(May 2, 1903–March 15, 1998)
Baby and Child Care [1945]

A History of Managed Health Care and Health Insurance in the United States

PETER D. FOX AND PETER R. KONGSTVEDT

STUDY OBJECTIVES

- Understand the evolution of health insurance and managed health care, including the forces that drove this evolution
- Understand current trends in managed health care, including how market dynamics continue to change over time
- Understand the public policy and market performance issues faced by managed health care in the past
- Understand the current environment for health insurance and managed health care in the United States

DISCUSSION TOPICS

1. Discuss why proto-HMOs were formed in the first place.
2. Discuss how managed care activities by non-HMO health plans seek to constrain health care costs and promote wellness.
3. Discuss how important it is that managed health care plans demonstrate that they offer quality care, and why that is the case.
4. Discuss the salient forces leading to the rise and fall of various types of managed health care plans. Speculate on how current and future forces might lead to further changes.
5. Discuss how the relationship between the government and the managed health care industry changed over the years.

■ INTRODUCTION

Health insurance and managed health care are inventions of the 20th century. In the late 19th century, a few insurers offered insurance policies to cover the cost of care for workplace accidents and for employee disability. Some of these insurance policies eventually evolved into coverage for care unrelated to a workplace accident but not until several decades later.

More so than other types of insurance, health insurance and managed care also have been in a never-ending state of change and turbulence, a state of "permanent whitewater."

This chapter explores the historical roots and evolutionary forces that have resulted in today's system. The reader should note that dates are concrete for such events as the passage of laws or the establishment of organizations, but only approximate time periods apply to trends.

■ 1910 TO THE MID-1940S: THE EARLY YEARS

The years before World War II saw the appearance of two distinct models of providing and paying for health care besides purely out-of-pocket. The first of these were early forms of what we would now call a health maintenance organization (HMO), a term that was not coined until the early 1970s. The other was the appearance of the first Blue Cross and Blue Shield (BCBS) plans. The key characteristic of these proto-HMOs was that it combined the functions of insurance and the health care delivery system, while the key characteristic of the early BC and BS plans was their exclusive use of existing hospitals and privately practicing physicians.

Prepaid Medical Group Practices

The Western Clinic in Tacoma, Washington, is sometimes cited as the first example of prepaid medical group practice. Started in 1910, the Western Clinic offered, exclusively through its own providers, a broad range of medical services in return for a premium payment of $0.50 per member per month.[1] The program was available to lumber mill owners and employees. It served to assure the clinic a flow of patients and revenues. A similar program was developed by a Dr. Bridge, who started a clinic in Tacoma that later expanded to 20 sites in Oregon and Washington.

As shall become apparent, 1929 was a remarkable year in the history of health plans of all types. In that year, Michael Shadid, MD, established a rural farmers' cooperative health plan in Elk City, Oklahoma, by forming a lay organization of leading farmers in the community. Participating farmers purchased shares for $50 each to raise capital for a new hospital in return for receiving medical care at a discount.[2] For his troubles, Dr. Shadid lost his membership in the county medical society and was threatened with having his license to practice suspended. Some 20 years later, however, he was vindicated by the out-of-court settlement in his favor of an antitrust suit against the county and state medical societies. In 1934 the Farmers Union assumed control of both the hospital and the health plan.

Also in 1929, Drs. Donald Ross and H. Clifford Loos established a comprehensive prepaid medical plan for workers at the Los Angeles Department of Water and Power. The plan covered physician services and hospitalization, and from the beginning had a focus on prevention and health maintenance.[3] For that reason, some consider it to be the first real HMO, although as noted previously, that term was not in use at the time. Drs. Ross and Loos were also expelled from their local medical society. The Ross-Loos Clinic was purchased in 1980 by the Insurance Company of North America, a forerunner of the CIGNA insurance company, and was closed when CIGNA divested its owned medical facilities in the late 1990s.

In 1932 the American Medical Association (AMA) adopted a strong stance against prepaid group practices,[*] favoring, instead, indemnity type insurance, which had minimal presence at the time. The AMA's position was in response to both the small number of prepaid group practices in existence at the time and the findings in 1932 of the Committee on the Cost of Medical Care—a highly visible private group of leaders from medicine, dentistry, public health, consumers, and so forth—that recommended the expansion of group practice as an efficient delivery system. The AMA's stance at the national level set the tone for state and local medical society opposition to prepaid group practice, which continued for many years.

Despite this opposition, prepaid group practices continue to emerge, reflecting a diversity of origins with the initial impetus coming, variously, from employers, providers seeking patient revenues, consumers seeking access to improved and affordable health care, and even a housing lending agency seeking to reduce the number of foreclosures. They encountered varying degrees of opposition from local medical societies. Two prominent examples are the Kaiser Foundation Health Plan and the now defunct Group Health Association of Washington, D.C.

The organization that evolved into the Kaiser Foundation Health Plan was started in 1937 by Dr. Sidney Garfield at the behest of the Kaiser Construction Company. It sought to finance medical care, initially for workers and families who were building an aqueduct in the southern California desert to transport water from the Colorado River to Los Angeles and, subsequently, for workers who were constructing the Grand Coulee Dam in Washington state. A similar program was established in 1942 at Kaiser ship-building plants in the San Francisco Bay area.

In 1937 the Group Health Association (GHA) was started in Washington, D.C., at the behest of the Home Owner's Loan Corporation to reduce the number of mortgage defaults that resulted from large medical expenses. It was created as a nonprofit consumer cooperative with a board that was elected by the enrollees.[†] The District of Columbia Medical Society vehemently opposed the formation of GHA. It sought to restrict hospital admitting privileges for GHA physicians and threatened expulsion from the medical society. A bitter antitrust battle ensued, culminating in the U.S. Supreme Court's ruling in favor of GHA. In 1994, faced with insolvency despite an enrollment of some 128,000, GHA was acquired by Humana Health Plans, a for-profit, publicly traded corporation. It was subsequently divested by Humana and incorporated into Kaiser Foundation Health Plan of the Mid-Atlantic.

The Blues

In 1929, the same year that saw the establishment of both the Ross-Loos Clinic's prepaid health plan and Dr. Shadid's rural farmers' cooperative health plan, Baylor Hospital in Texas agreed to provide some 1,500 teachers with prepaid

---

[*]The AMA was also generally opposed to multispecialty groups of any kind, prepaid or not.

[†]Its governance structure was quite similar to that required for the new consumer-owned and -operated plans (CO-OPs) enabled under the Patient Protection and Affordable Care Act (ACA) of 2010.

inpatient care at its hospital, an arrangement that represented the origins of Blue Cross. The initial single-hospital program was subsequently expanded to include the participation of other employers and hospitals. Hospitals and state hospital associations elsewhere followed suit by creating other Blue Cross plans. These new plans were usually sponsored by a local or regional hospital association and included all of its member hospitals. Their motivation was to establish a revenue stream for participating providers during the Great Depression.

The forerunner of Blue Shield appeared in the Pacific Northwest in 1939 and offered coverage of physician services, stimulated in part by lumber and mining companies that wanted to provide medical care for injured workers. It made arrangements with physicians, who were paid a monthly fee for their services through a service bureau.[4] State medical societies soon began to emulate the model across the country.

The earliest BC and BS plans thus resembled other early types of prepaid care, except that they relied on providers in independent private practices rather than having dedicated delivery systems. Because they included more than one hospital or one medical group, providers could not each be paid on an equal prepayment basis, so payment was typically based on charged fees. In order to define the payment terms between a Blue Cross plan and a hospital, hospitals created cost-based charge lists, the forerunners of today's hospital chargemaster (the price list a hospital creates for all services for which it charges, discussed in Chapter 5). Blue Shield plans developed payment rates for defined procedures.[*] Unlike the early prepaid group practices, BCBS plans paid for, but did not provide, the care, which is why we consider them an early form of health insurance, although technically speaking they are "service plans," as described in Chapter 2.

Over time many Blue Cross plans merged with their local Blue Shield counterparts, although some remain separate even now. Most of these were statewide, although there were (and still are) notable exceptions, for example, in Pennsylvania and New York State, both of which have several BC and BS plans. These early BCBS plans, collectively referred to as the "Blues," operated independently from each other and continue to do so. Today, however, a state's BCBS plan may be part of a single larger entity, which can be either a for-profit company or a nonprofit or noninvestor-owned company.

In a few cases the Blues plans competed with each other, but mostly they respected each other's geographic boundaries. Increasingly, they have entered each other's territory and do compete, although only one may use the

BCBS logo in a defined territory. Hospitals and physicians retained control of the various Blues plans until the 1970s when they changed to a community governance model, a customer-owned model (e.g., a mutual insurer), and in recent decades some have converted to publicly owned, for-profit corporations. The formation of the various BCBS plans in the midst of the Great Depression, as well as that of many HMOs, reflected not consumers' demanding coverage or nonphysician entrepreneurs' seeking to establish a business, but rather providers' wanting to protect and enhance patient revenues.

■ THE MID-1940s TO MID-1960s: THE EXPANSION OF HEALTH BENEFITS

World War II generated both inflation and a tight labor supply, leading to the 1942 Stabilization Act. That Act imposed wage and price controls on businesses, including limiting their ability to pay higher wages to attract scarce workers. However, the Act did allow workers to avoid taxation on the employer contribution to certain employee benefits plans, including health benefits, which gave impetus to the growth of commercial health insurance. Before World War II, only 10% of employed individuals had health benefits from any source, but by 1955 nearly 70% did, although much of it was for hospitalizations only.

HMO formation also continued, albeit at a slow pace. For example, two large HMOs were created that remain prominent today:

- In 1944, at the behest of New York City, which was seeking coverage for its employees, the Health Insurance Plan (HIP) of Greater New York was formed. In 2006 HIP and New York-based Group Health Incorporated (GHI) merged to form EmblemHealth.
- In 1947 consumers in Seattle organized 400 families, who contributed $100 each, to form the Group Health Cooperative of Puget Sound. Predictably, opposition was encountered from the Kings County Medical Society.

The 1950s also saw the appearance of HMOs resembling today's independent practice association (IPA) model, in which the HMO contracts with physicians in private fee-for-service (FFS) practices rather than having dedicated providers. These were a competitive reaction to group practice-based HMOs. The basic structure was created in 1954 when the San Joaquin County Medical Society in California formed the San Joaquin Medical Foundation to compete with Kaiser. The foundation established a relative value fee schedule for paying physicians, heard grievances against physicians, and monitored quality of care. It became licensed by the state to accept enrollee premiums and, like other HMOs, performed the insurance function. However, HMOs and insurance companies faced different regulatory

---

[*]Current Procedural Terminology (CPT) charge codes, which define the procedures for which doctors and other providers bill, was finally created by the AMA in 1966. The AMA has updated and maintained it ever since.

requirements in most states and were often regulated by different state agencies because HMOs both provided or contracted for the delivery of care and had risk for medical expenses, whether the HMO was based on a medical group or doctors in independent practice. That remains the case today.

The other noteworthy event in this time period occurred in 1945 with the passage of the McCarran-Ferguson Act, which exempted insurance companies from federal oversight, resulting in the obligation falling to the states. It also provided limited antitrust immunity for certain activities such as pooling of claims data for underwriting purposes as long as these activities were regulated by the state. This exemption was used primarily by property/casualty and disability insurers. It may also have been used by early health insurers, but by the 1970s and 1980s, states did not allow them to do so.

■ THE MID-1960s TO THE MID-1970s: THE ONSET OF HEALTH CARE COST INFLATION

In the early 1960s President John F. Kennedy proposed what eventually became Part A of Medicare, financed through taxes on earned income similar to Social Security, that would cover mostly hospital services. The Republicans in Congress subsequently proposed to cover physician services as well in what became Part B of Medicare. It was financed through a combination of general revenues and enrollee premiums. Following Kennedy's assassination, President Lyndon B. Johnson worked aggressively to achieve some of the late president's goals, including covering persons age 65 and over. In 1965 Congress passed two landmark entitlement programs: Medicare for older adults (Title XVIII of the Social Security Act) and Medicaid (Title XIX of the Social Security Act) for selected low-income populations (i.e., those who met income, asset, and family composition requirements).* The benefits and provider payment structures of Medicare were similar to those of BCBS plans of the time, with separate benefits for hospital and physician services, a bifurcation that still characterizes Medicare today.

The combination of Medicare, Medicaid, private insurance (whether by commercial carriers or BCBS plans), and other programs that pay for medical care (e.g., workers' compensation and Veterans Administration) resulted in the majority of health care being paid for by third-party payers. To illustrate, in 1960, 55.9% of all health care costs

nationally, regardless of source of coverage, were paid out of pocket, a figure that declined steadily as follows:

- 1965 – 42.9%;
- 1970 – 33.3%;
- 1980 – 22.9%;
- 1990 – 19.1%; and
- 2000 – 14.2%.[5]

The third-party payment system severs the link between who provides, who receives, and who pays for medical care, thereby generating both increased fees and greater utilization. The question often is whether the additional services are always medically necessary. This was often attributed primarily to Medicare, but, in fact, it was the total of all third-party payments that was inflationary, particularly when added to the impact of advances in technology and rising expectations regarding the health care sector. As an illustration, national health expenditures as a percent of Gross Domestic Product (GDP) rose from 5.2% in 1960 to 5.8% in 1965, the year before Medicare was implemented, and reached 7.4% in 1970.[6]

There are, however, isolated examples of early attempts to control costs beyond seeking discounts, including the following:†

- In 1959 Blue Cross of Western Pennsylvania, the Allegheny County Medical Society Foundation, and the Hospital Council of Western Pennsylvania performed retrospective analyses of hospital claims to identify utilization that was significantly above the average.[7]
- Around 1970 California's Medicaid program initiated hospital precertification and concurrent review in conjunction with medical care foundations in that state, typically county-based associations of physicians who elected to participate, starting with the Sacramento Foundation for Medical Care.
- The 1972 Social Security Amendments authorized the federal Professional Standards Review Organization (PSRO) to review the appropriateness of care provided to Medicare and Medicaid beneficiaries. Although the effectiveness of the PSRO program has been debated, it established an organizational infrastructure and data capacity upon which both the public and private sectors can rely. In time the PSRO became known as the Peer Review Organization (PRO) and, subsequently, the Quality Review Organization (QRO), which continues to provide oversight of clinical services on behalf of the federal and many state governments. In some cases the QRO entered into contracts to provide review services for employers or health plans. While the methods used by these organizations evolved along

---

*The original Medicaid Act covered only families with dependent children (as well as individuals with disabilities and older adults), while excluding childless singles and married couples. Eligibility has since been expanded over time. Also, the 1972 Social Security amendments extended Medicare coverage to individuals with work histories who were considered disabled, although there was a waiting period of more than 2 years after the onset of disability.

---

†What these activities are and how they are performed is described in Chapter 7.

with their acronyms, their focus remained essentially the same.

- In the 1970s a handful of large corporations initiated precertification and concurrent review for inpatient care, much to the dismay of the provider community. Some companies took other measures such as promoting employee wellness, sitting on hospital boards with the intent of constraining their costs, and negotiating payment levels directly with providers.[8]

Although unrelated to costs and initially only peripherally related to health insurance, another significant event occurred at the end of this period: the passage in 1974 of the Employee Retirement Income Security Act (ERISA). Although the focus of ERISA was initially on retirement benefits, it addressed employers' pretax employee benefits. Among other things, ERISA established appeal rights for denial of benefits and established new regulations for employers that self-funded their benefits plans in order to avoid state regulation and taxes. ERISA is discussed periodically throughout this book and more fully in Chapter 29.

The problem of health care costs' rising faster than the economy as a whole, thereby absorbing an increasing share of the GDP, increasingly became a subject of public discussion. Throughout the 1960s and into the early 1970s, HMOs played only a modest role in the finance and delivery of health care, although they were a significant presence in a few communities such as the Seattle area and parts of California. In 1970 the total number of HMOs was in the 30s, the exact number depending on one's definition. That would soon change.

■ THE MID-1970s TO MID-1980s: THE RISE OF MANAGED CARE*

Between 1970 and 1977, national health expenditures as a percent of GDP rose from 7.4% to 8.6%. The acceleration in health care costs, driven at least in part by the third-party FFS payment system, became a widely discussed problem. For example, the cover of the May 28, 1979, issue of *Time* magazine features a photo of a surgeon wearing an outsized dollar bill for a surgical mask, with the headline "Medical Costs: Seeking the Cure."[†] Seeking the cure led to the next major development: managed care as we know it today. In particular, this period saw the growth of HMOs; the appearance of a new model, the preferred provider organization (PPO); and a broad increase in utilization management by insurers.

---

*This section assumes the reader knows what an HMO and a PPO is. If that is not the case, the reader may wish to first review Chapter 3 or at least look the terms up in the Glossary.

[†]The cover story itself was a very lucid distillation of many of the causes of health care cost inflation, which by then had risen to 9.5% of the GDP (half what it is at the time of this book's publication). The story also makes approving note of a new approach: HMOs.

HMOs

The HMO Act was passed in 1973.[9] It authorized startup grants and loans and, more importantly, ensured access to the employer-based insurance market. It evolved from discussions that Paul Ellwood, MD, had in 1970 with the political leadership of the U.S. Department of Health, Education, and Welfare (which later became the Department of Health and Human Services).[10] Ellwood had been personally close to Philip Lee, MD, Assistant Secretary for Health during the presidency of Johnson and participated in designing the Health Planning Act of 1966.

Ellwood, sometimes referred to as the father of the modern HMO movement, was asked in the early Nixon years to devise ways to constrain the rise in the Medicare budget. Out of those discussions evolved both a proposal to capitate HMOs for Medicare beneficiaries (which was not enacted until 1982) and the laying of the groundwork for what became the HMO Act of 1973. The desire to foster HMOs reflected the perspective that the fee-for-service system, by paying providers based on their volume of services, incorporated the wrong incentives. Also, the term "health maintenance organization" was coined as a substitute for prepaid group practice, principally because it had greater public appeal.

The main features of the HMO Act were the following:

- Grants and loans were available for the planning and startup phases of new HMOs as well as for service area expansions for existing HMOs.
- State laws that restricted the development of HMOs were overridden for HMOs that were federally qualified, as described below.
- Most important of all were the "dual-choice" provisions, which required employers with 25 or more employees that offered indemnity coverage to also offer two federally qualified HMOs, one of each type: (1) the closed panel or group or staff model and (2) the open panel or IPA/network model, if the plans made a formal request of the employer.[‡]

Some HMOs were reluctant to exercise the mandate, fearing that doing so would antagonize employers, who would in turn discourage employees from enrolling. However, the dual-choice mandates were used by most HMOs of the time to get in the door of employer groups to at least become established. Because the federal mandate only applied to one HMO of each type, opportunities to exercise the mandate became scarce. The federal dual-choice provision expired in 1995 and is no longer in effect.

The statute established a process under which HMOs could elect to be federally qualified. Plans had to satisfy a series of requirements, such as meeting minimum benefit

---

[‡]Types of HMOs are described in detail in Chapter 2.

package standards set forth in the Act, demonstrating that their provider networks were adequate, having a quality assurance system, meeting standards of financial stability, and having an enrollee grievance process. Some states emulated these requirements and adopted them for all state-licensed HMOs.

Obtaining federal qualification had always been at the discretion of the individual HMO, unlike state licensure, which is mandatory. Plans that requested federal qualification did so for four principal reasons:

- First, it represented the equivalent of a "Good Housekeeping Seal of Approval" that was helpful in marketing.
- Second, the dual-choice requirements ensured access to the employer market.
- Third, the override of state laws—important in some states but not in others—applied only to federally qualified HMOs.
- Fourth, federal qualification was required for the receipt of federal grants and loans that were available during the early years of the Act.

Federal qualification no longer exists, but it was important when managed care was in its infancy and HMOs were struggling for inclusion in employment-based health benefits programs, which account for most private health coverage in the United States.

The HMO Act also contained provisions that, at the time, retarded HMO growth. This stemmed from it being a compromise in Congress between members having differing objectives. One camp was principally interested in fostering competition in the health care marketplace by promoting plans that incorporated incentives for providers to constrain costs. The second camp, while sharing the first objective, saw the HMO Act as a precursor to health reform and sought a vehicle to expand access to coverage for individuals who were without insurance or had limited benefits. Imposing requirements on HMOs but not on indemnity carriers, however, reduced the ability of HMOs to compete.

Of particular note were requirements with regard to the comprehensiveness of the benefit package as well as open enrollment and community rating. The open enrollment provision required that plans accept individuals and groups without regard to health status. The requirement for community rating of premiums (see Chapter 22 for a discussion of community rating) limited the ability of plans to relate premium levels to the health status of the individual enrollee or employer group. Both provisions represented laudable public policy goals; the problem was that they had the potential for making federally qualified HMOs noncompetitive because the same requirements did not apply to the traditional insurance plans against which they competed. This situation was largely corrected in the late 1970s with the enactment of amendments to the HMO Act that reduced some of the more onerous requirements. Other provisions of

the HMO Act have been revised over time as well, but there is no need to delve into them here.

Politically, several aspects of this history are of interest. First, although differences arose on specifics, the congressional support for legislation promoting HMO development was bipartisan. Also, there was no widespread state opposition to the override of restrictive state laws. In addition, most employers did not actively oppose the dual-choice requirements, although many disliked the federal government telling them to contract with HMOs.* Perhaps most interesting was the positive interaction between the public and the private sector, with government fostering HMO development both through its regulatory processes and also as a purchaser under its employee benefits programs. The federal government in effect promoted competition in health care financing and delivery by instituting a regulatory process.

HMOs focused on both managing utilization and changing the payment system to better align the goals of the HMO with those of providers. Group and staff model HMOs relied primarily on salaried doctors, thus eliminating FFS incentives to increase utilization. HMOs that contracted with private physicians rather than using its own physicians often used capitation in which the physician received a set monthly payment for each member enrolled in their panel of patients, regardless of how many services were provided. This approach was used principally for primary care physicians (PCPs), who, in addition either individually or collectively, had other financial incentives to control referrals to specialists. In this way, the FFS incentives to increase utilization were replaced with financial incentives to control utilization. Provider payment in managed health care is discussed in Chapter 5.

In all types of HMOs, members were required to go through their PCP in order to receive coverage for specialty or hospital care. HMOs routinely required precertification for all elective hospital admissions and actively monitored inpatient stays with the goal of reducing the amount of unnecessary utilization. By avoiding unnecessary admissions, increasing the use of outpatient surgery in place of inpatient stays for the same procedure, and reducing the average length of stay, HMOs wrung considerable unnecessary utilization out of the system.

As HMOs grew, hospitals that had provided discounts to BCBS plans now offered similar or superior discounts to HMOs in return for the HMOs' directing patients their way. In markets in which hospitals competed, some hospitals feared losing business if they did not contract with HMOs. New forms of payment emerged such as per diem payments,

---

*If an employer offered an HMO but that HMO had not exercised the mandate, another HMO could do so. As a result, employers would sometimes ask their preferred HMO to go ahead and mandate them so as to avoid having yet another plan to offer.

capitation, and case rates, as described in Chapter 5. HMOs, with their narrower networks, were the most aggressive in using these new forms of payment, and negotiations between payers and hospitals became more sophisticated. A similar dynamic played out with other providers, including physicians. Structural aspects of payer networks, including HMOs, are discussed in Chapter 4.

The HMO Act was largely successful. During the 1970s and 1980s, HMOs grew and began displacing traditional health insurance plans. What was not anticipated when the original HMO Act was passed was that it was the IPA model HMOs that grew the fastest, having greater enrollment by the late 1980s than group and staff model HMOs, a difference that has increased over time. This dynamic accelerated as commercial insurers and BCBS plans acquired or created their own HMOs.

In 1982 Congress passed the Tax Equity and Fiscal Responsibility Act (TEFRA), which authorized the Medicare program to pay HMOs on a capitated basis provided that they met Medicare's participation requirements. The intent, largely achieved, was that these HMOs, by virtue of their ability to control health care costs, could offer more comprehensive benefits than Medicare. For example, these new Medicare HMOs typically offered lower amounts of cost-sharing than did traditional Medicare, as well as coverage of prescription drugs and selected preventive services that traditional Medicare didn't cover at all. However, there has been considerable debate over whether the ability of HMOs to offer additional benefits within the Medicare capitation amount was due to efficiencies or to their attracting disproportionately healthy patients.[*]

Also in 1982, the federal government addressed the other major entitlement program when it issued a waiver to the state of Arizona that allowed it to rely solely on capitation, and not have a FFS alternative, in their Medicaid program.[11] A number of states had previously made major efforts, in some cases under federal demonstration waivers, to foster managed care in their Medicaid programs, but had not done so for the entire program.

HMOs were increasingly accepted by consumers, particularly due to the added benefits such as coverage of preventive services, child and women's preventive health visits, and prescription drugs, none of which were typically covered by traditional insurance or BCBS plans of the time.[†] In response, the traditional carriers and BCBS plans began adding prevention and drug coverage to their non-HMO products.

Preferred Provider Organizations and Utilization Management

Other managed care developments also occurred during the 1970s and early 1980s. Of note was the evolution of preferred provider organizations (PPOs). PPOs are generally regarded as having originated in Denver, where in the early 1970s Samuel Jenkins, a vice president of the benefits consulting firm of The Martin E. Segal Co., negotiated discounts with hospitals on behalf of its Taft-Hartley trust fund clients.[12] Hospitals did so in return for the health plans' having lower cost sharing for its users, thereby attracting patients who would otherwise have used competitor hospitals that were not in the network.

The concept soon expanded to include physicians and other types of providers. The term PPO came about because hospitals and doctors who agreed to discounted fees were therefore considered to be "preferred." People covered under the PPO faced lower cost-sharing if they saw a PPO provider than an "out-of-network" provider. In most cases they did not need authorization from a PCP "gatekeeper" to access care from other providers. This was in contrast to the typical HMO in which there was no coverage for benefits for nonemergency services from health care providers who were not in the network (with the exception that services were covered if the enrollee was temporarily outside of the HMO's service area), and all specialty care required PCP authorization.

PPO providers also agreed to certain cost-control measures such as complying with precertification requirements for elective hospitalizations, meaning that the doctor must notify the PPO before any elective admission and the patient must meet clinical criteria in order for the stay to be covered. Precertification programs remain common today. Second-opinion programs were also instituted, which entailed requiring a patient to obtain a second opinion from a different surgeon for certain elective procedures before they would be covered. Second-opinion programs are rarely mandated anymore.

Another development in indemnity insurance, mostly during the 1980s, was the widespread adoption of large case management, that is, the coordination of services for persons with expensive conditions such as selected accident patients, cancer cases, chronic illness causing functional limitations, and very low birth-weight infants. Utilization review, the encouragement of second opinions, and instituting large case management all entailed at times questioning physicians' medical judgments, something that had been rare outside of the HMO setting. These activities, further discussed in Part III of this book, were crude by today's standards of medical management but represented a radically new role of insurance companies in managing the cost of health care at the time.

Finally, the utilization controls in HMOs contributed to major practice pattern changes, including shifting care from

---

[*] More recently, Medicare adopted "risk adjustors" to health plan payments that relate the payment amount to the estimated health status of a plan's individual enrollees.
[†] The comprehensive benefits, including preventive services that HMOs were required to provide, were unique at the time, but HMOs were not required to offer coverage of prescription drugs. They did so to attract enrollees.

the inpatient to the outpatient setting and shortening the length of hospital stays. Shortening length of stay was also strongly encouraged by legislation enacted in 1982 mandating that Medicare change its payment mechanism in the traditional program from cost-based to paying a fixed amount per admission within a given class or grouping of diagnoses. This, and other methods of paying hospitals, is discussed in Chapter 5.

■ THE MID-1980s TO 2000: GROWTH, CONSOLIDATION, MATURATION, AND BACKLASH

From the mid-1980s through the mid-1990s, managed health care experienced rapid growth, expanding into all health sectors as traditional indemnity health insurance declined, creating a new set of strains on the health care sector. At the same time, new organizational forms appeared, companies began to specialize in certain managed care activities, and the industry began to consolidate.

Managed Care Expands Rapidly

HMOs and PPOs grew rapidly, with commercial HMO enrollment increasing from 15.1 million in 1984 to 63 million in 1996 and 104.6 million in 1999.[13] Initially PPOs lagged behind, but by the early 1990s enrollment was roughly equal, and by 1999 PPOs had 39% market share compared to HMOs at 28%. In the mid-1980s traditional indemnity insurance accounted for three-quarters of the commercial market; by the mid-1990s it was less than one-third of the market and would decline to single digits by 2000.[14]

A new product was also introduced during this period, the point of service (POS) plan, which combined elements of an HMO but with limited payment when out-of-network providers were used. Typically, a POS plan was like a PPO except that enrollees were required to select a single PCP (although they could change at any time), who authorized most referral services if the member wanted full coverage instead of the cost-sharing associated with out-of-network or nonauthorized services. Initially very popular, POS plans would stall out due to high costs and never exceeded HMO growth. These and other hybrid products make statistical compilations difficult, however. As new types of plans appeared, the taxonomy of health plan types both grew and blurred when the term managed care organization (MCO) came to represent HMOs, POS plans, PPOs, and multiple hybrid arrangements.*

Medicare and Medicaid also witnessed significant managed care growth. Medicare managed care (see Chapter 24) grew from 1.3 to 6.8 million between 1990 and 2000.[15] During the same time period, Medicaid managed care (see Chapter 25) grew from 2.3 million, or 10% of Medicaid beneficiaries, to 18.8 million, or 56%.[16] These two programs would show a different pattern subsequently, however.

As is the case with dandelions, rapid growth is not always good. Some HMOs outstripped their ability to run the business, overburdening management and their IT systems. In those MCOs, service eroded and mistakes increased. More ominously, the industry began to see a few health plan failures or near-failures.

Consolidation Begins

Beginning in the early 1990s consolidation increasingly occurred among both MCOs and health systems. Entrepreneurs, sensing financial opportunities, began to acquire or start HMOs. Consolidation took place as those entrepreneurs cashed out their investments. In other cases, they acquired smaller plans in order to build a regional or national company, enhancing their ability to have their stocks publicly traded. Financially troubled MCOs made good acquisition targets, allowing larger plans to acquire market share without spending much money. Although uncommon, MCOs that were getting close to failure might be seized by a state insurance commissioner who would then either sell it to another company or liquidate it and divide the membership up among the remaining, healthier MCOs.

Smaller plans were at a disadvantage. Large employers with employees who are spread geographically increasingly favored national companies at the expense of local health plans. For smaller plans, the financial strain of having to upgrade computer systems continually and to adopt various new technologies mounted. In addition, unless they had a high concentration in a small market, smaller plans found themselves unable to negotiate the same discounts as larger competitors, exacerbating the financial strain. At some point many of them simply gave up and sought to be acquired.

Not all mergers and acquisitions were large companies acquiring small ones. It also occurred among large companies. To illustrate, Aetna acquired U.S. Healthcare in 1996, NYLcare in 1998, and Prudential's health insurance business in 1999, all companies with a large presence in the market.[17] By 1999 the multistate firms, including Kaiser Permanente and the combined BCBS plans, accounted for three-quarters of national enrollment.

Another trend was health plans' converting from not-for-profit to for-profit status. United Health Care, the second largest health plan nationally with 34 million enrollees in 2011,[18] started as a nonprofit health plan in Minnesota. WellPoint, the largest health plan with 34.2 million enrollees in 2011, originated when Blue Cross of California converted to for-profit status and subsequently acquired several other Blues plans, which also converted to for-profit status. The Blues plan in Indiana also converted, renaming itself Anthem, and subsequently acquired other Blues plans. These conversions required the creation and funding of foundations, commonly

---

*The acronym "MCO" is itself now in decline, including its use in this book.

known as "conversion foundations," with the assets of the nonprofit plan, many of which are among the largest grant-giving foundations in their respective states. In 2004 Anthem combined with WellPoint, which effectively doubled the size of the merged for-profit BCBS plan. Today, the for-profit/not-for-profit split in the health payer sector is roughly 50-50, with the two largest nonprofit plans being Health Care Services Corporation, part of the Blues structure,* with 12.4 million enrollees, and Kaiser Permanente, with 8.8 million.[19]

Among physicians a slow but discernable movement away from solo practice and toward group practice also occurred. An increasing amount of consolidation among hospitals also occurred on a regional or local level in the 1990s, with over 900 mergers and acquisitions taking place during this period.[20] Hospital consolidation was commonly justified in terms of its potential to rationalize clinical and support systems.

A clearer impact, however, has been the increased market power to negotiate favorable payment terms when negotiating with commercial health plans, as is discussed in Chapters 4 and 5. Consolidation reached the point where a significant number of systems in effect had local hegemonies, usually for most services but sometimes only in selected services that health plans needed to offer. By being willing to enter only into comprehensive contracts with health plans for all services that the system offered, not just those that were unique or dominant in the area, considerable leverage in negotiations was gained. The result of consolidation by both health plans and providers was competition became muted. Instead of competition among multiple buyers and sellers, what evolved was closer to what economists call "bilateral monopolies," with both health plans and providers in local markets having little choice but to reach agreements with each other.

Integrated Delivery Systems Appear

Provider consolidation was not the only response to managed care. In many communities hospitals and physicians collaborated to form integrated delivery systems (IDSs), principally as vehicles for contracting with MCOs and with HMOs in particular. Types of IDSs are discussed in Chapter 2 and therefore are not described in detail here.

Most IDSs were created as rather loose organizations made up of a hospital and its medical staff, the most common of which was the physician-hospital organization (PHO). Most PHOs, and IDSs generally, allowed all physicians with admitting privileges at the hospital in question to participate rather than selecting the more efficient ones. Indeed, under the FFS method of payment, physicians with high utilization benefited the hospital financially and, thus, could not be excluded. Conversely, physicians were commonly required to

use the hospital for outpatient services (e.g., for laboratory tests) that might be obtained at lower cost elsewhere, also hurting the ability of the IDS to be price competitive. Most IDSs of the time suffered at least initially from organizational fragmentation, payment systems to individual doctors that were misaligned with the goals of the IDS, inadequate information systems, management that was inexperienced, and a lack of capital.

That would not stop many of them from wanting to "cut out the middleman" and become risk-bearing organizations themselves, a decision they would soon regret. Provider organizations lobbied hard to be allowed to accept risk and contract directly with Medicare. The Balanced Budget Act of 1997 (BBA 97)[†] allowed them to do so as provider-sponsored organizations (PSOs) if they met certain criteria (see Chapter 2). Large provider systems and physician practice management companies also accepted global capitation risk from HMOs. With a few exceptions they failed spectacularly, losing millions of dollars in a few short years. The federal waiver program for PSOs expired, although not until well after most had failed, and only a handful exist today as state-licensed entities that are also "grandfathered" by Medicare. Outside of California, the number of provider systems contracting to accept full risk for medical costs has dropped dramatically.

IDSs and provider systems often pursued another route to accepting full risk by forming a licensed HMO. The existence of a hospital or hospitals, physicians, and a licensed HMO and/or PPO under one corporate umbrella is called vertical integration, and for a while it was touted as the future of health care. Like so many futures confidently predicted by pundits, it mostly didn't come to pass because provider-owned HMOs mostly failed for the same reasons PSOs failed. But not all of them failed. Some health systems managed their subsidiary HMOs just like a stand-alone HMO would be managed, and did quite well. HMOs started by large, well-run medical groups also did quite well and continue to do well today. The rest sold, gave away, or closed their HMOs.

Utilization Management Shifts Focus

The focus of utilization management, which had been almost exclusively on inpatient care, shifted to encompass the outpatient setting as well, including prescription drugs, diagnostics, and care by specialists. Perhaps even more important is that the high concentration of costs in a small number of patients with chronic conditions resulted in significantly more attention being paid to high-cost cases and on disease management, as discussed in Chapters 7 and 8. The health plan focus on these patients was new, although

---

*HCSC encompasses, among other companies, the BCBS plans in Illinois, Texas, Oklahoma, and New Mexico.

†The BBA 97 also reduced payments to Medicare HMOs, and many believe this is what led to a decline in Medicare HMO enrollment in the early 1990s.

the extent of concentration of costs (i.e., the proportion of costs represented by the most expensive patients) has remained relatively stable over the years.

The role of the PCP also changed. In a traditional HMO, that role was to manage a patient's medical care, including access to specialty care. This proved to be a mixed blessing for PCPs, who at times felt caught between pressures to reduce costs and the need to satisfy the desires of consumers, who may question whether the physician has their best interests at heart in light of a perceived financial incentive to limit access to services. The growth of PPOs as compared to HMOs also led to a shift away from PCP-based "gatekeeper" types of plans under which a referral had to be obtained to access nonemergency specialty care. However, most plans (including PPOs) continued to have lower copays if members received care from a PCP than if they received care from a specialist, thus retaining a primary care focus.

The focus of utilization management was also sharpened through the growth of carve-out companies, which are organizations that have specialized provider networks and are paid on a capitation or other basis for a specialized service. Among services that lend themselves to being "carved out" are pharmaceutical benefits (Chapter 11), mental and behavioral health (Chapter 12), disease management (Chapter 8), chiropractic, and dental. The carve-out companies market principally to payers and large self-insured employers because they are generally not licensed as insurers and thus are limited in their ability to assume risk. In recent years some of the large health plans that contracted for such specialty services have reintegrated them back into the health plan in part because the carved-out services made it difficult to coordinate services (e.g., between physical and mental health).

Industry Oversight Spreads

Health insurance and managed care have always been subject to oversight by state insurance departments and (usually) health departments. The 1990s saw the spread of new external quality oversight activities. Starting in 1991 the National Committee for Quality Assurance (NCQA; see Chapter 15) began to accredit HMOs. The NCQA had been launched by the HMO's trade associations in 1979 but became independent in 1990 with the majority of board seats being held by employer, union, and consumer representatives. Interestingly, this board structure was proposed by the Group Health Association of America, which represented closed-panel HMOs at the time. Many employers require or strongly encourage NCQA accreditation of the HMOs with which they contract, and accreditation came to replace federal qualification as the "seal of approval." NCQA, which initially focused only on HMOs, has evolved with the market to encompass, for example, managed behavioral health care organizations (MBHOs), PPOs,

physician credentialing verification organizations, primary care medical homes, and more. They will likely accredit new organizational types as they appear. This is also the case with the two other bodies that accredit managed health care plans as described in Chapter 15, URAC* and Accreditation Association for Ambulatory Health Care (AAAHC), also known as the Accreditation Association.

Performance measurement systems (report cards) also came about, the most prominent being what was once called the Health Plan Employer Data and Information Set (HEDIS®),† which was developed by the NCQA at the behest of several large employers and health plans. The HEDIS data set has evolved over time. A summary of the data set current at the time of publication is in Chapter 15, and the most current version is available on NCQA's website at www.ncqa.org. Other forms of report cards also appeared and continue to evolve as a result of the market demanding increasing levels of sophistication.

At the federal level, Congress passed the Health Insurance Portability and Accountability Act of 1996 (HIPAA). A decade earlier a provision in the Consolidated Omnibus Budget Reconciliation Act of 1985 (COBRA) allowed individuals who lost eligibility for group coverage to continue group coverage for up to 18 months, although they could be required to pay the full cost plus 2% themselves. The initial focus of HIPAA was to provide a means for individuals to have continued access to coverage once they exhausted their COBRA benefit. It was only partially successful because the coverage was usually expensive, particularly for a young person who could commonly obtain coverage as an individual for less than the group rate, which reflected all individuals in the group, including older ones. Furthermore, having to pay the full cost of coverage often occurred as a result of someone losing his or her job, resulting in diminished income. More important to the industry, however, were the standards that HIPAA created for privacy, security, and electronic transactions. The standards are discussed in Chapters 18, 23, and 29.

The Managed Care Backlash[21]

Anti-managed care sentiment, commonly referred to as the "managed care backlash," became a defining force in the industry. As a society, we expected managed care to reduce the escalation of health care costs but became enraged at how it did it. In retrospect, why that happened is obvious because managed health care was the only part of the health care sector that ever said "no." The emotional overlay accompanying health care outstrips almost any other aspect of

---

*URAC is its only name and is no longer an acronym. At one time it stood for Utilization Review Accreditation Commission.
†HEDIS now stands for the Healthcare Effectiveness Data and Information Set.

life. The health problem of a spouse or child causes feeling in ways that a house fire or losing one's employment does not.

The roots of the backlash date back to the early 1990s. Most employers heretofore had allowed their employees to choose between an HMO and a traditional health insurance plan but required them to pay a substantially higher payroll deduction if they chose the traditional health plan. However, to control costs, many employers began putting all or most employees into a single managed care plan without offering the choice of an indemnity plan.

One source of contention with some consumers, particularly those who had not chosen to be in an HMO, was the requirement that they obtain authorization from their PCP in order to access specialty care. Arguably, this provision both reduces costs and increases quality by assuring that PCPs are fully appraised of the care that their patients receive. Conversely, consumers under the care of a specialist who was not in the HMO's network were required to transition their care to an in-network doctor, which was resented by individuals who had not voluntarily chosen to be in an HMO.

But there was more to the backlash. As noted earlier, rapid growth increased the risk of problems arising. Some of the problems were largely irritants, such as mistakes in paperwork or claims processing in health plans with IT systems that were unable to handle the load. Rapid growth also affected the ability to manage the delivery system. Where clinically oriented decisions on coverage were once done with active involvement of medical managers, some rapidly growing health plans became increasingly bureaucratic and distant from their members and the providers, causing them to be seen as cold and heartless, and the errors and delays in payment as intentional.

Rapid growth also sometimes led to inconsistencies in coverage decisions. The public's perception that decisions regarding coverage of clinical care being made by "bean counters" or other faceless clerks may not have been fair or accurate in the opinion of managed care executives, but neither was it always without merit. Some HMOs, particularly those whose growth outstripped their ability to manage, did delegate decision-making authority to individuals who lacked adequate training or experience and were not supported by the comprehensive algorithms that are common today. Furthermore, some plans were accused of routinely and intentionally denying, or delaying payment of, certain types of claims, caving in only when the member appealed, a charge vigorously disputed by the plans. In the turbulence created by rapid growth, entrepreneurial for-profit plans, and ragged administrative functions, it is simply not possible to know how often this occurred, if it did. Regrettably, the managed care industry during this period did a poor job of self-policing and lost the confidence of large segments of the public. Other problems were emotional and not a threat to health, such as

denial of payment for care that was not medically necessary,* for example, an unnecessary diagnostic test. For doctors and patients who are unaccustomed to *any* denial of coverage, it was easy to interpret this as overzealous utilization management, and in some instances utilization management was, indeed, overzealous. How often this occurred is impossible to know, not only because of the turbulence of the era but also because standard practices were only first coming into being and there are no studies on which to rely.

Finally, while uncommon, some problems did represent potential threats to health, such as denial of authorization for payment of a covered benefit for truly necessary medical care or difficulties in accessing care, thereby causing subsequent health problems. In some cases the denial of coverage was due to its not being a covered benefit; certain experimental transplants would not be covered, for example. This occurred with indemnity health insurance as well, but it was not viewed the same way. The public expects low premiums but coverage for all medical-related services, including ones that might be judged unnecessary or outside of the scope of the defined benefits.

Furthermore, whether a service is medically necessary or simply a convenience can be a matter of interpretation or dispute. Is a prescription for a drug to help with erectile dysfunction medically necessary? What about a growth hormone for a child who is short because his or her parents are short, not from a hormonal deficiency? Should fertility treatments be unlimited? Some interventions may be medically necessary for some patients but not for others; for example, in a patient with droopy eyelids but no impairment of vision, surgery is primarily cosmetic, although it often progresses until it is medically necessary because vision is impaired. Issues such as these potentially arise with each new and expensive medical intervention.

The most damning of all accusations was that health plans were *deliberately* refusing to pay for necessary care in order to enrich executives and shareholders, a perception enhanced by media stories of multimillion-dollar compensation packages of senior executives. Putting aside the fact that financial incentives drive almost all aspects of health care to varying degrees, as discussed in Chapters 5 and 9, this charge was particularly pernicious for health plans, particularly given the increasing number of for-profit plans.

When there are enough instances of serious problems, they make good fodder for news using the well-proven reporting technique of "identifiable victim" stories in which actual names and faces are associated with anecdotes of poor care or benefits coverage problems. That problems portrayed in the news may or may not have been represented fairly from the viewpoint of the health plan was

---

* The term "medical necessity" in the context of benefits coverage is discussed in Chapters 7 and 20.

irrelevant. When added on top of disgruntlement caused by minor or upsetting (though not dangerous) irritants caused by health plan operations, the public is not liable to be sympathetic to managed care, particularly with the consensus that few insurance companies are loved.

Politicians were quick to jump on the bandwagon, especially during the debate over the Health Security Act of 1993, proposed by President Bill Clinton but not enacted. Many states passed "patient protection" legislation such as prudent layperson standards for emergency care, stronger appeal and grievance rights, and requirements for HMOs to contract with any provider willing to agree to the HMO's contractual terms and conditions. (Whether the so-called "any willing provider" provision protects consumers is, at best, debatable.)

A good example of these laws was the prohibition of a "gag clause" in an HMO contract with a physician in which an HMO's contract supposedly prevented a physician from telling a patient what their best medical options were. So prevalent was that belief that it made the cover of the January 22, 1996, edition of *Time* magazine, showing a surgeon being gagged with a surgical mask and the headline reading "What Your Doctor Can't Tell You. An in-depth look at managed care—and one woman's fight to survive."[*] The Government Accountability Office (GAO), a part of the U.S. Congress, investigated the practice at the request of then-Senators Trent Lott, Don Nickles, and Larry Craig and issued their report on August 29, 1997. The GAO reviewed 1,150 physician contracts from 529 HMOs and could not find a single instance of a gag clause or any reported court cases providing guidance on what constitutes a gag clause.[22] This had no impact on public perception.

The popular press continued to run regular "HMO horror stories." For example, the cover of the July 12, 1998, issue of *Time* magazine shows a photo of a stethoscope tied in a knot and a headline that read "What Your Health Plan Won't Cover . . ." with the word *Won't* in bold red letters. In another example, the November 8, 1999, cover of *Newsweek*

magazine featured a furious and anguished woman in a hospital gown, with the words "HMO Hell" displayed across the page. HMOs were disparaged in movies, cartoons, jokes on late-night TV, and even the comics sections of newspapers. The number of lawsuits against HMOs increased, many alleging interference in doctor's decision making and practice of medicine. Many also alleged that capitation incented physicians to withhold necessary care, although this charge is refutable based on a series of research studies, as discussed in Chapter 5.

In a futile attempt to counter the rising tide of antipathy, the managed care industry kept trying to point out the good things it was doing for members such as coverage for preventive services and drugs, the absence of lifetime coverage limits, and coverage of highly expensive care, but there was nothing newsworthy about that. A reporter for a major newspaper, who did not himself contribute to the backlash, said at the time to one of this chapter's authors, "We also don't report safe airplane landings at La Guardia."

HMOs expanded their networks and reduced how aggressively they undertook utilization management. Some HMOs eliminated the PCP "gatekeeper" requirement, thereby allowing members open access to any specialist, albeit at higher copayment levels than applied visits to their PCP. To borrow words used a decade earlier by President George H.W. Bush in his inaugural address, HMOs became "kinder and gentler," with a concomitant increase in health care costs.

The managed care backlash eventually died down. The volume of HMO jokes and derogatory cartoons declined, news stories about coverage restrictions or withheld care became uncommon, and state and federal lawmakers moved on to other issues. But the HMO's legacy of richer benefits, combined with the general loosening of medical management and broad access to providers, collided with other forces by the end of the millennium, and health care costs once again began to rise. As they rose, the cost of health benefits coverage rose as well, leading to an increase in the uninsured and greater cost-sharing for those with coverage.

---

[*]The cover story was called "Medical Care: The Soul of an HMO" and was about a woman's fight with a California HMO over coverage for a procedure known as autologous bone marrow transplantation for her disseminated breast cancer. Coverage authorization was denied because it was considered experimental and investigational by a majority decision of a committee of the HMO's private oncologists. The story reported a considerable amount of communication, meetings, phone calls, medical visits, and so forth, as well as the salaries and bonuses of HMO executives. It does not mention a "gag clause" or any similar term.

The woman succeeded in getting the procedure covered and an arbitration panel awarded her family punitive damages from the HMO, one of a number of lawsuits that finally forced HMOs and insurers to pay for this procedure. Unfortunately, the woman died soon after the procedure was done. Rigorous scientific study of autologous bone marrow transplantation eventually found that it was worse than conventional treatment alone, and it is no longer performed. The story highlights another dynamic in the U.S. health system: the practice of medicine by judge and jury.

■ 2000 TO 2010: COSTS RISE AND COVERAGE DECLINES

HMO commercial enrollment market share peaked in 1999 at 104.6 million, or 28% of the market. It declined thereafter, reaching 78.5 million in 2004 (24% market share) and hovering between that and 76 million (21% market share) since then. POS plans, which had enjoyed 24% market share in 1999, also steadily declined, down to 8% by 2010. PPOs, on the other hand, gained market share—from 39% in 1999 up to 58% by 2010.[23] Commercial market shares are shown in **Figure 1-1**.

Medicare managed care enrollment reversed itself and declined to 5.3 million by 2003, largely as a result of a provision in the Balanced Budget Act of 1997 that reduced what

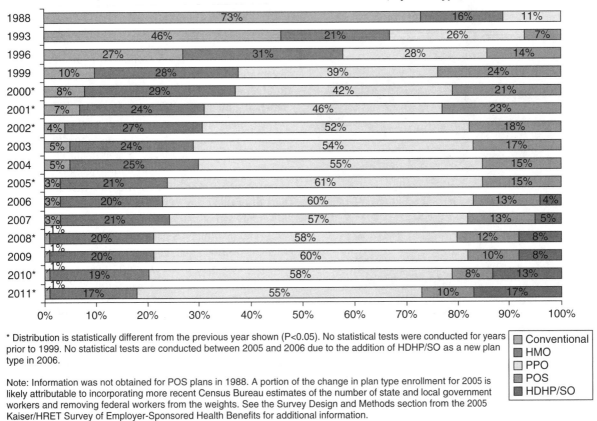

FIGURE 1-1 Distribution of Health Plan Enrollment for Covered Workers, by Plan Type, 1988–2011

Source: "Employer Health Benefits 2011 Annual Survey, (#8225)," p. 61. http://ehbs.kff.org/pdf/2011/8225.pdf. The Henry J. Kaiser Family, September 2011. This information was reprinted with permission from the Henry J. Kaiser Family Foundation. The Kaiser Family Foundation is a nonprofit private operating foundation, based in Menlo Park, California, dedicated to producing and communicating the best possible analysis and information on health issues.

Medicare paid the health plans. That changed as a result of the enactment in 2001 of the Medicare Modernization Act (MMA). The MMA created the first major benefit expansion in Medicare since its initial passage in 1965: the Part D drug benefit. It also changed the name of the Medicare managed care program from Medicare + Choice to Medicare Advantage (MA) and changed substantially the methodology for payment to private Medicare plans (MA is discussed in detail in Chapter 24). New MA plans began enrolling members in 2004, reversing the decline and growing to over 12 million by 2011.[24] HMOs remain the largest form of MA plans, however, as illustrated in **Figure 1-2**. The principle effect of the MMA was to increase payment from several percentage points below what standard Medicare would have paid in the fee-for-service system to several points above. For 2010, it is estimated that MA plans will receive payments that are an average of 8.7 percent above what Medicare would have spent had the enrollees remained in standard Medicare.[25] The Patient Protection and Affordable Care Act (ACA), discussed later, reduces payment levels over a several-year period to closer to parity with the Medicare FFS program.

Medicaid had a much smoother trajectory. Cash-strapped states increasingly turned to private managed Medicaid organizations, and Medicaid plans grew from 18.8 million enrolled in 2000 to 26.9 million people by 2004, representing 61% of all Medicaid beneficiaries.[26] Managed Medicaid is discussed in detail in Chapter 25.

Health Care Costs Again Exceed Economic Growth

By 2003 national health expenditures as a percent of GDP had reached 15.9%, a huge increase since 1977, when they amounted to 8.6%. They rose slowly until 2007, reaching 16.2%, but as the economy declined the amount consumed by health care rose to 17.6% in 2009, only 2 years later. However, even before then, rising health care costs became a major political and economic issue because of the percent of government spending going to health care generally and Medicare and Medicaid specifically, the reduced affordability of private insurance, and the impact on the overall economy stemming from health care representing an ever increasing share of GDP.

The health economy is too complex to ascribe the persistent rise in health care to any single attribute or even a

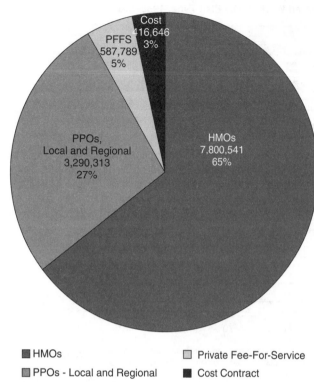

HMOs
PPOs - Local and Regional
Private Fee-For-Service
Cost Contract

FIGURE 1-2 Medicare Advantage Enrollment, Totals and Percent February 2011

Source: Created by authors using CMS Monthly Enrollment by Plan Report as of March 3, 2011. www.cms.gov/MCRAdvPartDEnrolData/EP/list.asp#TopOfPage.

constellation of attributes. At its most basic, health care costs are the results of price × volume (i.e., utilization). Price increases by large health systems and by drug and device manufacturers have been substantial in recent years, as discussed in Chapters 4, 5, and 11, respectively. Increased utilization of both existing and new technologies has also been a major factor, especially in the area of outpatient procedures, as discussed in Chapter 7. Increased demand for services has also played a major role. In some cases that demand is created by consumers, although how much of that results from direct-to-consumer advertising, billboards, news stories, and the like is difficult to determine. In any event, consumers have heightened expectations, appropriate or not. There is also compelling evidence that provider-induced demand occurs when physicians own or otherwise benefit financially from a technology that they can order such as imaging, as discussed in Chapters 4 and 7.

New and expensive technologies—often of largely unknown effectiveness—appear regularly. Because the third-party payment system insulates the provider and patient from costs, such new technologies are usually priced to deliver high margins. The practice of defensive medicine, due to the threat and reality of malpractice suits, contributes to cost increases, although various analyses indicate that it is

a minor factor in the aggregate. The aging of the population has an increasing role to play, one that is magnified by our ability to sustain life through more aggressive treatments.

Another factor, the authors believe, is that the managed care backlash discussed earlier led to health plans' being more reticent to question the necessity of procedures or to intervene in any way that could have the appearance of practicing medicine. While hard to quantify, we are paying a price for telling managed health care to "back off." One area where plans have continued to innovate and intervene is in the care of patients with significant chronic illnesses because these patients account for a disproportionately high percentage of medical expenses, as discussed further in Part III of this book.

Finally, administrative costs in both provider organizations and health plans have always been a factor, something that will be ameliorated by electronic medical records and by the availability of information on health plans that will facilitate comparison shopping and the purchase of insurance in new ways, such as over the Internet, that will, in particular, reduce spending on insurance agent commissions. And as of 2011, the ACA placed limits on the percentage of the premium that can be used for sales, administration, governance, and profit. These factors are explored in Parts III and IV of this book.

Out-of-Pocket Spending Increases

As health care costs increase, so does the cost of insurance coverage. In the commercial market, employers continue to pay approximately 70% of the cost, with the remainder coming from payroll deductions, as illustrated in **Figure 1-3**.

Increasing payroll deductions were not the only way in which costs to consumers rose. In an effort to limit premium increases, employers also began to increase deductibles (the amount an individual must pay before any coverage goes into effect). By 2010 more than 17% of large firms and nearly half of all small firms had an annual deductible of $1,000 or more.[27] Cost-sharing also increased for routine visits and prescriptions. Where once the typical office copayment was $5, it is now $20 for visits to a PCP and $40 for visits to specialists. In addition, coverage of prescription drugs usually had a single copayment regardless of the drug in question, but drug benefits are now typically subject to complex tiered copayments, depending, for example, on whether the drug is generic or brand and whether or not it is on the formulary. This reversed the downward trend in the percentage of total costs paid out of pocket that was noted earlier in the chapter.

The middle of this decade also saw the appearance of consumer-directed health plans (CDHPs), also known as high-deductible health plans (HDHPs), which confer savings in federal income taxes. They take several forms, including health savings accounts (HSAs), health care payment accounts (HPAs), and HDHPs without such accounts. The

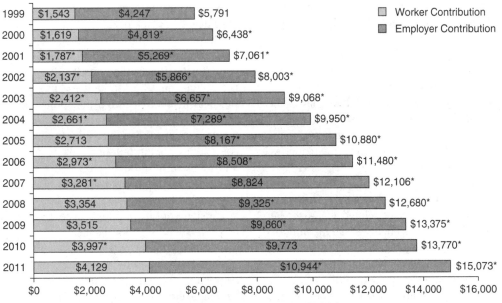

| | | Worker Contribution |
| | | Employer Contribution |

1999 $1,543 $4,247 $5,791
2000 $1,619 $4,819* $6,438*
2001 $1,787* $5,269* $7,061*
2002 $2,137* $5,866* $8,003*
2003 $2,412* $6,657* $9,068*
2004 $2,661* $7,289* $9,950*
2005 $2,713 $8,167* $10,880*
2006 $2,973* $8,508* $11,480*
2007 $3,281* $8,824 $12,106*
2008 $3,354 $9,325* $12,680*
2009 $3,515 $9,860* $13,375*
2010 $3,997* $9,773 $13,770*
2011 $4,129 $10,944* $15,073*

$0 $2,000 $4,000 $6,000 $8,000 $10,000 $12,000 $14,000 $16,000

*Estimate is ststistically different from estimate for the previous year shown (P<0.05).

FIGURE 1-3 Average Annual Worker and Employer Contributions to Premiums and Total Premiums for Family Coverage, 1999–2011
Source: "Employer Health Benefits 2011 Annual Survey, (#8225)," p.69. http://ehbs.kff.org/pdf/2011/8225.pdf. The Henry J. Kaiser Family, September 2011. This information was reprinted with permission from the Henry J. Kaiser Family Foundation. The Kaiser Family Foundation is a nonprofit private operating foundation, based in Menlo Park, California, dedicated to producing and communicating the best possible analysis and information on health issues.

main benefit to the enrollee is savings in both taxes and premiums. HDHPs and CDHPs, which are more fully discussed in Chapter 2, have deductibles equal to or higher than $1,200 for singles and $2,400 for families in 2011.*

Embedded in CDHPs is the notion that consumer choice and accountability need to be enhanced. The initial focus was to provide members with better information regarding quality and cost of care along with information to help them understand their health care. However, they are controversial because, whatever the resulting savings, people with high incomes disproportionately benefit, and persons with high medical expenses, notably those with chronic conditions, face higher out-of-pocket expenses, often year after year.

Managed care has not ceded the field to sole reliance upon the use of cost-sharing combined with improved information to assist in decision making. For example, pay-for-performance programs have been implemented to align financial incentives to providers with quality goals, as discussed in Chapter 5. Also, the concept of value-based insurance design (VBID; also referred to as value-based insurance benefits design, or VBIBD) has come to the fore. As discussed in Chapter 7, it refers to lowering the economic barriers to access created by cost-sharing for treatment of people with selected chronic conditions, for example, eliminating any copayments for certain drugs

for a member with congestive heart failure in order to increase compliance and avoid clinical deterioration resulting in hospitalization.

Increasing Numbers of Uninsured

The maximum level of cost-sharing is 100%, which is what the uninsured face, and their numbers have increased throughout the decade as a result of many factors, including fewer small employers offering coverage, the decline in the number of manufacturing jobs, an increase in the number of individuals who declined employer-based coverage because of increasing payroll deductions, and people unable to get coverage because of medical conditions or increasingly high premiums. The percentage of Americans without health insurance rose from 14% in 1999 to 17% in 2009.[28] This was a specific problem addressed by Congress in 2010.

The Patient Protection and Affordable Care Act

The ACA was signed into law on March 23, 2010. It is nearly a thousand pages long and is the most sweeping health care law since 1965 when Medicare and Medicaid were enacted. It affects the entire health care sector, but its greatest impact is on the payer industry and on access to health benefits coverage for all Americans. Because the ACA is so sweeping, it is not possible to cover it all within the confines of this book. Provisions of the ACA that are important to understand are addressed throughout this book, and Chapter 30 is specifically focused on it.

---

*Federal tax law prescribes that the deductible be at least at these levels in order to qualify for tax benefits, with the actual dollar amount being set by the Treasury Department each year.

Some provisions of the new law were already in effect at the time of publication, although the major coverage expansions will not occur until 2014. However, passage of the ACA does not mean that Congress will have no more to say. Members of Congress are divided on the topic of health reform, and changes in the balance of power are likely to have an impact on the ACA just as it has had on all major laws since our nation was founded. It is, therefore, possible that aspects of the ACA described in this book will be changed significantly by the time you read it. Consequently, the reader will need to keep up to date through other sources. There is no shortage of opinions about the ACA, and a great deal of information and misinformation exists everywhere one turns. The Kaiser Family Foundation (not related to Kaiser Permanente), in particular, is an excellent source for unbiased information that is easily accessible. It can be accessed by navigating to www/kff.org and clicking on the appropriate links, or directly by navigating to http://healthreform.kff.org (current at the time of publication). Access to that and other useful links are also available by going to www.kongstvedt .com and choosing "Useful Links" or directly by navigating to www.kongstvedt.com/useful_urls.html.

■ CONCLUSION

Managed health care has made significant contributions to the delivery system, many positive but also some negative. HMOs, for example, were the source of considerable evidence that many procedures that were once performed on an inpatient basis only could be performed in an outpatient setting with favorable outcomes. HMOs also showed that inpatient length of stay could be reduced without deleterious effect. These changes over time became the norm of practice. Likewise, their early emphasis on prevention is laudable and is now the law. Of note, the early HMOs were the source of considerable research on quality of care, far more so than the unmanaged fee-for-service medical system. This research contributed to policymakers and large employers becoming comfortable contracting with them. Furthermore, it helped accelerate the overall broadening of quality measurement and management beyond the hospital setting to which it had been confined earlier.

Related to that, the initial and ongoing public and regulatory mistrust of managed health care and health insurers in general led to the creation of standard measures such as HEDIS and the Consumer Assessment of Healthcare Providers and Systems (CAHPS®) survey (both are discussed in Chapters 14 and 15). CAHPS began as a consumer satisfaction survey solely for Medicare HMOs but has become more widely used. The focus on quality and the increasing use of measurement also led to the concept of value-based payment such as pay-for-performance and other models, described in Chapter 5. A related concept is data transparency for consumers, allowing individuals to see the performance scores for both providers and health plans, something once considered a "black box."

Despite these contributions, managed health care plans have often been described as managing cost rather than care. To the extent that this accusation is valid, some of the blame must be ascribed to large employers to which the health plans are highly responsive, as they must be. Employers facing erosion in their own financial condition due to rising health care costs demand that health plans do something about it, but then seek plans with large networks and focus only minimally on health care processes. As a result, many large employers look to constrain costs by increasing enrollee cost-sharing and having employees pay a larger share of the premium. Recently, however, a few large employers with high local concentrations of employees have been looking to narrower networks once again.

On a negative note, the managed care industry did not respond well to the backlash. It did not at the time make sufficient efforts at self-regulation, although many health plans were supportive of the NCQA. But at first, it handled the backlash primarily as a public relations problem. In opposing legislation introduced to address the backlash, it also opposed what most people viewed as sensible legislation, notably the layperson emergency rule and the right to appeal coverage denials to an independent body, resulting in the impression that it was putting money ahead of patient care. This impression was exacerbated by ongoing examples of spectacular wealth derived by entrepreneurs when they sold their HMOs to the public or to a larger company.

One other disappointment was the result of managed health care's response to the market. Many, including the authors of this chapter, historically promoted competition among health plans as a means to restrain the ever-rising health care costs by using different systems of care that would compete on quality as well as costs. However, this potential has gone substantially unrealized as PPOs, as well as open-panel or IPA types of HMOs, have dominated the market as health plans sought very broad networks in order to be attractive to consumers. The effect is that, in most markets, the overlap in participating providers among health plans is so great that the provider network becomes a matter of lesser importance to the enrollee.

Rising costs meant rising levels of uninsured, and was the impetus behind the passage of the ACA in 2010, the most sweeping health care legislation since Medicare and Medicaid. Whether or not the ACA will accomplish its intended goals is unknown, but it is fair to say that its primary and initial focus is on access to health insurance, and not on restraining costs. As this book goes to press, the issue of cost containment is again being featured prominently in the media. Unfortunately, everyone has his or her "silver bullet"; for example, if we could only solve the malpractice problem *or* if we could only get patients to pay higher cost-sharing so that they would be more inclined to seek efficiencies in services delivery *or* if provider payment could be changed to avoid the incentives in fee-for-service to deliver more, and more expensive, care *or* fill-in-your-favorite-solution-here. Each of these has a place as part of a comprehensive strategy, as do other approaches such as promoting wellness and addressing the problem of untested, questionable, expensive, and marginally effective technologies. Little addressed, however, is the significant problem of each part of the health care system seeking to protect its turf and income, commonly resorting to political processes to do so.

Is the American public prepared to tackle the cost issues? Health plans can only do so much on their own. In the short run they must respond to the desires of their customers—individuals, employers, or unions—who themselves may neither be willing to address the issues nor be well informed. They must also respond to state and federal regulators, a requirement rapidly evolving under the ACA, and those regulators also may be unwilling or unable to address the issues. Managed health care has and will continue to make important contributions but it is not the panacea some had hoped for. However, panacea or not, we are not likely to return to a world of unmanaged and unexamined health care. Managed health care, like the entire health sector and our society overall, will continue to evolve.

Endnotes

1   Mayer TR, Mayer GG. HMOs: Origins and Development. *N Engl J Med.* 1985; 312(9):590–594.

2   MacLeod GK. An overview of managed care. In: Kongstvedt PR, ed. *The Managed Care Handbook.* 2nd ed. Gaithersburg, MD: Aspen; 1993:3–11.

3   Starr P. *The Social Transformation of American Medicine.* New York: Basic Books; 1982:295–310.

4   Blue Cross and Blue Shield Association. *Blue Beginnings.* Available at www.bcbs.com/about/history/blue-beginnings.html. Accessed April 23, 2011.

5   Calculation by the authors from CMS national health expenditure data in the file "National Health Expenditures by type of service and source of funds, CY 1960–2009," www.cms.gov/NationalHealthExpendData/. Accessed May 14, 2011.

6   Calculation by the authors from CMS national health expenditure data in the file "NHE summary including share of GDP, CY 1960–2009," www.cms.gov/NationalHealthExpendData/. Accessed May 14, 2011.

7   Fielding JE. *Corporate Cost Management.* Reading, MA: Addison-Wesley; 1984.

8   Ibid., and Fox PD, Goldbeck WB, Spies JJ, *Health Care Cost Management, Private Sector Initiatives.* Ann Arbor, MI: Health Administration Press; 1984.

9   HMO Act of 1973, 42 U.S.C. § 300e.

10   Strumpf GB. Historical evolution and political process. In: Mackie DL, Decker DK, eds. *Group and IPA HMOs.* Gaithersburg, MD: Aspen; 1981:17–36.

11   Kaiser Family Foundation. *Medicaid: A Timeline of Key Developments.* Kaiser Family Foundation website; 2011. Available at www.kff.org/medicaid/timeline/pf_entire.htm. Accessed April 4, 2011.

12   Spies JJ, Friedland J, and Fox PD. Alternative health care delivery systems: HMOs and PPOs. In: Fox PD, Goldbeck W, and Spies, JJ, eds. *Health Care Cost Management: Private Sector Initiatives.* Ann Arbor, MI: Health Administration Press; 1984:43–68.

13   Created by authors using data from the Centers for Disease Control and Prevention, National Center for Health Statistics, and the Agency for Healthcare Research and Quality, Medical Expenditure Panel Survey.

14   Kaiser/HRET Survey of Employer-Sponsored Health Benefits, 1999–2010; KPMG Survey of Employer-Sponsored Health Benefits, 1993, 1996; the Health Insurance Association of America (HIAA), 1988; and the Sanofi-Aventis Managed Care Digest Series, HMO–PPO Digest 2010–2011. *Data sources:* SDI and the Centers for Medicare and Medicaid Services.

15   Ibid.

16   Ibid.

17   Aetna. *Aetna History.* Aetna website; 2001. Available at www.aetna.com/about-aetna-insurance/aetna-corporate-profile/aetna-history/index.html. Accessed March 2, 2011.

18   MCOL Quarterly Reports, May 2011, used for 2011 enrollment levels for both United Health Care and WellPoint; http://healthsprocket.com/hs/node/756. Accessed August 1, 2011.

19   Alliance for Advancing Nonprofit Health Care. *Basic Facts and Figures: Nonprofit Health Plans.* Alliance for Advancing Nonprofit Health Care website. Available at www.nonprofithealthcare.org/resources/BasicFactsAndFigures-NonprofitHealthPlans9.9.08.pdf. Accessed March 25, 2011.

20   Vogt WB. *Hospital Market Consolidation: Trends and Consequences.* NIHCM Expert Voices; November 2010. Available at www.nihcm.org/pdf/EV-Vogt_FINAL.pdf. Accessed March 27, 2011.

21   The description of the managed care backlash is based on the author's own experiences as well as many academic papers, including:

● Blendon R, Brodie M, Benson J, et al. Understanding the Managed Care Backlash. *Health Affairs.* 1998;17(4):80–94.

● Rodwin M. Backlash: As Prelude to Managing Managed Care. *J Health Politics Pol Law.* 1999;24(5):1115–1126.

● Draper D, Hurley R, Lesser CS, et al. The Changing Face of Managed Care. *Health Affairs.* 2002;21(1):11–23.

22 Government Accountability Office publication, "GAO HEHS-97-175 HMO Gag Clauses."

23 Kaiser Family Foundation and Sanofi-Aventis Managed Care Digest, op cit.

24 Calculated by authors using CMS Monthly Enrollment by Plan Report. Accessed March 3, 2011.

25 Biles B, et al., "Medicare Advantage in the Era of Health Reform: Progress in Leveling the Playing Field," Commonwealth Fund pub. 1491, vol. 5, March 31, 2011.

26 Kaiser/HRET Survey, op cit.

27 Kaiser/HRET Survey, op cit.

28 U.S. Census Bureau. Health Insurance Coverage Status and Type of Coverage All Persons by Age and Sex: 1999 to 2009. Health Insurance Historical Tables. Available at: www.census.gov/hhes/www/hlthins/data/historical/index.html. Accessed May 13, 2011.

CHAPTER

2

Types of Health Insurers, Managed Health Care Organizations, and Integrated Health Care Delivery Systems

Eric R. Wagner and Peter R. Kongstvedt

STUDY OBJECTIVES

- Understand the different types of health insurers and managed health care organizations
- Understand key differences between these types of organizations
- Understand the inherent strengths and weaknesses of each model type
- Understand the difference between insured and self-funded health plans
- Understand the new payer envisioned in the Patient Protection and Affordable Care Act (ACA)
- Understand the basic forms of integrated delivery systems (IDSs) and how they are evolving
- Understand the major strengths and weakness of each type of IDS, initially and how they have played out as the markets developed
- Understand the roles of physicians and hospitals in each type of IDS
- Understand new IDS models being formed due to passage of the ACA

DISCUSSION TOPICS

1. Describe the continuum of health insurer and managed health care plans and key differences for each, using examples of each.
2. Discuss the primary strengths and advantages and weaknesses and disadvantages of each type of managed care plan.
3. Discuss in what type of market situations might each type of managed care plan be the preferred model.
4. Describe how a managed care plan of one type might evolve into another type of plan over time.
5. Discuss the key elements of the different types of integrated delivery systems.
6. Describe the conditions under which a managed care plan would desire to contract with an integrated delivery system or conversely, avoid it; describe these conditions for each model type.
7. Discuss the challenges and opportunities facing new types of payers and IDSs due to the ACA.

■ INTRODUCTION

Describing the types of payer and provider organizations in a field as dynamic as managed health care is much like describing what a cloud looks like on a breezy day—it looks like a lot of different things to different people, and it keeps changing right before your eyes. This is no surprise because as was shown in Chapter 1, the health care system in the United States evolves continually and change is the only constant. With the passage of the Patient Protection and Affordable Care Act of 2010 (ACA), the American health care system faces more significant change than any time since the passage of Medicare and Medicaid during the 1960s.[1] Included among ACA's many provisions are several that add new acronyms to the managed care lexicon. Because of the size and complexity of the ACA and of our system as a whole, it is not possible to predict with certainty which elements or new organizational forms will endure and which ones will not.

Originally, health maintenance organizations (HMOs), preferred provider organizations (PPOs), and traditional forms of indemnity health insurance were easily distinguishable, mutually exclusive products and mechanisms for providing coverage of health benefits. Point of service (POS) plans appeared, combining HMO-like features with indemnity coverage, blurring the landscape. Managed care elements migrated to all product types, but didn't necessarily carry the same labels. Even newer types of plans such as high-deductible health plans (HDHPs) and related consumer-directed health plans (CDHPs) with pretax savings accounts, easily distinguishable at first, became less so as traditional PPO deductibles rose to five figures.

The reality is that health insurance and managed care have, for all practical purposes, merged, whether we see it or not. And mostly we don't. Research done back in 2002 during the latter portion of the managed care backlash (discussed in Chapter 1) found that most of the commercially insured American public, the vast majority of whom were in fact enrolled in a managed care plan, did not believe that they received their health care coverage through managed care.[2]

Further confusing the taxonomic landscape are different types of provider organizations collectively referred to as integrated health care delivery systems (IDSs)* that initially appeared in reaction to managed care, and to HMOs in particular. Just like managed care organizations (MCOs), IDSs evolved, morphed, and lurched from one form to another.† This dynamic continues today. For example, under

pressure from the Centers for Medicare and Medicaid Services (CMS), the federal agency that oversees the Medicare program, new IDS models have come about, including primary care medical homes (PCMHs) and accountable care organizations (ACOs), which were also specifically given impetus in the ACA. Another example of continuing change is the striking degree to which physicians are no longer practicing independently, but are being hired by hospitals, a topic discussed briefly in this chapter and in more depth in Chapter 4.

The blurring of distinctions between types of health plans is a result of the adoption of managed care activities by different types of plans. When HMOs first appeared, for example, no other types of plans focused on managing inpatient utilization, so that activity was considered an attribute of HMOs. Because of the rising cost of inpatient care, however, most types of plans also began to address inpatient utilization. The same dynamic occurred in most medical management, covered in Part III of this book.

Despite this, very real distinctions between different types of managed care plans remain, and are worth understanding. Doing so means focusing not on particular processes or activities, but on how the plans are organized; what their relationship is with hospitals and, in particular, with physicians; what requirements are placed upon members and providers around health benefits coverage; and how they are licensed and regulated. For example, HMOs are licensed differently than are health insurers or PPOs, and have unique regulatory requirements.

■ TAXONOMY

It's bad enough that we must sometimes struggle to distinguish an HMO from a PPO from a POS plan or a CDHP. We must struggle equally with how we name these things. Recall that the term "MCO," which came to mean any kind of HMO, POS, or PPO as an indirect result of the managed care backlash discussed in Chapter 1, is now being used less often than it once was. It is now more or less interchangeable with another generic term, "payer,"‡ referring to any organization that administers health benefits and pays providers.

The term "health plan" is often used colloquially as interchangeable with MCO, payer, and health insurer. That colloquial use occurs in this chapter as well as throughout the book, but is technically incorrect. The health plan is actually the health benefits plan, and that means the entity responsible for setting the benefits and bearing the risk for medical costs. As discussed next, a considerable amount of

---

* No reason that the "H" doesn't get used in this acronym other than "IDS" rolls off the tongue better, but IDS is the term commonly used.
† Just to add to the confusion, some of these types of IDSs are even required to be licensed by the state if they accept risk for medical costs. In California, for example, HMOs must have a Knox-Keene license, and IDSs that accept risk must have a "limited" Knox-Keene license.

---

‡ "Payer" as applied to a managed health care organization or a health insurer, in turn used to be spelled "payor," and is still used that way by many. On behalf of its editor, this book accepts its share of the blame for once pushing it that way, and now pushing it back.

coverage in this country is through employer-sponsored self-funded benefits plans in which the employer sets the benefits and bears the risk for medical costs, not the insurer. Legally speaking, the health plan is the employer while the payer organization is only an administrator, although it's still the payer because it actually processes claims payments. It's an important distinction for many purposes, but unimportant for others. It is therefore used interchangeably with MCO and payer except when it's necessary to make the distinction.

Some also use the term "health insurer" or even "insurer" to mean any kind of payer. Technically that too is incorrect because HMOs are licensed differently than are insurers, and an insurer may only administer the benefits for a self-funded benefits plan, but not hold the insurance risk for medical costs as just noted. This chapter, like the book, will use the terms "health insurer" or "insurer" broadly and will only distinguish by plan type or between being the insurer and being the administrator of a self-funded benefits plan when necessary to do so.

From a legal and regulatory standpoint, there is no difficulty with taxonomy. All of these different organizations are defined under laws, licensed accordingly if subject to licensure, and regulated as unique types of entities. That aspect is explored in Chapters 28–30. Because the content of this chapter and the rest of the book is from an operational standpoint, taxonomy is used consistent with the industry overall, not regulators. That's the reason for all of these terms sometimes being used differently depending on whatever point is being made.

To recap: For purposes of this chapter, the reader may assume that anytime the terms "MCO" or "payer" are used, it applies to all types of payer organizations. When the term "health plan" is used, it too is interchangeable with MCO and payer unless it's necessary to distinguish between an insured and a self-funded benefits plan. When describing a particular feature or function specific to a specific type of plan such as an HMO, POS, PPO, CDHP or self-funded health benefits plan, those specific terms will be used.

Along similar lines, the term "IDS" is also used generically, with more specific IDS types identified as appropriate. But that can wait until later in the chapter.

■ INSURED VERSUS SELF-FUNDED BENEFITS PLANS

Before delving into the different types of payers, it is worth looking at the differences between insured and self-funded benefits plans. Less than half of all employer group health benefits plans actually are covered under health insurance. As of 2010, over 59% of all group health coverage was through employer self-funded group health benefits plans, a percentage that has been slowly increasing, as shown in **Table 2-1**. The larger the employer group, the more likely it is to self-fund its plan. The proportion of insured to self-funded business will vary from payer to payer. National companies have a lot of self-funded accounts, and local or regional companies have more insured business. HMOs also tend to have more insured accounts than self-funded ones, but that too varies.

In health insurance, employers or individual subscribers pay premiums and the health plan is at risk for the cost of covered medical services. But under provisions in the Employee Retirement Income Security Act (ERISA; see Chapter 29), employers are allowed to self-fund their benefits plans. In a self-funded plan, the employer is at risk for the cost of covered medical services, and the money used to pay claims is provided by the employer only at the time claims are paid on its behalf, not from premiums paid to an insurer or HMO.

By self-funding an employer avoids paying state premium taxes or complying with most (though not all) state laws and mandated benefits. It also means keeping any profit an insurer would make on the premiums. On the other hand, the level of risk is high and only predictable when looking at large numbers of covered lives. A small risk pool, meaning a small number of individuals covered

TABLE 2-1	**Percentage of Covered Workers in Partially or Completely Self-Funded Plans, by Firm Size, 1999–2010**											
	1999	**2000**	**2001**	**2002**	**2003**	**2004**	**2005**	**2006**	**2007**	**2008**	**2009**	**2010**
3–199 workers	13%	15%	17%	13%	10%	10%	13%	13%	12%	12%	15%	16%
200–999 workers	51	53	52	48	50	50	53	53	53	47	48	58*
1,000–4,999 workers	62	69	66	67	71	78	78	77	76	76	80	80
5,000 or more workers	62	72	70	72	79	80	82	89	86	89	88	93
ALL FIRMS	**44%**	**49%**	**49%**	**49%**	**52%**	**54%**	**54%**	**55%**	**55%**	**55%**	**57%**	**59%**

Source: "Employer Health Benefits 2010 Annual Survey (#8085), p.170. http://ehbs.kff.org/pdf/2011/8225.pdf." The Henry J. Kaiser Family, September 2010. This information was reprinted with permission from the Henry J. Kaiser Family Foundation. The Kaiser Family Foundation is a non-profit private operating foundation, based in Menlo Park, California, dedicated to producing and communicating the best possible analysis and information on health issues.

under the plan, is subject to chance more than anything else; for example, an employer with 23 healthy marathon-running employees may have very low costs, until one of those runners is hit by a bus, has four surgical repairs and a new hip, and spends 8 months in rehabilitation. For that reason, typically it's only the large employers that self-fund, but the number of mid-sized firms that self-fund has been increasing recently.

Self-funded employer groups typically purchase reinsurance to protect themselves against very high costs. Some large health insurers and Blue Cross Blue Shield (BCBS) plans in fact sell reinsurance to self-funded customers, but a substantial portion of reinsurance is purchased from commercial reinsurance firms, both domestic and international. Some companies even use what is called a "captive" insurance or reinsurance company, meaning one they own themselves and use primarily for their own purposes. Captives are often domiciled offshore where they are regulated differently than U.S. Insurers.

Reinsurance, however, is not health insurance. It is not required to provide the same breadth of coverage, and is not subject to the ACA or ERISA. For example, an employer with a self-funded plan will be required to provide certain benefits and may not discriminate among employees, but a reinsurer may decline to cover certain benefits (e.g., transplants) or even certain individuals in the plan (e.g., a severely ill neonate). This is known as "applying a laser" or "lasering" the reinsurance policy, meaning a highly focused exclusion or exclusions. Not all reinsurers use lasers, but when they do, it's typically upon renewal after the condition(s) have been identified, not when the initial policy was sold, so the restriction(s) only applies going forward. The employer, however, is still responsible for covering employee benefits, but will have no reinsurance protection for excluded high-cost conditions or cases and will be unable to buy affordable reinsurance from another carrier.

Another difference between reinsurance and health insurance is the period during which a cost may be covered, and under what conditions. In health insurance, coverage begins when a member is both eligible and enrolled, and coverage may be retroactive. It ends when the member is either no longer eligible or leaves the plan. Costs incurred during that period of time are covered subject to the types of terms such as compliance with utilization management (UM), discussed later in this chapter and in Chapter 7. This is also applicable to self-funded benefits plans.

That is not the case with reinsurance. Reinsurance is typically one of several forms, including:

- **Claims made**, meaning the reinsurer has liability only when the event occurred and the insurer was informed of the potential for liability while the insurance is in force. If informed after the policy has lapsed, the insurer has no liability.
- **Claims paid**, meaning coverage is only for medical claims paid by the health benefits plan in a specific time period (e.g., 1 year). The coverage is for any claims paid during the contract period, regardless of when the costs were actually incurred. After the period of coverage has ended, there is no further coverage for costs even if they were incurred during the period when the reinsurance was in force and the reinsurer was notified, but no claims were paid by the benefits plan.
- **Occurrence**, meaning coverage applies if the policy was in force when the event occurred, regardless of whether or not the reinsurer was notified or a claim was paid. This is most like actual health insurance, and is also either the most expensive or unavailable.

Because of the guaranteed issue requirement in the ACA, an employer that cannot obtain unrestricted reinsurance will still be able to purchase actual health insurance beginning in the year 2014. However, only premiums for small employer groups are pooled together under community rating (see Chapter 22). Large groups may be experience rated. In other words, beginning in 2014, a large employer with high costs but a lasered reinsurance policy will be able to purchase unencumbered health insurance—but it won't be cheap.

From an operational point of view, self-funded employer groups contract with an administrator to manage their plans on a day-to-day basis under an administrative services only (ASO) contract. The administrator is paid only to administer the benefits plan on behalf of the plan sponsor, but is not paid to assume risk for medical costs and does not hold the money used for claims payment. Self-funded employers usually (but not always) contract with payers such as HMOs, commercial insurers, or BCBS plans to administer their benefits plan, and the payer's logo will appear on ID cards and correspondence. Doing so allows the self-funded plan to take advantage of a payer's network (the topic of Part II in this book), medical management (Part III), and claims adjudication and member services capabilities (Part IV). To everyone except the employer and the plan administrator, there is no obvious difference between insured or self-funded.

Health insurers have few barriers to being the administrators of self-funded plans. But HMO regulations of some states preclude HMOs from offering self-insured benefits plans. HMOs avoid these prohibitions by incorporating related corporate entities that use the HMO's negotiated provider agreements, management systems, utilization protocols, and personnel to service the self-insured line of business. They also use contract amendments or appendices that add the HMO-related entity to the contractual terms, and typically use a logo that is nearly indistinguishable from the regular logo.

There are several reasons to discuss self-funding in the context of this chapter. The first reason is to dispel the notion that every time a payer does something to lower medical costs, they pocket the money. But when savings apply to self-funded business, it lowers the amount the employer pays but has no impact on the payer's administrative fees.* The second reason is to explain why certain inconsistencies may appear in how medical benefits are covered. ERISA allows an employer with a self-funded plan a great deal of latitude in benefits design; they will be more limited beginning in 2014 under the ACA (see Chapter 30), but still allowed to differ from insured benefits in some regards. This latitude means they can choose to cover a benefit differently than how the payer typically does, although as a practical matter they usually go with existing payer policy. Finally, because ERISA defines the self-funded employer as the plan sponsor (the payer organization is simply the administrator), they can and sometimes do set up their own unique health plans, and on occasion even "private label" them. ERISA is discussed further in Chapter 29.

■ THE MANAGED CARE CONTINUUM

Before discussing each specific type of insurer or managed health care plan, it helps to look at how the most common types of payers array along the continuum illustrated in **Figure 2-1**. This is done by looking at a combination of structural and functional differences, bearing in mind that the functional differences are less pronounced than they once were.

On one end of the continuum is managed indemnity with simple precertification of elective admissions and

large case management, superimposed on a traditional indemnity insurance plan. Similar to indemnity is the service plan, which has contractual relationships with providers addressing maximum fee allowances, prohibiting balance billing, and using the same UM techniques as managed indemnity. Indemnity or service plans typically remain the licensed entity upon which other types of managed health care plans other than HMOs are built, however.

Further along the continuum are PPOs, POSs, open-panel (both direct contract and individual practice association [IPA] types) HMOs, and finally closed-panel (group and staff model) HMOs. Progressing from one end of the continuum to the other, new and broader elements of management and accountability are added, the complexity and the associated overhead increases, and the potential for control of cost and quality increases as well.

CDHPs, which combine a high-deductible insurance policy with a PPO network and a unique pretax medical savings plan, do not fit neatly on this continuum, although they are closer to PPOs than the other traditional types. Because of that, as well as their continued evolution, they are separately described later in the chapter. Even further afield from this model are third-party administrators (TPAs) that provide á la carte, barebones services to self-funded plans, and they too are separately addressed later in the chapter.

Types of IDSs, including new organization models and approaches envisioned in the ACA such as ACOs and PCMHs, have some attributes applicable to this continuum, but are even less easy to classify than different types of MCOs. Furthermore, they are primarily in the business of providing health care, not managing the health care benefit. Therefore, they are addressed separately later in the chapter. The last major topic addressed in this chapter is vertical integration.

■ TYPES OF HEALTH INSURERS AND MANAGED CARE ORGANIZATIONS

With the clear understanding that functional features of one type of plan often appear in another, what follows is a

---

*Typical ASO contracts do not pay the administrator—the payer organization—for medical savings. Performance requirements are usually limited to claims payment speed, member services responsiveness, and so forth.

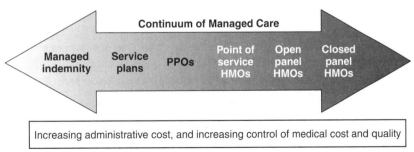

FIGURE 2-1 Continuum of Managed Care

discussion of the broad types of health insurers and managed care organizations. As noted earlier, the terms "insurer," "MCO," "payer," or "health plan" may be used to cover the whole array of plan types. But distinctions between types of MCOs are not mere historic relics; there are differences that matter, and the terms themselves still enjoy wide usage (or misusage in some cases).

Unless one works in the industry, it's hard to grasp just how many different legal designations exist for payer organizations. It is common for a single company to be made up of multiple variants, each licensed under different sets of laws and regulations. States also usually require HMOs and insurers to be licensed as a state corporation. As of 2011, for example, a partial list of company names used by the national payer company Aetna included:

- Aetna Health of [State]* Inc. (HMO corporations in the states in which they operate);
- Aetna Health Insurance Company;

----
* [State] means the name of each individual state, where applicable.

- Aetna Life Insurance Company;
- Aetna Life Insurance Company HMO;
- Aetna Health Inc. Preferred Provider Benefit Plans; and
- Aetna Dental of [State] Inc.[3]

There are also distinctions that are important for reasons that may have little or nothing to do with what the payer sells and manages. To the average consumer, for example, there is no difference between a not-for-profit insurance company and one organized as a mutual insurer; neither pays dividends to stockholders. To take it further, a mutual uses financial surpluses to the benefit of its policyholders (usually putting it toward premiums) because policyholders technically "own" the company, similar to a health care cooperative (co-op). These types of distinctions will only be referenced if it's important to do so, but will otherwise not be discussed further.

Figure 2-2 shows how the major different types of plans have grown or declined between 1988 and 2010. This section is not confined to only these, however, and many types of plans, such as HMOs, have many variants of their own.

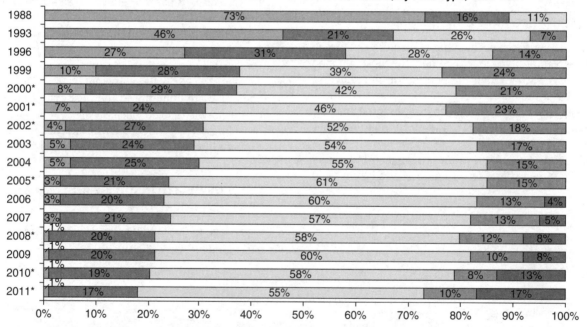

Distribution of Health Plan Enrollment for Covered Workers, by Plan Type, 1988–2011

* Distribution is statistically different from the previous year shown (P<0.05). No statistical tests were conducted for years prior to 1999. No statistical tests are conducted between 2005 and 2006 due to the addition of HDHP/SO as a new plan type in 2006.

Note: Information was not obtained for POS plans in 1988. A portion of the change in plan type enrollment for 2005 is likely attributable to incorporating more recent Census Bureau estimates of the number of state and local government workers and removing federal workers from the weights. See the Survey Design and Methods section from the 2005 Kaiser/HRET Survey of Employer-Sponsored Health Benefits for additional information.

FIGURE 2-2 Distribution of Health Plan Enrollment for Covered Workers, by Plan Type, 1988-2011

Source: "Employer Health Benefits 2011 Annual Survey, (#8225)," p. 61. http://ehbs.kff.org/pdf/2011/8225.pdf. The Henry J. Kaiser Family, September 2011. This information was reprinted with permission from the Henry J. Kaiser Family Foundation. The Kaiser Family Foundation is a nonprofit private operating foundation, based in Menlo Park, California, dedicated to producing and communicating the best possible analysis and information on health issues.

Indemnity Insurance or Indemnity Coverage

Indemnity type of health insurance is simply that: it indemnifies the beneficiary from financial costs associated with health care. Indemnity insurance and service plans (see later) were the main type of health plan prior to the advent of managed health care, with notable exceptions, as discussed in Chapter 1. Originally, few controls were in place to manage cost, and coverage was only for illness, not for wellness; preventive services such as immunizations; or prescription drugs. The insurance company usually paid based on billed charges, but it might also determine what a maximum appropriate charge should be for a professional visit, and base coverage on that rather than the billed amount. Providers were free to bill the beneficiary for anything not paid by the insurance company. In some cases, the insurance company paid the money directly to the beneficiary and the provider was required to collect unpaid amounts from the beneficiary.

Rising health care costs hit traditional indemnity health insurance hard during the 1980s and early 1990s. Their initial response was to add a managed care overlay, which is discussed shortly. But overall, as managed care grew, indemnity insurance shrank. It now makes up only 1% of the market, making it rare but not quite extinct. It may also be a component of another type of plan such as a POS plan.

But the disappearance of traditional health insurance does not mean the disappearance of the health insurance industry. Traditional health insurance was (and for the tiny amount still in the market is) a product, not a company. Health insurers consolidated as most traditional health insurance carriers exited the business by selling the health insurance book of business to another insurer or by being acquired. The remaining carriers built PPOs on their insured products, using their existing licenses, along with building or acquiring various other types of managed health care plans.

Service Plans

Service plans, the majority (though not all) of which are Blue Cross and Blue Shield (BCBS) plans, have their origins with the providers themselves, as discussed in Chapter 1. Traditional service plans are similar in some ways to indemnity insurance from a benefits standpoint, but differ in a very important way: they have a contracted provider network. The contract brings several highly significant elements found in all managed care plans (Chapter 6), elements that grow stronger further down the continuum:

- The plan contracts directly with providers (physicians, hospitals, and so forth);
- Provider contracts specify that the plan will pay them directly and they may only bill the patient (member) for coinsurance, copays, or deductibles;

- The plan has a method of calculating
    - The maximum professional fee(s) for all procedures or provider visits, and
    - The appropriate payment to hospitals;
- As long as a member receives services from a contracted provider, the member is protected from balance billing; that is, a provider cannot bill the member for
    - Charges denied by the plan, or
    - For any differences between the amount the provider charged and what the service plan determined is the maximum allowable amount, referred to as "allowed charges."

Unmanaged service plans were subject to the same pressures as indemnity insurance in regard to medical costs, and suffered the same fate. The difference is that their traditional insurance products may have disappeared but the service plan itself did not. Like the traditional health insurance carriers, service plans easily evolved into PPOs, but they also continue to exist as distinct contracted networks alongside the PPO. In that case, a service plan contracted provider that chooses not to participate in the service plan's PPO will still be bound by the terms of the service plan contract when seeing PPO members. The other major legacy of service plans is that they often had, and still have, the largest networks in a community, which provides a competitive advantage even now, although not for the original traditional product.

Managed Indemnity

As HMOs began to succeed in controlling the utilization and cost of health services, traditional carriers responded by developing managed care overlays that could be combined with traditional indemnity insurance, service plans, or indemnity-like self-funded benefits plans (the term *indemnity insurance* is being used to refer to all three forms of coverage in this context). These managed care overlays were intended to provide some measure of cost control for indemnity plans, while retaining the individual's freedom of choice of provider, and coverage for out-of-plan services.

These managed care overlays are also still present in the market, having evolved to be applicable to other types of products. Although traditional indemnity health insurance is now rare because of the high cost, other forms of nonhealth indemnity health coverage exist in which they are used, such as workers' compensation.[*] They are also used by large self-funded plans that choose which services to overlay on their plan and which they may forgo. The services are provided by the payer or by separate companies

---

[*]Workers' compensation benefits are regulated under labor laws. When insured rather than self-funded, the insurance is a form of property/casualty insurance, not health insurance.

that specialize in that service, and more than one company may provide services to a self-funded account.

The following are the most common types of managed care overlays:

- *General utilization management.* These companies offer a menu of UM activities that can be selected by individual employers or insurers.
- *Large case management.* Some firms have developed to assist employers and insurers with managing very costly cases, also called large or catastrophic cases, regardless of the type of care involved. This service includes screening to identify catastrophic cases, collection of information required for timely notification of a reinsurer, ongoing monitoring of the treatment, providing assistance in managing the case, and negotiating provider payments for high-cost cases.
- *Specialty utilization management.* Firms that focus on utilization review for specialty services have become common. Behavioral health (see Chapter 12) and dental care are two examples of specialty UM overlays.
- *Disease management.* Free-standing disease management (DM) companies or an insurer's internal program may focus on specific common, chronic diseases such as diabetes rather than on utilization more broadly. See Chapter 8 for a detailed discussion of DM.
- *Rental networks.* Some offer networks of contracted providers within individual markets and bear strong resemblances to PPOs (discussed later and in Chapter 4).
- *Workers' compensation utilization management.* In response to the rapid increases in the cost of workers' compensation insurance, firms have developed managed care overlays to address both standard UM and some unique aspects involved with workers' compensation benefits.

Indemnity insurance companies that remained in the business of health insurance typically carried these concepts several steps farther along the continuum by transforming themselves into PPOs, and through acquisitions of HMOs and other managed care companies. In fact, all of the major indemnity insurance companies that existed at the beginning of the 1990s have either sold their health insurance business lines to other companies or acquired major managed care companies.

Preferred Provider Organizations

PPOs, which are currently the dominant type of managed care plan, are entities that contract with a network of participating providers, who are therefore considered "preferred." Participating providers contractually agree to accept the PPO's payment structure and payment levels, and the PPO agrees to pay the provider directly rather than send the check to the member. In these two ways, PPOs are similar to service plans. However, PPO providers also agree to abide by stronger UM requirements and other procedures implemented by the PPO, and any consequences of failing to abide by those requirements is borne by the provider, not the member. Payment terms also usually represent a greater discount than those found in service plans.

In return, members who see PPO providers for care have higher levels of coverage; for example, an in-network office visit may require a $20 copayment, but an out-of-network office visit is subject to the deductible, then 40% coinsurance once the deductible is met, plus the nonparticipating provider will balance bill for the entire amount of billed charges. PPOs may limit the size of the network in order to provide more business to participating providers, but many states passed "any willing provider" laws (see Chapter 28) requiring the PPO to accept any provider meeting its credentialing criteria (see Chapter 4) who also agrees to the PPO's terms. PPOs can be broad or they can be specialty-only (e.g., behavioral health, chiropractic, or dental).

PPOs vary in how they perform UM. In many PPOs, the PPO itself is responsible for UM. Other PPOs agree to work with third-party companies that perform UM, or the PPO may own a UM company. PPOs not owned and operated by health insurers or BCBS plans typically also agree to comply with an employer's or a payer's UM program. Specialty PPOs more often perform their own UM, however. Quality management (QM) has, until recently, been almost an afterthought in PPOs, as was accreditation (see Chapter 15), but that has been changing.

PPOs may be owned by many different types of organizations, as illustrated in **Table 2-2**. Furthermore, a PPO may be operated solely for the benefit of its owner—for example, a PPO created by a BCBS plan that provides services only to BCBS members—or it may be a so-called rental PPO that was formed to offer services to any health plan under an administrative fee agreement (which may be limited to an access fee alone, or may include fees for other activities such as UM, claims repricing, etc.). Rental PPOs are discussed in more detail in Chapter 4.

When PPO coverage is insured, it is through a health insurer licensed in the states in which it operates, while single-employer self-funded PPO plans are not subject to state licensure. States may have laws limiting benefits differences between in-network and out-of-network coverage (e.g., no more than a 20% difference). Some states go further and require PPOs to be licensed as PPO entities, and a few states such as Pennsylvania further differentiate between a provider-sponsored PPO and an insurer-sponsored PPO, under the reasonable assumption that a provider-sponsored PPO is typically not in the risk business.

Like most other parts of the health care industry, the PPO segment has experienced substantial consolidation during the last decade. The number of PPO companies declined by more than half to 476 from 2000 to 2009, even as enrollment increased from approximately 100 million enrollees at

TABLE 2-2	PPO Ownership—2009		
Type of owner	Number of eligible employees (millions)	Percentage of eligible employees	Number of PPOs
Employer or employer coalition	0.7	0.5	3
HMO	6.0	4.1	34
Hospital	0.2	0.1	2
Hospital alliance	8.7	6.0	51
Independent investor	29.5	20.1	36
Insurance company	90.9	62.0	304
Multi-ownership	7.3	5.0	25
Physician/hospital joint venture	2.4	1.6	9
Physician/medical group	0.6	0.4	7
Third-party administrator	0.3	0.2	2
Other	0.1	<0.1	3
Total	**146.8**	**100%**	**476**

Source: Sanofi-Aventis Managed Care Digest Series, *HMO-PPO Rx Digest 2010–2011.* www.managedcaredigest.com, accessed May 21, 2011. Used with permission.

the turn of the century to almost 150 million during 2009.[4] Since the last edition of this book, enrollment has become much more concentrated in PPOs owned by insurance companies, growing from 47.9% of enrollment in 2004 to almost 62.0% of enrollment in 2009. This also meant that in the same period, PPOs owned by investors saw their share of enrollment cut in half, from 40.4% to 20.1%. Some of this change was because insurers bought previously independent PPO companies, while some is due to insurers needing less rental PPO coverage as a result of having expanded their own networks.

Exclusive Provider Organizations

Exclusive provider organizations (EPOs) are similar to PPOs in their organization and purpose. Unlike PPOs, however, EPOs limit benefits coverage only to services provided by participating providers, except urgent or emergency services. Because EPOs typically do not otherwise cover services received from nonparticipating providers, they share at least one similarity to HMOs. EPOs typically are not licensed as HMOs, but use an existing PPO network for in-network services and most often are used by self-funded employer groups or governmental benefits plans not subject to typical state regulation. In some cases the EPO was created specifically for a single employer, but most PPOs and national insurers offer EPO plans to employers using their existing PPO networks. Unlike HMOs, EPOs typically do not require a member to coordinate all specialty and facility-based care by going through a primary care provider (PCP) "gatekeeper," as described later in this chapter.

EPOs typically are implemented by self-funded employers whose primary motivation is cost-saving. These employers are less concerned about the reaction of their employees to severe restrictions on the choice of health care provider and offer the EPO as a replacement for traditional health insurance or PPO coverage. State and local governments may take the same approach for the same reasons.*

Recently, a few large employers combined EPO-type health plans for their employees and coupled them with onsite primary care centers.† Under some of these programs, the employees and covered dependents are not only limited to the EPO's provider network, they also are required to receive their primary care (and sometimes their prescription drugs too) through the onsite centers. These onsite primary care centers also usually serve as the providers of occupational medicine for the employers who implement them. In the view of the employers who offer this hybrid plan, they are striving for both higher quality care and lower costs of providing benefits. While a number of employers have expressed interest in implementing these types of EPO plans, the actual number of plans and covered individuals remains small.

_____
*Under ERISA, state and local governmental benefits plans, as well as church-sponsored benefits plans, are technically not considered self-funded, but may administer their plans as though they are a single-employer self-funded plan. Federal employee health benefits plans are subject primarily to regulation only through the Office of Personnel Management.

†As an example, Cerner Corporation, which is a large health care information technology company, offers such a health benefit plan to its Kansas City–based employees and dependents.

Point-of-Service Plans

POS plans essentially combine an HMO (or HMO-like health plan) with indemnity-type coverage for care received outside of the HMO. HMO members covered under POS benefit plans may decide whether to use HMO benefits or indemnity-style benefits for each instance of care. In other words, the member is allowed to make a coverage choice at the *point of service* when medical care is needed.

They originated in the second half of the 1980s as a way for large self-funded employers to provide a managed care plan that would combine the cost savings of an HMO without completely losing coverage for care provided out of network. This would address the fears of individuals who worried they might need care from a renowned specialist for a rare (and expensive) disorder and that the HMO would not authorize it or cover the cost.

POS plans also provided a way for HMOs to broaden their appeal and gain enrollment. It was also very appealing for large insurers that owned HMOs, but who never were completely comfortable with the concept. Soon nearly all insurers with HMOs offered POS plans. Independent HMOs were slower to adopt POS plans, however. Because HMOs are licensed differently than are health insurers, freestanding HMOs needed to obtain a health insurance license to offer such coverage. As the managed care backlash grew (Chapter 1) a few states even passed laws mandating that all HMOs provide out-of-network coverage, effectively converting their HMOs to POS plans in a stroke.[*]

The indemnity coverage available under point-of-service options from HMOs typically incorporates high deductibles and coinsurance to encourage members to use HMO services within-network instead of out-of-plan services. Payment may also be limited to the amount the HMO would have paid an in-network provider, which typically is much less than the amounts charged by out-of-network providers. Members who use the non-HMO benefit portion of the benefit plan may also be subject to utilization review such as preadmission certification and continued stay review (Chapter 7).

POS plans and PPOs both provide differing benefits coverage levels for in-network and out-of-network services, but they are not equivalent. **Table 2-3** provides a comparison between them.

Once touted as yet another wave of the future, they grew in the mid-1990s, only to decline in popularity as their hoped-for cost savings failed to materialize, as charted in Figure 2-2.

Health Maintenance Organizations

HMOs are classified primarily by the type of relationship it has with the physicians who provide services to

TABLE 2-3	Differences between Typical PPOs and POS Plans		
Feature		**PPO**	**POS**
Licensed as HMO		No	Yes
Licensed as insurer		Yes	Yes
Level of benefits when provided by in-network providers		Good	Comprehensive
Must go through PCP "gatekeeper" for highest level of benefits for nonemergency care		No	Yes
Deductible prior to any coverage for in-network, facility-based services		Yes	Usually not
Coinsurance versus copay for in-network services		Varies	Copay
Differential between in-network and out-of-network benefits limited to 20%		Yes	Varies, but often higher
Confined to HMO service area		No	Yes

Source: Copyright P. R. Kongstvedt. Used with permission.

its members, which was codified in the HMO Act of 1973 (Chapter 1). Early forms of HMOs such as prepaid group practices, co-ops, and early foundation model (IPA-like) HMOs existed prior to 1973, but most coverage at the time was through traditional indemnity insurance or service plans with no coverage restrictions related to who provided medical services. HMOs had such restrictions, so the Act required HMOs to have a health care delivery system in place that members would use for most health care services. Specifically, the Act defined an HMO as: "...a public or private entity which is organized under the laws of any State and which [...]provides basic and supplemental health services to its members[†] in the manner prescribed by subsection (b) of this section."

Subsection (b) referenced in that definition went on to describe a set of comprehensive benefits, fixed payments to the HMO, and a number of other provisions, including the requirement that:

"...at least 90 percent of the services of a physician which are provided as basic health services shall be provided through

(i) members of the staff of the health maintenance organization,
(ii) a medical group (or groups),
(iii) an individual practice association (or associations),
(iv) physicians or other health professionals who have contracted with the health maintenance organization for the provision of such services, or

---

[*]This only applied to HMO coverage for which the HMO was at risk. Under ERISA, self-funded HMO coverage is not subject to such state laws.

[†]Members were defined as an "enrolled population," similar to how all health plans view members.

(v) any combination of such staff, medical group (or groups), individual practice association (or associations) or physicians or other health professionals under contract with the organization."[5]

In other words, HMOs are not only responsible for handling the financial aspect of benefits coverage, which is also what traditional health insurers and service plans did, but they were also responsible for creating and maintaining a health care delivery system to provide those covered services. The provisions of Subsection (b) defined the basic types of HMO health care delivery systems, and we continue to define them that way today. In discussing them in this section, however, the order of subprovisions (iv) through (i) will be reversed for two reasons: (1) it more closely aligns with the continuum of managed care shown in Figure 2-1 and (2) it aligns with decreasing market presence.

Almost all HMOs contract directly with hospitals and health systems, with some rare exceptions, so the relationship between an HMO and the hospitals in its network has traditionally had no bearing on what type of HMO it is. In the short term, the rapid increase in health systems employing large panels of physicians, as well as the appearance of new IDS structures such as PCMHs and ACOs, is unlikely to have much impact on plan type. Whether or not this remains the case is hard to predict, especially for IDSs and HMOs heavily involved in Medicare and/or Medicaid. Furthermore, issues germane to closed-panel HMOs can and do resonate with issues faced by health systems with large panels of employed physicians.

It is worth emphasizing one particular HMO feature: with limited exceptions, states allow only HMOs to share risk with providers. That once was a true statement for Medicare as well, but some of the payment reform models described in the ACA for traditional fee-for-service (FFS) Medicare contain language that implicitly and explicitly have elements of financial risk, although not the full-risk model that sank the PSOs. States may well adopt some of these to help ameliorate their growing Medicaid costs and allow them for non-HMO health plans as well. Risk-sharing and other payment topics are addressed in Chapter 5.

All HMOs, regardless of model type, share a few things in common that differentiate them from health insurers. There are also a few things common to almost all HMOs, but exceptions exist. Both are listed here, and the appropriate chapter in the book is identified in brackets.

Important differentiating elements common to *all* HMOs include:

- Licensed by states under different laws and statutes than health insurers are, and are subject to more stringent rules and regulations [Chapter 28].
- Must provide adequate access to providers within its service area, defined by states and/or Medicare as appropriate [Chapter 4].

- Must include "no balance billing" clauses in all provider contracts that are stronger than those found in non-HMOs, in which a provider agrees to never bill a patient covered under the HMO for charges that the HMO is obligated to pay, even if disagreements arise between the provider and the HMO or the HMO goes out of business altogether [4].
- Must allow direct access to PCPs and ob/gyn physicians [Chapters 5, 7, and 30].
- Must have written policies and procedures for
  - Physician credentialing [Chapter 5];
  - UM [Chapter 7]; and
  - QM [Chapter 14].
- Must maintain defined minimum levels of capital reserves (called claims reserves) to be able to continue to pay claims even if they are losing money [Chapter 21].

Elements common to *most* HMOs include:

- Usually share some level of financial risk with some physicians [Chapter 6]
  - Usually only with primary care
  - Can be with a medical group
  - Can be with the entire physician network or an independent practice association (IPA)
  - Level of financial risk usually modest, and limited by law for Medicare HMOs.
- Most require members to see a PCP for routine services and to access specialty care [Chapter 7].
- Most are accredited by one of three accreditation organizations [Chapter 15]:
  - The National Committee on Quality Assurance (NCQA);
  - URAC*; or
  - The Accreditation Association for Ambulatory Health Care (AAAHC).

Types of Health Maintenance Organizations

Broadly speaking, HMOs may be viewed as either open-panel plans or closed-panel plans. Open-panel HMOs contract with private physicians who agree to provide care to the HMO's members, and are therefore considered open to private physicians who agree to the HMO's terms and conditions and who meet the HMO's credentialing criteria (see Chapter 4). In other words, open-panel HMOs do not themselves provide care to members, but rely on private physicians to do so.

Closed-panel HMOs provide most of the care to members through either a single medical group associated with the HMO or through physicians employed by the HMO, and are therefore considered closed to private physicians. In other

---

*URAC used to stand for Utilization Review Accreditation Commission, but URAC is now simply URAC.

words, closed-panel HMOs do provide care to members, although even closed-panel HMOs contract with private physician specialists for some services. A third category is the true network model HMO, found primarily in the western United States. HMOs also may employ more than one model type.*

There are two types of open-panel HMOs and two types of closed-panel HMOs. Most HMOs use more than one approach but one will predominate, and that is typically how the HMO is classified. Their distribution as of 2009 is shown in **Table 2-4**. Each is addressed in more detail next.

Independent Practice Association Model

IPA model HMOs make up almost half of all operating HMOs in the country, as shown in Table 2-4. In this model, the HMO contracts with an association of physicians—the IPA—to provide physician services to their members. The HMO does not contract with the IPA physicians directly. The IPA is a distinct legal entity, and its physician members are independent private practitioners. IPA physicians continue to see their non-HMO patients and maintain their own offices, medical records, and support staff. The term "independent" relates only to the relationship the physician has with the HMO and with the IPA; in other words, the physicians are not employees of the HMO or the IPA, but are independent contractors. Physicians in an IPA can, however, be employees of medical groups or health systems.

IPAs typically seek to contract with physicians from all specialties. Broad participation of physicians allows the IPA to provide all necessary physician services through participating physicians and minimizes the need for IPA

---

*NB: The terms "open panel" and "closed panel" are useful for understanding HMO structure, but are used in less often in general discussions than they once were, in favor of more specific HMO identifiers.

physicians to refer HMO members to nonparticipating physicians for care. The IPA also performs credentialing[†] and network management (see Chapter 4) and often some medical management such as referral authorizations (see Chapter 7).

IPAs usually follow one of two different approaches in relationship to HMOs: (1) the IPA has been independently established by community physicians and it contracts with more than one HMO in the community or (2) the HMO works with community physicians to create the IPA, which then contracts with the HMO on an exclusive basis. As health systems grow their base of employed physicians, they may form health systems–specific IPAs that would resemble nonexclusive IPAs in their approach to HMO contracting.

Physician payment is discussed in detail in Chapter 5, but is briefly addressed here to show that the payment methodology used by an HMO may not always align with how practicing physicians are actually paid.[‡] Most (though not all) HMOs pay the IPA through capitation for all physician services. Independent IPAs typically use the capitation money to pay participating physicians using either FFS or a combination of FFS for specialists and capitation for PCPs, although an IPA may also capitate certain specialists. When using FFS, IPAs typically pay all their participating physicians using a fee schedule, but withhold a portion of each payment for incentive and risk-sharing purposes. An IPA made up predominantly of employed physicians, one associated with a health system, for example, may pay physicians a salary with a productivity bonus.

Unlike the direct contract model described next, the IPA provides a vehicle for otherwise independent physicians to negotiate as a group with the HMO. While it provides the physicians with some of the negotiating benefits of belonging to a group practice, it differs in that individual members of an IPA retain their ability to negotiate and contract directly with the HMO. Because of their acceptance of combined risk through capitation payments, IPAs are generally immune from antitrust restrictions on group activities by physicians as long as they do not prevent or prohibit their member physicians from being able to contract directly with an HMO. As a practical matter, it is uncommon for physicians to bypass the IPA.

Direct Contract Model

As the name implies, direct contract model HMOs contract directly with independent physicians or medical groups to provide physician services to their members. Because there is no IPA, the HMO does the credentialing (an HMO could

---

TABLE 2-4	Distribution of Enrollment by HMO Model Type, 2009				
	Operating HMO plans		**HMO enrollment**		
Model Type	**Number**	**Percentage**	**Number (Millions)**	**Percentage**	
IPA	218	49.9%	34.8	46.2%	
Network/direct contract	170	38.9%	23.8	31.6%	
Group	36	8.2%	15.1	20.1%	
Staff	13	3.0%	1.5	2.1%	
TOTAL	**437**	**100.0%**	**75.3**	**100.0%**	

Source: Managed Care Digest Series, HMO-PPO Digest 2011, data source SDI. Copyright Sanofi-Aventis U.S., LLC and SDI. www.managedcaredigest.com. Used with permission.

[†]The IPA performs credentialing on behalf of the HMO, using the HMO's standards.
[‡]If the reader has no knowledge about different payment terms, it will be useful to return to this section after reviewing Chapter 5, which describes varied approaches to provider payment.

still delegate to a credentialing verification organization, as discussed in Chapter 4), network management, and UM. Direct-contract HMOs pay physicians through capitation and FFS, in various combinations. Payment to the physicians is also direct, although a medical group or health system may still pay their physicians through a methodology different from what the HMO uses. Direct contracting is the second most common type of HMO model.

Because the network of both the direct contract model HMO and an IPA model HMO is composed of independent physicians, they appear similar to an outside observer. It is, therefore, common for this type of model also to be referred to as an IPA, despite the lack of the legal entity of an IPA. Like so many terms in managed health care, there is little purity of taxonomy. However, the reader should be aware of the differences because the presence or absence of an actual IPA has an effect on the HMO and its management needs.

Group Model

In pure group model HMOs, the HMO contracts with a multispecialty medical group practice to provide all physician services to the HMO's members. The physicians in the group practice are employed by the group practice and not by the HMO, and share facilities, equipment, medical records, and support staff. Medical offices often have ancillary services such as laboratory and X-ray. Some may have full or limited pharmacies, and larger centers may have additional services such as physical therapy. The group may contract with the HMO on an all-inclusive capitation basis to provide physician services to HMO members. Alternatively, the group may contract on a cost basis to provide its services, in which case it shares attributes of the staff model, as described next.

In group model HMOs, the medical group may be captive to the HMO, or the HMO may be captive to the group. There are significant cultural differences between the two, although they share many similar attributes as well, including strong physician leadership and a physician management structure, having enough physicians on staff to provide for most of the care typically needed by members, having an internal peer review and QM function, more ability to invest in and use support systems such as an electronic medical record system, and the adoption of similar practice behaviors.

In the captive group model, the group practice exists solely to provide services to the HMO's beneficiaries. In some cases, the HMO originally formed the group practice to serve its members and provides administrative services to the group. The most prominent example of this type of HMO is the Kaiser Foundation Health Plan, where the Permanente Medical Groups provide most physician services for Kaiser's members. The Kaiser Foundation Health Plan, as the licensed HMO, is responsible for marketing the benefit plans, enrolling members, collecting premium payments, and performing other HMO functions. The Permanente Medical Groups are responsible for rendering physician services to Kaiser's members under an exclusive contractual relationship with Kaiser. Kaiser is sometimes mistakenly thought to be a staff model HMO because of the close relationship between it and the Permanente Medical Groups. Although not the only example, Kaiser is clearly the most robust, particularly in California.

In the captive HMO model, an established independent medical group is the sponsor or owner of the HMO. An example of this is the Geisinger Health Plan based in Danville, Pennsylvania. The Geisinger Clinic, which is a large, multispecialty physician group practice, is a long-established independent medical group that provides medical care to members of the Geisinger Health Plan as well as non-HMO patients. The HMO also contracts with independent physicians to ensure adequate coverage of its entire service area, focusing mainly on primary care, ob/gyn, and similar specialties, while having the entire network refer complex cases to the group. Physicians in the group are paid a salary plus incentives based on their performance and productivity.

Staff Model

In a staff model HMO, the physicians who serve the HMO's covered beneficiaries are employed by the HMO. These physicians typically are paid on a salary basis and usually also receive bonus or incentive payments. Like group models, staff model HMOs must employ physicians in all the most common specialties to provide for the health care needs of their members, but unlike large established medical groups, these HMOs are more likely to contract with private physician specialists as well.

Health systems employing a large panel of PCPs and specialists such as ob/gyns, general surgeons, and other high-volume specialists are also staff models, though not HMOs. However, if such systems contract with an HMO under capitation or a similar risk-based payment model, they will face most of the same management issues faced by a staff model plan; for example, physician productivity is usually much lower than it is for private physicians. This is partially offset by their ability to use their leverage to negotiate high payment rates, however. There were once a number of staff model HMOs, but most of them are either gone or have since shed their physician components. Examples included Harvard-Pilgrim Health Plan (the physicians became an independent medical group that is no longer exclusive to Harvard-Pilgrim), Group Health Association of Washington, DC (no longer in existence), FHP (no longer in existence), HealthAmerica (sold several times), and others.

Insurance companies dabbled off and on with creating staff model systems, usually abandoning them after a while. But recent problems with access to primary care, exacerbated by the growing shortage of PCPs, once again led some payers to experiment with establishing primary care centers. In these new experiments, centers may be staffed with a combination of PCPs and mid-level practitioners (see Chapter 4).

Advantages and Disadvantages of Open- and Closed-Panel HMOs

The advantages of open-panel HMOs are:

- They are much more easily marketed and sold because they include a large panel of private physicians;
- Because participating physicians are located throughout the HMO's service area, it's easier for members to find one that is conveniently located;
- Routine medical management functions may be delegated to the IPA in IPA model HMOs; and
- They are much easier and less costly to set up and maintain.

The disadvantages of open-panel HMOs are:

- Because the HMO is not involved with providing medical care itself, it has little ability to manage the care being provided and must rely primarily on the use of benefits determinations and medical necessity criteria; and
- Premiums are often somewhat higher than those of closed panels.

The advantages of closed panel HMOs are:

- The ability to more closely manage the medical care provided by the medical group;
- Delegation of many routine medical management functions to the group, thereby reducing administrative costs; and
- The convenience of "one-stop shopping" for members as most group and staff model HMOs use large office buildings that house doctors' offices and small procedure rooms, and often have basic X-ray and pharmacy services, for example.

The disadvantages of closed-panel HMOs are:

- They are not as easily marketed to new members when people already have an established relationship with a doctor and do not want to change it;
- Locations of the HMO's medical offices may not be convenient for all members;
- Closed-panel HMOs are really only feasible in medium to large cities where the market is large enough; and
- They are more complex and costly to set up and maintain compared to any other form of health plan.

True Network Model

The term "network model" is often applied to any open-panel plan, or sometimes is used synonymously with the direct contract model. But it is useful to differentiate a "true" network model in which the HMO contracts with more than one large medical group or physician organization. To an outside observer, it looks like an open-panel HMO with a large community-based network. But structurally, the HMO is not limited to a single IPA or medical group, but does not have thousands of individual contracts either. Operationally, it more resembles a capitated group or strong IPA model in which the physicians take on a significant portion of utilization and QM.

The group practices may be broad-based, multispecialty groups; large group practices without walls (GPWWs); IPAs; physician-hospital organizations (PHOs); or some combination of these (all are described later in this chapter and in Chapter 4). One example of this type of HMO is the Tufts Area Health Plan in Massachusetts, which contracts with multiple PHOs; another is HealthNet in California, which contracts with several large GPWWs and IPAs. True network models predominate in California where there are a number of existing large medical groups (with and without walls), unlike most other parts of the country where groups tend to be smaller. Recently, they have been associated with high costs despite low utilization due to the group's ability to demand high rates of payment.[6]

As noted previously and discussed in more detail in Chapter 4, health systems are increasingly employing primary and specialty care physicians. At some point this creates the infrastructure for a true network model plan. For example, two or three large health systems with many employed physicians could form a true network model plan, either by contracting with an HMO or other payer, or perhaps even as a "private label" network for large employers. They could also be the delivery system for a true network model Medicare Advantage plan (see Chapter 24), leveraging that experience to improve their performance under the new Medicare FFS and bundled payment models used for ACOs and PCMHs. The true network model may well play a larger role in coming years.

Mixed Model HMOs

As the term describes, many HMOs or MCOs are actually mixes of different model types. It is far more common for closed-panel types of MCOs to add open-panel components to their health plan than the reverse, but there are examples of large open-panel HMOs adding a staff model component through a contract with an IDS, for example.

Open-Access HMOs

Open access usually refers to a benefits plan most closely resembling a hybrid of a POS plan and an EPO. Like a POS plan, the member selects a PCP and gets the highest level of benefits by using the HMO system, but may bypass that system and access specialty care directly, albeit with less coverage. Like an EPO, however, only services provided by in-network providers are covered, regardless of whether accessed through the PCP "gatekeeper" or by going directly to a specialist. Some open-access HMOs dispense with the PCP "gatekeeper" approach entirely and simply require a higher copayment for specialist care, but still restrict any coverage to services from in-network providers. Open-access HMOs are not as common as PCP-based HMOs. Many were created in the 1970s and 1980s and then abandoned. However, new ones appeared in the late 1990s and were reasonably successful.

Consumer-Directed Health Plans

CDHPs combine an HDHP with some form of individually based, pretax savings account. They are often associated with a PPO network as well. At its most basic, health care costs are paid first from the pretax account and when that is exhausted, any additional costs up to the deductible are paid out of pocket by the member. Preventive services are not subject to the deductible, however, both by convention and now under requirements in the ACA for all qualified health plans.

There are two basic forms of CDHP benefits plans: employer-based using a health payment account (HRA) and individual-based using a health savings account (HSA). A simplified example of a CDHP benefit design for an individual is illustrated in **Figure 2-3**.

HRAs are funded solely by the employer on a pretax basis, and are not considered taxable income to the employee. The employer determines how much pretax money to put into the account and how much of any unused money in an HRA may be rolled over from year to year. An HRA is also considered a group health plan subject to COBRA continuation requirements (see Chapter 29) if and when an employee leaves the company.

HSAs for individuals were created as part of the Medicare Modernization Act. As of 2011, only individuals covered by a HDHP with an annual deductible of at least $1,200 (or $2,400 if it's family coverage) may make tax-deductible contributions to an HSA. The HDHP is also limited to maximum

out-of-pocket expenses of less than $5,950 (or $11,900 if it's family coverage). Both of these amounts are determined on an annual basis by the Treasury Department. Individuals eligible for Medicare, claimed as a dependent on somebody else's tax return, or covered under another policy are not eligible to contribute to an HSA. Any money left in an HSA at the end of the year may be rolled into the next year. Banks charge fees for holding the HSA, however, so funds can go down even if never used for medical expenses.

CDHPs are not considered managed health care plans by some, who consider them as more akin to simpler indemnity-type insurance plans from the past. This is because of the presence of a high-deductible health insurance policy as the primary product, combined with new pretax funding mechanisms for at least a portion of the costs. Furthermore, one of the initial tenets behind CDHPs is that the consumer has become shielded by traditional managed care plans as to how much health really costs; in other words, consumers have come to believe that an office visit really only costs $20 or that a sophisticated diagnostic test only costs $20. The CDHP is therefore constructed to make cost a factor in consumer decision making through the use of both the pretax fund and the bridge, with the CDHP providing information to consumers to help them make decisions based on cost and quality of services.

CDHPs have not entirely shed all aspects of managed health care, however. Most are associated with a PPO to provide the value of the negotiated discount to the consumer. From the provider viewpoint, this is a mixed blessing at best because while the provider's fee is discounted, they must still collect any amounts due under the deductible from the member. As discussed earlier in regard to service plans,

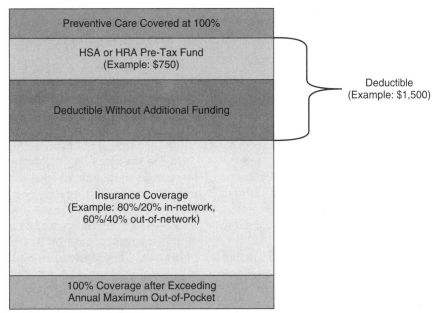

FIGURE 2-3 Example Construct of a Basic CDHP Individual Benefit

collecting from individuals is far harder than getting paid directly by the payer, which was the major attraction of the service plan in the first place.

This problem is not confined to CDHPs. As noted in Chapter 1, the average deductible for PPOs has risen dramatically in recent years, often exceeding $1,000, blurring the line between a basic PPO and a CDHP.

Payers have tried to address this collection problem in several ways. Integrating the functions of the HRA or HSA through a debit card or attaching a credit facility to the HRA or HSA are two approaches. These have not been entirely satisfactory, but have helped. Most large payers are also able to provide real-time information about any remaining deductible amounts so the provider can collect at the time of service, but not all providers are able to access this or it may only be available through certain channels. Some payers also allow a member to authorize a direct provider payment from their HRA or HSA at the time the claim comes in. Also, the ACA requires ID cards to be machine readable in 2013, including eligibility and cost-sharing information.

Simply integrating with an existing PPO is the most common but not the only aspect of managed care that CDHPs retain. Integration of medical management into the new plan designs remains an evolving aspect as well, particularly with CDHPs offered by the larger and more established companies. Basic PPO-level UM and DM are most frequently applied because even in CDHPs a small proportion of the membership accounts for a disproportionately high percentage of medical costs. In those cases, medical costs can quickly move past the pretax fund and the bridge and trigger the high-deductible insurance, where focus on managing chronic disease is exactly the same as it is for any other type of managed health care plan. Having said that, how a CDHP applies DM in the early stages of a chronic disease, when costs are still applicable to the pretax fund and the bridge, is still evolving.

Third-Party Administrators

A TPA is a company that administers benefits for a self-funded employer group, but does not have all the capabilities of a major payer organization. They are not considered managed care plans per se, although they may provide some managed care services. Services may be barebones, such as enrollment and claims processing only, and the employer purchases other services such as UM or access to a rental PPO (see Chapter 4) on an á la carte basis from one or more companies. In some cases, the TPA is able to provide many of these additional services, but they are sold as separate services.

TPAs are not licensed insurers, and the TPA itself assumes no risk. It often has arrangements with reinsurers and may assist the employer group in obtaining it. In other cases, a reinsurer may bring the business to the TPA. TPAs have well-defined responsibilities to administer the employer group's health plan. Although TPAs are not licensed insurers, more than 30 states require TPAs to be licensed in their own right and have regulations that govern a TPA's written agreement with a reinsurer. States may also regulate the TPA's provider payment methodology and timeliness of claims payments.

Consumer Operated and Oriented Plans

Section 1322 of the ACA (see Chapter 30) created a "Federal program to assist establishment and operation of nonprofit, member-run health insurance issuers" to be called a ". . . Consumer Operated and Oriented Plan (CO-OP)."[7] These are new payer organizations, not existing health care cooperatives like Group Health Cooperative of Puget Sound, although the concept of member ownership is the same. The ACA specifically calls for the CO-OPs to offer coverage to small groups and individuals through the new state health insurance exchanges (see Chapters 16 and 30).

The ACA further requires that a CO-OP not be run by a state or local government, and that neither it nor any related entity was a health insurance issuer on July 16, 2009. It will need to be licensed by the state and comply with all state insurance laws. Although a CO-OP may not have been a payer before, it can purchase certain administrative services such as claims processing services, information technology, and so forth. A CO-OP must be governed by a board that is subject to the majority vote of its members, as further described in Chapter 3.

At the time of publication, no CO-OP has been created. Small new payer organizations do not have a good track record of survival, though, so it is unclear how many will be created, if any, and of those how many will survive.

■ INTEGRATED HEALTH CARE DELIVERY SYSTEMS

Just as there are myriad types of MCOs, there are myriad types of IDSs. Because there is such wide variation in IDS structures, only the more common forms are discussed here. With a few exceptions, types of IDSs are also difficult to label, so terms or identifiers may not always match up to an IDS's structural or organizational design.

At the very least, an IDS represents providers coming together in some type of legal structure for the purposes of managing health care and contracting with health plans such as HMOs, PPOs, or health insurance companies. Some IDSs even combine different types of IDSs as well. The common denominator, however, is the physician; many types of organizations can exist in health care for purposes of managing health care and contracting with health plans that do not involve physicians, but unless there is a significant physician component, it would not be considered an IDS.

The presence of the four most common types of IDSs is shown in **Figure 2-5** later in the chapter.

Independent Practice Association

IPAs have been discussed earlier in this chapter and in Chapter 4, so will not be repeated here except to note it may be a component of another type of IDS.

Physician Practice Management Companies

Physician practice management companies (PPMCs) arrived on the integration scene in the mid-1990s. They typically were publicly traded companies, placing great pressure on the need to report positive earnings. Hospitals were not involved. Most failed and some went bankrupt, while others exited the business altogether. A few do remain, or reemerged as smaller and more focused companies, however.

Several reasons contributed to their failure. One common problem was decreased physician productivity. PPMCs purchased physician practices only to find that once the physician had "cashed out" his or her practice, there was no longer sufficient incentive for them to be highly productive. PPMCs also found that there was in fact little profit margin to be had in practices in which the primary cost was for compensation, despite small improvements in practice overhead costs from economies of scale. Most of them also entered into full-risk capitation arrangements with HMOs, and did no better managing it than PSOs did for Medicare.

The PPMCs that thrived were more specialty-focused than the massive PPMCs that had acquired primary and specialty care practices alike, for example, a PPMC focusing solely on neonatal critical care, or one focused on radiology. Unlike a group practice, the physicians were (and are) employees of the PPMC, which not only manages the practice but provides managed care services as well. Some PPMCs that focused solely on managing the office and that also remained relatively small in scope also managed to survive.

Group Practice Without Walls

The GPWW, also known as the clinic without walls, is a step toward greater integration of physician services. The GPWW does not require the participation of a hospital and, indeed, is often formed as a vehicle for physicians to organize without being dependent on a hospital for services or support. In some cases, GPWW formation has occurred to leverage negotiating strength not only with MCOs but with hospitals as well. In other cases, a hospital sponsors and supports a GPWW as a component of the IDS.

The GPWW is composed of private practice physicians who agree to aggregate their practices into a single legal entity, but the physicians continue to practice medicine in their independent locations. In other words, the physicians appear to be independent from the view of their patients, but from the view of a contracting entity such as an HMO, they are a single group. This is differentiated by two salient features from the for-profit, physician-only management services organizations (MSOs) described later. First, the GPWW is owned solely by the member physicians and not by any outside investors. Medical groups can and do hire physicians as employees, however, so not all physicians providing care are owners of the group. Second, the GPWW is a legal merging of all assets of its member physicians' practices rather than the acquisition of only the tangible assets (as is often the case in an MSO).

To be considered a medical group, the physicians must have their personal income affected by the performance of the group as a whole. Although an IPA will place a defined portion of a physician's income at risk (that portion related to the managed care contract held by the IPA), the group's income from any source has an effect on the physician's income and on profit-sharing in the group. That being said, it is common in this model for an individual physician's income to be affected most by individual productivity.

The GPWW is owned by the member physicians, and governance is by the physicians. The GPWW may contract with an outside organization to provide business support services. Office support services are generally provided through the group, although as a practical matter the practicing physicians may notice little difference in what they are used to receiving.

The GPWW model continues to exist in markets with substantial amounts of full-risk capitation such as California, where it can represent a significant amount of revenue. But even when capitation is for direct services only, the GPWW can potentially achieve enhanced revenues through pay-for-performance programs, as discussed further in Chapter 5. Outside of such markets, the GPWW model is currently much less common. Overall market consolidation, combined with pressures on Medicare payments and new performance-based payment models, may lead to a renewed interest.

Physician–Hospital Organizations

The PHO is an entity that, at a minimum, allows a hospital and its physicians to negotiate with payers. PHOs may do little more than provide for such a negotiating vehicle, although this could pose an antitrust risk. PHOs may actively manage the relationship between the providers and payers, or they may provide more services, to the point where they may more aptly be considered MSOs, as discussed next. Some PHOs even accept capitation and function as small IPAs.

By definition, a PHO requires the participation of a hospital and at least some portion of the admitting physicians. They are considered the easiest type of integrated system to develop (although they are not actually that easy, at least if done well). They also are a vehicle to provide some integration while preserving the independence and autonomy of the physicians. In the mid-1990s, PHOs were formed primarily as a defensive mechanism to deal with an increase in managed care contracting activity. Even then, it was not uncommon for the same physicians who joined the PHO already to be under contract with one or more managed care plans. Since then, fewer PHOs were created, though existing ones continue to operate. The weakest form of PHO is the messenger model. This means that the PHO analyzes the terms and conditions offered by an MCO and transmits its analysis and the contract to each physician, who then decides on an individual basis whether to participate.

More commonly, the PHO participants develop model contract terms and payment levels and use those terms to negotiate with payers. The PHO usually has a limited amount of time to negotiate the contract successfully (e.g., 90 days). If that time limit passes, then the participating physicians are free to contract directly with the payer; if the PHO successfully reaches an agreement with the payer, then the physicians agree to be bound by those terms. The contract is still between the physician and the payer, or between the hospital and the payer. In some cases, contracts between the providers and the payer are relatively brief and incorporate the contract between the PHO and the payer by reference.

The reader should note that the "PO" portion of a PHO may be a different model entirely. As an example, a GPWW or an IPA could represent the physician portion of the PHO, although most commonly the physicians remain independent and contract individually with the PHO.

One final note concerning PHOs and other types of physician organizations: the Federal Trade Commission (FTC) toughened its scrutiny of such organizations during the early 2000s. Physician organizations that are not paid on a capitation basis, or that do not accept substantial financial risk through some other mechanism, now find it much more difficult to operate within the FTC's antitrust safety zone. Although it is beyond the scope of this chapter, those interested in physician organizations are urged to consult with competent antitrust counsel during the formation and operational stages.[*]

Within the last several years, some PHOs began to take advantage of *clinical integration* as a rationale under the antitrust laws to justify negotiation with MCOs on behalf of otherwise unrelated physicians and other providers. Because of the public benefit associated with improving health care quality and reducing unnecessary utilization, federal antitrust agencies established an exemption to allow PHOs to negotiate payment terms with MCOs provided that those

financial terms were an essential component of the PHO's achievement of defined quality or utilization objectives. In other words, an antitrust exemption was deemed appropriate for organizations whose providers are clinically integrated even if they are not financially integrated. Advocate Healthcare in the Chicago area has been one of the more prominent examples of a clinically integrated PHO through its Advocate Physician Partners organization.

One of the hallmarks of clinically integrated organizations is their focus of the same types of metrics used by more traditional managed care organizations. For example, such organizations often set targets for and publicly report performance against the Healthcare Effectiveness Data Information Set (HEDIS®) quality measures used by NCQA to evaluate HMOs and PPOs. In addition, clinically integrated organizations may set utilization goals, such as reducing emergency department visits or hospital inpatient readmissions. Their focus on these efforts can help the payers with which they contract to achieve their own quality goals, which is why some payers have embraced them. Finally, the same accreditation organizations used by HMOs have created recognition standards for clinically integrated IDSs such as PHOs.

Management Services Organizations

An MSO represents the evolution of the PHO into an entity that provides more services to the physicians. Not only does the MSO provide a vehicle for negotiating with MCOs, but it also provides additional services to support the physicians' practices. The physician, however, usually remains an independent private practitioner. MSOs are typically based around one or more hospitals, but there are some physician-only MSOs that are closer to PPMCs than hospital-based MSOs.

In its simplest form, the MSO operates as a service bureau, providing basic practice support services to member physicians. These services include such activities as billing and collection, administrative support in certain areas, electronic data interchange such as electronic billing, and other services. Recently, existing MSOs are being considered excellent vehicles to provide the electronic backbone for the electronic medical record and other forms of electronic connectivity addressed in Chapter 23.

The physician can remain an independent practitioner, under no legal obligation to use the services of the hospital on an exclusive basis. The MSO must receive compensation from the physician at fair market value, or the hospital and physician could incur legal problems. The MSO should, through economies of scale as well as good management, be able to provide those services at a reasonable rate.

An MSO may also be considerably broader in scope. In addition to providing all the services described earlier, the MSO may actually purchase many of the assets of the physician's practice; for example, the MSO may purchase the

---

[*] Interested readers may also want to review the FTC's opinion in the Matter of North Texas Specialty Physicians and other resources on this case. A summary with further links may be found at: www.ftc.gov/opa/2005/12/ntsp.shtm, accessed August 2, 2011.

physician's office space or office equipment (at fair market value). The MSO can employ the office support staff of the physician as well. MSOs can further incorporate functions such as QM, UM, provider relations, member services, and even claims processing in those markets where there is significant full-risk capitation. This form of MSO is usually constructed as a unique business entity, separate from a PHO. These too show overlap with PPMCs, as earlier described.

Like PHOs, MSOs do not always have direct contracts with health plans, or the contract does not take the place of direct contracts between a payer and the MSO's providers. This is for two reasons: (1) many plans insist on having the provider be the contracting agent and (2) many states will not allow health plans (especially HMOs) to have contracts with any entity that does not have the power to bind the provider. The physician may remain an independent private practitioner under no contractual obligation to use the hospital on an exclusive basis.

Foundation Model

A foundation model IDS is one in which a hospital creates a not-for-profit foundation and actually purchases physicians' practices (both tangible and intangible assets) and puts those practices into the foundation. This model usually appears when there is a legal or regulatory barrier, for example, a state law against the corporate practice of medicine, meaning a hospital cannot employ the physicians directly or use hospital funds to purchase the practices directly. It must be noted that to qualify for and maintain its not-for-profit status, the foundation must prove that it provides substantial community benefit. Once more common than today, they are now mostly confined to a few states.

A second form of foundation model does not involve a hospital. In that model, the foundation is an entity that exists on its own and contracts for services with a medical group and a hospital. Recall from Chapter 1 that in the early days of HMOs, many open-panel types of plans that were not formed as IPAs were formed as foundations; the foundation held the HMO license and contracted with one or more IPAs and hospitals for services.

The foundation itself is governed by a board that is not dominated by either the hospital or the physicians (in fact, physicians may represent no more than 20% of the board) and includes lay members. The foundation owns and manages the practices, but the physicians become members of a medical group that, in turn, has an exclusive contract for services with the foundation; in other words, the foundation is the only source of revenue to the medical group. The physicians have contracts with the medical group that are long term and contain noncompete clauses.

Although the physicians are in an independent group, and the foundation is also independent from the hospital, the relationship in fact is close among all members of the triad. The medical group, however, retains a significant measure of autonomy regarding its own business affairs, and the foundation has no control over certain aspects, such as individual physician compensation.

Provider-Sponsored Organizations

A provider-sponsored organization (PSO) is an archaic use of the acronym that now stands for today's Patient Safety Organization. It is included primarily to illustrate a very important lesson from the past. As discussed in Chapter 1, PSOs were a cooperative venture of a group of providers who controlled an integrated provider system engaged in *both* delivery and financing of health care services. On its surface, that sounds like a co-op HMO or similar type of early closed-panel HMO. And on its surface, that was true. The problem lay beneath the surface.

The anti–managed care backlash was building rapidly, and one expression of that was a firmly held belief by many providers that HMOs were meddlesome "middlemen" that extracted a big chunk of the money but provided no value. Under considerable pressure from organized provider organizations, PSOs were authorized by Congress under a Medicare demonstration waiver as part of the federal Balanced Budget Act of 1997, and were created so as to allow provider organizations to contract directly with Medicare on an at-risk basis for all medical services, bypassing entirely existing Medicare HMOs (called Medicare+Choice at that time). As a grand experiment, it failed miserably. Providers found to their detriment that taking on full risk for the health care costs of older adults involved more than taking the money and providing the services. In other words, "cutting out the middleman" in the form of bypassing experienced Medicare HMOs was a fast route to deep financial losses, mostly absorbed by the hospitals. They found, for example, that medical costs were made up of more than the services delivered by members of the PSO; considerable expense was also associated with care delivered by non-PSO providers, medical technology costs, and so forth. Most PSOs also continued to use existing FFS payment or otherwise failed to spread the financial risk sufficiently.

PSOs were adverse risk magnets too. Physicians and hospitals see individuals as patients, while HMOs see individuals as members, not all of whom are patients. Having a patient-centric view of the market is an excellent approach as a provider, but it also means that the patients who were seen the most often were the first ones to be signed up for coverage under the PSO. The payment model for HMOs at the time made no adjustments for acuity, so payment for a healthy 68-year-old male was the same as for a 68-year-old male with advanced heart and kidney disease.

Of equal importance as adverse risk, PSOs also typically were unable to conduct the type of UM and DM that HMOs routinely used, because part of the reason the physicians

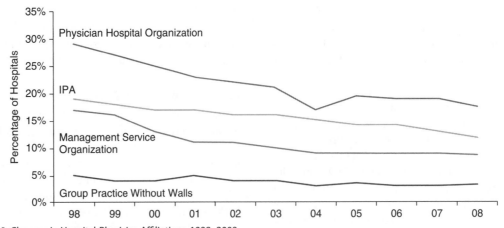

FIGURE 2-4 Changes in Hospital-Physician Affiliations, 1998–2008

Source: Avalere Health analysis of American Hospital Association Annual Survey data, 2008, for community hospitals in the AHA's TRENDWATCH CHARTBOOK 2010. www.aha.org/research/reports/tw/chartbook/index.shtml. Used with Permission.

and hospital formed the PSO was to get out from under what they perceived of as undue interference by HMOs. This was often exacerbated when the most prominent members of the PSO's medical staff were also the heaviest utilizers. Under traditional FFS, that meant they were a good source of revenue for the hospital, but under full risk they became a liability. Any attempt to restrain their utilization, however, risked having them leave entirely and take their entire (mostly profitable FFS) caseload with them.

The failure of nearly all PSOs meant that they essentially disappeared from the managed health care landscape. The federal waiver authority for PSOs quietly expired in 2002 with few survivors to mourn its passing. The small handful of PSOs that did manage to succeed were allowed to continue under a "grandfathering" provision as long as they met state financial and licensure requirements similar to those of an HMO. They exist today as organizations that look much like a type of successful provider-sponsored HMO described in Chapter 1, except for having no three-letter acronym.

PSOs may be gone, but there is much to learn from their demise, particularly for new organizations accepting performance-based payments under the ACA. There is a theoretical argument that PSOs may have survived if paid under today's acuity-adjusted payment method (described in Chapter 24) that is now used for MA plans (and proposed as an element for ACO payment). But adverse risk was only part of the problem. Of equal weight was their serious inability to manage utilization by their member physicians.

Health systems today that employ large groups of physicians, or new ACOs composed of hospitals and private medical groups, looking to participate in the new Medicare payment programs would do well to study the failure of PSOs with a cold and analytical eye. Participation in ACOs and PCMHs today is voluntary, but only PCMHs are a demonstration project under a waiver. ACOs are written into

the ACA, as is a mandate for changing Medicare payment models. PSOs did not have to fail; rather, they had to change the way they functioned.

Hospitals with Employed Physicians

Regardless of type, IDSs created to align private physicians with hospitals has been declining for over a decade, as illustrated in **Figure 2-4**. The other way hospitals and physicians come together is when the hospital employs PCPs and specialists. The employed-physician type of IDS first appeared in the mid to late 1990s when hospitals acquired PCP practices as a response to HMOs, most of which used a PCP "gatekeeper" model. In most, but not all, cases this was followed by serious financial losses as physician productivity plummeted. Hospitals then divested their physician service lines, sending the PCPs back out into their own practices. It is essentially the same time period, same dynamic, and same outcome as that described earlier for the giant PPMCs.

Beginning in the early 2000s, hospitals once again began to employ physicians, but now they are employing both PCPs and specialists. Hospitals both acquire practices and directly hire physicians in steadily increasing numbers. An article published in March 2011 reported a 75% increase in the number of physicians employed by hospitals since 2000, and the percentage of practices owned by hospitals now exceeds those owned by physicians.[8] Related to that, a press release by the Medical Group Management Association in June 2010 about physician placement reported that 65% of established physicians and 49% of physicians hired out of residency or fellowship were placed in hospital-owned practices in 2009.[9]

Figure 2-5 shows the rise in the number and percentages of medical groups in IDSs from 2001 to 2010. This trend will only continue. As of 2010, 65% of hospitals said they were

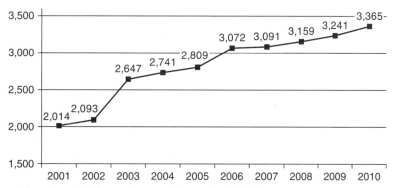

FIGURE 2-5 Number of Medical Groups in Integrated Delivery Systems, 2001–2010

Source: SDI © 2011 in the Sanofi-Aventis Managed Care Digest Series® / Hospitals/Systems Digest 2011. www.managedcaredigest.com/. Used with permission.

making efforts to increase the number of employed physicians, PCPs, hospitalists, medical specialists, and surgeons.[10]

There are several forces fueling this trend. In some cases, physicians can't keep up with costs and requirements such as electronic records; they see income stagnate or they seek a better lifestyle, and turn to their hospital for help. In other cases the hospital wants to prevent physicians from becoming competitors, by opening up a high-margin ambulatory procedure facility, for example. In either case, both the hospital executives and the physicians have a more realistic attitude than they did back in the 1990s.

In almost all cases, employing a large number of physicians also substantially increases the hospital's negotiating leverage, a dynamic that can only increase as demand for access to primary care increases under the ACA. This exacerbates the problem payers now have in negotiating and contracting with health systems that dominate a local area or region, described in Chapters 4 and 5. Because IDSs with a large number of employed physicians encompass aspects of contracting for facilities as well as professionals, it is further discussed in Chapter 4.

There are also positive aspects of this trend, however. One major one is discussed in the next section. Other positive aspects include professional management, better electronic transactional systems such as claims and authorizations, a more rapid adoption of electronic medical records, greater ability to coordinate care across a system, greater ability to observe and manage practice behavior, better communications, and a more stable physician base.

■ **ORGANIZATIONS EMERGING UNDER HEALTH REFORM**

The time leading up to consideration and passage of the ACA was a period of experimentation and articulation of "new" concepts for transforming the health care system in the United States. Well before the ACA, sustained increases in health care spending that outstripped the general inflation rate generated interest among policymakers to find methods of "bending the cost curve" to bring costs more in line with their views of the appropriate amount to be spent nationally on health care.*

Some of the new concepts did not wait for enactment of ACA, while others were given a direct boost by its passage. The intent here is not to suggest that these concepts are dependent on the ACA, but rather that they are an outgrowth of the directional movement toward health reform. The ACA specifically references four types of organizations: ACOs, PCMHs, bundled payment programs (not an organization per se, but a payment model that requires at least some type of de facto organization), and CO-OPs. CO-OPs were discussed earlier, and bundled payments are discussed in Chapter 5. ACOs and PCMHs are briefly discussed next.

Accountable Care Organizations

ACOs are among the few types of organizations specifically written into the ACA to concretely address bending the cost curve in the traditional Medicare program.[11] The ACA specifically requires their promotion unless Congress amends that portion of the Act. Seldom has a term or concept become so widespread and become such a repository of hope with so little in the way of "proof of concept." Most published studies demonstrating positive results and used in support of ACOs actually demonstrate the value of existing and closely managed provider systems or medical groups with significant experience in managed health care.

Where did this concept originate and what are ACOs? While it may be difficult to pinpoint the precise coinage of the ACO terminology, one of the earliest articulations of the concept and the term appeared in a *Health Affairs* "Web-exclusive" article by Elliott Fisher, Mark McClellan, and colleagues in January 2009.[12] They proposed "a new

---

* The health care journals and blogs from the time were full of articles and dialogue on "bending the cost curve," with many recommendations but little consensus.

approach to help achieve more integrated and efficient care by fostering local organizational accountability for quality and costs through performance measurement and 'shared savings' payment reform." The authors explicitly recognized that organizations with the strongest accountability—closed-panel HMOs—were likely to be unacceptable to most Medicare beneficiaries. In other words, ACOs were formulated as a pragmatic solution to the problem that most Medicare beneficiaries (and, indeed, most Americans) are unwilling to enroll in a traditional closed-panel HMO because of the restrictions such organizations place on their choice of provider and access to health care services, and to address costs in the traditional FFS Medicare program.

CMS published the final rule regulating ACOs on October 20, 2011.[13] In addition to addressing several related initiatives and pilot programs, the final rule defined what kind of entities are eligible to form an ACO, what structural and financial requirements an ACO would have to meet, how performance would be measured, and the shared savings program. At the time of publication, ACOs have not been implemented. Therefore the following discussion is based on what the final rule provides for, not what actually exists.

ACO Structural Requirements

According to the final rule, the following ACO participants or combinations of ACO participants are eligible to form an ACO that may apply to participate in a shared savings program:

1. ACO professionals in group practice arrangements,
2. Networks of individual practices of ACO professionals,
3. Partnerships or joint venture arrangements between hospitals and ACO professionals,
4. Hospitals employing ACO professionals,
5. Rural health clinics (RHCs),
6. Federally qualified health centers (FQHCs), and
7. Critical access hospitals (CAHs).

The final rule also requires the ACO to be a legal entity that is authorized to conduct business in each state in which it operates, and an ACO formed by two or more otherwise independent ACO participants must be a legal entity separate from any of its ACO participants. The ACO specifically must be formed for the purposes of:

1. Receiving and distributing shared savings;
2. Repaying shared losses or other monies determined to be owed to CMS; and
3. Establishing, reporting, and ensuring provider compliance with health care quality criteria, including quality performance standards.

The governing body of the ACO must include a Medicare beneficiary who does not have a conflict of interest with the ACO or have an immediate family member who has a conflict of interest. At least 75% of the ACO's board seats must be held by ACO participants. The ACO must have a management structure in place that is similar to what is found in a nonprofit health plan, in which management is under the governance of the board. ACO participants must demonstrate a meaningful commitment, which is broadly defined in the final rule as a sufficient financial or human investment such that ACO losses would be considered to be a significant motivator.

Shared savings programs, including the potential for financial risk, are at the heart of the ACO concept. The shared saving payment methodology is discussed in Chapter 5 along with other approaches to payment. Because the model includes some risk for repayment of a percentage of claims paid, for purposes of qualification, an ACO must show that it can repay losses equal to at least 1% of the total per capita Medicare Parts A and B FFS expenditures for its assigned beneficiaries during the most recent performance year (or benchmark if there is no history). Alternatively, an ACO may demonstrate its ability to repay losses by obtaining reinsurance, placing funds in escrow, obtaining surety bonds, establishing a line of credit (as evidenced by a letter of credit that the Medicare program can draw upon), or establishing another appropriate repayment mechanism that will ensure its ability to repay the Medicare program.

Patient-Centered Medical Home

Strictly speaking, PCMHs are not a concept that was born during the lead-up to enactment of the ACA. Some commentators believe, in fact, that the PCMH concept "represents more of a change in labels than a real change in the model."[14] Indeed, the PCMH concept had its roots in 1967 when the American Academy of Pediatrics (AAP) described a "medical home" as an ideal approach for caring for children with special health care needs.

Subsequently, and after much work by researchers and medical professional societies, the AAP joined with the American Academy of Family Physicians, the American College of Physicians, and the American Osteopathic Association in February 2007 to publish "Joint Principles of the Patient Centered Medical Home." This statement of principles articulates the key characteristics of PCMHs as viewed by their proponents and as implemented by most of those organizations that have pursued their development:

- Patients have ongoing relationships with a *personal physician* who provides first contact, continuous, and comprehensive care.
- Patients receive *care from a team* of individuals at the practice level, led by the personal physician, who take collective responsibility for providing care.
- Personal physicians take responsibility for *providing or arranging all of the health care needs* for the patient, including all types of care at all stages of life.

- The patient's care is *coordinated or integrated across all elements* of the health care continuum and across the patient's community.
- *Quality and safety are key parts* of the PCMH, enhanced by evidence-based medicine, continuous quality improvement, active patient engagement in decision making, use of information technology, and a voluntary "recognition process" by an accrediting group.
- Patients have *enhanced access to care* through open scheduling, expanded hours, and better communication between practices and their patients.
- Payment to PCMHs should appropriately *recognize the "added value" provided to patients*, including recognition of services outside of face-to-face visits, payment for coordination of care, recognition of case-mix differences, and provision of incentive payments associated with reduced hospitalization and quality improvement.[15]

There are many similarities between these PCMH principles and the roles envisioned for PCPs in the traditional "gatekeeper" PCP model HMOs discussed earlier. The PCMH concept, however, has some differences with that traditional role. First, like today's closed-panel HMOs but unlike open-panel HMOs, it explicitly recognizes and embraces the concept of a care team aligned around the primary care PCP. The team is used both to leverage the number of patients who can receive care from an individual PCP as well as to use nonphysicians to provide support in roles that don't require the skills and training of a physician. Some effective PCMHs include medical assistants, LPNs, RNs, advanced practice nurses and other mid-level practitioners (Chapter 4), and pharmacists on their teams to support (and be led by) the PCP.[16]

Second, also like HMOs, there is an enhanced focus on the quality monitoring and improvement aspects of the PCP's role in a PCMH. This is reinforced with the suggestion that PCMHs should be subject to some type of accreditation. In 2008, NCQA established a recognition program for PCMHs with standards designed to assess the extent to which individual practices meet the PCMH principles described previously. Those familiar with NCQA's health plan accreditation programs would see many similarities in approach to the PCMH recognition program. Similarly, URAC and AAACH have established review criteria for PCMHs. All three have similarities but are not the same.

Third, the value of patient engagement and participation in the decision-making process is explicitly a part of the PCMH concept. The role of the patient was not always clear under the traditional "gatekeeper" PCP model or even in closed-panel HMOs. In line with the Institute of Medicine's recommendations, PCMHs are viewed as one of the key mechanisms through which patients can become more engaged in how and when they are treated. The ACA also allows a qualified health plan participating in a state health insurance exchange (see Chapters 16 and 30) to provide coverage through a qualified PCMH* as long as it meets criteria defined by the Secretary, creating the potential for an HMO-like hybrid plan.[17]

While the early evidence from implementation of PCMHs has been encouraging, there are not yet sufficient examples to know whether they will be effective or appropriate in most or all settings, particularly because most of those early successes occurred in well-established systems that already had a track record (e.g., the Geisinger Clinic). These are also the same examples used to demonstrate the potential value of ACOs, further blurring the already convoluted taxonomy of IDSs.

Many organizations are actively testing PCMHs and ACOs, including large payers and BCBS plans, as well as statewide multipayer pilot programs. The next several years should provide a wealth of information to help future policymakers understand whether PCMHs are the "real deal" and can actually help bend the cost curve or, alternatively, are nothing more than a rebranding of the old PCP concept. One thing is clear, however: PCMHs as envisioned represent a true incarnation of the best principles of "managed care."

■ VERTICAL INTEGRATION

The last major topic is vertical integration. Most of the IDSs described so far could be considered vertically integrated if they combined physicians and hospitals. But for this section, vertical integration refers to a concept once thought to be the future of the health care sector in the United States: physicians, hospitals, and insurance or benefits administration all came together under a single corporate entity. The thinking was that by so doing, all incentives would be aligned and efficiencies would prevail. This charming notion was proven to be incorrect, sometimes disastrously so, by organizations that tried it in the 1980s and early 1990s.

Vertically integrated systems of the past were made up primarily of hospitals and managed care organizations, although a few included physicians. However, executives running hospitals looked to maximize revenues, particularly for high margin services, while executives running the insurance or managed care operations looked for maximum savings. Because savings to a payer equates to less revenue to a provider, a natural conflict occurred in almost all cases where vertical integration was attempted. Physicians, generally suspicious of managed care anyway, resented what they believed to be interference in their practices (see Chapter 7).

Examples include Humana, a Kentucky-based company that began as a national hospital company, added HMOs

---

*Referred to in the ACA as a "primary care medical home."

and managed care services, and ultimately divested the hospital business. Tennessee-based Equicor began as a joint venture between the Equitable Life Insurance Company and Hospital Corporation of America, but internal tensions between the hospitals and the insurer (including their HMOs) were never far below the surface, and the company was sold to the national health insurer CIGNA. Bucking the trend was Allina in Minnesota, but that state's attorney general forced it to separate the payer company from the provider company, so it is no longer integrated. Attempts at so-called "virtual integration" involving contracts and agreements quickly either disappeared or morphed into more traditional payer–provider types of relationships.

Examples of successful vertical integration do exist, however. They are typically configured around a strong regional provider such as a health system or large medical group. In most cases, the provider system or group is the dominant feature, and it is they who own and operate the HMO or PPO.

Related to that, two new developments may see forms of vertical integration reappear. The first is the rapid increase in employment of physicians by large hospital systems discussed earlier and in Chapter 4. This creates a form of integration, but has also led to payers purchasing practices to both offset the hospital system's increased leverage and to improve access for members. That too is a recurrence of a form of integration that had diminished in the past. By way of example, at the time of publication, Highmark, a Pennsylvania-based BCBS company, filed papers with the Commonwealth to merge with the West Penn Allegheny Health System in order to compete more effectively with the University of Pittsburgh Medical Center, a massive system that employs physicians and has its own health plan.[18] Other examples include the purchase of practices by payers in certain parts of the country. While not yet a trend, it may represent the beginnings of one.

The ACA provides the other impetus. As noted earlier, it calls for payment changes in Medicare and new organizational approaches such as ACOs and PCMHs, discussed above. These new organizations would be paid through shared savings, but the overall trend will be downward pressure. An alternative to ACOs for health systems is found in MA (see Chapter 24) in which both upward and downward risk exists. The dismal experience of PSOs described earlier may not be replicated because the physicians are employed and not private, and health systems are not necessarily looking to take all the risk are exploring ways to partner with experienced MA plans. The creation of health insurance exchanges and new payer models under the ACA may also lead to new forms of vertical integration. It is simply not possible to predict any of these things with certainty at this time.

■ **CONCLUSION**

Managed health care is on a continuum, with a number of plan types offering an array of features that vary in their abilities to balance access to care, cost, quality control, benefit design, and flexibility. The rise and evolution of integrated health care delivery systems has paralleled the industry. During the last three decades, managed health care has gone from being a relatively small part of the health care system synonymous with "alternative delivery system" to being a mainstream manner in which individuals covered under employer-based health benefits plans, individuals with health insurance, and many government beneficiaries obtain their care. Managed health care will continue to evolve, with features from one type of plan appearing in others and new features continually being developed. As consolidation in the marketplace continues, it will blur the lines further. The recent appearance of new designs such as consumer-directed health plans and the as-yet-untested ACOs makes taxonomy an even greater challenge than it was before. And although there is no one single definition of the term *managed health care* that has endured and gone unchanged from the past or will survive into the future, the basic tenets of managed health care will continue to evolve in pace with market demands and requirements, and with legal and regulatory change.

Endnotes

1   The Patient Protection and Affordable Care Act (P.L. 111-148) as amended by the Health Care and Education Reconciliation Act of 2010 (P.L. 111-152), which was signed into law on March 30, 2010. For purposes of this chapter, the Affordable Care Act (ACA) includes both laws.

2   According to the 2002 Health Confidence Survey conducted by the Employee Benefit Research Institute, only 30% of the respondents think they have ever been in a managed care plan. In contrast, almost 90% of the public has been covered by managed care. See 2002 Health Confidence Survey posted results, www.ebri.org/pdf/surveys/hcs/2002/hcs02pq.pdf, accessed May 15, 2011. See also "Health Confidence Survey: Managed Care Confusion," Employee Benefits Research Institute, October 2001.

3   Aetna Company Names web page at http://www.aetna.com/legal-notices/aetna_company_names.html, accessed August 1, 2011.

4   Sanofi-Aventis Managed Care Digest Series, HMO-PPO Rx Digest 2010–2011. Available at www.managedcaredigest.com, accessed May 21, 2011.

5   HMO Act of 1973, 42 U.S.C. § 300e.

6   Berenson RA, Ginsburg PB, Kemper N. Unchecked Provider Clout in California Foreshadows Challenges to Health Reform. *Health Affairs* 2010; 29(4).

7   42 U.S.C. 18042, The Patient Protection and Affordable Care Act.

8   Kocher R, Sahni, NR. Hospitals' Race to Employ Physicians: The Logic behind a Money-Losing Proposition. March 30, 2011. Available at: http://healthpolicyandreform.nejm.org/?p = 14045. Accessed April 27, 2011.

9   Medical Group Management Association (MGMA). MGMA Physician Placement Report: 65 Percent of Established Physicians Placed in Hospital-Owned Practices. June 3, 2010. Press Release. Available at: www.mgma.com/press/default.aspx?id = 33777. Accessed April 27, 2011.

10 American Hospital Association. The State of America's Hospitals—Taking the Pulse: Results of AHA Survey of Hospital Leaders. March/April 2010. Available at: www.aha.org/aha/research-and-trends/health-and-hospital-trends/2010.html. Accessed May 9, 2011.

11 ACA Section 3022.

12 Fisher ES, et al. Fostering Accountable Health Care: Moving Forward in Medicare. *Health Affairs* 2009; 28: w219–w230.

13 42 CFR Part 425 §1345-F.

14 Kilo CM, Wasson JH. Practice Redesign and the Patient-Centered Medical Home: History, Promises, and Challenges. *Health Affairs* 2010; 29(5):775.

15 "Joint Principles of the Patient Centered Medical Home," published by the Patient Centered Primary Care Collaborative, www.pcpcc.net, accessed May 23, 2011. While the principles are summarized here, serious students may wish to read the originals to ensure that the nuances contained therein are understood.

16 For example, Group Health Cooperative in Seattle has reported good success with this type of care team. See Reid RJ, et al. The Group Health Medical Home at Year Two: Cost Savings, Higher Patient Satisfaction, and Less Burnout for Providers. *Health Affairs* 2010; 29(5):835–843 for a good description of their program and results.

17 Section 1301, 42 U.S.C. 18021 (a)(3).

18 http://www.cbsnews.com/8301-505245_162-57320474/highmark-files-west-penn-merger-papers-with-state//. Accessed November 13, 2011.

CHAPTER

3

Elements of the Management and Governance Structure

Peter R. Kongstvedt

STUDY OBJECTIVES

- Understand the basic elements of governance and control of a managed care organization
- Understand governance requirements for new consumer operated and oriented plans (CO-OP) in the Patient Protection and Affordable Care Act (ACA)
- Understand risk management at the board level
- Understand the typical key executive roles in a managed health care plan
- Understand the typical committees in a managed health care plan

DISCUSSION TOPICS

1. Describe and discuss the most important functions of a board of directors.
2. Describe and discuss how a typical board can lower their risk profile.
3. Discuss the governance requirements for CO-OPs in the ACA and the benefits and risks of those requirements.
4. Describe and discuss the key executive positions and their functions.
5. Describe and discuss typical operating committees and their functions.

■ INTRODUCTION

It is not really possible to deal comprehensively with the topic of the management and governance structure in one chapter of a book. Myriad courses, texts, and other learning resources that deal with the basic elements of management are available to readers. For the purposes of this chapter, it is assumed that the reader has a working knowledge of business and management, so certain fundamental aspects of management are not discussed here; for example, how to read a balance sheet, write a job description, or construct an organizational chart.

With a few exceptions, there is no standardization of management governance or control structure in managed care; for example, the function, or even the very presence, of a board of directors varies from plan to plan. The exceptions are the board makeup for nonprofit companies, for cooperatives (co-ops, as the acronym has traditionally been used), and the ownership and governance requirements for CO-OPs (as used for the new consumer operated and oriented plans) written into the ACA.[1]

The function of key officers or managers, as well as of committees, likewise varies depending on the type of organization, ownership of the organization, and the motivations and skills of the individuals involved. Furthermore, provider organizations have their own unique governance and control aspects. This chapter focuses primarily on health insurers and managed care organizations, although a brief discussion on provider-based managed care is also included when appropriate.

Because each plan constructs its own management control structure to suit its needs and meet regulatory requirements, only a few of the most common elements are described in this chapter. Also, legal and regulatory requirements (state and federal) may vary depending on other aspects, including:

- For-profit status
- Not-for-profit status
- State of domicile
- Product types such as
  - Commercially insured
  - Self-funded
  - Medicare
  - Medicaid
- Provider-owned insurers, health maintenance organizations (HMOs), and/or preferred provider organizations (PPOs)
- CO-OPs as defined under the Patient Protection and Affordable Care Act (ACA)
- Provider organizations such as
  - Integrated delivery systems (IDSs) and their variants
  - Patient centered medical home (PCMH) organizations
  - Accountable care organizations (ACOs)

As described in Chapter 1, consolidation has been a defining feature within the health care sector. Because of this, traditional elements of governance and management control either do not exist or exist on paper only for many health plans unless they are free-standing organizations. State laws and regulations may require certain governance structures, but that does not translate into a free-standing board, for example. Likewise, management control in national companies is far more likely to be exerted at the national or regional level than at a local level. Nevertheless, it is important to understand this aspect of how a health plan works because regardless of size, or whether it is organizationally structured as a subsidiary or a free-standing health plan, the broad areas of governance and control still exist.

Specific legal and regulatory elements are addressed in context in the following chapters, and not otherwise broken out here except as they specifically apply to governance:

- Chapter 19 (fraud control)
- Chapter 20 (member services, including the formal appeals process)
- Chapter 21 (finance)
- Chapter 22 (underwriting and rating)
- Chapter 24 (Medicare Advantage)
- Chapter 25 (managed Medicaid)
- Chapter 28 (state regulation)
- Chapter 29 (federal regulation)
- Chapter 30 (the ACA)

Detailed discussions of operational activities are likewise the topics of most chapters in this book. What follows in this chapter is a brief overview of certain management control elements specifically applicable to health insurance and managed health care plans.

■ BOARD OF DIRECTORS

Many, although not all, types of managed care plans have a board of directors. The makeup and function of the board are influenced by many factors, but the board has the final responsibility for governance of the operation. Boards are also required under state laws for most types of corporations, including insurance companies and health maintenance organizations (HMOs).

Plans or Organizations without a Board

Before discussing board makeup and responsibilities, it is worth noting that not all plans or managed care organizations are always required to have one, or at least one that actually governs it. Examples include:

- Preadmission certification and medical case management operations of insurance companies;
- PPOs developed by large insurance companies;
- PPOs developed for single employers by an insurance company;
- An HMO set up by a single company for purposes of serving only the employees of that company;
- Employer-sponsored or developed plans or managed care functions; and
- HMOs or exclusive provider organizations (EPOs) set up as a line of business of an insurance company.

With one exception, these operations or plans are subsidiaries of larger companies; those companies do have boards of directors, but their boards are involved with oversight of the entire company and not the subsidiary operation. Preferred provider organizations (PPOs) or HMOs that are divisions of insurance companies may be required to list a board on their licensure forms, but that board may have little real operational role, as discussed later. The one exception noted earlier is an HMO set up by a single company for purposes of serving only the employees of that company, which is considered a form of self-funded benefits administration and is regulated by federal labor laws, not state insurance or HMO laws.

Provider organizations such as risk-bearing IDSs, PCMH organizations, and ACOs may or may not have their own boards, although PCMHs and ACOs participating in Medicare must at least have an organizational structure capable of distributing payment.

An IDS with an existing board does not necessarily need to create a new one. In any case, the inclusion of providers who are not all employees of the organization but who will nevertheless participate in the shared savings program make it more likely that it will be structured in a similar fashion as a physician-hospital organization (PHO). PHOs and other organizational structures for IDSs are discussed in Chapter 2.

Board Makeup

All HMOs have boards (except single-employer plans, which is not discussed further), although not all those boards are particularly functional. This is typically the case with HMOs that are part of large national companies or even subsidiaries of large regional plans such as a statewide Blue Cross and Blue Shield plan. Each local HMO is incorporated and required to have a board, but it is not uncommon for the chains to use the same two corporate officers (perhaps with one local representative) as the board for every HMO. Again, the board fulfills its legal function and obligation, but the actual operation of the HMO is controlled through the management structure of the parent company (which typically does have a board) rather than through a direct relationship between the plan's administrators and the board.

The legal requirements for boards, particularly for HMOs, are spelled out in each state's laws and regulations. In the past, it was common for states to require an HMO to have at least one-third of the board be consumer representatives, but this is no longer necessarily the case. The same requirement used to exist for federal qualification, but that no longer exists either.

Board makeup also varies depending on whether the plan is for-profit, in which case the owners' or shareholders' representatives may hold the majority of seats, or not-for-profit, in which case there will be broader community representation. The use of outside directors rather than plan officers as directors is dictated by local events, company bylaws, and laws and regulations (including the tax code for not-for-profit health plans). It is common, however, for plan officers to have at least one board seat, typically held by the chief executive officer (CEO), and possibly several others; however, except for a privately held for-profit company, officers cannot hold the majority of seats.

A very few not-for-profit health plans are organized as cooperatives, in which case the board members are all members of the plan. Not-for-profit plans that are not cooperatives are generally best served by board members who are truly independent and who have no potential conflicts of interest. In many states, provider-sponsored not-for-profit payers may be restricted to no more than 20% of board seats being held by participating providers. Provider-sponsored for-profit plans may have majority representation by providers, and must therefore take special precautions to avoid antitrust problems.

Cooperatives, Consumer Operated and Oriented Plans, and Accountable Care Organizations

Three specific organizational structures are addressed here, and then not addressed further in this chapter. Cooperatives have existed for over a century, but CO-OPs and ACOs as defined in the ACA are new. Each has specific requirements for their boards, but the regulations for CO-OPs and ACOs have not been finalized at the time of publication.

Cooperatives

Recall from Chapter 1 that the very first proto-HMOs were cooperatives (co-ops, in lowercase letters), and a few exist even today (e.g., Group Health Cooperative of Puget Sound). Two aspects of structure and governance are found in co-ops: they are nonprofit and they are governed by the members of the co-op. Managed health care plans that are co-ops are also closed-panel HMOs, combining the financing and provision of health care, usually through a medical group or an employed physician staff. They may or may not also have one or more hospitals.

There are other medical-related co-ops too. The most common use of the term "medical co-op" is for medical marijuana distribution organizations. Like other co-ops, they are member-based. There are also a few examples of co-ops that provide health care services to members that are not comprehensive; for example, a physician or medical group may provide their services to co-op members on a prepaid basis, but they do not provide or pay for services they do not themselves provide. A health care co-op could also provide nonphysician services, a co-op for purchasing medical supplies, for example.

Co-ops have generally not been involved in providing comprehensive health insurance except as closed-panel HMOs. The closest similar structure is the mutual insurance company, in which the policyholders technically own the company and financial surpluses are used either for business purposes or to keep premiums lower. They are neither for-profit nor nonprofit companies, and are better defined as "non-investor-owned."

CO-OPs

CO-OPs are defined in the ACA as a new type of health payer that can offer coverage through the new state health insurance exchanges. It is to focus on the individual and small group market

Like traditional co-ops, the ACA requires that the CO-OPs governance "be subject to a majority vote of its members...;" unlike traditional co-ops, the ACA goes on to require that governance "...incorporate ethics and conflict of interest standards protecting against insurance industry involvement and interference...."[2] In other words, to be a CO-OP as defined in the ACA, and be eligible for startup assistance, the bylaws and board must protect itself from contamination by the existing health insurance and managed health care industry. This is reinforced in another provision that specifically prohibits CO-OPs based on organizations that were health insurers as of July 2009, or an organization sponsored by a state or local government.[3]

In selecting from an organization to develop a CO-OP and be eligible for startup assistance, states are to give priority to applicants that will offer qualified health plans on a statewide basis, will utilize integrated care models, and have significant private support;[4] in other words, CO-OPs that have some kind of relationship with an IDS. Although no regulations have been issued at the time of publication, the law also appears to support a traditional closed-panel model, though it does not necessarily have to be an HMO. CO-OPs will be required to meet state requirements for health insurers, however. If a state does not set up one or more CO-OPs, the ACA gives the federal government the authority to do it for them.[5]

ACOs

ACOs, which are specifically addressed in the ACA, are designed to provide coordinated care in the traditional fee-for-service (FFS) Medicare program, although they may also provide services to commercial payers. The ACA requires an ACO to "have a formal legal structure that would allow the organization to receive and distribute payments for shared savings" to "participating providers of services and suppliers," and to have a "mechanism for shared governance" in order to participate in the program.[6] CMS published the Final Rule regulating ACOs on October 20, 2011, including the specifics around governance and management.[7] As previously noted in Chapter 2, for purposes of contracting with CMS for the shared savings program, the following ACO participants or combinations of ACO participants are eligible to form an ACO:

1. ACO professionals in group practice arrangements,
2. Networks of individual practices of ACO professionals,
3. Partnerships or joint venture arrangements between hospitals and ACO professionals,
4. Hospitals employing ACO professionals,
5. Rural Health Clinics (RHCs),
6. Federally Qualified Health Centers (FQHCs), and
7. Critical Access Hospitals (CAHs).

The final rule also requires the ACO to be a legal entity that is authorized to conduct business in each State in which it operates, and an ACO formed by two or more otherwise independent ACO participants must be a legal entity separate from any of its ACO participants. The ACO specifically must be formed for the purposes of:

1. Receiving and distributing shared savings;
2. Repaying shared losses or other monies determined to be owed to CMS; and
3. Establishing, reporting, and ensuring provider compliance with health care quality criteria, including quality performance standards.

The governing body of the ACO must include a Medicare beneficiary who does not have a conflict of interest with the ACO or have an immediate family member who has a conflict of interest. At least 75% of the ACO's board seats must be held by ACO participants. The ACO must have a management structure in place that is similar to what is found in a nonprofit health plan, in which management is under the governance of the board. ACO participants must demonstrate a meaningful commitment, which is broadly defined in the Final Rule as a sufficient financial or human investment such that ACO losses would be considered to be a significant motivator.

The ACA also requires that an "ACO shall have in place a leadership and management structure that includes clinical and administrative systems," but does not specify the elements that the governance, the accompanying leadership, or management structures must have.[8] The Final Rule is a bit more specific, but still provides for a great deal of flexibility. It states, in part, that "The ACO's operations must be managed by an executive, officer, manager, general partner, or similar party whose appointment and removal are under the control of the ACO's governing body and whose leadership team has demonstrated the ability to influence or direct clinical practice to improve efficiency processes and outcomes.

Clinical management and oversight must be managed by a senior-level medical director who is a physician and one of its ACO providers/suppliers, who is physically present on a regular basis at any clinic, office, or other location participating in the ACO, and who is a board-certified physician and licensed in a State in which the ACO operates."[9] As a practical matter, except for marketing and sales and any issues around benefits, the governance and management roles described in the chapter serve for ACOs as well as different types of payer plans.

In Medicare, ACOs can face many of the same potential pitfalls of any provider-owned and -controlled health plan even though they are not traditional state-licensed plans. Sharing financial incentives between providers, particularly in ACOs accepting a single payment for all services, can put them at risk of violating federal anti-kickback laws that govern physician self-referral for Medicare patients, as well as federal health care fraud and abuse laws and regulations (commonly referred to as the "Stark laws"). The ACA does not create specific safe harbors or exceptions that address the operation of ACOs under current laws. It does, however, allow the Secretary of Health and Human Services (HHS) to waive the requirements of the anti-kickback, Stark, and civil monetary penalty laws as necessary. At the time of publication, CMS and the Office of the Inspector General have issued only an interim Final Rule addressing waivers of certain fraud and abuse laws in connection with the shared savings program.

Function of the Board

The remainder of this section addresses boards that are either free-standing or that function as though they were. As stated earlier, the function of the board is governance: overseeing and maintaining final responsibility for the plan. In a real sense, the buck stops with the board. Final approval authority of corporate bylaws rests with the board. It is the bylaws that govern the basic structure of management, authority, and control not only for the plan officers but for the board itself.

The fiduciary responsibility of the board in an operating plan is clear. General oversight of the profitability or reserve status rests with the board, as does oversight and approval of significant fiscal events such as a major acquisition or a significant expenditure. In a for-profit plan, the board has fiduciary responsibility to protect the interests of the stockholders. In the wake of recent accounting scandals such as the Enron debacle, Congress enacted the Sarbanes–Oxley Act of 2002 to significantly tighten accounting standards as well as provide for far greater accountability on the part of both boards of directors (the audit committee in particular) and senior management for financial reporting.[10] The Sarbanes–Oxley Act is discussed further in Chapter 21.

Legal responsibilities of the board may also include review of reports and document signing. For example, a board officer may be required to sign the quarterly financial report to the state regulatory agency, the board chairperson may be required to sign any acquisition documents, and the board is responsible for the veracity of financial statements to stockholders.

Setting and approving policy is another common function of an active board. This may be as broad as determining the overall policy of using a "gatekeeper" system, or it may be as detailed as approving organizational charts and reporting structures. Although most policies and procedures are the responsibility of the plan officers, an active board may set a policy regarding what operational policies must be brought to the board for approval or change.

In HMOs and many other types of managed care plans, the board has a special responsibility for oversight of the quality management (QM) program and for the quality of care delivered to members. Usually this responsibility is discharged through board (or board subcommittee) review of the QM documentation (including the overall QM plan and regular reports on findings and activities) and through feedback to the medical director and plan QM committee. In free-standing plans, the board also has responsibility for hiring the CEO of the plan and for reviewing that officer's performance. The board in such plans often sets the CEO's compensation package, and the CEO reports to the board.

Board Committees

Active boards generally have committees to take up certain functions. Common board committees may include:

- An executive committee for rapid access to decision making and confidential discussions;

- A compensation committee to set general compensation guidelines for the plan, set the CEO's compensation, and approve and issue stock options;
- A finance committee or audit committee to review financial results, approve budgets, set and approve spending authorities, review the annual audit, review and approve outside funding sources, and so forth;
- A QM committee as noted above; and
- A corporate compliance committee to oversee the organization's compliance requirements, as discussed later in this chapter.

Board Liability Issues

Any board faces the problem of liability for its actions. This is especially so in a board made up of outside directors and in a board of a not-for-profit organization. This is not to say that a board must always make correct decisions—it may make an incorrect decision, but do so in good faith—although being right is often considered better than being wrong. Rather, it is to say that a board should act in ways to reduce its own liability, and such actions will also be consistent with good governance. It is beyond the scope of this chapter to fully discuss board liability and prevention, but a few general comments may be made. Examples given in this section do not constitute legal opinions but are simply provided to help illustrate possible issues. The reader is urged to consult competent legal counsel as needed to understand board liability fully.

It is of paramount importance that board members exercise their duties to the benefit of the plan and not in their own self-interest. Conflict of interest is a very difficult problem and can surface more readily than one might suppose. Examples of such conflicts would include actions that preferentially profit the board member or actions that are more in the interest of the board member than the plan, for example, influencing how services are purchased by the plan or taking advantage of proprietary information for personal profit. It is certainly possible for an action to benefit both the plan and the board member, but extra care must be taken to ensure that the action is first in the interest of the plan. In many cases, a board member with an obvious conflict of interest will abstain from voting on an issue or may even recuse themselves from being present when the board discusses it.

The board must also take care that it operates within the confines of the plan bylaws. In other words, the board cannot take any action that is not allowed in the bylaws of the organization. Examples of such actions might include payment to an individual beyond the normal payment policies, entering into an unrelated line of business, and so forth. Board members must also perform their duties with some measure of diligence. For example, if plan management provides board members with information needed to properly decide on a course of action or a policy, it is incumbent on the board members to understand what is being provided and to ask the necessary questions to gain an adequate understanding to make an informed decision. Related to this is a duty to actually attend board meetings; although this might seem obvious, some board members may be so lax in their attendance as to provide virtually no governance or oversight. In all events, thorough documentation of the decision-making process is valuable, and those records should be maintained for an appropriate length of time. And, as noted earlier, the audit committee in particular has added responsibility as a result of Sarbanes–Oxley.

While the board's primary responsibility is to the plan or organization and to the shareholders in the event that the plan is for-profit, it may also have some measure of responsibility to other individuals or organizations if the plan acts in such a way as to harm the other party illegally. For example, if a health plan knowingly sets a policy not to credential physicians, and a panel physician commits malpractice, it is possible that the board (which either agreed to the policy or failed to change it) may have some liability. Regardless of how the board is made up, it is important for there to be adequate director and officer liability insurance as well as insurance for errors and omissions. The need for such insurance may be attenuated by certain provisions in the company's or plan's bylaws holding the board members and officers harmless from liability. This issue requires review by legal counsel.

■ KEY MANAGEMENT POSITIONS

The roles and titles of the key managers in any plan vary depending on the type of plan, its legal organization, its line of business, its complexity, whether it is free-standing or a satellite of another operation, and the local needs and talent. There is little consistency in this area from plan to plan. How each key role is defined (or even whether it will be present at all) is strictly up to the management of each plan. What follows, then, is a general overview of certain key roles.

Executive Director/Chief Executive Officer

Most plans have at least one key manager. Whether that individual is called a CEO, an executive director, a general manager, or a plan manager is a function of the items mentioned earlier in this chapter such as scope of authority, reporting structure of the company, and so forth. In a free-standing health plan, that individual is truly the chief executive officer with significant authority and responsibility. In most cases, like that of a health plan being the subsidiary of a larger company, this key manager will often be referred to as an executive director. An IDS with a considerable amount of risk- or performance-based business typically will also have somebody focused on overall performance.

The executive director has responsibility for general administrative operations and public affairs. The executive director is also normally responsible for all the operational aspects of the plan, although increasingly this is not the case for subsidiaries of larger companies. For example, some large companies have marketing reporting vertically to a regional marketing director rather than through the plan manager. A few companies take that to the extreme of having each functional area reporting vertically to regional managers rather than having all operations coordinated at the local level by a single manager. There is little standardization in the industry. Generally speaking, however, the further along the managed care continuum a health plan is, the more likely it is that the executive director will have greater responsibilities.

In free-standing plans such as a traditional HMO, the CEO is responsible for all areas. The other officers and key managers report to the CEO, who in turn reports to the board (or to a regional manager in the case of national companies that have relatively autonomous HMO subsidiaries). In a free-standing plan, the CEO also has heightened responsibilities for financial reporting under Sarbanes–Oxley, including personally attesting to the accuracy of the financial statements (along with the chief financial officer).

Medical Director/Chief Medical Officer

Almost by definition, managed care plans have a medical director or chief medical officer. Whether that position is a full-time manager or a community physician who comes in a few hours per week is determined by the needs of the plan and the plan type. Although part-time medical directors were once common in the early period of managed care, that is now relatively uncommon. In smaller and free-standing plans or IDSs, the medical director reports to the CEO. In regional or national companies, the medical director(s) may report to an executive director, but more often reports through another senior officer.

The chief medical officer typically is responsible for QM, utilization management (UM), and medical policy. Only the smallest plans or managed care IDSs have only one medical director to carry out all of these responsibilities, however. Smaller local or regional plans usually have a medical director and several associate medical directors. Large local or regional plans expand on that concept, with the senior medical officer responsible for many other medical directors who in turn are each responsible for specific functions such as basic UM, QM, disease and case management, or some other defined function. In plans that are subsidiaries of national or regional companies, care management functions are often provided through a centralized organization.

The medical director may have responsibility for provider relations, provider recruiting, and network maintenance, but many large health plans and most national companies have chosen to place network management activities under a nonphysician officer under the belief that network contracting and management is less a clinical function than it is a business function. This is borne out by Chapters 4 and 5 that address network structure and contracting and payment.

Finance Director/Chief Financial Officer

In free-standing plans or large operations, it is common to have a finance director or chief financial officer (CFO). That individual is generally responsible for oversight of all financial and accounting operations, fiscal reporting, and budget preparation. In some smaller plans, rating and underwriting also report to this function. This position usually reports to the executive director, although once again some national companies use vertical reporting.

Large plans and national companies always have a CFO. In those cases, the CFO has ultimate responsibility for all of the financial management and reporting. But duties or functions are frequently grouped into distinct areas that are in turn managed by their own leaders, who report to the CFO. Examples of such distinct areas include:

- Operational finance—responsible for monitoring and managing the budget process, day-to-day financial management, reporting, and the like;
- Treasury—responsible for managing cash and the movement of money in and out of the organization, and for managing statutory reserve levels or risk-based capital (see Chapter 21);
- Investment or portfolio management (if separate from the Treasury function)—responsible for managing the plan's investments; and
- Internal audit—responsible for ensuring adherence to proper internal financial controls and to applicable laws and regulations.

Marketing Director

The marketing director is responsible for marketing the plan. Responsibility generally includes oversight of marketing representatives, market strategy, advertising, client relations, and enrollment forecasting. In small or free-standing plans, this position reports to the CEO. In larger plans, it may report vertically. Large companies also typically separate marketing from sales, having marketing focusing on areas such as strategy, production of supporting collateral material, public relations, product design, advertising, and so forth. Sales then focuses on the different distribution channels such as direct sales, sales through brokers, or sales through benefits consultants. Sales is often further subdivided into particular types of markets such as large self-funded employer groups, small groups, Medicare Advantage, and so forth. Eventually it comes together, but often not until it reaches corporate headquarters.

Operations Director

In larger plans, it is not uncommon to have an operations director. This position usually oversees claims, enrollment, underwriting (unless finance is doing so), member services, office management, and any other traditional back-room functions. In small plans, the information technology (IT) function may also be overseen by the operations director. This position usually reports to the executive director in smaller plans.

Large organizations often divide the senior-most positions into those of CEO and plan president. When this occurs, the CEO is responsible for working with the board, external relations, shareholder relations (in for-profit plans), finance, and strategy. The president is the chief operating officer (COO) and is responsible for all internal operations, sales and marketing, and medical management. Some large organizations, particularly not-for-profit ones, may appoint the COO to the position of executive vice president rather than president.

Chief Information Officer

Most plans separate out the chief information officer function from operations because IT supports virtually all other functions. This officer is responsible for all of the computer hardware and software and often other technology support systems as well such as telecommunications. This position may also be called a chief technology officer.

Corporate Compliance Officer

Health plans must have a corporate compliance officer to ensure that the plan operates in compliance with applicable regulatory requirements under Medicare Advantage (see Chapter 24), if applicable; Medicaid (see Chapter 25), if applicable; the Health Insurance Portability and Accountability Act (HIPAA; see Chapter 29); Sarbanes–Oxley; and a plethora of other federal and state laws. Examples of typical corporate compliance requirements include:

- Maintain operations in compliance with laws and regulations
- Make legal and policy changes quickly in response to identified compliance needs
- Increase organizationwide vigilance of legal and regulatory requirements
- Develop training programs for employees around compliance requirements such as privacy and security, false claims, and so forth
- Perform internal audits of compliance requirements
- Maintain a function for employees to report noncompliance without fear of retaliation
- Provide information to the board of directors and appropriate committees
- Respond appropriately to investigations, audits, and other compliance issues that may arise

- Monitor administrative, technical, and physical safeguards to protect the privacy of protected health information (PHI), including procedures for verifying the identity and authority of requestors of information
- Create detailed specifications of what must be documented to ensure compliance with the regulation
- Decrease the likelihood of civil liability

Corporate compliance is discussed further in the chapters on fraud and abuse (Chapter 19), finance (Chapter 21), Medicare Advantage (Chapter 24), managed Medicaid (Chapter 25), and on state and federal laws and regulations (Chapters 28 and 29).

◼ MEDICAL MANAGEMENT COMMITTEES

Again, there is little consistency from plan to plan regarding committees, especially in the case of managed care subsidiaries of national or large regional companies. Medical management committees are distinct from committees of the board, in that they are concerned with functional activities rather than governance.

In medical management, committees serve to broaden some elements of responsibility and allow important input from the field into procedure and policy, or even into case-specific interpretation of existing policy. Some examples of common medical management committees are given here. The actual formation, role, responsibility, and activity of any committee vary from plan to plan. These examples of committees are from the viewpoint of an HMO, and may or may not be used in other types of payers. More information about each of these areas may be found in the pertinent chapters of this book.

Credentialing Committee

Credentialing refers to the review of a professional provider's ability to meet the plan's standards for participation, being board certified, for example. The credentialing committee sets those standards, although standards typically are similar from one HMO to another. A provider that does not meet credentialing criteria is usually not offered a contract, but should the provider wish to appeal that decision, it is usually the credentialing committee that reviews the case and makes the decision. Occasionally such provider appeals are handled by the peer review committee.

Quality Management Committee

This is one area where a committee is essential for oversight of the QM activity, setting of standards, review of data, feedback to providers, follow-up, and approval of sanctions. See Chapter 14 for further discussion.

Peer Review Committee

Peer review refers to the confidential process in which a committee of physicians reviews complaints or concerns about a specific participating physician that are brought to its attention by the plan's medical managers. The peer review committee may perform the same function in reviewing problematic utilization behavior of individual physicians. The peer review committee may be a subset of the QM committee, but is typically separate.

Medical Advisory Committee

Some plans, particularly smaller ones, have a medical advisory committee whose purpose is to review general medical management issues brought to it by the medical director. Such issues may include changes in the contract with providers, compensation, changes in authorization procedures, and so on. This committee serves as a sounding board for the medical director. Occasionally it has voting authority, but that is rare because such authority is really vested with the board. In national companies, this committee may have input to local medical management issues, but medical issues that cross all plans (e.g., medical policy for new technology) are generally provided from a corporate-level medical policy committee.

Denial of Coverage Appeal Committee

The review processes for appeals of a denial of benefits coverage is addressed by law in both the Employee Retirement Income Security Act (ERISA) and the ACA, as described in Chapters 20 and 30. The processes include both an internal and an external review process. The internal review process does not necessarily require a committee, only physician reviewers whose specialty is appropriate for the clinical issues involved, and were neither involved in the member's care nor in the initial coverage denial decision.

Most plans, however, do have an appeals review committee. This committee is typically made up various specialists who may attend meetings only if their specialty is related to the type of appeal being reviewed. The committee is also staffed by nonvoting nonphysicians, as described further in Chapter 20. External review is usually conducted by companies or organizations specializing in that function.

Pharmacy and Therapeutics Committee

As discussed in Chapter 11, plans often have a pharmacy and therapeutics (P&T) committee. Because almost all prescription drug benefits are administered by a pharmacy benefits management company (PBM; also discussed in Chapter 11) that has a P&T committee of its own, a plan's P&T committee does not typically develop the formulary. In closed-panel plans with their own pharmacies, that may not be the case. P&T committees usually recommend local or plan-specific changes to the overall formulary, and review abnormal prescription utilization patterns by providers.

Management Control Structure

The management control structure refers to issues such as reporting responsibility, spending (and other commitment) authority, hiring and firing, the conduct of performance evaluations of employees, and so forth. Each plan will set these up to fit its situation and needs. Although these issues are too diverse to be addressed in this chapter, a wealth of material on all of these functions can be found in the general management literature. One item that is of special significance is the operating report, which may be called by a variety of terms such as executive dashboard, because (to paraphrase an old saying) you can't manage what you don't measure. Most tightly run managed care plans develop an operating report to use as the basic management tool, and it typically reports the month- and year-to-date utilization, operational, and financial status of the plan. Those data are backed up with details regarding membership, premium revenue, other revenue, medical costs (usually total and broken down into categories, such as hospital, primary care, referral care, ancillary services, and so forth), marketing costs, administrative costs (including key operating metrics), other expenses, taxes (if appropriate), and the bottom line. Results are generally reported in terms of whole dollars and per member per month or similar types of metrics.

How much detail is reported routinely or on an ad hoc basis is a local call. The point here is that managed care, especially in tightly run plans, is so dynamic that managers cannot wait for quarterly results. Managers must have current and reliable data from which to manage. Sutton's Law dictates that you must "go where the money is," and that can only be done if the operating report tells you where to look.

■ CONCLUSION

The basic functions of governance and control in HMOs and other managed care plans are similar to those in any business, although the specifics regarding the board of directors, plan officers, and responsibilities of key managers vary tremendously from plan to plan. With the market consolidation of the managed health care industry, governance and management control functions that were routine in free-standing health plans have now become more vertical, coming together not at the local level but rather at the level of regional or corporate officers. Nevertheless, the management and governance needs remain, even if the form and structure continues to evolve under legal, regulatory, and market pressures.

Endnotes

1　The Patient Protection and Affordable Care Act (P.L. 111-148) as amended by the Health Care and Education Reconciliation Act of 2010 (P.L. 111-152), which was signed into law on March 30, 2010. For purposes of this chapter, the Affordable Care Act (ACA) includes both laws.

2　ACA Section 1322(c)(3).

3　ACA Section 1322(c)(2)(A) and (B).

4　ACA Section 1322(b)(1)(A)(ii).

5　ACA Section 1322(b)(1)(B)

6　ACA Section 1899(b)(2)(C) and Section 1899(b)(1), respectively.

7　42 CFR Part 425 CMS-1345-F.

8　ACA Section 1899(b)(2)(F).

9　42 CFR Part 425 CMS-1345-F §425.108.

10　P.L. 107-204, 116 Stat. 745. Also known as the Public Company Accounting Reform and Investor Protection Act of 2002 and commonly called SOX or SarbOx.

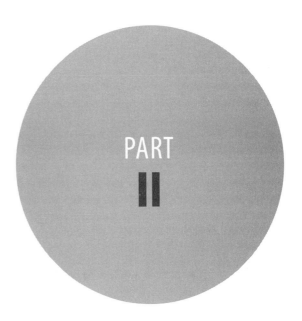

PART

II

Network Contracting and Provider Payment

"When one's all right, he's prone to spite
The doctor's peaceful mission.
But when he's sick, it's loud and quick
He bawls for a physician."

Eugene Field
(1850–1895)
Doctors, *st. 2 [1890]*

The Provider Network

Peter R. Kongstvedt

STUDY OBJECTIVES

- Understand network development methodologies
- Understand the role of primary care physicians, specialty care physicians, and nonphysician providers in different types of managed care plans
- Understand the unique attributes of hospital-based physicians
- Understand the increasing role of hospital-employed physicians
- Understand different types of contracting approaches or methods for physicians and for hospitals
- Understand basic credentialing
- Understand issues of network maintenance
- Understand critical differences between inpatient and outpatient services and how that relates to contracting
- Understand basic contracting approaches to different types of ancillary services and which approaches work best under what circumstances

DISCUSSION TOPICS

1. What are the most important issues to focus on in network maintenance?
2. Discuss differences in network development and management for different types of health plans.
3. What proactive steps can a managed care plan take to improve provider relations? How might these steps differ between different types of health plans?
4. Discuss different approaches a health plan might take to developing and maintaining a network under differing conditions such as a rural area, a medically underserved area, or a community in which there is little competition between certain types of specialists.
5. Discuss market attributes that might make contracting with a hospital more or less difficult for a health plan.

■ INTRODUCTION

The backbone of any managed health care plan is the provider network, consisting of contracted physicians, hospitals and health systems, nonphysician professionals, ancillary and therapeutic services and facilities, and any other providers of care. In this chapter, the focus is on the structure of the network because except for a few differences that will be noted as appropriate, the structural issues are the same regardless of type of plan. Provider payment is addressed in the next chapter. Topics applicable to the provider network as a whole are addressed first, followed by sections focusing on physicians, hospitals and health systems, other facilities, ancillary services, and ambulance and medical transportation.

■ WHY CONTRACT?

In Chapter 2, the presence of a contract between a payer and a provider was one of the first differentiating elements distinguishing all types of health plans from the basic indemnity type of health insurance. Obviously a contract requires the willing participation of both parties. But why do the parties want to enter into a contract at all? There are really multiple answers to that question, and the reasons a provider wants to contract are related to, but not the same as, the reasons a health plan contracts. Although discussed throughout this book, it is worthwhile simply listing some of the more important ones here.

From the viewpoint of a health plan, examples of reasons to contract include:

- Obtaining favorable (less than full) pricing (discussed in Chapter 5)
- Agreement that the provider will provide services to the plan's members
- Meet service area access standards required by states and Medicare (discussed in the next section)
- As discussed in Chapter 6, obtain contractual agreement for several clauses, many of which are required by states (and Medicare if the payer has a Medicare Advantage [MA] plan), including:
  - Direct submission of claims—the provider agrees to send claims directly to the payer, not to the member;
  - No Balance Billing—the provider agrees to not bill the plan's members for any amount above the agreed-upon payment terms except for applicable deductible, coinsurance, and/or copayment amounts;
  - Hold Harmless—the provider agrees to not bill members for any amounts owed to it by the plan under any circumstances, including nonpayment or payer bankruptcy (applicable primarily to health maintenance organizations [HMOs] and MA plans); a strong Hold Harmless clause obviates the need for a No Balance Billing clause because it covers that as well;

  - The provider agrees to cooperate with the plan's utilization management (UM) program;
  - The provider agrees to cooperate with the plan's quality management (QM) program;
  - The provider agrees to the plan's right to audit clinical and billing data for care provided to plan members; and
  - The provider agrees to not discriminate and other similar requirements.

Reasons for a provider to contract include:

- Obtain favorable (higher) pricing when in a strong negotiating position (discussed in Chapter 5);
- Ensure that it will not be excluded from the network of a large payer, thereby losing business to a competitor;
- Direct payment by the payer, thereby avoiding the need to collect from the patient, a process that is difficult and has a poor success rate;*
- Timely payment, meaning getting paid within a defined time period, usually 30 days or less, which is much faster than Medicare or Medicaid;
- Have plan members be preferentially directed or steered to contracting providers, including specialists and hospitals;
- Not lose business as a payer steers members to contracted providers and away from noncontracted providers, or in the case of an HMO, not get paid at all for nonemergency services to HMO members; and
- Defined rights around disputing claims and payments.

■ THE SERVICE AREA

The service area is a fundamental concept in managed health care. It is defined by state laws and regulations for HMOs, point-of-service (POS), and managed Medicaid plans,† and by federal laws and regulations for MA plans. State laws and regulations are discussed in Chapter 28, and MA and managed Medicaid are discussed in Chapters 24 and 25, respectively.

The service area is simply the defined geographic area in which the plan provides access to primary and specialty care, hospital care and other health services; in other words, the geographic area of an HMO's provider network. If an HMO cannot provide sufficient access to providers in a geographic area, it will not be licensed to sell in that area either. Indemnity-type health plans are licensed to sell their products and services anywhere throughout the state in which they are

---

* The value of being paid directly is so high that in some states, the physician and hospital associations applied enough pressure to require it, even in the absence of a contract. Also, Medicare now requires Medicare Advantage plans to directly pay at least the amount covered under fee-for-service Medicare.
† As discussed in Chapter 3, POS plans are nearly always HMOs that have some level of coverage for out-of-network services.

licensed. Preferred provider organizations (PPOs) may or may not face similar service area requirements. Because PPOs are typically offered by health insurers licensed to sell business anywhere in the state, in some states a PPO plan could be offered in areas with few or no contracted providers.

Service areas are usually designated by counties and typically must be contiguous, meaning there may not be any gaps in the network as a result of deliberately avoiding a particular geographic area, also referred to as redlining. If an HMO is operating in different, noncontiguous geographic areas within a state, it usually has to do so as a separate type of plan through a subsidiary. MA plans once had a similar requirement, but noncontiguous service areas are now allowable.

State laws define minimum access requirements for service areas, as does Medicare for all MA PPOs and HMOs. Most large employers have access requirements as well, and these are similar to requirements set by states. Minimum access requirements are often defined by distance and number of providers, for example, at least two primary care physicians within 3 miles of each zip code in an HMO's licensed service area. A similar common requirement uses average travel time instead of distance; for example, no more than a 15-minute drive time to access a primary care physician (PCP), or a 30-minute drive time to an acute care hospital. Minimum HMO access requirements usually differ for PCPs, specialty care physicians (SCPs), and behavioral health care providers, recognizing that it's reasonable to travel a little further to see a specialist. Distance requirements for rural areas allow for greater travel time; for example:

- Two PCPs within 30 miles,
- Specialists within 100 miles, and
- A basic-services hospital within 30 miles of a rural zip code.

Medicare uses formulas to calculate the minimum number of hospitals and physicians an MA plan must have under contract for each specialty on a county-by-county basis.

HMO access requirements may also differentiate between the presence of contracted providers and the presence of contracted PCPs with open practices. Having PCPs under contract allows the HMO to continue to operate in a particular area, but a lack of any PCPs with practices open to new members could result in the HMO's not being allowed to sell new business there. HMO contracts therefore typically require PCPs to accept a defined number of new HMO members before they can close their practice.

Recently, California began to mandate HMO access standards based on the average length of time it takes a member to get an appointment with a provider. The new standards are 10 days or less for a PCP appointment and 15 days or less for an appointment with a specialist.[1] Such standards are difficult to measure, and are heavily influenced by factors such as the shortage of PCPs in some parts of the country.

■ THE NATIONAL PROVIDER IDENTIFIER

Under a provision of the Health Insurance Portability and Accountability Act (HIPAA), the National Provider Identifier (NPI) was phased in during 2007–2008. It replaced all other forms of provider identifiers such as the old Medicare Universal Provider Identification Numbers (UPINs), Blue Cross and Blue Shield numbers, health plan provider numbers, TRICARE (see Chapter 26) numbers, Medicaid numbers, and so forth. The NPI is a 10-digit number, with the 10th digit being a checksum. There is no embedded intelligence in the NPI. Nothing in the 10 digits will provide any additional information about the provider other than identifying who or what the provider is. The only provider numbers that were not affected were the taxpayer identifying number and the Drug Enforcement Administration (DEA) number for providers who prescribe or administer prescription drugs. The employer identification number was not affected either, to the extent that a provider is also an employer.

The NPI is unique and never ending in that once assigned a NPI, the provider will use that identifier for all transactions regardless of location, plan type, or anything else. This works reasonably well for hospitals and facilities, although health systems can have different NPI numbers for different units. For physicians, however, it is not uncommon for a physician to work on some days for a clinic that has its own NPI, on other days for a group with its own NPI, or as an independent practitioner.

■ CONTRACT MANAGEMENT

A typical mid-sized or large payer organization[*] may have thousands of provider contracts. If the organization encompasses different model types such as an HMO, POS, and PPO, it may have different contracts for each product, or a master contract with different appendices for each product (contracts are discussed in detail in Chapter 6). Contracts change over time, but prior versions must be kept in case of disputes at a later date. Payment rates likewise change on a regular basis and differ by plan type, but this is usually managed by the claims department (see Chapter 18). Other common changes a payer must track include changes in a provider's address or contact information, physicians joining or leaving a practice, hospitals adding or moving facilities, and so forth. Credentialing information such as licensure status, board certification, and other elements discussed later in the chapter must be tracked and managed according to credentialing standards in place for that particular type of plan.

---

[*]For purposes of simplification, unless plan type matters, health insurers and managed care plans will be referred to generically as payers or health plans.

Contract Management Systems

While it's possible to do this through a basic structured query language (SQL) relational database manager to address these issues, it's cumbersome and still prone to perpetuating errors. Therefore, many payers use software called a contract management system (CMS*) to handle it. A robust CMS will also perform validity checks and force the reconciliation of any potential errors, duplicates, or multiple versions. A CMS capability is often included in the payer's main information technology (IT) system on newer systems, but organizations using older or home-grown systems must use a free-standing but more capable CMS and integrate its use into the main system.

Larger and more sophisticated organizations are more likely to take full advantage of the capabilities of a CMS. A CMS must be secure because it contains some information that is private or proprietary to the health plan. With that in mind, examples of capabilities of a well-functioning CMS include many, if not all, of the following:

- Identify network gaps or where provider recruiting is most needed (this function uses data from the CMS, but often is carried out elsewhere and is included here for completeness)
- Track recruiting efforts, provide reminders, and generate recruiting reports
- Generate new contract blanks and new contracts with information filled in (e.g., the provider's name, address)
- Store copies of different versions of any provider's contract
- Track and report contract changes for each provider, including when changes occurred and for what reason, for any substantial variant from the standard such as:
  - Changes in language
  - Exceptions to certain contract clauses that are otherwise standard
  - New clauses that are not in the standard contract
- Track and manage permissions and sign-offs on:
  - Standard contracts
  - Contracts with nonstandard terms
- Store images of signed documents and convert imaged documents such as PDF files into machine-readable formats using optical character recognition
- Support an entirely paperless contracting process (not a typical feature yet, but will be eventually)
- Early notification or reminders for upcoming actions such as recredentialing or renegotiations
- Direct electronic feed of required demographic information to other internal functions described above

---

* Not to be confused with the federal Centers for Medicare and Medicaid Services.

- Direct electronic feed of market-facing systems such as Internet portals where members can search for physicians using various search criteria
- Be searchable on multiple attributes

The CMS may also support contract modeling, meaning the ability to analyze the potential impact of changes in contract terms. Modeling may also be done through different systems in which data from past claims history, changes in plan demographics and/or utilization, and other data elements are used to populate a modeling program or even a spreadsheet. Modeling is applicable to payment terms, which are discussed in Chapter 5, but is also discussed in this chapter in the context of the negotiating process.

Maintaining and tracking provider demographic and credentialing information, which is discussed later in this chapter, is not the only thing a good CMS must do. Provider files and physician files in particular are often a mess; for example, there may be duplicate records, multiple versions, or out-of-date versions for the same physician. In many older claims systems, the provider information would be entered and if the system could not immediately and correctly identify the provider, a new provider file would be created; for example, there might be a record for McCoy, L MD; a second record for McCoy, Leonard MD; and a third record for Leonard, McCoy MD. Different payment schedules might be applied depending on which record the system accessed.

Finally, other functions in a health plan routinely access provider information, including care and medical management (Chapter 7), prescription drug benefit management (Chapter 11), quality management (Chapter 14), marketing and sales (Chapter 16), HMO enrollment (Chapter 17), claims (Chapter 18), fraud and abuse detection (Chapter 19), member services (Chapter 20), and member self-service functions.

Outsourcing Contracting and Network Maintenance

Until recently, all health plans carried out recruiting, contracting, and network maintenance functions using their own personnel. While not yet the common practice, outsourcing it has been slowly increasing in recent years, and for two different reasons. The first and perhaps most common reason is simply cost. Continual pressures to reduce administrative costs, exacerbated by new medical loss ratio (MLR) restrictions in the Patient Protection and Affordable Care Act (ACA; see Chapter 30), have led payers to look at any approach to reducing costs, including outsourcing. Plans that do outsource this function may only outsource part of it (e.g., network maintenance).

The other reason for an increase in outsourcing recruiting and network management is for specialized products such as MA and managed Medicaid. Outsourcing in this case might be confined to recruiting, either because the plan's network managers are not sufficiently familiar with those products, or because they do not have the staff to undertake a major recruiting effort. In other cases outsourcing is for recruiting and maintenance because a substantial part of an MA plan's payment is now based on their star rating (see Chapter 24), and providers have an impact on that.

Rental Networks

No payer has a network in place in all parts of the United States. The Blue Cross and Blue Shield (BCBS) system addresses this through their BlueCard® system in which a member of one BCBS plan is able to see providers in another BCBS plan's service area as though they were a member of that plan as well. Non-BCBS plans must take a different approach, as do third-party administrators (TPAs; see Chapter 2) that have no network of their own: they rent one or more networks.

A rental network, which is also briefly described in Chapter 2, is a commercial PPO that builds and maintains a network of contracted physicians, hospitals, and (sometimes) ancillary service providers, and makes it available to payers or self-funded employers for a fee. In the case of a payer supplementing its own network through a rental network, if a member receives services from a physician or hospital that is not in the payer's own network but is in the rental PPO, then the payment terms of the rental PPO are in force. Rental PPOs generally charge an access fee and separate fees for conducting UM within their network. In many cases, the rental PPO's providers send the claims to the PPO, which then re-prices them and sends them to the payer for payment. The rental PPO is then paid a percentage of the difference between the full charges and the discount.

There are national rental PPO companies as well as many local ones, and local PPOs frequently also contract with the national companies. In some cases a local or regional payer with a good network will rent it to another payer, although one it does not compete with. Some local or regional HMOs have also contracted with other HMOs along the same lines, and a few large regional HMOs have negotiated exclusive agreements with a national insurer for their HMO and PPO products. BCBS plans typically do not use rental networks because they have no need to. In past years, health plans did not always make it clear that it had such contracts with rental PPOs, and a provider that contracted with the rental PPO but not the payer would find itself receiving the PPO payment and not the billed charges, requiring it to write down the difference, even in an area in which the payer had its own network. This was known as a stealth or silent PPO, but is now uncommon following several lawsuits. Payers that use rental PPOs now put the logo of the rental PPO someplace on the member's identification card.

■ PHYSICIANS AND OTHER PROFESSIONALS

Overall, the majority of practicing physicians in the United States do contract with managed care plans to varying degrees. Data Bulletin No. 35, issued in September 2009 by the Center for Studying Health System Change, reported that 87.6% of all physicians had at least one managed health care contract, distributed as follows:

- 87.9% of internists
- 89.9% of family practitioners
- 95.2% of pediatricians
- 86% of medical subspecialists
- 90.1% of surgeons
- 90.4% of ob/gyns.[2]

The turnover rate is a much more difficult figure to come by. At least one study found that the median PCP turnover rate was 7.1% (but a wide range of 0–53.3%).[3] This is close to the 2010 national medical group physician turnover rate of 6.1% reported by the American Medical Group Association.[4] Reasons for turnover in managed health care plans were not noted, for example, voluntary versus involuntary departure or change in location. Turnover did have an impact on selected measures of quality, however. For every 10% increase in the PCP turnover rate, 0.9% fewer members reported being highly satisfied with their health care. Higher primary care turnover was also associated with lower ratings of preventive care, including lower rates of childhood immunization, lower rates of well-child visits in the first 15 months of life, lower rates of cholesterol screening, and lower rates of cervical cancer screening,[5] all of which support the need to manage the network to keep turnover as low as practical.

Access Needs

A plan's access needs share similarities with the concept of the service area discussed earlier, but service areas are the minimum acceptable levels of access defined by laws and regulations, while a plan's access needs take into consideration both marketing and overall levels of service. Broadly speaking, access needs revolve around whether or not PCPs are accepting new members and how long members must wait to get appointments for either primary or specialty care. Both HMOs (including POS plans) and PPOs must address access, but HMOs are much more affected due to the member's need to use contracted providers. Examples of what could affect a plan's access needs include:

- The need to improve the network's size to effectively compete against a larger plan,
- An expansion of an HMO's service area,
- The need to recruit new PCPs in areas where the plan's current PCPs have closed their practices to new members,
- The need to improve access in areas with high concentrations of members,
- The need to have a network for an entirely new type of plan such as an MA or managed Medicaid plan (Chapters 24 and 25),

- To satisfy a state or federal requirement to improve access to PCPs following a market conduct survey, and
- The need to contract with physicians who use a newly contracted hospital.

Access needs are far less complex for PPOs because they provide in-network levels of coverage as long as a member sees any contracted provider, although copayments for PCP visits are usually lower than for SCPs. For PPOs, simply having sufficient numbers of contracted providers representing all major specialties is of primary interest, although PPO managers typically monitor access problems as well.

Closed-panel HMOs, large medical groups with a significant HMO patient base, or integrated delivery systems (IDSs) with employed physicians and a substantial managed health care membership must assess access needs in a far more focused way. The earliest days of HMOs, when group and staff model plans were much more prevalent, provides some data about physician staffing and these data may be relevant to newly emerging IDSs, particularly those with a large panel of employed physicians.

While good data exists for health system staffing, similar data for closed-panel HMOs is old, although potentially still useful. Data published in 1991 about large closed-panel HMOs that primarily served a commercial population reported the following average staffing ratios:

- The overall physician-to-member staffing ratio was 1.3 physicians per 1,000 members (i.e., 1.3 physicians of all specialties combined for every 1,000 commercial members)
- The PCP-to-member staffing ratio was 0.8:1,000, distributed as:
  - 0.3 for full-time general/family practice
  - 0.3 for internal medicine
  - 0.2 for pediatrics
- The ob/gyn-to-member staffing ratio was 0.1:1,000.[6]

Data published in 1995 reported some differences in staffing ratios between "large" and "small" closed-panel HMOs, with the difference occurring at approximately 80,000 members. The study reported the following data:

- Closed-panel HMOs with less than 80,000 members:
  - Overall physician-to-member ratio was 2.8:1,000
  - PCP-to-member staffing ratio was 0.89:1,000
- Closed-panel HMOs with more than 80,000 members:
  - Overall physician-to-member ratio was 1.2:1,000
  - PCP-to-member staffing ratio was 0.66:1,000
- Staffing ratios for physicians to Medicare managed care members in either case increased to 1.6:1,000.[7]

Another source a few years later cited two mature staff model HMOs with 1.8 total physicians per 1,000 members, which was a more generous staffing level than earlier "lean"

HMO staffing ratios and was close to the national average physician-to-population ratios.[8]

Types of Physicians and Other Professional Providers

There are many different types of professionals that a typical health plan will have in its contracted network. For purposes of this chapter, this includes any professional health care provider whose services are paid for separately from any payments to a facility. All professional providers discussed must be licensed by the state in which they practice. Physicians have an MD or DO degree, while other types of providers have a variety of different degrees.

Primary Care and Specialty Care Physicians

Most managed care organizations divide the physician network into PCPs and SCPs, although in reality such distinctions are not always clear. This is because in all types of health care delivery and health plans, the role of the PCP is important. Even in the absence of a health plan design that requires enrollees to access their PCP in order to obtain either direct care or referral authorization for specialty care (so-called "gatekeeper" types of health plans), a great deal of the regular health care of Americans is via PCPs.

In virtually all systems, physicians specializing in family practice, internal medicine, and pediatrics are considered PCPs. Unfortunately, there has been a decline in the number of graduating medical students who identify generalist and primary care as their chosen specialty. The percentage of graduating medical students reporting specialty choices in generalist and primary medicine has decreased from 60.7% in 1997 to 42.1% in 2006.[9] General practitioners (i.e., physicians who have not obtained full residency training beyond their internships) may also be considered PCPs, but their use by MCOs is quite low except in rural or underserved areas where there may not be sufficient residency-trained PCPs.

Many obstetrics/gynecology (ob/gyn) specialists feel that they too deliver primary care to their patients. They make the valid point that they are often the only physician a young woman sees for many years, at least in the case of generally healthy young women. Even prior to passage of the ACA, almost all plans, including HMOs, allowed direct access to ob/gyn physicians. Under the ACA it is now required of all plans.

While it is most common for PCPs to be trained in primary care, many internists are also trained in an additional specialty (e.g., pulmonary medicine or gastroenterology). Unless such a specialist restricts his or her practice to only specialized conditions or procedures (e.g., a gastroenterologist who focuses primarily on scoping procedures), it is common to have a practice mix of both specialty patients and primary care. In the early days of managed care, it was more common for HMOs to adhere more strictly to a definition of primary care than it is now when most health plans consider most internists with specialties to also act as PCPs. This theoretically could lead to adverse selection in which the sicker patients of that specialist actively seek to join an HMO that allows them to access the specialist as a PCP, but as a practical matter that is no longer an issue given the broad nature of most networks and the fact that physicians generally participate with multiple plans if they participate at all.

For traditional HMOs, the distinction between PCP designation and SCP designation is very important in regard to how specialty services are authorized and paid for. In a traditional HMO in which the PCP acts as the care coordinator and must authorize any visits to a specialist (a so-called "gatekeeper" type of HMO), the HMO cannot allow a specialist to be able to see a member for primary care, then refer that member back to him- or herself at a later time for specialty services (i.e., get paid first to see the member as a PCP, then get paid a second time to see the same member as a SCP). It is uncommon and foolhardy to allow a physician to be able to authorize referrals back to themselves and get paid twice to provide care for the same member. It is possible, however, for a physician to be a PCP for their own panel of members, but take referrals as a SCP from other PCPs who are not associated with that physician in some way, such as in the same multispecialty group.

In those plans that provide for open access (i.e., do not require a member to receive authorization from his or her PCP in order to see a specialist), it is enough to determine whether or not the SCP meets the credentialing criteria (discussed below) and to simply ask the physician if he or she would like to be included in the directory as both general internal medicine and his or her specialty, or specialty alone. The only other reason to differentiate is to apply the correct copayment requirement to the benefit when copays for PCP visits are less than for SCP visits.

Hospital-Based Physicians

A very unique type of specialist is the hospital-based physician (HBP). Broadly speaking, HBPs fall into one of five specialties:

- Radiology;
- Anesthesiology;
- Pathology;
- Emergency Medicine; and
- Hospitalist.

The first three—radiology, anesthesiology, and pathology—are traditional types of HBPs that have been associated with hospitals for over half a century. They are frequently in a single medical group, which is typically the only group providing those services, although exceptions exist. Emergency departments (EDs) have been staffed by specialists in emergency medicine for many decades now, and those specialists also may be part of a medical group with exclusive rights, or may be employed directly by the hospital.

In most cases, neither a patient nor a payer has the option to use a different HBP.* And because of their exclusivity, HBPs may resist contracting with a payer from which they have been accustomed to getting their full charges because contracting will not bring them increased business. Payers, on the other hand, are very reluctant to contract with hospitals if the HBPs do not also contract because that means that the plan and its members are exposed to the HBP's higher charges and balance billing, as discussed in the next section. In situations in which there is any significant volume of cases, a payer may not contract with a hospital that cannot ensure the participation of the HBPs.

Hospitals argue that HBPs are independent physicians and not under the control of the hospital. While that is true for nonemployed HBPs, the hospital is still the only party with enough leverage to bring the HBPs to the negotiating table because by definition the hospital is the only place the HBPs practice, for all practical matters, although some large HBP groups may serve more than one hospital system. A refusal by an HBP to contract with a payer means the HBP is placing his or her economic interests ahead of those of the hospital and those medical staff that have contracted with the payer. Once this becomes clear, the hospital is often successful in bringing the HBPs into the negotiation.

Furthermore, nonemployed HBPs may have a professional services agreement (PSA) that obligates the HBPs to "negotiate in good faith" with health plans that are negotiating their contract with the hospital. Some PSAs provide that if the HBP group cannot come to an acceptable agreement with the payer, the group must notify the hospital and give it an opportunity to negotiate on behalf of the group. Although it is not unusual for hospital contracts with their HBPs to be of 2–3 years' duration, most have a 90- or 120-day "termination without cause" clause. Thus, anything that causes problems for a hospital can result in immediate pressure on the HBPs that provide service to that hospital under the usual PSA, although this is clearly something a typical hospital executive would only do if no other options were available.[10] Conversely, if a hospital has no near competitors, it may choose not to make the effort, or at least not for any payer with which it does relatively little business. HBPs may also provide services in outpatient settings such as diagnostic imaging facilities and ambulatory surgery centers. As these are all elective, a plan would most probably not contract with an ambulatory or diagnostic center unless the HBPs associated with the center also contracted with the plan.

Hospitalists are different from the other four types of HBPs. Hospitalists are physicians, usually internal medicine

*There are rare instances where a hospital may have two or even more competitive groups. This may be seen where a hospital has both an academic and private practice group coexisting in the same institution, or when a large multispecialty group has a significant presence and demands that their patients be seen by their own HBPs.

specialists, who concentrate solely on the day-to-day management of inpatient care. In some cases, the hospitalist may concentrate solely on critical care and is also then referred to as an intensivist or less commonly as a comprehensivist. In other cases, the hospitalist manages most types of inpatient cases, excluding certain focused types of cases such as childbirth or transplantation. A hospitalist that covers inpatients only at night, to relieve attending physicians of their on-call burden, is referred to as a nocturnist.

Hospitalists are not present in all hospitals, but their presence has been growing since the mid-1990s. According to a 2007–2008 survey by the Society of Hospital Medicine, 58% of all hospitals use them, including 83% of hospitals with more than 200 beds, and hospitalists are employed as follows:

- 40% employed by hospitals
- 18% by academic hospital medicine programs
- 14.5% by local hospitalist-only medical groups
- 14.5% by multispecialty or primary care medical groups
- 13% by multistate hospitalist-only medical groups.[11]

If a hospitalist is employed or is part of an independent group holding a PSA with the hospital, then contracting issues are the same as with other HBPs. Hospitalists may also be members of a medical group, in which case they contract with that group.

Nonphysician or Mid-level Practitioners that Provide Primary Care

Nonphysician clinicians (NPCs) or mid-level practitioners (MLPs) in primary care include physician assistants (PAs) and nurse practitioners (NPs). There are several different types of NP designations, each having a different focus and training; those include advanced practice registered nurses (APRNs), nurse-midwives (NMs), nurse anesthetists (NAs), and clinical nurse specialists (CNSs). The use of NPCs in health care is quite widespread, with one study reporting an increase in the proportion of patients who saw NPCs from 30.6% to 36.1%; this includes a mix of patients who saw both an NPC and a physician along with patients who saw only an NPC for care, and includes types of NPCs such as psychologists, optometrists, and chiropractors that are not generally considered MLPs.[12]

Staffing rations vary in managed care plans regarding use of such NPCs. For example, in 1995 Dial et al. reported, "The median enrollment-weighted ratio of FTE APNs per 100,000 members in those plans was 19.7, with an interquartile range of 15.9 to 21.5. Almost two-thirds (63.4 percent) of responding HMOs employed PAs. With two exceptions, these were the same HMOs that reported having APNs on staff. The median weighted ratio of FTE PAs per 100,000 members was 8.1, with an interquartile range of 8.1 to 14.8."[7]

As of 2008, there were 158,348 NPs in the country, including 18,492 NMs, 34,821 NAs, and 59,242 CNSs.[13] Scope of practice varies from state to state, although all must be certified by the states in which they work. The supply of NPs ranged from 356 in North Dakota to 15,614 in California.[14] A 2007 report by the University of California, San Francisco, identified the following scope of practice characteristics for NPs:

- Eleven states permit NPs to practice independently, without physician involvement
- Twenty-seven states require NPs to practice in collaboration with a physician and use written practice protocols
- Ten states require physician supervision of NPs
- NPs in all states may prescribe medications, but physician involvement is generally required in varying degrees
- Specific practice authorities are sometimes articulated, although states may require physician involvement for any task:
  - Forty-four states explicitly authorize NPs to diagnose (sometimes limited in scope, however)
  - Thirty-three states explicitly authorize NPs to refer
  - Twenty states explicitly authorize NPs to order tests[15]

The American Academy of Physician Assistants estimates that as of May 2010, there were 88,771 PAs, of which 74,469 were in clinical practice.[16] The supply of PAs ranged from 87 PAs in Mississippi to 7,723 in New York.[17] Approximately 38% work in hospitals, 35% in medical group practices, 9% in solo physician practices, 8% in rural settings, and the remainder worked in several other settings.[18] PAs are allowed to write prescriptions in all states.

Although the data are old, closed-panel (group and staff model) health plans are more likely to use nonphysician providers to deliver some medical care to their members. In a previously cited study, 65% of closed-panel plans reported the use of nonphysician providers, with a mean ratio of 0.08:1,000.[7] In a 1992 report, fully 86% of closed-panel plans reported using nonphysician providers (compared with 48% of open-panel plans), 52% of plans used PAs, 52% of plans used NPs, and 28% of plans used certified NMs.[19]

Well-qualified NPCs are generally found to be a great asset in managed care in that they are able to deliver excellent primary care, provide more health maintenance and health promotion services, tend to spend more time with patients, and receive generally good acceptance from most members. NPCs may also play an important role in the management of chronically ill patients. They may provide the primary locus of coordination of care or case management for patients with diseases such as chronic asthma, diabetes, and the like. In a similar vein, NPCs may take a key role in managing high-risk patients, using practice protocols for prevention and health maintenance in this population. Certified nurse-midwives may not only provide services for routine deliveries, but may in fact provide primary gynecological care using practice guidelines and protocols.

NPs and, less frequently, PAs may be paid directly by a health plan under certain circumstances. Their services are more frequently paid for through a bundled fee to a facility (a topic discussed in Chapter 5) or under the charges from the supervising physician. With the increase in demand expected under the ACA beginning in 2014, this may change as MLPs become an increasingly important portal of access for primary care.

Mental Health Providers

There is a wide array of professionals that provide mental health and substance abuse services. Many practice independently and may be under a direct contract with a payer, while others provide services as employees of an organization that has the contract with the health plan.

Psychiatrists are physicians specializing in mental health, are able to prescribe drugs, and are considered a specialist like any other. Nonphysician mental health providers include:

- Psychologist—has a doctoral degree in psychology, such as a PhD, PsyD, or EdD from an accredited doctoral program, and 2 years of supervised professional experience
- Clinical social worker (LCSW)—a counselor with a master's degree in social work from an accredited graduate program
- Licensed professional counselor (LPC)—a counselor with a master's degree in psychology, counseling, or a related field
- Certified alcohol and drug abuse counselor—a counselor with specific clinical training in alcohol and drug abuse and providing individual and group counseling
- Psychiatric nurse practitioner or nurse psychotherapist—a registered nurse practitioner with special training in psychiatric and mental health nursing, and in many states may also prescribe psychiatric medications
- Marital and family therapist—a counselor with a master's degree and special training in marital and family therapy

Other Professionals

Other types of professionals are also usually found in a health plan's network, although considerable variation exists from plan to plan and state to state. Examples of licensed professionals that may either contract directly or work for an organization that has a contract with a plan include:

- Podiatrists
- Dentists, orthodontists, and oral surgeons
- Optometrists
- Chiropractors
- Physical therapists
- Other rehabilitation therapists

- Occupational therapists
- Nutritionists
- Acupuncturists
- Audiologists
- Respiratory therapists
- Home health care providers

For purposes of this chapter, all further discussion about the professional network will address only the physician network.

Types of Physician Contracting Situations

There are a number of possible types of contracting situations with which an open panel may have to deal in developing a network. Contracts are addressed in Chapter 6 in detail, as is payment in Chapter 5. This discussion focuses on the types of situations that may present themselves, regardless of specific contracting and payment issues.

Individual Physicians

This is the most common category of contracting in open panels, which is not surprising given the large number of solo practitioners in many parts of the country. In this model, the physician contracts directly with the health plan and not through any third party or intermediary. The advantage to the plan is that there is a direct relationship with the physician, which makes it clearer and simpler to interact. The disadvantage is that it is only one physician, and therefore the effort to obtain and maintain that relationship is disproportionately great.

Medical Groups

Not substantially different from individual physicians, small groups (i.e., 2–10 physicians) usually operate relatively cohesively. Most plans will refuse to contract with physicians in a group unless the entire group contracts. The advantage to the plan is that the same amount of effort to obtain and maintain a small group yields a higher number of physicians. Plans generally prefer to contract with medical groups for that reason. The disadvantage is that, if the relationship with the group needs to be terminated (for whatever reason, theirs or the health plan's), then there is greater disruption in patient care because managed health care plans typically will not contract with a group unless all of its members meet credentialing criteria and agree to the contract's terms and conditions.

Medical groups can be single specialty (e.g., all primary care internists or all orthopedic surgeons), or multispecialty. Relatively uncommon in certain parts of the country, medical groups in general and multispecialty groups in particular are occasionally the dominant practices in certain areas. The advantage of contracting with multispecialty groups is that the plan obtains not only PCPs but SCPs as well. This provides for broader access (including specialists to whom other PCPs may refer) and allows for existing referral patterns to continue.

One potential disadvantage of multispecialty groups is that sometimes they are dominated by the SCPs in the group, which may lead to inappropriate overutilization of referral services. Another potential disadvantage is the case where, by accepting the group, the plan is forced to accept a specialist whose cost or quality is not what is desired (although not so bad as to prevent contracting with the group).

Finally, a medical group may be a group practice without walls (GPWW), as described in Chapter 2. In that case, the contracting situation has attributes of both a true medical group and an independent practice association (IPA), as discussed next.

Independent Practice Associations

In the early 1970s, it was envisioned that open-panel plans would all be IPA model plans (or the similar foundation model). In this situation, there is actually a legal entity of an IPA, which contracts with physicians, and the IPA in turn contracts with the health plan. The advantage to the plan is that a large number of providers come along with the contract. Furthermore, if relations between the IPA and the health plan are close, there may be a confluence of goals, which benefits all parties. An integrated delivery system (IDS; see Chapter 2) may also use an IPA for the physician portion of the integrated delivery system. Most IPAs encompass all or most specialties, including primary care, but some single-specialty IPAs do exist. A payer may need to contract with more than one IPA in order to provide adequate coverage for the entire service area. Lastly, some relationships between IPAs and payers, and with HMOs in particular, are exclusive, while others are not.

The primary value to contract with an IPA is that it brings a large number of physicians into the health plan at one time. Only one negotiating focus is required because the IPA physicians all agree to abide by terms agreed to between the IPA and the payer. The IPA may also be willing and able to accept more financial risk than could a solo physician or small group. In addition, some IPAs also carry out functions such as network management, credentialing, and even medical management (both UM and QM) on behalf of the payer, thereby allowing for lower administrative costs. The medical loss ratio requirements of the ACA make delegation of certain administrative functions like these more desirable.

There are two primary disadvantages to contracting with IPAs. The first is that an IPA can function somewhat as a union, and the IPA can hold a considerable portion (or perhaps all) of the delivery system hostage to negotiations. This fact has not been lost on the Justice Department of the federal government. IPAs that function as anticompetitive forces may encounter difficulties with the law.

The second disadvantage is that the plan's ability to select and deselect individual physicians is much more limited when contracting through an IPA than when contracting directly with the providers. If the IPA is at risk for medical expenses, there may be a confluence of objectives between the plan and the IPA to bring in cost-effective and high-quality providers and to remove those providers whose cost or quality is not acceptable. Unfortunately, the IPA has its own internal political structure, so that defining who is cost effective or high quality, as well as dealing with outliers, may not match exactly between the plan and the IPA. If the plan has the contractual right to refuse to accept or to de-participate (i.e., remove) individual providers in the IPA, that obstacle may be avoided, although the purely political obstacles remain.

Faculty Practice Plans

Faculty practice plans (FPPs) are medical groups that are organized around teaching programs, primarily at university hospitals. An FPP may be a single entity or may encompass multiple entities defined along specialty lines (e.g., cardiology or anesthesiology). Plans generally contract with the legal group representing the FPP rather than with individual physicians within the FPP, although that varies from plan to plan.

FPPs represent special challenges for various reasons. First, many teaching institutions and FPPs tend to be less cost effective in their practice styles than private physicians. This probably relates to the primary missions of the teaching program: to teach and to perform research. Cost effectiveness is only a secondary goal (if a goal at all).

A second challenge is that an FPP, like a medical group, comes all together or not at all. This again means that the plan has little ability to select or deselect the individual physicians within the FPP. Related to that is the lack of detail regarding claims and encounter data. Many FPPs simply bill the plan, accept capitation, or collect encounter data in the name of the FPP rather than in the name of the individual provider who performed the service. This means that the plan has little ability to analyze data to the same level of detail that is afforded in the rest of the network.

A third major challenge is the use of house officers (interns and residents in training) and medical students to deliver care. In teaching hospitals, the day-to-day care is actually delivered by house officers rather than by the attending faculty physician, who functions as a teacher and supervisor. Medical residents and medical students, because they are learning how to practice medicine, tend to be profligate in their use of medical resources; they are there to learn medicine, not simply to perform direct service to patients. Furthermore, experience does allow physicians to learn what is cost effective, and residents and medical students have yet to gain such experience. Nevertheless, there is some evidence that intensive attention to UM by faculty can have a highly beneficial effect on house staff.[20] That type of focus remains the exception and not the rule, but there has been a slow acceptance of the need to manage utilization even within teaching programs.

The last major issue with teaching programs and FPPs is the nature of how they deliver services. Most teaching programs are not really set up for case management. It is far more common to have multiple specialty clinics (e.g., pulmonary, cardiology, or vascular surgery) to which patients are referred for each specific problem. Such a system takes on the characteristics of a medical pinball machine, where the members ricochet from clinic to clinic, having each organ system attended to with little regard for the totality of care. This can lead to run-ups in cost as well as continuity problems and a clear lack of control or accountability, although proponents of the electronic medical record hope that this will diminish as real-time access to all clinical information becomes available.

Despite these difficulties, there are good reasons for health plans to contract with teaching programs and FPPs other than the societal good derived from the training of medical practitioners. Teaching programs and FPPs provide not only routine care but tertiary and highly specialized care as well, care that the plan will have to find means to provide in any event. Teaching programs also add prestige to the plan by virtue of their reputation for providing high-quality care, although that can be a two-edged sword in that the participation of a teaching program may draw adverse selection in membership.[*] Most teaching programs and FPPs recognize the problems cited above and are willing to work with plans to ameliorate them.

Physicians in Integrated Delivery Systems

There are two basic types of physician contracting situations found in IDSs:

- IDSs that are primarily made up of the hospital system and affiliated privately practicing physicians, and
- IDSs that are primarily made up of hospital systems that employ a large number of physicians.

They are not mutually exclusive and it's increasingly common to see both at the same health system. Even then, one tends to factor more heavily than the other, so they are discussed separately.

As described in Chapter 2, hospitals and physicians created organizations to legally and structurally come together through various affiliation models such as physician-hospital organizations (PHOs) and management services organizations (MSOs), or an affiliation with an IPA or a GPWW. The positive and negative ramifications that apply to IPAs are similar to those for affiliation types of IDSs (including their antitrust risk) and have been discussed already. In certain states, HMOs are not allowed to contract solely with the IDS in an affiliation model, but must have direct contracts with the physicians. The individual physician contract may be brief and encompass no more than standard "hold harmless" language (see Chapter 6) and then reference the con-

tract between the IDS and the physician, and in turn the contract between the IDS and the plan. This requirement is meant to ensure that each and every individual physician understands and agrees to certain provisions required under state law, such as the prohibition on balance billing (discussed in Chapters 1 and 6). As discussed in Chapter 2, regardless of model type the percentage of hospitals with physician affiliations has been declining for over a decade, and hospitals have increasingly been employing physicians.

The employed-physician type of IDS first appeared in the mid to late 1990s when hospitals acquired PCP practices as a response to managed health care, and HMOs in particular. In most, but not all, cases this was followed by serious financial losses as physician productivity plummeted. Hospitals then divested their physician service lines, sending the PCPs back out into their own practices.

When a hospital employs a sufficiently large number of PCPs and specialists, it substantially increases its negotiating leverage, a dynamic that can only increase as demand for access to primary care increases under the ACA. This exacerbates the problem of negotiating and contracting with health systems that dominate a local area or region. There are also positive aspects of this trend. Because IDSs with a large number of employed physicians encompass aspects of contracting for facilities as well as professionals, it is further discussed in the section on the hospital network.

Patient Centered Medical Home Organizations[†]

Primary care medical home (PCMH) organizations (see Chapter 2) are at least theoretically based on an organizational structure built around PCPs. Whether that structure is actually physician-centric or centered on an IDS is not, in fact, a fixed concept. Both providers and payers are creating various organizational and/or compensation models and applying the label of PCMH. Accountable care organizations (ACOs), a similar model, are more likely to be facility-based, though not exclusively so, so they are discussed later in the chapter. Of note, the ACA has specific provisions allowing a PCMH to provide coverage as a qualified health plan, as long as it meets criteria defined in the ACA, which means it could also compete with a payer that offers through state health insurance exchanges beginning in 2014.[21]

As noted in Chapters 2 and 7, PCMH organizations are supposed to coordinate all care for a group of patients, but, unlike in an HMO, the patients receiving care via the PCMH or ACO are not locked in. Originally conceived as a model for traditional fee-for-service (FFS) Medicare, the idea spread to the commercial sector where it has been mutating into many different forms. For purposes of contracting, credentialing, and so forth, the most appropriate models to consider are either the IPA or an IDS with employed physicians.

---

[*]In other words, people with serious illnesses will choose a plan that provides access to highly specialized care, while avoiding plans that do not.

[†]An earlier term, Primary Care Medical Home, has been displaced by the broader term Patient Centered Medical Home to allow the same services to be provided by different organizations.

Specialty Management Companies

Although not common, there exist companies that focus on managing very specialized services using physicians. In some cases, these companies are physician practice management companies (PPMCs; see Chapter 2) that manage the specialty medical group and technically it is the medical group that contracts with the payer even though it is managed by the PPMC. In other cases, the physicians work for the specialty management company and it is the company that contracts with the payer.

Two examples out of many are single-specialty case management such as neonatal care and emergency and critical care using non-hospital-based physicians. The physicians working for these companies obtain privileges at all hospitals in a defined service area, and are then responsible for providing care for all of an HMO's cases that fall within certain criteria; for example, in the neonatal intensive care unit or patients seen in the emergency department who must be evaluated for possible hospital admission.

Physician Credentialing

It is not enough to get physicians to sign contracts. Without performing proper credentialing, the plan has no knowledge of the quality or acceptability of physicians. Furthermore, in the event of a legal action against a physician, the plan may expose itself to some liability by having failed to carry out proper credentialing. In the past, for example, one well-known study reported that up to 5% of physicians applying for positions in ambulatory care clinics had misrepresented their credentials on their applications.[22] Because of changes in reporting boards (discussed later) and in how sophisticated credentialing verification organizations (CVOs) operate, as discussed in the next paragraphs, the problem of fraudulent credentials has been diminished, though not eliminated.

Regulatory requirements for credentialing are variable. At the state level, some states prescribe the minimum requirements to credential physicians, while other states simply require network-based health plans to conduct credentialing and recredentialing without specifying what data is to be collected and/or verified. Credentialing requirements may also vary depending on the type of plan, with HMO credentialing requirements usually being more stringent than other types. Accreditation organizations (see Chapter 15) have defined relatively similar minimum credentialing data and process requirements as part of health plan accreditation, and an accredited health plan is "deemed" to also meet applicable requirements for Medicare and most states.

The responsibility for credentialing typically resides with either the medical director or a vice president overseeing networks. Regardless of where the responsibility lies, the requirements are the same. Plans also commonly have a credentialing committee for purposes of governance of that activity, as discussed in Chapter 3. If a provider fails to meet clear-cut credentialing standards such as board certification or license restrictions, most plans simply do not contract with him or her. In cases that are less than clear-cut, or when a provider makes a case for appeal, it is typically the credentialing committee that reviews the case.

The initial credentialing process is carried out during the recruiting process, prior to adding new physicians in a group or hospital already under contract, or rarely, after a contract or letter of intent is signed. Medicare Advantage plans must also determine if a physician has been sanctioned by Medicare or Medicaid, and as a practical matter this is often done even for non-Medicare plans. HMOs typically require recredentialing every 36 months, although it is less extensive than primary credentialing. Most, but not all, PPOs also require recredentialing. In the past, some regulators and outside accreditation agencies required that the health plan (in particular HMOs) conduct primary source verification (i.e., obtain the information directly rather than relying on another party to obtain it). Fortunately, the industry has evolved and accredited CVOs (i.e., CVOs accredited by an accreditation organization; see Chapter 15) may be relied upon to conduct much of the data collection and verification on behalf of a health plan.

In 2002, in response to the ever-growing burden on both health plans and (especially) providers created by the credentialing process, as well as increasing and more complex new sources of data, a coalition representing the health plans, with the support of providers and others, created the CAQH®* Universal Provider Datasource® (UPD®) to provide significant improvements in efficiency and efficacy of the credentialing process. While UPD is not used by every payer organization in the United States, it is used by a substantial number of them, including most of the major commercial companies and a majority of BCBS plans. Given the scope and size of UPD, it is worth making note of it and briefly describing what it does in regard to credentialing.

The UPD allows a provider to self-report their required credentialing data to one source, either online or via fax or mail, at no cost; the cost to access the UPD is borne by the health plans, hospitals, and credentialing entities that subscribe to it. Providers maintain control of and regularly reattest to their information in the UPD, authorizing which organizations are able to access their data. Primary source verification (PSV), required as a condition of accreditation, is performed externally by a contracted CVO, a delegated credentialing entity such as a hospital or IPA, or internally by credentialing staff.

CAQH monitors data from sources that are not necessarily sampled by regional payers or even CVOs: data regarding sanctions and discipline actions from across all states and the District of Columbia, and the Office of Inspector General (OIG) and Office of Personnel Management (OPM). Not all sanctions and disciplinary actions merit action on the part of the plan, but either a pattern of sanctions or disciplinary actions or an egregious problem, including deceiving the plan

---

*Formerly the Council for Affordable Quality Healthcare, they formally changed their name to CAQH.

regarding such actions, typically results in the plan terminating that physician's contract. Ongoing monitoring of this type of information is important for maintaining the quality and integrity of the network and is a requirement for accreditation.

Table 4-1 lists the elements of a typical credentialing application. **Table 4-2** lists Credentialing Verification Sources (to be used by the payer, CVO or IPA). **Table 4-3** provides examples of elements for ongoing monitoring.

■ THE DATA BANK

The federal Data Bank consists of two special databases: the National Practitioner Data Bank (NPDB), which was established in 1986 and operationalized in 1989, and the Healthcare Integrity and Protection Data Bank (HIPDB),

which was established in 1996 and operationalized in 1999. Both data banks have an impact on how health plans credential providers, and their use is standard practice for credentialing and recredentialing. Although these data banks have recently been merged, they are described separately for purposes of clarity.

The National Practitioner Data Bank

The NPDB was created by the Health Care Quality Improvement Act of 1986 (HCQIA),[23] with final regulations published in 1989.[24] The HCQIA provides for qualified immunity from antitrust lawsuits for credentialing activities as well as professional medical staff sanctions when the terms of the Act are followed. To be eligible, such entities must both provide health care services and have a formal peer review process for

---

TABLE 4-1	**Elements of a Typical Credentialing Application**

• Demographics, licenses, and other identifiers
  —Full name
  —Date of birth, place of birth, country of birth, gender
  —Social Security number
  —Home address
  —Medical license
  —Drug Enforcement Agency (DEA) registration
  —State Controlled Substance Registration
  —National Provider Identifier (NPI)
  —Educational Commission for Foreign Medical Graduates (ECFMG) number
  —United States Medical Licensing Examination (USMLE) number
  —Workers' compensation number
  —Universal provider identification number (UPIN) for Medicare and state identification number for Medicaid*
 	
• Education, training, and specialties
  —Professional education
  —Undergraduate education
  —Internship, residency, fellowship
  —Primary specialty, secondary specialty
  —Certifications
  —Other interests
 	
• Practice details
  —Credentialing, business, billing office contact information
  —Practice general information
  —Office hours
  —Accepted patients
  —Covering colleagues
  —Partners/associates
  —Phone coverage
  —Practice limitations, age limitations, handicap accessibility
  —Practice services
 	
• Billing and remittance information
	• Hospital privileges
	  —Hospital contact information
	  —Admitting privileges
	
	• Professional liability insurance
	  —Carrier contact information
	  —Coverage
	
	• Work history and references
	  —Current and previous work history (past 10 years or since graduation)
	  —Gaps in work history (3 months or more)
	  —Military service
	  —Professional references
	
	• Disclosure questions
	  —Limitations or suspension of privileges
	  —Suspension from government programs
	  —Malpractice cancellation
	  —Felony conviction
	  —Drug and alcohol abuse
	  —Chronic or debilitating illness
	
	• Images of supporting documents
	  —Current Professional Liability Insurance Policy Fact Sheet
	  —DEA Registration
	  —Educational Commission for Foreign Medical Graduates (ECFMG) Certificate, if applicable
	  —State Controlled Dangerous Substance Certificate, if applicable
	  —State License Certificate
	  —Internal Revenue Service Form W-9: Request of Taxpayer Identification Number and Certification
	  —Workers' Compensation Certificate of Coverage
	  —Curriculum vitae
	  —U.S. Department of Defense (DOD) DD214 Certificate of Release or Discharge from Active Duty, if applicable
	  —Visa, if applicable
	  —Specialty Board Certificate

*Medicare and Medicaid identifiers, despite being replaced by the NPI in 2007–2008, may still need to be obtained for any providers being newly credentialed in order to determine sanctions by those government payers. This would not apply, however, to a provider newly in practice.
Source: CAQH, used with permission. http://www.caqh.org/.

TABLE 4-2	Credentialing Data Verification Sources

Graduation from medical school (any one of the following):
- Confirmation from the medical school
- American Medical Association Master File of Physicians in the United States
- Confirmation from the Association of American Medical Colleges
- Confirmation from the Educational Commission for Foreign Medical Graduates, for international medical graduates licensed after 1986
- Confirmation from state licensure agency, if the agency performs primary verification of medical school graduation

Valid license to practice medicine (any one of the following):
- State licensure agency
- Federation of State Medical Boards
- Primary admitting facility if the facility performs primary verification of licensure

Completion of residency training (any one of the following):
- Confirmation from the residency training program
- American Medical Association Master File of Physicians in the United States
- Confirmation from the Association of American Medical Colleges
- Confirmation from state licensure agency, if the agency performs primary verification of residency training

Board certification (any one of the following):
- American Board of Medical Specialties Compendium of Certified Medical Specialists
- American Osteopathic Association Directory of Osteopathic Physicians
- Confirmation from the appropriate specialty board
- American Medical Association Master File of Physicians in the United States
- Confirmation from state licensure agency, if the agency performs primary verification of board status

TABLE 4-3	Examples of Elements for Ongoing Network Monitoring

Elements	Examples of external sources
• Disciplinary actions from licensing boards	• State licensing boards
• Expiration of medical license	• HHS Office of Inspector General Exclusions Database
• Expiration of specialty certification	• Office of Personnel Management Debarment List
• Expiration of malpractice insurance	• NPDB/HPBD (discussed next)
• Malpractice events	• UPD
• Medicare debarment	• American Board of Medical Specialties
• Member complaints and grievances	• Federation of State Medical Boards
• Utilization review	• Office of Foreign Assets Control

the purpose of furthering the quality of health care. Information reported to the NPDB is considered confidential and may not be disclosed except as specified in the regulations.

Hospitals are required to query the NPDB every 2 years. Health care entities such as HMOs, PPOs, and group practices may query under the following circumstances:

1. When entering an employment or affiliation arrangement with a physician, dentist, or other health care practitioner;
2. When considering an applicant for medical staff appointment or clinical privileges; or
3. When conducting peer review activity.

The Act also states that any hospital, HMO, PPO, or group practice may contact the NPDB to obtain information about a physician and that, if the hospital or health plan fails to do so, it will be assumed that it did so anyway. In other words,

there is a potential for liability on the part of the plan if it fails to check with the NPDB and contracts with a physician who has a poor record as reported in the NPDB, and there is a malpractice problem later on.

The Healthcare Integrity and Protection Data Bank

The Secretary of the U.S. Department of Health and Human Services (DHHS), acting through the Office of Inspector General (OIG), was directed by HIPAA (see also Chapter 29) to create the HIPDB to combat fraud and abuse in health insurance and health care delivery. The HIPDB is a national health care fraud and abuse data collection program for the reporting and disclosure of certain final adverse actions (excluding settlements in which no findings of liability have been made) taken against health care providers, suppliers, or practitioners.

The HIPDB is a tracking system that serves as an alert function to users, indicating that a comprehensive review of the past actions of practitioners, providers, or suppliers may be prudent. HIPDB information should be used in combination with information from other sources to make determinations on acceptance or rejection of a provider into the network. In addition to federal and state agencies that purchase health care services (Medicare, Medicaid, the Department of Defense, and so forth), health plans are also eligible to query the HIPDB. For purposes of this database, a health plan is defined as:

- A policy of health insurance.
- A contract of a service benefit organization.
- A membership agreement with an HMO or other prepaid health plan.
- A plan, program, agreement, or other mechanism established, maintained, or made available by a self-insured employer or group of self-insured employers; practitioner, provider, or supplier group; third-party

administrator; integrated health care delivery system; employee welfare association; public service group or organization; or professional association.

- An insurance company, insurance service, or insurance organization licensed to engage in the business of selling health care insurance in a state and that is subject to state law that regulates health insurance.[25]

■ ON-SITE OFFICE EVALUATION

As discussed in Chapter 15, an initial on-site office evaluation of PCPs, ob/gyns, and high-volume behavioral health providers is required for accreditation by the National Committee for Quality Assurance (NCQA). NCQA also merged PPO and POS accreditation with their HMO accreditation, so any PPOs or

TABLE 4-4	The Data Bank at a Glance: NPDB versus HIPDB	
NPDB		**HIPDB**
Background		
The National Practitioner Data Bank was established under Title IV of Public Law 99-660, the Health Care Quality Improvement Act of 1986, and is expanded by Section 1921, as amended by section 5(b) of the Medicare and Medicaid Patient and Program Protection Act of 1987, and as amended by the Omnibus Budget Reconciliation Act of 1990. NPDB is an information clearinghouse to collect and release all licensure actions taken against all health care practitioners and health care entities, as well as any negative actions or findings taken against health care practitioners or organizations by peer review organizations and private accreditation organizations.		The Healthcare Integrity and Protection Data Bank was established under Section 1128E of the Social Security Act as added by Section 221(A) of the Health Insurance Portability and Accountability Act of 1996. HIPDB was implemented to combat fraud and abuse in health insurance and health care delivery and to promote quality care. HIPDB alerts users that a more comprehensive review of past actions by a practitioner, provider, or supplier may be prudent.
Who Reports?		
• Medical malpractice payers		• Federal and state government agencies
• State health care practitioner licensing and certification authorities (including medical and dental boards)		• Health plans
• Hospitals		
• Other health care entities with formal peer review (HMOs, group practices, managed care organizations)		
• Professional societies with formal peer review		
• State entity licensing and certification authorities		
• Peer review organizations		
• Private accreditation organizations		
What Information Is Available?		
• Medical malpractice payments (all health care practitioners)		• Licensing and certification actions
• Any adverse licensure actions (all practitioners or entities)		• Revocation, suspension, censure, reprimand, probation
• Revocation, reprimand, censure, suspension, probation		• Any other loss of license or right to apply for or renew a license of the provider, supplier, or practitioner, whether by voluntary surrender, nonrenewal, or otherwise
• Any dismissal or closure of the proceedings by reason of the practitioner or entity surrendering the license or leaving the state or jurisdiction		• Any negative action or finding by a federal or state licensing and certification agency that is publicly available information
• Any other loss of license		• Civil judgments (health care–related)
• Adverse clinical privileging actions		• Criminal convictions (health care–related)
• Adverse professional society membership actions		• Exclusions from federal or state health care programs
• Any negative action or finding by a state licensing or certification authority		• Other adjudicated actions or decisions (formal or official actions, availability of due process mechanism and based on acts or omissions that affect or could affect the payment, provision, or delivery of a health care item or service)
• Peer review organization negative actions or finding against a health care practitioner or entity		
• Private accreditation organization negative actions or findings against a health care practitioner or entity		

continues

TABLE 4-4	*(Continued)*

NPDB	HIPDB
Who Can Query?	
• Hospitals	• Federal and state government agencies
• Other health care entities, with formal peer review	• Health plans
• Professional societies with formal peer review	• Health care practitioners/providers/suppliers (self-query)
• State health care practitioner licensing and certification authorities (including medical and dental boards)	• Researchers (statistical data only)
• State entity licensing and certification authorities*	
• Agencies or contractors administering Federal health care programs*	
• State agencies administering state health care programs*	
• State Medicaid fraud units*	
• U.S. Comptroller General*	
• U.S. Attorney General and other law enforcement*	
• Health care practitioners (self-query)	
• Plaintiff's attorney/pro se plaintiffs (under limited circumstances)**	
• Quality improvement organizations*	
• Researchers (statistical data only)	
Who Cannot Query?	
The Data Bank is prohibited by law from disclosing information on a specific practitioner, provider, or supplier to a member of the general public. However, persons or organizations can request information in a form that does not identify any particular organization or practitioner.	

*Eligible to receive only those reports authorized by Section 1921.
**Eligible to receive only those reports authorized by HCQIA.
Source: The Data Bank, Health Resources and Services Administration, U.S. Department of Health and Human Services; www.npdb-hipdb.com/topNavigation/aboutUs.jsp. Accessed April 19, 2011.

non-HMO POS plans seeking NCQA accreditation must meet the same standards. URAC, another of the three accreditation organizations discussed in Chapter 15, requires HMOs to conduct an initial on-site office evaluation on all physicians as part of the initial credentialing process. The third accreditation organization, the Accreditation Association for Ambulatory Health Care (AAAHC), also conducts on-site office evaluations, but almost all of those are on provider facilities.*

The actual on-site office evaluation may be delegated as long as standards are met. For example, if the plan has contracted through an IDS or IPA, all credentialing, including on-site office evaluations, may be delegated to the IDS, though still requiring that accreditation standards be met. PPOs may not perform an office evaluation, but typically otherwise adhere to physician minimum credentialing requirements for documentation described above, at least for initial credentialing. Some PPOs may conduct an office

evaluation to determine the overall acceptability of the practice environment, but not as part of an accreditation process.

There are two main items to evaluate in a physician's office: capacity to accept new members and office ambiance. In addition, the plan or IDS may review the office from the standpoint of a quality management process, compliance with Occupational Safety and Health Administration (OSHA) guidelines, presence of certain types of equipment (e.g., a defibrillator), and so forth. Depending on the scope of the on-site evaluation, a review may be performed in one fairly short visit or, as is the case for evaluations as part of the accreditation process, a more detailed review may require a trained health professional, usually a nurse, and may take an hour or two.

The number of new members a physician will accept into his or her practice is usually written into the contract. But to better determine actual capacity, the reviewer may ask to examine the appointment system (or appointment book in some small offices) to see how much appointment availability the physician has. For example, if there are no

---

* As noted in Chapter 15, as of April 2011, AAAHC accredits only 18 managed health care plans, all but one of which are in Florida.

available appointment slots for a physical examination for 6 weeks or more, the physician may be overestimating his or her ability to accept more work.

The recruiter can also get an idea of how easy it is for a patient with an acute problem to be put on the schedule. This may be examined by looking at the number of acute slots left open each day and by looking at the number of double-booked appointments that were put in at the end of each day. In addition, the recruiter can assess less tangible items such as cleanliness of the office, friendliness of the staff toward patients, and general atmosphere. Hours of operation can be verified, as can provisions for emergency care and in-office equipment capabilities.

Finally, accredited plans must have policies and procedures in place to conduct on-site office evaluations if member complaints reach a defined threshold, for example, a defined actual number or a defined level of seriousness (assuming the plan does not have good reason to simply dismiss the complaint). As a practical matter, even nonaccredited network-based plans have such policies. As with credentialing overall, such ad hoc on-site reviews may be delegated, or a plan that delegates basic credentialing and office evaluation may choose to conduct complaint-based evaluations itself.

■ MEDICAL RECORD REVIEW

As part of the recruiting process in the past, the medical director of an HMO may have reviewed a sample of a physician's medical records to ensure that physicians already practiced high-quality, cost-effective medicine. This practice is now rarely done for a variety of reasons, the most important being the privacy requirements under HIPAA (Chapter 29) because plans only have the right to review medical records on plan members, and then only when there is "a need to know." Medical record review is routinely undertaken for defined services provided to plan members in accordance with the plan's quality management program, however, as discussed in Chapter 14.

Orientation

Because managed health care has been around as long as it has, on-site orientation is less common than in the past, but some payers may still do it for new practices. In many cases, a physician new to the plan has joined an existing practice or organization already under contract, so orientation material provided by the contracted practice contains already understood policies and procedures. For the sake of efficiency, orientation of physicians new to the plan may also be done through self-service via the Web. In the event that an on-site orientation is undertaken, a well-planned approach will pay off in improved compliance with the plan's procedures and policies, in increased professional satisfaction on the part of the physician, and in increased member satisfaction.

TABLE 4-5	**Examples of Topics for Physician Orientation**

- Plan subscription agreement and schedule of benefits
- Authorization policies and procedures
- Committees and meetings
- Quality management program and peer review
- Credentialing and recredentialing requirements
- Forms and paperwork
- Web portals and self-service
- Utilization and financial data, to the degree it is supplied by the plan
- Member transfer in or out of practice (HMOs)
  - Member initiated
  - Physician initiated
- Plan member grievance procedure
- Payment rates and schedule
- Payer contact information
  - By functional need (e.g., physician services, precertification, claim or authorization appeals)
  - Hours of operation
- Network information such as:
  - Affiliated providers
  - Contracted hospitals and other facilities
  - Ancillary services (e.g., lab, imaging)
  - Formulary and contracted pharmacies
  - Identified "Centers of Excellence" for selected procedures

Orientation, whether on-site, virtual via the Web, or through distributed manuals and forms (paper or electronic), is aimed at two audiences: the physician and the physician's office staff. **Table 4-5** lists some topics to consider in orienting physicians and **Table 4-6** lists some topics for orienting their office staff.

Physician Directories

It has become common for payers to provide provider directories to members via the Internet. In the simplest case, this means a static look-up function whereby a member can search the directory to find a physician that meets specialty and geographic needs. In more advanced settings, this may include more detailed information such as a photo, cultural information (e.g., languages spoken or a special focus on certain cultural needs), the ability to create and print out a map to the office, and other useful information. HMO members may also choose or change their PCP online. Some payers also report whether or not a provider meets certain other standards such as compliance with electronic medical records.

Many of the larger payers also provide a designation about which physicians meet certain criteria for adherence to defined evidence-based medical practice and for

TABLE 4-6	Examples of Topics for Physician Practice Office Staff Orientation

- Plan subscription agreement and schedule of benefits
- Network information such as:
  - Affiliated providers
  - Contracted hospitals and other facilities
  - Ancillary services (e.g., lab, imaging)
  - Formulary and contracted pharmacies
  - Identified "Centers of Excellence" for selected procedures
- Authorization policies and procedures
- Forms and paperwork
- Plan member grievance procedure
- Member identification card and eligibility verification
- Current member list and eligibility verification
- Payer contact information
  - By functional need (e.g., eligibility checking, claims status, precertification)
  - Hours of operation
- Electronic data exchange requirements
- Web portals and self-service

cost management. Sometimes directories will report other measures such as reported member satisfaction rates. In other cases, payers contract with third parties to provide such information as can be compiled from public sources and provide members access to that information via the Web. And it is not only payers that have such websites. There are several private companies that provide consumers with access to similar information, as well as a listing of the health plans in which the physician participates.

Network Maintenance

Maintenance of the physician network remains key to any health plan's success. Physician attitudes toward managed health care, health insurance, or any third-party payers remain dismal in many cases, although most often when physicians are in an open-panel direct-contract HMO or PPO, and they mostly contract as individuals or small groups. In cases where they are in large groups or are employed by a dominant IDS, they are able to exercise greater negotiating leverage to achieve higher payment rates.

Network maintenance as addressed in this section refers to managing the network from a business point of view, not from a clinical one, although there are obvious overlaps. If medical management is broadly considered to be onerous by the physicians, for example, no amount of efficient business transactions will completely make up for generated ill will. There are also going to be management issues that are unique to a particular physician and do not represent larger management issues—inappropriate behavior, for

example—that would not create broad management intervention across the network.

How plans approach network maintenance is continually changing. For example, the increase in self-service capabilities via the Web allows physician office staff to take care of many routine needs such as submitting authorizations, checking on claims status, or reconciling submitted and paid claims. Another example would be when a plan contracts with an IDS with many employed physicians, in which case maintenance of the physician network is something the IDS handles, not the plan. Even then, plan managers should remain in close touch with the IDS in order to address physician concerns.

In most plans, provider service representatives are responsible for maintaining communications with independent physicians in the network panel as well as the physician's office staff, and to assist with routine and regularly occurring needs not met via self-service. Representatives typically rely on the CMS discussed at the beginning of the chapter to help track contacts and issues, but if the CMS is not robust, they may also use a customer relationship management (CRM) system for issue tracking, contact information maintenance, storing images of paper documents (e.g., contracts and correspondence), and the like.

Some care must be taken in selecting the individuals who will fill this role. Unless a provider relations representative is mature and experienced, he or she may be prone to forgetting for whom they are actually working. It is appropriate and necessary for them to represent the physician's point of view to plan management, but it is inappropriate if they find themselves siding against the health plan in the event of a dispute unless the plan is truly at fault. The provider relations staff must seek to prevent rifts, not to foster them.

The plan should have a well-developed early warning system for troubleshooting. Such a system could include regular on-site visits by provider relations staff (and occasionally by the medical director, at least in the case of larger medical groups) and regular two-way communications vehicles. Regular meetings with groups of participating physicians, attended by senior-level representatives (possibly including physicians representing the health plan) are also good vehicles for keeping current with network attitudes and issues.

Bringing network physicians into projects, and paying them for the effort, is beneficial and helps the plan achieve its goals. For example, simply thrusting a complex pay-for-performance program (Chapter 5) upon the network will likely generate ill will. But having the participation of representative network physicians usually results in both a stronger program and greater acceptance.

At the level of individual physicians, changes in patterns, particularly patterns in utilization and compliance with plan policy and procedure, will often be a sign that the relationship is going awry. Last, close monitoring of the member services complaints report can yield crucial information; physicians will often tell their patients what they think and what they intend to do long before they tell the plan.

Removing Physicians from the Network

Beyond the elements referred to previously, another function of network maintenance is the determination of who not to keep in the plan. In any managed care plan, there will be physicians who simply cannot or will not work within the system and whose practice style is clearly cost ineffective or of poor quality. It is not common to remove a physician from the network and must not be taken lightly for many reasons, including disruption to the network and the risk of legal liability.

Sanctions for reasons of poor quality are the most serious, and health plans must work closely with legal counsel to establish proper processes for doing so. Removal of a physician from the network for quality reasons must also follow the process described in the HCQIA, including reporting such removal to the NPDB, as well as the medical licensure boards in many states.

In the case of an unacceptably costly practice style, the plan must develop a mechanism for identification of such practitioners that uses a combination of claims and utilization data (see Chapter 10) and then have a program for providing that physician with data and information to assist with performance improvement. A performance improvement program should also provide for direct interactions with one of the plan's medical directors. If identified providers are reluctant to change, even after the medical director has worked closely with them, then serious consideration should be given to terminating them from the network. In that case, the plan, IPA, or IDS should have a formal performance evaluation system, including peer review by a panel of physicians with no conflict of interest regarding the physician being reviewed (Chapter 3).

There are several common objections to removing a physician from the network. Asking the members to change physicians is not easy or pleasant, benefits managers get upset, and invariably it seems the physician in question is in a strategic location. The decision often comes down to whether the plan wants to continue to subsidize that physician's poor practice behavior from the earnings of the other physicians (in capitated or risk/bonus types of payment systems) and from the plan's earnings, or drive the rates up to uncompetitive levels. If those are unacceptable alternatives, then the separation must occur.

Various states, though not all, have enacted legislation that requires "due process" or "fair procedure" protection for instances when a provider is terminated from participating in a health plan. This type of legislation also requires health plans to show cause, provide reasons in writing, and/or allow for appeal or review of criteria for practice profiling or utilization/cost performance when providers are terminated from participation in a health plan's network.

There is little uniformity, however, from state to state in regard to such laws.

Some HMOs contractually require a physician to participate until the entire membership has had a chance to change plans (which may take a year unless the physician's member panel is small), but that option can be quite costly because the physician will have no incentive to control cost once he or she has been notified of termination. In those cases, the HMO contract usually also allows the plan to increase the amount of withhold, if present (e.g., from 20% up to 50%) to cover excess costs. In PPOs there is usually no need for such arrangements because the member may still see that physician, albeit at a higher level of coinsurance.

◼ HOSPITALS AND AMBULATORY FACILITIES

As discussed earlier, an HMO, MA, or managed Medicaid plan must have adequate hospital coverage in its service area as a condition of licensure, as well as marketplace acceptability. PPOs generally do not have as stringent a requirement or any requirement at all in some states, but market demand still requires an adequate hospital network. And as a practical matter, a health plan's physician and hospital networks need to be complimentary.

In decades past, recruiting hospitals into a new plan's network was a primary area of focus. In today's more mature market, network maintenance and periodic renegotiation of existing contracts is the predominant activity, although recruiting still does take place. Beyond market maturity, this is also driven by the fact that there are fewer hospitals now than there once were. Ambulatory facilities, on the other hand, have grown in number and scope.

The approach to hospital and facility network development and maintenance will be affected to some degree by the type of health plan. An HMO is more likely to have a restricted network than a PPO, for example. In past decades, HMOs did indeed seek to contract with a sharply limited number of hospitals in order to obtain significant discounts in return for channeling patients, but that dynamic eroded due to market demand for broad networks. As costs have escalated, however, interest in narrower networks has resurfaced.

Types of Facilities and Contracting Situations

There are many different types of facilities that a payer may have in its contracted network. These are primarily hospitals and hospital-based health systems. In the early days of managed health care, most hospitals were independent. Many still are, but they have not been in the majority for many years now. Hospitals may be for-profit or nonprofit, owned either by investors or the community. Hospitals also vary in their focus, including general acute care, tertiary care, or single specialty.

Ambulatory facilities are even more widely varied. They include ambulatory surgical centers (ASCs), facilities focused on specific types of procedures such as endoscopy centers, dialysis centers, urgent care centers, and so forth. They may be owned by a health system, the physicians, a for-profit company, or jointly.

Community-Based Single Acute Care Hospitals

Once the dominant type of hospital, the numbers of community-based single acute-care hospitals (i.e., nonprofit hospitals that are not part of a larger system) have been in a slow decline for decades, with some closing and many more merging with larger health systems. At the time of publication, it is still the dominant form of hospital in rural areas, although how long that will remain the case is difficult to predict.

Contracting with rural free-standing acute-care community hospitals can be difficult if there are no viable alternatives. They are also far less likely to negotiate payment terms beyond the basic forms described in Chapter 5. Fortunately, rural hospitals are usually among the least expensive inpatient facilities because they have fewer high-tech services and are located in low-cost areas. A payer may agree to a minimal discount in order to obtain agreement on the rest of the contract's terms, if that hospital is necessary to have in its service area. MA plans also have the option of declaring them an "essential" provider, as discussed in Chapter 24, and pay Medicare rates.

Hospitals surrounded by larger competitors, on the other hand, are usually very eager to contract as they feel the pressures from the larger systems. In earlier times, large systems sometimes exerted their negotiating leverage by insisting on exclusivity, at least in the geography they served, leaving smaller acute-care hospitals out in the cold. But antitrust concerns have diminished this in recent years. Given the higher costs associated with large systems, as discussed next, having lower-cost alternatives is usually desirable for a health plan.

Multihospital Systems

Consolidation in the hospital industry has been significant, as shown in **Figure 4-1**. From the mid-1990s through the mid-2000s, the total number of hospitals dropped as struggling hospitals closed. That trend reversed by mid-decade as new hospitals were built to meet increasing demand. But growth did not occur through the creation of new free-standing acute-care hospitals, but through expansion by large multihospital systems (MHSs). MHSs also acquired free-standing hospitals, and beginning in 2006, the number of hospitals in MHSs began to exceed the number of free-standing hospitals, and the gap has only increased since then.

Hospital consolidation has had a profound impact on the hospital networks of health plans. As hospitals merged into regional MHSs and thereby eliminated competition, they have been able to use their market power to obtain significant ongoing increases in payments, a topic addressed in Chapter 5. Large MHSs also typically require that all hospitals in their system be included in all products a payer sells as a condition of contracting with the system's flagship hospitals.

As noted earlier, the increasing trend of hospitals employing physicians not only improves their negotiating position, but also adds another dynamic affecting costs when employed physicians send patients only to the ambulatory, diagnostic, and therapeutic services offered by the MHS instead of lower-cost alternatives available in the community. In some cases, the MHS offers to waive the difference in a patient's coinsurance, or even waive it entirely so the patient

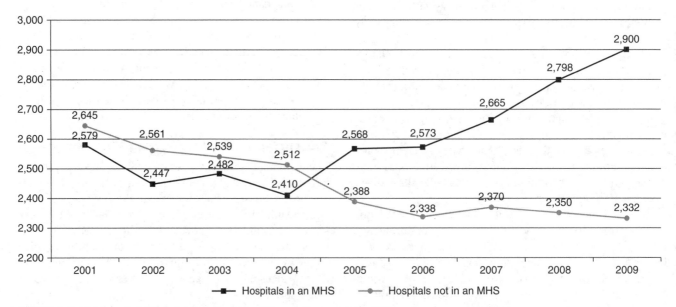

FIGURE 4-1   Total number of hospitals in and out of multihospital systems, 2001–2009

Source: SDI © 2010 in The Sanofi-Aventis Managed Care Digest Series® / Hospitals/Systems Digest 2011. www.managedcaredigest.com. Used with permission.

has no financial incentive to not go along. Coinsurance or copay waivers are generally prohibited under Medicare, and many states consider it a form of fraud,[*] but that is not consistent from state to state. In any event, it creates an additional challenge for UM, as discussed in Chapter 7.

There is potential value to payers in such systems as well, although it has not yet been expressed to the same degree as price increases. For example, health systems with large numbers of employed physicians are better positioned to address access needs for those payers they contract with. They also are able to have more professionally managed administrative services, electronic medical records (EMRs), and electronic data interchange.

Systems with a large panel of employed physicians and strong physician leadership are potentially better able to work with payers on new models of care, including the new payment structures encouraged in the ACA. Under payment models in which the MHS, including its physicians, have a substantial performance component, much of the UM could be done by the MHS and would be considered medical benefits costs, not subject to the ACA's limits on medical loss ratio costs for health insurers. Finally, working with MHSs that have a large panel of primary and specialty physicians, payers could create a "private label" network product.

For-Profit National Hospital Companies

A report issued by the U.S. Center for Health Statistics in 2010 using data supplied by the American Hospital Association, as of 2008 there were 982 for-profit hospitals, compared to 2,923 nonprofit community hospitals, 1,106 state or local hospitals, and 213 federal hospitals.[26] Most, but not all, of the for-profit hospitals belonged to companies that owned hospitals in many different locations. The purchase of nonprofit hospitals by for-profit hospital companies accelerated between the mid-1980s and mid-1990s, then leveled off until around 2005 when it once again began to rise.

Nonprofit hospitals usually agree to be purchased by a for-profit company because they don't have the capital or resources to modernize, or are unable to generate sufficient margin to continue operations. This dynamic occurs in the mergers of nonprofits leading to MHSs as well. The national chains, however, may not have the same type of regional presence as do many MHSs, although in some communities they clearly do.

Because national companies are organized much like any business, individual hospitals have much less local autonomy. Negotiating and contracting are more likely to be done

at the national level when the payer is also national or a multistate regional health plan. The national hospital companies also usually have a strong regional management structure, so local or state health plans, and sometimes multistate health plans, are more likely to contract at that level. But in all cases, contracting by the hospital company is supported by their national resources, such as a legal department.

Specialized Hospitals

Some hospitals specialize in providing care to only a certain type of patient. They fall into two broad categories: hospitals able to provide care for serious complex conditions and hospitals that provide care for less intense and/or chronic conditions.

Children's hospitals are an example of hospitals that not only focus on providing care to children but on complex conditions as well. Women's hospitals, focusing on conditions specific to women, and obstetrics in particular, are less common than they once were, but are otherwise similar, as are the even less common eye and ear hospitals. Examples of hospitals providing less intense or chronic care include rehabilitation hospitals and those providing psychiatric care or substance abuse treatment.

Hospitals specializing in complex care usually have few if any competitors that can provide the same very specialized care. As a result, health plans will usually be able to obtain a contract, but payment terms are typically high. Hospitals providing chronic or long-term care are much more likely to agree to favorable rates.

Physician-Owned Single-Specialty Hospitals

According to the trade association Physician Hospitals of America, as of 2011 there were 275 physician-owned hospitals in 33 states. These hospitals include acute care, long-term acute care, emergency medicine, specialty, women's, children's, rehabilitation and psychiatric.[27] Not to be confused with specialized hospitals, physician-owned single-specialty hospitals are facilities owned, at least in part, by the physicians who use it, and they have been subject to criticism, especially by community and tertiary hospitals who accuse them of "skimming" off the most lucrative cases, referring to healthy patients who require fewer resources and who also have private insurance or Medicare.

Because they restrict themselves to elective procedures within a single specialty, these hospitals do not have emergency departments nor are they equipped to handle patients with multiple and severe medical conditions, for example, a cardiac patient with poorly controlled diabetes that might require a fully staffed medical intensive care unit. As a result, regular hospitals are left to deal with sicker patients, less remuneration, and a requirement to provide a broad array of services.[28] Some studies also found a strong relationship between physician and high utilization; one study, for example, found that ownership by orthopedic surgeons

---

[*] By waiving cost-sharing, a provider is actually charging lower fees. For example, if a provider charges $10,000 and the member is responsible for paying 20% as coinsurance, the member should pay $2,000. If the provider waives that $2,000, then the actual charge is $8,000, not $10,000. As discussed in Chapter 6, the reverse applies as well, and a payer cannot require a member to pay a percentage of billed charges if it has negotiated lower actual payment rates.

was associated with 54–129% increases for carpal tunnel repair, 33–100% increases for rotator cuff repair, and 27–78% increases for arthroscopy.[29] This topic is discussed in more detail in Chapter 7.

The Medicare Modernization Act of 2003 (MMA) placed a moratorium on allowing physicians to self-refer to *new* single-specialty hospitals (existing ones were not included) in which they had an equity interest,[30] but that moratorium expired in August 2006 and development of new hospitals resumed. In 2010, however, passage of the ACA significantly limited any possible expansions of the number of operating rooms, procedure rooms, and beds beyond those existing as of March 23, 2010, and new physician-owned facilities that are not certified as Medicare participants by December 31, 2010, will not be allowed into the program. The ACA also requires hospitals to disclose any physician ownership interest to Medicare and to patients.

Commercial payers differ widely in their approach to physician-owned single-specialty hospitals. Some avoid them because of concerns about overutilization noted above. Others choose to contract with them because they offer prices significantly lower than the typical general hospital, and are often willing to accept capitation from HMOs (see Chapter 5). When a payer does contract with a single-specialty hospital, the general and tertiary hospitals in the network may seek an increase in payment because presumably those cases not done at the single specialty hospital will be sicker and require more resources.

Accountable Care Organizations

Accountable care organization (ACO) is a term coined by the Medicare Payment Advisory Commission (MedPAC), adopted by CMS and incorporated into the ACA, to describe an organized group of providers that coordinates the care for designated beneficiaries in the traditional Medicare FFS program and that will participate in a shared savings program. As described in Chapters 2 and 3, the ACA provides for a wide array of possible models, but they must all meet certain requirements. Commercial health plans have also contracted with ACOs, but their definitions of ACOs are flexible and not consistent between payers or with CMS. These commercial pilot programs are much more akin to contracting with IDSs, both those with employed physicians and those working with private physicians. Because Medicare ACOs are paid by CMS, it is the IDS models that are most appropriate to consider for purposes of contracting.

Government Hospitals

Hospitals may be controlled by local and state governments or the federal government. County-run community hospitals are little different from any other nonprofit acute care hospital. State-run hospitals most often provide specialized care, such as long-term psychiatric care, although many have closed over the years. Hospitals run by the federal government include those of the Departments of Veterans Affairs, the Defense Department, the U.S. Public Health Service, and the Indian Health Service. They rarely contract with commercial payers because there is no need to.

Subacute Care: Skilled or Intermediate Nursing Facilities

In addition to contracting with acute-care hospitals, payers usually contract with at least one subacute facility (i.e., a skilled or intermediate nursing facility) and/or rehabilitation facility within the service area. Subacute facilities are well suited for prolonged convalescence or recovery cases (e.g., a patient requiring prolonged traction, a frail patient requiring prolonged intravenous antibiotics for a deeply seated infection, or a patient requiring prolonged stroke rehabilitation), if home therapy is not appropriate for some reason, because the cost for a bed day in a subacute facility will be much less than in an acute-care hospital. In other cases, a patient may be able to be cared for at home, but it is still more cost effective to deliver the therapy in the subacute facility due to more favorable pricing achievable through economies of scale.

Ambulatory Surgical and Procedure Centers

As noted earlier, most communities have free-standing ASCs for outpatient surgery and other invasive procedures. In some cases, ambulatory facilities are highly specialized such as dialysis centers or chemotherapy centers. Similar to single-specialty hospitals, they are typically equipped to handle only routine cases. Many are equipped to do general anesthesia. Some are owned by health systems, others by physicians or by independent for-profit or nonprofit organizations not associated with a health system. Payers view physician-owned ASCs much the same as physician-owned single-specialty hospitals.

Unlike hospitals, which have consolidated into MHSs, there is usually more competition between ambulatory facilities. Health systems, particularly MHSs, typically require a payer to contract with their ambulatory facilities as a condition of contracting overall. But a demand to exclude competing ambulatory facilities may be seen as anticompetitive, so payers often contract with multiple facilities. This allows them to obtain more favorable pricing, which is important because simply changing from inpatient to outpatient does not, in itself, necessarily reduce costs.

Hospice

Hospice is a broad term referring to health care services provided at the end of life. It may be an inpatient facility, an ambulatory facility, or a program that has no facilities of its own. Hospice is increasingly provided by national for-profit companies. In all cases, however, a contract between a payer and the hospice organization will be similar to those for hospitals or ambulatory facilities.

Retail Health Clinics

Retail health clinics, also called convenient (or convenience) care clinics (CCCs), are essentially small clinics, usually associated with a retail store such as a grocery store or pharmacy. They are typically staffed by MLPs such as NPs and PAs. They are discussed in this section instead of the section on physicians and other professionals because most contracting situations are with the facility, which in turn employs the professionals. As of 2009 there were approximately 1,200 retail clinics around the country, 73% of which are operated by three for-profit retail chains: CVS [MinuteClinic], Walgreens [Take Care Clinics], and Target [TargetClinic].[31] The remaining clinics are operated by physician groups or hospital chains, partners of a retail chain, or are stand-alone clinics. It is a dynamic sector, so who owns what is likely to change regularly.

Over 95% of retail clinics provide basic primary care services including sore throat and cough (100%); treatment of minor skin conditions (99.7%); immunizations (98.9%); routine preventive health examinations or preventive screening, such as cholesterol testing or diabetes screening (96.2%); pregnancy testing (96.0%); or treatment of allergies (95.6%).[31] Retail clinics often provide basic health services at a substantially lower price than other health care settings. One study found that the overall costs at retail clinics for three common illnesses were substantially lower than the care that was provided in physician offices, urgent care centers, and emergency departments. An article from 2009 reported that the average overall cost at a retail clinic was $110, compared to $166 at a physician office, $156 at an urgent care center, and $570 at an emergency department.[32]

Nearly all retail clinics have contracts with managed care companies including Medicare. In a sample of 98 clinics in 2008, 97% accepted private insurance, 93% accepted Medicare, and 60% accepted some form of Medicaid.[31] Because it costs the payer or employer less for a retail health clinic visit than a physician visit for a minor condition, some health plans reduce the amount of cost-sharing a member has when using one.

Physicians, particularly PCPs, have mixed attitudes regarding retail health clinics. On the one hand, it may ease some capacity pressures on a very busy practice. On the other hand, it is lost revenue to the PCP (or the ED, but EDs are so overcrowded these days that it's welcome relief to most). Physicians also raise the concern that use of retail health clinics does not provide for continuity of care, may not provide adequate quality, and contain the possibility of missing a serious condition. Research has shown, however, that quality is at least as good as typical physician care, but the impact on continuity is not clear.[33]

Urgent Care Centers

Urgent care centers, or urgi-centers, at first appear to be similar to retail clinics, but they are not. They more closely resemble a hybrid of a Level V (i.e., low-level) emergency department or a PCP practice. They are staffed by physicians as well as nurses and MLPs, and are able to provide a wider array of care. Like ASCs, they may be owned by health systems, by a medical group, or by independent for-profit or nonprofit organizations not associated with a health system. Some payers, especially closed-panel HMOs, often run their own urgent care centers.

Free-standing, private for-profit urgent care centers typically do not accept private insurance because it means discounting their charges, although this is not always the case. Urgent care centers run by health systems usually include them in their overall contract. HMOs in particular may contract with one or two in a community so as to provide an alternative to the emergency room.

Other Types of Ambulatory Facilities

Payers may also contract with other types of ambulatory facilities, some examples of which are listed here but not further discussed because they are typically treated the same as other ambulatory facilities:

- Birthing centers;
- Community health centers;
- Diagnostic imaging centers;
- Endoscopy centers;
- Lithotripsy centers;
- Occupational health centers;
- Pain management centers;
- Radiation oncology centers;
- Surgical recovery centers; and
- Women's health centers.

Negotiating and Contracting with Hospitals and Health Systems

Typical negotiating and contracting practices around multimillion-dollar contracts between payers and hospitals are similar to multimillion-dollar negotiating and contracting in other business in that they are complex, must address many elements in detail, and are often drawn out over time. Because of their scope, size, and importance, only hospital and health system negotiations and contracting are addressed here.

The magnitude of such agreements necessitate that negotiating and contracting between payers and hospitals be business to business and carried out at arm's length, just as it is for any large and sophisticated business. Because payers contract with many hospitals and hospitals contract with many payers, contract terms and dates for each may vary considerably from contract to contract, and it's not uncommon for each to be continually negotiating with one organization or another. Therefore, payers and hospitals alike typically have staff that specialize and focus primarily on negotiating such contracts, supported by external actuarial and consulting firms to assist as needed.

Goal Setting and the Use of Data

Unlike the majority of physician contracts, payment and contract terms are negotiated with each individual hospital or health system. Each part has its own reasons for wanting to contract with the other, so each has their own goals. Typical payer goals would include:

- Obtain the most favorable (defined as lowest) pricing and provider participation possible on behalf of their customers and members
  - For all hospital inpatient and outpatient services;
  - For hospital-related ancillary services; and
  - For HBP services.
- Obtain payment terms that contribute to having an overall underwriting margin on their insured business
- Meet access standards required by states and Medicare
- Ensure that the hospital will send claims directly to the payer, not to the member
- Obtain contractual agreement for several clauses required by states (and Medicare if the payer has an MA plan), as described in Chapter 6, including:
  - No Balance Billing—the provider agrees to not bill the plan's members for any amount above the agreed-upon payment terms except for applicable deductible, coinsurance, and/or copayment amounts;
  - Hold Harmless—the provider agrees to not bill members for any amounts owed to it by the plan under any circumstances, including nonpayment or payer bankruptcy (applicable primarily to HMOs and MA plans);
  - Cooperation with the plan's QM system;
  - The right to audit clinical and billing data for care provided to plan members; and
  - Nondiscrimination and other requirements.

Typical hospital goals would include:

- Obtain the most favorable (defined as highest) payment terms possible;
- Ensure that it will not be excluded from the network of a large payer, thereby losing business to a competitor;
- Have plan members be preferentially directed to use the hospital, thereby increasing business;
- Not losing medical staff to a competitor if those physicians provide care to the payer's members;
- Direct payment by the payer, which very important to hospitals because if they do not participate in the payer's network, the payer has no obligation to pay the hospital directly and may instead send the check to the member, and hospitals generally have a very difficult time getting that money;
- Timely payment, meaning getting paid within a defined time period, usually 30 days or less, which is much faster than Medicare or Medicaid; and
- Defined rights around disputing claims and payments.

Focusing on financial goal setting, each organization typically determines its overall goal such as achieving a certain percentage increase or decrease in the aggregate. Each organization will also determine the point where terms would be so unacceptable that it would be better to walk away. Both the overall financial goal and the point of walking away may change over the course of negotiations.

The overall goal must then be translated into proposed concrete payment rates for specific types of services, as discussed in Chapter 5. This is typically done by using financial models.

The Negotiating and Contracting Process

Before beginning the negotiation and contracting process, plan management must first decide how much they are willing to limit the choices in the plan. A large local plan, in particular an HMO, that is willing to limit the number of participating hospitals will have greater negotiating leverage. Limiting the number also means a competitive disadvantage in the marketplace because prospective members and accounts often use hospitals as a means of judging whether to join the plan. (PPOs may also limit the size of their network, but are at least theoretically less likely to do so than HMOs.) The marketplace reality is that most plans seek to contract with most hospitals, although that may be turning back as employers become more willing to limit network size to better control costs.

The typical negotiating process usually involves multiple rounds of back-and-forth proposals. Either party may make the first proposal, which may then set the scene for ongoing negotiations or, less commonly, be rejected out of hand. The initiating party often presents their proposal along with any commentary to support changes that are the most likely to be resisted by the other party. For example, a hospital may tell a payer that it's losing money on a particular service line* or a payer may tell a hospital that it can no longer preferentially refer members to the facility for a particular procedure (e.g., heart surgery) unless the hospital offers more competitive rates.

It is unusual for the parties to come to agreement quickly if any substantial changes are proposed, for example, hospital demands for double-digit rate increases or payer demands for a substantial change in payment methodology. Typically the party receiving the new proposal models the potential impact of that proposal and compares it to the goals they had set. This usually leads to a counterproposal or, less commonly, an outright rejection.

In all cases, each party uses its own proprietary data to model the impact of proposed payment terms. As this process is a business-to-business negotiation, neither party is under any obligation to share its proprietary data set or

---

*Since commercial payers cover underpayments by Medicare and Medicaid, "losing" may actually mean not getting enough money in the aggregate, not achieving revenue targets, or *actually* losing money on payment rates from the payer.

models or its analysis of any particular scenarios with the other. Any disclosure of data and modeling by one party or the other is strategic in nature and done to support the party's goals in the negotiation. Such strategic disclosures are typically confined to a single issue; for example, a hospital may show data to support the need for higher than average case rates for a specific service such as maternity, or a payer may show data to support the contention that a procedure costs 20% less at a comparable hospital. Each party is expected to have the expertise and capabilities to understand the impact of the proposed terms or to obtain professional assistance in the event those capabilities are lacking, for example, either party may engage a consulting or actuarial firm to assist in analyzing the data and creating models.

Assuming the two parties come to agreement over terms, and given the drawn out nature of many of these negotiations, the hospital and payer often use the first year as a "base" year and negotiate a percentage increase for each year of a multiyear contract.

Credentialing of Hospitals and Ambulatory Facilities

Hospital credentialing refers to the requirement that the hospital meets applicable accreditation standards. Payers depend on state licensure agencies to ensure that a facility meets required standards, and typically also depend on accreditation by an appropriate organization. This differs from credentialing of PCPs and other physicians for several reasons, the most important of which is that payers simply do not have the resident knowledge to adequately credential the many types of facilities in a community.

Hospital accreditation is almost always carried out by the Joint Commission (JCI or JC; formerly the Joint Commission on Accreditation of Health Care Organizations, or JCAHO). For community hospitals, this is usually sufficient and no further credentialing is done. Ambulatory facilities are credentialed in a similar fashion, although the accreditation agency may be one other than JCI. For example, the Accreditation Association for Ambulatory Health Care (AAAHC) focuses on ambulatory facilities such as ASCs, endoscopy centers, dialysis centers, and so forth.

Other organizations besides JCI and AAAHC that provide accreditation of facilities and services that are deemed acceptable by CMS, and therefore by private payers, include:

- The Healthcare Facilities Accreditation Program (HFAP), focusing on osteopathic hospitals;
- Det Norske Veritas (DNV), a Norwegian firm whose hospital accreditation program was deemed by CMS in 2008 as meeting Medicare requirements;
- The American Association for Accreditation of Ambulatory Surgery Facilities Accreditation Program (AAAASF), focusing on ASCs;

- The Community Health Accreditation Program (CHAP), focusing on community services such as home health, hospice, and similar programs; and
- The Accreditation Commission for Health Care (ACHC), which also focuses on community services similar to those accredited by CHAP.

Accreditation programs focusing on PCMHs and ACOs are under development or being provided by several organizations, including NCQA, URAC, and JCI.

Nonphysician professionals employed by the facility (e.g., nurses or clinical nurse anesthetists) do not contract with the payer because they work either for the facility or for a physician group. As such, responsibility for credentialing is with the facility or physician group employing them, and those standards are addressed by the facility accreditation organization. In some cases, a health plan will set further criteria applicable to certain types of care; for example, cardiac surgery, or obesity surgery. Examples of such criteria include:

- A minimum number of cardiac bypass operations each year;
- A percentage of patients that meet defined outcomes following obesity surgery;
- A staffing ratio of nurses and physicians for an intensive care unit; and/or
- Participation in National Cancer Institute protocol studies.

A hospital meeting the appropriate criteria for a defined set of procedures would be considered a "center of excellence," and the health plan would, at a minimum, selectively refer those types of cases to it. PPOs and POS plans would provide higher levels of coverage for care provided in those facilities, and HMOs might only provide coverage for care when received at a designated center.

■ ANCILLARY SERVICES

They are broadly divided into diagnostic and therapeutic services. Examples of diagnostic ancillary services include:

- Laboratory;
- Imaging, such as
  - Routine radiology (X-rays),
  - Nuclear imaging,
  - Computed tomography (CT),
  - Magnetic resonance imaging (MRI),
  - Magnetic resonance angiography (MRA),
  - Positron emission tomography (PET) scans;
- Electrocardiography;
- Cardiac testing, such as
  - Plain and nuclear stress testing,
  - Cardiac nuclear imaging and other invasive imaging,

- ■ Echocardiography,
- ■ Holter monitoring; and
- ● Other diagnostic testing.*

Examples of therapeutic ancillary services include:

- ● Cardiac rehabilitation,
- ● Noncardiac rehabilitation,
- ● Physical therapy (PT),
- ● Occupational therapy (OT),
- ● Speech therapy, and
- ● Other long-term therapeutic services.

Pharmacy services are a special form of ancillary services that account for a significant measure of cost and this topic is discussed in detail in Chapter 11. Mental health and substance abuse services may also be considered ancillary from a health plan's standpoint, but are really core services, albeit discreetly defined; those services are discussed in Chapter 12.

Contracting for Ancillary Services

Because ancillary services are elective and nonurgent (if an ancillary service is urgently needed, it will be in conjunction with an outpatient visit), payers often contract with a rather limited number of them, often through a national or regional chain. They also rely far more heavily on favorable contracting terms to manage the cost of ancillary services than they do on managing utilization, but there has been an increased focus on utilization, as discussed in Chapter 7.

Ancillary services are unique in that they are rarely sought out by the patient unless ordered by a physician. There are, however, diagnostic services companies that do not require a physician order, such as a free-standing cardiac testing company or one offering "comprehensive" testing to consumers. Payers rarely, if ever, contract with such companies, even when they are owned by a contracted facility or medical group.

Physician-Owned Ancillary Services

Ancillary services may be provided by a hospital or health system or by an independent company, which may be locally owned or, as is frequently the case, owned by a regional or national company. In some cases, they are owned by the same physicians that order their use, a practice called self-referral. Self-referral represents a unique and significant problem in managed health care because there is compelling evidence that physician ownership of diagnostic or therapeutic equipment or services, whether owned individually or through joint ventures or partnerships, can lead to significant increases in utilization of those services. (This

*When these services are provided as part of an inpatient stay or during an ambulatory procedure, they are not considered to be ancillary.

topic is explored more fully in Chapter 7 in the context of UM.)

From a contracting perspective, it is neither practical nor desirable to completely restrict physicians' ability to use appropriate services or equipment that they own in order to deliver routine care within their specialty, for example, orthopedists cannot properly care for their patients if they cannot take radiographs. When contracting, however, physician-owned services should not be allowed to become a lucrative profit center because it is subject to abuse.

Managed care plans deal with this issue in a number of ways. One method is to have an outright contractual ban on self-referral other than for specifically designated services. For example, a cardiologist may be paid for performing in-office exercise tolerance testing but not be paid when referring to a free-standing cardiac diagnostic center in which he or she has a fiduciary relationship or performing the test in-office. Another method is to pay for self-referred services at a rate low enough to minimize any profit. HMOs may also choose to include it in the capitation payment.

Credentialing of Ancillary Service Providers

Providers of ancillary services are credentialed in a similar manner to facilities, relying on state licensure and, in some cases, external accreditation as well, although this is less common. Some payers such as HMOs may also evaluate the provider for things such as accessibility and availability, adequate office space, ability to produce reports on quality, and so forth. This approach may also be taken for ancillary services provided in physician's offices, such as radiology; offices failing to meet privileging criteria do not receive payment for those services.

Ambulance and Medical Transportation Services

Ambulance and transportation services are a unique type of ancillary service. Ambulance services (both ground and air) are typically in response to an accident, trauma, or a serious medical condition such as a heart attack or an acute illness. In some cases, ambulances are summoned when they're not necessary, but that's an issue of medical necessity, not contracting. In an urgent or emergency situation, an ambulance might be dispatched after a person calls 911, be requested by a law enforcement officer or fire fighter, ordered by a physician, or through some other channel. Regardless of how it's summoned, there is rarely a choice among competing ambulance services.

There is no uniformity about who actually operates the ambulance service. Local fire departments typically provide ambulance services in urban areas, but there are exceptions. Ambulance service may also be provided by a health system, by a local health authority, or by a for-profit ambulance company. In some communities, most of the costs for services to uninsured individuals are borne by taxpayers, although charging is now common. Medicare and Medicaid pay set fees, but fees charged to private payers vary widely. The same services may cost twice as much (or more) when provided by one ambulance service compared to another.

Some payers contract for ambulance services, but not all do. Even when contracts exist, ambulance services are often provided out of area, especially for motor vehicle accidents and other traumatic injuries, in which case there is no contract. Payment of such services is addressed in Chapter 5. Payers also often contract with a medical transportation company for nonurgent services such as medical transport of chronically ill people.

■ CONCLUSION

One of the hallmarks of managed health care is the existence of a provider network. Managed health care plans such as PPOs and HMOs are dependent on their networks to deliver medical care to their subscribers; even closed-panel HMOs depend to some degree on a network of private physicians and hospitals. Networks are subject to heavy regulatory terms as well as marketplace demands. As a result, much attention is focused and refocused on the network.

Endnotes

1   Helfand D. California limits HMO wait times. *Los Angeles Times*. January 19, 2010. Available at: http://articles.latimes.com/2010/jan/19/news/sns-health-obama-cali-hmo. Accessed February 3, 2011.

2   Boukus E, Cassil A, O'Malley AS. A Snapshot of U.S. Physicians: Key Findings from the 2008 Health Tracking Physician Survey. *Center for Studying Health System Change*. Data Bulletin No. 35, September 2009.

3   Plomondon ME, Magid DJ, Steiner JF, et al. Primary care provider turnover and quality in managed care organizations. *Am J Manag Care*. 2007;13(8):465–472.

4   Flatt T. Physician turnover rates mirror economic conditions and housing market. *American Medical Group Association*. April 18, 2011. Available at: www.amga.org/AboutAMGA/News/article_news.asp?k = 508. Accessed April 22, 2011.

5   Plomondon ME, op cit.

6   Group Health Association of America (GHAA), *HMO Industry Profile, Vol. 2: Physician Staffing and Utilization Patterns* (Washington, DC: GHAA, 1991). No longer in print.

7   Dial TH, Palsbo SE, Bergsten, et al. Clinical staffing in staff- and group-model HMOs. *Health Affairs*. 1995;14(2): 168–180.

8   Hart LG, Wagner E. Physician staffing ratios in staff-model HMOs: A cautionary tale. *Health Affairs*. 1997;16(1): 55–70.

9   Jeffe DB, Whelan AJ, Andriole DA. Primary care specialty choices of United States medical graduates, 1997–2006. *Acad Med*. 2010;85(6):947–958.

10 Personal communication with Lawrence R. Muroff, MD, FACR; CEO of Imaging Consultants, Inc., Tampa, FL.

11 Society of Hospital Medicine 2010 Media Kit. Available at: www.hospitalmedicine.org/AM/Template.cfm?Section = Home&CONTENTID = 23077&TEMPLATE = /CM/ContentDisplay.cfm. Accessed April 27, 2011.

12 Druss BG, Marcus SC, Olfson M, et al. Trends in care by nonphysician clinicians in the United States. *N Engl J Med*. 2003;348(2):130–137.

13 U.S. Department of Health and Human Services Health Resources and Services Administration. *The Registered Nurse Population: Findings from the 2008 National Sample Survey of Registered Nurses*. September 2010. Available at: http://bhpr.hrsa.gov/healthworkforce/rnsurvey/2008/. Accessed April 22, 2011.

14 Kaiser Family Foundation. *Providers and Service Use*. September 24, 2010. Available at: www.statehealthfacts.org/comparecat.jsp?cat = 8&rgn = 6&rgn = 1. Accessed April 21, 2011.

15 Christian S, Dower C, O'Neil E. *Overview of Nurse Practitioner Scopes of Practice in the United States*. Center for the Health Professions, University of California, San Francisco, 2007.

16 American Academy of Physician Assistants. *About Physician Assistants: FAQ*. Available at: www.aapa.org/about-pas/faq-about-pas. Accessed April 22, 2011.

17 Kaiser Family Foundation, Providers and Service Use, op cit.

18 American Association of Physician Assistants. *National Physician Assistant Census Report*. 2009. Available at: www.aapa.org/images/stories/Data_2009/National_Final_with_Graphics.pdf. Accessed April 22, 2011.

19 Packer-Thursman J. The role of midlevel practitioners. *HMO Magazine*. March/April 1992: 28–34.

20 Woodside JR, Bodne R, Tonnesen AS, Frazier J. Intensive, focused utilization management in a teaching hospital: An exploratory study. *Qual Assur Util Rev*. 1991;6(2):47–50.

21 The Patient Protection and Affordable Care Act (P.L. 111-148) Section 1301, 42 U.S.C. 18021 (a)(3).

22 Schaffer WA, Rollo FD, Holt CA. Falsification of clinical credentials by physicians applying for ambulatory staff privileges. *N Engl J Med*. 1988;318(6):356–357.

23 Health Care Quality Improvement Act of 1986, Public Law 99-660, November 14, 1986.

24 Federal Register 45 CFR Part 60.

25 Section 1128E of the Social Security Act (P.L. 104-191, the Health Insurance Portability and Accountability Act of 1996).

26 National Center for Health Statistics. Health, United States, 2010: With Special Feature on Death and Dying. Hyattsville, MD. 2011.

27 www.physicianhospitals.org, accessed May 30, 2011.

28 Greenwald L, Cromwell J, Adamache W, et al. Specialty versus community hospitals: Referrals, quality and community benefits. *Health Affairs* 2006;25(1):106–118.

29 Mitchell JM. Effect of physician ownership of specialty hospitals and ambulatory surgery centers on frequency of use of outpatient orthopedic surgery. *Arch Surg.* 2010; 145(8):732–738.

30 42 U.S.C. 1395nn (d)(3)(B).

31 Rudavsky R, Pollack CE, Mehrotra A. The geographic distribution, ownership, prices, and scope of practice at retail clinics. *Ann Intern Med.* 2009;151(5):315–320.

32 Mehrotra A, Liu H, Adams JL, et al. Comparing costs and quality of care at retail clinics with that of other medical settings for 3 common illnesses. *Ann Intern Med.* 2009;151(5):321–328.

33 Weinick RM, Pollack CE, Fisher MP, Gillen EM, Mehrotra A. *Policy Implications of the Use of Retail Clinics*. Santa Monica, CA: RAND Corporation, TR-810-DHHS, 2010. Available at: www.rand.org/pubs/technical_reports/TR810. Accessed April 28, 2011.

Provider Payment

PETER R. KONGSTVEDT

STUDY OBJECTIVES

- Understand the different methods of paying primary care physicians (PCPs) and specialty care physicians (SCPs) in different types of health plans
- Understand the variations of the most common forms of each method
- Understand the strengths and weaknesses of each method and each variation
- Understand regulatory constraints on payment methodologies, and the circumstances that bring those constraints into effect
- Understand the basic forms of payment for hospitals, and the most common modifiers
- Understand the basic forms of payment for ambulatory facilities and ancillary services
- Understand the basic approaches to pay for performance (P4P)
- Understand critical differences between hospital and physician-focused P4P programs
- Understand the challenges in administering such programs

DISCUSSION TOPICS

1. Discuss the key differences between different types of payment methodologies, and when each type would be the preferred approach.
2. Discuss what conditions would make a particular type of payment methodology either undesirable or prohibited.
3. Describe the key elements in most capitation programs in open-panel health maintenance organizations.
4. Describe the difference between service risk and financial risk in capitation.
5. Describe the market and/or network environment that would favor using capitation versus fee-for-service, and vice versa.
6. Discuss the key advantages and disadvantages of the various payment methodologies for hospitals from the point of view of a managed care plan, by type of plan. Perform the same exercise, but from the point of view of the hospital.
7. Discuss the new payment methodologies reference in the Patient Protection and Affordable Care Act.
8. Discuss what a health plan must do to increase the effectiveness of a P4P program.
9. Discuss how P4P programs might evolve in the future.

■ INTRODUCTION

This chapter provides an overview of the common (and a few uncommon) methods used to pay providers, including physicians, hospitals and other facilities, and ancillary services. Payment for pharmaceuticals is addressed separately in Chapter 11. Most of these payment methods are used by the types of payers discussed in Chapter 4, including health insurers, preferred provider organizations (PPOs), third-party administrators (TPAs), point of service (POS) plans, and health maintenance organizations (HMOs). Traditionally, HMOs were the only payer type that used all available payment methodologies, including those that shared financial risk with providers.* But new payment models such as "shared savings" approaches by Medicare and some private payers, as well as new methodologies referenced in the Patient Protection and Affordable Care Act (ACA), begin to blur that distinction.

Provider payment in the context of this chapter refers only to direct payment by private payers to health care providers for the provision of care for a covered service or services. It does not refer to payment by individuals to out-of-network providers in which no contract exists, although that topic is briefly addressed in regard to out-of-network hospitals. Payment models used by the governmental payers Medicare and Medicaid are discussed only peripherally or in the context of methods also used by commercial payers.

---

*As in many other chapters, the word "payer" is used as a generic term referring to all types of payers, rather than the older term "managed care organization" or MCO, the use of which is diminishing. Specific types of payers are identified in the text when it is appropriate to do so.

■ IT IS PAYMENT, NOT REIMBURSEMENT

As a general (and obvious) concept, payers wish to control how much they pay out to providers, and providers want to receive as much payment as possible. In the emotionally charged health care sector, those fundamental concepts are either not expressed overtly, or are expressed as pejoratives. For example, "All the insurer cares about is profit, so they're not going to pay what they should" or "That hospital system is gouging us, jacking up their rates because they know they have no competitors." The irony of such epithet-hurling is that hospitals and payers make about the same margins on average: 4.8% and 4.3%, respectively, as of May 27, 2011, as shown in **Figure 5-1**. Of course, there will be individual payers or health systems with margins higher or lower, but rarely with the types of margins found in pharmaceutical, biotechnology, or device manufacturers.

To mask the unpleasantness associated with words like "profit" or even "margin," the term commonly used for provider payment is "reimbursement," but it is an incorrect usage of the word. The definition of reimbursement found on Princeton University's online dictionary, for example, is:

"(n) Reimbursement—compensation paid (to someone) for damages or losses or money already spent etc. 'He received reimbursement for his travel expenses'."[1]

Reimbursement is applied to everyone the same way; for example, out-of-pocket travel expenses for a vice president or a sales representative are reimbursed equally. Aside from somebody padding their expense account, reimbursement

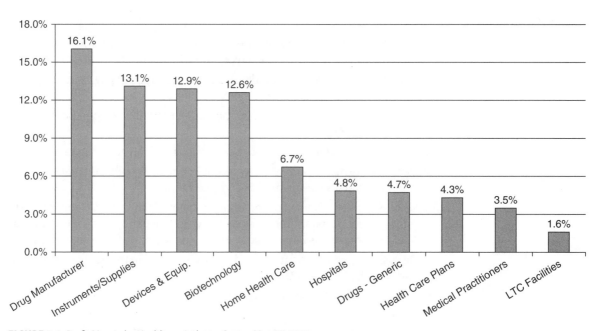

FIGURE 5-1 Profit Margin by Healthcare Industry Sector, May 27, 2011
Source: Data from http://biz.yahoo.com/ic/ind_index.html. Accessed May 27, 2011.

does not drive behavior. In other words, reimbursement implies fairness and equity.

Payment, on the other hand, has far less implications of fairness or equity. Payment is what one gets when cashing a paycheck—and not everyone is paid the same. This holds true in health care. For the same service or procedure, Medicaid pays less than Medicare, Medicare pays less than private payers, and for hospitals at least, private payers do not pay the same amount. Specialty care physicians (SCPs) are paid more than primary care physicians (PCPs), large medical groups often demand higher payment rates than allowed for independent physicians, and employed physicians typically negotiate their salaries.

Payment for pass-through costs (e.g., a hospital including the cost of a medical device in its charges) is reimbursement, but it is for payment to the device manufacturer, adding a buffer between who pays and who gets paid. If the device cost is marked up by the provider, then both the provider and manufacturer are being paid. But if a hospital receives a manufacturer rebate or payment for a failed device under warranty but does not pass it along to the payer, then the hospital and the hospital alone was paid twice.

No person or organization does not want to be paid well, and will look to increase pay when possible. In other words, payment, unlike reimbursement, does drive behavior. This reasonable behavior is neither bad nor good. It simply is. The value of firmly understanding the difference between payment and reimbursement is that it makes it far easier to understand not only the payment methodologies themselves, but the impact of payment on behavior, whether explicitly acknowledged or not.

◼ THE IMPACT OF PAYMENT METHODOLOGIES

It is seductively easy to embrace the idea that simply "fixing" how providers are paid will achieve any goal other than rearranging how dollars are divvied up. At worst, payment policies cause higher utilization and costs. At best, payment policies do not cause higher utilization and costs, and better align the financial goals of who pays and who gets paid. But payment policies alone will not cause costs to go down or even change if not accompanied by actively managing the health care delivery system, which is the focus of Part III of this book. This is particularly the case when a new approach to payment appears that is so complex, it becomes nearly impossible to determine the effect of any one element within it.*

There also are qualitative differences between hospitals and physicians around payment. Hospitals typically analyze their sources of payment, compared to costs as best they can determine, to analyze the financial margins of their services; in other words, whether they make money or lose money for various services such as obstetrics or nuclear imaging services. This is usually done for each different payer, or at least those accounting for most of their volume. Said another way, hospitals and health systems look at payment just as any business would.

The impact of payment methods on physicians is different. As discussed in Chapter 9, how a physician is paid—or not paid—influences physician behavior, but it is not the sole influence or even necessarily the strongest. Believing that changing how physicians are paid will, by itself, solve anything is naive and unproductive. The typical physician is not an entrepreneur and is not primarily focused on income. More often than not, physicians are target income-driven professionals who focus first on providing medical care.[†]

◼ HETEROGENEITY IS THE NORM

Providers are often paid through different methodologies by different payers at the same time, potentially making the impact of any approach difficult to assess. But when different payment models compete, one usually wins. In hospitals, for example, high profits from payment by commercial payers can actually induce losses on a hospital's Medicare business because lowering costs would lower profits on the commercial business.[2] Physicians are also unlikely to change how they care for one patient versus another based on differing payment methods applicable to each patient.[3]

Managed care is marked by a high degree of continual change and variation, and that has always been the case. Change occurs through market forces, changes in managed health care practices, new laws or regulations (especially in Medicare and Medicaid), the ACA, and other forces. As a result, the divisions by provider type and the payment approach described here are not always found in a pure state. Also, the same payer often uses different payment methods in different locations, or even in the same location. For example, a national company may capitate physicians in its HMO in one state, but pay fee-for-service (FFS) in another; or in the same community a payer may pay one hospital under Medicare Severity adjusted diagnosis-related groups (MS-DRGs) and another hospital under per diems.[‡]

Payment methodologies used for different types of providers also overlap, but may be expressed differently. Payments may also be subject to modifiers so that in certain circumstances, a payment is changed or a different type of payment is made. Payers may also use different payment methodologies at different times for the same providers.

---

*Payers, providers, policy analysts, and consultants tinker endlessly with payment methodologies, many of which can only be called "OWAs," or other weird arrangements.

[†]With some exceptions such as physician self-referral, a topic discussed further in Chapters 6 and 7.
[‡]MS-DRGs and per diems are described later. The point here is only to illustrate varied usage of payment approaches.

With that understanding, provider payment is discussed in the following order:

- Payment of physicians;
- Payment of hospitals, health systems, and ambulatory procedure facilities;
- Combined payment of hospitals and physicians
    - Global fees and bundled pricing,
    - Global capitation, and
    - Combined payment of hospitals and physicians using "shared savings";
- Pay for performance (P4P);
- Payment of ancillary service providers; and
- New models of payment under the ACA.

■ PAYMENT OF PHYSICIANS

There are many different methodologies used to pay physicians. The use of different payment models varies based on multiple factors including the type of payer organization, product design, geographic location, type of specialty, physician organizational structure, and state and federal laws and regulations. Whatever payment method is used, not all services provided by a physician may be paid for by a commercial payer. Issues of medical necessity come into play, but also payment policies. For example, typical payer medical policy is to pay a second surgeon attending an operation only half the fee paid to the primary surgeon. Overall, the effect of pricing and payment on physician behavior and use of services is complex and subject to other economic, psychological, and organizational issues.[4]

It is also important to understand that the payment methodology used by a payer may not always be the way the physicians themselves are actually paid. For example, an HMO may capitate* an Independent Practice Association (IPA; Chapter 4), but the IPA uses the capitation money to pay its physicians through FFS, which has actually been the case for decades.[5, 6] In fact, as shown in **Table 5-1**, less than 20% of practicing physicians are paid through a share of practice revenue, despite the common belief that it is the prevailing method. On the other hand, how a payer pays a medical group or IPA will certainly catch the attention of its medical leaders, so the change in payment model from a payer through to individual physician compensation is not a complete disconnect. In all events, compensation of individual physicians is beyond the reach of this chapter.

Any payer, including an HMO, may use any type of nonrisk method of payment, but with a few exceptions, only HMOs may use payment methodologies that incorporate financial risk-sharing with providers. However, the ACA created a new Center for Medicare and Medicaid Innovation

TABLE 5-1	Physician Compensation Arrangements, 2008	
Performance-adjusted salary		43.8%
Fixed salary		24.7%
Shift, hourly, or other time-based payment		6.2%
Share of practice revenue		19.5%
Other compensation		5.8%

Source: 2008 Health Tracking Physician Survey, Center for Studying Health System Change, Washington, D.C. www.hschange.com. Used with permission.

(CMMI) charged with introducing new payment models in the traditional Medicare FFS program that look very much like risk-sharing.[7] As of yet, it is hard to predict how much commercial payers may adopt these approaches for their non-HMO commercial business.

Table 5-2 lists nonrisk physician payment methodologies, and **Table 5-3** lists risk-based physician payment methodologies that HMOs may also use. Many types of payment methodologies also incorporate potential modifiers under certain circumstances, and those are discussed as they appear. Physician payment methodologies that are combined with facility payment methodologies are discussed in the section on payment of facilities.

Non-Risk-Based Physician Payment

All types of payers, including HMOs, may use physician payment methods that do not share financial risk with the physicians. Even HMOs that use risk-based payment approaches, discussed later, also use non-risk-based methods for at least some participating physicians, with the exception of HMOs, which capitate an IPA for all professional services, including care from out-of-network providers. The predominant form of payment today is FFS, which is discussed next. Case rates can be said to contain some element

TABLE 5-2	Nonrisk Physician Payment Used by All Types of Payers

- Fee-for-service
    - Straight charges
    - Usual customary or reasonable (UCR)
    - Percentage discount on charges
    - Fee schedule
    - Relative value scale (RVS)
    - Resource-based relative value scale (RBRVS)
    - Percent of Medicare RBRVS
    - Special fee schedule or RVS multiplier
    - Facility fee add-on
- Case rates and global fees

---

*Capitation is a type of fixed monthly payment described later in the chapter.

TABLE 5-3	Risk-Based Physician Payment Also Used by HMOs

- Capitation
  - Variation factors
    - Age and sex
    - Acuity
    - Other
  - PCP only
    - With a withhold
    - Without a withhold
  - Individual versus pooled risk
  - Specialist
  - Global
  - Independent practice association
  - Contact capitation
- At-risk FFS
  - Fee percentage withhold
  - Budgeted FFS

of risk-sharing because the same fee is paid regardless of the ease or difficulty of any one case, but that is usually addressed through outlier protection so is included in this section. The related concept of bundled pricing, combining physician and hospital payments, is discussed in the section on hospitals and facilities.

Fee for Service

There are some veterans of managed health care who hold that the FFS system of American medicine is the root of all the problems we have historically faced with high costs. Although that is simplistic, there is truth to it, particularly when there are few or no controls in place. In a system where economic reward is predicated on how much one does, particularly if procedural services pay more than cognitive ones, it is only human nature to do more since it pays more. The reward is immediate and tangible: A bill is made out, and it usually gets paid (though often at a discount if paid by a health plan). Doing less results in getting paid less. FFS is also more easily manipulated than risk-based payment. For example, if the in-network payment for a particular procedure or visit code is held down, physicians may simply "upcode," a term referring to billing based on a higher-paying code associated with a more complex procedure or visit. FFS also rewards "churning," a term referring to having a patient come back more often than necessary. Because FFS pays based on billing codes, and there are nearly 8,000 of them for physicians alone, FFS also encourages "unbundling," a term referring to using several billing codes for a procedure. Upcoding, churning, and in some cases unbundling are considered forms of billing abuse, as described in Chapter 19.

On the other side of the argument, FFS results in distribution of payment with at least some relationship to

expenditure of resources. In other words, a physician who is caring for sicker patients will be paid more, reflecting that physician's greater investment of time, energy, and skills. FFS also produces better data since physicians will be more careful to enter all applicable billing codes, something that a capitated physician has little incentive to do. FFS is nearly universal in PPOs, CDHPs, Blue Cross and Blue Shield (BCBS) service plans, and TPAs. Risk-sharing FFS can be used by HMOs or IPAs, but that is discussed later.

Determination of Fees

The term "prevailing fees" refers to the fact that the fees billed for professional services are not uniform across geographic areas or type of physician specialty, and payers typically take those differences into account; for example, it is costlier to practice in an urban area than in a rural one. It is necessary for a health plan to know what the prevailing fees are in order to determine its own fee schedule, as well as when paying for care delivered by out-of-network physicians, as discussed in the next section. However, as will also be discussed, fees vary so widely that most payers do not rely only on prevailing fees when determining how much to pay.

The historical method of determining prevailing fees is known as the usual, customary, or reasonable (UCR) fee. Where once it was defined as "usual, customary, *and* reasonable," it is now often defined as "usual, customary, *or* reasonable." The definition of reasonable is in the eye of the beholder, however, and payers often determine certain charges to be grossly overpriced. For example, when the charges for a procedure like cataract removal and lens implantation were first set, it was a new and complex procedure, took a long time to do, and required skills in rare supply. Now it is a highly routine and high-volume procedure, takes little time, and is performed by a great number of ophthalmologists; the historical basis for the charge is therefore no longer valid. In consequence, payments for that procedure are lower than they once were. The opposite dynamic occurs with new technology, for which billed charges are frequently higher than it was for whatever technology it replaced.

The traditional approach to determining prevailing fees is to collect data for charges by current procedural terminology (CPT) code in a defined region (e.g., a city); calculate the 25th, 50th, and 75th percentiles; and then choose which percentile represents a reasonable prevailing fee. Another common type of coding system that is used is the Healthcare* Common Procedural Coding System (HCPCS) for certain

---

*The "H" once stood for Health Care Financing Administration, the old name of the Centers for Medicare and Medicaid Services. HCPCS includes some CPT codes, but also includes codes for billing for other types of services such as ambulance and durable medical equipment.

services, such as providing infusion. The use of CPT and HCPCS will not change in 2013 even though the new *International Classification of Diseases*, 10th Edition (ICD-10), which will become mandatory then, replaces some HCPCS codes; it affects primarily facility-based billing.

Payers typically do not have enough fee data to be able to determine UCR unless they are very large in a geographic area, such as a BCBS plan with a high market penetration in a single state, in which case they can achieve statistically meaningful numbers. Even large national health insurance companies may have a large amount of data, but it is spread across wide geographic areas and there may be sufficient data to set the maximum for certain CPT codes, but not others.

For this reason, many health plans purchase a commercially available database. Two companies that provide these are Ingenix® (www.ingenix.com)* and Emdeon® (www.emdeon.com). Both companies provide information based on charge data in various geographic regions as well as additional information including conversion factors based on a relative value scale (discussed later). Actuarial firms also commonly use proprietary prevailing fee databases.

In 2009, under significant pressure from (then) New York State Attorney General Andrew Cuomo, Ingenix agreed to a settlement in which it admitted that its database was not statistically valid because, in part, claims data were not gathered from all possible sources and claims were not audited. The focus of the suit was payment of out-of-network claims, not in-network fee schedules as discussed below. The settlement also called for UnitedHealth Group (UHG), Ingenix's corporate parent, to pay $50 million into a state fund to create a new nonprofit physician fee database called FAIR Health,™ and settled with other payers for $50 million more. The governor subsequently required its use by New York State payers. Shortly after that settlement, UHG agreed to a $350 million settlement of three class-action lawsuits filed in federal court by the American Medical Association, UnitedHealth Group members, health care providers, and state medical societies, all pertaining to payment amounts for out-of-network services.

If UCR alone is used to determine fees, the result is fee inflation since higher charges result in higher fee percentiles and higher payments, with nothing to stop a provider from continually inflating his or her charges. This is the crux of why many consider FFS to contribute to cost inflation. The wide spread in charged fees also skews the percentiles since significant outliers pull the percentiles toward the skewed end. If a payer relies on percentiles to calculate payment, increasing charges necessarily lead to increasing payments that in turn encourage more charge increases. Therefore, payers typically combine UCR data with other sources of fee informa-

tion, often Medicare payment rates, to create fee schedules for payment to in-network providers, which is discussed later.

Out-of-Network Fees

The way a health plan determines fees to be paid to noncontracting providers is not the primary focus of the chapter, but it is still important. In any service plan—PPO, POS, CDHP, or even HMO—members will sometimes incur out-of-network charges (i.e., from providers that do not contract with the health plan). In the case of HMOs, that will generally only occur in emergencies or when the member is traveling far from the service area and needs care. For other types of plans, out-of-network care is expected and is part of the benefits package. In the case of HMOs that do not have out-of-network benefits, costs for true emergencies or out-of-network care authorized by the HMO are usually paid in full.

Other than for pure HMO products, what a payer will typically pay for out-of-network charges is not simply based on UCR. This was the issue at the heart of the Ingenix suit. The contention was that a benefits plan purporting to cover a percentage of out-of-network costs was actually covering less than that by not relying only on an area's prevailing fees or UCR, regardless of how high or low it was, instead relying on a commercial database that often determined UCR at a lower rate. This also potentially exposed a member to higher amounts of balance billing from noncontracted providers.

Prior to the lawsuit, for example, a POS plan might have provided for a 30% coinsurance for out-of-network care, but that didn't mean that the plan would actually pay 70% of the charge. Unless the benefits state specifically that the plan will pay at those levels, which it almost never did, the most common approach was to pay at 70% of what the POS plan considered reasonable using the commercial prevailing fee or UCR schedule. That approach is still used by some, but many payers have tightened the language used for out-of-network benefits coverage.

In some cases, coverage is based on the fee schedule that the plan uses to pay in-network providers. Because the in-network fees are typically discounted, the difference between the "allowed" fee and what the patient was charged can be considerably more than 30%. In other cases, the payer will combine UCR data and the Medicare payment rates to determine the allowed fee, or simply base it on a percentage of the Medicare allowed fee, typically somewhere between 100% and 150% of Medicare.

Using Medicare as the basis for determining payment on out-of-network charges has a significant impact when applied to the highest out-of-network fees. For example, in August 2009 the payer trade organization America's Health Insurance Plans (AHIP) issued the results of a survey of out-of-network physician charges compared to Medicare-allowed fees in 30 states. Listing the 10 most expensive charges in each state, they found that the highest charges

---

*In past decades, health plans commonly used the MDR® database and the Prevailing Healthcare Charges System®. Both were purchased by Ingenix, which has since combined and supplemented them.

TABLE 5-4   **Examples of High Charge Fees Compared to Medicare Allowed Fee**

State	CPT code	Service description	Amount billed	Medicare allowed fee	Charge as a pct. of Medicare
California	29881	Minimally invasive knee meniscus surgery	$20,120.00	$584.98	3,439%
Colorado	47562	Laparoscopic gallbladder removal	$26,100.00	$625.94	4,170%
Florida	99215	Outpatient office visit of moderate to high severity requiring two out of three: comprehensive history, comprehensive exam, and high complexity medical decision making	$4,150.00	$119.75	3,466%
New Jersey	22612	Lower back spinal fusion	$72,000.00	$1,628.96	4,420%
New York	43239	Upper GI endoscopic visual exam diagnostic exam with biopsy	$29,998.00	$388.64	7,719%*

*Of the 10 examples from New York, the state where the Ingenix lawsuit was filed, the lowest was 2,287% more than Medicare.
Source: Data from the "The Value of Provider Networks and the Role of Out-of-Network Charges in Rising Health Care Costs," AHIP Center for Policy and Research, August 2009. www.ahipresearch.org/ValueofProviderNetworksSurvey.html. Accessed June 15, 2011. Used with permission.

for many procedures and office visits exceeded Medicare's allowed fees by thousands of percent, as illustrated in **Table 5-4** by five examples from that report. Regardless of whether or not one considers Medicare's fees low, or AHIP's report too sensational, there is no possible justification for such exorbitant charges. And because the report does not contain statistical quartiles, it does not illustrate the prevalence of exorbitant fees.

Straight Charges and Discount on Charges

On rare occasion, an HMO would contract with a physician on the basis of paying full charges. The reason was to gain the physician's agreement to the other contract terms such as the no balance billing clause. This allowed the HMO to fill in any critical lacunae in its network. Even then, the HMO would try to contractually limit how much the physician could raise fees each year by tying it to some index.

Payment using a simple discount on charges has also been used by both HMOs and PPOs. Though not common, it still occurs, but only when a physician or group is the only option an HMO or PPO has; however, it is more likely with an HMO since a PPO does not necessarily have to comply with access standards to all major specialties. Because of fee inflation, payment of full or discounted charges is uncommon.

Fee Schedules

A fee schedule is simply a list of the maximum amount that a health plan will pay for each and every type of encounter or procedure based on the coding methodologies noted earlier. If the plan is using its own historical payment schedules, or is relying on a prevailing fee database and simply selecting a percentile to use, then each encounter or procedure will be associated with a maximum payment amount.

In the past, the negotiated payment rate to contracted providers might simply have been a percentage discount off of the reasonable prevailing fee or the submitted claim,

whichever is lower. The advantage to using this approach is that it is extremely easy to obtain. Most physicians will gladly accept a discount on fees if it ensures rapid and direct payment. The two problems with this are the relentless upward pressure of fees described earlier, and that there is nothing to prevent a physician whose fees are below the maximum from increasing their fees up to the maximum, which they will promptly do unless they are totally asleep at the wheel. It is now rare for any physician to charge less than the maximum allowed payment.

Relative Value Scales

The use of a relative value scale (RVS) in one form or another has been widely used in FFS. In a basic RVS, each procedure or billing code, as defined in CPT, has a relative value associated with it called a relative value unit (RVU). The physician is paid on the basis of a monetary multiplier for the RVS value. For example, if a procedure has a value of 4 and the multiplier is $12, the payment is $48. In the past, RVS's reflected prevailing fees or UCRs, but had the advantage of allowing for easy modifications to all fees by simply changing the multiplier. This could be done uniformly for all types of billing codes, or differently for classes of procedures; for example, the multiplier for office visits could be raised more than the multiplier for cataract removal and lens implantation.

A classic problem in using a UCR-based RVS and negotiating the value of the multiplier is the imbalance between procedural and cognitive services. As in FFS in general, procedures have higher charges than cognitive services. In other words, there is less payment to a physician for performing a careful history and physical examination and thinking about the patient's problem than for doing a procedure involving needles, scalpels, or machines. This is why the simple UCR-based RVS has given way to the slightly more complex resource-based relative value scale (RBRVS).

TABLE 5-5	Illustration of RBRVS Calculation for CPT Code 99213, Expanded Office Visit	
Metric		**Value**
Work RVU		0.97
Practice Expense RVU		0.99
Malpractice Insurance Cost RVU		0.07
TOTAL RVUs (0.97 + 0.99 + 0.07)		2.03
RBRVS Payment Rate (2.03 × $27.00)		$54.81

Note: Values are for illustrative purposes only, and do not reflect payment rates by Medicare or commercial payers.
Source: Copyright P.R. Kongstvedt Company, LLC. Used with permission.

Resource Based Relative Value Scale

The most well-known RBRVS was developed for Medicare on behalf of the Health Care Financing Administration (HCFA), which is now called the Centers for Medicare and Medicaid Services (CMS). RBRVS was created to address the imbalance between cognitive and procedural services by lowering the value of invasive procedures (e.g., cataract surgery) and raising the value of cognitive ones (e.g., office visits).

In RBRVS, each CPT code is associated with three RVUs. The first and largest RVU is supposed to reflect the difficulty of the procedure, and the amount of time, training, and the relative skills required to provide it. A second RVU reflects the practice cost such as materials, clinical settings, and so forth. The third RVU reflects the cost of medical malpractice insurance associated with the type of procedure and the location. The three RVUs are added together, and the multiplier is applied to that sum. This is illustrated in **Table 5-5** with a hypothetical example of a payment rate calculation for a primary care expanded office visit.

CMS uses the RBRVS to pay all physicians for services to Medicare beneficiaries. For Medicare participating physicians, the payment is the RBRVS rate. Nonparticipating physicians are subject to a complex maximum limiting charge, which is 115% of the Medicare-allowed payment amount; however, the Medicare-allowed payment amount for services furnished by nonparticipating physicians is 95% of the normal fee schedule amount, so the maximum allowed charge is actually only 107.25% of the fee schedule amount (i.e., 115% of 95%).

The weights placed on the relative values are reviewed by the Relative Value Update Committee (RUC) of the American Medical Association every 5 years, and the RUC's recommendations are used by CMS. In the 2002 update, at the request of several specialty societies several hundred specialty procedures were revised upward, resulting in an increase in pay for specialty procedures and a decrease in payment for primary care office visits. In the 2007 review, the RUC recommended a 20% upward revision for primary care and office

visits, but federal budget limitations held it to only 6.5%.[8] Around the same time, resource values for many procedures were lowered, resulting in decreases in payment for certain cardiac and imaging services. Under the ACA, payment to PCPs in Medicare (and Medicaid) is also increased.

The Medicare RBRVS is not the only one in use. For example, the RBRVS used for determining fees in workers' compensation programs in California was modified to include physician psychological stress when a bad outcome has serious consequences. Commercial RBRVS systems are also available and widely used to fill in RVUs for codes not regularly used by CMS for Medicare.

When FFS is used for physician payment in commercial plans, payment rates are commonly determined through RBRVS with a higher dollar value multiplier. In some markets, an MA plan will contract for the same payment rate that Medicare uses, but it is more common to contract for the Medicare rate plus a small percentage increase; for example, the Medicare RBRVS fee plus 5%. If the physician participates in Medicare, this represents an actual increase in payment, which is why they typically agree to it. Some commercial plans contract using Medicare's payment rate plus a larger percentage, similar to an approach described earlier for determining a reasonable out-of-network charge. The percent above Medicare will vary from market to market.

Variation Based on Location of Service

Because the facility costs make up part of the total cost of a procedure, many health plans pay attention to where a procedure is performed. For example, the same procedure performed in a hospital facility is often far more expensive than when performed in a free-standing ambulatory surgical center, due solely to the differences in what each type of facility charges (unless the plan has negotiated equivalent charges for each type of location). In order to lower aggregate costs, the plan may reduce the fees paid to the physician if the procedure is performed in a hospital or other high-cost location, but increase the fees paid if the physician uses a low-cost facility.

Special Fee Schedules or RVS Multipliers

Payers typically apply the same payment rates for all physicians in a community, but have increasingly found themselves having to negotiate with particularly strong medical groups or with health systems employing large numbers of physicians. As a result, such large groups or systems are able to demand and obtain higher payment rates. They're generically referred to as "special" rates because they are higher than the general fee schedule. It may apply to a fee schedule or, more commonly, the multiplier on relative values. Special rates are also costly to administer, since they usually require manual processing or intervention because many claims systems are unable to handle such exceptions.

Special payment rates were once relatively uncommon. But as the percentage of physicians employed by hospitals has grown, along with an increase in medical group size, the percentage of special payments has also grown. Anecdotally, in at least a few parts of the country the percentage of special rates has gone from less than 10% to over 40%.[9]

Add-On Facility Fee

Another increasing trend is the add-on facility fee, in which a hospital that runs the clinics or offices used by physicians bills a separate fee. It is actually a payment to a facility, not a physician, but is included here because payments to physicians practicing in their own offices are inclusive of all the costs associated with providing care, and no extra fee is paid for office space or support. Since the add-on facility fee is not offset by a lower physician charge, this is nothing more than another bite of the apple by the hospital. It may occur when the hospital employs the physicians, or at a teaching hospital with a physician faculty practice plan, or when the hospital or integrated delivery system (IDS) is running a management services organization (MSO; see Chapter 2) that includes practice management.

When payers contract with hospitals that charge an add-on fee, they typically negotiate that fee out of the payment and require the participating hospital to not balance bill the member. But when the payer does not have enough negotiating leverage to do so, or if the system is not in the payer's network, members find themselves facing an unexpected additional cost that is usually not covered in their benefits.

Electronic Visits

Electronic visits, or e-visits, are also known as online visits. This refers to a clinical interaction between a physician and a patient that takes place via the Internet, not on a face-to-face basis. This is usually done through a specialized form of secure e-mail, or through the use of a more structured application that automatically filters requests for e-visits via branched chain algorithms and access to medical self-help. Some payers are now paying physicians for providing care via e-visits, though at a rate usually lower than that of a standard office visit. The member may be required to pay their usual copayment based on plan design, and is so informed prior to using the service. There is no uniformity of either fees or coding for such visits, but eventually that will change.

The Impact of Fee Schedules on Coinsurance

For any benefits plan in which the member must pay coinsurance (a percentage of the total) to a contracted FFS provider, the amount is based on the payment rate the payer uses, not the physician's charges. This policy is the result of numerous lawsuits in the 1980s by states' attorneys general.

It applies only to coinsurance, and not to fixed copayments or fixed deductibles.

Prior to those lawsuits, some insurers and BCBS plans that contracted with providers for reduced fees or charges calculated the member's coinsurance requirement on the charged amount, not on the negotiated amount. For example, if a member was subject to a 20% coinsurance requirement and a physician charged $100 but the plan's negotiated fee was $75, the member had to pay 20% of $100 (or $20), not 20% of $75 (or $15). This was determined to be fraudulent by the courts because the member was required to pay a percentage of the total cost, not of charges that exceeded the total. As illustrated above, the member was in fact paying more than the designated percentage of the total required payment to the contracted provider.

This issue only applies to payments to contracted providers whose charges are higher than the total payment they agree to accept as payment in full. It does not apply to any charges by noncontracted providers, even when the plan's payment is less than the charges, as discussed earlier.

Case Rates and Global Fees

A case rate or a global fee is a single payment that encompasses all professional services delivered in an episode. Common examples of case rates include obstetrics, in which a single fee covers all prenatal visits, the delivery itself, and at least one postnatal visit, and certain surgical procedures, in which a single surgical fee pays for preoperative care, the surgery itself, and postoperative care. Case rates are similar to FFS in that they are event-based, but they significantly reduce the ability to unbundle charges or to churn visits. A case rate may be subject to additional outlier fees if significant complications occur, in which case payments are typically based on a discount on charges.

The term "global fee" is easily confused with the related term "global payment." The concept is the same except it includes the facility payment along with the professional. For that reason, it is best to avoid its use in favor or case rate for professional payment, and bundled payment or even package pricing for combined single payment for facility and professional services. Bundled payment is discussed later in the chapter.

Fees for Physician-Owned Ancillary Services

Physician-owned ancillary services refers to physicians who purchase, lease, or invest in a significantly expensive device such as a sophisticated cardiac imaging device or a magnetic resonance imaging (MRI) machine, and refers also to the physicians that order its use on their patients. Related to this is the issue of physician-owned hospitals and facilities, discussed in Chapter 4. The topic is noted here as a placeholder, only to remind the reader that payment of physicians can come through many channels. It is discussed in more detail in the section on payment for ancillary services and in Chapter 7.

Price Transparency

The term "price transparency" or "pricing transparency," sometimes also referred to as "cost transparency," simply refers to making information about the cost or price of health care services available to consumers. This is a central tenet of CDHPs: inform consumers about the cost and quality of services and empower them to make their own decisions. It is also a concept cautiously advocated in a 2008 report to Congress by the Congressional Research Service.[10] Price transparency has had no impact on pricing variability in New Hampshire however, one of the few states to require it.[11] There are also cogent arguments that in health care, price transparency could actually result in price increases, not decreases.[12]

As a practical matter there are some difficulties with using price transparency such as people needing services on an urgent or acute basis, whether or not a consumer is capable of distinguishing between differing services, fears that lower cost care must be inferior care, and so forth. But the concept has taken root and is being implemented, both by health plans and by some providers as well.

Pricing transparency is usually done by posting pricing information on the Internet, often by the health plan. It is typically available only to registered members of the plan. Some private companies also provide access to pricing information to consumers, and charge a small fee for it. What information is actually being posted is not necessarily straightforward, however.

Information about physician pricing is usually how much the plan pays contracted physicians for certain things (e.g., office visits, delivering a baby, and the like), and in some cases, what the local prevailing charges are. This allows the consumer to understand how much more they will have to pay if they see a noncontracting physician. At the time of publication, most health plans that post information at all are not posting pricing information specific to individual physicians, but rather using an aggregate type of data.

Many CDHPs and health plans also provide assistance with a type of calculator that allows the consumer to figure out what their out-of-pocket responsibility will be and the effect on their health payment account or health savings account (discussed in Chapter 2). A few take into account the actual benefits plan the member has, but most do not. What the ultimate impact of this approach will be is not known.

Risk-Based Physician Payment

Risk means that a physician's income from an HMO can vary based on utilization and/or medical care cost. Capitation is the most well-known type of risk-based payment, but risk-based FFS is also common. Because of a concern in the past that capitation could incentivize a physician to withhold necessary services, state laws typically only allowed HMOs to capitate providers, which was part of the reason HMOs were required to have more stringent rules about utilization and quality management. That concern proved to be unfounded, as is discussed later, but it is still the case that only HMOs can use risk-based payment. However, there is a caveat to that statement: some new and experimental payment models in the ACA, as well as new "shared savings" approaches to payment, have at least some of the attributes of risk-based payment. Those are discussed toward the end of the chapter.

Capitation of Primary Care Physicians[*]

Capitation is prepayment for services on a per-member per-month (PMPM) basis. In other words, a physician is paid the same amount of money every month for every member in their patient panel regardless of whether that person receives services or not, and regardless of how extensive those services are. Capitation is typically used only by HMOs because only HMOs can use a PCP "gatekeeper" system in which a member selects a single PCP or primary care group for services, and to access specialty care. Because of this, utilization and costs can be attributed—directly or indirectly—to that PCP. For example, if a PCP is paid $20.00 PMPM and his patient panel has an average visit rate of four visits per year, that is roughly the equivalent of $60 per visit (($20.00 × 12 months) ÷ 4 visits per year = $60.00 per visit).

The same concept applies to any capitated provider, including specialists, multispecialty medical groups, hospitals, laboratories, and so forth. The key requirement is that members are "locked in" to that provider and are not covered for services from another provider of the same type under most circumstances. Plan types in which members are free to access any network provider make it difficult at best to attribute costs and utilization.

Financial Risk versus Service Risk   There are two broad categories of risk for capitated physicians: financial risk and service risk. Financial risk refers to actual income placed at risk, regardless of whether or not the physician has a service risk as well. Financial risk is usually confined to capitated PCPs, though it can easily be applied to performance-based FFS as well. Furthermore, an identical system may be put in place for a capitated contract with an IPA in which all participating physicians, both PCPs and SCPs, bear an equal amount of financial risk. There are two common forms of financial risk: withholds and capitated pools

---

[*]Resist the temptation to refer to a capitated physician leaving an HMO's network as "decapitation." The last time that was considered even faintly humorous, Spiro Agnew was Vice President of the United States.

for non-primary care services. Financial risk is discussed in more detail later.

Service risk refers to the physician receiving a fixed payment for his or her own professional services, but not being at risk in the sense of having potentially to pay money out (or conversely, not receive money due to them). In other words, service risk is essentially the fact that if service volume is high, then the physician receives relatively lower income per encounter, and vice versa. While the physician may not be at obvious financial risk, the physician does lose the ability to sell services to someone else for additional income in the event that their schedule fills up with capitated patients at a rate that is higher than that used to calculate the capitation. This issue is irrelevant if the physician has slack time in his or her schedule, but can be an issue if the physician is extremely busy. It is common for physicians, primarily PCPs with large panels of capitated members, to feel that their capitation patients are "abusing" the service by coming in too frequently, but the perception is always more grievous than the reality.

There are many different forms and variants of capitation, the most common of which are discussed in the sections that follow. Capitation may be used to pay either PCPs or SCPs, but is more commonly used for PCPs. There are also differences in how PCPs and SCPs are typically paid under capitation. Therefore, general elements of capitation are described first, followed by issues specific to PCP capitation and then to SCP capitation.

Prevalence of Capitation The data about the prevalence of capitation do not always match, but are still generally consistent. Differences are secondary to sampling methodologies and differences in focus, but are useful to better understand the prevalence of capitation and its variants. The two reports that are used, with permission, are:

1. The Sanofi-Aventis Managed Care Digest Series®/ HMO-PPO Digest 2010 that uses data from their 2009 survey, including state insurance departments and telephone and paper surveys of licensed HMOs (responses less than 100%).
2. The 2009 American Medical Group Association (AMGA) report *Capitation and Risk Contracting Survey* that uses data from 75 members of AMGA member medical groups of varying configurations and ownership, but not individual physicians.

As of 2009, over half of the HMOs in the country capitated their PCPs, and about one-third had at least some capitated SCPs.[13] There were some differences based on plan size, as shown in **Figure 5-2**, and age of the HMO, as shown in **Figure 5-3**, but they are not significant.

The prevalence of capitation varies by region, however, with the western United States having the highest levels while the east having the lowest, as seen if **Figure 5-4**.

As is discussed shortly, the capitation methodology can vary; for example, an HMO may primarily only capitate PCPs, another capitates for all professional services, while a provider-owned HMO pays the medical group a percent of the premium. The actual numbers used to calculate capitation may also vary, most commonly by age and sex of an enrolled panel, but also by acuity or level of illness. A sample distribution of these differences for medical groups in the AMGA study are illustrated in **Figure 5-5**, and all are discussed in this section.

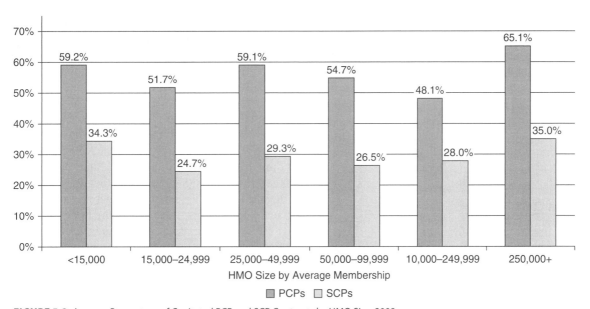

FIGURE 5-2 Average Percentage of Capitated PCP and SCP Contracts by HMO Size, 2009

Source: SDI © 2010 in The Sanofi-Aventis Managed Care Digest Series®/HMO-PPO Digest 2010. www.managedcaredigest.com. Used with permission.

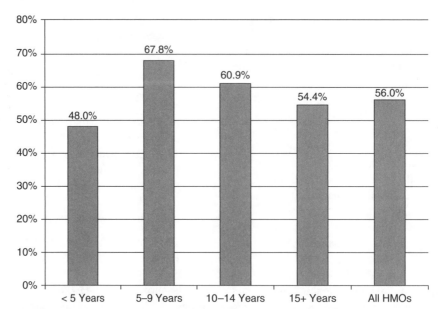

FIGURE 5-3 Percentage of HMOs with Capitated PCP Contracts by HMO Age, 2009

Source: SDI © 2010 in The Sanofi-Aventis Managed Care Digest Series®/HMO-PPO Digest 2010. www.managedcaredigest.com/. Used with permission.

Most capitated physicians are also paid through FFS by other payers, and there is great variability in what amount of an individual physician's revenue comes from capitation. In 2007, for example, one study reported that approximately 29% of California and 18% of Oregon physician office visits were paid through capitation, compared to only 4% in other parts of the country.[14] Percentages reflected the average of all physicians, however, even those that do not have a capitation contract with an HMO. And market forces also have an impact; in certain markets, for example, physicians and medical groups that were once capitated are now paid under FFS, in some cases unwillingly.[15]

Scope of Covered Services   The first step in determining an appropriate capitation is to define what is covered in the scope of services and what is not. This forms the basis

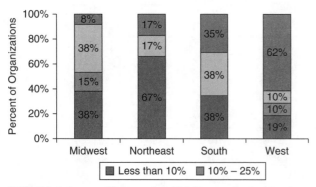

FIGURE 5-4 Percent of Revenue from Risk Contracts by Region, 2008

Source: American Medical Group Association and ECG Management Consultants, © 2008. ECG/AMGA Capitation and Risk Contracting Survey, Alexandria, VA. www.amga.org. Used with permission.

for estimating the total costs of primary care or costs for a specific specialty. If a plan does not have sufficient credible data on primary or specialty care service usage, a national actuarial firm can provide the necessary detail as well as help calculate capitation rates.[*]

All services that the PCP or SCP will be expected to provide, including preventive services, outpatient care, and hospital visits,[†] must be defined, as illustrated in Chapter 6. Certain definitions require special attention such as diagnostic testing, prescriptions, and surgical procedures. For example, selected diagnostic testing (e.g., office urinalysis or electrocardiograms) may be included in the capitation, but other lab testing must be sent out to an outside reference lab (Chapter 7) and the capitation covers only blood-drawing, unless, as is common, the patient is sent to a free-standing outside reference lab for all routine services, including blood-drawing.

Surgical and endoscopic procedures are a particularly difficult area to define if the same procedure is performed by some PCPs and by SCPs, or not all SCPs perform the procedure. For example, a capitated PCP may be incented to refer the patient out rather than incur the expense; however, paying the PCP FFS for that procedure (referred to as a carve-out, and discussed later) also carries the risk of overutilization.

Other services such as immunizations are easy to define, but still may or may not be covered by the capitation

---

[*]For example, the authors of Chapter 22, "Underwriting and Rating," are principals with one such actuarial firm, Milliman, Inc. (www .milliman.com).

[†]It is now rare for PCPs to provide care to hospitalized patients, as discussed in Chapter 7, but should be taken into account nonetheless.

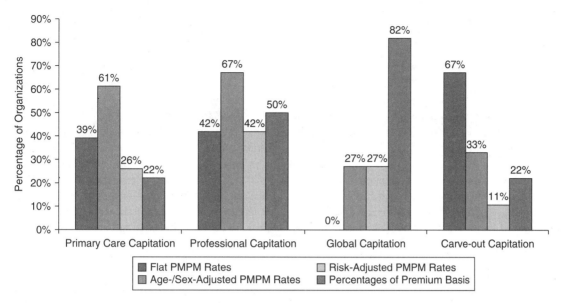

FIGURE 5-5 Capitation by Contract Type, 2008

Source: American Medical Group Association and ECG Management Consultants, © 2008. ECG/AMGA Capitation and Risk Contracting Survey, Alexandria, VA. www.amga.org. Used with permission.

payment if the cost of the service is volatile. The schedule of immunizations frequently changes as new vaccines are released, and the cost of the vaccine may fluctuate as well. Therefore, many HMOs include the cost to administer the vaccine in the capitation, but the cost of the vaccine itself is passed through at cost. A similar approach is used for specialty infusions. The cost is determined by the HMO, not the physician, typically by using a reference price, meaning the cost at which the HMO can purchase the vaccine or drug.

Calculation of Capitation Payments   Most plans use an actuary to set capitation cost categories on the basis of the plan's geographic area, the benefits plans in place, network pricing, and the HMO's medical management capability. Large payers typically have actuaries on staff, while smaller HMOs use outside actuarial firms. If the plan has been in operation for some time, is sufficiently large, and has a data system capable of tracking the details, estimating annual capitation amounts is a matter of collating the existing data, to which the actuary applies an expected trend.

The following illustrates by working backward rather than forward as the earlier illustration did, and using slightly different numbers. If a PCP is paid approximately $65.00 per visit (collected, not charged) and the average primary care visitation rate is 4.2 care visits per member per year (PMPY), then multiplying 4.2 × $65.00 and dividing the result by 12 (to get the revenue per month) yields $22.75 PMPM. This would approximate the capitation rate before taking cost-sharing into account.[*]

HMOs that also use a risk/bonus arrangement often demonstrate to physicians that if utilization is managed they will receive more than they would have under FFS. For example, using the same capitation PCP rate of $22.75 PMPM and 4.2 visits PMPY, if good utilization management yields a bonus of $4.50 PMPM from the risk pools (discussed later), then the physician receives a year-end reconciliation that blends out to $27.25 PMPM or $77.86 per visit. Also, pure luck (good or bad) will have an effect on the ultimate per-visit payment, as discussed later.

Variations by Age and Gender   Capitation systems routinely vary PCP capitation by the age and gender of the enrolled member to take into account the differences in average utilization of medical services in those categories. For example, the capitation rate for a member younger than 18 months of age might be $70.00 PMPM to reflect the high utilization of services by newborns. The capitation rate may then fall to $10.00 PMPM for members 1–2 years of age, $9.00 PMPM for members 2–18 years of age, $8.00 PMPM for male members 18–45 years of age, and $35.00 PMPM for female members 18–45 years of age (reflecting the higher costs for women in their childbearing years), and so forth. As an end result of this, the actual PMPM payment to a physician may fluctuate each month depending on the demographics of their enrolled panel of members. As with most factors that are used to vary capitation amounts, the larger the enrolled panel of capitated members a physician

---

[*]This simple crude example is entirely fabricated, plus it does not take into account any particular definition of scope of covered services, actual visitation rates for an area, visit rate differences by age and sex, average collections by a physician, effect of copayments, or differences in mean fees among different specialties. Neither this figure nor any other capitation amount used in this chapter should be considered accurate.

has, the more likely that adjustments will accurately reflect expected utilization.

SCP capitation is less likely to vary based on age and gender. Where an HMO will need many PCPs to provide care to members, it needs fewer SCPs for any given specialty because the use rate is lower; for example, more people go in for coughs and colds than go in for abdominal surgery. As a result, SCPs typically have a much larger panel of members, resulting in greater predictability.

Variations by Acuity Levels or Case Mix Adjustment Beyond adjusting capitation for age and sex, some HMOs adjust it based on health status or clinical acuity. It is not as common as one would expect for several reasons. First, premium revenue rates for commercial HMOs typically did not take group experience into account. That changed several years ago, but only for large groups. Under the ACA, experience rating will be restricted to larger groups only. The practical outcome is that only a small portion of an HMO's premiums will reflect experience, and it is difficult to adjust capitation for only a small portion of any PCP's members, but not the rest.

The second reason is that until recently, systems used to classify members based on burden of illness were difficult to use and not always accurate. Related to this, the cost of making acuity-based capitation adjustments can add considerably to administrative costs because most still require manual intervention at some point, though that is slowly changing. Also, communicating the reasons for acuity-based adjustments to physicians can present a challenge since all physicians will welcome an upward adjustment, but few will happily accept one that's downward.

Unlike commercial health plans, however, individuals covered under Medicare typically do have a history of using medical care, and their average PMPM costs are significantly higher. Many of the problems associated with using acuity level to adjust capitation for commercial members exists for Medicare except for premium payment. CMS now pays MA plans based on the acuity or level of illness of individual members (Chapter 24), eliminating a very serious barrier to acuity-based capitation adjustment. CMS will also account for acuity in its new payment approaches, as discussed in the last part of this chapter. And as hospitals hire more physicians or physicians create larger groups, the problem of small numbers is also attenuated. All of these mean it is reasonable to expect acuity adjustments to become more mainstream in the future.

Finally, in all health plans there will be a very small percentage of members who are seriously ill with multiple complex conditions. Adjusting a capitation payment for these people compounds generic problems in performance measurement related to case-mix adjustment, size of treatment effects, availability of adequate standards and metrics, and more.[16] Because the percentage of members are very high risk and high cost, HMOs sometimes either make special

provisions for payment to the PCP or SCP, or do not even include those members in the physician's capitated panel.

Variations by Other Factors Another relatively easily analyzed factor is geography. Even in the same statistical metropolitan area, there may be considerable differences in utilization and in prevailing fees, as discussed earlier. Therefore, HMOs typically factor geography into calculating capitation rates. Practice type may occasionally be a legitimate capitation factor. For example, internists argue that the case mix they get is different from the case mix family practitioners get, and some cardiologists perform cardiac procedures whereas others do not. Medical specialists who also provide primary care also have patients who are sicker than patients of general internists, even in the same strata of age and sex.[17]

There may be straightforward business adjustments to capitation as well. As noted earlier, very strong medical groups or health systems with large panels of employed physicians may demand and get capitation payments higher than the rest of the network. It is also possible for the opposite to occur. An HMO may pay a higher capitation rate to those physicians who do not sign up with any other HMOs (an exclusivity bonus usually does not apply to participating with non-HMO payers). Such arrangements could raise a potential antitrust problem depending on the particular situation, so legal counsel must be involved.

Effect of Copayment Levels Copayment levels have a direct impact on capitation rates, both for direct physician capitation and for PCP risk pool allocations (discussed under PCP capitation). This is illustrated through the following example, in which the member copayment is changed from $20.00 per visit to $25.00.

The original capitation rate was $15.75 PMPM, calculated using these assumptions: $65.00 per visit in total, an average of 4.2 visits PMPY, and a $20.00 per visit member copayment:

- $65.00 per visit
  - $20 per visit from member copayment
  - $45.00 per visit from HMO direct payment
- $45.00 per visit × 4.2 visits PMPY = $189.00 PMPY
- $189.00 PMPY ÷ 12 months = $15.75 PMPM

A new capitation rate of $14.00 PMPM uses the same assumptions, but changes the copayment to $25.00:

- $65.00 per visit
  - $25.00 per visit from member copayment
  - $40.00 per visit from HMO direct payment
- $40.00 per visit × 4.2 visits PMPY = $168.00 PMPY
- $168.00 PMPY ÷ 12 months = $14.00 PMPM

While copayment amounts are routinely used to calculate initial capitation amounts, as a practical matter, some health plans do not actually reduce the capitation amount when they increase required copays, preferring instead to inform the physicians that instead of an adjustment to their capitation, they are getting a fee increase through the ability to double the amount of copayment collected at the time of service. This, ironically, reintroduces an element of FFS into a capitated system, though not enough to actually have much of an effect, if any. The same adjustments apply to calculating contributions to referral and hospital risk pools, which are discussed in the section on PCP capitation.

Adjusting capitation rates for copays is less easy if there are widespread differences in copay amounts among different accounts. For example, if 60% of the members have a $20.00 copay, 15% have a $25.00 copay, and 25% have a $40.00 copay for primary care services (not to mention differential copays for specialty services), calculating the appropriate capitation can be a challenge both to carry out and to explain to the physicians. Even so, it is worth doing unless the variations are minor or infrequent, and automated tools can make the calculations painless.

Effect of Benefits Reductions   Changes in benefits design in response to marketplace demands will change the actuarial assumptions used to build capitation rates, but except for changes in cost-sharing, the impact is usually limited. For example, limitations on infertility treatments or on durable medical equipment are usually not great enough to warrant changing previously acceptable capitation rates, but that is not an absolute.

Behavioral Shift   Commercial actuaries have proprietary models for what they term "behavioral shift," which refers to members altering their use of medical (or any other) services in response to economic stimuli or barriers. Those models are not generally available in the public literature, however. Whether or not capitation payments should be changed because of behavioral shift is difficult to know, but it probably should not be used.

The reason is that the effect of copays and cost-sharing on utilization is difficult to predict, with some studies demonstrating a reduction in spending but others showing increases in total costs. A synthesis of cost-sharing research created by the Robert Wood Johnson Foundation shows that, at best the impact is a mixed bag, with results differing based on multiple medical and socioeconomic factors.[18] Studies of CDHPs, which are designed to require high levels of cost-sharing, appear to show a reduction in member-imitated demand,[19] but that may be a result of positive selection (i.e., healthier people choose the less expensive CDHP when given a choice).[20]

Point-of-Service Plans

As discussed in Chapter 2, POS plans are those that allow members to obtain a high level of benefits by using the HMO or "gatekeeper" system while still having insurance-type benefits available if they choose to use providers without going through the managed care system. POS plans were very popular when they were first introduced, but declined due to higher costs. Nevertheless, HMOs that offer POS, including those required to do so under state laws, must take the benefits design into account. The plan may be able to actuarially determine the level of in-network and out-of-network use for the entire enrolled group, which cannot be said for an individual physician's member panel. This has an obvious impact on capitation rates. When POS plans were first introduced in the 1980s, some plans attempted to adjust capitation rates on the basis of prospective in-network utilization. The capitation rate was thus reduced, further exacerbating the problem of luck (good or bad). Because of the problem of small numbers noted earlier, when one adds the probability of out-of-network usage, chance becomes an even greater force. One PCP might find that all of his or her members access services exclusively via the PCP (resulting in underpayment via the reduced capitation), whereas another PCP may find that the majority of his or her members go out-of-network (resulting in overpayment via the low visit rate).

Other plans attempted to make adjustments on a retrospective basis, actually asking a PCP to refund a percentage of the capitation payment they had received all year (corresponding to the percentage of out-of-network costs above that predicted actuarially), or increasing the withhold to high levels to recover the money. These two approaches created terribly difficult exercises in provider relations, were generally perceived as unfair (a perception shared by this author), and are now uncommon or perhaps nonexistent except in some very large IPAs or medical groups.

The problem of using capitation with POS became so difficult that many plans chose to capitate PCPs for pure HMO (i.e., not POS) members and pay FFS (without using any risk pool) for POS members. This created new problems due to the schizophrenic payment systems, and resulted in what psychologists refer to as cognitive dissonance. In most cases, HMOs with high levels of POS membership simply changed to FFS for everything.

Primary Care Capitation

As noted earlier, PCP capitation is used only when a PCP "gatekeeper" structure is in place. In other words, the member may access the PCP whenever he or she needs to do so, but will only be covered for services by SCPs upon referral by their PCP, with notable exceptions such as direct access to ob/gyn physicians, as discussed in Chapter 4; direct access to PCPs and ob/gyn physicians is also now a requirement under the ACA. Plans that capitate PCPs may not necessarily capitate ob/gyns, however, and women covered by gatekeeper-type HMOs typically also select an internist or family physician to be their PCP. Issues specific to PCP capitation are discussed next.

Capitation systems usually allow for certain services to be carved out of the PCP capitation payment. A common example noted earlier is immunizations, which are not paid under capitation but instead are paid on a fee schedule or cost pass-through. As a general rule, carve-outs should only be used for those services that are not subject to discretionary utilization. In the case of immunizations, the medical guidelines for administering them are clear-cut but subject to change (e.g., there may be an increase in the number of immunizations that are to be given in the first years of life, or new vaccines are approved for use), and there is little question about their use. That would not be the case, for example, for office-based diagnostic imaging in which there is a high degree of discretion about when imaging is necessary, particularly if it is a profit center for the physician, as in the section on payment for ancillary services.

Many capitation systems also hold the PCP accountable for non-primary care services, either through risk programs or through positive incentive programs, both of which are discussed next.

Withholds and Physician Risk Pools

Some HMOs that capitate PCPs also have additional forms of capitation-related PCP financial risk and reward through withholds and capitation risk pools[*] for non-primary care. When used, the HMO conducts the same exercise of defining services and estimating costs for whatever specialty

---

[*]Not to be confused with the same term as applied to a market segment such as the small employer group market in which all small employer groups are in the same risk pool. It is the same concept, but applied differently.

TABLE 5-6	HMO Use of Physician Withholds/Risk Pools, Nation, 2006–2010	
Year	Percentage of HMOs using physician withholds/risk pools	Enrollment in HMOs using physician withholds/risk pools
2006	30.3%	24,855,970
2007	29.2%	25,581,087
2008	29.9%	24,121,540
2009	32.0%	21,317,302
2010	28.9%	18,714,180

Source: Sanofi-Aventis Managed Care Digest Series®/*HMO-PPO/Medicare-Medicaid Digest 2010–2011.* www.managedcaredigest.com. Used with permission.

services, institutional care, or ancillary services will be included in the risk pools. How withholds and risk pools are typically administered is discussed next. But before that it is worth noting that, as shown in **Table 5-6**, the prevalence of HMOs using withholds and risk pools has been in steady decline for several years, reaching approximately 30% as of 2010. By comparison, over half of HMOs use PCP capitation for direct services, as shown earlier in Figure 5-2.

Also, as noted earlier and illustrated in Table 5-1, individual physicians within a medical group may not be subject to an individual withhold, even if the medical group is subject to a withhold. This is shown in **Figure 5-6**.

A withhold is simply a percentage (e.g., 20%) of the primary care capitation that is withheld every month and

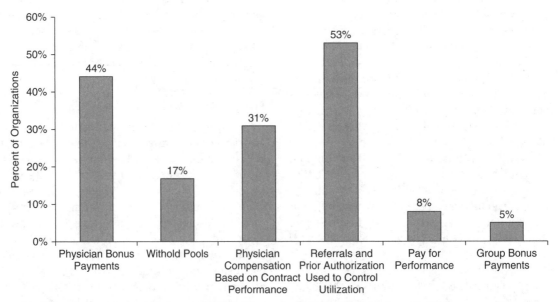

FIGURE 5-6 Physician Incentives Reported for Medical Groups in the AGMA Capitation Survey, 2008
Source: American Medical Group Association and ECG Management Consultants, © 2008. ECG/AMGA Capitation and Risk Contracting Survey, Alexandria, VA. www.amga.org. Used with permission.

used to pay for cost overruns in referral or institutional services. In the earlier example of $20.00 PMPM, a 20% withhold would be $4.00. Each month, the PCP would actually be paid the capitation minus the withhold amount; in the example, the monthly payment would be based on $16.00 PMPM. The withhold money is held by the plan and used at year end to pay for cost overruns for services allocated to the risk pool or pools, with the remainder returned to the PCP, as discussed below.

While rare (and even more rarely used), some plans also have a clause in their physician's contract that states that the plan may increase the amount of withhold in the event of cost excesses beyond what is already being withheld. For example, the withhold amount can be increased from 20% to 30% if referral costs are out of control. This method is ill-advised since it has little positive effect on utilization and only serves to reallocate a small amount of money from payment of PCPs to payment of other providers. While generating a great deal of ill will, the total dollars saved by the plan in such cases are best described as "decimal dust." As MCOs have become more sophisticated in medical management, there is far less reliance on financial incentives to control or influence utilization.

When capitation exists for primary care services and the PCP is also on a bonus/risk program for other medical costs, payment for referral services and institutional services is often made from capitation funds or pools as well. The services themselves may be paid for under a number of mechanisms (FFS, per diem, capitation, and the like), but the expense is drawn against a capitated fund or pool. There are a variety of ways that HMOs handle these types of risk pools, and some common methods are described here.

It must be stressed that the illustration that follows generally no longer exists in the real world exactly as it appears here. In HMOs that use this approach, there is considerable variation, and there is no uniformity as to whether or not an HMO will put the PCP at some level of risk for either or both of these types of service. The illustration also reflects models that were more prevalent roughly a decade ago, while mature HMOs have undergone considerable changes since then. Nevertheless, the illustration provides a common basis for understanding this type of model. **Figure 5-7** illustrates schematically how some of these risk pools operate.

There are three broad classes of non-primary care risk pools: referral (or specialty care); hospital or facility care, regardless of whether or not it is inpatient, outpatient, or emergency department; and ancillary services such as laboratory, radiology, pharmacy, and so forth. Pharmacy may also be considered a separate risk pool. Many HMOs also have a fourth "other" pool in which they accrue liabilities for such things as stop loss or malpractice, but the physicians have no stake in it (see later). Some HMOs combine

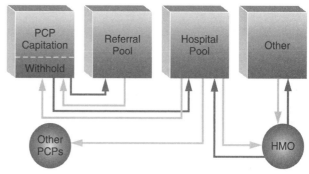

FIGURE 5-7 Capitation Risk Pools

the ancillary services into the "other" pool, which is the model illustrated in Figure 5-3. It is not uncommon for these risk pools to be handled in different ways regarding the flow of funds and levels of risk and reward for the physicians and the plan.

As an example, the PCP receives a $25.00 PMPM blended capitation rate for primary care services (in other words, the blend of all the age and sex capitation rates for that physician's membership base comes out to $25.00 PMPM). For each member, $60.00 PMPM is added to a capitated pool for all specialty referral services, and $300.00 PMPM is added to a capitated pool for inpatient and ambulatory facility-based services.* The PCP does not actually receive the money in those pools; the plan holds on to it. Any medical expenses incurred by members in that PCP's panel will be counted against the appropriate pool of funds. At the end of the year, a reconciliation of the various pools is made, as discussed below.

As with primary care, the scope of covered services must first be defined. For example, will home health be covered under institutional or referral (probably institutional because it reduces institutional costs), and will hospital-based physicians (e.g. radiology, pathology, and anesthesia) be covered under institutional or referral? The same exercise is carried out with any category for which capitated funds will be accrued in a risk pool.

If not all the withhold is used or there is a surplus in either the referral pool or the institutional services pool, then often any surplus in a pool is first used to pay for any excess expenses in the other pool. For example, if there is money left in the referral pool but the institutional pool has cost overruns, the extra funds in the referral pool are first applied against the excessive expenses in the hospital pool, and vice versa.

After both funds are covered, any excess money is paid to the physicians. In some cases only those physicians with positive balances in their own risk pools receive any money.

*The reader is reminded that these numbers are presented for illustrative purposes and do *not* represent accurate capitation rates.

For example, a PCP has referral services funds tracked for his or her own patients. If the cost of services for those members leaves a positive balance in the referral pool, and if there is money left in the institutional services pool on a plan-wide basis, the PCP receives a pro rata share of the money. In other words, risk is shared with all physicians in the plan, but reward may be tracked individually. In another example, some plans disburse positive balances in referral and institutional funds on the basis of both utilization and measures of quality and member satisfaction.

The degree to which an individual PCP's pools will have an impact on year-end bonus payments may vary. If the decision is to minimize risk to individual PCPs but not eliminate the risk pools entirely, then a low stop loss protection level must be set (see later) to minimize or even stop tracking expenses against an individual PCP's pools while those expenses are still low. For example, if a PCP has a member with an expensive chronic disease, the referral expenses will be paid either out of the plan-wide referral capitation pool, out of a separate fund for disease management costs, or out of a separate stop-loss fund, and will not count against the individual PCP's referral risk fund after referral expenses have reached, for example, $5,000. In this way, high-cost cases, which could wipe out an individual PCP's risk pool, will have less effect than that PCP's ability to management overall referral expenses in the rest of the member panel.

In plans where both a referral and hospital risk pool is used, some plans pay out all extra funds in the referral pool but only half the funds in the hospital pool. In other cases there may be an upper limit on the amount of bonus a PCP can receive from the hospital pool. The justification for this is that the plan stands a considerably greater degree of risk for hospital services and therefore deserves a degree of reward. Furthermore, it is often a combination of utilization management and effective negotiating that yields a positive result, and the plan does most or all of the negotiating, and usually manages utilization as well.

Pharmacy Costs   A specific category of expense is an area of both focus and disagreement: the risk for the cost of pharmaceuticals. Payers have employed a variety of means to manage drug costs. Examples include changing the benefit to a three-tier or four-tier copay, replacing copays with deductibles and/or coinsurance, increased use of drug utilization review, precertification of selected drugs, the use of formularies, contracting for favorable terms, and other techniques, as discussed in detail in Chapter 11. Pertinent to this chapter though is a brief discussion around the use of financial risk/incentives based on drug costs. As noted earlier, some MCOs do not include drug costs in any financial risk/incentive programs, though most do at least provide data and feedback to network physicians on drug utilization and cost.

There is no evidence that the presence or absence of financial incentives has a negative effect on quality or has led to inappropriate prescribing. One can debate whether or not the use of financial risk/incentives has any real effect on drug costs, but two older studies failed to show such an association.[21,22] With the high levels of variation in prescribing patterns and habits, it is theoretically sound to place drug costs into a risk/incentive program along with the other aspects of managing this benefit cost since it is the physician who prescribes the drug. Unfortunately, it may not be the PCP, but rather the SCP that writes the prescription, although that issue is not markedly different from any diagnostic or other therapeutic interventions by an SCP. The cost of the drug benefit is also influenced heavily by the prices a payer is able to negotiate with drug manufacturers.

For all of these reasons, drug costs may not be a component of a capitated risk pool. It is appearing more frequently in pay-for-performance programs in all types of plans, as discussed later in the chapter.

Medical Expenses Not Typically Applied to Primary Care Physician Risk Pools   As noted earlier, even in plans that use withholds and physician risk pools, there are certain medical expenses for which PCPs will not be at risk. For example, a plan may negotiate a capitated laboratory contract; laboratory capitation is then backed out of the referral and primary care capitation amounts and accounted for separately. If the PCP orders laboratory services from another vendor, that cost is deducted from his or her referral pool; otherwise, lab cost and use has no effect on the PCP's compensation.

Other examples of such nonrisk services include any type of carved-out services, for example, if the HMO has negotiated a capitated carve-out contract for behavioral health care (see Chapter 12). Other exceptions typically include a rider benefit such as vision or dental, or services over which PCPs have no control, such as obstetrics. Another example would be defined catastrophic conditions where the PCP is taken out of the case management function by the plan and the plan's case management system takes over the coordination of care. It is important to use clear and consistent definitions of what types of cases will be treated this way. Otherwise, there will be pressure from PCPs to include too much in this category, thereby eroding the entire concept of capitation. Once a service has been taken out of the at-risk category, it is exceedingly difficult to put it back in.

Stop-Loss Protection   The degree of risk to which any physician is exposed needs to be defined. As mentioned earlier, it is common for an HMO to stop deducting expenses against an individual PCP's pool after a certain threshold is reached for purposes of the year-end reconciliation. There are two forms of stop-loss protection: costs for individual members and aggregate cost protection.

As an example of individual case cost protection, if a PCP has a member with leukemia, after the referral expenses reach $5,000, it will no longer be counted against the PCP's referral pool, or perhaps only 20% of expenses in excess of $3,500 will be counted against the referral pool; the uncounted expenses will be paid either from an aggregate pool or from a specially allocated stop-loss fund.

It is possible to vary the amount of stop-loss protection by the size of a PCP's member base to reduce the element of chance. For example, if a PCP has fewer than 300 members, the stop loss is $2,000; if the PCP has more than 800 members, the stop loss is $5,000. It is equally common for a stop loss to exist for hospital services, although the level is much higher (e.g., $50,000). As alluded to earlier, the lower the stop loss, the less the effect of high-cost cases on individual capitation funds and the greater the effect of overall medical management by the PCP. On the other hand, if it is too low there may be a perverse incentive to run up expenses to get them past the stop loss. Multitiered stop loss also creates an artificial barrier to the PCPs' acceptance of new members. For example, if the stop loss for 300 members or fewer is less than that for 301 members or more, PCPs may resist adding members above the 300 limit so as to protect the lower stop-loss level. Tiered stop loss can be time limited to prevent this problem.

As an example of aggregate protection, the plan may reduce deductions to 20% or even stop deducting referral expenses after total expenses for an individual PCP reach 150% of the capitation risk pool amount. Providing aggregate stop-loss protection on the basis of a percentage of total capitation allows such protection to be tied to the membership base of the PCP. Since most HMOs limit the total risk at which a PCP is placed (e.g., 20% of the PCP's capitation amount, as noted above), as well as regulatory limits in Medicare and Medicaid HMOs as noted below, aggregate stop loss is useful primarily in large groups or IDSs.

The combination of stop-loss protection and risk-sharing across the physician panel (discussed later) serves to reduce any individual PCP's exposure to events outside his or her control. It is frustrating to manage properly all your cases but receive no incentive because one seriously ill patient had high expenses.

In any case, providing stop-loss protection to an individual physician is important, and the plan must budget for its cost. Although such stop-loss protection can be paid from the aggregate of all the physician's referral funds, that ensures that there will be a draw on the withhold (if there is one). Because positive referral balances will be paid back to PCPs, negative balances will need to be funded through the withhold, so there can never be a full return of the withhold. Therefore, it is preferable to budget a line item for stop-loss expense and to reduce the referral allocations by that amount.

Lastly, only the largest HMOs can afford to carry the total cost of stop-loss protection, and provider groups that accept full or global risk (discussed below) are rarely able to do so. Provider groups or IDSs at full risk as well as small to mid-sized HMOs therefore purchase commercially available reinsurance that protects the health plan or provider organization from the cost of catastrophic claims, also referred to as shock claims. Reinsurance is usually for both individual highly expensive claims and for excessively high aggregate costs.

Individual versus Pooled Risk   All forms of financial risk are affected by how the HMO handles the issue of individual risk versus pooled risk. In other words, to what degree is an individual physician at risk for their own performance, versus the degree that that risk is shared with some or all other PCPs? It is human nature to wish to share the downside risk (and pain) with others, but keep the upside (profit) for oneself. In those plans that do track risk pools individually, it is more common for only one pool (usually referral), if any, to be tracked on an individual basis while the withhold, if any, and hospital pool are aggregate. It is very rare for the hospital risk pool, when it exists, to be at the individual physician level.

As discussed in Chapter 4 and noted earlier in this chapter, HMOs may contract directly with PCPs, or through an IPA, a physician hospital organization (PHO), a management services organization (MSO), or other form of IDS (Chapter 2). The HMO capitates the IPA, or IDS, but that organization may or may not capitate the PCPs. In fact, some of these organizations pay the PCPs on a FFS basis, using one or more of the FFS payment methods (performance-based or not) described later.

Even when there is no intervening organization, the issue of actually who is being capitated, and for what, still remains. Is it the individual PCP? A subset of the total network of PCPs or pools of doctors (PODs)? Is it the entire network of PCPs? The answers may not be the same for each category or risk. For example, a plan may wish to capitate PCPs individually for their own services, combine them into PODs for purposes of referral services, and use the performance of the entire network for purposes of hospital services.

A plan can also choose to use different categories for risk and for reward. For example, a plan may spread risk across the entire network, but only reward a subset of PCPs. An example was given earlier in which positive balances in withholds or referral pools were used to offset deficits in the hospital pool; any remaining surplus balance would only be paid to those PCPs with a positive balance.

There are common and predictable problems with individual risk. The majority of those problems relate to the issue of small numbers. As noted earlier, luck can have as much or more of an impact on utilization as does good management, at least in small member panels. As a PCP's panel grows to over 500 members, this problem starts to lessen, but still persists. This is one of the most important reasons that HMOs typically require PCPs to not close their practice to the HMO until that PCP has at least 250 or more members (see Chapters 4 and 6); it is also the identical reason that a PCP should desire to have a large panel enrolled. When a PCP has good utilization results, they generally desire to keep the reward for their hard labors; when results are poor, they frequently feel that they have been dealt an abnormally sick population of members, and should not be held accountable for the high medical costs. This is a common and usually unfounded complaint, but a sophisticated practice profiling system is able to quantify this (see Chapter 10).

The larger the dollars at stake, the more danger the problem of small numbers becomes to an individual PCP. While stop loss and reinsurance somewhat ameliorate the problem, the problem remains. This is the very reason that plans may be willing to use individual pools for referral services, but will not do so for hospital services, where the dollars are substantially higher.

The other major problem with individual risk is the ability of some PCPs to game the system. In other words, in order to enhance income, the PCP manages to get their sickest patients to transfer out of the practice, with a resulting improvement in that individual PCP's medical costs. While all plans prohibit a PCP from kicking a member out of his or her practice due to medical condition, the rare unethical PCP can find a way to do so and remain undetected. Related to that is the concern that individual risk incents a PCP to withhold necessary medical care. While this charge has been leveled at the HMO industry for many years, it has never been demonstrated, and is discussed later.

If the plan chooses to pool risk across the entire network, then the flip side of individual risk occurs: the impact of any individual PCP's actions are diluted so much as to be undetectable. If a PCP is having good results, then they may resent having to cover for the problems of colleagues with poor results (of course, no one objects to being helped out when one's own results are poor). If the plan does not track individual results, then it will have little capability of providing meaningful data to individual physicians to help them better manage medical resources. Also, there is some evidence from older studies that individual risk/bonus arrangement elicits behavior changes, while aggregated risk/bonus arrangements do not.[23]

Because of these two extremes, many plans have chosen to use PODs for at least some financial risk management. PODs are a subset of the entire network, although there is no standard size. PODs may be a large medical group, an aggregation of 10–15 physicians, or may be made up of all participating PCPs in an entire geographic area. A POD could also be made up of the physicians in a PHO or MSO that accepts risk. The common denominator is that there are sufficient members enrolled in practices in the POD to allow for statistical integrity, but small enough to still allow the POD to make changes that will be seen in utilization results. The chief risk is that PODs require support from the plan in the form of data and utilization management.

Specialty Physician Capitation

SCP capitation is typically simpler than PCP capitation. As with PCP capitation, it is a fixed-payment PMPM for services to a defined population of members. The capitation payment may be adjusted for age, sex, and product type, but not as universally as is found in PCP capitation. Severity adjustment, as discussed earlier, is also possible, although may be needed less due to a larger panel of members, which allows for greater actuarial integrity. In all events, the capitation amount will be calculated based on the expected volume of referrals, the average cost, the ability to manage utilization, and the relative negotiating strengths of each party. A large plan may have past data to guide it, but even then it is common to use an outside actuary to derive the correct capitation amount.

As with PCP capitation, the services covered by the capitation payment must be clearly defined, including those procedures to be carved out, meaning not paid through capitation. The reason for this is that those SCPs that perform high-cost procedures will be relatively disadvantaged compared to SCPs that perform only less expensive office-based care, even if both SCPs are in the same specialty. The risk of such carve-outs is obvious: There is no incentive to not perform the procedure, and every financial incentive to do it. Alternatively, the capitation of an SCP that performs such procedures may be adjusted upward to reflect the additional capability, while also allowing that SCP to bill the plan FFS when performing the procedure upon referral from another physician.

Though now rare, the capitation amount may be based on a percent of premium revenue, rather than a hard PMPM dollar amount. In Medicare and Medicaid plans this is not unreasonable, since the premium revenue is set by the government, and presumably has the appropriate mix of specialty services already in the total. For commercial plans, however, it is now rarely done, if ever.

While theoretically the same utilization issues apply to specialty care as well as primary care, the numbers involved in SCP capitation are often significantly smaller for any given specialty (even though specialty PMPM costs as a whole is usually one and a half to two times higher than primary care). For example, PCP capitation may average $27.00 PMPM, while the capitation for neurology may be $1.05. Thus, adjustments based on demographic variables become very small indeed, and may not be worth the effort. Because the numbers can be smaller, a SCP requires a much higher number of members in order for capitation to have meaning. Where a PCP may achieve relative stability in capitation at a membership level of 400–600, a SCP may require triple that number or more in order to avoid the problem of random chance having more effect than medical management on utilization.

Directly capitating SCPs as individuals or as specialty groups (or multispecialty groups) is the easiest approach, though a specialty IPA or a single-specialty management company may also be the vehicle for contracting and capitating, as noted in Chapter 4. Unless the SCP group, IPA, or other contracting vehicle is able to cover the entire service area, however, the plan must create procedures for the PCPs to know to which SCP they should refer those patients who are actually covered under the capitation.

Unusual Approaches to Specialty Capitation   Specialty capitation has been subject to numerous different approaches, most of which were touted at the time as the best way to do it. The following methodologies were used at one time or another, and still exist here and there, but are now quite uncommon. They may have some relevancy to the new methods of payment under consideration through the ACA, however.

Disease Management Companies and Specialty Institutions   Another variation on single group capitation is capitation for single specialty services to a specialty company that specializes in specific types of care, such as cancer or cardiac care. As discussed in Chapter 4, this is most commonly a company or corporation that employs physicians and support staff, and provides facilities and ancillary services, or may be a professional group in those states that have corporate practice of medicine acts prohibiting physicians from being employees of corporations for purposes of practicing medicine. It can also be an organization created by a large, comprehensive provider system as an internal unit. The organization is then responsible for providing all specialty services within the HMO's service area. This approach may also be applied to emergency department care if the vendor's physicians are on staff at all of the HMO's participating hospitals.

This can also be done for single-specialty services through a single institution; for example, the HMO contracts with a local university faculty practice plan for all cardiology services. The contracted institution is then responsible to arrange for specialty services that it cannot provide itself. The primary specialty contract holder receives the capitation payment, and must then administer payment to subcontractors. This approach is still used on occasion, and may increase where health systems now employ a large panel of physicians.

Either way, the focus is on those chronic conditions in which a broad, integrated approach can make a difference in outcomes and/or cost of care. Because they are more comprehensive, the capitation calculation must take into account a somewhat larger set of factors such as:

- Inpatient cost and utilization;
- Outpatient costs and utilization;
- By service type;
- By location;
- Physician costs and utilization;
- Non-acute-care costs;
- Inpatient facilities such as skilled nursing facilities;
- Outpatient or alternative settings such as hospice;
- Pharmaceutical costs and utilization;
- Those agents included as a routine part of medical–surgical benefits such as injectables;
- The cost of outpatient or chronic drugs if the disease management organization is to be at risk for their use;
- Frequency of the disease state;
- New occurrences expected by age and sex categories; and
- Existing cases.[24]

Contact Capitation   Contact capitation is an odd and now very uncommon form of SCP capitation, but it warrants brief discussion since it has similarities to new forms of payment under consideration by CMS, and payment reforms considered in the ACA. Like any other form of payment, contact capitation does not have a single definition of how it works, and is subject to a variety of local variations. Furthermore, while it once elicited interest (at least on the West Coast) as a sophisticated way of capitating, it turned out to be too complex to be widely adopted.

Contact capitation begins with a budgeted PMPM capitated pool of money for each major specialty. Like other forms of capitation, provision in the calculations are made for product design, the effect of copays and coinsurance, the effect of stop-loss insurance for catastrophic cases, and the effect of other-party liability offsets must also be accounted for, as discussed earlier as well as later.

The plan then tracks each unique member contact with each specialist; that is, regardless of whether that member/patient sees the SCP once or 100 times, it is counted as a single contact. This is tracked over a set period of time, such as a year, a quarter, or semi-annually. Once the period is over, the counters are reset to zero and it begins again. The plan pays out the total capitated pool of money to the SCPs based on the distribution of the contacts. For example, if one cardiologist has 8% of the total number of cardiology contacts (i.e., unique, nonduplicated patients), that cardiologist receives 8% of the total capitation pool. It is usually assumed that once a patient makes contact with that SCP, the patient will remain with the SCP. Of course, this is not something that can be guaranteed, and so provision must be made for patients that change SCPs during the course of the tracking period.

The timing of payouts under contact capitation is highly variable, unlike more common forms of capitation. Since the payout is a factor of the total percentage of contacts in a period of time, it cannot occur until adequate encounters have occurred to allow for a calculation. The few systems that still use contact capitation usually use an entire 12-month period to make the adjustments, though some may do so on a quarterly or semi-annual basis. In any case, some form of interim payment mechanism must therefore be in place since even an IPA run by Darth Vader would not expect physicians to receive no payment for a year. This interim payment may be a form of discounted FFS, it may be a monthly "capitation" payment based on the distribution of contacts each month or to-date, or some other means. In all cases, this adds a layer of complexity to the ultimate calculation and, in the dreaded event it requires an actual refund of money from a SCP, very hard feelings will follow.

Contact capitation strongly resembles some of the new value-based payment approaches envisioned for traditional Medicare by CMS and addressed within the ACA.

Pros and Cons of Capitation

Because physician capitation engenders a great deal of opinion, informed or not, it is worth discussing the major positives and negatives about capitation before moving on to risk-based FFS. In past decades, a lack of understanding by physicians would have been relatively high on the list of problems related to capitation, but that is no longer the case, as illustrated in **Figure 5-8**.

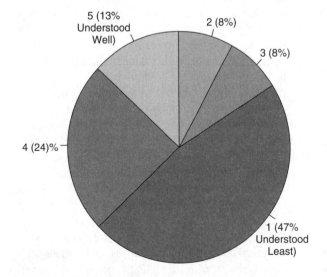

FIGURE 5-8 Physician Understanding of Risk Contracts, 2008.
Note: 1, least understood; 5, well understood
Source: American Medical Group Association and ECG Management Consultants, © 2008. ECG/AMGA Capitation and Risk Contracting Survey, Alexandria, VA. www.amga.org. Used with permission.

Pros   The first and most powerful reason for an HMO to capitate providers is that capitation puts the provider at some level of risk or incentive for medical expenses and utilization. Capitation eliminates the FFS incentive to over-utilize, and brings the financial incentives of the capitated provider in line with the financial incentives of the HMO. Under capitation, costs are more easily predicted by the health plan (though not absolutely predictable because of problems of out-of-network care). Capitation is also easier and less costly to administer than FFS (e.g., fewer claims to adjudicate), thus resulting in lower administrative costs in the HMO and potentially lower premium rates to the member.

The most powerful reasons for a provider to accept capitation from an HMO are financial. Capitation ensures good cash flow: the capitation money comes in at a predictable rate, regardless of services rendered, and comes in as pre-payment, thus providing positive cash flow. Also, for physicians who are effective medical case managers as well as cost-effective providers of direct patient care, the profit margins under capitation can exceed those found in FFS, especially as FFS fees come under continued pressure.

Cons   In an unmanaged FFS system, there is a direct and immediate relationship between doing something and getting paid for it; under capitation, the reward is temporally remote from the action. In other words, the capitation check does not change each month depending on services. Furthermore, by carefully constructing a stop-loss protection program, the effect of high-cost cases on capitation funds is attenuated. Spreading the risk over more than one physician can lower the effect of single cases on a physician's payment, but at the cost of not recognizing individual performance. In other words, the immediate incentive of FFS is not replaced with an immediate incentive through capitation.

The most common actual problem with capitation involves chance. As mentioned earlier, a significant element of chance is involved when there are too few members in an enrolled base to make up for bad luck (or good luck, but nobody ever complains about that). Physicians with fewer than 100 members may find that the dice simply roll against them, and they will have members who need bypass surgery or have cancer, AIDS, or a host of other expensive medical problems. The only way to assuage that is to spread the risk for expensive cases through common risk-sharing pools for referral and institutional expenses and to provide stop-loss protection for expensive cases.

The biggest argument against capitation was that it promoted inappropriate underutilization; in other words, capitation incentivizes a physician to withhold necessary care. Once a very hot topic, the preponderance of literature demonstrated that managed care actually provided equal or better care to members than uncontrolled FFS systems, even while lowering costs. There were so many studies on the topic that rather than include them as endnotes, they are listed in Appendix 5-1.

As experience with capitation grew while at the same time the market penetration of HMOs declined, this argument against capitation lost any real sense of urgency, but it could resume if provider risk-based payment increased. For example, in research published a decade ago, when consumers were asked if a 10% cost control/quality physician incentive program was a good or bad idea, 73% said that a cost control incentive was a bad idea and only half responded that a quality incentive program was a good idea.[25]

Risk-Based Fee-for-Service

Capitation is only one type of risk-based HMO physician payment. The other way uses FFS, typically through the use of withholds, but sometimes by the application of mandatory fee reductions or budgeted FFS.

Fee-for-Service PCP Withholds   Similar to gatekeeper-type HMOs that use PCP capitation withholds, HMOs or IPAs that use FFS to pay PCPs often withhold a certain percentage of the fee to cover medical cost overruns. For example, the HMO or IPA may withhold 20% of the fee in a risk pool until the end of the year. In effect, physicians receive only 80% of the allowed fee, but may receive the other 20% at the end of the year if there were no excess medical costs. HMOs that do not use a "gatekeeper" model typically return remaining withhold funds on a straight pro rata basis, although some plans return withhold on a preferential basis to PCPs as opposed to SCPs.

Mandatory Fee Reductions   In an HMO where risk for medical cost is shared with all the physicians and payment is on a FFS basis, there must be a mechanism whereby fees may be reduced unilaterally by the HMO in the event of serious cost overruns. This draconian measure is no longer found in HMOs that are not provider-sponsored since such plans long ago failed and either disappeared or were acquired by healthier plans. A provider-sponsored plan usually does not have access to deep financial resources, however, so cannot allow itself to drop into a serious financial deficit. For example, the plan may be using a fee schedule that is equivalent to a 20% discount on the most common fees in the area. In the event that medical expenses are over budget and there is not enough money in the risk withhold fund to cover them, all physicians' fees are reduced by a further percentage, say an additional 10%, to cover the expenses. At this point, the effective discount is 30%, although this would really be 50% in the event that a withhold system was in place, all of the withhold funds had been used, and there were still excess medical liabilities. The major policy decision to be made when things go south is setting how low fee reductions will go before they will not be further reduced. For example, the

plan may set the lowest possible fees at 60% of Medicare, although, if the plan reaches that point, there may not be many physicians left in the network to pay.

Budgeted FFS   Related to mandatory fee reductions, budgeted FFS is used in a few plans. In this variation, which is much like contact capitation, briefly discussed earlier, the plan budgets a maximum amount of money that may be spent in each specialty category. This maximum may be expressed either as a PMPM amount (e.g., $7.50 PMPM) or as a percentage of revenue (e.g., 5.6% of premium revenue). As costs in that specialty category approach or exceed the budgeted amount, the withhold amount in that specialty and only that specialty is increased. In addition, the fees for that specialty, but not all specialties, may be reduced.

This approach has the advantage of focusing the payment changes on those specialties in which excess costs occur rather than on all specialties in the network. The disadvantage is that this is not individual provider specific; in other words, all SCPs are treated the same, and there is no specific focus on individual outliers. It can also drive some specialists out of the network. This approach was once somewhat popular in HMOs that did not use PCPs to manage care, but is now uncommon.

Legislation and Regulation Applicable to Risk-Based Physician Payment

Beginning in the 1990s, many states and the federal government passed laws and created regulations that affected physician incentive programs, especially risk-based payment. While capitation and/or incentive programs have not been found to have a negative effect on quality, as addressed earlier, the intent was to protect beneficiaries from the potential harm that the politicians and regulators perceived existed. In general, while adding an extra layer of bureaucracy (and therefore a bit of extra cost), health plans have had little or no problem complying.

Not all states have passed such laws or promulgated such regulations, and those that have show little consistency from one state to another. In general, when states do have such laws, they focus on disclosure of financial incentives, as noted in Chapter 28. Because of this lack of consistency and stability at the state level, the reader will have to research each state individually as needed.

The remainder of this section focuses on the federal regulations, since those are consistent and also serve to illustrate the approaches taken by some states. Beginning in 1987, CMS (then called HCFA) implemented regulations that placed limits on physician incentive programs in Medicare and Medicaid MCOs. These regulations have been modified several times since then. The reader is also referred to Chapter 24 for further discussion of Medicare Advantage and to Chapter 25 for a discussion of Medicaid and managed health care.

"Significant Financial Risk"

Congress passed legislation placing certain requirements on Medicare HMOs with risk-based physician contracts (at the time they were called Medicare+Choice, but are now called MA-HMOs). Those requirements were based on whether or not the contract placed the physician or medical group at "significant financial risk"[*] (SFR) for medical costs. The legislation applies only to Medicare and Medicaid HMOs.

The Federal Register defines SFR as follows:

"The amount at risk for referral services is the difference between the maximum potential referral payments and the minimum potential referral payments. Bonuses unrelated to utilization (e.g., quality bonuses such as those related to member satisfaction or open physician panels) should not be counted towards referral payments. Maximum potential payments is defined as the maximum *anticipated* total payments that the physician/group could receive. If there is no specific dollar or percentage amount noted in the incentive arrangement, then the PIP [*payment incentive plan*] should be considered as potentially putting 100% of the potential payments at risk for referral services. The SFR threshold is set at 25% of 'potential payments' for covered services, regardless of the frequency of assessment (i.e., collection) or distribution of payments. SFR is present when the 25% threshold is exceeded.

"The following incentive arrangements should be considered as SFR:

- Withholds greater than 25% of potential payments.
- Withholds less than 25% of potential payments if the physician or physician group is potentially liable for amounts exceeding 25% of potential payments.
- Bonuses that are greater than 33% of potential payments minus the bonus.
- Withholds plus bonuses if the withholds plus bonuses equal more than 25% of potential payments. The threshold bonus percentage for a particular withhold percentage may be calculated using the formula: Withhold % = -0.75 (Bonus %) + 25%.
- Capitation arrangements, if the difference between the maximum potential payments and the minimum potential payments is more than 25% of the maximum potential payments; or the maximum and minimum potential payments are not clearly explained in the physician's or physician group's contract.
- Any other incentive arrangements that have the potential to hold a physician or physician group liable for more than 25% of potential payments."[26]

---

[*]The definition of "significant" is a legislative one, not one based on any particular research.

TABLE 5-7	Limits on Referral Costs Based on Patient Panel Size in Medicare or Medicaid HMOs		
Patient panel size	Single combined limit	Separate institutional limit	Separate professional limit
1–1,000	$6,000	$10,000	$3,000
1,001–5,000	$30,000	$40,000	$10,000
5,001–8,000	$40,000	$60,000	$15,000
8,001–10,000	$75,000	$100,000	$20,000
10,001–25,000	$150,000	$200,000	$25,000
>25,000	None	None	None

Source: 42 CFR 422.208.

Any service that a physician does not provide him- or herself, or that is not provided by another member of the physician's group, should be considered a referral service. If the physician group refers patients to other providers (including independent contractors to the group) to perform the ancillary services, then those services are considered referral services. If the physician group performs ancillary services, then those services are not considered referral services. Whether or not such referrals contribute to the financial risk borne by the physician will depend on whether his or her compensation arrangements are such that referrals for those services or supplies could impact upon the physician's income.

Stop-loss protection must be in place to protect physicians and/or physician groups to whom SFR has been transferred by an HMO. Either aggregate or per patient stop loss may be acquired. The rule specifies that if aggregate stop loss is provided, it must cover 90% of the cost of referral services that exceed 25% of potential payments; physicians and groups can be held liable for only 10%. If per patient stop loss is acquired, it must be determined based on the physician or physician group's patient panel size and cover 90% of the referral costs, which exceed the per patient limits noted in **Table 5-7**.

CMS has also set criteria for when an HMO, physician, or physician group may pool their patients for purposes of determining stop-loss levels. To determine the patient panel size in Table 5-7, specific criteria are stated in the regulations. Any entity that meets all five criteria required for the pooling of risk will be allowed to pool that risk in order to determine the amount of stop loss required by the regulation. Those five criteria are:

1. Pooling of patients is otherwise consistent with the relevant contracts governing the compensation arrangements for the physician or group (i.e., no contracts requiring risk can be segmented by HMO or patient category);

2. The physician or group is at risk for referral services with respect to each of the categories of patients being pooled;

3. The terms of the compensation arrangements permit the physician or group to spread the risk across the categories of patients being pooled (i.e., payments must be held in a common risk pool);

4. The distribution of payments to physicians from the risk pool is not calculated separately by patient category (either by the Medicare HMO or by Medicaid, Medicare, or commercial HMO); and

5. The terms of the risk borne by the physician or group are comparable for all categories of patients being pooled.[27]

Pooling and stop-loss requirements applicable to a group cannot be extended to a subcontracting level. In other words, if a group meets pooling requirements for a high stop loss, but subcontracts with physicians who are at SFR with smaller patient panels, then the stop-loss requirements for the smaller panels apply to those subcontracted physicians. If an HMO uses PODs, as described earlier in this chapter, then the pooling criteria may still be met by the POD if the incentive program for the POD physicians meets the criteria noted above, even though the POD is not an actual legal entity. In other words, the concept of sharing risk and reward via a POD system may be considered pooling for this purpose.

An HMO, medical group, or physician may combine commercial membership with Medicare and Medicaid membership for purposes of pooling if the financial risk is applicable to all members, but may not do so if the risk arrangements are different between those types of patients. If such pooling is appropriate but stop loss is still required, then the stop-loss arrangement need only cover Medicare and Medicaid members, not commercial members. Although Table 5-7 does indicate what constitutes SFR for small panel sizes (i.e., 500–1,000 members), HMOs typically avoid putting a physician at that level of risk. As discussed earlier in this chapter, the degree of financial risk for medical costs that a physician with a small panel would face is usually limited by the HMO in any event. In cases where a physician with a small panel might be placed at SFR, the HMO can provide stop-loss protection by adjusting the capitation payment or fee schedule so as to budget for the cost of the stop loss (in other words, treat it as an insurance premium).

Finally, for those medical groups with large panels of enrollees, or for IDSs that pool risk, either the HMO may provide stop-loss coverage at a competitive premium rate or commercial stop-loss insurance is available from third parties.

Disclosure Requirements

CMS requires disclosure to both CMS itself and to members or beneficiaries of the Medicare or Medicaid HMO. This disclosure applies to all providers in the network if they are at any financial risk. For example, if an HMO capitates an IPA, and the IPA in turn capitates a medical group, then both financial arrangements are subject to disclosure. If that medical group in turn subcapitates other medical groups, that too is subject to disclosure. IPAs that contract only with individual physicians and not with physician groups are considered physician groups under this rule.

The following pieces of information are required by the regulation to be provided to CMS:

- Whether referral services are covered by the PIP. If only services furnished directly by the physician or group are addressed by the PIP, then there's no need for disclosure of other aspects of the PIP;
- Type of incentive arrangement (e.g., withhold, bonus, capitation);
- Percent of total income at risk for referrals;
- Amount and type of stop-loss protection;
- Panel size and whether enrollees were pooled in order to achieve the panel size; and
- If the MCO is required by this regulation to conduct a customer satisfaction survey, a summary of the survey results.[28]

At Medicare or Medicaid beneficiaries' request, HMOs must provide information indicating whether the HMO or any of its contractors or subcontractors use a PIP that may affect the use of referral services, the type of incentive arrangement(s) used, and whether stop-loss protection is provided. If the HMO is required to conduct a survey, it must also provide beneficiary requestors with a summary of survey results.

Medicare HMOs with SFR were also required to use the Consumer Assessment of Health Plans Study (CAHPS®), which was focused solely on Medicare managed care plans for any plan that put physicians at SFR. That has since evolved, however, and CAHPS® now stands for Consumer Assessment of Health Providers and Systems and is designed to look at Medicare managed care, Medicare FFS, Medicare providers, and Medicare drug plans. It is under the purvey of the Agency for Healthcare Research and Quality (AHRQ*) and is far more broadly administered. In fact, health plans typically now use it to meet one of the requirements for external accreditation (see Chapter 15).

The HMO is only required to provide to a beneficiary a summary statement or letter outlining all of the incentive arrangements in place throughout the HMO. A beneficiary won't necessarily be able to tell from the required HMO disclosure whether or not a specific physician has a PIP, or the amount or type of risk that individual physician might experience. However, there is nothing in federal statute or

---

*www.cahps.ahrq.gov.

regulation to prevent an HMO or individual physician from providing physician-specific information to a beneficiary who requests it.

Civil Liability for Physician Compensation Programs

In cases where an HMO, IDS, or medical group does not have Medicare or Medicaid risk business, and there are no state laws or regulations governing physician compensation or incentives, managers should note that potential liability still remains in civil court. Physician incentives in managed health care have largely withstood legal challenges in the past, but that is no guarantee that they cannot be successfully challenged in a jury trial.

Regardless of the facts or merits of incentive systems, some judges and juries have expressed their opinion in judgment that financial incentives to manage utilization or cost are injurious to patients. In the late 1990s, it did not even require that a member had been injured; the very existence of an incentive program was reason enough.

For example, in 1999, two states, Texas and Georgia, passed legislation to make it easier for members to sue HMOs. In another example from 1999, Harris Methodist Health Plan in Texas reached a $4.7 million settlement with plaintiffs' attorneys who had filed two class-action lawsuits against the HMO because it did not disclose that capitation payments included prescription costs; thus, they argued, physicians were incented to limit prescribing. The settlement is believed to be the first in the nation in which uninjured patients recovered cash (approximately $50 per member) because the HMO failed to disclose such incentives.[29] Exposure to lawsuits regarding financial incentives is not necessarily confined solely to individual plaintiffs. In 1998, the former attorney general of Texas, citing a 1997 state law prohibiting financial incentives "that act directly or indirectly as an inducement to limit medically necessary services," filed a suit in a state district court, asking the court to fine six HMOs and prevent them from offering financial incentives to physicians. Harris Methodist Health Plan of Texas, the same HMO cited above, was fined $3.5 million in that action. On the other hand, other lawsuits have rejected any linkage between physician incentives and the care provided.[30]

For benefits plans that are self-funded under the Employee Retirement Income Security Act (ERISA; see Chapter 29), the supreme court provided limits against lawsuits for incentive programs and other activities, which is often referred to as the "ERISA shield."[31] In recent years, civil actions alleging injury from risk-based physician payment methodologies are now typically part of an overall pot of allegations, rather than being singled out.

Shared Savings

Payment using a shared savings methodology combines elements of risk and nonrisk payment, and is used by payers other than HMOs. It is relatively rare but will soon grow based on CMS desire to use it in the traditional Medicare FFS program, as well as commercial payer interest. It may apply only to physician payment or to combined hospital-physician payment, so is discussed in the section on combined payment.

■ PAYMENT OF HOSPITALS, HEALTH SYSTEMS, AND AMBULATORY FACILITIES

Hospitals, health systems, and ambulatory procedure facilities refer to the physical facilities in which care is provided, not to the physicians providing that care, and this section examines payment to facilities alone, not in combination with physician payment, which is discussed later. Facilities are referred to generically as "hospitals" unless there is a need to differentiate them, for example, physician-owned facilities versus nonprofit facilities. Two issues are discussed before discussing types of payments: (1) hospital payer mix and its impact on cost-shifting and (2) hospital price inflation for commercial payers.

Hospital Payer Mix and Cost-Shifting

Hospitals derive revenue from many different sources, and all commercial payers combined usually accounts for less than one half of a typical nonprofit hospital's total revenue, with any one commercial payer accounting for only a portion of that. In some states, the local BCBS plan accounts for the largest share of commercial revenue, and typically two or three non-BCBS commercial payers account for most of the rest. Other markets are more evenly distributed. The average payer mix for nonprofit community hospitals in 2008 is illustrated in **Figure 5-9**.

Not all payers pay the same amount. Differences exist between commercial payers for any one hospital, but generally speaking, all pay more than Medicare or Medicaid because Medicare and Medicaid do not pay the full cost of care, as shown in **Figure 5-10**. This is referred to as "cost-shifting." Because of cost-shifting, revenue from commercial payers is higher as a percent than are bed-days; for example, commercially insured bed-days may be 36% of total bed-days, but revenue from commercial payers (including out-of-pocket cost sharing by patients) is typically closer to 40% or more of total revenues.

Hospital Price Inflation

Like many health sectors, hospital cost inflation has continually outstripped general inflation. Part of the reason is that hospitals found themselves facing ever more contracting challenges as payers, and HMOs in particular continued to seek ways of controlling costs and blunting price increases. The movement from inpatient to outpatient care,

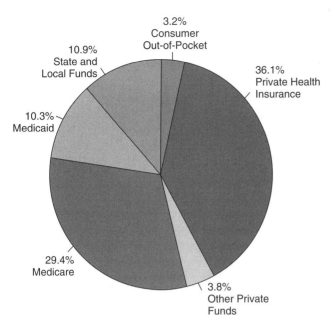

FIGURE 5-9 U. S. Hospital Payer Mix, 2008

Source: Data from the CMS Office of the Actuary, www.cms.gov/
NationalHealthExpendData/02_NationalHealthAccountsHistorical.asp#TopOfPage/
nhe2009nhe2009.zip.

which at first threatened hospital revenues, was addressed by increasing charges for outpatient care. But the move to outpatient also meant that new competitors sprang up, such as free-standing ambulatory surgical centers that were often partially owned by the physicians who used it. Patients with few medical complications and good coverage were drawn off, leaving the hospital with sicker patients and a higher percentage of noncovered care.

Competition from these new centers and from other hospitals also led to a "medical arms race" in which hospitals

had to have the latest and greatest devices and services in order to attract and retain the medical staff, and surgeons in particular because surgical care provides better margins than nonsurgical care does. Movement from inpatient to outpatient care also meant that patients that were admitted were on average sicker and required a greater intensity of care. And drug pricing has seen serious price inflation, affecting many inpatient stays. Hospitals also faced increasing problems with cash flow. Payrolls must be met, the facility must be maintained, and the drugs and devices for patient care must be paid for. The nursing shortage meant rising nursing salaries and increasing staffing pressures.

Hospitals cannot negotiate prices with Medicare or Medicaid, however, only with commercial payers. This means that except for other minor sources of revenue, commercial payers are the only place hospitals can go to increase their revenues to deal with pressures such as those described earlier. In other words, hospitals seek to maximize margins on commercial payment.

This was often difficult to do in the past because in most communities, hospitals competed with each other. But that began to change as hospitals consolidated on a local and a regional basis, as described in Chapter 4. By 2003 almost 90% of all metropolitan areas were considered "highly consolidated hospital markets."[32] As multihospital systems gained market power, they were able to demand and receive increased prices from commercial payers.[33-38] The result is displayed in **Figure 5-11**, which shows a sharp increase in hospital prices to commercial payers beginning around 2002.

Hospital pricing is not the only factor leading to hospital cost inflation, of course. For example, the average number of procedures on a per capita basis has also sharply increased. Utilization issues, however, are addressed in Chapter 7. The focus of this chapter is on payment.

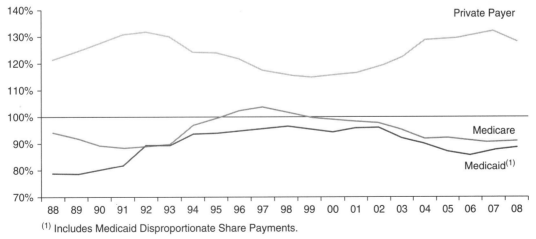

(1) Includes Medicaid Disproportionate Share Payments.

FIGURE 5-10 Aggregate Hospital Payment-to-Cost Ratios for Private Payers, Medicare and Medicaid, 1988–2008

Source: Avalere Health analysis of American Hospital Association Annual Survey data, 2008, for community hospitals in the AHA's TRENDWATCH CHARTBOOK 2010. www.aha.org/research/reports/tw/chartbook/ch4.shtml. Used with permission.

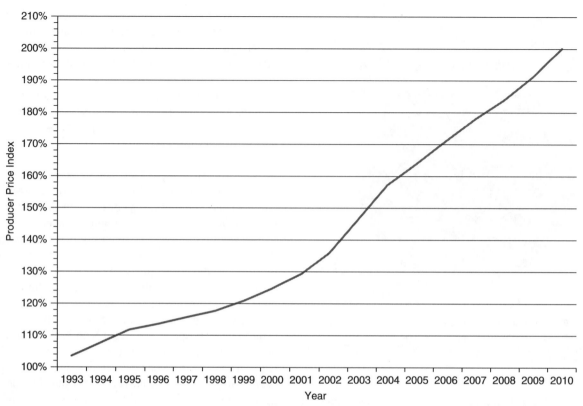

FIGURE 5-11 Producer Price Index for Hospital Prices to All Payers Other than Medicare and Medicaid, 1993–2010

Source: Data from the U.S. Bureau of Labor Statistics Database, Producer Price Index by Industry, General Medical and Surgical Hospitals by Payer Type, All Payers Other than Medicare and Medicaid; Series ID PCU62211A62211A6.

Negotiating Hospital Payment

Although network contracting is addressed primarily in Chapter 4, negotiating prices is addressed here. Common issues in negotiating and contracting for hospital payment are discussed first, followed by a brief discussion of ad hoc negotiating with non-contracted facilities.

Negotiating Payment to a Contracted Hospital

As noted earlier, payers prefer to use the same payment method for all physicians in a community, or perhaps mix a few together such as PCP capitation and SCP FFS. Hospitals with large panels of employed physicians and large medical groups are increasingly able to negotiate special fee schedules, but payers typically do not negotiate with individual physicians. This is not the case with hospitals.

Typical negotiating and contracting practices around multimillion-dollar contracts between payers and hospitals are similar to multimillion-dollar negotiating and contracting in other business in that they are complex, must address many elements in detail, and are often drawn out over time. The magnitude of such agreements necessitate that negotiating and contracting between payers and hospitals be business to business and carried out at arm's length, just as it is for any large and sophisticated

business. Because payers contract with many hospitals and hospitals contract with many payers, contract terms and dates for each may vary considerably from contract to contract, and it is not uncommon for each to be continually negotiating with one organization or another. Therefore, payers and hospitals alike typically have staff that specialize and focus primarily on negotiating such contracts, supported by external actuarial and consulting firms to assist as needed.

Focusing on financial goal-setting, each organization typically determines its overall goal such as achieving a certain percentage increase or decrease in the aggregate. Each organization will also determine the point where terms would be so unacceptable that it would be better to walk away. Both the overall financial goal and the point of walking away may change over the course of negotiations.

The typical negotiating process usually involves multiple rounds of back-and-forth proposals. Either party may make the first proposal, which may then set the scene for ongoing negotiations or, less commonly, be rejected out of hand. The initiating party often presents their proposal along with any commentary to support changes that are the most likely to be resisted by the other party. For example, a hospital may tell a payer that it is losing money on a particular service line,* or a payer may tell a hospital that it can no longer preferentially refer members to the facility for a particular procedure (e.g., heart surgery) unless the hospital offers more competitive rates.

It is unusual for the parties to come to agreement quickly if any substantial changes are proposed, for example, hospital demands for double digit rate increases or payer demands for a substantial change in payment methodology. Typically the party receiving the new proposal models the potential impact of that proposal and compares it to the goals they had set. This usually leads to a counterproposal or, less commonly, an outright rejection.

In all cases, each party uses its own proprietary data to model the impact of proposed payment terms. As this process is a business-to-business negotiation, neither party is under any obligation to share its proprietary data set or models or its analysis of any particular scenarios with the other. Any disclosure of data and modeling by one party or the other is strategic in nature and done to support the party's goals in the negotiation. Such strategic disclosures are typically confined to a single issue; for example, a hospital may show data to support the need for higher than average case rates for a specific service such as maternity, or a payer may show data to support the contention that a procedure costs 20% less at comparable hospitals. The overall goal must then be translated into proposed concrete payment rates for specific types of services. This is typically done by using financial models.

As a general rule, payers seek to avoid charge-based payment methodologies such as charges or discounts on charges because the payer cannot control how high or how often a hospital will increase charges. Payers usually prefer more fixed types of payment terms such as per diems, MS-DRGs, case rates, or capitation (HMOs only).† For the same reason, the typical payer will seek to reduce the number of carve-outs, or eliminate them if possible. If the payer is completely unable to avoid charge-based terms, it will typically seek to negotiate limits on how much those charges can rise from year to year.

Ad Hoc Negotiations

Before discussing contractually agreed-upon payment methodologies, it is worthwhile briefly discussing the role of ad hoc negotiations. This simply refers to the fact that members will sometimes receive care from an out-of-network hospital. For example, a member may have a heart attack or a motor vehicle accident while outside of the plan's service area. In such cases, the hospital will bill full charges.

Most payers have a department that is responsible for negotiating with noncontracted providers for individual,

highly expensive cases. In the case of emergency care, the health plan clearly has an obligation to provide coverage, but it is in the financial interest of the health plan, the member, and the provider to agree to what will be charged and what will be paid. This lowers the financial exposure of the health plan for obvious reasons, but it also lowers the member's financial exposure to balance billing for any charges not covered by the plan or due to having to pay a percentage coinsurance. The provider in turn is paid quickly and directly, which is of great benefit as noted earlier.

Types of Hospital Payment for Inpatient Services

How hospitals are paid parallels how physicians are paid in many respects, but significant differences exist as well. Like physicians, there are a few dominant forms of payment, but experimentation has produced many variations on those common approaches, as well as creating entirely new methodologies. The exception to this wide variety is in Maryland, where hospital payment rates are regulated. On the federal front, even before passage of the ACA, CMS had been looking at pilot programs for new methods of payment, though most involved combining physician and hospital payment into one program, as discussed later in the chapter.

Table 5-8 lists common hospital payment methodologies. Sometimes only one method is used, but occasionally the same payer will have different payment methods in place

TABLE 5-8	**Common Hospital Payment**		
Common hospital and facility payment methods		**Inpatient**	**Outpatient**
Straight charges		X	X
Discounted charges		X	X
Per diem		X	
Diagnosis-related groups (DRGs)		X	
MS-DRGs (Medicare Severity-DRGs)		X	
Percent of Medicare		X	X
Case rates—facility only or bundled with professional		X	X
Capitation (HMOs only)		X	X
Ambulatory surgical center (ASC) rates under the Medicare Hospital Outpatient Prospective Payment System (HOPPS)			X
Ambulatory payment classifications (APCs)			X
Ambulatory Payment Groups® (APGs)			X
Other		X	X

Source: Copyright P.R. Kongstvedt Company, LLC. Used with permission.

---

*Since commercial payers cover underpayments by Medicare and Medicaid, "losing" may actually mean not getting enough money in the aggregate, not achieving revenue targets. It may or may not mean *actually* losing money on payment rates from the payer.

†As in the section on physician payment, these are described later in this section.

TABLE 5-9	Common Hospital Payment Modifiers		

Common hospital and facility payment modifiers	Inpatient	Outpatient
Volume-related sliding scale—applicable to all but full charges or capitation	X	X
Carve-outs—applicable to:		
• Discount on charges	X	X
• Per diem	X	
• DRGs and MS-DRGs	X	
• Percent of Medicare	X	X
• Case rates	X	X
• Capitation	X	X
• APCs and APGs		X
Credits—applicable to all types of facility payment	X	X
Differential by service type—applicable to per diem	X	
Differential by Day—applicable to:		
• Discount on charges	X	
• Per diem	X	
Outlier or stop loss—applicable to:		
• DRGs and MS-DRGs	X	
• Percent of Medicare	X	X
• Case rates	X	X
• Capitation	X	X
• APCs and APGs		X

Source: Copyright P.R. Kongstvedt Company, LLC. Used with permission.

for the same hospital. Payment methods may vary by type of product (e.g., HMO vs. PPO), but not always. Payers also often use different approaches or payment terms for their MA products than they do for their commercial products, and likewise if they also have a Medicaid product. In most cases outpatient facility payments differ from inpatient payments. Finally, there are many possible ways of modifying payments, for example, increasing the discount as volume goes up, or receiving extra payments for highly expensive cases. Commonly used payment modifiers are listed in **Table 5-9**.

Although risk-based payment exists for hospitals, just as it does for physicians, it is almost entirely service risk rather than financial risk. Therefore, risk-based payment will not be separate from nonrisk payment. Further detail on specific types of payment follows a discussion of two aspects of hospital payment than can potentially affect nearly all types of payment: the chargemaster and the two payment modifiers, carve-outs and outliers.

The Chargemaster

All of a hospital's charges are listed in a master document called the chargemaster. The typical chargemaster now lists over 5,000 separate billing codes and their associated charges, and continues to grow as new technology and procedures appear. Both the chargemaster and the prices for each code may differ from hospital to hospital. The chargemaster is used to generate bills to self-pay individuals or noncontracted payers, and will usually be made up of hundreds of different charge codes. It is also what a hospital typically uses to determine if it is making or losing money on a service or from a specific payer, and as the basis for negotiations.

The actual charges typically have only a passing relationship with actual costs, however. Because cost accounting is so difficult in the hospital environment, only costs associated with purchased drugs or devices that are used only once can be accurately tracked; for example, the chargemaster may list a price of a drug as its cost plus a markup. This is particularly the case for implantable devices that can make up over half the cost of an inpatient or ambulatory procedure, as is discussed shortly. For the rest, the chargemaster only reflects a relative difference in the amount of resources used, and costs are spread to all the charge codes.* Of particular importance, other than

---

*This is what accounts for anecdotes such as a $20.00 acetaminophen tablet.

in Maryland, hospitals are generally free to charge whatever they want in their chargemaster. This bears both on contracted pricing and on the topic of outliers, which is discussed shortly as well.

Carve-Outs, Credits, and Outliers

There are two ways that the amount actually paid for a case may be modified that can potentially affect any types of payment except straight, nondiscounted charges, and those are carve-outs and outliers. Credits, a third modifier related to carve-outs, may be applicable to any type of facility payment.

Carve-Outs

Hospitals typically seek to carve expensive surgical implants or drugs out of its payment, and pass the cost through, often with a markup. Depending on volume, this may or may not be reasonable, but it also eliminates any incentive for the hospital to negotiate prices with its own vendors or to get the physicians to agree to use a single manufacturer. Payers seek to limit the number of carve-outs to provide that incentive, and to better control case costs. This is particularly the case when the volume of the implantable device or the drug is high, and therefore predictable.

The pass-through cost of implants is considerable. An analysis by the Wall Street advisory firm Barclay's capital, for example, found that implant pricing accounted for up to half of the total case cost in very common inpatient procedures, as seen in **Table 5-10**. In the event a payer agrees to a carve-out, the payment is usually limited to a reference price, not simply a pass-through with a markup; meaning payment is based on the lowest available price, regardless of what the hospital paid for it. As a fallback, a payer might agree to the pass-through charge, but restrict any markup. They also typically require audit rights.

TABLE 5-10	Implant Pricing as a Percent of the Total DRG for Selected Orthopedic and Cardiac Procedures		
Orthopedic procedures	**Percent of DRG**	**Cardiac procedures**	**Percent of DRG**
Hip/knee implant	51%	Pacemaker	41%
Hip/knee revision	45%	Intracoronary dilation w/ catheterization	68%
Lumbar fusion	50%	Coronary stent	28%
Cervical fusion	38%	Heart valve	14%

Source: Barclays Capital estimates, based on corporate filings, 2011. www.barcap.com/. Used with permission.

Credits

Credits are a modifier that is the exact opposite of carve-outs, and should be incorporated into any carve-out terms. All implantable devices come with a warranty, and should the device fail or require removal ("de-implantation") for any reason such as a bad reaction, manufacturers provide a full or partial refund to the hospital or ambulatory facility. Warranties typically run from 3–5 years, and the amount may be prorated based on how old the device is when it needs to be removed or replaced.

Because almost any situation involving a warranty takes place after the initial implantation, it is almost always too late to apply to payment for the procedure on a prospective basis. Hospitals and ambulatory facilities also do not necessarily link the refund with a specific case, at least at the time it is received. However, they are required to rebate Medicare for these credits when they are associated with a case paid under traditional Medicare FFS, so CMS and the Office of the Inspector General have been increasing their scrutiny of how well hospitals are complying with that requirement. For that reason, facilities participating in Medicare, which is almost all of them, have been developing the means to do so.

As was just seen in Table 5-10, the high cost of implantable joints and devices makes this something that should not be ignored. The best approach to addressing this in the contract is to follow the processes used by Medicare. This provides the full value of the credit and requires the hospital or ambulatory facility to do what they must do in any case for Medicare. Like Medicare, payers should also secure audit rights and exercise them on a periodic basis.

Outliers

Outliers or outlier cases refer to extra payment if a patient's costs exceed certain thresholds. It is less likely to come up when the payment type is based on charges, which is discussed next, and most likely to come up in every other type of payment. Whether or not an inpatient or outpatient case is classified as an outlier is based on "costs," which in turn is based on the hospital's chargemaster. That means that price increases in the chargemaster result in more cases being considered as outliers.

Payment for outlier cases is typically a combination of the original payment, plus discounted charges beginning at the point the outlier threshold was crossed. Depending on the type of payment and on negotiated terms, up to a third or even nearly half of all inpatient cases get classified as outliers. Payers have become increasingly focused on negotiating outlier terms, though those terms are also subject to the same market power forces that affect all hospital pricing. Because of chargemaster inflation, commercial payers frequently negotiate not only the percent discount on charges for outliers, but limitations on how much of each year's chargemaster increase can be used for both calculating whether or not a case is an outlier and for determining the level of discount.

Charges

There are several ways that charges may be the basis of payment to hospitals, including straight charges, discounted charges, and a sliding scale on charges. Charge-based payment is also combined with non-charge-based payment under certain circumstances that will be identified as appropriate.

Straight Charges

The simplest (albeit least desirable) payment mechanism in health care is straight charges. It is also obviously the most expensive, after the option of no contract at all. This is a fallback position to be agreed to only in the event that the MCO is unable to obtain any form of discount at all, since it is still desirable to have a contract with a no-balance-billing clause in it (Chapter 6) for purposes of reserve requirements and licensure. Contracts that pay straight charges for all care are very uncommon in managed care.

Straight Discount on Charges

A straight percentage discount on charges is a contract in which the hospital submits its claim in full and the plan discounts it by the agreed-to percentage, which is considered payment in full other than any applicable coinsurance or copay. The amount of discount that can be obtained will depend on the factors discussed above. This type of arrangement is not infrequent in markets with low levels of managed care penetration and in rural markets, but is very uncommon in markets with high levels of managed care.

When this type of arrangement does exist, a payer will usually at the least require that no single charge from the chargemaster can exceed a certain degree of inflation from year to year for purposes of payment. The payer cannot tell the hospital what it can charge others, however. In other words, the hospital is free to raise chargemaster fees as much as they like, but the payer's exposure is limited to a certain percentage increase.

Sliding Scale Discount on Charges

Sliding scale discounts are another option, again in markets with low managed care penetration but some level of competitiveness between hospitals. With a sliding scale, the percentage discount is reflective of total volume of admissions and outpatient procedures. Whether to lump the two categories together or deal with them separately is not as important as making sure that the parties deal with them both. With the rapidly climbing cost of outpatient charges,

savings from reduction of inpatient utilization could be negated by an unanticipated overrun in outpatient charges.

An example of a sliding scale is a 20% reduction in charges for 0–200 total bed-days per year, with incremental increases in the discount up to a maximum percentage. An interim percentage discount is usually negotiated, and the parties reconcile at the end of the year based on the final total volume. The time periods for measurement are also negotiable. For example, the discount could vary on a month-to-month basis rather than yearly. The sliding scale could track total bed-days, number of admissions, or whole dollars spent. The most important thing is to be sure that it is a clearly defined and easily measurable objective. Similar to straight discount, payers seek to limit their degree of exposure to increases in the chargemaster.

Carve-Outs from Discount on Charges

While not as common as carve-outs in other types of payment, hospitals sometimes seek to exclude certain pass-through charges from discounting. Payers seek to have no carve-outs since discounted charges are so high to begin with, but it is a common demand.

Inpatient versus Outpatient Charges and Discounted Charges

Unlike types of payment per diems and DRGs, which are discussed next, charges-based payment is applicable for both inpatient and outpatient services. In fact, hospitals that negotiate different payment terms often seek to be paid a discount on charges for ambulatory facility services. It may also seek different discount or carve-out terms for inpatient and outpatient as well, but that's relatively uncommon.

Per Diems

Unlike straight charges, a negotiated per diem is a single charge for a day in the hospital regardless of any actual charges or costs incurred. In this very common type of arrangement, the plan negotiates a per diem rate with the hospital and pays that rate without adjustments. For example, the plan will pay $1,000 for each day regardless of the actual cost of the service. The key to making a per diem work is predictability. If the plan and hospital can accurately predict the number and mix of cases, then they can accurately calculate a per diem. The per diem is simply an estimate of the charges or costs for an average day in that hospital minus the level of discount. The larger the volume of business between the hospital and the MCO, the more predictable the average daily cost will be. Per diems also provide savings for shorter lengths of stay, unlike other types of payment such as DRGs, which are described later. Finally, per diems typically apply only to inpatient services, not outpatient.

Flat Per Diems

Once more common than it is now, flat per diems means a single per diem rate is negotiated and applied to any type of inpatient day. In other words, the payment for an intensive care day is the same as a day for a routine medical patient. Because of the high differences in cost, service-specific per diems are more common in acute-care hospitals. But hospitals without costly services or specialized hospitals such as rehabilitation facilities are good candidates for flat per diems.

Service-Specific Per Diems

Service-specific per diems refer to multiple sets of negotiated per diems based on service type; examples include different per diems for medical–surgical, obstetrics, intensive care, neonatal intensive care, rehabilitation, and so forth. Service-specific per diems also diminish the need to negotiate outlier provisions.

Per Diem Differential by Day in Hospital

This simply refers to the fact that most hospitalizations are more expensive on the first day. For example, the first day for surgical cases includes operating suite costs, the operating surgical team costs (nurses and recovery), and so forth. This type of payment method is generally combined with a per diem approach, but the first day is paid at a higher rate. For example, the first day may be $1,800 and each subsequent day is $850.

Sliding Scale Per Diems

Like the sliding scale discount on charges discussed above, the sliding scale per diem is also based on total volume. In this case, the plan negotiates an interim per diem that it will pay for each day in the hospital. Depending on the total number of bed-days or admissions in the year, the plan will either pay a lump-sum settlement at the end of the year or withhold an amount from the final payment for the year to adjust for an additional reduction in the per diem from an increase in total bed days or admissions. It may be preferable to make an arrangement whereby on a quarterly or semiannual basis the plan will adjust the interim per diem so as to reduce any disparities caused by unexpected changes in utilization patterns.

Per Diem Carve-Outs

Payment using per diems is frequently subject to carve-outs, and the approach of most payers has already been described.

Per Diem Outliers

Outliers typically only become an issue with per diems if the parties have negotiated a single flat per diem rate, which is no longer common. But even when service-specific per diems are negotiated, a hospital may negotiate to have some cases such as transplants or other very costly types of cases be considered as outliers. The approach to outliers has been discussed already.

Diagnosis-Related Groups and Medicare-Severity Diagnosis-Related Groups

DRGs were developed for Medicare, and are broadly referred to as inpatient prospective payment. It is a flat per-discharge payment that varies based on diagnoses, procedures, and (under MS-DRGs) burden of illness. DRGs place responsibility on the hospital to manage the inpatient stay. Savings from shorter stays do not go to the payer. DRGs are applicable only to inpatient care, not outpatient. Payment under DRGs typically includes provisions for added payment for outlier cases, which is addressed first.

Straight DRGs

The original DRG systems classified each admission into one of 467 different groups based on diagnostic and procedure billing codes. Patients with multiple diagnoses or having multiple procedures are grouped together, resulting in a final payment amount. Many payers relied on the CMS DRG schedules, while others purchased commercial DRGs or combined the two. Because charge codes are an element in determining DRGs, they are subject to miscoding, leading many payers (and Medicare) to periodically audit cases.

Outliers

Outliers have nearly overwhelmed traditional straight DRGs. In one multistate payer organization, outliers made up over 40% of all cases when it was paying straight DRGs.[39] This serious rise in cases considered to be outliers also affected Medicare, leading to the creation of MS-DRGs.

MS-DRGs

Medicare had been working to incorporate severity of illness and complications into DRGs for several years, as the number of outlier cases rose. This led CMS to change to MS-DRGs for all cases. MS-DRGs take into consideration how sick a patient is upon admission, and adjust payments to reflect both severity of illness and complications during an admission. Many, but not all, payers have also changed. But it has not eliminated the outlier problem. In 2010, the same payer referenced that had experienced 40% outliers under DRGs experienced approximately 30% of all commercial admissions classified as outliers, despite having converted entirely to MS-DRGs.[40]

DRG and MS-DRG Carve-Outs

Like per diems, hospitals may seek to carve certain costs or services out of the DRG payment. Payers use the same approach to this that they do for per diems.

Percent of Medicare

Some commercial payers negotiate rates based on a percentage markup of whatever Medicare would pay for similar services. It may vary from as low as Medicare + 5% (usually for an MA plan) to as high as Medicare + 60% (usually for a commercial plan). Cases that are not typically paid by Medicare or where there are no Medicare rates (e.g., neonatal care) must be defined and terms agreed upon. MA plans often use this approach since even a small percentage increase is valuable to a hospital. All of the potential modifiers applicable to DRGs and MS-DRGs are applicable to percent of Medicare.

Facility-Only Case Rates

Similar to DRGs, facility-only case rates are a flat payment for a defined service. This refers only to the facility fee, not to a bundled price including payment to the physician. All of the potential modifiers applicable to DRGs and MS-DRGs are applicable to facility case rates. Facility-only case rates can be used for both inpatient and outpatient services.

The most common type of facility-based case rate is for obstetrics, negotiating a flat case rate for a normal vaginal delivery and a flat rate or case rate for a cesarean section, or a blended rate for both. In the case of blended case rates (which are much preferred over separate rates for the two types of deliveries), the expected payment for each type of delivery is multiplied by the expected (or desired) percentage of utilization. Case rates for specialty procedures at tertiary hospitals are also common, for example, coronary artery bypass surgery, heart transplants, or certain types of cancer treatment. These procedures, although relatively infrequent, are tremendously costly. They are often combined with some other type of payment system. For example, inpatient care may be paid through MS-DRGs, but knee replacement surgery is paid using a flat case rate.

Capitation

Hospital capitation, like physician capitation, refers to paying the hospital on a PMPM basis to cover all institutional costs for a defined population of members. As with physician payment, capitation is generally used only by HMOs, though HMOs usually do not use capitation exclusively. The payment may be varied by age and sex but does not fluctuate with premium revenue. Severity-adjusted capitation is still relatively uncommon, but as CMS fully converts to severity-adjusted payments to MA plans (see Chapter 24), those plans may also begin to adjust capitation payments to hospitals. Severity adjustments for commercial members are also feasible using existing methodologies.

Capitation can be used to pay for both inpatient and outpatient services. If a hospital owns the HMO, or the HMO is owned by a medical group that also controls the hospital, both inpatient and outpatient hospital services are likely to be capitated. Approximately one-third of all HMOs have at least one hospital capitation contract, as seen in **Figure 5-12**. Hospital capitation overall has declined even more than physician capitation, except in select locations in the western United States.[*]

Capitation Outliers and Stop Loss

Some capitation contracts will contain outlier terms similar to those discussed earlier, but outliers are typically classified at much higher trigger points. Health systems that either own the HMO or that have a substantial portion of their revenue coming from capitation may instead purchase commercial stop loss or reinsurance. In that case, the cost of reinsurance is usually included by the hospital when it models capitation rates.

Capitation Carve-Outs   Carve-outs in capitation are no different than those for other forms of payment. As with the other payment models, hospitals seek to carve out various devices and drugs, and HMOs seek to limit them. The exception to that is when a capitated hospital does not actually provide a particular service, in which case it is not included in the capitation buildup.

Contract Capitation   Contract capitation of hospitals is similar to contract capitation for specialty physicians, as discussed earlier, and it too is very uncommon now. In brief, the capitation is tied to the percentage of admissions to a hospital, with adjustments for the type of service, for example, the amount of capitation applied to obstetrics will differ from that applied to cardiac surgery.

Such adjustments can quickly become complicated, particularly when there are more than two types of service adjustments to be made. And, like contract capitation for specialty physicians, this system requires sophisticated information systems and is often not an automated function, thus requiring manual administration. Unlike specialty physician contract capitation, however, the number of participants is lower and therefore at least theoretically more manageable. Contract capitation can also be combined with case rates or other types of payment, and may be modified by carve-outs and outliers. Overall, however, it is typically costly to administer and prone to error, so, like its physician counterpart, it is rare.

---

[*]The data in Figure 5-12 may be skewed somewhat by the presence of health systems that also own HMOs. That would have more of an impact on this figure than on one for physicians since an HMO owned by a health system will typically capitate itself, but must still contract with private physicians. At least for now.

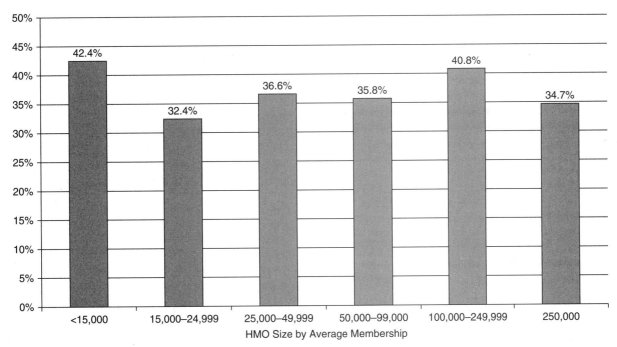

FIGURE 5-12 Percent of HMOs with Capitated Hospital Contracts by HMO Size, 2009

Source: SDI © 2010 in The Sanofi-Aventis Managed Care Digest Series®/HMO-PPO Digest 2010. www.managedcaredigest.com/. Used with permission.

Percent of Revenue

In the past, some hospitals were paid a percentage of the premium revenue, but that has become rare for the same reasons discussed earlier: it subjects the hospital to bearing the full insurance risk as well as absorbing any premium revenue shortfalls. As noted already, it most closely resembles capitation, but its flaws make it less suitable for the typical hospital system unless it owns the health plan. In the event a hospital is paid through this approach, having adequate reinsurance is critical.

◼ PAYMENT FOR AMBULATORY FACILITY SERVICES

As care has shifted, so have costs. It is not uncommon to see outpatient charges exceeding the cost of an inpatient day unless steps are taken to address that imbalance. As already noted, charge-based payments, facility-based case rates, and capitation can be used for both inpatient and outpatient services, although not always together. Per diems and DRGs are used only for inpatient services, and this section discusses payment methodologies applicable only to facility-based outpatient or ambulatory services.

Hospitals, as discussed earlier, frequently seek payment for ambulatory services using a different payment type than inpatient care. Hospitals most frequently seek payment through a discount on charges, subjecting it to greater inflation than typical inpatient payments. Only in recent

years have payers become more aggressive about using non-charge-based payment approaches.

Payment for facility-based ambulatory services is very important because of the dramatic rate of growth in both the total number of procedures performed and in the rate of growth itself. This has also been accompanied by a shift from hospital-based ambulatory surgery centers (ASCs) to free-standing ASCs, which may also be owned in whole or in part by physicians (physician-ownership is discussed in all three chapters of Part II). Figures 7-4–7-7 in the next chapter provide an illustration of the growth and shift in ambulatory procedures.

Ambulatory Payment Classification and Ambulatory Patient Groups

There are two classification systems developed and used in the payment of ambulatory visits or encounters: ambulatory patient groups (APGs) and ambulatory payment classifications (APCs). APGs were developed by 3M[41] as a forerunner similar to APCs, and continues to maintain and update them. Medicare uses only APCs, but APCs and APGs both are used by state Medicaid agencies and commercial payers.

CMS pays ASCs using a methodology broadly referred to as the ambulatory services hospital outpatient prospective payment system (OPPS), classifying the thousands of different procedures into hundreds of different APC treatment groups. It includes all ancillary costs, but certain items are carved out such as particular drugs, the cost to acquire transplanted tissue, and so forth. Medicare APC payments are also adjusted for geography and complexity of the procedure. APCs (and less commonly APGs) are also now used by many payers and by Medicaid agencies.

APGs and APCs are to outpatient services what DRGs are to inpatient ones, although APGs and APCs are based on procedures rather than simply on diagnoses, contain a greater degree of adjustment for severity, and are considerably more complex. They are superior to using charges as a basis of payment for outpatient services because they are inherently less subject to price inflation. There are now several commercial systems that support these for both payers and provider systems.

Outliers and Carve-Outs for Ambulatory Services

Outliers are not a significant problem in payment for ambulatory services, but occasionally provisions are negotiated when a hospital provides very complex care on an outpatient basis. Carve-outs, on the other hand, are a substantial topic in ambulatory services because so many procedures involve an implant (e.g., lens and cochlear implants). This is an area that payers must focus on during negotiations, even when charge-based payment terms are agreed to.

Payment for Emergency Departments

Except in some cases of capitation, payment for emergency department (ED) services differs from both inpatient and ambulatory care payment, but is always negotiated as part of the inpatient contract.

Unlike other services, hospitals have a legal requirement regarding emergency services. In 1986 the federal government passed the Emergency Medical Treatment and Active Labor Act (EMTALA) to prevent transfer or "dumping" of uninsured patients by private hospitals to public hospitals.[42] EMTALA requires that all patients presenting to any hospital ED must have a medical screening exam performed by qualified personnel, usually the emergency physician. The medical screening exam cannot be delayed for insurance reasons, either to obtain insurance information or to obtain preauthorization for examination.

One unique aspect of the ED is its function as a gateway to admission to the hospital. In the case of trauma or other obvious significant medical conditions, this is a proper and expected use of the ED. But because of concerns about legal liability, many EDs have established chest pain protocols that result either in an admission to the cardiac care unit or in an observation stay (see the next section), regardless of how serious the patient's condition appears to be. This results in substantially increased costs to the plan, as well as to the member if they have coinsurance. Some plans have addressed this problem by negotiating special rates for such admissions when there is no subsequent evidence of a heart attack. Other plans actually contract with specialty

management companies to assume responsibility for the evaluation and disposition of these cases at each hospital's ED, as discussed briefly in Chapter 7.

Finally, the ACA requires that emergency services must be covered at the same in-network level of benefits, even if the member goes to a noncontracted hospital and/or is treated by noncontracted physicians, and without the need for prior authorization.[43] The ACA goes on to craft specific "prudent layperson" language to apply to medical necessity for coverage, and links it to emergency services required under EMTALA.[44] This obviously does not protect the member from balance billing, however. In response, some states have required similar coverage, but also prohibited noncontracting facilities and physicians from balance billing the patient. It is not known how many states will adopt similar provisions.

Payment for Observation Stays

As a result of commercial and government payers refusing to pay for an overnight stay for certain conditions, as well as liability concerns about ED visits in certain cases, most hospitals have created observation stays. Such stays are usually 23 hours or less, though it is possible to twist the definition at times to cover more than that. The purpose of an observation stay is just what it implies: to keep an eye on a patient in order to determine if full admission is warranted or not. On the one hand, the resources used for an observation stay are similar to those used for a single day of an inpatient stay (usually the first day, which is front-loaded with costs, as noted earlier), so the payer and the hospital may choose to treat it as a single day under the payment methodology. On the other hand, it may be argued that the patient is not as sick as one that clearly requires admission and therefore an observation stay should be paid at a lesser rate. The latter is more commonly the case when negotiating payment for observation stays.

Price Transparency

Price transparency as applied to hospitals is theoretically no different than that for physicians, except a contract between a payer and a hospital typically requires the terms to remain confidential. Payers may post pricing history for noncontracted hospitals if they have it, however. An alternative is to provide information to consumers about their out-of-pocket cost differences between different hospitals. Public data about Medicare payments is also available.

Refusal to Pay at All

There are two cases in which a payer typically refuses to pay a hospital, and the hospital may not balance bill the member: (1) costs associated with inefficiencies or nonclinical errors and (2) serious medical errors, often referred to as "never events."

Refusal to Pay for Inefficiencies or Nonclinical Errors

Many payers refuse to pay for services that are incurred due to hospital inefficiencies or nonclinical errors. For example, if a patient is admitted for a routine surgical procedure but surgery is delayed due to scheduling problems, the payer will not pay for the extra day. Similarly, if a patient is admitted on a weekend and the hospital is unable to perform certain necessary diagnostic tests (e.g., radiology specialty procedures is not open on weekends), the payer will not pay for the weekend days that the patient spends. This policy often extends to any extra days in the hospital due either to a physician not ordering the discharge or to a hospital's not performing the discharge in a timely manner.

Refusal to Pay for Serious Reportable Events or "Never Events"

The term "never events" was coined in 2001 by Dr. Ken Kizer, former CEO of the National Quality Forum (NQF), to apply to medical errors that should never occur (e.g., wrong-site surgery). NQF formally calls them serious reportable events. In 2002, the NQF defined 27 such events, expanding the list in 2006 and again in 2011. As of 2011, there are now 29, grouped into six categories and listed in **Table 5-11**.

Medicare will no longer pay anything for costs associated with "never events," and the ACA specifically requires that policy, broadening it to hospital-acquired conditions more generally, though with exceptions under certain conditions.[45] Most commercial payers have been doing this as well.

Medicare Hospital Payment and Excess Readmissions under the ACA

Beginning in 2013, the ACA calls for hospitals with higher-than-expected readmission rates will experience decreased Medicare payments, excluding critical access hospitals or hospitals with only a small number of readmission cases.[46] Hospital performance will be evaluated based on the 30-day readmission measures for heart attack, heart failure, and pneumonia that are currently part of the Medicare pay-for-reporting program and reported on Hospital Compare. Planned readmissions and readmissions that are unrelated to the first admission are excluded.

CMS will calculate hospitals' actual readmission rates and compare them to hospitals' expected readmission rates. Those hospitals with higher than expected readmission rates will be required to pay back to the Medicare program the payments they received for those readmissions deemed to be excessive. To recoup the money, CMS will determine an adjustment factor for each hospital with excessive readmissions that will decrease the hospital's Medicare payment rate across all discharges. There is a ceiling as to how large the reduction can be. In FY 2013, the reduction cannot be greater than 1%. In FY 2014, it cannot be larger than 2% and in FY 2015 and beyond, it cannot be greater than 3%.

Beginning in FY 2015, CMS may expand the list of conditions to include chronic obstructive pulmonary disorder and several cardiac and vascular surgical procedures, as well as any other condition or procedure the agency deems appropriate. At the time of publication, CMS had not yet published proposed rules for the readmissions payment penalty. Once CMS implements this program, commercial payers are likely to follow suit.

■ COMBINED PAYMENT OF HOSPITALS AND PHYSICIANS

Since the early days of HMOs, there have been instances in which the HMO contracted with both the hospital and the physicians for a defined type of service using a single payment. It would be up to the hospital and physicians to determine how best to share that payment. For example, when the author first became the medical director of a small group model HMO in 1983, the HMO had a contract with a highly regarded heart center for a single all-inclusive rate for cardiac bypass surgery. The rate was different for different types of bypasses, but the HMO paid the center the single rate and no more. PPOs began to adopt this approach as well, often under a "centers of excellence" benefits design.

Two broad types of combined payments have existed for years: global fees, also known as bundled pricing, and global capitation. A newer third type using a shared-savings approach appeared some years ago, but recent pressure by CMS as well as changes under the ACA are accelerating interest in this model. There is quite a lot of crossover between these three, but each has at least one unique element. Global capitation is discussed first because bundled pricing and shared savings have considerable overlap.

Global Capitation

Global capitation simply means HMO payment of a single entity for all medical services; in other words, the complete or near-complete transfer of risk to the providers through a provider organization. It requires a single entity to accept the single capitation and manage all care. Large medical groups or provider systems that own an HMO in effect are paid through global capitation since they own the payer that holds the risk, but global capitation for purposes of this section refers to an HMO globally capitating an independent provider entity. Global capitation for all medical costs is now uncommon, but where it does exist, it usually carves out some medical costs such as pharmacy.

Global capitation, like bundled pricing, requires the hospital and physicians to have predetermined policies about how the payment will be shared, and payment methods should be aligned. For example, paying physicians using FFS creates potential losses for a globally capitated IDS unless physicians are part of an experienced IPA. Adequate reinsurance is also a requirement.

TABLE 5-11	Serious Reportable Events as of 2011

1. SURGICAL OR INVASIVE PROCEDURE EVENTS
- Surgery or other invasive procedure performed on the wrong site
- Surgery or other invasive procedure performed on the wrong patient
- Wrong surgical or other invasive procedure performed on a patient
- Unintended retention of a foreign object in a patient after surgery or other invasive procedure
- Intraoperative or immediately postoperative/postprocedure death in an ASA Class 1 patient

2. PRODUCT OR DEVICE EVENTS
- Patient death or serious injury associated with the use of contaminated drugs, devices, or biologics provided by the health care setting
- Patient death or serious injury associated with the use or function of a device in patient care, in which the device is used or functions other than as intended
- Patient death or serious injury associated with intravascular air embolism that occurs while being cared for in a health care setting

3. PATIENT PROTECTION EVENTS
- Discharge or release of a patient/resident of any age, who is unable to make decisions, to other than an authorized person
- Patient death or serious injury associated with patient elopement (disappearance)
- Patient suicide, attempted suicide, or self-harm that results in serious injury while being cared for in a health care setting

4. CARE MANAGEMENT EVENTS
- Patient death or serious injury associated with a medication error (e.g., errors involving the wrong drug, wrong dose, wrong patient, wrong time, wrong rate, wrong preparation, or wrong route of administration)
- Patient death or serious injury associated with unsafe administration of blood products
- Maternal death or serious injury associated with labor or delivery in a low-risk pregnancy while being cared for in a health care setting
- Death or serious injury of a neonate associated with labor or delivery in a low-risk pregnancy
- Patient death or serious injury associated with a fall while being cared for in a health care setting
- Any Stage 3, Stage 4, and unstageable pressure ulcers acquired after admission/presentation to a health care setting
- Artificial insemination with the wrong donor sperm or wrong egg
- Patient death or serious injury resulting from the irretrievable loss of an irreplaceable biological specimen
- Patient death or serious injury resulting from failure to follow up or communicate laboratory, pathology, or radiology test results

5. ENVIRONMENTAL EVENTS
- Patient or staff death or serious injury associated with an electric shock in the course of a patient care process in a health care setting
- Any incident in which systems designated for oxygen or other gas to be delivered to a patient contains no gas, the wrong gas, or is contaminated by toxic substances
- Patient or staff death or serious injury associated with a burn incurred from any source in the course of a patient care process in a health care setting
- Patient death or serious injury associated with the use of physical restraints or bedrails while being cared for in a health care setting

6. RADIOLOGICAL EVENTS
- Death or serious injury of a patient or staff associated with the introduction of a metallic object into the MRI area.

7. POTENTIAL CRIMINAL EVENTS
- Any instance of care ordered by or provided by someone impersonating a physician, nurse, pharmacist, or other licensed health care provider
- Abduction of a patient/resident of any age
- Sexual abuse/assault on a patient or staff member within or on the grounds of a health care setting
- Death or serious injury of a patient or staff member resulting from a physical assault (i.e., battery) that occurs within or on the grounds of a health care setting

Source: National Quality Forum, © 2011. Used with permission. www.qualityforum.org/Publications/2011/02/National_Voluntary_Consensus_Standards_for_Public_Reporting_of_Patient_Safety_Event_Information.aspx.

As discussed in Chapter 1, the rapid growth of HMOs in the 1990s was associated with a rapid growth in capitation. Capitation of physicians and hospitals has already been discussed, but global capitation also appeared in the late 1990s on a large scale when many physician practice management companies (PPMCs; see Chapters 1 and 2) and IDSs sought out global capitation for all medical costs, believing that substantial profits were to be had by "cutting out the middleman." Most PPMCs failed, as also discussed in earlier chapters. A few IDSs failed as well, but more often they suffered substantial losses and now no longer accept global risk. There remain exceptions, mostly in California, but global capitation is no longer as prevalent as it once was, though it was never a dominant form of payment.

The difficulties associated with global capitation in the past affected managed care payment today in two ways. First and most obvious, there are fewer provider organizations that seek or accept global risk. Second, when the PPMCs failed, the HMOs had to pay the physicians and cover the loss in order to keep the network intact, and that resulted in a very high degree of hesitation by HMOs in even considering delegation of global risk.

Bundled Payment, Package Pricing, and Global Payment

Bundled payments (newer term), package pricing (older term), and global payment* (also an older term) all refer to the same thing: a single fee covering all facility and professional services related to a particular episode of care; only the term bundled payment is in current use. Common examples include various procedures used to treat coronary artery disease, including the example provided above. The bundled payment might cover multiple types of procedures or there might be a different bundled payment for each type of procedure. Bundled pricing that includes many different types of interventions requires a high volume of procedures in order to have a predictable mix of cases. Bundled payment for procedures are paid only for services provided, not month in and month out like capitation. In most cases, the bundled payment precludes upcoding and, as its name makes clear, unbundling.

To illustrate, think of a major university medical center and its faculty contracting to provide all cardiac testing, coronary angiography, and interventional cardiac procedures under a single global fee. The bundled payment would only be paid when an intervention was involved, not necessarily if a patient was simply referred. In some cases, the diagnostic work-up will be uncomplicated and the patient will have a stent placed, or perhaps a coronary angioplasty; in other cases, the patient will have a complex disease and require multivessel coronary artery bypass graft (CABG) surgery. In all cases, the bundled payment is the same, though extremely complex or costly cases would typically be treated as outliers, as discussed earlier for other hospital payment models. More commonly, bundled payment is more focused. For example, the university medical center might be paid one bundled payment for placing stents, a different bundled payment for angioplasties, and a separate bundled payment for CABGs. Each bundled payment would include all facility and professional diagnostic and postprocedure care, however. Bundled payment is also common for ambulatory procedures and is similar to that just described.

Bundled payment can be used for chronic care as well. One example where it may be used by a commercial payer is for acquired immunodeficiency syndrome (AIDS), but it could be used for other chronic conditions requiring specialized care. In the case of bundled payment for chronic care, the bundled payment is either for an episode of care or paid as a fixed fee on a regular basis. While surgical episodes of care are relatively easy to define, it is more difficult for medical care, in which some credible methodology must be used to define an episode. An example of one such methodology that is often used by commercial payers is Episode Treatment Groups® (ETGs) by Ingenix.† ETGs use a methodology that takes medical and pharmaceutical claims data to classify medical conditions by combining related services into a medically relevant and distinct unit—a complete episode of care.[47]

As with all types of payment, the services to be covered by the bundled payment must be well defined. Plans may use their own data to calculate the bundled payment, or they may use outside data. The approach to outliers must also be explicitly addressed, including how an outlier will be determined, what will be paid, and how the payment amount is to be determined. Costs associated with never events are typically excluded from payment.

Successful bundled payment contracts all have one thing in common: the hospital and physicians have a predetermined way of dividing the payment, and all involved providers agree to its terms. The payer is not involved in this. When bundled payment contracts fail, it is typically because this aspect is not rock solid. Provider systems best able to deal with this are academic medical centers with a unified faculty practice plan, a very strong multispecialty medical group with an affiliated medical center, or a health system with an already successful HMO. Health systems with employed physicians also have the potential to succeed at bundled pricing, but will be handicapped if the physicians function autonomously or if their compensation remains bound to tradition.

A bundled payment pilot by Medicare in the 1990s for CABG surgery produced savings of 12–27%, although CMS did not extend the program due to local opposition.[48] But Medicare sets its own prices, which commercial payers cannot do. As a result, bundled pricing does not, by itself, necessarily achieve savings for a commercial health plan beyond whatever might be associated with unbundling. As already discussed, health system consolidation and its accompanying market power drives prices up, and that can negate the potentially positive impact of bundled pricing.[49]

Finally, the ACA specifically requires a bundled payment pilot program for FFS Medicare.[50] The pilot is to be conducted by selecting 10 common and expensive conditions that are also associated with relatively high levels of com-

---

*A payment term easily confused with a global fee, which refers to a fixed fee to a specialist for a defined type of service such as maternity or cardiac bypass surgery.

†www.ingenix.com.

plications and avoidable readmissions. The episode span begins at least 3 days prior to admission and extends to at least 30 days after discharge, and the bundled payment applies to all care provided during the episode. At the time of publication, CMS had not published any rules for this program.

Shared Savings

Shared savings refers to a noncapitation payment methodology in which cost savings compared to a targeted cost are shared between the payer and a provider organization. CMS had been exploring potential models for the traditional FFS Medicare program, and when the ACA was passed, it included language directing CMS to implement it through accountable care organizations (ACOs).[51] In other words, shared savings programs in Medicare do require waiver or pilot programs like most other new payment models do, but are implemented through regulation. Commercial payers have also been piloting shared savings programs, but their implementation is far from uniform and the results are not yet known.

Earlier versions of shared savings focused only on the potential for bonus payments or gain-sharing, similar to P4P as discussed later in the chapter. New models incorporate the potential for payment reductions or a return of money. In other words, it may contain elements of both risk-based and non-risk-based payment, making it the exception to the rule that only HMOs are able to contract with providers using risk-based payment. How often downside risk will be paired with upside bonus is impossible to predict. And while CMS payment methods are not subject to state regulation, it is possible that states will regulate both payment and network structures when shared savings incorporating risk is used for commercial payers. Also, pilot programs by commercial payers have included supplemental payments for care coordination, and commercial pilot programs have also typically been upside-only since providers would otherwise decline to participate. When or if that will change is unknown.

CMS published the final rule regulating shared savings and ACOs in traditional FFS Medicare on October 20, 2011.[52] As described in Chapters 2 and 3, the rule defined the types of organizations that could potentially qualify to be ACOs, as well as ACO governance, organizational, and financial requirements, at least in broad terms. The shared savings methodology was also defined, and what follows is a summary of that program. At the time of publication, it had not actually been implemented, so only the provisions of the rule are provided here.

Performance Measurement and Shared Savings

In the final rule, savings are defined as performing better than a benchmark overall cost target for a group of specific Medicare beneficiaries covered under traditional FFS Medicare.[*] For purposes of measuring performance, an ACO must have at least 5,000 assigned Medicare beneficiaries. ACOs are not HMOs, however, meaning that beneficiaries in FFS Medicare who are assigned to the ACO for purposes of measuring performance are not restricted to using only ACO providers. They can see any provider they want.

The assignment process is not irrational, however, since it looks at whether or not a beneficiary receives primary care from an ACO participating PCP, or else the majority of charges come from ACO participants. Assignment will also use a preliminary prospective-assignment method with beneficiaries identified quarterly, with a final reconciliation after each performance year based on patients served by the ACO. The assignment process itself involves two steps:

- Step 1: for beneficiaries who have received at least one primary care service from a physician, use plurality of allowed charges for primary care services rendered by primary care physicians.
- Step 2: for beneficiaries who have not received any primary care services from a primary care physician, use plurality of allowed charges for primary care services rendered by any other ACO professional.

In the first year of ACO operations, ACO performance around quality measurements will be subject to pay for reporting. Beginning the second year, it will be subject to pay for performance, which is discussed later. Quality performance measures will likely grow over time as they have in other managed health care organizations. Initially, however, quality performance will be assessed using 33 measures in four domains: patient experience, care coordination and patient safety, preventive health, and caring for at-risk populations.

From a day-to-day payment perspective, ACO providers will continue to be paid under traditional Medicare. But ACO performance against benchmarks will determine whether or not the ACO participants receive an additional bonus from shared savings, or be required to repay a percentage of what they were paid.

CMS will create cost benchmarks for each ACO by first using the most recent 3 years of Medicare Part A and Part B weighted claims data attributable to beneficiaries assigned to the ACO. Those data are then adjusted for severity and case mix, and further adjusted for certain types of care such as end-stage renal disease or dual eligibles (those eligible for both Medicare and Medicaid), and for historical trend. The benchmark and performance measurement also use a methodology to protect against catastrophically high cost cases, although it differs from that typically used for capitated risk pools described earlier.

---

[*] In other words, Medicare beneficiaries enrolled in a Medicare Advantage plan cannot be attributed to an ACO as well, although enrollment in a Medicare Part D prescription drug plan can.

In its first 3 years of operation, a new ACO can elect to share only in savings, and bear no risk. A new ACO can also elect to share both savings and losses (which CMS calls the "two-sided model"), in which case the potential amount of savings it is eligible to share is higher. After the first 3-year period, all ACOs must share both savings and losses. In the two-sided model, an ACO that meets all requirements will receive shared savings up to a maximum of 60% of all savings, not to exceed 15% of the total updated benchmark target, beginning with the first dollar.

Shared losses means the ACO would be required to actually refund the CMS some portion of what it was paid in the aggregate for the assigned members. Payment of shared losses may not exceed 60% of the total losses, and are further limited to a percentage of the overall updated benchmark as follows: 5% in the first performance year, 7.5% in the second performance year, and 10% in the third and any subsequent performance years.

CMS will share data with the ACO about each assigned beneficiary, and allow the ACO to market itself in order to facilitate having beneficiaries actively choose to be assigned to it. Finally, the amount of shared savings is also affected by the ACO's performance in the four quality domains noted earlier.

The jury is very much out on whether ACOs will achieve the promise envisioned by their proponents. However, the ACA is clear in its intent that overall payment levels be reduced or at least flattened, and that payment be tied to improvements in performance that include quality and cost. Additional specifics can be found at www.cms.gov/ACO.*

The Source and Use of Savings

Because shared savings are meant to lower costs, setting and resetting the goals must occur on a regular basis, accounting for changes in performance. Almost all savings come from reducing facility services, and most shared savings programs at the time of publication do not replace that reduction in facility revenue, making it an overall reduction in payment. If traditional FFS payment becomes increasingly less acceptable, shared savings could become more popular. But health systems with market power can simply resist its use by commercial payers, though not Medicare.

How savings are used is not straightforward in commercial health plans. Medicare, Medicaid, and fully insured commercial accounts can share savings since they are all at risk for medical costs. But self-funded commercial accounts must agree to share savings, which they do not always do. This poses a significant challenge to these programs because providers have no way of knowing which patients are in self-funded plans and which are not, and in any event, they are not likely to treat them differently. Therefore, if

a self-funded employer will not agree to a shared savings payment method, the payer administering the plan would most likely not identify those members as eligible for the program.

Pilots of various bundled pricing and shared savings programs have yielded mixed results. For example, one large system with multiple facilities and a large panel of physicians did demonstrate savings, but the health system lost money as a consequence.[53] Results from a Medicare 5-year shared savings pilot program found that large and highly experienced medical groups were able to achieve or even beat savings targets, but groups or systems with less experience were not able to meet or sustain savings targets.[54] Others have determined that net of the cost of implementation and the modest amount of shared savings, especially compared to lost revenues, that shared savings demonstrations have had negative financial results.[55] Providing a more positive example, a large commercial payer collaborated with regional health systems and physicians to focus on a set of defined conditions, resulting in reduced complications and millions in savings.[56] The most likely course will be for shared savings payment to increase over time, supported by improved provider care coordination and organizational capabilities.

PAY FOR PERFORMANCE

P4P refers to payment methods used to incent providers around issues other than managing utilization, though some payers combine utilization-based incentives into their P4P programs. A reasonable definition developed at a P4P Design Principles conference in November 2004, sponsored by American Healthways, Inc. and Johns Hopkins University, is: "The use of incentives to encourage and reinforce the delivery of evidence-based practices and health care system transformation that promotes better outcomes as efficiently as possible."[57]

Another useful description that was written for P4P, applicable to physicians but is relevant to hospitals as well, is:

"The goal of incorporating financial incentives for quality into physicians' payments is not simply to reward 'good' physicians or punish 'bad' ones. The goal is to change the status quo by stimulating both immediate and long term improvements in performance."[58]

Under various labels, P4P has been present in many HMOs for at least three decades. For example, in group and staff model HMOs where it is easier to observe behavior, formal performance evaluations of physicians were used in the 1970s.[59] In open-panel HMOs, including direct-contract models and IPAs, incentive programs that included quality-based goals such as compliance with clinical protocols, in addition to utilization-based goals, have existed since the 1980s.[60, 61] P4P hospital contracts have likewise existed since

*Current at the time of publication.

TABLE 5-12	Examples of Differences between Pay for Performance and Shared Savings	
Attribute	Pay for performance	Shared savings
Type of payment	Fixed percentage payments	Percent of savings against target costs
Adjusted for acuity	Affects which processes are evaluated, affects outcome measures	Often used to adjust cost targets
Focus on defined conditions	Yes	Often, but not always
Focus of measures	Compliance with evidence-based medical practice	Total episode costs
Quality focus: Structure, process, or outcomes	Mostly on clinical processes, some on clinical outcomes	Mostly on cost outcomes, some on clinical outcomes
Ability to use with self-funded commercial accounts	Moderate	Difficult
Industry experience with approach	Decades	New

Source: Copyright P.R. Kongstvedt Company, LLC. Used with Permission.

the late 1980s.[62] The last broad survey of P4P by HMOs was published in 2006, reporting that over half of the HMOs surveyed, representing more than 80% of persons enrolled, used P4P, of which 90% had programs for physicians and 38% had programs for hospitals. [63]

P4P programs focus primarily on clinical performance, mainly adherence to evidence-based clinical practice and patient safety, although some include a utilization-related component such as the prescription rate for generic drugs. Some include nonclinical performance measures such as electronic health records (EHRs), electronic connectivity, electronic decision support, and patient satisfaction. A useful way to view clinical performance in P4P programs is the classic approach to measuring quality first described by Avedis Donabedian, discussed in Chapter 14 and paraphrased here:[64]

> **Structure**: The physical and programmatic support for care. Examples would include existence of computerized order entry systems, appointment availability, electronic medical records (EMRs) or electronic health records (EHRs), and the like. The financial incentive system itself is also an example of structure. Many performance measures that are considered nonclinical would fall into this category, though some clinical ones do as well.
>
> **Process**: How care is actually delivered, regardless of the outcome of that care. Examples include adherence to evidence-based clinical protocols, the processes used by hospital nursing staff to dispense medications, and so forth.
>
> **Outcome**: The clinical outcome of how care is delivered. Examples include improved blood test results for diabetics, fewer safety errors in a hospital, improved quality of life for a patient with

a chronic and debilitating disease, and patient satisfaction with care.

Distinguishing P4P from other payment incentive programs, particularly shared savings, is not always easy. For example, a shared savings program that achieves positive results by lowering complication for a defined set of procedures appears to differ from P4P only in how the amount of money is calculated. But unless the shared savings program rewards many process measures, it differs from the typical P4P approach. The easiest way to think about P4P versus shared savings is to note the differences listed in **Table 5-12**, recognizing that it is usually far less clear in the real world.

Except in California, there is neither stability nor commonality in how P4P programs are created and used by health plans and governmental payers. In California, the Integrated Healthcare Association (IHA),* representing employers, providers, consumers, and all of the major payers have created a common set of measures for use in P4P, but currently that is the exception.

Measures and Goals

There are a plethora of measures being used in P4P programs across the country. No one program uses all possible measures since that would be overwhelming and would also dilute the effect of measurement on any individual type of care. One of the most important lessons learned as P4P evolved was the importance of focus. Choosing exactly what measures to target created focused attention on a defined process and (possible) outcome. For example, prior to early P4P efforts focused on improving the use of beta blockers following an acute heart attack, compliance was dismal, but improved considerably after several years of attention.

_____
*www.iha.org.

Measures may be complex or they may be simple, although as a general rule simpler measures are both more understandable, more likely to be implemented, and more likely to be accepted. It is possible to be too simple, however, and the program will need to contain sufficient complexity to account for variations that are outside the abilities of the providers to control. Acuity adjustments reflecting overall levels of illness sometimes affect which particular processes are measured as well as outcomes. In general, however, because most P4P programs apply to broad populations, and because typical P4P measures are not focused on costs, adjusting for severity is not routinely used.

Lastly, parameters must be set around the population of members for which data will be collected. For example, a member may be required to be continuously enrolled with the health plan for at least 2 years in order for data regarding breast cancer screening to be used.[*] So-called "anchor dates" are usually set so that identical time periods are used for certain measures. In programs that measure individual performance, the program may also choose not to even collect data from a provider if the number of members subject to the measure is too small (e.g., 30 or fewer members). Of course, data should only be collected for clinical services that are covered under the payers' schedule of benefits.

Sources of Data

Data must be reliable, consistent, and valid. In other words, data collected to create measurement results need to mean what the program understands it to mean, the data need to mean the same thing when reported by different providers, and the data need to actually represent what happened. It should be as easy to collect and report as possible, though the more sophisticated the program becomes, the more complex the data-reporting aspect becomes. Hospitals that have installed highly functional clinical support systems are more able to report more complex data, and increasing use of EHRs should enhance physicians' reporting capabilities.

The typical sources of data used to create P4P performance measures are:

- Medical claims
- Pharmacy claims
- Laboratory results
- Clinical chart or medical record audits
  - Inpatient episodes
  - Outpatient procedures
  - Medical office chart reviews
- Facility or medical office audits
- Nonstandardized patient surveys

Data that is not routinely captured by the claims systems, meaning data other than medical and pharmacy claims, are the most likely to slip through the cracks. For example, a common measure in P4P focusing on care for diabetes is a regular test for sugar in the urine, but many PCPs do this through a simple dipstick instead of sending the patient to a laboratory. PCPs typically do not submit a claim for a dipstick urine test since it is part of a routine office visit for a diabetic patient, so the PCP may be seen as noncompliant with that measure in a P4P program that relies primarily on claims data.

Sources of Evidence-Based Clinical Process Measures

Measures used in a P4P program may be created by the payer, but more often begin by using nationally recognized standards for evidence-based medicine and accepted patient safety requirements. In order to gain support, the providers need to "buy in" to the program, so measures must also be seen as valid by the providers. This is done through involvement of the providers via their appropriate representatives. The use of nationally recognized standards also makes it more appealing to providers and examples of where those measures may be found are shown in **Table 5-13**.

One specific nationally recognized set of measures, the Healthcare Effectiveness Data and Information Set (HEDIS®) is worth singling out. HEDIS was created and is continually upgraded by NCQA, is a mature and widely accepted set of measures that are commonly used by HMOs and other payers, and is often incorporated, in whole or in part, in a P4P program. The entire HEDIS data set can be found in Chapter 15.

Incorporation of consumer perspectives on quality can be relatively complex,[65] although very simple measures such as overall satisfaction, while not as useful as more rigorously constructed survey instruments, at least have the advantage of ease of administration. The most commonly used standardized set of measures is the CAHPS, available from the AHRQ[66]; CAHPS's initial focus was on health plans, but versions focusing on hospitals and on ambulatory care are also now used. CAHPS has also been incorporated by reference into the HEDIS measures.

Table 5-13 provides examples of nationally recognized sources for specific clinical measurements.

Medicare however, does use a type of P4P in traditional FFS Medicare called the Physician Quality Reporting System (PQRS). As of 2011, it had 240 measures that eligible physicians would be assessed on based on their claims submissions as well as claims submitted by other providers, facilities, and ancillary services.[67] Physicians can also submit data extracted from their electronic medical record (EMR) system. Other measures include the use of an EMR, e-prescribing, keeping registries of patients by condition, and more. The PQRS can apply to an individual physician or to a bona fide medical

---

[*]Short gaps in enrollment may be allowed, for example, 45 days or less in a year and only one such gap.

TABLE 5-13	Examples of Sources for P4P Evidence-Based Clinical Measurements
Organization	**URL**
Agency for Healthcare Research and Quality	www.ahrq.gov
Ambulatory Care Quality Alliance (AQA)	www.ambulatoryqualityalliance.org
Bridges to Excellence®, including the Prometheus® P4P System	www.bridgestoexcellence.org
Centers for Medicare and Medicaid Services (CMS)	www.cms.hhs.gov
Hospital Quality Alliance (HQA; sponsored by the American Hospital Association)	www.aha.org/aha/key_issues/qualityalliance/index.html
Integrated Healthcare Association (IHA)	www.iha.org
Leap Frog Group	www.leapfroggroup.org
National Committee on Quality Assurance (NCQA)	www.ncqa.org
National Guidelines Clearinghouse	www.guideline.gov
National Quality Forum (NQF)	www.qualityforum.org
State-based organizations (e.g., the Massachusetts Health Quality Partnership)	www.mhqp.org
URAC	www.urac.org

Sources also include professional associations such as the American College of Physicians, the American College of Surgeons, the American College of Cardiology, the American Diabetes Association, etc.

Source: Compiled by author from websites current as of June 2011.

group. The total incentive is up to 1% of that year's total Medicare payments to the physician or group.

The ACA has a specific section called the Value-Based Payment Modifier under the Physician Fee Schedule in Medicare that is to be based on measures of quality, outcomes, and costs.[68] It is not clear at the time of publication how this will differ from the PQRS except for the requirement that it be focused on the quality of the care provided compared to the cost, as the PQRS does not address cost.

Goals

P4P requires the measures to be translated into achievable goals that can be tied to actual incentive payment. The goals can be fixed or relative. Fixed goals are measures such as the percentage of diabetic patients having their blood tested annually for HbA1c levels, a marker for control of long-term blood sugar levels. Relative goals are measures or improvement over past performance such as a 10% improvement of a PCP's immunization rate. Both may work equally well in the early stages when there is a large gap between actual and desired performance. Relative goals become problematic as performance improves, however, as incremental improvements of good performance become harder to achieve.

Specific incentives are then tied to specific goals. P4P programs typically focus on more than one goal, but vary on the number of goals included under P4P. If HEDIS measures are used, goals may also be set for aggregate compliance rates, for example, 90% compliance with five clinical measures. It is common to set goal thresholds below which no incentive is paid, and incentives are often paid based on the degree to which the thresholds were exceeded.

P4P Payment

How measurements are used in P4P payment is highly variable from payer to payer, and also differs for hospitals and physicians. The same measures used in P4P may also be used in creating tiered networks, which are discussed in Chapter 4. Broadly speaking, payment under P4P may come through adjustments to payment rates, or be paid out as bonuses. In all cases, the amount of P4P payment is typically based on levels of compliance with the program's measures, not on a percent of cost savings.

The amount of P4P incentive payment also varies. Hospitals typically are able to receive between 0.4% and 4% of total payment in the form of P4P, while physician incentives range from 5% up to 10% of total payments, although there are a few programs that reach 20%.[69] For physicians, at least, the amount of incentive payment has a strong and linear correlation with how willing they are to participate.[70] However, as discussed earlier and shown in Table 5-1, individual physicians in any case are frequently insulated from specific payment methodologies.

Adjustment of Payment Rates

A common approach to P4P payment is to use it to adjust provider payment rate schedules, usually by adjusting the multipliers for either DRGs or the monetary value assigned to RBRVS units. HMOs that use a withhold may base part of the withhold return on meeting or exceeding P4P clinical goals, not just on utilization. The timing of when to make such adjustments must be taken into consideration; annual adjustments are the most common, but it is possible to make adjustments on a more frequent basis. Funding adjustments to payment allowances requires no defined source of money, since medical claims are a benefits cost.

Bonus Payments

Bonus payments are separate from any direct payment for services, and may be paid out in full for meeting a threshhold, may be graduated based on the degree to which a goal has been met, or a combination of the two. Timing of bonus payments varies from program to program. Paying incentives on a frequent basis, quarterly for example, does not provide enough data or a long enough period of time to detect actual trends, and the amount of the bonus may be perceived as too small to have a significant impact. Annual bonus payments have the problems of being more remote from the events that are being measured, but this can be countered by providing regular performance reports.

P4P Bonus Payment Funding Sources

Bonus payments by commercial payers require a defined source of money because of the differences in fully insured versus self-funded accounts. A payer can budget for P4P bonus payments and include that cost in the premiums paid by all fully insured accounts. In self-funded accounts, the employer is at risk, even though the payer is performing the administration, including processing the claims payment. Any claims costs or savings go to the employer, not the payer, so it is not built into any premium. There is little publicly available information about how commercial payers fund P4P bonus programs, so how often payers use the following alternatives is unknown.

HMOs that use PCP capitation can fund bonus payments simply by creating a bonus pool, similar to a risk pool. The amount is budgeting in dollars PMPM, $1.25 PMPM for example, which is a medical benefits cost like any other capitated risk pook but is not funded through any withhold of the PCP's capitation payment.

Administrative services only (ASO) contracts are negotiated between the employer and the payer* on a service-specific basis, and each type of service is priced separately. That means that the payer must negotiate with the employer to fund a P4P program as a separate item. This may be done as a discrete fund, or it may be done as a percentage of the employer's actual medical costs. If only some self-funded accounts agree to fund P4P, that means the others are "free riders" in economic terms, enjoying the benefit of something they didn't pay for. A payer could also choose to fund P4P bonuses using only money from insured business, making all self-funded accouts free riders; at least two payers do this.[71]

Alternatively, a payer can hold back a small percentage of an increase in payment schedules used for both insured and self-funded accounts, and set that aside to fund a bonus program. CMS does this for their P4P-type programs. Funding could also come from an increase in fees, but the increase is held as a type of withhold. For example, a payer could budget a 4% increase but pay claims based on a 2% increase, using the other 2% to fund P4P bonuses. This is similar to the capitation withhold described earlier, but payments are not based primarily on costs. In all events, P4P bonus payments still represent legitimate medical claims costs, although they are paid as part of the P4P program.

Measuring Individual versus Group Performance

Hospitals are usually measured on their own in P4P programs. This is because hospitals provide a lot of care, meaning a lot of measurable events. By focusing on common types of care such as community-acquired pneumonia, heart attacks, strokes, and patient safety, sufficent credible data can be collected. Furthermore, care provided by the hospital is attributable to the hospital.

This is not necessarily the case with physicians. One complaint about performance measures for individual physicians is that more than one physician may be involved with the care of any particular patient; for example, a cardiologist and a family practitioner may both provide care to a patient with coronary artery disease. This is the same issue encounted with shared savings, but amplified when applied to a single physician rather than a care system. Weakness in measures also arise due to the small numbers of measurable events. For example, a physician may only have 120 patients with a particular health plan, many of whom do not have signficant medical problems and seek little care; those that do seek care have a variety of conditions, so only a handful of patients receive care that is the focus of the P4P program. For example, one study looking at diabetes, a very common chronic condition, projected that a physician would need to have over 100 patients with diabetes before the reliability of an individual physician report card would be 80 percent.[72] Since the incidence of diabetes is 11.3% in adults over the age of 20, that means that a PCP would need to have about 900 members† covered by a single payer just to achieve an

---

†In a commercial plan it would actually be more, since the 11.3% incidence rate includes adults aged 65 and older who make up 13% of the population, but have a 26.9% incidence rate for diabetes.

80% confidence level. Other articles support the difficulties inherent with measuring performance when there many variables but insufficient credible data.[73]

There is also the problem of patient compliance. A physician may practice with strict adherence to evidence-based medicine, but if he or she is the physician for a large cohort of alcoholic, cigarette-smoking, motorcycle-riding drug dealers with authority problems, poor outcomes are more likely to be due to noncompliance by patients, not physician performance.

One way to address these problems is to incent performance of a large group of physicians such as a large medical group, an IPA, or the entire local network instead of individual physicians; in other words, collect the data from each physician, but measure aggregate performance. Assuming the care being measured is relatively common or frequent, this allows measurements to be statistically significant and patient compliance traits even out. The weakness of measuring the group is that the impact on individual performance is only indirect. How the group distributes the incentive compensation to individual physicians is likely to be unrelated to individual performance.

Another approach is to focus on process and structure, but not outcomes. Examples of measurable processes might include documenting that appropriate tests, prescriptions, or preventive services were ordered, even if the patient fails to follow through. Other examples of measurable structure would include the use of e-prescribing or an EHR. The only type of outcome study that would at least theoretically be valid at the level of individual physicians would be measures related to patient satisfaction.

Finally, P4P can also be applied to an IDS that combines payment of hospitals and physicians. At this point it begins to become difficult to distinguish it from some form of value based payment, which after all is a form of P4P.

Impact of Pay-for-Performance Programs

Since P4P has existed in one form or another for so many years, results about its effectiveness should be clear. Unfortunately, it is anything but. Older studies report success, lack of success, and/or lack of sustained success. [74–76] Even long-established and well-run programs such as California's IHA have reported both great success[77] and then tempered it by reporting improvements in performance but without any breakthrough changes.[78]

Remarkably, there is one study published in 2005 that is cited by proponents of P4P as demonstrating superior metrics for providers under P4P than for a similar set of providers that were not under P4P; however, that same study is cited by critics of P4P as showing that most of the incentives went to providers that were already providing better quality of care, thus concluding that P4P did not actually change any behavior.[79] Similarly, researchers looking at P4P in Massachusetts concluded that P4P was not associated with a greater improvement in quality compared to a rising secular trend.[80]

P4P may also have a "halo" effect in which improvements in a system under P4P lead to similar improvements in other systems that are not under P4P. For example, a study of 260 hospitals in a Medicare P4P demonstration project compared to a control group of 780 hospitals not in the demonstration project found that more than half of the P4P hospitals achieved high performance scores, compared to fewer than one-third of the control hospitals. However, after 5 years, the two groups' scores were virtually identical.[81] Another study found that hospitals in P4P programs had better performance compared to hospitals that publicly reported data but were not in a P4P program.[82]

Aside from administrative frustrations that come from any type of record-keeping, especially manual, P4P has no real negative impact on quality, and either adds to quality improvement or at least aligns provider payment with quality goals. Once a subject of intense interest, enthusiasm, and hope, P4P is no longer seen as as yet another example of "the answer" to lowering costs and improving quality, but it continues to be used by HMOs and other payers.

■ PAYMENT FOR ANCILLARY SERVICES

To recap from Chapter 4, ancillary services are broadly divided into two major categories and one minor one. One major category is diagnostic services such as laboratory, imaging, cardiac studies, and the like. The other major category is therapeutic services such as physical or occupational therapy. The minor category is transportation, including ambulance and scheduled medical transportation. Payment methodologies are similar, so payment as applied to the types of service will only distinguish between them if necessary.

Unlike the type of service, ownership of an ancillary services provider can have a significant impact on payment policies, something that has already been noted several times.[*] This is because use of ancillary services is almost always ordered by a physician, not simply sought out by a patient. In other words, physicians usually control the use of ancillary services. The three main types of ownership are owned by a free-standing or independent company, hospital owned, and physician owned. Each is briefly discussed following the description of types of payment.

Many ancillary services are amongst the first to be "carved out" of the main medical delivery system to take advantage of cost reductions based on economies of scale. This type of economic steering provides for volume increases to the contracting provider. Carving out an ancillary service also allows an HMO to more easily use a risk-based payment approach such as capitation. Unlike physician

---

[*]And is addressed yet again in Chapter 7.

services, ancillary services are typically limited to a small subset of providers, which allows for greater leverage in negotiating payment and service terms. It is also reasonable to require members to travel further for nonurgent ambulatory ancillary services.

Depending on the type of payer, this is an area where there are often relatively strict limits on benefits coverage. A payer may, for example, pay a member only the negotiated in-network rate for services incurred out-of-network, except for emergency care, and the differences between charges and negotiated rates can be tenfold or higher. Most HMOs and a substantial number of non-HMO payers, particularly self-funded plans, will only provide coverage for in-network ancillary services.

In certain areas, however, there may be little competition between ancillary service providers; for example, a rural area or a very small town, in which case a payer has less negotiating leverage. Ambulance services are another area where there is typically little competition, plus ambulances are frequently summoned on a non-elective basis, both of which have an impact on payment policies.

Types of Payment

There are no significantly unique types of payment applicable only to ancillary services, although some are less suitable than others. A brief description of common methodologies follows.

Discounted FFS or a Fee Schedule

Many routine diagnostic ancillary services such as laboratory are high-volume services, so it is not difficult to obtain substantial discounts, usually in the form of a fee schedule.

Flat Rates

Similar to per diem payments to hospitals, flat rates simply mean that the ancillary provider is paid a fixed single payment rate regardless of the number of visits or resources used in providing services. For common high-volume services such as laboratory or routine radiology, this means a fixed fee that does not change regardless of what is ordered.

For therapeutic ancillary providers, case rates can be tiered, similar to differing per diem rates based on type of service in a hospital. For example, for home health care that is inclusive of high-intensity services such as chemotherapy or other high-technology services, the plan may pay different levels of case rates depending on which category of complexity the case falls into.

Capitation

In HMOs or plans that have absolute limitations on out-of-network benefits, ancillary services are frequently capitated, although only if members have acceptable access to the ancillary services provider. HMOs with out-of-network benefits such as a POS plan may still capitate, and simply provide

little or no coverage for nonemergency services from a noncontracted provider. The benefit to the provider of the ancillary service is a guaranteed source of referrals and a steady income. Capitation also removes the FFS incentives that may lead to overutilization of provider-owned services.

Certain types of ancillary services are easier to capitate than others. If an ancillary service is highly self-contained, then it is easier to capitate; for example, physical therapy usually is limited to therapy given by the physical therapists, and does not involve other types of ancillary providers. Home health, on the other hand, is often a combination of home health nurses and clinical aids, durable medical equipment (DME), home infusion and medication delivery (which includes the cost of the drug or intravenous substance as well as the cost to deliver it), home physical therapy, and so forth. A number of plans have successfully capitated for home health services, although those have tended to be larger plans with sufficient volume to be able to accurately predict costs in all of these different areas. Other plans have been able to capitate only parts of home health, home respiratory therapy for example, but have had less success in other forms. In those cases, a combination of capitation and fixed case rates is useful, for example, capitating for basic home care, but paying case rates for a course of chemotherapy.

A relatively uncommon variant on capitation is similar to the single-specialty organization discussed in Chapter 4. In this case, a single entity accepts capitation from the plan for all of a particular ancillary service and then serves as a network manager. Service is provided from the organization's providers, if it has them, and from participating ancillary services providers under a subcontract with the network manager. The subcontracted providers are paid through subcapitation, some form of FFS or case rates, but in all events, the network manager is at risk for the total costs of the capitated service.

Some plans that capitate for ancillary services also use P4P or service-level risk programs to ensure high levels of quality and satisfaction. For example, a plan may withhold 10% of the capitation or set up an incentive pool to ensure compliance with service standards such as accessibility, member satisfaction, turnaround time for results, responsiveness to referring physicians, documentation, and so forth.

Ancillary Services from a Contracted Hospital

The discussion to this point has been about payment for ancillary services from an independent or free-standing company. Negotiating business terms is done on a business-to-business basis at arm's length, and the issues are straightforward. But ancillary services owned by a hospital or by a physician are another matter.

Medical–surgical hospitals uniformly provide some types of ancillary services, and frequently most of them.

The chargemaster fees associated with these are typically quite high compared to free-standing companies. They are also used for inpatient care, of course, but payment in that case is negotiated as part of the overall inpatient payment.

Ancillary services can become a sore subject in the relationship between a payer and a hospital. Payers typically contract with free-standing companies to get far lower prices, and steering patients is part of that equation. But hospitals usually seek to be paid for all such services and to have no benefits differentials that would steer patients to another provider. Hospitals, therefore, often include ambulatory ancillary services in the overall negotiation. It would not be the norm for a hospital to allow a major contract to lapse over this issue, but neither do they ignore it.

Even when terms are agreed to, it is not unusual for a payer to agree to payment terms but not to stop steering members to another, less expensive provider, and that is usually what they do. With the rapid increase in hospitals employing physicians, however, the dynamic has changed in some cases. Physicians who once would simply send patients to whatever ancillary services provider was in a payer's network may find that being employed by a hospital also means being directed to only use the hospital's services. Hospitals may waive any additional cost-sharing by the member as an inducement, although many payers consider this fraud, as has been noted elsewhere. This is a recent development in terms of magnitude, so how payment may change over time because of it is hard to know at this point.

Physician-Owned Ancillary Services

There have long been data demonstrating that physician ownership[*] of any type of service provider—hospitals, ambulatory procedure facilities, or ancillary services—is strongly associated with marked increases in utilization when compared to the use of those same services by physicians with no ownership interest. In other words, physicians who own diagnostic equipment have a conscious or subconscious pressure to use it to not only make it pay for itself, but to be a profit center. The general term for this is "physician self-referral."

Self-referral for imaging, especially costly types of imaging such as MRIs, and nuclear or cardiac scanning is a particularly serious problem. It has been documented since the 1980s, for example, that physician ownership of imaging equipment led to a fourfold increase of its use compared to physicians who referred such studies to radiologists.[83] Little has changed in 30 years, and more recent examples of studies demonstrating the strong link between physician

self-referral for imaging and increased utilization and costs include:

- Highly compensated in-office myocardial perfusion imaging by cardiologists occurs six times more often than when the procedure is referred to a radiologist;[84]
- Physician ownership of MRI machines drives up its use and overall costs;[85]
- Imaging self-referral is associated with higher costs but limited impact on duration of illness;[86]
- There is a boom in self-referral, but no consensus on how to stop it;[87] and
- The argument that self-referral offers convenient, same-day, one-stop service to patients and allows treatment to start sooner is false; for example, an analysis of 2006 and 2007 Medicare data showed that self-referral provided same-day imaging for 74% of low-cost types of X-rays, but only 15% of costly and advanced procedures such as CT and MRI.[88]

Self-referral demonstrably increases utilization and costs not only for imaging but for laboratory services[89] and a wide variety of other ancillary services.[90] Similarly, physician-ownership in ambulatory surgical centers is linked to a doubling of surgical volume.[91] Medicare placed an outright ban on billing for certain physician-owned services to address this, but then created an enormous "loophole" in the form of the In-Office Ancillary Services Exemption (IOASE) that allows for direct payments to providers for a large number of specialized services as long as they are performed in the physician's office. As a result, there are some mighty big offices out there, as well as a push by manufacturers to make equipment and devices ever more compact.

The ACA did not significantly tighten restrictions on physician ownership limitations. It simply froze development of new physician-owned specialty hospitals while grandfathering existing ones, and it requires greater transparency in reporting ownership. In the past few years, CMS has begun to reduce payments for IOASE imaging, reducing its value as a profit center. Paradoxically, that may be driving even more increases in utilization and costs as physicians who own or have long-term leases on these devices cost-shift to the private sector.

Commercial payers must use a combination of contracting terms and benefits designed to address this rising source of costs. Some refuse to pay for self-referral services other than low-cost ones such as simple X-rays or ultrasounds, but it is not widespread yet. Other payers use reference pricing, and only cover up to the amount it pays to a contracted free-standing or hospital-owned provider. Because of the need to bring in enough revenue to cover the loan or lease cost plus yield a profit, some physicians who own equipment contractually agree to the same lower payment terms, and make it up on volume through high utilization. In

---

[*]Ownership covers both actual outright ownership as well as leasing of equipment. The underlying elements are the same: the physician invests a certain amount of money and looks for a return on the investment, just like any business does.

other cases, they waive the difference in cost-sharing, so the member has no economic disincentive. HMOs that capitate specialists routinely add any self-referral services to what is defined as covered under the capitation payment. This also requires the physician to only use his or her device in order to prevent having to pay twice. HMOs are also better able to place strict requirements on contracted providers prohibiting self-referral, although how many actually do is not known.

■   **OTHER NEW MODELS OF PAYMENT UNDER THE PATIENT PROTECTION AND AFFORDABLE CARE ACT**

The ACA addresses some approaches to payment for FFS Medicare, and possibly Medicaid, by specifically calling them out. Examples that have already been identified and discussed include:

- No payment for never events;
- Payment reductions for hospitals with higher than average avoidable readmissions;
- The bundled payment pilot;
- Shared savings for ACOs;
- Value-based payments for ACOs and PCMHs; and
- The value-based payment modifier to the physician fee schedule.

The ACA has even more provisions around payment reforms in Medicare that do not fit neatly into specific payment methodologies discussed to this point.* One major provision in the ACA created the new Center for Medicare and Medicaid Innovations (CMMI) to test, evaluate, and expand different payment methodologies in Medicare and Medicaid.[92] The law specifically describes 20 possible models for testing, which are listed in **Table 5-14**.

The ACA does not restrict the CMMI to experimenting only with the payment methodologies listed in Table 5-14, but directs it to look at other approaches as well. At the time of publication, no rules or regulations have been issued for any new payment methodology for Medicare and Medicaid other than shared savings. Because of that, little more can be said at this time other than to make two observations:

1. Because Medicare makes up such a high percentage of the total payments to hospitals and most physicians, any changes it makes in payment methodologies will affect private payers, often in unknown or unpredictable ways.
2. Where CMS goes, private payers often follow.

The reader can keep up to date on the status of any new payment methodologies under consideration by the CMMI

_____

*This point being the end point.

TABLE 5-14	**Experimental Payment Methodologies Described in the CMMI Section of the ACA**
Patient-centered medical homes for high-need individuals, for women's health care, and to move primary care practices from FFS toward comprehensive payment or salary-based payment	Permission for states to test integrated care for dual eligibles
Direct contracting with provider groups to promote delivery models through risk-based comprehensive payment or salary-based payment	Permission for states to test all-payer payment reform
Geriatric assessments and comprehensive care plans to coordinate care	Evidence-based guidelines for cancer care aligned with payment incentives
Coordination of care to move providers from FFS toward salary	Post-acute care improved through rehabilitation centers, long-term care hospitals, and home care
Use of health information technology, including home telehealth technology, to coordinate care of high-risk chronically ill people	Home health providers paid to work with interdisciplinary teams
Physician payment for advanced diagnostic imaging tied to appropriateness criteria	Collaborative high-quality, low-cost institutions disseminate and implement best-practices and assist other institutions in implementing them
Utilization of medication therapy management services	Electronic monitoring used by specialists to facilitate inpatient care at IDSs
Community-based health teams to support small-practice medical homes	No referrals for many outpatient services, such as physical therapy
Encouragement of providers to use patient decision-support tools to improve understanding of treatment options	Comprehensive payments to IDSs that include a teaching hospital and physicians, and that try new methods for training health care professionals

Source: Compiled by author from the ACA Sec. 3021 42 U.S.C. §1315a (b)(2)(B)(i-xx).

by periodically checking their website at http://innovations
.cms.gov.*

■ CONCLUSION

Provider payment is payment, it is not reimbursement.
Payment has the potential to affect behavior, while true
reimbursement does not. Therefore, to the degree possible,
payment methodologies should align the financial incentives and goals of the health plan and the network providers
who deliver the care. Capitation for HMOs, P4P for all types
of payers, and probably shared savings approaches do that
in ways that traditional FFS does not.

But any payment methodology is a tool, and like any tool
it has limitations. Just as a hammer is the correct tool for
pounding and removing nails, it is poor for cutting wood,
and, if used without at least a modicum of skill, will result
in a painful self-inflicted injury. Payment may be a powerful and often effective tool, but can only be effective in
conjunction with other managed care functions: utilization
management, quality management, network contracting,
provider relations, and the many other activities of a well-
run managed health care plan.

■ APPENDIX 5-1

Examples of Research on the Impact of Managed Care or Capitation on Quality or Outcomes

Baker LC, Cantor JC. Physician satisfaction under managed
care. *Health Affairs.* 1993;12 Suppl:258–270.

Berwick DM. Quality of health care. Part 5: Payment
by capitation and the quality of care. *N Engl J Med.*
1996;335(16):1227–1231.

Braveman P, Schaaf M, Egerter S, et al. Insurance-related
differences in the risk of ruptured appendix. *N Engl J
Med.* 1994;331(7):444–449.

Braveman P, Schaaf VM, Egerter S, Bennett T, Schecter W.
Insurance related differences in the risk of ruptured
appendix. *N Engl J Med.* 1994;331(7):444–449.

Brook RH. Managed care is not the problem, quality is.
JAMA. 1997;278(19):1612–1614.

Bruno R, Gilbert B. In California, Medi-Cal managed care
is superior to Medi-Cal fee-for-service. *Manag Care Q.*
1998;6(4):7–14.

Carlisle D, Siu AL, Keeler EB. HMO vs. fee-for-service care of
older persons with acute myocardial infarction. *A J Public
Health.* 1992;82(12):1626–1630.

Clancy CM, Hillner BE. Physicians as gatekeepers—the
impact of financial incentives. *Arch Intern Med.*
1989;149(4):917–920.

Dudley RA, Miller RH, Korenbrot TY, Luft HS. The impact of
financial incentives on quality of health care. *Milbank Q.*
1998;76(4):649–686.

Hellinger FJ. The effect of managed care on quality. *Arch
Intern Med.* 1998;158(8):833–841.

Lurie N, Christianson J, Finch M, Moscovice I. The effects
of capitation on health and functional status of the
Medicaid elderly: A randomized trial. *Ann Intern Med.*
1994;120(6):506–511.

Michael D, Weiss MD. Capitation can be beneficial
to providers and patients. *Maryland Med J.*
1997;46(4):170–171.

Miller RH, Luft HS. Does managed care lead to better or
worse quality of care? *Health Affairs.* 1997;16(5):7–25.

Murray JP, Greenfield S, Kaplan SH, Yano EM. Ambulatory
testing for capitation and FFS patients in the same
practice setting: Relationship to outcomes. *Med Care.*
1992;30(3):252–261.

Relman A. Medical insurance and health: What about
managed care? *N Engl J Med.* 1994;331(7):471–472.

Riley G, Potosky AL, Lubitz JD, Brown MC. Stage of cancer at
diagnosis for Medicare HMO and fee-for-service enrollees.
Am J Public Health. 1994;84(10):1598–1604.

Seidman JJ, Bass EP, Rubin HR. Review of studies that
compare the quality of cardiovascular care in HMO verses
non-HMO settings. *Med Care.* 1998;36(12):1607–1625.

Sloss EM, Keeler EB, Brook, et al. Effect of a health
maintenance organization on physiologic health. *Ann
Intern Med.* 1987;106(1):130–138.

Udvarhelyi IS, Jennison K, Phillips RS, Epstein AM.
Comparison of the quality of ambulatory care for FFS
and prepaid patients. *Ann Intern Med.* 1991;115(5):
394–400.

Ware JE, Brook RH, Rogers WH, et al. Comparison of health
outcomes at a health maintenance organization with
those of FFS care. *Lancet.* 1986;1(8488):1017–1022.

Whitmore H. Comparing outcomes in managed care. *HMO
Magazine.* 1996;37(1):75-76.

𝓔𝓃𝒹𝓃𝓸𝓉𝓮𝓼

1   WorldNet Search: Reimbursement. Available at: http://
    wordnetweb.princeton.edu/perl/webwn?s = payment.
    Accessed June 12, 2011.

2   Stensland J, Gaumer ZR, Miller ME. Private-payer
    profits can induce negative Medicare margins. *Health
    Affairs.* May 2010;29(5):1045–1051.

3   Conrad DA, Maynard C, Cheadle A, et al. Primary care
    physician compensation method in medical groups.
    JAMA 1998;279(11):853–858.

4   Health Care Financing and Organization. Physician
    payment and physician behavior: A complex interaction.
    *The Changes in Health Care Financing and Organization
    Initiative.* December 2010. Washington, DC: 1-5. Available
    at: www.hcfo.org/publications/physician-payment-
    and-physician-behavior-complex-interaction. Accessed
    December 17, 2010.

---

*Current at the time of publication.

5   Robinson JC. Blended payment methods in physician organizations under managed care. *JAMA*. 1999;282(13): 1258–1263.

6   Rosenthal MB, Frank RG, Buchanan JL, Epstein AM. Transmission of financial incentives to physicians by intermediary organizations in California. *Health Affairs*. 2002;21(4):197–205.

7   The Patient Protection and Affordable Care Act (P.L. 111–148) Section 3021, 42 U.S.C. §1315(a).

8   Ginsburg PB. Rapidly evolving physician-payment policy—More than the SGR. *N Engl J Med*. 2011;364(2): 172–176.

9   Personal communications with chief medical officers and vice presidents for network management, conducted April–June 2011.

10 Austin AD, Gravelle JG. Does price transparency improve market efficiency? Implications of empirical evidence in other markets of the health sector. Congressional Research Service Report. April 29, 2008; Order Code RL34101. Available at: www.fas.org/sgp/crs/misc/ RL34101.pdf. Accessed June 22, 2011.

11 Tu HT, Lauer J. Impact of health care price transparency on price variation: The New Hampshire experience. Issue brief no. 128. Washington, DC: Center for Studying Health System Change, 2009. Available at: www.hschange.com/ CONTENT/1095/1095.pdf. Accessed June 22, 2011.

12 Ginsburg PB. Shopping for price in medical care. *Health Affairs*. 2007;26(2):w208–w216.

13 Sanofi-Aventis. Managed Care Digest Series®: HMO-PPO/Medicare-Medicaid Digest 2010. Available at: www.managedcaredigest.com.

14 Zuvekas SH, Cohen JW. Paying physicians by capitation: Is the past now prologue? *Health Affairs*. 2010;29(9): 1661–1666.

15 Super N. From capitation to fee-for-service in Cincinnati: A physician group responds to a changing marketplace. *Health Affairs*. 2006;25(1):219–225.

16 Landon BE, Normand SL, Blumenthal D, Daley J. Physician clinical performance assessment: Prospects and barriers. *JAMA*. 2003;290(9):1183–1189.

17 Kravitz RL, Greenfield S, Rogers W, et al. Differences in the mix of patients among medical specialties and systems of care: results from the medical outcomes study. *JAMA*. 1992;267(12):1617–1623.

18 Swartz K. Cost-sharing: Effects on spending and outcomes. Robert Wood Johnson Foundation Synthesis Report No. 20. December 2010.

19 Fronstin P, MacDonald J. Consumer-driven health plan participants display cost-conscious behavior, utilize wellness programs. Employee Benefit Research Institute. December 1, 2009.

20 Beeuwkes Buntin M, Damberg C, Haviland A, et al. Consumer-directed health care: early evidence about effects on cost and quality. *Health Affairs*. 2006;25(6): w516–w530.

21 Popovian R, Johnson K, Nichol M, Liu G. The impact of pharmaceutical capitation to primary medical groups on the health-care expenditures of medicare HMO enrollees. *J Manag Care Pharm*. 1999;5(5):438–441.

22 Hillman AL, Pauly MV, Escarce JJ, et al. Financial incentives and drug spending in managed care. *Health Affairs*. 1999;18(2):189–200.

23 Debrock L, Arnould RJ. Utilization control in HMOs. *Q Rev Econ Financ*. 1992;32(3):31–53.

24 LaPensee KT. Pricing specialty carve-outs and disease management programs under managed care. *Manag Care Q*. 1997;5(2):10–19.

25 Gallagher TH, St. Peter RF, Chesney M, Lo B. Patients' attitudes toward cost control bonuses for managed care. *Health Affairs*. 2001;20(2):186–192.

26 Federal Register 42 CFR 422.208/210, June 26, 1998.

27 Ibid.

28 Ibid.

29 *Ingram vs. Harris Health Plan*, No. 98-CV-179 (USDC E.D. Texas, settlement filed Oct. 12, 1999).

30 *Shea v. Esensten*, Minn. Ct. App. No. 949878 (2/6/01).

31 Jost TS. The Supreme Court limits lawsuits against managed care organizations. *Health Affairs*. 2004;Suppl Web Exclusive:w4-417–426.

32 Vogt WB (RAND Corp.). Hospital market consolidation: Trends and consequences. Report to the NIHCM Foundation. November 2009.

33 Devers KJ, Casalino LP, Rudell LS, Stoddard JJ, Brewster LR, Lake TK. Hospitals' negotiating leverage with health plans: How and why has it changed? *Health Serv Res*. 2003;38(1, Pt. 2):419–446.

34 United States Government Accountability Office. *Differences in health care prices across metropolitan areas linked to competition and other factors*. Pub. No. GAO-06-281T. December 2005. Available at: www.gao. gov/new.items/d06281t.pdf. Accessed July 14, 2006.

35 Berenson RA, Ginsburg PB, Kemper N. Unchecked provider clout in California foreshadows challenges to health reform. *Health Affairs*. 2010;29(4):699–705.

36 Oberlander J, White J. Public attitudes toward health care spending aren't the problem, prices are. *Health Affairs*. 2009;28(5):1285–1293.

37 Reinhardt E. The pricing of U.S. hospital services: Chaos behind a veil of secrecy. *Health Affairs*. 2006;25(1): 57–69.

38 Vladeck BC, Rice T. Market failure and the failure of discourse: Facing up to the power of sellers. *Health Affairs*. 2009;28(5):1305–1315.

39 Personal communications with the chief medical officer; the identification of the organization is confidential.

40 Ibid.

41 3M Health Information Systems. Available at: www.3m.com/ us/healthcare/his/products/outpatient/ambulatory .jhtml. Accessed July 16, 2006.

42 P.L. 99-27242 U.S.C. §1395dd.

43   ACA Section 2718, 42 U.S.C. §300gg-19a (b)(1).

44   ACA Section 2718, 42 U.S.C. §300gg-19a (b)(2).

45   ACA Section 3008, 42 U.S.C. §1395ww.

46   ACA Section 3025, 42 U.S.C. §1395ww.

47   Ingenix website. Episode treatment groups. 2011. Available at: www.ingenix.com/about/ETG/etgoverview/. Accessed June 27, 2011.

48   Liu CF, Sujha S, Cromwell J. Impact of global bundled payments on hospital costs of coronary artery bypass grafting. *J Health Care Financ.* 2001;27(4):39–54.

49   Examination of Health Care Cost Trends and Cost Drivers Pursuant to G.L. c. 118G, § 6½(b), Report for Annual Public Hearing, Office of [Massachusetts] Attorney General Martha Coakley, June 22, 2011.

50   ACA Section 3023, 42 U.S.C. §1395cc-4.

51   ACA Section 3022, 42 U.S.C. §1395 et seq.

52   42 CFR Part 425 §1345-F.

53   Pham HH, Ginsburg PB, McKenzie K, Milstein A. Redesigning care delivery in response to a high-performance network: The Virginia Mason Medical Center. *Health Affairs.* 2007;26(4):w532–w544.

54   Kaiser Health News. Mixed signals on Medicare pilot savings projects. October 28, 2010. Available at: www.kaiserhealthnews.org/stories/2010/october/28/ft-mixed-signals-on-medicare-pilot-savings-projects.aspx. Accessed June 28, 2011.

55   Haywood TT, Kosel KC. The ACO model—a three-year financial loss? *N Engl J Med.* 2011;364(14):e27–e27.

56   Share DA, Campbell DA, Birkmeyer N, et al. How a regional collaborative of hospitals and physicians in Michigan cut costs and improved the quality of care. *Health Affairs.* 2011;30(4):636-645.

57   Outcomes-Based Compensation: Pay-for-performance design principles. Available at: www.rewardingquality.com. Accessed July 18, 2006.

58   Epstein AM, Lee TH, Hamel MB. Paying physicians for high-quality care. *N Engl J Med.* 2004;350(4):406–410.

59   Cooper RM. Formal physician performance evaluations. *J Ambul Care Manage.* 1980;3:19–33.

60   Schlackman N. Integrating quality assessment and physician incentive payment. *Qual Rev Bull.* 1989;15(8): 234–237.

61   Traska MR. HMO Uses Quality measures to pays its physicians. *Hospitals.* 1988;62(13):34–36.

62   Sennett C, Legorreta AP, Zata SL. Performance-based hospital contracting for quality improvement. *J Qual Improv* 1993;19(9):374–383.

63   Rosenthal MB, Landon BE, Normand SLT. Pay for performance in commercial HMOs. *N Engl J Med.* 2006; 355(18):1895–1902.

64   Donabedian A. *The Definition of Quality and Approaches to its Assessment.* Ann Arbor, MI: Health Administration Press; 1980.

65   Cleary PD, Edgman-Levitan S. Health care quality: Incorporating consumer perspectives. *JAMA.* 1997; 278(19):1608–1612.

66   Agency of Healthcare Research and Quality (AHRQ). The Consumer Assessment of Healthcare Providers and Systems (CAHPS) program. Available at: www.cahps.ahrq.gov/default.asp. Accessed July 21, 2006.

67   www.cms.gov/PQRS/Downloads/2011_PhysQualRptg_MeasuresList_033111.pdf. Accessed August 31, 2011.

68   ACA Section 3007 42 U.S.C. §1395w-4.

69   Author's review of multiple programs described in public documents.

70   De Brantes FS, D'Andrea BG. Physicians respond to pay-for-performance incentives: Large incentives yield greater participation. *Am J Manage Care.* 2009;15(5): 305–310.

71   Confidential personal communications with author.

72   Hofer TP, Hayward RA, Greenfield S, et al. The unreliability of individual physician "report cards" for assessing the costs and quality of care of a chronic disease. *JAMA.* 1999;281(22):2098–2105.

73   Mehrotra A, Adams JL, Thomas JW, McGlynn EA. Cost profiles: Should the focus be on individual physicians or physician groups? *Health Affairs.* 2010;29(8):1532–1538.

74   Dudley RA. Pay-for-performance research: How to learn what clinicians and policy makers need to know. *JAMA.* 2005;294(14):1821–1823.

75   Rosenthal MB, Frank RG. What is the empirical basis for paying for quality in health care? *Med Care Res Rev.* 2006;63(2):135–157.

76   Dudley RA, Miller RH, Korenbrot TY, Luft HS. The impact of financial incentives on quality of health care. *Millbank Q.* 1998;76(4):649–685.

77   www.iha.org/071306.htm. Accessed July 23, 2006

78   Damberg CL, Raube K, Teleki SS, de la Cruz E. Taking stock of pay-for-performance: A candid assessment from the front lines. *Health Affairs.* 2009;28(2): 517–525.

79   Rosenthal MB, Frank RG, Epstein AM. Early experience with pay-for-performance: From concept to practice. *JAMA.* 2005;294(14):1788–1793.

80   Pearson SD, Schneider EC, Kleinman KP, et al. The impact of pay-for-performance on health care quality in Massachusetts, 2001–2003. *Health Affairs.* 2008;27(4): 1167–1176.

81   Werner RM, Kolstad JT, Stuart EA, Polsky D. The effect of pay-for-performance in hospitals: Lessons for quality improvement. *Health Affairs.* 2011;30(4):690–698.

82   Lindenauer PK, Remus D, Roman S, et al. Public reporting and pay for performance in hospital quality improvement. *N Engl J Med.* 2007;356(5):486–496.

83   Hillman BJ, Joseph CA, Mabry MR, et al. Frequency and costs of diagnostic imaging in office practice—a

comparison of self-referring and radiologist-referring physicians. *N Engl J Med*. 1990;323(23):1604–1608.

84 Levin DC, Rao VM, Parker L, Frangos AJ, Intenzo CM. Recent payment and utilization trends in radionuclide myocardial perfusion imaging: Comparison between self-referral and referral to radiologists. *J Am Coll Radiol*. 2009;6(6):437–441.

85 Baker LC. Acquisition of MRI equipment by doctors drives up imaging use and spending. *Health Affairs*. 2010;29(12):2252–2259.

86 Hughes DR, Bhargavan M, Sunshine JH. Imaging self-referral associated with higher costs and limited impact on duration of illness. *Health Affairs*. 2010;29(12):2244–2251.

87 Hillman BJ, Goldsmith J. Imaging: The self-referral boom and the ongoing search for effective policies to contain it. *Health Affairs*. 2010;29(12):2231–2236.

88 Sunshine J, Bhargavan M. The practice of imaging self-referral doesn't produce much one-stop service. *Health Affairs*. 2010;29(12):2237–2243.

89 Office of the Inspector General. Financial arrangements between physicians and health care businesses: Report to Congress. Washington, DC: U.S. Department of Health and Human Services; 1989. U.S. Dept of Health and Human Services Publication OAI-12-88-01410.

90 State of Florida Health Care Cost Containment Board. Joint ventures among health care providers in Florida. Tallahassee, FL: State of Florida; 1991;2.

91 Hollingsworth JM, Ye Z, Strope SA, et al. Physician-ownership of ambulatory surgical centers linked to higher volume of surgeries. *Health Affairs*. 2010;29(4):683–689.

92 ACA Section 3021, 42 U.S.C. §1315a.

Legal Issues in Provider Contracting

MARK S. JOFFE AND KELLI D. BACK

CHAPTER

6

STUDY OBJECTIVES

- Understand the necessary steps and considerations in negotiating a managed care contract
- Understand the typical format of a managed care contract
- Understand common clauses and provisions in managed care contracts
- Understand the key issues underlying the terms of a managed care contract

DISCUSSION TOPICS

1. Discuss the differences between a letter of intent and an agreement. What is the purpose of each?
2. Discuss why the "definitions" section of a contract is important and name a few definitions that should be carefully reviewed or drafted and why.
3. Describe and discuss important issues relating to payment that should be addressed in a managed care agreement.
4. Describe and discuss the importance of the "hold harmless" clause in managed care contracts.
5. Discuss the two general categories of termination grounds typically included in a managed care contract. Describe the advantages of each from a provider perspective and the types of instances in which they might be evoked.
6. Describe and discuss four provider obligations commonly included in managed care contracts.

■ INTRODUCTION

The purpose of a managed care organization is to provide or arrange for the provision of health care services. Most managed care organizations (MCOs, also commonly referred to as health plans or payers*) such as health maintenance organizations (HMOs), preferred provider organizations (PPOs), and Medicare Advantage (MA) plans are network based, meaning they provide their services through arrangements

with individual physicians, individual practice associations (IPAs), medical groups, hospitals, and other types of health care professionals and facilities. The provider contract formalizes the MCO–provider relationship. A carefully drafted contract accomplishes more than mere memorializing of the arrangement between the parties. A well-written contract can foster a positive relationship between the provider and the MCO. Moreover, a good contract can provide important and needed protections to both parties if the relationship sours.

This chapter is intended to offer to the MCO and the provider a practical guide to reviewing and drafting a provider

---

*The terms *MCO* and *payer* are used interchangeably to refer to any type of network-based payer organization unless otherwise specified.

contract. In the appendices that follow the chapter are a MCO–primary care physician agreement and a MCO–hospital agreement. The authors have annotated these contracts, which have been provided solely for illustrative purposes. The operational aspects of network development (physician, hospital, and ancillary services), credentialing, payment issues, and the like are addressed in Chapters 4 and 5, and issues related to utilization management (UM) and quality management (QM) are addressed in Chapters 7 and 14, respectively.

Contracts need not be complex or lengthy to be legally binding and enforceable. A single-sentence letter agreement between a hospital and an MCO that says that the hospital agrees to provide access to its facility to enrollees of the MCO in exchange for payment of billed charges is a valid contract. If a single paragraph agreement is legally binding, why is it necessary for MCO–provider contracts to be so lengthy? The answer is twofold. First, many terms of the contract, although not required, perform useful functions by articulating the rights and responsibilities of the parties. Because commercial payers are an important revenue source to most providers, a clear understanding of these rights and responsibilities is important. Second, many contractual provisions are required by state licensure regulations (e.g., a hold harmless clause; see Chapter 28) or by government payer programs such as Medicare and Medicaid (see Chapters 24 and 25, respectively).

An ideal contract or contract form does not exist. Appropriate contract terms vary depending on the issues of concern and objectives of the parties, each party's relative negotiating strength, and the desired degree of formality. Although the focus of this chapter is explaining key substantive provisions in a contract, the importance of clarity cannot be overstated. A poorly written contract confuses the parties, and increases substantially the likelihood of disagreements over the meaning of contract language. A contract should not only be written in simple, commonly understood language but should be well organized so that either party is able to find and review provisions as quickly and easily as possible.

The need for clarity has become more important as contracts have become increasingly complex. Many MCOs may act as an HMO, a PPO, and a third-party administrator. Those types of payer organizations will frequently enter into a single contract with a provider to provide services in all three capacities. In addition, this single contract may obligate the provider to furnish services not only to the MCO enrollees but also to enrollees of a number of affiliates or nonaffiliates of the MCO.

The following discussion is designed to provide a workable guide for MCOs and providers to draft, amend, or review contracts. The discussion is cast at some times from the perspective of the MCO and at other times from the provider's perspective. Most of the discussion relates to contracts directly between the MCO and the provider of services. When the contract is between the MCO and an IPA or medical group, the MCO needs to ensure that the areas discussed below are appropriately addressed in both the MCO's contract and the contract between the IPA or medical group and the provider.

■ GENERAL ISSUES IN CONTRACTING

Before discussing specific provisions, it is worth looking at general issues that contracts between health plans and providers typically address.

Key Objectives

Both the MCO and the provider should divide key objectives into two categories: those that are essential and those that, although not essential, are desirable. Throughout the negotiations process each party needs to keep in mind both the musts and the desirable objectives. Not infrequently, an MCO or a provider will suddenly realize at the end of the negotiation process that it has not achieved all its basic goals. The MCO's key objectives will vary. If the MCO is in a community with a single provider of a particular specialty service, merely entering into a contract on any terms with the provider may be its objective. On the other hand, the MCO's objectives might be quite complex, and it may demand carefully planned negotiations to achieve them.

"Must" objectives may derive from state and federal regulations, which may require or prohibit particular clauses in contracts. MCOs need to be aware of these requirements and make sure that their contracting providers understand that these provisions are required by law.

Beyond the essential objectives are the desirable ones. Before commencing the drafting or the negotiation of the contract, the MCO should list these objectives and have a good understanding of their relative importance. This preliminary thought process assists the MCO in developing its negotiating strategy.

Annual Calendar

Key provider contracts may take months to negotiate. If the contemplated arrangement with the provider is important to the MCO's delivery system, it will want to avoid the diminution of its bargaining strength as the desired effective date approaches.

The MCO should have a master schedule identifying the contracts that need to be entered into and renewed. This schedule should include timelines that identify dates by which progress on key contract negotiations should take place. Although such an orderly system may be difficult to maintain, it may protect the MCO from potential problems that may arise if it is forced to operate without a contract or to negotiate from a weakened position. The use of an automated contract management system, as described in Chapter 4, can greatly facilitate this aspect of contracting.

Letter of Intent Compared to Contract

The purpose of a letter of intent is to define the basic elements of a contemplated arrangement or transaction between two parties. A letter of intent is used most often when the negotiation process between two parties is expected to be lengthy. A letter of intent is a preliminary, nonbinding understanding that allows the parties to ascertain whether they are able to agree on key terms. If the parties agree on a letter of intent, the terms of that letter serve as the blueprint for the contract. Some people confuse a letter of intent with a letter agreement. Because a letter of intent is not a legally binding agreement, regulators will not consider the provider in evaluating whether an MCO, especially an HMO, has made available and accessible the full range of services required to meet access standards described in Chapter 4. Therefore, the use of a letter of intent should be limited to identifying the general parameters of a future contract.

■ CONTRACT STRUCTURE

As mentioned earlier, clarity is an important objective in drafting a provider contract. A key factor affecting the degree of clarity of a contract is the manner in which the agreement is organized. In fact, many MCO contracts follow fairly similar formats. The contract begins with a title describing the instrument (e.g., "Primary Care Physician Agreement"). After this is the caption, which identifies the names of the parties and the legal action taken, along with the transition, which contains words signifying that the parties have entered into an agreement. Then, the contract includes the recitals, which are best explained as the "whereas" clauses. These clauses are not intended to have legal significance but may become relevant to resolve inconsistencies in the body of the contract or if the drafter inappropriately includes substantive provisions in them. (The use of the word "whereas" is merely tradition and has no legal significance.)

The next section of the contract is generally the definitions section, which includes definitions of all key contract terms. The definitions section precedes the operative language, including the substantive health-related provisions that define the responsibilities and obligations of each of the parties, representations and warranties, and declarations. The last section of the contract, the closing or testimonium, reflects the assent of the parties through their signatures. Sometimes, the drafters of a provider contract decide to have the signature page on the first page for administrative simplicity.

Contracts frequently incorporate by reference other documents, some of which will be appended to the agreement as attachments or exhibits. As discussed further later, MCOs frequently reserve the right to amend some of these referenced documents unilaterally.

The contract's form or structure is intended to accomplish three purposes: to simplify a reader's use and understanding of the agreement, to facilitate amendment or revision of the contract where the contract form has been used for many providers, and to streamline the administrative process necessary to submit and obtain regulatory approvals.

Clarity and efficiency can be attained by using commonly understood terms, avoiding legal or technical jargon, using definitions to explain key and frequently used terms, and using well-organized headings and a numbering system. The ultimate objective is that any representative of the MCO or the provider who has an interest in an issue be able to find easily the pertinent contract provision and understand its meaning.

Exhibits and appendices are frequently used by MCOs to promote efficiency in administering many provider contracts. The MCO, to the extent possible, could design many of its provider contracts or groups of provider contracts around a core set of common requirements. Exhibits may be used to identify the terms that may vary, such as payment rates and provider responsibilities. This approach has several advantages. First, it eases the administrative burden in drafting and revising contracts. Second, if an appendix or exhibit is the only part of the contract that is being amended and it has a separate state insurance department or health department provider number, the MCO need only submit the amendment for state review. Third, when a contract is under consideration for renewal and the key issue is the payment rate, having the payment rate listed separately in the appendix lessens the likelihood that the provider will review and suggest amending other provisions of the contract.

■ COMMON CLAUSES, PROVISIONS, AND KEY FACTORS

Most provider contracts contain a number of common clauses and provisions. Ones most commonly found are discussed next.

Names

The initial paragraph of the contract will identify the names of the parties entering into the agreement. It is always a good idea to ensure that the parties named in the opening paragraph are the parties who are signing the agreement. If one organization is signing the agreement on behalf of affiliates, the organization's authority to do so needs to be clearly conveyed in the agreement. In addition, the other organization may want to have the signing party represent and warrant that it is authorized to sign on behalf of the nonsigning party or parties. This is also the case where a physician group or intermediate entity is signing on-behalf of its member physicians. If the nonsigning party is much stronger financially than the signing party, it would be worthwhile to have a representation directly from the nonsigning party that the signing party may enter into the agreement on its behalf. In reviewing a contract, providers should be particularly sensitive to the responsibilities of nonparties to the agreement. For example, since most payers administer benefits on behalf of self-insured employer groups, are there assurances that self-insured employers will fulfill their responsibilities under the agreement?

Recitals

A contract will typically contain in rather legalistic prose a series of statements describing who the parties are and what they are trying to accomplish. These statements are called "recitals" and are relatively unimportant because they should not contain substantive contractual obligations. However, MCOs and providers should review these statements to confirm their accuracy and that each party is not assuming any unintended responsibilities.

Table of Contents

Although a table of contents has no legal significance, the reader will be greatly assisted in finding pertinent sections in a long contract. One common failing in contract renegotiations is neglecting to update the table of contents after the contract has been amended.

Definitions

The definitions section of a contract plays an essential role in simplifying the structure and the reader's understanding of a contract. The body of the contract often contains complicated terms that merit amplification and explanation. The use of a definition, although requiring the reader to refer back to an earlier section for a meaning, simplifies greatly the discussion in the body of the agreement. A poorly drafted contract will define unnecessary terms or define terms in a manner that is inconsistent with their use in the body of the agreement.

Defined terms are frequently capitalized in a contract to alert the reader that the word is defined. Definitions are almost essential in many contracts, but their use may complicate the understanding of the agreement. Someone who reads a contract will first read a definition without knowing its significance. Later, when he or she reads the body of the contract, he or she may no longer recall a term's meaning. For this reason, someone reviewing a contract for the first time should read the definitions twice: initially and then in the context of each term's use. Definitions sections tend to err on the side of containing too many definitions. A term that is used only once in a contract need not be defined. On the other hand, a critical reader of a contract will identify instances in which the contract could be improved by the use of additional definitions.

In reviewing a contract, MCOs and providers should not underestimate the importance of the definitions section. A provider's right to payment may depend on how such terms as *emergency, covered services,* or *medical necessity* are defined. Moreover, the population to which the provider is agreeing to furnish services for the rates set forth in the agreement is often defined under terms such as *member, beneficiary,* or *benefit plan.* It is very important to review the definitions section of a contract initially as well as in the context of the terms usage in the body of the contract.

An occasional defect in some contracts is that the drafter includes substantive contract provisions in definitions. A definition is merely an explanation of a meaning of a term and should not contain substantive provisions. This does not mean that a definition that imposes a substantive obligation on a party is invalid. In reviewing a contract, if a party identifies a substantive provision in a definition, the party should ensure that its usage is consistent with the corresponding provision in the body of the contract.

Terms that are commonly defined in a managed care context are *member, subscriber,* or *beneficiary; medical director; provider* and specific types of providers as necessary such as *inpatient facility, ambulatory facility,* and *hospital-employed physicians; payer* and specific types of payer as necessary such as *HMO, PPO,* and *MA plan; physician; primary care physician; emergency; medically necessary* or *medical necessity;* and *utilization review (UR), UM,* and *QM.* Some of these terms, such as *medically necessary,* are very important to readers' understanding of the parties' responsibilities and should be considered carefully in the review of a contract. In many managed care agreements, payers other than the MCO are responsible for payment under the contract. In this case, who a payer is and how they are selected and removed become very important to the provider. The definition of member or enrollee is also important. The contract should convey clearly who is covered under the agreement and whom the MCO can add in the future. The MCO and provider should ensure that these terms are consistent, if appropriate, with those in other contracts (e.g., the group enrollment agreement).

It is important to note that a number of the definitions in the contract may be controlled by state or federal law and may specifically reference such law or laws. For example, Medicare and Medicaid law and a number of state laws set forth a definition of emergency services, and Medicare law and an increasing number of states set forth standards for "medical necessity." And, as noted earlier, states typically have specific requirements around "hold harmless" and "no balance billing" clauses, which may vary depending on the type of payer such as an HMO or PPO. The Patient Protection and Affordable Care Act of 2010 (ACA) also contains certain provisions that qualified health plans must adhere to, although the ACA itself does not require specific contractual language. The contracting parties should be aware of the law and should, at a minimum, ensure that the definitions in the contract are consistent with such law.

■ PROVIDER OBLIGATIONS

The next major section to look at defines the obligations that the provider agrees to contractually.

Provider Qualifications and Credentialing

Provider contracts should include the provider's representations and warranties that the provider meets the managed care plan's applicable requirements for network participation. These representations and warranties should include, at a minimum, that the provider has a valid license, has not been excluded from participation in any federal health care program, and/or, in the case of an institutional provider, meets any relevant accreditation standards and Medicare conditions for participation. As discussed later in this chapter, it is important that the provider be obligated to notify the managed care plan if any of this information changes.

In addition, the contract should include a provision requiring the provider to comply with any of the managed care plan's policies and procedures for credentialing and recredentialing of providers.

Provider Services

Because the purpose of the agreement is to contract for the provision of health services, the description of those services in the contract is important. As mentioned above, the recitation of services to be furnished by the provider could be either set out in the contract or set out in an exhibit or attachment. An exhibit format frequently allows the party more flexibility and administrative simplicity when it amends the exhibited portion of the agreement, particularly when the change requires regulatory approval.

Contracts may use the term *provider services* to denote the range of services that are to be provided under the contract. Contracts frequently broadly define provider services as those services within the licensure, experience, and expertise of the provider. However, as MCOs increasingly look to specialty networks to manage and provide certain services, they may wish to more narrowly define provider services or may wish to retain flexibility to carve out certain services that are generally furnished by a range of providers and have them furnished exclusively through a specialty network.

The contract needs to specify to whom the provider is obligated to furnish services. Although the answer is that the provider furnishes services to covered enrollees, the contract needs to define what is meant by a covered enrollee. This definition is valuable as some payers "rent" their networks to other payers, third-party administrators, and/or self-insured employers, as described in Chapter 4. The definition of covered enrollee might be broader than a provider anticipates. The contract also needs to explain how the provider will learn who is covered and assign the responsibility for payment if services are furnished to a noncovered person. MCOs and providers frequently disagree on this issue. The providers' view is frequently that, if the MCO represented that the individual was covered, the MCO should be responsible for payment. In contrast, the MCO frequently asserts that it should not be responsible for the costs of services provided to noncovered enrollees and that the provider should seek payment directly from the individual. This issue is particularly important when the enrollee population includes Medicaid beneficiaries who are unlikely to be able to pay the provider for services. Oftentimes, the issue is resolved based on relative negotiating strength.

Provider contracts should also cover adequately a number of other provider responsibilities, including their responsibilities to refer or to accept referrals of enrollees, the days and times of days the provider agrees to be available to provide services, and substitute on-call arrangements, if appropriate. Provider contracts may also specify the qualifications necessary for the provider of back-up services when the provider is not available. Some of these requirements may be posed as conditions of participation in public programs, such as the MA program.

If the provider is a hospital, the contract will include language identifying the circumstances in which the MCO agrees to be responsible or not responsible for servicesprovided to nonemergency patients. A fairly common provision in hospital contracts states that the hospital, except in emergencies, must have as a prerequisite before admission the order of the participating physician or other preadmission authorization. The hospital contract also should have an explicit provision requiring that the MCO be notified within a specified period after an emergency admission.

A particularly sensitive issue is whether the MCO's coverage of emergency medical services meets state and/or federal requirements for such coverage. Medicare, Medicaid, the ACA, and a number of state laws require managed care plans to pay for screening and stabilization services in situations in which a prudent layperson reasonably believed that an emergency medical condition existed. A related policy and contracting issue is whether such a law automatically entitles a hospital to payment for performing the initial screen that is required when a patient goes to the emergency room.

A good provider contract should be supplemented by a competent provider relations program to resolve problems that arise and so providers have a means to answer questions about their contract responsibilities. A common example is the opportunity to appeal claim denials by the MCO. Technically, a denial of coverage is only applicable to the member since it is a benefits issue. However, denial of payment based on noncompliance by the provider that has no impact on a member is a different matter.

Nondiscriminatory Requirements

Provider agreements frequently contain clauses obligating the provider to furnish services in the same manner as the provider furnishes services to patients who are not members of the MCO (i.e., not to discriminate on the basis of payment source). In addition, a clause is used to prohibit other types of discrimination on the basis of race, color, sex, age, disability, religion, and national origin. Government contracts may require the use of specific contract language, including a reference to compliance with the Americans with Disabilities Act and the Rehabilitation Act of 1973. As an alternative, the MCO and provider may want to add a second contract clause that requires compliance with all applicable nondiscrimination requirements under federal, state, and local law. These obligations may also apply to subcontractors of the provider.

Compliance with UM and QM Programs

One key factor affecting the success of the MCO is its providers being able and willing to appropriately manage the utilization of services. To do so, the providers need to follow the UM guidelines of the MCO as described in detail in Chapter 7. An exception may be if the provider is assuming substantial financial risk, in which case the provider may be expected to adopt and implement its own UM procedures. The contract needs to set out the provider's responsibilities in carrying out the MCO's UM program.

The MCO's dilemma is how to articulate this obligation in the contract when the UM program may be quite detailed and frequently is updated over time. One option used by a few MCOs is to append the utilization review program to the contract as an exhibit. Another option is merely to incorporate the program by reference or to generally require the provider to comply with the managed care plan's policies and procedures and to include utilization review requirements in those policies and procedures. In either case, it is important for the MCO to ensure that the contract allows it to amend the UM standards in the future without the consent of the provider. If the MCO does not append a cross-referenced standard, the MCO should either give each provider a copy of the guidelines and any amendments, or make the guidelines available through means such as an Internet portal. Without this documentation, the provider might argue that he or she did not agree to the guidelines or subsequent amendments.

The contract needs to inform providers of their responsibilities to cooperate in efforts by the MCO to ensure compliance and the implications of the provider not meeting the guidelines. Contracts differ on whether the MCO is seeking the provider's "cooperation" or "compliance." Providers generally favor an obligation to cooperate rather than to comply with these programs because a requirement to comply with the programs' decisions seems to preclude the right to disagree.

The same basic concepts and principles apply to the provider's acceptance of the MCO's QM program. A few MCOs equate their UM and their QM programs. This attitude not only reflects a misunderstanding of the objectives of the two programs but is likely to engender the concern or criticism of government regulators who view the two programs as being separate. In the last several years, as MCOs have placed greater emphasis on their QM programs, provider compliance responsibilities have correspondingly increased. The contract should include a provision requiring the provider to cooperate both in furnishing information to the MCO and in taking corrective actions to fix deficiencies, if appropriate.

Acceptance of Enrollee Patients

A provider contract, particularly with a physician or physician group, will need a clause to ensure that the provider will accept enrollees regardless of health status. This provision is more important when the payment model uses risk-sharing, as described in Chapter 5, in which the physician has an incentive to dissuade high utilizers from becoming part of his or her panel. Some provider contracts with primary care physicians (PCPs) also include a minimum number of members that the physician will accept into his or her panel (e.g., 250 members). The contract should also include fair and reasonable procedures for allowing the provider to limit or stop new members added to his or her panel (at a point after the provider has accepted at least the minimum number of members initially agreed upon) and a mechanism to notify the MCO when these changes take place. The MCO needs to have data regarding which providers are limiting panel size in order to comply with regulatory requirements concerning access to care.

The contract should also specify the circumstances in which the provider, principally in the case of a PCP, can cease being an enrollee's physician. Examples may be abusive behavior or refusal to follow a recommended course of treatment. This contract language would need to be consistent with language in the member subscriber agreement and in compliance with licensure requirements and/or federal health care program requirements, which frequently identify the grounds in which a physician may end the physician–enrollee relationship.

Provider Network Issues

As described in Chapter 2, PPOs use contracts in which the provider would be a "preferred provider." That meant that enrollees would be given financial incentives to see the provider and the provider would offer a discount to the MCO in exchange for increased patient traffic caused by the financial incentives to use the provider. Such network arrangements are sometimes also called "primary networks."

Some point of service (POS) or narrow-network plans that offer out-of-network coverage may also contract with providers to create a "secondary network" to help contain their costs for services furnished by nonpreferred providers. Similarly, many national or large regional payers have a primary network, but must also address costs for services provided in areas where they do not have a primary network at all. The usual approach they take is to "rent" a network from a national PPO network company, for which they pay an access fee and typically a percentage of the discount, as described in Chapter 4. In other cases, they may contract for access to another commercial insurers network, meaning a network that was not specifically created in order to rent to various payers.

Secondary networks are also known as "wrap" or "complementary networks." A secondary network allows health plans to access discounts when their members receive services from nonpreferred providers (i.e., those not in the plan's primary network). Providers participating in secondary networks have a written contract with an MCO or network administrator obligating them to furnish discounts to organizations with which the MCO or administrator contracts. Secondary network providers are not considered "preferred providers" and their services are usually subject to the "out-of-network" level of coinsurance or copayment under the health plan.

Contractual provisions obligating physicians to participate in such networks have generally not been obvious. Such obligations are frequently keyed to the definition of "enrollees" to whom providers are obligated to provide services at a discounted rate. However, MCOs should be aware that an increasing number of states have adopted legislation that requires plans to clearly specify whether they rent their networks or otherwise allow other organizations to access their provider network discounts.

Another trend in provider network is "tiered networks." MCOs using tiered networks provide financial incentives for enrollees to use a subset of providers in the provider network, for example, by providing for lower cost sharing when an enrollee uses a "tier one" provider as compared to a "tier two" provider. Such an arrangement may allow a MCO to steer enrollees to providers favorable to the organization by having lower costs or providing higher-quality services. In order to allow for the use of a tiered network, an MCO must ensure that its provider contract does not include language that would prohibit it from treating one network provider differently than another. MCOs should carefully consider the criteria they use to assign providers to different tiers. Providers have brought litigation seeking to ensure that such criteria are based on legitimate and objective grounds.

Enrollee Complaints and Appeals

The contract should require the provider to cooperate in resolving enrollee complaints and appeals of benefits coverage denials, and to notify the MCO within a specified period of time when any complaints are conveyed to the provider. Since the ACA and many state licensure laws require specific member denial of coverage appeals processes as described in Chapters 20 and 30, the language in the contract should be written sufficiently broadly to ensure provider cooperation with those procedures.

Maintenance and Retention of Records and Confidentiality

Provider contracts should require the provider to maintain both medical and business records for specified periods of time. For example, these agreements could provide that the records must be maintained in accordance with federal and state laws and consistent with generally accepted business and professional standards as well as whatever other standards are established by the MCO. If the contract contains this general language, it is desirable for the managed care plan to inform its network providers separately of these timeframes. Furthermore, if the MCO participates in any public or private payer program that establishes certain specific records retention requirements, those requirements should be conveyed to the providers. The contract should state that these obligations survive the termination of the contract.

The MCO also needs a legal right to have access to books and records. The contract will want to state that the MCO, its representatives, and government agencies have the right to inspect, review, and make or obtain copies of medical, financial, and administrative records. The provider would want the availability of this information to be limited to services rendered to enrollees, and during normal business hours. The issue of reasonable notice may also be addressed; providers will want reasonable notice for any inspection of records, but payers will want the ability to access records with little or no notice for purposes of auditing suspect claims. A potential compromise might define reasonable notice under different conditions. The cost of performing these services is often an issue of controversy. If there are no fees for copying these records, the contract should so state. When the MCO is acting on behalf of other payers, it is desirable to have language acknowledging that the other payers have agreed to comply with applicable confidentiality laws.

In addition to the availability of books or records, the MCO might also want the right to require the provider to prepare reports identifying statistical and descriptive medical and patient data and other identifying information as specified by the MCO. If such a provision is included in the contract, the MCO should inform the provider of the types of reports it might request to minimize any future problems. Finally, the provider should be obligated to provide information that is necessary for compliance with state or federal law. A related provision almost always included in provider contracts is a requirement that the provider maintain the confidentiality of medical records.

An often neglected legal issue is how the MCO obtains the authority to access medical records. Provider agreements periodically contain an acknowledgment by the provider that the MCO is authorized to receive medical records. The problem with this approach is that the MCO might not have the right to have access to this information and, if it does not, an acknowledgment of that right in the contract has no legal effect. While the Federal Health Insurance Portability and Accessibility Act (HIPAA; see Chapter 29) gives providers and managed care plans the right to use and disclose protected health information (PHI) for purposes of treatment, payment, and health care operations without obtaining individual authorization, some state laws may limit the right that insurers and HMOs, as payers, may have to access medical records.

It is also important to remember that HIPAA requires that only the minimum necessary PHI to achieve the intended task be used or disclosed; in other words, the different types of PHI may be required for a claims review, a disease or case management program, peer review, and quality management (see Chapters 3, 5, 8, and 14). MCOs should review their state law provisions, and any applicable federal law provisions, on these issues and their plans' procedures for obtaining the appropriate consents of their members to have access to this information. Many MCOs obtain this information through signatures that are part of the initial enrollment materials. These consents could also be obtained at the time health services are rendered. MCOs and providers need to be particularly sensitive to confidentiality concerns with regard to minors, incompetents, and persons with communicable diseases for which there are specific state confidentiality statutes governing disclosure of information.

MCOs and their providers should also be aware of any agreements that might further limit their ability to use or disclose information regarding enrollees or patients. For example, MA plans enter into a data use agreement with the Centers for Medicare and Medicaid Services (CMS) that limits their ability to use or disclose information obtained from CMS for the purpose of administering the MCO's MA contract. Thus, an MA plan faces restrictions that go beyond those set forth in HIPAA and state law.

If an MCO delegates to a provider responsibilities other than simply furnishing health care services to its members and the MCO is disclosing to the provider protected health information or the provider is obtaining such information on the MCO's behalf, the contract between the parties must include a "business associate agreement." Under HIPAA, a business associate agreement is required if a party will perform services involving the use or disclosure of PHI on behalf of an entity subject to the HIPAA provisions concerning privacy and security of PHI (known as a covered entity). Such services may include, but are not limited to, credentialing or claims processing, tasks often performed by IPAs. Due to limits the ACA places on the percentage of premium that may be used for sales, governance, administration, and profit or surplus, payers may increase the amount of delegation to providers when such delegation would be considered a medical cost. Both health care providers and managed care plans are covered entities under HIPAA. Furthermore, recent amendments to HIPAA make business associates directly subject to HIPAA provisions. A model business associate agreement is included at the end of this chapter.

■ **PAYMENT**

The payment terms of the agreement often represent the most important provision for both the provider and the MCO. As mentioned earlier, payment terms are frequently set forth in an exhibit appended to the contract and are cross-referenced in the body of the agreement. A number of payment issues should be covered in the contract; for example, who will collect the copayments. Another issue concerns the MCO's payment responsibilities for uncovered services. A provision needs to state that unauthorized or uncovered services are not the responsibility of the MCO. To avoid members receiving unexpected bills from providers for noncovered services, contracts may say that in order to bill a member for noncovered services, the provider must first inform the member that a service will not be covered by the health plan prior to providing the service. Moreover, to avoid any debates about whether a member was informed that the service would not be covered, the best practice is to require the provider to obtain the member's written acknowledgment of financial liability before the services are rendered. In addition, the contract will frequently contain a provision that precludes the provider from ever billing an enrollee when the MCO has determined that the service is not medically necessary. Such a provision may be required by state law.

From the provider's perspective, he or she needs a clear understanding of what is necessary for a service to be authorized. If the provider submits claims to the MCO, the contract should set out the manner in which the claim is to be made and either identify the information to be provided in the claim or give the MCO the right to designate or revise that information in the future. If the contract specifies the information to be included in a claim, the MCO should also have the unilateral right to make changes in the future. If the provider submits claims electronically, both the provider and the MCO will be obligated to comply with the provisions of HIPAA concerning standard transactions, as discussed in Chapters 18 and 23.

The agreement should also obligate the provider to submit claims within a specified period and the MCO to pay claims within a certain number of days. The latter requirement should not apply to contested claims, claims that have errors, duplicate claims, or claims that are missing required data. The parties should ensure that the number of days for claims payment set forth in the contract is consistent with any applicable state or federal laws regulating such payment. While MA law does not set forth a specific timeframe in which contracting providers must be paid, it does require that MA plans set forth in their provider contracts a "prompt payment" provision as negotiated by the contracting parties.

The contract needs also to address reconciliations to account for overpayments or underpayments. There are a number of reasons that an MCO may wish to recoup previously paid amounts from a provider; for example, the payment amount was incorrectly calculated or the plan discovered that the individual was not eligible to be a member of a health plan at the time the service was rendered. A provider may also request additional payment if the provider determines that it has been underpaid by the MCO. A number of states have laws limiting the time period during which an MCO can recoup previously paid amounts from its providers or providers can request additional payment. Even in instances where such laws are not applicable, the contract should set forth the period during which a reconciliation or recoupment may be requested, in order for the parties to avoid liability for claims they thought were settled years ago. Provider contracts frequently provide that the MCO can subtract overpayments to providers from amounts due to the provider. From a provider's perspective, it is important that the contract require the managed care plan to provide prior notice of its intent to recoup, specifying the basis for the recoupment and notifying the provider they may appeal a recoupment decision.

Risk-Sharing Arrangements*

The most complex aspects of provider contracts are often the risk-sharing arrangements such as those discussed in Chapter 5, and which are typically done only by HMOs. However, various incentive programs have come and gone over the years that may be used by payers other than HMOs. The concept of risk-sharing has become even more complex with the passage of the ACA. Payment reform in the traditional Medicare fee-for-service (FFS) program was already underway by CMS, beginning with a pilot program for patient-centered medical homes (PCMHs), when the ACA was passed. But the ACA provided a significant boost to it by authorizing accountable care organizations (ACOs), and by creating the Center for Medicare and Medicaid Innovation and the Independent Medicare Advisory Board, all of which are discussed in Chapter 30. Under the applicable provisions in the ACA, several of the payment reform approaches contain elements of risk-sharing for traditional FFS Medicare, and commercial payers, both HMOs and non-HMOs, are looking to adopt them as well. Therefore, while the rest of this section specifically addresses provisions in a risk-sharing contract between an HMO and a provider, elements may apply to new payment models as well. At the time of publication, CMS had issued the final rule for only one of these payment models, the ACO shared savings model for the traditional Medicare FFS program. The reader is referred to Chapters 2 and 3 for a discussion on the structure and governance of ACOs, and to Chapter 5 for a description of payment under shared savings.

Risk can be shared with providers in significantly varying degrees depending on the initial amount of risk transferred, the services for which the provider is at risk, and whether the HMO offers stop-loss protection. Risk pools with complicated formulas determining distributions are frequently used when services are capitated or when payments are based on a fee schedule with or without withholds. Although the primary objective of these arrangements is to align incentives to discourage unnecessary utilization, the complexity of many of these arrangements can confuse providers and engender distrust when their distribution falls below expectations. For that reason, some HMOs that had complex risk-sharing arrangements revised them to be simpler and more understandable. If the risk-sharing approach is complex, the provider's understanding will be greatly enhanced by the use of examples that illustrate for providers the total payments they will receive in different scenarios.

HMOs should be aware of and comply with any state and/or federal laws that regulate risk-sharing arrangements.

---

*Risk-sharing payment methodologies such as capitation, withholds, risk pools, stop loss, and the like are all described in Chapter 5. If the reader is not familiar with any of these terms, it may be useful to return to this section after reading that chapter.

For example, Medicare and Medicaid HMO-based plans must comply with the requirements for physician incentive plans (PIPs). The PIP requirements impose stop-loss obligations on when payment arrangements for the provision of services to Medicare or Medicaid beneficiaries put a physician or physician group at risk for more than 25% of total potential payments for services the physician or group does not directly provide (i.e., referral services); under federal laws, this is considered to be a significant financial risk (SFR). (Details are provided in Chapter 5.) Moreover, managed care plans providing services to commercial enrollees with Medicare as a secondary payer may also need to comply with PIP obligations in order to qualify for an exception from the compensation prohibitions under the personal services exception to the federal physician self-referral law.

Risk-Sharing and Integrated Delivery Systems

In some situations, an HMO capitates an integrated delivery system (IDS; see Chapter 2) to provide all or a substantial portion of the IDSs' health care services. In developing these relationships, the parties need to identify very carefully the obligations of the IDS. The agreement needs to clearly identify the services that will be covered and not be covered under the agreement. A variety of other specific issues must also be carefully defined as well as any exceptions. Very importantly, if the IDS is made up of a hospital and private physicians rather than employed physicians, the contract must be clear as to the obligations of the various parties and how payments will actually be made, as well as who will make them. Global or bundled payment methodologies in which a single payment is made for the combined hospital and physician services should be approached in a similar manner. (Details on these and other specific issues are found in Chapters 4 and 5.)

Pay for Performance

For many years now, payers have been using pay for performance (P4P) to pay incentives to providers based on their performance on specified measures. Performance measures can be based on a range of measures including the Healthcare Effectiveness Data and Information Set (HEDIS®; see Chapter 15) scores. They may also include measures of patient satisfaction such as the Consumer Assessment of Healthcare Providers and Systems (CAHPS®; see Chapter 15) from the Agency for Healthcare Research and Quality used by Medicare and HEDIS. MA plans are particularly incented to reward their participating providers for performance as those organizations can increase their revenue by scoring high on CMS plan performance measures, referred to as the Stars program (see Chapter 24). P4P is discussed in detail in Chapter 5, and whatever details are applicable are to be addressed in the contract.

Because P4P programs change regularly, they are usually addressed through an appendix rather than the body of the contract. The terms should balance the payer's ability to refine the measurement mechanisms as information on P4P evolves. However, it should provide enough information for the provider to predict the potential range of payment and the general types of measures on which the payment will depend.

Value-Based Payment

Value-based payment (VBP) is specifically written into the ACA for traditional FFS Medicare. For that reason, some commercial payers have been implementing it as well. VBP is described in Chapter 5, but in general it is a form of risk and incentive payment to both a hospital and physicians that is based on defined performance for specific conditions such as heart attack or community-acquired pneumonia. Measures include overall inpatient costs, early or preventable readmissions, and overall episode of care or condition costs, all adjusted for level of illness. In this way it is similar to P4P; what sets it apart from P4P is the presence of a risk corridor instead of only an incentive plan.

VBP terms in contracts between commercial payers and providers should be approached in a similar manner to P4P or bundled pricing. If it is applied to all payments, then it is best addressed like any risk-sharing arrangement. At the time of publication, CMS had not yet finalized any rules or regulations for VBP, so little else can be said about it here.

Coordination of Benefits, Other-Party Liability, and Subrogation

This is generally referred to a coordination of benefits (COB) and other party liability (OPL), as described in Chapter 18. COB and OPL is best addressed using a balanced approach. The provider should be required to inquire about whether or not the patient has coverage from any other insurers, and transmit that information to the MCO under defined circumstances such as an inpatient admission. A claim subject to COB or OPL would allow for a 2-month period for collection from the purported primary carrier after submission. If unsuccessful, the MCO would pay while awaiting resolution of the dispute. COB is discussed again later in this chapter.

Provider contracts should contain provisions to address situations in which a party other than the enrollee or MCO is financially responsible for all or part of the services provided to an enrollee. There are three forms, as described in detail in Chapter 18:

- COB in which a plan member also has coverage through another health plan;
- OPL in which a plan member's medical costs are the responsibility of a non–health insurer such as workers' compensation or an automobile insurance policy; and
- Subrogation in which a managed care plan is entitled to recovery of medical costs it has already paid for, but which were included in the calculation of a damages

award in a lawsuit. Subrogation is typically not an issue in payer–provider contracts, however.

Such provisions should set forth the provider's obligation to assist the MCO in identifying other parties that are responsible for paying for, or providing, services to an enrollee. In addition, the provision should identify the party with the responsibility for billing another payer and indicate the party to which the payment belongs. Some MCOs allow their providers to collect and keep third-party recoveries, whereas others will require that the information be reported and deducted. Often, the specific procedure depends on how the provider is paid (e.g., on an FFS basis, a capitation basis, or by some other mechanism).

A sensitive issue is the potential liability of an MCO if a provider collects from Medicare inappropriately when the MCO had primary responsibility under the Medicare secondary payer rules. This applies primarily to non-MA plans since MA plans typically do not encounter this situation. Under CMS regulations, the MCO is legally responsible and may be forced to pay back CMS even if the payment was received by the provider without the knowledge of the MCO. MCOs should include a contract provision transferring the ultimate financial liability to the provider in this circumstance.

Another issue that should be addressed in the contract is the responsibility of the MCO as a secondary carrier when the provider is paid by the primary carrier. The payment may be an amount greater than the amount the provider would have received from the MCO, or it may be less, and may include cost-sharing on the patient's part. A general set of rules was created by the National Association of Insurance Commissioners (NAIC), and while those rules are not laws, they are typically followed by most payers. Some states also have specific laws pertaining to COB, OPL, and subrogation, and a contract should comply with the applicable regulations. In the absence of a state law, and because state laws about COB and OPL do not apply to self-funded benefits plans in any event, the contract should address payment policies in cases of COB and OPL.

HOLD HARMLESS AND NO BALANCE BILLING CLAUSES

Virtually all provider contracts contain a hold harmless clause under which the provider agrees not to sue or assert any claims against the enrollee for services provided that are covered under the contract, but not paid for by the plan, even if the MCO becomes insolvent or otherwise fails to meet its obligations, as discussed in Chapters 2 and 4.

A related no balance billing clause, if separate in the contract, applies to the amount of the payment, also called the allowed charge, as discussed in Chapters 4 and 5. The no

balance billing clause prohibits the provider from billing a member for any difference between billed charges and the allowed charge. It does not prohibit billing for any applicable cost-sharing such as deductibles or coinsurance, or for non-covered services such as cosmetic surgery. For example, if a contracted physician charges $100 for a visit but the health plan's fee schedule pays $70, the physician may not bill the member for the $30 difference between the two. Many contracts combine hold harmless and no balance billing in the same clause since the hold harmless provision applies equally to the difference between payment of the allowed charge and the billed charge. Further details on payment terms that relate to no balance billing are provided in Chapter 5.

State insurance departments (or other agencies having regulatory oversight in this area) typically will not approve a provider contract form without inclusion of hold harmless and no balance billing clauses, and frequently require specific language. Providers under contract that do not contain these clauses are also typically not considered to be network providers by regulators, meaning they cannot be listed in a health plan's directory as participating providers or as meeting access requirements further discussed in Chapter 4. CMS also requires these clauses for MA plans, using model language created by the NAIC.

RELATIONSHIP OF THE PARTIES

Provider contracts usually contain a provision stating that the MCO and the provider have an independent contractual arrangement. The purpose for this provision is to refute an assertion that the provider serves as an employee of the MCO. The reason is that under the legal theory of respondeat superior the MCO would automatically be liable for the negligent acts of its employees. Although MCOs typically include a provision such as this in their provider contracts, it may or may not be of value. In a lawsuit against the MCO by an enrollee alleging malpractice, a court or jury may consider other factors, as can occur in any civil suit.

A related clause frequently used in provider contracts states that nothing contained in the agreement shall be construed to require physicians to recommend any procedure or course of treatment that physicians deem professionally inappropriate. This clause is intended, in part, to affirm that the MCO is not engaged in the practice of medicine and to protect the MCO from liability arising from a provider's negligence.

USE OF NAME AND PROPRIETARY INFORMATION

Many provider contracts limit the ability of either party to use the name of the other. This is done by identifying the circumstances in which the party's name may or may not be used. Contract clauses may allow the MCO the right to use the name of the provider in the provider directory or other documents listing the plan's participating providers. They may furnish the provider with the right to advise patients of their affiliation with the health plan. Since health plans and providers usually contract in order to do business together, a mutual agreement to use each other's name, marks, and signs for purposes of marketing and sales is common.

An agreement allowing use of the name of the other party should be clear that any use of the name does not mean one party is representing or speaking on behalf of the other, although that may be addressed through the relationship of the parties clause just discussed. Beyond these uses and limitations, one party needs the written approval of the other party to use the name and any symbol, trademark, and service mark of the entity.

In addition, the MCO and the provider will want to ensure that proprietary information is protected. The contract should require that the provider keep all information about the MCO confidential and prohibit the use of the information for any competitive purpose after the contract is terminated. This typically applies to all terms for which there are no legal or regulatory disclosure requirements.

■ NOTIFICATION

The MCO needs to ensure that it is advised of a number of important changes that affect the ability of the provider to meet his or her contractual obligations. The contract should identify the information that needs to be conveyed to the MCO and the timeframes for providing that information.

For example, a physician might be required to notify an MCO within 5 days or less upon loss or suspension of his or her license or certification, loss or restriction of hospital privileges, issuance of any formal charges brought by a government agency, change in or loss of liability insurance coverage, and/or the initiation of a civil action by an enrollee. Although specific events should be identified in the contract, a broad catch-all category should also be included, such as an event that if sustained would materially impair the provider's ability to perform the duties under the contract. The contract should require immediate notification if the provider is sanctioned under a federal health care program. If an MA or managed Medicaid plan contracts with a provider who has been sanctioned, or continues to have a sanctioned provider in its network, the plan may be subject to penalties or even removal from the program. In a hospital contract, the corresponding provisions would be when the hospital suffers from a change that materially impairs its ability to provide services or if action is taken against it regarding certifications, licenses, or federal agencies or private accrediting bodies.

The provider should ensure that the contract requires the plan to provide prior notification of any substantive changes to policies and procedures with which the provider is bound to comply, for example, to the plan's provider manual for other than trivial changes not affecting the provider. Similar to notification provisions for providers, plans must typically notify providers if it becomes financially impaired or has lost its license.

The contract should specify for each party the manner and the place where any notices required under the contract must be sent. The typical information includes:

- Address used as the primary business address;
- Fax number, if applicable;
- E-mail address used for business, preferably an address capable of receiving secure e-mails; and
- Website address.

In the past, many contracts required delivery to be made by registered first class mail to the attention of a specific person or department. Delivery of hard copy may also be allowed for a delivery service that obtains a signature on receipt. With the expansion of electronic communications, MCOs and providers may secure e-mail that also provides for acknowledgment of receipt.

■ INSURANCE AND INDEMNIFICATION

Insurance provisions in contracts are fairly straightforward. The obligations in the contract may be for both professional liability coverage and general liability coverage. The MCO wants to ensure that the provider has resources to pay for any eventuality. The contract will state particular insurance limits, provide that the limits will be set forth in a separate attachment, or leave it up to the MCO to specify. A hospital agreement may require only that the limits be commensurate with limits contained in policies of similar hospitals in the state. From the MCO's perspective, it will probably want a specific requirement in order to ensure adequate levels of insurance. A provision should also be included requiring the provider to notify the MCO of any notification of cancellations of the policy. Another needed notification in a physician context is notification of any malpractice claims. From the provider's perspective, it is also important to ensure that the MCO maintains adequate insurance to cover its liabilities.

Cross-indemnification provisions in which each party indemnifies the other for damages caused by the other party are common in contracts. These clauses may also be used to assign to the losing party the responsibility to pay attorneys' fees of the prevailing party. One weakness of the cross-indemnification clause is that some professional liability carriers will not pay for claims arising from these clauses because of general exclusions in their policies for contractual claims. Although these clauses are frequently used, this limitation and the fact that the provider and the plan should still be liable for their own negligent acts suggest that these indemnification clauses are not essential.

■ TERM, SUSPENSION, AND TERMINATION

One section of most contracts identifies the term of the contract and the term of any subsequent contract renewals. Many contracts have automatic renewal provisions if no party exercises its right to terminate within a specified time period before the renewal date. In some cases, the contracts do not technically renew since they remain in force until one or the other party gives notice of cancellation; this is referred to as an "evergreen" contract, and rather than define a renewal date, it only defines termination terms. This is most often the case with physician contracts.

Hospital contracts typically renew automatically every year, but payment rates change upon renewal, and only for a defined period of time. Given how lengthy the negotiating process is these days, and the number of contracts that hospitals and MCOs both must manage, it is common to negotiate multiyear terms, usually by negotiating the payment rates for the first year, and then a multiplier for each subsequent year. Three years is a common time period for payment rates in multiyear hospital contracts.

Some contracts give a right of suspension to the MCO. In suspension, the contract continues, but the provider loses specific rights. For example, if a provider fails to follow UM protocols a specified number of times, the provider will not be assigned new members or perhaps will receive a reduction in the amount of payment. The advantage of a suspension provision is that total termination of a contract might be counterproductive for the MCO, but a suspension might be sufficiently punitive to persuade the provider to improve.

Termination provisions fall into two categories: termination without cause and termination with cause. From the MCO's perspective, the value of having a termination without cause provision is that the MCO need not defend a challenge by the provider on the substantive issue of whether the specified grounds for termination were met. From a provider's perspective, it allows a provider to get out of the agreement when the provider is unhappy with how the contract is administered but there has been no specific breach of the contract's terms.

One important issue is when the contract may be terminated. Some contracts allow termination without cause only upon the end of the contract's term, which is seen more often in contracts with hospitals and far less often in physician contracts. Other contracts allow it following notification by the terminating party. A common notice period is 90 days for termination without cause. However, it

is important to note a number of issues: Is it possible to terminate without cause during the first term of the contract? Can the contract be terminated at any time or only at the end of a term when 90 days' notice is provided prior to the renewal date? In addition, state or federal law may affect a managed care plan's ability or procedures for terminating without cause. For example, the Medicare Advantage regulations require at least 60 days' prior notice before terminating without cause. If the MCO has the right to terminate without cause, frequently the provider will also be given that right.

Another related issue to be aware of is the terms that survive termination of the agreement. For example, some state laws require providers to continue to provide services for a specified period of time after their contract has terminated. Such provisions commonly apply where the providers is furnishing a course or treatment to an individual with a terminal or chronic illness or to a pregnant woman. Such provisions are intended to ensure continuity of care for persons being treated by a provider at the time of the provider's termination.

Continuation of care requirements may also relate to the state's requirements for the MCO to have protections against insolvency and have to be reflected in the contract. If a managed care plan includes a requirement to continue care in the contract, it should ensure that the provider will continue meeting the contractual requirements with regard to the services for which the plan continues to cover after the termination. Specifically, the provider must continue to meet the managed care plan's hold harmless requirements, reporting requirements, and QM requirements.

Terminations with cause may allow the health plan to terminate faster and should be used in situations where the MCO needs to act quickly. The contract might establish two different categories: one for immediate termination upon notice and another for termination 30 days after written notice is provided. Many contracts give either party a right to cure any contract violations during the notification period prior to termination. This time period, although useful to an MCO if it has allegedly violated the agreement, extends the period of time before a contract termination is effective. Grounds for termination of a provider for cause other than immediate may be temporary loss of hospital privileges, breach of contract, failure to meet accreditation and credentialing requirements, failure to provide services to enrollees in a professionally acceptable manner, bankruptcy, and refusal to accept an amendment to the contract agreement.

A provision allowing for termination if the provider takes any actions or makes any communications that undermine or could undermine the confidence of enrollees in the quality of care provided by the MCO may be included in a provider contract. However, a managed care plan should be aware that such provisions are sensitive and may be interpreted as a "gag clause." So-called gag clauses, which supposedly prohibited physicians from fully discussing a patient's treatment options and medical conditions, are prohibited under federal health care programs and a number of state laws.* If the managed care plan elects to use such a provision, the clause should make clear that the intent is to prohibit disparagement of the managed care plan and that a physician remains free to advise his or her patients regarding all medically indicated treatment options, regardless of whether such treatments are covered under the managed care plan, to discuss the patient's medical condition and to make medical recommendations within the scope of the provider's licensure.

The contract should be clear that a provider, upon termination, is required to cooperate in the orderly transfer of enrollee care, including records, to other providers. The provider also should agree to cooperate in resolving any disputes. Finally, the provider should continue to furnish services under the terms of the contract until the services being rendered to enrollees are complete or the MCO has made appropriate provisions for another provider to assume the responsibility. The contract should also be clear that the provider is entitled to compensation for performing these services. In general, too little consideration has been given to preparing for contract terminations. When the provider and the MCO enter into a contract, little thought is given to what will occur when the contract ends. Often, relationships end acrimoniously, and it is in both parties' best-interest to consider how their interests will be protected in the event the contract is terminated.

The contract should give the managed care plan the right to immediately terminate the contract upon the occurrence of certain events including the provider's loss of licensure or accreditation; a significant restriction on their license, including their Drug Enforcement Agency permit to prescribe or dispense controlled medications; commitment of a felony; or exclusion from a federal health care program. A good contracting practice is to include a general provision, which allows for immediate termination of the contract if, in the opinion of the MCO, continuation of the contract would endanger the health or well-being of the managed care plan's members. Such a clause would allow the MCO the flexibility to terminate the contract immediately in the case of an unforeseen contingency of sufficient gravity to endanger the managed care plan's enrollees.

Medicare Advantage law requires an MA plan to furnish physicians with detailed written notice of an adverse participation decision (i.e., a termination or suspension) and the right to appeal. The notice must specify the grounds for the action and the majority of the panel that decides the appeal must be peers of the affected physician. Some states also have laws furnishing providers with the right to appeal MCO terminations and set forth requirements for such appeal procedures.

■ "FLOW DOWN" CLAUSES AND PROVIDER SUBCONTRACTS

A managed care plan may be obligated to "flow down" certain clauses that are included in the contract between the managed care plan and the payer. For example, if a MCO has a contract with the federal government or a state Medicaid agency, the managed care plan is obligated to include in its provider contracts or policies a clause recognizing that the payments the provider receives from the managed care plan to provide services to enrollees under the applicable federal health care program are, in whole or part, from federal funds and that the provider and any of its subcontractors are therefore subject to certain laws that are applicable to individuals and entities receiving federal funds, including but not limited to Title VI of the Civil Rights Act of 1964, the Age Discrimination Act of 1975, the Rehabilitation Act of 1973, and the Americans with Disabilities Act. The managed care plan should be aware of any contract provisions that must be "flowed down" to its contractors. Moreover, the managed care plan should carefully note whether those provisions must be included in the contracts of all downstream providers, meaning subcontractors entering into agreements to provide services to the MCO's members.

In addition to clauses that must be "flowed down" from the plan/payer contract, if a provider will be a subcontractor to another provider that contracts directly with the managed care plan, the contract between the managed care plan and the first-tier provider should include a provision that sets forth the requirements that must be included in the downstream subcontracts. This provision may set forth the terms of the provider's contract that must be included in any of the provider's subcontracts. Medicare Advantage policy specifically identifies a number of contract provisions that must be included in downstream contracts to provide services to members of MA plans. Managed care plans should make sure that they comply with similar requirements under other federal or state law.

In addition, if the provider will be subcontracting, the contract should specify whether the managed care plan or the provider will credential any subcontracting providers. If the managed care plan delegates its credentialing

---

*Recall from Chapter 1 that in 1997 at the request of the U.S. Senate, the General Accountability Office (GAO) reviewed 1,150 physician contracts from 529 HMOs and could not find a single instance of a gag clause or any reported court cases providing guidance on what constitutes a gag clause [GAO HEHS-97-175 HMO Gag Clauses]. Still, a clause preventing disparagement must be carefully written nevertheless.

function, it should generally state the standards under which the provider will be credentialing its subcontractors. The managed care plan may want to reserve the right to approve, suspend, or deny the participation of any of the provider's subcontractors. Medicare Advantage law requires MA plans to reserve this right and to specify it in their contracts.

DECLARATIONS

In declarations, the parties provide answers to a number of "what if" questions. These clauses are common to all contracts.

A force majeure clause relieves a party of responsibility if an event occurs beyond its control. In a provider contract this instance is more likely to arise if the provider is no longer able to provide services. In considering force majeure clauses, the parties need to distinguish between events that are beyond a party's control and those that disadvantage a party but for which the party should still be obligated to perform the contract's responsibilities.

A choice of law provision identifies the law that will apply in the event of a dispute. Absent a violation of public policy in the state in question, a court will apply the agreed-upon law. Frequently, lawyers draft contracts using the state in which their client is located without consideration of the advantages and disadvantages of the underlying law. In provider contracts where the MCO and the provider are located in the same state, this clause has little relevance.

A merger clause specifies that only the language in the agreement shall constitute the contract. Such a clause prevents a party from arguing that oral conversations or other documents not included in the contract modify the contract's terms.

A provision allowing or not allowing parties to assign their rights is frequently included in contracts. Provider contracts usually prohibit a provider from assigning its rights under a contract. Some contracts are silent on the right of the MCO to assign the contract. Silence would generally allow the MCO to assign the contract. An option is to allow the MCO to assign the contract only to an affiliate or a successor without the written consent of the provider.

A clause identifying how the contract will be amended is almost always included in a provider contract. A contract will frequently give the MCO the unilateral right to amend the contract absent an objection by the provider. This procedure is valuable to the MCO if it has a large provider panel and it is administratively difficult to obtain the signatures of all the providers. If a provider is unwilling to accept such a broad term, an MCO may wish to address potential administrative difficulties by including a clause to allow for amendment through notice to the provider if the amendment is required in order to comply with applicable state or federal law.

A severability clause allows the contract to continue if a court invalidates a portion of the contract. This is a common provision in a contract, but it is unlikely that the problem will arise. Contracts also set forth a notice requirement identifying how notices are provided to parties and to whom. The manner in which notice is provided is important. If a notice requires that the communication be conveyed by certified mail with return receipt requested, an alternative form of delivery is not valid. Parties should consider what is administratively feasible before agreeing on how notice will be given.

CLOSING

Both parties need to confirm that the parties identified at the beginning of the contract are the parties that sign the contract. Also, if a corporation is one of the parties, the signatory needs to be authorized on behalf of the corporation to sign the agreement.

CONCLUSION

The provider contract establishes the foundation for the working relationship between the MCO and the provider. A good contract is well organized and clearly written and accurately reflects the full intentions of the parties. In drafting and reviewing provider contracts, the MCO and the provider need to keep in mind their objectives in entering the relationship, the relationship of this contract to other provider contracts and agreements, and applicable regulatory requirements.

APPENDICES

The appendices to this chapter contain two sample provider contracts and a sample business associate agreement. The business associate agreement is necessary when the plan delegates to the provider services beyond the provision of care that require access to identifiable health information. Such services may include credentialing or claims payment. In the sample provider contracts, the authors have annotated each contract to point out strengths and weaknesses of the provisions. Both provider contracts are based on an HMO since those tend to be the most complex. Non-HMO plans typically have similar terms and conditions, but do not require HMO-only clauses such as that pertaining to a PCP panel size. These two contracts are provided for illustrative purposes and are not represented as ideal agreements.

■ APPENDIX 6-1: SAMPLE PHYSICIAN AGREEMENT

AGREEMENT BETWEEN

_____

HEALTH MAINTENANCE ORGANIZATION

And

_____

PRIMARY CARE PHYSICIAN

THIS AGREEMENT, made and entered into the date set forth on the signature page hereto, by and between _____, a health maintenance organization [Alternative: _____, Inc., a _____corporation] (hereinafter referred to as "HMO"), which is organized and operated as a health maintenance organization under the laws of the State of _____ and the individual physician or group practice identified on the signature page hereto (hereinafter referred to as "Primary Care Physician").

WHEREAS, HMO desires to operate a health maintenance organization pursuant to the laws of the State of _____;

WHEREAS, Primary Care Physician is a duly licensed physician (or if Primary Care Physician is a legal entity, the members of such entity are duly licensed physicians) in the State of _____, whose license(s) is (are) without limitation or restriction;[*] and

WHEREAS, HMO has as an objective of the development and expansion of cost-effective means of delivering quality health services to Members, as defined herein, particularly through prepaid health care plans, and Primary Care Physician concurs in, actively supports, and will contribute to the achievement of this objective; and

WHEREAS, HMO and Primary Care Physician mutually desire to enter into an Agreement whereby the Primary Care Physician shall provide and coordinate the health care services to Members of HMO.

NOW, THEREFORE, in consideration of the premises and mutual covenants herein contained and other good and valuable consideration, it is mutually covenanted and agreed by and between the parties hereto as follows.

[*] Although there is nothing wrong with having a statement here that the PCP's license is not restricted, the body of the contract, as is the case in this contract in Section IV.H, needs to contain this requirement and provide that the failure to maintain the license is grounds for termination.

PART I. DEFINITIONS

A. Covered Services means those health services and benefits to which Members are entitled under the terms of an applicable Evidence of Coverage which may be amended by HMO from time to time.[†]

B. Emergency Services means those Medically Necessary services provided in connection with an "Emergency," defined as a sudden or unexpected onset of a condition requiring medical or surgical care which the Member secures after the onset of such condition (or as soon thereafter as care can be made available but which in any case not later than twenty-four (24) hours after onset) and in the absence of such care the Member could reasonably be expected to suffer serious physical impairment or death. Heart attacks, severe chest pain, cardiovascular accidents, hemorrhaging, poisonings, major burns, loss of consciousness, serious breathing difficulties, spinal injuries, shock, and other acute conditions as HMO shall determine are Emergencies.[‡]

C. Encounter Form or Electronically Transmitted Data means a record of services provided by Primary Care Physician to Members in a format acceptable to the HMO.[§]

D. Evidence of Coverage means a contract issued by HMO to a Member or an employer of Members specifying the services and benefits available under the HMO's prepaid health benefits program.[¶]

[†] This definition notes the HMO's right to revise the covered services that the PCP is required to provide. If the physicians were capitated for those services, a mechanism would need to be available to revise the capitation rate accordingly. Furthermore, if the HMO wishes to "carve out" any services for provision by a specialty network, the HMO may wish to list in an attachment the range of covered services it authorizes the physician to provide or the exceptions from those services within the physician's licensure.

[‡] The definition for emergency services would be coordinated with the definition used in the HMO's group enrollment agreement. In many instances, the definition of emergency services is regulated under state or federal law and may set forth a prudent layperson standard for determining whether an emergency medical condition exists. Examples are a useful method of illustrating the types of conditions that are considered emergencies. Some contracts will exclude deliveries during the last month of pregnancy while the mother is traveling outside the service area.

[§] By stating that the encounter form must be acceptable to the HMO, the contract allows the HMO to change its requirements in the future. Electronically transmitted data refers to the use of electronic transactions that conform to standards required under HIPAA.

[¶] If the provider's obligation to furnish services under the agreement is not limited to HMO enrollees (e.g., covered persons under an administrative services only [ASO] arrangement with a self-insured employer or other HMOs to which the organization subcontracts its network providers), this definition would have to be written more broadly and conforming changes would need to be made to the agreement.

E. Health Professionals means doctors of medicine, doctors of osteopathy, doctors of podiatric medicine, dentists, nurses, chiropractors, optometrists, physician assistants, clinical psychologists, social workers, pharmacists, occupational therapists, physical therapists, and other professionals engaged in the delivery of health services who are licensed, practice under an institutional license, or are certified or practice under other authority consistent with the laws of the State of _____.

F. Medical Director means a physician designated by HMO to monitor and review the provision of Covered Services to Members.

G. Medically Necessary services and/or supplies means the use of services or supplies as provided by a hospital, skilled nursing facility, physician, or other provider that are required to identify or treat a Member's illness or injury and that, as determined by HMO's Medical Director or its utilization review committee, are: (1) consistent with the symptoms or diagnosis and treatment of the Member's condition, disease, ailment, or injury; (2) appropriate with regard to standards of good medical practice; (3) not solely for the convenience of the Member, his or her physician, hospital, or other health care provider; and (4) the most appropriate supply or level of service which can be safely provided to the Member.[*] When specifically applied to an inpatient Member, it further means that the Member's medical symptoms or condition requires that the diagnosis or treatment cannot be safely provided to the Member as an outpatient.[†]

H. Member means both a Subscriber and his or her eligible family members.[‡]

I. Participating Physician means a physician who, at the time of providing or authorizing services to a Member, has contracted with or on whose behalf a contract has been entered into with HMO to provide professional services to Members.

J. Participating Provider means a physician, hospital, skilled nursing facility, home health agency, or any other duly licensed institution or Health Professional under contract with HMO to provide professional and hospital services to Members.

K. Primary Care Physician means a Participating Provider who is a duly licensed doctor of medicine or osteopathy who provides primary care services to Members (e.g., general or family practitioner, internist, pediatrician, or such other physician specialty as may be designated by HMO) and is responsible for referrals of Members to Referral Physicians, other Participating Providers, and, if necessary, non-Participating Providers. Each Member shall select or have selected on his or her behalf a Primary Care Physician.

L. Referral Provider means a Participating Health Professional who is responsible for providing certain services upon referral by a Primary Care Physician.

M. Service Area means those counties in _____ set forth in Attachment A and such other areas as may be designated by HMO from time to time.

N. Subscriber means an individual who has contracted, or on whose behalf a contract has been entered into, with HMO for health care services.

PART II. OBLIGATIONS OF HMO

A. Administrative Procedures. HMO shall make available to Primary Care Physician a manual of administrative procedures (including any changes thereto) in the areas of record-keeping, reporting, and other administrative duties of the Primary Care Physician under this Agreement. Primary Care Physician agrees to abide by such administrative procedures including, but not limited to, the submission of HMO Encounter Forms documenting all Covered Services provided to Members by Primary Care Physician.[§]

B. Compensation. For all Medically Necessary Covered Services provided to Members by Primary Care Physician, HMO shall pay to Primary Care Physician the compensation set forth in Attachment B.[¶] Itemized claims for all Covered Services rendered by Primary Care Physician must be submitted to HMO within ninety (90) days of the date the service was rendered in order to be compensated by HMO. The purpose of the risk-sharing/incentive compensation arrangement set forth in Attachment B is to monitor utilization, control costs of health services, including hospitalization, and to achieve utilization goals while maintaining quality of care.

C. Processing of Claims. HMO agrees to process Primary Care Physician claims for Covered Services rendered to Members. HMO will make payment within thirty (30) days from the date the claim is received with sufficient documentation. Where a claim requires

---

[*] This clause gives the HMO the authority to deny coverage for a medically appropriate procedure where another procedure is also appropriate. Although this clause does not explicitly address the subject, it is intended to give the HMO the right to cover the most cost-effective, medically appropriate procedure. An alternative way of addressing the issue is to state explicitly as one of the criteria that the procedure performed is the least costly setting or manner appropriate to treat the enrollee's medical condition.

[†] This last sentence is a good addition to the definition. It makes clear the preference of outpatient care over inpatient care.

[‡] Member is usually regarded as synonymous with enrollee. The definition of member should be consistent with the definition used in the group enrollment agreement.

[§] This paragraph allows the HMO to designate and amend the information, including the claims form, that the PCP provides the HMO without obtaining the prior approval of the PCP.

[¶] This contract pays PCPs on a FFS basis. Attachment B also sets forth alternative language if an HMO pays its PCPs on a capitated basis.

additional documentation, HMO will make payment within thirty (30) days from date of receipt of sufficient documentation to approve the claim.[*]

D. Eligibility Report. HMO shall provide Primary Care Physician with a monthly listing of eligible Members who have selected or have been assigned to Primary Care Physician.

E. Reports. HMO will provide Primary Care Physician with periodic statements with respect to the compensation set forth in Attachment B and with utilization reports in accordance with HMO's administrative procedures. Primary Care Physician agrees to maintain the confidentiality of the information presented in such reports.

PART III. OBLIGATIONS OF PRIMARY CARE PHYSICIAN

A. Health Services. Primary Care Physician shall have the primary responsibility for arranging and coordinating the overall health care of Members, including appropriate referral to Participating Providers, and for managing and coordinating the performance of administrative functions relating to the delivery of health services to Members in accordance with this Agreement. In the event that Primary Care Physician shall provide Member non-Covered Services, Primary Care Physician shall, prior to the provision of such non-Covered Services, inform the Member:
1. of the service(s) to be provided,
2. that HMO will not pay for or be liable for said services, and
3. that Member will be financially liable for such services.[†]

For any health care services rendered to or authorized for Members by Primary Care Physician for which HMO's prior approval is required and such prior approval was not obtained, Primary Care Physician agrees that in no event will HMO assume financial responsibility for charges arising from such services, and payments made by HMO for such services may be deducted by HMO from payments otherwise due Primary Care Physician.[‡]

B. Referrals. Except in Emergencies or when authorized by HMO, Primary Care Physician agrees to make referrals of Members only to Participating Providers, and only in accordance with HMO policies. Primary Care Physician will furnish such Participating Providers complete information on treatment procedures and diagnostic tests performed prior to such referral. In the event that services required by a Member are not available from Participating Providers, non-Participating Providers may be utilized with the prior approval of HMO. HMO will periodically furnish Primary Care Physician with a current listing of HMO's Participating Providers.

C. Hospital Admissions. In cases where a Member requires a non-Emergency hospital admission, Primary Care Physician agrees to secure authorization for such admission in accordance with HMO's procedures prior to the admission. In addition, the Primary Care Physician agrees to abide by HMO hospital discharge policies and procedures for Members.[§]

D. Primary Care Physician's Member Panel. Primary Care Physician may request that he/she does not wish to accept additional Members (excluding persons already in Primary Care Physician's practice that enroll in HMO as Members) by giving HMO written notice of such intent thirty (30) days in advance of the effective date of such closure. Primary Care Physician agrees to accept any HMO Members seeking his/her services during the thirty- (30-) day notice period. Primary Care Physician agrees to initiate closure of his/her practice to additional Members only if his/her practice, as a whole, is to be closed to additional patients or if authorized by HMO. A request for such authorization shall not be unreasonably denied. HMO may suspend, upon thirty (30) days prior written notice to Primary Care Physician, any further selection of Primary Care Physician by Members who have not already sought Primary Care Physician's services at the time of such suspension.

E. Charges to Members. Primary Care Physician shall accept as payment in full, for services which he/she provides, the compensation specified in Attachment B. Primary Care Physician agrees that in no event, including, but not limited to, non-payment, HMO insolvency, or breach of this Agreement, shall Primary Care Physician bill, charge, collect a deposit from, seek compensation, remuneration or payment from, or have any recourse against Subscriber, Member, or persons other than the HMO acting on a Member's behalf for services provided pursuant to this Agreement. This provision shall not prohibit collection of copayments on HMO's behalf made in accordance with the terms of the Health Maintenance Certificate between HMO and Subscriber/Member.

Primary Care Physician agrees that in the event of HMO's insolvency or other cessation of operations,

---

[*] Prompt payment timeframes are usually set forth in state law. The timeframes in the contract must meet those legal requirements. This paragraph allows the HMO to delay payment to the physician while waiting for sufficient documentation.

[†] This prior notification requirement is an important requirement and often required by state law.

[‡] It is important for the HMO to make sure that the physicians know the circumstances or conditions for which prior HMO approval is required.

[§] Here, again, it is important for the HMO to ensure that the PCPs have full notice of all the requirements for prior authorization and discharges.

services to Members will continue through the period for which the premium has been paid and services to Members confined in an inpatient hospital on the date of insolvency or other cessation of operations will continue until their discharge.

Primary Care Physician further agrees that:

1. this provision shall survive the termination of this Agreement regardless of the cause giving rise to termination and shall be construed to be for the benefit of the HMO Member, and that

2. this provision supersedes any oral or written contrary agreement now existing or hereafter entered into between Primary Care Physician and Member, or persons acting on their behalf.[*]

F. Records and Reports.

1. Primary Care Physician shall submit to HMO for each Member encounter a claim that shall contain such statistical and descriptive medical and patient data as specified by HMO. Primary Care Physician shall maintain such records and provide such medical, financial, and administrative information to HMO as the HMO determines may be necessary for compliance by HMO with state and federal law, as well as for program management purposes. Primary Care Physician will further provide to HMO and, if required, to authorized state and federal agencies, such access to medical records of HMO Members as is needed to assure the quality of care rendered to such Members. HMO shall have access at reasonable times, upon request, to the billing and medical records of the Primary Care Physician relating to the health care services provided Members, and to information on the cost of such services, and on copayments received by the Primary Care Physician from Members for Covered Services. Utilization and cost data relating to a Participating physician may be distributed by HMO to other Participating physicians for HMO program management purposes.

2. HMO shall also have the right to inspect, at reasonable times, Primary Care Physician's facilities pursuant to HMO's credentialing, peer review, and quality assurance program.

3. Primary Care Physician shall maintain a complete medical record for each Member in accordance with the requirements established by HMO. Medical records of Members will include the recording of services provided by the Primary Care Physician, specialists, hospitals, and other reports from referral providers, discharge summaries, records of Emergency care received by the Member, and such other information as HMO requires.[†] Medical records of Members shall be treated as confidential so as to comply with all federal and state laws and regulations regarding the confidentiality of patient records.[‡]

G. Provision of Services and Professional Requirements.

1. Primary Care Physician shall make necessary and appropriate arrangements to assure the availability of physician services to his/her Member patients on a twenty-four (24) hours per day, seven (7) days per week basis, including arrangements to assure coverage of his/her Member patients after-hours or when Primary Care Physician is otherwise absent, consistent with HMO's administrative requirements. Primary Care Physician agrees that scheduling of appointments for Members shall be done in a timely manner. The Primary Care Physician will maintain weekly appointment hours which are sufficient and convenient to serve Members and will maintain at all times Emergency and on-call services. Covering arrangements shall be with another physician who is also a Participating Provider or who has otherwise been approved in advance by HMO. For services rendered by any covering physician on behalf of Primary Care Physician, including Emergency Services, it shall be Primary Care Physician's sole responsibility to make suitable arrangements with the covering physician regarding the manner in which said physician will be paid or otherwise compensated, provided, however, that Primary Care Physician shall assure that the covering physician will not, under any circumstances, bill HMO or bill Member for Covered Services (except copayments), and Primary Care Physician hereby agrees to indemnify and hold harmless Members and HMO against charges for Covered Services rendered by physicians who are covering on behalf of Primary Care Physician.

2. Primary Care Physician agrees:

   (a) not to discriminate in the treatment of his/her patients or in the quality of services delivered to HMO's Members on the basis of race, sex, age, religion, place of residence, health status, disability, or source of payment, and

   (b) to observe, protect, and promote the rights of Members as patients. Primary Care Physician

---

[*] State regulatory agencies often dictate the precise language of this clause.

[†] This paragraph contains an important requirement. The PCP serves as a gatekeeper and the coordinator of care for this HMO. To serve this function, the PCP needs information from referral providers. There, of course, needs to be a requirement in the contracts with referral providers that this information be provided to the applicable PCP.

[‡] For this sentence to be effective, the HMO needs to ensure that its staff and the PCP understand state and federal confidentiality laws. Special requirements often arise in some areas, such as for acquired immunodeficiency syndrome and mental health and substance abuse services.

shall not seek to transfer a Member from his/her practice based on the Member's health status, without authorization by HMO.

3. Primary Care Physician agrees that all duties performed hereunder shall be consistent with the proper practice of medicine, and that such duties shall be performed in accordance with the customary rules of ethics and conduct of the applicable state and professional licensure boards and agencies.

4. Primary Care Physician agrees that to the extent he/she utilizes allied Health Professionals and other personnel for delivery of health care, he/she will inform HMO of the functions performed by such personnel and that such personnel shall meet applicable licensure or certification and supervision requirements applicable to the services performed.

5. Primary Care Physician shall be duly licensed to practice medicine in _____ and shall maintain good professional standing at all times. Evidence of such licensing shall be submitted to HMO upon request. In addition, Primary Care Physician must meet all qualifications and standards for membership on the medical staff of at least one of the hospitals which have contracted with HMO and shall be required to maintain staff membership and full admission privileges in accordance with the rules and regulations of such hospital and be otherwise acceptable to such hospital. Primary Care Physician agrees to give immediate notice to HMO in the case of suspension or revocation, or initiation of any proceeding that could result in suspension or revocation, of his/her licensure, hospital privileges, or participation under a federal health care program (as defined in 42 U.S.C. §1320a-7b(f)) or the filing of a malpractice action against the Primary Care Physician.

H. Insurance. Primary Care Physician, including individual physicians providing services to Members under this Agreement if Primary Care Physician is a legal entity, shall provide and maintain such policies of general and professional liability (malpractice) insurance as shall be necessary to insure the Primary Care Physician and his/her employees against any claim or claims for damages arising by reason of personal injuries or death occasioned, directly or indirectly, in connection with the performance of any service by Primary Care Physician. The amounts and extent of such insurance coverage shall be subject to the approval of HMO. Primary Care Physician shall provide memorandum copies of such insurance coverage to HMO upon request.* Primary Care Physician

agrees to notify HMO within five (5) days of any reduction to or cancellation of such insurance coverage.

I. Administration.

1. Primary Care Physician agrees to cooperate and participate in such review and service programs as may be established by HMO, including utilization and quality assurance programs, credentialing, sanctioning, external audit systems, administrative procedures, and Member and Participating Provider appeals and grievance procedures. Primary Care Physician shall comply with all determinations rendered through the above programs.

2. Primary Care Physician agrees that HMO may use his/her name, address, phone number, picture, type of practice, applicable practice restrictions, and an indication of Primary Care Physician's willingness to accept additional Members, in HMO's roster of physician participants and other HMO materials. Primary Care Physician shall not reference HMO in any publicity, advertisements, notices, or promotional material or in any announcement to the Members without prior review and written approval of HMO.

3. Primary Care Physician agrees to provide to HMO information for the collection and coordination of benefits when a Member holds other coverage that is deemed primary for the provision of services to said Member and to abide by HMO coordination of benefits and duplicate coverage policies. This shall include, but not be limited to, permitting HMO to bill and process forms for any third-party payer on the Primary Care Physician's behalf for Covered Services and to retain any sums received. In addition, Primary Care Physician shall cooperate in and abide by HMO subrogation policies and procedures.

4. Primary Care Physician agrees to maintain the confidentiality of all information related to fees, charges, expenses, and utilization derived from, through, or provided by HMO.

5. In the event of:
   (a) termination of this Agreement,
   (b) the selection by a Member of another Primary Care Physician in accordance with HMO procedures, or
   (c) the approval by HMO of Primary Care Physician's request to transfer a Member from his/her practice.

   Primary Care Physician agrees to transfer copies of the Member's medical records, X-rays, or other data to HMO when requested to do so in writing by HMO, at the reasonable, customary, and usual fee for such copies.

6. Upon termination of the Agreement, the Primary Care Physician shall not use any information

---

* The HMO should have this insurance information on file. Thus the HMO, as a matter of course, should request this information and require notification of changes in the insurance coverage.

obtained during the course of the Agreement in furtherance of any competitors of the HMO.

7. Primary Care Physician warrants and represents that all information and statements given to HMO in applying for or maintaining his/her HMO Primary Care Physician Agreement are true, accurate, and complete. The HMO Participating Provider application shall be incorporated by reference into this Agreement. Any inaccurate or incomplete information or misrepresentation of information provided by Primary Care Physician may result in the immediate termination of the Agreement by HMO. Primary Care Physician shall notify HMO as soon as possible, but no more than five (5) days after, of any changes to the information provided in the Participating Provider application.

8. Primary Care Physician shall cooperate with HMO in complying with applicable laws relating to HMO.

9. HMO or its designee shall have the right to conduct periodic audits of Primary Care Physician claims and records and may audit its own records to determine if amounts have been properly paid under this Agreement. HMO shall provide Primary Care Physician with the results of any such audits. Any amounts determined to be due and owing as a result of such audits shall be promptly paid or, at the option of HMO, offset against other amounts due to Primary Care Physician, subject to the right of appeal as set forth in HMO's policies and procedures.*

PART IV. MISCELLANEOUS

A. **Modification of This Agreement.** This Agreement may be amended or modified in writing as mutually agreed upon by the parties. In addition, HMO may modify any provision of this Agreement upon thirty (30) days' prior written notice to Primary Care Physician. Primary Care Physician shall be deemed to have accepted HMO's modification if Primary Care Physician fails to object to such modification, in writing, within the thirty- (30-) day notice period.†

B. **Interpretation.** This Agreement shall be governed in all respects by the laws of the State of _____. The invalidity or unenforceability of any terms or conditions hereof shall in no way affect the validity or enforceability

of any other terms or provisions. The waiver by either party of a breach or violation of any provision of this Agreement shall not operate as or be construed to be a waiver of any subsequent breach thereof.

C. **Assignment.** This Agreement, being intended to secure the services of and be personal to the Primary Care Physician, shall not be assigned, sublet, delegated, or transferred by Primary Care Physician without the prior written consent of HMO.

D. **Notice.** Any notice required to be given pursuant to the terms and provisions hereof shall be sent by certified mail, return receipt requested, postage prepaid, to HMO or to the Primary Care Physician at the respective addresses indicated herein. Notice shall be deemed to be received 5 days after the date mailed (as indicated on the date of the notice), but notice of change of address shall be effective upon receipt.‡

E. **Relationship of Parties.** None of the provisions of this Agreement is intended to create nor shall be deemed or construed to create any relationship between the parties hereto other than that of independent entities contracting with each other hereunder solely for the purpose of effecting the provisions of this Agreement. Neither of the parties hereto, nor any of their respective employees, shall be construed to be the agent, employer, employee, or representative of the other, nor will either party have an express or implied right of authority to assume or create any obligation or responsibility on behalf of or in the name of the other party. Neither Primary Care Physician nor HMO shall be liable to any other party for any act, or any failure to act, of the other party to this Agreement.

F. **Gender.** The use of any gender herein shall be deemed to include the other gender where applicable.

G. **Legal Entity.** If Primary Care Physician is a legal entity, an application for each physician who is a member of such entity must be submitted to and accepted by HMO before such physician may serve as a Primary Care Physician under this Agreement.

H. **Term and Termination.** The term of this Agreement shall be for three (3) years from the "effective date" set forth on the signature page. This Agreement may be terminated by either party at any time without cause by prior written notice given at least sixty (60) days in advance of the effective date of such termination. This Agreement may also be terminated by HMO effective immediately upon written notice if Primary Care Physician's (or if a legal entity, any of the entity's physicians') medical license, participation

---

* State law may regulate the period of time during which an HMO may retrospectively adjust claims and/or recoup any overpayments.
† This is a common provision and useful in simplifying the administrative work associated with amending the agreement. Needless to say, it is important for the HMO to explain clearly the nature of the amendment to the PCP. From a provider's perspective, it is desirable to obtain a provision that allows the provider to object to any unilateral amendment. Furthermore, providers should obtain an exception that would not allow the HMO to unilaterally decrease the payment rate set forth in the agreement.

---

‡ Before adopting this paragraph, an HMO should consider whether it is necessary to require that all notifications be sent by certified mail, return receipt requested. If the HMO has a large provider panel, it might prefer the right to send information by regular mail or secure e-mail.

under a federal health care program, or hospital privileges are suspended, limited, restricted, or revoked, or if Primary Care Physician violates Part III (E), (G)(3), (G)(5), (H), (I)(1), or (I)(4) herein. Upon termination, the rights of each party hereunder shall terminate, provided, however, that such action shall not release the Primary Care Physician or HMO from their obligations with respect to:

1. payments accrued to the Primary Care Physician prior to termination;
2. the Primary Care Physician's agreement not to seek compensation from Members for Covered Services provided prior to termination; and
3. completion of treatment of Members then receiving care until continuation of the Member's care can be arranged by HMO.

In the event of termination, no distribution of any money accruing to Primary Care Physician under the provisions of Attachment B shall be made until the regularly scheduled date for such distributions. Upon termination, HMO is empowered and authorized to notify Members and prospective Members, other Primary Care Physicians, and other persons or entities whom it deems to have an interest herein of such termination, through such means as it may choose. In the event of notice of termination, HMO may notify Members of such fact and assign Members or require Members to select another Primary Care Physician prior to the effective date of termination. In any event, HMO shall continue to compensate Primary Care Physician until the effective date of termination as provided herein for those Members who, because of health reasons, cannot be assigned or make such selection during the notice of termination period and as provided by HMO's Medical Director.

IN WITNESS WHEREOF, the foregoing Agreement between _____ and Primary Care Physician is entered into by and between the undersigned parties, to be effective this ____ day of _____, 20___.

PRIMARY CARE PHYSICIAN

_____

_____

By: _____

(Name of Individual Physician or of Group Practice—Please Print)

_____

(Date)

_____

(Mailing Address)

_____

(City, State, ZIP)

_____

(Telephone Number)

_____

(National Provider Identification Number(s)) – Use a separate sheet of paper if necessary.

_____

(Taxpayer Identification Number)

_____

(Drug Enforcement Agency Number)

_____

(Signature)

_____

(Name and Title if signing as authorized representative of Group Practice)

_____

(Date)

■ APPENDIX 6-2

ATTACHMENT B

COMPENSATION SCHEDULE

PRIMARY CARE PHYSICIAN AGREEMENT

I. Services Rendered by Primary Care Physicians

For Covered Services provided by Primary Care Physician in accordance with the terms of this Agreement, HMO shall pay Primary Care Physician his/her Payment Allowance, less any applicable copayment for which the Member is responsible under the applicable Evidence of Coverage, and less the Withhold Amount, as described below. "Payment Allowance" shall mean the lower of (i) the usual and customary fee charged by Primary Care Physician for the Covered Service, or (ii) the maximum amount allowed under the fee limits established by HMO.

II. Withholds from Payment Allowance

HMO shall withhold from each payment to Primary Care Physician a percentage of the Payment Allowance ("Withhold Amount") and shall allocate an amount equal to such withhold to an HMO Risk Fund. HMO shall have the right, at its sole discretion, to modify the percentage withheld from Primary Care Physician if, in its judgment, the financial condition, operations, or commitments of the HMO or its expenses for particular health services or for services by any particular Participating Providers warrant such modification.

III. Withhold Amount Distributions

HMO may, at its sole discretion, from time to time distribute to Primary Care Physician Withhold Amounts retained by HMO from payments to Primary Care Physician, plus such additional amounts, if any, that HMO may deem appropriate as a financial incentive to the provision of cost-effective health care services. HMO may, from time to time, commit or expend Withhold Amounts, in whole or in part, to assure the financial stability of or commitments of the HMO or health care plans or payers with or for which the HMO has an agreement to arrange for the provision of health care services, or to satisfy budgetary or financial objectives established by HMO.

Subject to HMO's peer review procedures and policies, a Primary Care Physician may be excluded from any distribution if he/she does not qualify for such distribution, for example, if he/she has exceeded HMO utilization standards or criteria. No Primary Care Physician shall have any entitlement to any funds in the HMO Risk Fund.

IV. Accounting

Primary Care Physician shall be entitled to an accounting of Withhold Amounts from payments to him/her upon written request to HMO.

■ APPENDIX 6-3

ATTACHMENT B (ALTERNATE)

CAPITATION PAYMENT

PRIMARY CARE PHYSICIAN AGREEMENT

Compensation

I. Capitation Allocation

The total monthly amounts paid to Primary Care Physician will be determined as follows:

For each Member selecting Primary Care Physician ("selecting" also includes Members assigned to a Primary Care Physician), 90 percent of the monthly Primary Care Service capitation set forth below for Primary Care Services shall be

paid by HMO to Primary Care Physician by the 5th day of the following month. The capitation shall be set according to the particular benefit plan in which each Member is enrolled. Where the capitation is not currently adjusted for age and/or sex, HMO reserves the right to make such age and/or sex adjustment to the capitation rates upon thirty (30) days' notice. In consideration of such payments, Primary Care Physician agrees to provide to Members the Primary Care Services set forth in Attachment C hereto. Health Plan shall allocate the remaining 10 percent of the monthly capitation payments to a Risk Reserve Fund which is subject to the further provisions of this Attachment. The capitation payments to Primary Care Physician for Primary Care Services, subject to the above withhold, are as follows:

Coverage Plans

Age/Sex[*]	Commercial Plan__ Capitation Payment	Commercial Plan__ Capitation Payment	Commercial Plan__ Capitation Payment
0–24 months/M/F	$ ____	$ ____	$ ____
2–4 years/M/F	$ ____	$ ____	$ ____
5–19 years/M/F	$ ____	$ ____	$ ____
20–39 years/F	$ ____	$ ____	$ ____
20–39 years/M	$ ____	$ ____	$ ____
40–49 years/F	$ ____	$ ____	$ ____
40–49 years/M	$ ____	$ ____	$ ____
50–59 years/F	$ ____	$ ____	$ ____
50–59 years/M	$ ____	$ ____	$ ____
>60 years/F	$ ____	$ ____	$ ____
>60 years/M	$ ____	$ ____	$ ____

Primary Care Physician is financially liable for all Primary Care Services rendered to Members under the above capitation. If Primary Care Physician fails to do so, HMO may pay for such services on behalf of Primary Care Physician and deduct such payments from any sums otherwise due Primary Care Physician by HMO.

■ APPENDIX 6-4: SAMPLE HOSPITAL AGREEMENT

HEALTH MAINTENANCE ORGANIZATION

---

[*] Capitation rate cells may be calculated using acuity adjustments to include disease factors or other factors that could more accurately predict costs.

PARTICIPATING HOSPITAL AGREEMENT*

THIS AGREEMENT, made and entered into the date set forth on the signature page hereto, by and between _____ (the "Hospital"), a facility duly licensed under the laws of the State of _____ and located at _____, and _____ ("HMO"), a health maintenance organization [Alternative: a _____ corporation] organized under the _____ law, and located at _____.

WHEREAS, HMO provides a plan of health care benefits (the "Plan") to individuals and their eligible family members and dependents who contract with HMO or who are the beneficiaries of a contract with HMO for such benefits ("Members"), and in connection with such Plan, arranges for the provision of health care services, including Hospital Services, to such Members; and

WHEREAS, the Hospital desires to provide Hospital Services to Members in accordance with the terms and conditions of this Agreement as hereinafter set forth; and

WHEREAS, HMO desires to arrange for the services of the Hospital for the benefit of the Members of the Plan.

NOW, THEREFORE, in consideration of the foregoing recitals and the mutual covenants and promises herein contained and other good and valuable consideration, receipt and sufficiency of which are hereby acknowledged, the parties hereto agree and covenant as follows:

PART I. DEFINITIONS

A. Covered Services means those health services and benefits to which Members are entitled under the terms of the applicable Evidence of Coverage, which may be amended by HMO from time to time.

B. Emergency Services means those Medically Necessary services provided in connection with an "Emergency," defined as a sudden or unexpected onset of a condition requiring medical or surgical care which the Member receives after the onset of such condition (or as soon thereafter as care can be made available but not more than twenty-four (24) hours after onset) and in the absence of such care the Member could reasonably be expected to suffer serious physical impairment or death. Heart attacks, severe chest pain, cardiovascular accidents, hemorrhaging, poisonings, major burns, loss of consciousness, serious breathing difficulties, spinal injuries, shock, and other acute conditions as HMO shall determine are Emergencies.

C. Evidence of Coverage means a contract issued by HMO to a Member or an employer of Members specifying the services and benefits available under the HMO's prepaid health benefits program.

D. Hospital Services means all inpatient services, emergency room, and outpatient hospital services that are Covered Services.

E. Medical Director means a physician designated by HMO to monitor and review the provision of Covered Services to Members.

F. Medically Necessary services and/or supplies means the use of services or supplies as provided by a hospital, skilled nursing facility, physician, or other provider required to identify or treat a Member's illness or injury and which, as determined by HMO's Medical Director or its utilization management committee, are: (1) consistent with the symptoms or diagnosis and treatment of the Member's condition, disease, ailment or injury; (2) appropriate with regard to standards of good medical practice; (3) not solely for the convenience of the Member, his/her physician, hospital, or other health care provider; and (4) the most appropriate supply or level of service which can be safely provided to the Member. When specifically applied to an inpatient Member, it further means that the Member's medical symptoms or condition requires that the diagnosis or treatment cannot be safely provided to the Member as an outpatient.

G. Member means both an HMO subscriber and his/her enrolled family members for whom premium payment has been made.

H. Participating Physician means a physician who, at the time of providing or authorizing services to a Member, has contracted with or on whose behalf a contract has been entered into with HMO to provide professional services to Members.

I. Participating Provider means a doctor of medicine, doctor of osteopathy, doctor of podiatric medicine, hospital, skilled nursing facility, home health agency, or any other duly licensed institution or health professional under contract with HMO to provide health care services to Members. A list of Participating Providers and their locations is available to each Member upon enrollment. Such list shall be revised from time to time as HMO deems necessary.

J. Primary Care Physician means a Participating Provider who is a doctor of medicine or doctor of osteopathy who provides primary care services to Members (e.g., general or family practitioner, internist, pediatrician,

_____

*For consistency, the HMO has used the same definitions for this agreement and the preceding PCP agreement. This agreement also uses some of the same provisions as in the PCP agreement. Comments made to those provisions in the PCP agreement will not be repeated here.

or such other physician specialty as may be designated by HMO) and is responsible for referrals of Members to referral physicians, other Participating Providers, and, if necessary, non-Participating Providers.

PART II. HOSPITAL OBLIGATIONS

A. Hospital shall provide to Members those Hospital Services that Hospital has the capacity to provide. Such services shall be provided by Hospital in accordance with the provisions of its Articles of Incorporation and bylaws and medical staff bylaws and the appropriate terms of this Agreement.

B. Hospital shall render Hospital Services to Members in an economical and efficient manner consistent with professional standards of medical care generally accepted in the medical community. Hospital shall not discriminate in the treatment of members and, except as otherwise required by this Agreement, shall make its services available to Members in the same manner as to its other patients.* In the event that an admission of a Member cannot be accommodated by Hospital, Hospital shall make the same efforts to arrange for the provision of services at another facility approved by HMO that it would make for other patients in similar circumstances. In the event that Hospital shall provide Member non-Covered Services, Hospital shall, prior to the provision of such non-Covered Services, inform the Member:
   1. of the service(s) to be provided,
   2. that HMO will not pay for or be liable for said services, and
   3. that Member will be financially liable for such services.

C. Except in an Emergency, Hospital shall provide Hospital Inpatient Services to a Member only when Hospital has received certification from HMO in advance of admission of such Member. Services which have not been so approved or authorized shall be the sole financial responsibility of Hospital.

D. HMO agrees to pay for medical screenings required under law to determine if an emergency medical condition exists. However, HMO reserves the right to determine if any such services were medically necessary.†

E. If, and to the extent that, the Hospital is not authorized to perform preadmission testing, the Hospital agrees to accept the results of qualified and timely laboratory, radiological and other tests and procedures that may be performed on a Member prior to admission. The Hospital will not require that duplicate tests or procedures be performed after the Enrollee is admitted, unless such tests and procedures are Medically Necessary.

F. In an Emergency, Hospital shall immediately proceed to render Medically Necessary services to the Member. Hospital shall also contact HMO within twenty-four (24) hours of the treatment of the emergency treatment visit or emergency admission. HMO has twenty-four- (24-) hour on-call nurse coverage for notification of Emergency Services or admits.
   If Hospital fails to notify HMO within the required time period, neither HMO nor the Member shall be liable for charges for Hospital Services rendered subsequent to the required notification period that are deemed by HMO not to be Medically Necessary.‡

G. Hospital shall cooperate with and abide by HMO's programs that monitor and evaluate whether Hospital Services provided to Members in accordance with this Agreement are Medically Necessary and consistent with professional standards of medical care generally accepted in the medical community. Such programs include, but are not limited to, utilization management, quality assurance review, and grievance procedures. In connection with HMO's programs, Hospital shall permit HMO's utilization management personnel to visit Members in the Hospital and, to the extent permitted by applicable laws, to inspect and copy health records (including medical records) of Members maintained by Hospital for the purposes of concurrent and retrospective utilization management, discharge planning, and other program management purposes.

H. Hospital shall cooperate with HMO in complying with applicable laws relating to HMO.

I. HMO or its designee shall have the right to conduct periodic audits of Hospital claims and records and may audit its own records to determine if amounts have been properly paid under this Agreement. HMO shall provide Hospital with the results of any such audits. Any amounts determined to be due and owing as a result of such audits shall be promptly paid, or, at the option of HMO, offset against other amounts due to Hospital, subject to the right of appeal set forth in HMO's policies and procedures.

PART III. LICENSURE AND ACCREDITATION

Hospital represents that it is duly licensed by the Department of Health of the State of _____ to operate a hospi-

---

* This requirement serves the same purpose as its counterpart in the PCP agreement of requiring the hospital to treat HMO members in the same manner as FFS patients.
† This provision addresses the HMO's responsibility for hospital charges incurred to provide a medical screening examination, as required by Section 1867 of the Social Security Act, to enrollees seeking care from the hospital's emergency department.

---

‡ To avoid disputes, the hospital and HMO need a common understanding of the meaning of the term Medically Necessary. The definition of that term used in this contract favors the HMO by allowing for its interpretation.

tal, is a qualified provider under the Medicare program, and is accredited by the Joint Commission on the Accreditation of Healthcare Organizations ("Joint Commission"). Hospital shall maintain in good standing such license and accreditation and shall notify HMO immediately should any action of any kind be initiated against Hospital which could result in:

1. the suspension or loss of such license;
2. the suspension or loss of such accreditation; or
3. the imposition of any sanctions against Hospital under a federal health care program as defined in 42 U.S.C. 1320a-7b(f).

Hospital shall furnish to HMO such evidence of licensure, Medicare qualification, and accreditation as HMO may request.

PART IV. RECORDS

A. Hospital shall maintain with respect to each Member receiving Hospital Services pursuant to this Agreement a standard hospital medical record in such form, containing such information, and preserved for such time period(s) as are required by the rules and regulations of the _____ Department of Health, the Medicare program, and the Joint Commission. The original hospital medical records shall be and remain the property of Hospital and shall not be removed or transferred from Hospital except in accordance with applicable laws and general Hospital policies, rules, and regulations relating thereto; provided, however, that HMO shall have the right, in accordance with paragraph (B) below, to inspect, review, and make copies of such records upon request.
B. Upon consent of the Member and a request for such records or information, Hospital shall provide copies of information contained in the medical records of Members to other authorized providers of health care services and to HMO for the purpose of facilitating the delivery of appropriate health care services to Members and carrying out the purposes and provisions of this Agreement, and shall facilitate the sharing of such records among health care providers involved in a Member's care. HMO and, if required, authorized state and federal agencies shall have the right upon request to inspect at reasonable times and to obtain copies of all records that are maintained by Hospital relating to the care of Members pursuant to this Agreement.

PART V. INSURANCE AND INDEMNIFICATION

A. Hospital shall secure and maintain at its expense throughout the term of this Agreement such policy or policies of general liability and professional liability insurance as shall be necessary to insure Hospital, its agents and employees against any claim or claims for damages arising by reason of injury or death, oc-casioned directly or indirectly by the performance or nonperformance of any service by Hospital, its agents or employees. Upon request, Hospital shall provide HMO with a copy of the policy (or policies) or certificate(s) of insurance which evidence compliance with the foregoing insurance requirements. It is specifically agreed that coverage amounts in general conformity with other similar type and size hospitals within the State of _____ shall be acceptable to HMO and be considered satisfactory and in compliance with this requirement.*
B. Hospital and HMO each shall indemnify and hold the other harmless from any and all liability, loss, damage, claim, or expense of any kind, including costs and attorney's fees, arising out of the performance of this Agreement and for which the other is solely responsible.

PART VI. MEDICAL STAFF MEMBERSHIP

Notwithstanding any other provision of this Agreement, a Participating Physician may not admit or treat a Member in the Hospital unless he/she is a member in good standing of Hospital's organized medical staff with appropriate clinical privileges to admit and treat such Member.†

PART VII. HMO OBLIGATIONS

A. HMO shall provide to or for the benefit of each Member an identification card which shall be presented for purposes of assisting Hospital in verifying Member eligibility. In addition, HMO shall maintain other verification procedures by which Hospital may confirm the eligibility of any Member.
B. HMO will, whenever an individual, admitted or referred, is not a Member, advise Hospital within thirty (30) days from the date of receipt of an invoice from Hospital for services to such an individual. In such cases, Hospital shall directly bill the individual or another third party payer for services rendered to such individual.
C. In the event continued stay or services are denied after a patient has been admitted, HMO or its representative shall inform the patient that services have been denied.

PART VIII. USE OF NAME

Except as provided in this paragraph, neither HMO nor Hospital shall use the other's name, symbols, trademarks,

---

*This paragraph reflects the difference in relative bargaining strength that the HMO has with hospitals and physicians. Although the HMO–PCP agreement gives the HMO the right to approve malpractice coverage, no such right is contained in the HMO–participating hospital agreement. Another factor may be that the concern of inadequate coverage may be greater for a physician than a hospital.
†Requiring the HMO's physicians to comply with the hospital's medical staff requirements is important and reasonable.

or service marks in advertising or promotional material or otherwise. HMO shall have the right to use the name of Hospital for purposes of marketing, informing Members of the identity of Hospital and otherwise to carry out the terms of this Agreement. Hospital shall have the right to use HMO's name in its informational or promotional materials with HMO's prior approval, which approval shall not be unreasonably withheld.

PART IX. COMPENSATION

Hospital will be compensated by HMO for all Medically Necessary Covered Services provided to Members in accordance with the provisions of Attachment A annexed hereto and incorporated herein.*

PART X. PAYMENT TO HOSPITAL BY HMO

For Hospital Services rendered to Members, Hospital shall invoice HMO at Hospital's current charges. [Alternative: For Hospital Services rendered to Members, Hospital shall invoice HMO.†] Except for Hospital Services which HMO determines require further review under HMO's utilization management procedures, or when there are circumstances which are beyond the control of HMO, including submission of incomplete claims, HMO shall make payment of invoices for Hospital Services within thirty (30) calendar days after the HMO's receipt thereof. HMO authorized copayments shall be collected by the Hospital from the Member and the Member shall be solely responsible for the payment of such copayments. All billings by Hospital shall be considered final unless adjustments are requested in writing by Hospital within sixty (60) days after receipt of original billing by HMO, except for circumstances which are beyond the control of Hospital.‡ No payment shall be made unless the invoice for services is received within sixty (60) days after the date of discharge of the Member or date of service, whichever occurs later. Hospital shall interim bill HMO every thirty (30) days for patients whose length of stay is greater than thirty (30) days.

PART XI. PROHIBITIONS ON MEMBER BILLING

Hospital hereby agrees that in no event, including, but not limited to, nonpayment by HMO, HMO's insolvency or

---

*Attachment A provides for payment as a percentage of Medicare rates. By structuring the agreement in this manner, the HMO is able to negotiate different payment arrangements with hospitals without revising the body of the agreement.

†This broader alternative language along with the cross-reference to Attachment A in the preceding paragraph allows the body of the contract to be used for any type of payment arrangement. An alternative Attachment A is offered that establishes per diem rates for inpatient stays and a percentage of charges for outpatient services.

‡To avoid potential disputes, the hospital and the HMO should have some general understanding of the meaning of the term beyond the control of Hospital.

breach of this Agreement, shall Hospital bill, charge, collect a deposit from, seek compensation, remuneration or payment from, or have any recourse against a Member or persons other than HMO acting on a Member's behalf for services provided pursuant to this Agreement. This provision shall not prohibit collection of copayment on HMO's behalf in accordance with the terms of the Health Maintenance Certificate between HMO and Member. Hospital agrees that in the event of HMO's insolvency or other cessation of operations, services to Members will continue through the period for which the premium has been paid and services to Members confined in an inpatient hospital on the date of insolvency or other cessation of operations will continue until their discharge.

Hospital further agrees that:

1. this provision shall survive the termination of this Agreement regardless of the cause giving rise to termination and shall be construed to be for the benefit of the Member; and
2. this provision supersedes any oral or written contrary agreement now existing or hereafter entered into between Hospital and Member, or persons acting on their behalf.

PART XII. INSPECTION OF RECORDS

Upon request, and at reasonable times, HMO and Hospital shall make available to the other for review such books, records, utilization information, and other documents or information relating directly to any determination required by this Agreement. All such information shall be held by the receiving party in confidence and shall only be used in connection with the administration of this Agreement.

PART XIII. COORDINATION OF BENEFITS

Hospital agrees to cooperate with HMO toward effective implementation of any provisions of HMO's Evidence of Coverage and policies relating to coordination of benefits and claims by third parties. Hospital shall forward to HMO any payments received from a third-party payer for authorized Hospital Services where HMO has made payment to Hospital covering such Hospital Services and such third-party payer is determined to be primarily obligated for such Hospital Services under applicable Coordination of Benefits rules. Such payment shall not exceed the amount paid to Hospital by HMO. Except as otherwise required by law, Hospital agrees to permit HMO to bill and process forms for any third-party payer on Hospital's behalf, or to bill such third party directly, as determined by HMO. Hospital further agrees to waive, when requested, any claims against third-party payers for its provision of Hospital Services to Members and to execute any further documents that reasonably may be required or appropriate for this purpose. Any such waiver shall be contingent upon HMO's payment to Hospital of its (HMO's) obligations for charges incurred by Member. This para graph shall not be interpreted as a waiver of Medicare beneficiary cost-sharing obligations to the extent that such waiver is in violation of federal law.

PART XIV. TERM AND TERMINATION

A. This Agreement shall take effect on the "effective date" set forth on the signature page and shall continue for a period of one year or until terminated as provided herein.
   1. Either party may terminate this Agreement without cause upon at least ninety (90) days' written notice prior to the term of this Agreement.
   2. Either party may terminate this Agreement with cause upon at least thirty (30) days' prior written notice.
B. HMO shall have the right to terminate this Agreement immediately by notice to Hospital upon the occurrence of any of the following events:
   1. the suspension or revocation of Hospital's license;
   2. the suspension, revocation, or loss of the Hospital's Joint Commission accreditation or Medicare qualification; or
   3. breach of Part II(E) or Part XI of this Agreement.
C. HMO shall continue to pay Hospital in accordance with the provisions of Attachment A for Hospital Services provided by Hospital to Members hospitalized at the time of termination of this Agreement, pending clinically appropriate discharge or transfer to an HMO-designated hospital when medically appropriate as determined by HMO. In continuing to provide such Hospital Services, Hospital shall abide by the applicable terms and conditions of this Agreement.

PART XV. ADMINISTRATION

Hospital agrees to abide by and cooperate with HMO administrative policies including, but not limited to, claims procedures, copayment collections, and duplicate coverage/subrogation recoveries. Nothing in this Agreement shall be construed to require Hospital to violate, breach, or modify its written policies and procedures unless specifically agreed to herein.

PART XVI. MEMBER GRIEVANCES

Hospital agrees to cooperate in and abide by HMO's grievance procedures in resolving Member's grievances related to the provision of Hospital Services. In this regard, HMO shall bring to the attention of appropriate Hospital officials all Member complaints involving Hospital, and Hospital shall, in accordance with its regular procedure, investigate such complaints and use its best efforts to resolve them in a fair and equitable manner. Hospital agrees to notify HMO promptly of any action taken or proposed with respect to the resolution of such complaints and the avoidance of similar complaints in the future. The Hospital shall notify the HMO after it has received a complaint from an HMO Member.

PART XVII. MISCELLANEOUS

A. If any term, provision, covenant, or condition of this Agreement is invalid, void, or unenforceable, the rest of the Agreement shall remain in full force and effect. The invalidity or unenforceability of any term or provision hereof shall in no way affect the validity or enforceability of any other term or provision.
B. This Agreement contains the complete understanding and agreement between Hospital and HMO and supersedes all representations, understandings, or agreements prior to the execution hereof.
C. HMO and Hospital agree that, to the extent compatible with the separate and independent management of each, they shall at all times maintain an effective liaison and close cooperation with each other to provide maximum benefits to Members at the most reasonable cost consistent with quality standards of hospital care.
D. No waiver, alteration, amendment, or modification of this Agreement shall be valid unless in each instance a written memorandum specifically expressing such waiver, alteration, amendment, or modification is made and subscribed by a duly authorized officer of Hospital and a duly authorized officer of HMO.
E. Hospital shall not assign its rights, duties, or obligations under this Agreement without the express, written permission of HMO.
F. None of the provisions of this Agreement are intended to create nor shall be deemed to create any relationship between HMO and Hospital other than that of independent entities contracting with each other hereunder solely for the purpose of effecting the provisions of this Agreement. Neither of the parties hereto nor any of their respective employees shall be construed to be the agent, employer, employee, or representative of the other.
G. This Agreement shall be construed in accordance with the laws of the State of _____.
H. The headings and numbers of sections and paragraphs contained in this Agreement are for reference purposes only and shall not affect in any way the meaning or interpretation of this Agreement.
I. Any notice required or permitted to be given pursuant to the terms and provisions of this Agreement shall be

sent by registered mail or certified mail, return receipt requested, postage prepaid, to:

_____

_____

_____

_____

_____

_____

and to Hospital at:

_____

_____

_____

_____

_____

All notices shall be deemed received 5 days after the date of mailing (as indicated by the date on the notice).

IN WITNESS WHEREOF, the foregoing Agreement between _____ and Hospital is entered into by and between the undersigned parties, to be effective the ____ day of _____, 20___.

By: _____

Title: _____

Date: _____

HOSPITAL

By: _____

Title: _____

Date: _____

ATTACHMENT A

PARTICIPATING HOSPITAL COMPENSATION

Subject to the terms and conditions set forth in this Agreement, HMO shall pay Hospital _____ (____%) of the applicable Medicare payment rate, for Medically Necessary Covered Services provided to Members.

ATTACHMENT A (ALTERNATE)

PARTICIPATING HOSPITAL COMPENSATION

Subject to the terms and conditions set forth in this Agreement, HMO shall pay Hospital, as follows:

Service	Type of Payment	Payment per Day
Inpatient care		
Non-maternity Per Diem		$_____
Secondary Non-maternity Per Diem		$_____
Tertiary Maternity Per Diem		$_____
Psychiatric Per Diem		$_____
Well Newborn Children Per Diem		$_____
Outpatient care		

Outpatient surgery Percentage of Medicare Payment Rate: ___%

Other than outpatient surgery Percentage of Medicare Payment Rate: ___%

▪ APPENDIX 6-5: SAMPLE BUSINESS ASSOCIATE ADDENDUM

BUSINESS ASSOCIATE ADDENDUM

I. DEFINITIONS

As used in this Addendum, the following terms have the meanings assigned to them below:

A. *Agreement.* Agreement shall mean the Provider Service Agreement.
B. *Breach.* "Breach" shall have the same meaning as the term "breach" in 42 CFR 164.402.
C. *Business Associate.* "Business Associate" shall mean Provider.
D. *Covered Entity.* "Covered Entity" shall mean HMO.
E. *Individual.* "Individual" shall have the same meaning as the term "individual" in 45 CFR § 160.103 and shall include a person who qualifies as a personal representative in accordance with 45 CFR § 164.502(g).
F. *Privacy Rule.* "Privacy Rule" shall mean the Standards for Privacy of Individually Identifiable Health Information at 45 CFR Part 160 and Part 164, Subparts A, D and E.
G. *Protected Health Information.* "Protected Health Information" shall have the same meaning as the term "protected health information" in 45 CFR § 160.103, limited to the information created or received by Business Associate from or on behalf of Covered Entity.

H. *Required By Law.* "Required By Law" shall have the same meaning as the term "required by law" in 45 CFR § 164.103.

I. *Secretary.* "Secretary" shall mean the Secretary of the Department of Health and Human Services or his designee.

J. *Unsecured Protected Health Information.* "Unsecured Protected Health Information" means Protected Health Information that is not rendered unusable, unreadable, or indecipherable to unauthorized individuals through the use of a technology or methodology specified by the Secretary in the guidance issued under section 13402(h)(2) of Public Law 111–5 on the HHS website.

Any other terms used, but not otherwise defined, in this Addendum shall have the same meaning as those terms in the Privacy Rule.

II. PERMITTED USES AND DISCLOSURES

A. Except as otherwise limited in this Addendum, Business Associate may use or disclose Protected Health Information to perform functions, activities, or services for, or on behalf of, Covered Entity as set forth in the Agreement, provided that such use or disclosure would not violate the Privacy Rule if done by Covered Entity.

B. Covered Entity shall not request Business Associate to use or disclose Protected Health Information in any manner that would not be permissible under the Privacy Rule if done by Covered Entity, except as set forth in Sections II.C and II.D herein.

C. Except as otherwise limited in this Addendum, Business Associate may use Protected Health Information for the proper management and administration of the Business Associate or to carry out the legal responsibilities of the Business Associate.

D. Except as otherwise limited in this Addendum, Business Associate may disclose Protected Health Information for the proper management and administration of the Business Associate, provided that disclosures are Required By Law, or Business Associate obtains reasonable assurances from the person to whom the information is disclosed that it will remain confidential and used or further disclosed only as Required By Law or for the purpose for which it was disclosed to the person, and the person notifies the Business Associate of any instances of which it is aware in which the confidentiality of the information has been breached.

E. Business Associate may use Protected Health Information to provide Data Aggregation services to Covered Entity as permitted by 45 CFR § 164.504(e)(2)(i)(B).

F. Business Associate may use Protected Health Information to report violations of law to appropriate Federal and State authorities, consistent with § 164.502(j)(1).

III. OBLIGATIONS AND ACTIVITIES OF BUSINESS ASSOCIATE

A. Business Associate agrees to not use or disclose Protected Health Information other than as permitted or required by this Addendum or as Required By Law.

B. Business Associate agrees to use appropriate safeguards to prevent use or disclosure of the Protected Health Information other than as provided for by this Addendum.

C. Business Associate agrees to report to Covered Entity any use or disclosure of the Protected Health Information not provided for by this Addendum of which it becomes aware.

D. Business Associate agrees to ensure that any agent, including a subcontractor, to whom it provides Protected Health Information received from, or created or received by Business Associate on behalf of, Covered Entity agrees to the same restrictions and conditions that apply through this Addendum to Business Associate with respect to such information.

E. Business Associate agrees to provide access to Covered Entity, within 10 business days of a request of Covered Entity, to Protected Health Information in a non-duplicative Designated Record Set, in order to meet the requirements under 45 CFR § 164.524. In the event that Business Associate uses or maintains an Electronic Health Record that includes Protected Health Information of or about an Individual, then Business Associate shall provide an electronic copy (at the request of Covered Entity, and in the reasonable time and manner requested by Covered Entity) of the Protected Health Information to Covered Entity in accordance with 42 U.S.C. § 17935(e) as of the compliance date of that section.

F. Business Associate agrees to make any amendment(s) to Protected Health Information in a Designated Record Set that the Covered Entity directs or agrees to pursuant to 45 CFR § 164.526 within 10 business days of a request from Covered Entity.

G. Business Associate agrees to make internal practices, books, and records, including policies and procedures and Protected Health Information, relating to the use and disclosure of Protected Health Information received from, or created or received by Business Associate on behalf of, Covered Entity available to the Covered Entity, or to the Secretary, in a reasonable time and manner requested by Covered Entity or the time and manner designated by the Secretary, for purposes of the Secretary determining Covered Entity's compliance with the Privacy Rule.

H. Business Associate agrees to document such disclosures of Protected Health Information and information related to such disclosures as would be required for Covered Entity to respond to a request by an Individual for an accounting of disclosures of Protected Health Information in accordance with 45 CFR § 164.528 and, for Business Associates that use or maintain Electronic Health Records with respect to services furnished to Covered Entity, 42 U.S.C 17935(c).

I. Business Associate agrees to provide to Covered Entity, within 10 business days of a request from Covered Entity, information collected in accordance with Section III.H. of this Addendum, to permit Covered Entity to respond to a request by an Individual for an accounting of disclosures of Protected Health Information in accordance with 45 CFR § 164.528 and in accordance with the requirements for accounting for disclosures made through an Electronic Health Record in 42 U.S.C. 17935(c).

J. Business Associate agrees to implement administrative, physical, and technical safeguards that reasonably and appropriately protect the confidentiality, integrity, and availability of the Electronic Protected Health Information that it creates, receives, maintains, or transmits on behalf of Covered Entity as required by 45 CFR 164 Subpart C and ensure that any agent, including a subcontractor, to whom Business Associate provides such information agrees to implement reasonable and appropriate safeguards to protect it.

K. Business Associate agrees to report to Covered Entity any security incident involving electronic Protected Health Information of which it becomes aware. For purposes of this agreement, "security incident" means the attempted or successful unauthorized access, use, disclosure, modification, or destruction of information or interference with system operations.

L. Business Associate agrees, following the discovery of a Breach of unsecured Protected Health Information, to notify Covered Entity of such Breach without unreasonable delay and in no case later than 60 calendar days after discovery of a Breach. A Breach shall be treated as discovered by Business Associate as of the first day on which such breach is known to Business Associate or, by exercising reasonable diligence, would have been known to Business Associate. Business Associate shall be deemed to have knowledge of a Breach if the Breach is known, or by exercising reasonable diligence would have been known, to any person, other than the person committing the Breach, who is an employee, officer, or other agent of Business Associate (determined in accordance with

the federal common law of agency). Notification of a Breach to Covered Entity shall include, to the extent possible, the identification of each Individual whose unsecured Protected Health Information has been, or is reasonably believed by Business Associate to have been, accessed, acquired, used, or disclosed during the Breach. Business Associate further agrees to provide to Covered Entity, at the time of notification or promptly thereafter as the information becomes available, any other information that Covered Entity is required to include in notification to Individuals under 42 CFR §164.404, including but not limited to:

(i)   A brief description of what happened, including the date of the Breach and the date of the discovery of the Breach, if known;

(ii) A description of the types of unsecured Protected Health Information that were involved in the Breach (such as whether full name, social security number, date of birth, home address, account number, diagnosis, disability code, or other types of information were involved);

(iii) Any steps Individuals should take to protect themselves from potential harm resulting from the Breach; and

(iv) A brief description of what the Business Associate is doing to investigate the Breach, to mitigate harm to Individuals, and to protect against any further Breaches.

M. Business Associate shall comply with 42 CFR 164.502(b) by requesting, using, and/or disclosing only the minimum amount of PHI necessary to accomplish the purpose of the request, use, or disclosure unless making an exempt use or disclosure and will use a Limited Data Set, as defined by the Privacy Rule, if practicable.

IV. OBLIGATIONS OF COVERED ENTITY

A. Covered Entity shall notify Business Associate of any limitation(s) in its notice of privacy practices of Covered Entity in accordance with 45 CFR § 164.520, to the extent that such limitation may affect Business Associate's use or disclosure of Protected Health Information.

B. Covered Entity shall notify Business Associate of any changes in, or revocation of, permission by Individual to use or disclose Protected Health Information, to the extent that such changes may affect Business Associate's use or disclosure of Protected Health Information.

C. Covered Entity shall notify Business Associate of any restriction to the use or disclosure of Protected Health Information that Covered Entity has agreed to in accordance with 45 CFR § 164.522, to the extent that such restriction may affect Business Associate's use or disclosure of Protected Health Information.

V. TERM AND TERMINATION

A. *Term.* The provisions of this Addendum shall terminate when all of the Protected Health Information provided by Covered Entity to Business Associate, or created or received by Business Associate on behalf of Covered Entity, is destroyed or returned to Covered Entity, or, if it is infeasible to return or destroy Protected Health Information, protections are extended to such information, in accordance with the termination provisions in this Section.

B. *Termination for Cause.* Upon Covered Entity's knowledge of a material breach by Business Associate, Covered Entity shall either:

a. Provide Business Associate 30 days to cure the breach or end the violation. If Business Associate fails to cure the breach within 30 days, this Addendum and all provisions of the Agreement that require the exchange of Protected Health Information to implement shall be terminated;

b. Immediately terminate this Addendum and all provisions of the Agreement that require the exchange of Protected Health Information to implement if Business Associate has breached a material term of this Addendum and cure is not possible; or

c. If neither termination nor cure are feasible, Covered Entity shall report the violation to the Secretary.

C. *Effect of Termination.*

a. Except as provided in paragraph (b) of this section V.C. of this Addendum, upon termination of this Addendum for any reason, Business Associate shall return or destroy all Protected Health Information received from Covered Entity, or created or received by Business Associate on behalf of Covered Entity. This provision shall apply to Protected Health Information that is in the possession of subcontractors or agents of Business Associate. Business Associate shall retain no copies of the Protected Health Information.

b. In the event that Business Associate determines that returning or destroying the Protected Health Information is infeasible, Business Associate shall provide to Covered Entity notification of the conditions that make return or destruction infeasible. Upon the Parties' agreement that return or destruction of Protected Health Information is infeasible, Business Associate shall extend the protections of this Addendum to such Protected Health Information and limit further uses and disclosures of such Protected Health Information to those purposes that make the return or destruction infeasible, for so long as Business Associate maintains such Protected Health Information.

VI. MISCELLANEOUS

A. *Regulatory References.* A reference in this Addendum to a section in the Privacy Rule means the section as in effect or as amended.

B. *Amendment.* The Parties agree to take such action as is necessary to amend this Addendum from time to time as is necessary for Covered Entity to comply with the requirements of the Privacy Rule and the Health Insurance Portability and Accountability Act of 1996, Pub. L. No. 104–191 as amended.

C. *Survival.* The respective rights and obligations of Business Associate under Section V.C. of this Addendum shall survive the termination of the Agreement and this Addendum.

D. *Interpretation.* Any ambiguity in this Addendum shall be resolved to permit Covered Entity to comply with the Privacy Rule.

E. *Indemnification.* Business Associate will indemnify and hold harmless Covered Entity and any of its officers, directors, employees, or agents from and against that portion of any claim, cause of action, liability, damage, cost, or expense, including attorneys' fees, arising solely out of any non-permitted or violating use, disclosure, or request for Protected Health Information or other breach of this Addendum by Business Associate.

Covered Entity will indemnify and hold harmless Business Associate and any of its officers, directors, employees, or agents from and against that portion of any claim, cause of action, liability, damage, cost, or expense, including attorneys' fees, arising solely out of any non-permitted or violating use, disclosure, or request for Protected Health Information or other breach of this Addendum by Covered Entity.

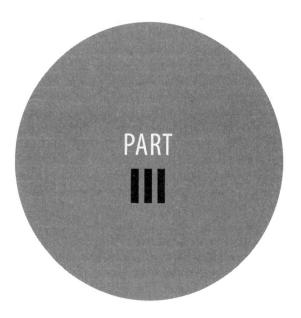

PART

III

Management of Utilization and Quality

"You can't always get what you want.
But if you try sometimes
You just might find
You get what you need."

Mick Jagger [1969]

Basic Utilization and Case Management

Peter R. Kongstvedt

STUDY OBJECTIVES

- Understand what managing utilization means
- Understand basic measurements of utilization
- Understand the basic categories of medical–surgical utilization management
- Understand the basic approaches to managing utilization in the inpatient, ambulatory, and ancillary services categories
- Understand what basic utilization management techniques are most useful in different situations
- Understand basic roles for different types of professionals in managing utilization
- Understand how approaches to managing utilization have changed over the years, and why those changes have occurred

DISCUSSION TOPICS

1. Discuss the key attributes of managing basic medical–surgical utilization in different types of managed care plans.
2. Discuss how basic utilization management has changed over the years, and why.
3. Discuss the types of data and reports that would be useful to the medical director for managing specialist utilization; discuss how this might differ in different types of plans.
4. Discuss how utilization management might change in the future, and why.
5. Briefly describe differences in managing utilization of acute care versus chronic care.
6. Discuss the unique challenges a provider or hospital-sponsored health maintenance organization has in managing utilization, and how those challenges might realistically be met.
7. Discuss the use of hospitalists for inpatient care, and how to improve the effectiveness of transmission care.
8. Discuss various policies and procedures for managing ancillary utilization in different types of managed care plans; be specific regarding the type of ancillary service.

INTRODUCTION

In its simplest form, overall health care costs are the product of price and volume; put another way, Total Cost = Provider Prices × Medical Utilization. Price is what is paid to providers for goods and services on behalf of covered members, and volume is how much goods and how many services are paid for. Once you get past the simple equation above, things get very complex very quickly, as is the case with almost every aspect of this industry.

The broad term utilization management (UM), also occasionally called care management, covers the many activities a payer or integrated delivery system (IDS) applies to reduce or manage overall medical costs other than negotiating prices, which was the subject of Chapter 5. For purposes of clarity, this chapter only uses UM so as to avoid confusing UM with case management. And again for purposes of clarity, even though the acronym CM can stand for both care management and case management, in this chapter CM will only be used to refer to case management.

There are three main areas of focus for UM. The first involves a variety of review functions to determine whether or not a medical service is or should be covered under the benefits plan, and under what circumstances it should be covered. The second is a set of activities designed to facilitate necessary services being provided for the lowest reasonable cost. The third is the reduction of unwarranted practice variation by establishing parameters for cost-effective utilization through adherence to evidence-based medical guidelines. All three overlap at times.

UM has evolved along with the market. In the early managed care era when utilization was high, basic approaches to UM produced rapid and impressive results, especially in reducing unnecessary hospital bed-days. However, as discussed in Chapter 1, the "managed care backlash" against health maintenance organizations (HMOs) and the desire of consumers to have both broad access to providers and fewer restrictions on access to care by eliminating, for example, the primary care physician (PCP) "gatekeeper" model, led many HMOs to reduce UM activities. HMOs also created point-of-service (POS) plans that allowed for out-of-network benefits with reduced UM requirements. At the same time, preferred provider organizations (PPOs) and consumer-directed health plans (CDHPs) grew, both of which are less likely to approach UM in as comprehensive an approach as a traditional HMO, and more likely to take a selective approach to UM.[1]

Chapter 1 described how the decline of HMOs and aggressive UM was accompanied by the growth of health care cost inflation, but not for the same reasons it had been high in earlier decades. The provider environment had changed as well over the years, and inpatient bed-days* remained low compared to the premanaged health care era. They've been rising again, as is shown later in the chapter, but not anywhere close to the levels they were at in the 1970s and 1980s. However, lower inpatient days did not and does not equate to lower costs.

---

* "Bed-days" is a measure of inpatient utilization that is defined later in the chapter.

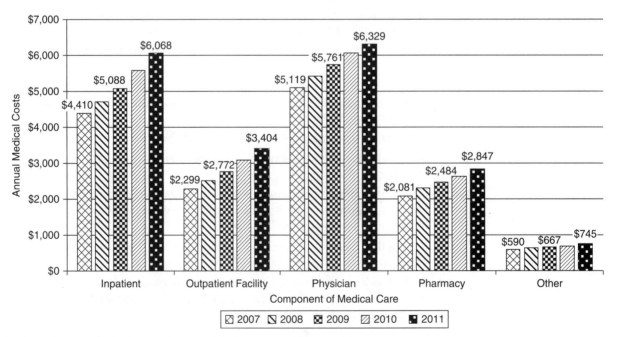

FIGURE 7-1 Milliman Medical Index Spending Growth by Component of Care, 2007–2011

Source: 2011 Milliman Medical Index, http://publications.milliman.com/periodicals/mmi/pdfs/milliman-medical-index-2011.pdf. Accessed July 7, 2011. Used with permission.

There are many sources of data, both detailed and summarized, on cost increases for different types of care, but one serves to illustrate the size of the issue. The actuarial services firm Milliman publishes an annual report on costs in the commercial marketplace, using a typical family of four covered under a PPO. Adding up the costs paid by the employer and the employee, including out-of-pocket cost-sharing, the total reached $19,393 by 2011, which is more than double the $9,235 annual cost per family reported in 2002. They further broke it down by the components of care, as seen in **Figure 7-1**.

The reasons health care costs are relentlessly inflationary are complex, and there is only partial agreement among experts and policymakers as to what are the most important causes. Some elements are simply factual and supported by data, such as pricing (Chapter 5), an absolute increase in the number of ambulatory procedures, increasing use of various diagnostic testing, and the appearance and increasing use of new drugs and technology where previously no alternative existed.* The fact of an increase in procedures or diagnostic testing sheds no light on whether or not the increase is inappropriate, however. We know that one reason for higher costs is an increase in the number of procedures, but we don't know all the reasons *why* the number of procedures is higher. Said another way, we may know why some costs go up, but sometimes we only know the intermediate cause, not the root cause.

Another factual element is the degree of cost concentration in a small percentage of individuals. As shown in **Figure 7-2**, only 1% of the nation's population accounts for over 20% of medical costs, 20% of the nation's population accounts for over 80% of costs; conversely, half of the nation's population accounts for only 3% of total medical costs.

---

*Each of these is documented and referenced at appropriate points in the chapter.

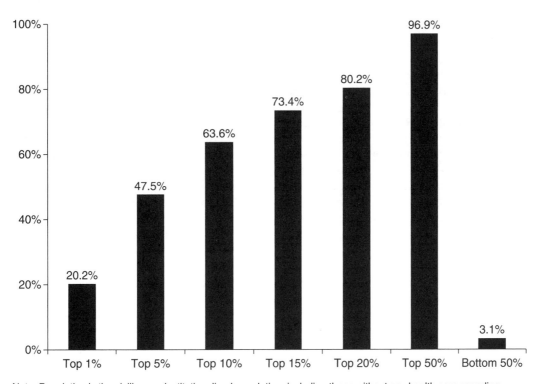

Note: Population is the civilian noninstitutionalized population, including those without any health care spending. Health care spending is total payments from all sources (including direct payments from individuals, private insurance, Medicare, Medicaid, and miscellaneous other sources) to hospitals, physicians, other providers (including dental care), and pharmacies; health insurance premiums are not included.

FIGURE 7-2 Concentration of Health Care Spending in the U.S. Population, 2008

Source: "Concentration of Health Care Spending in the U.S. Population, 2008," Kaiser Slides, The Henry J. Kaiser Family Foundation, February 2011, http://facts.kff.org/chart. aspx?ch=1344. This information was reprinted with permission from the Henry J. Kaiser Family Foundation. The Kaiser Family Foundation is a non-profit private operating foundation, based in Menlo Park, California, dedicated to producing and communicating the best possible analysis and information on health issues http://facts.kff.org/chart .aspx?ch=1344.

As one would expect, the presence of chronic medical conditions are associated with higher costs, and multiple chronic conditions with the highest of all. High costs associated with multiple chronic medical conditions come from higher usage of all types of care, not just hospitalizations. Details on utilization are available in a report on Medicare costs by the Johns Hopkins Bloomberg School of Public Health on behalf of the Robert Wood Johnson Foundation; the report also documents the relationship between the number of chronic medical conditions and costs, which is summarized as follows:

- 0 chronic conditions – 1% of Medicare expenditures,
- 1 chronic condition – 3%,
- 2 chronic conditions – 6%,
- 3 chronic conditions – 10%,
- 4 chronic conditions – 9%, and
- 5 chronic conditions – 79%.[2]

It is this concentration that led to the concept of disease management (DM; see Chapter 8). In combination with the decrease in obviously unnecessary utilization—long stays for routine services, for example—it also led to a shift in focus for most UM programs as well as the appearance of new provider organizational models promoted in the Patient Protection and Affordable Care Act (ACA)[3] such as patient-centered medical homes (PCMHs) and accountable care organizations (ACOs), as discussed in Chapter 2 and elsewhere.

Other elements also contribute to increasing costs, but their roles are less easily defined and their impact subject to ongoing debate. The use of evidence-based clinical guidelines is an example. There's a reason doctors go to college for 4 years, medical school for another 4 years, residency training for another 3–5 years, and, in many cases, a final 2 years of specialty training: the human body and the practice of medicine are complex. But medical care is also subject to scientific research, and that research can lead to the development of evidence-based medical practice guidelines.

There is general acceptance that deviations from those guidelines are at least one reason for inappropriate utilization, but it is not the only one and how it fits in to all the other causes is unclear. But where utilization guidelines, case management, condition management, and wellness/behavior modification health coaching are incorporated into health delivery, the degree of practice variation and the amount of inappropriate care are reduced. This affects even the nonmanaged care patients of physicians who have significant managed care practices; for example, lower inpatient utilization in nonmanaged care patients is observed when managed care presence is high.[4]

This chapter's purpose is to provide an overview of the various elements and functions that fall under the broad concept of UM. Much of what is discussed in this chapter is presented in greater detail and with more focus in other chapters, which underscores the fact that management of medical services is not made up of discrete and unrelated activities. The first third of the chapter explores topics generally applicable to medical utilization regardless of the type of any specific UM activities or type of health plan. The other two-thirds are taken up with detailed discussion of the various specific elements and activities of basic UM.

Finally, not all types of payers undertake all of the UM activities discussed in this chapter, but all are used in some type of combination by some type of payer. Generally speaking, HMOs have a greater focus on UM than do other types of payers, and some elements of UM are specific to HMOs only. Most, however, may be used by other types of payers as well.

■ MEASUREMENTS AND METRICS IN UTILIZATION MANAGEMENT

It is not possible to manage overall utilization well unless there is a means to measure it. Most of the metrics used in UM are also used to manage overall finances, predict and set rates, determine levels of risk, and so forth. But for the most part, only medical management uses these metrics on a daily, weekly, or monthly basis to guide day-to-day efforts.

The following basic types of utilization metrics are examples of some standard industry metrics:

- Units of measurement broadly applicable to most types of utilization or cost
  - Average cost per type of medical service or object; for example, the average cost per inpatient admission or the average cost per prescription
  - Percentages of types of services or objects; for example, the percent of procedures done at one facility versus another or the percent of prescriptions dispensed as generic rather than brand name drugs
- Metrics that take membership into account
  - Per member per month, or PMPM (e.g., 4.2 physician office visits PMPM or $29.17 PMPM for office visits)
  - Per member per year, or PMPY (e.g., 9.2 prescriptions PMPY, or $474.53 PMPY for prescription drugs)
- Units of measurement broadly applicable to facility-based utilization
  - Bed-days per thousand members per year, also referred to as bed-days per thousand or BD/K (e.g., 243.7 BD/K)
  - Admissions per thousand members per year
  - Ambulatory procedures per thousand members per year, or procedures per thousand
  - Length of stay (LOS) or average length of stay (ALOS) (e.g., 3.0 days ALOS)

Like most metrics, they are created by dividing one set of whole numbers by another set of numbers. For example, all premium revenue in whole dollars divided by the total number of members who are fully insured yields the premium revenue per member; or the cost of all prescription drugs in whole dollars divided by the total number of prescriptions yields the cost per prescription. Metrics also typically incorporate some measurement of time such as per month or per year. Metrics using a time period can also be averaged over a different time period, for example, the year to date average of a per month metric. The same type of metrics may be used for units of utilization or for costs.

Metrics also often take membership into account and are reported on a per member basis. Metrics that incorporate varying periods of time, which is most of them, must take into account that the number of members enrolled in the plan will vary from month to month, sometimes to a considerable degree. This is handled by using a running total of members for each month, which is referred to as "member months." For example, if a plan has 100,000 members in January, 110,000 in February, and 107,000 in March, the total member months for the first quarter is 317,000 member months. To calculate the average cost per member, then, the total whole dollars spent during a time period is divided by the total member months in that time period to yield the average cost per member. Metrics related to membership and adjusted for differences in monthly enrollment levels allow them to mean the same thing from month to month, which whole numbers would not.

Table 7-1 provides a hypothetical example of inpatient costs for a health plan with approximately 900,000 members, using whole dollars to calculate cost as PMPM and PMPY on a monthly and year-to-date (YTD) basis.

Numbers that are very large or very small are difficult to grasp and use on a day-to-day basis, so utilization metrics normally use a denominator that best allows the numerator to be more easily understood. Metrics whose numerators have two, three, or four integers are easier to handle than ones with ten or ones with small fractions, which is why metrics are not all reported using the same denominators. It is also easier to see the impact of any changes when the numerators use similar-appearing ranges.

Most metrics are understandable using common sense. Table 7-1 provides one example. Summary metrics such as these may be sufficient for calculating premium requirements, but not for actively managing utilization. UM requires metrics be further refined. In other words, the average PMPM cost of a broad category such as inpatient care does not provide enough information for managers to know what to focus on. That is accomplished by using the same approach to metrics, but at a finer level of detail, for example:

- Differences between hospitals;
- Differences between types of services such as general medical versus intensive care;
- Differences between the expected utilization and what is actually observed;

TABLE 7-1	Hypothetical Example of Overall Inpatient Costs in Whole Dollars, PMPM, PMPY, and Year End						
Month	Inpatient cost (whole dollars)	YTD inpatient cost (whole dollars)	Members	YTD member months	PMPM	YTD PMPM	YTD PMPY
January	$88,010,900	$88,010,900	901,263	901,263	$97.65	$97.65	$1,171.83
February	$91,121,080	$179,131,980	901,583	1,802,846	$101.07	$99.36	$1,192.33
March	$92,734,900	$271,866,880	901,784	2,704,630	$102.83	$100.52	$1,206.23
April	$93,357,300	$365,224,180	901,935	3,606,565	$103.51	$101.27	$1,215.20
May	$94,936,200	$460,160,380	902,739	4,509,304	$105.16	$102.05	$1,224.56
June	$93,924,830	$554,085,210	902,958	5,412,262	$104.02	$102.38	$1,228.51
July	$90,238,460	$644,323,670	905,927	6,318,189	$99.61	$101.98	$1,223.75
August	$88,472,603	$732,796,273	905,923	7,224,112	$97.66	$101.44	$1,217.25
September	$92,402,753	$825,199,026	905,102	8,129,214	$102.09	$101.51	$1,218.12
October	$91,840,254	$917,039,280	905,276	9,034,490	$101.45	$101.50	$1,218.05
November	$93,581,267	$1,010,620,547	905,712	9,940,202	$103.32	$101.67	$1,220.04
December	$88,372,956	$1,098,993,503	905,295	10,845,497	$97.62	$101.33	$1,215.98
Year-end average	$91,582,792		903,791		$101.33		$1,216.00
Year-end total		$1,098,993,503		10,845,497			

- Differences between the expected cost and what is actually observed; and
- Specific rates of inflation for the utilization and cost for defined types of care such as imaging or biopharmaceutical infusion.

Metrics Specific to Facility-Based Utilization

As seen in Figure 7-1, the cost of commercial coverage for inpatient and outpatient facility care accounts for a nearly half of the overall cost, but accounts for over 60% of the total increase from 2010 to 2011. And that does not even include the physician costs associated with inpatient stays or ambulatory procedures. Because facility-based utilization is so costly, in addition to the usual PMPM and PMPY costs, payers use specific standardized metrics based on inpatient LOS and units of utilization per 1,000 members per year to measure and manage it. LOS is typically measured for individual cases during concurrent review, as discussed later, and ALOS is used for overall medical management. Per thousand metrics are most often used for inpatient bed-days, inpatient admissions, and ambulatory procedures.

Utilization per thousand is measured based on a year. For example, an admission rate of 55 admissions per thousand means that for every 1,000 plan members, 55 will be admitted at some time during the year.* But it is not annual in the sense of needing to wait until year end; it is annualized, meaning that even if the time period being measured is less than a year, month to date for example, it is calculated as though that amount of utilization held steady for an entire year. This allows the numerator to fall within the same type of range as other utilization metrics.

Definition of the Numbers

Before providing the formula for calculating inpatient bed-days, admissions, or procedures per thousand, it is important to note that choosing and precisely defining what is to be measured is not always simple. The formula for calculating the metrics may be standard, but deciding what to count as a bed-day can vary a bit.

In past decades, some payers would count outpatient surgery as a single day in the hospital. But because payment for outpatient procedures is almost always different than for inpatient days (see Chapter 5), it is more appropriate to count outpatient procedures separately, though using the same approach to the calculation. A few plans count skilled nursing home days in the total, though most do not. While plans may add commercial, Medicare, and Medicaid into the total calculation, it is most common to separate those very different types of businesses and patient populations. In some plans, the day of discharge is counted; in most it is not unless the hospital charges for it.

How to count nursery days is not straightforward, and a decision must be reached on whether to count nursery days in the total when the mother is still in the hospital or only if the newborn is boarding over or in intensive care. The most reasonable approach is to count them if they are separately billed for and the rate is equivalent to a regular inpatient day, but if they are included with the mother's stay, then there is no real need. If the newborn requires a stay beyond the mother's discharge or if the neonate is in the intensive care unit, charges will be quite high and payers count them as neonatal intensive care unit (NICU) days.

Observation stays, or partial days, are another category that requires definition. Observation stays are deliberately designed to be less than 24 hours so as to avoid being considered an admission. But they are also typically less costly than an ambulatory procedure, putting them in between an inpatient day and an ambulatory procedure. Because observation stays have been increasing, particularly when emergency department chest pain protocols call for keeping any case in which a heart attack cannot definitively be ruled out, some large plans track them separately. Others include them as a single inpatient day, which can lead to a higher than normal admission rate and lower than normal ALOS.

Skilled nursing bed-days, or step-down units as discussed later, may be included as regular bed-days or tracked separately. There is no hard rule, just as there isn't for any of these types of bed-days, but payers typically count skilled nursing or step-down unit bed-days as a regular day if they are part of an acute stay and expected to be short term, and separately if expected to last more than a week or so.

Formulas to Calculate Institutional Utilization per Thousand

The standard formula to calculate utilization per thousand is relatively straightforward, and will be illustrated by looking at bed-days per thousand. The exact same formula is applicable to calculating admissions and ambulatory procedures per thousand. It may be calculated for any chosen time period (e.g., a single day, month to date, a quarter, or year to date). Because the measure is always annualized, the calculation of bed-days per thousand uses the assumption of a 365-day year as opposed to a 12-month year to prevent variations that are due solely to the length of a month.

The formula is: $[A \div (B \div 365)] \div (C \div 1,000)$

- **A** is the gross (meaning the total) number of bed-days (or admissions or ambulatory procedures) in the time period

---

*Actually, the admission rate only refers to the number of admissions, not whether or not each admission represented a different person. The same member could be admitted more than once, and each time would count as a separate admission.

- **B** is the number of days in the time period
- **C** is the average plan membership in the time period
  B can be the total number of days in any period of time, such as:
  - A single day
  - Month-to-date
  - Month
  - Year-to-date
  - Year

This calculation may be broken into steps. **Table 7-2** illustrates the calculation for bed-days per thousand on a single day, while **Table 7-3** illustrates the calculation for bed-days per thousand for a month to date after 3 weeks into the month.

Medical managers also want to know which hospitals are being used, and what each hospital's specific cost and utilization metrics are. This is especially important because of the high cost differences between hospitals, as discussed in Chapters 4 and 5. UM typically further divides these measurements by categories such as inpatient type of service and location. Type of service is the most common, and examples of typical inpatient categories include:

- Medical–surgical,
- Obstetrics,
- Intensive care,
- Neonatal intensive care,
- Psychiatric or substance abuse rehabilitation, and
- Skilled nursing or medical–surgical rehabilitation.

Examples of typical ambulatory procedure categories include:

- Scoping procedures
  - May be all types, or
  - May separate gastrointestinal, orthopedic, and other;
- Orthopedic procedures and implants;
- Cardiac procedures and implants;
- General surgical procedures;
- Cardiac imaging and diagnostic testing;
- Other costly imaging such as nuclear scans, magnetic resonance imaging (MRI), and positron emission tomography (PET) scans;
- Dialysis; and
- Chemotherapy and other infusion therapies.

Data about cost, quality, and utilization is used in many other ways besides the very basic metrics discussed here, as is apparent in most of the book's chapters. There are also other metrics payers commonly use. For example, Chapter 10 focuses specifically on the use of data and provider profiling in medical management, and most plans use and report on both the expansive Healthcare Effectiveness Data and Information Set (HEDIS®) and Consumer Assessment of Healthcare Providers and Systems (CAHPS®) data sets, which are described in Chapter 15.

TABLE 7-2	**Example Calculation of Bed Days for a Single Day**

Assume: Current hospital census = 300
          Plan membership = 500,000

Step 1: Gross days   = 300 ÷ (1 ÷ 365)
                       = 300 ÷ 0.00274
                       = 109,500

Step 2: Days per 1,000 = 109,500 ÷ (500,000 ÷ 1,000)
                       = 109,500 ÷ 500
                       = 219

Therefore, the days per thousand for that single day is 219.

TABLE 7-3	**Example Calculation of Bed-Days for the Month to Date (MTD), Three Weeks into the Month**

Assume: Total gross hospital bed-days MTD = 6,382
        Plan membership = 500,000
        Days in MTD = 21

Step 1: Gross days MTD   = 6,382 ÷ (21 ÷ 365)
                           = 6,382 ÷ 0.0575
                           = 110,925.24

Step 2: Days per 1,000 in MTD = 110,925.24 ÷ (500,000 ÷ 1,000)
                              = 110,925.24 ÷ 500
                              = 222 (rounded)

Therefore, the MTD days per thousand is 222.

■ REGIONAL VARIATIONS IN UTILIZATION AND COSTS

Not only are there variations between individual physicians in their use of evidence-based medical practice, but there is a substantial body of evidence that hospital utilization and procedure rates vary significantly from one geographic area of the country to another for unexplained reasons. In other words, utilization is not the same in different parts of the country, but relatively consistent within a locale. For example, states in the eastern United States have higher rates of inpatient care than western states do, and similar geographic differences may be demonstrated for almost all types of medical care.

As far back as 1982, Wennberg and Gittelesohn coined the term "surgical signature" to describe a regional practice pattern of surgical rates within an area that cannot be explained by differences in population morbidity or other market phenomena.[5] In 1985, Wennberg and Caper reported that the rate of some treatments did not vary much from one market to the next, but other treatments varied four- or fivefold across markets with no population-based explanation for the differences.[6]

Variations on utilization continued to be reported from then on, including research that revealed geographic variations in the type and use of different treatments by physicians across the country. Research also found significant variations not only by region, but sometimes on a hospital-to-hospital basis, including variations between academic facilities.[7, 8]

Currently, the most widely used national comparative data of geographic differences is a continuation of Dr. Wennberg's work, the *Dartmouth Atlas of Health Care*, which publishes an annual report of cost and utilization variations by geographic location and hospital, as well as self-service comparative tools and research reports.[*] In a study published in 2009, researchers at the Dartmouth Atlas of Health Care reported that only 18% of the variation was due to

medical conditions.[9] Other researchers, analyzing the same Medicare data but factoring in more individual health status indicators, reported that medical conditions accounted for approximately 30% of the difference, and when factoring in different payment methods by Medicare, the explainable portion of variation rose to 45%. But even under the best of circumstances, at least half the variation remained unexplained.[10, 11]

Interestingly, a different study examined variation by comparing claims data in the Dartmouth Atlas and claims data from commercial payers, and reported a modestly positive correlation between Medicare and commercial utilization, but not cost; high commercial costs correlated most strongly with hospital market concentration, as discussed in Chapter 5, and high Medicare costs correlated with markets that were less concentrated.[12]

Researchers looking at the local level may find reasons supporting differences, but when looking at the national level, the variation is striking. **Figure 7-3** shows admissions and bed-days per 1,000, and ALOS for all people in the United States regardless of age, sex, or benefits coverage. The differences are striking.

Differences in individual health status, and in price and payment methodologies, account for some amount of

_____

[*] www.dartmouthatlas.org.

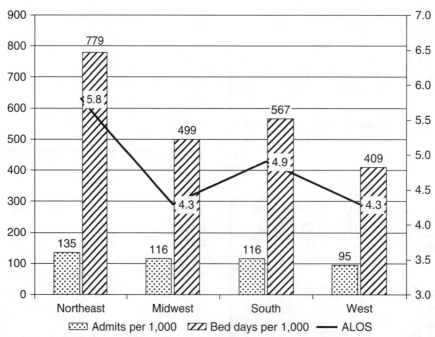

FIGURE 7-3 Regional Variation in Admissions per 1,000, Bed-Days per 1,000, and Average Length of Stay for U.S. Population Regardless of Age or Insurance Coverage, 2007

Source: Data from U.S. National Center for Health Statistics, Vital and Health Statistics, "Discharges, Days of Care, and Average Length of Stay in Nonfederal Short-Stay Hospitals, by Selected Characteristics: United States, selected years 1980–2007," www.cdc.gov/nchs/hus/contents2010.htm#table099. Accessed July 15, 2011.

variation, but that leaves a considerable amount unexplained and not fully understood. There is no consensus of opinions on why regional variation occurs, but possible explanations include:

- Physician enthusiasm for certain treatments or types of care;
- Preference-based care in which options exist but either the physician or the patient has a clear preference for one over the others;
- Local medical community norms, regardless of any basis in evidence-based practice;
- Over- or undersupply of specialists and/or hospitals;
- Over- or undersupply of costly diagnostic devices or centers;
- Physician ownership of hospitals, ambulatory procedure facilities, or costly diagnostic devices;
- Cultural or socioeconomic variations in patient populations;
- The profitability of different types of care or procedures;
- The prevalence of different types of payers, and the market share of HMOs in particular;
- The impact of cost-sharing on consumers;
- The impact of a state's regulatory environment;
- The practice of "defensive medicine" in areas with high rates of medical malpractice suits; and
- Anything else you can think of.

Before leaving the topic, it is worth placing the issue of variation in perspective. It is neither desirable nor possible to reduce variation to zero. The human body and the practice of medicine are far too complex to equate to an assembly line or a fast-food restaurant. A certain amount of variation is actually desirable because a lack of variation implies no change, and nobody will argue that medicine should be practiced now like it was in 1972, or even 2002. But variations caused by not practicing evidence-based medicine, by unwillingness to change, by force of habit or unsupported preference, or by inappropriate motives such as financial enrichment, those are the focus of UM.

■ BENEFITS DESIGN AND MEDICAL UTILIZATION

The primary focus of health benefits plan design is to create a product that can successfully compete in the market, but it can also have an impact on utilization, which is often taken into account during the design process. The broad topic of benefits design is discussed in Chapter 16 in the context of sales and marketing. It is also addressed in Chapter 30 because there are explicit benefits requirements in the ACA. Some went into effect almost immediately, prevention for example, while others are effective beginning

in 2014. Except for prevention benefits, the ACA allows for four tiers of cost-sharing,[13] making it generally compatible with existing benefits designs.[*]

Cost-sharing is often used by non-HMO payers to control premium inflation. In most cases, actuaries simply reduce the amount the plan will need to pay by the amount paid by the member. This is similar to adjusting capitation rates for copayments that was described in Chapter 5. But it is also used to get members to change how and even when they access care. This is called behavioral shift, and it means that the design of the benefit will cause at least some members to make different choices than they might if the benefits were designed in another way, including if there is no coverage at all. It has been studied for decades since the first publications from the seminal 1970s-era Rand Health Insurance Experiment began to appear in the early 1980s.[14]

The uses of benefits design is most obvious in HMOs that use PCP gatekeepers to manage access to specialty and facility care, since members are required to change behavior, in this case by not going directly to a specialist. Provider networks in both HMOs and PPOs also provide better benefits for members to induce them to get their care within the network. In the case of HMOs, but not HMOs with point of service (POS; see Chapter 2) plans, it is not cost-sharing so much as it is no coverage.

More subtly, network tiering, which is described in Chapter 4, is a benefits design that depends more on behavioral shift than on the member actually sharing much of the cost. In the case of hospital tiering, there may be a $500 or $1,000 increase in the deductible when using a non-tier-one hospital, but the actual cost difference between a tier-one and tier-two hospital may be closer to $10,000 or more. In other words, the difference in the deductible is far too low to cover the difference in cost, but it is high enough to induce an individual to choose the tier-one facility.

Consumer-Directed Health Plans

CDHPs were originally designed *specifically* to cause consumers to change how they used health services. The thinking was that by "having skin in the game" through more out-of-pocket cost-sharing, consumers would be more aware about the cost of care and would factor that in when seeking medical care. The same concept was part of the reason for having a pretax savings option that would ultimately

---

[*]The ACA also immediately prohibited lifetime maximum benefits for health coverage and requires the phase-out of annual benefits limitations by 2014. But while having no benefits does reduce utilization, it is not the same as managing utilization, so it is not discussed further.

cover at least part of the out-of-pocket costs, since they would still be exposed to the actual costs rather than being shielded from it by billing and payment taking place behind the scenes. The exception to increased cost-sharing in CDHPs was for prevention benefits, which were often covered in full even before that was required under the ACA.

The lower premiums associated with CDHPs resulting from lower levels of coverage make them increasingly attractive to employers. But the ability of CDHPs to lower overall costs in the long term is not clear. An early study reported that CDHPs were associated with both lower costs and lower cost increases, but also had modest favorable health selection, meaning people who signed up with a CDHP were healthier than average, and there was also evidence of both appropriate and inappropriate changes in care use.[15] A more recent study found that families enrolled in CDHPs did have lower costs than those enrolled in a traditional PPO, but only when the deductible was over $1,000 and the employer was not generous in funding a pretax savings account.[16] Conversely, another study looking at an employer offering both a CDHP and a traditional PPO reported that high deductibles led to lower use of prescription drugs, but not overall costs in the long term, particularly once the deductible was met.[17]

A very comprehensive synthesis of cost-sharing studies published by the Robert Wood Johnson Foundation in 2010* concluded that CDHPs were not necessarily effective, and were sometimes associated with negative consequences.[18] So at best, there is ambiguity about CDHP effectiveness in controlling costs long term, and no useful research on long-term outcomes or health status have been published, at least at the time of this book's publication.

Value-Based Insurance Benefit Design

Where CDHPs use higher cost sharing as a means of lowering utilization, lower cost sharing can be used as a means of deliberately increasing it. The two types of benefits design that have applied this are benefits for wellness and prevention and value-based insurance benefits design (VBID or VBBD).

First-dollar coverage for prevention was the most common type of positive inducement even before the ACA made it mandatory for all health benefits plans, and it is thoroughly addressed in Chapter 13 as well as summarized later in this chapter.

More recently, VBID has been applied to medical benefits for chronic conditions. It may be applied generally to induce the use of lower-cost alternatives, or it may be tailored to fit individuals. VBID is discussed here but not under cost-sharing because most types of VBID are technically a "waiver of

benefits," meaning the benefit normally requires cost-sharing through deductibles, coinsurance, or copayments.

The most common broad use of VBID has been by pharmacy benefits managers (PBMs; see Chapter 11) who may identify members taking an expensive brand-name drug and offer to waive any copayments if they change to an inexpensive generic alternative, but only if their doctor agrees with the change. It has also been used in case management to expedite an inpatient discharge or reduce the risk of admission, providing a hospital bed for home use, for example. In recent years, there has been an extension of the concept to common, potentially high-cost medical conditions such as congestive heart failure, diabetes, cardiovascular disease, chronic obstructive pulmonary disease, and so forth. The basic idea is to use VBID to improve compliance with treatment for individuals who might otherwise not comply due to out-of-pocket costs. When used, VBID is typically part of an overall DM program and usually applied to drug coverage, meaning the PBM would be directed to waive any cost-sharing for selected prescription drugs, even if they are not generic (although they typically are) for individuals identified by the DM clinical managers. A similar approach could be applied to office visit copayments or any other services or devices in which improved compliance could be linked to lower costs, reduced likelihood of hospitalization, and better outcomes.

While VBID has its enthusiastic supporters and is certainly logical in theory, there is not enough long-term research to know with any certainty how much impact it has, if any, on chronic conditions. But there is some indication that on a purely clinical basis, it does. In the short term, however, costs almost always go up due to an increase in the use and cost of prescription drugs. Savings come in the next year or two as VBID and other applicable DM approaches reduce the rate of avoidable hospitalizations in these individuals (see Chapter 8).

Finally, despite a great deal of talk about VBID, there are only a handful who are experimenting with it beyond prevention and wellness (which is now mandatory anyway). The cost to actually administer VBID is variable and potentially high because most claims systems are not able to alter benefits for individual members, or even subscribers,[†] although PBM claims systems are more likely than medical claims systems to be able to do so. Because of the relatively low level of take-up for VBID by employers, it may be some time before its true value can be assessed.

■   DEMAND MANAGEMENT

The term "demand management" in health insurance and managed health care is used much more narrowly than it is

---

*Any reader interested in the topic of the impact of cost-sharing in health benefits is strongly encouraged to read the synthesis report at www.rwjf.org/pr/synthesis.jsp at the time of publication.

†A subscriber is the family member with coverage through his or her employer, and members are all individuals with coverage, including the dependents of a subscriber.

in economic theory. Applied to health benefits, it refers to health plan activities that are designed to lower members' needs for health care services. Done well, it also may provide a competitive advantage to a health plan by enhancing its reputation for service and giving members additional value. HMOs typically provide the most demand management services compared to other types of payers, although most payers provide at least some. Demand management services fall into six broad and interrelated categories:

1. Nurse advice lines;
2. Self-care and self-evaluation programs;
3. Preventive services;
4. Health risk appraisals;
5. Shared decision-making programs; and
6. Personal health records and personal health management tools.

Nurse Advice Lines

Nurse advice lines provide members with access to advice regarding medical conditions, the need for medical care, health promotion and preventive care, and numerous other advice-related activities. They first came into common use in closed-panel HMOs, where they were once (and occasionally still are) referred to as "triage"[*] nurse lines, but are now common in most health plans. Plans may staff these lines with their own nurses, or they may purchase the service from any one of a number of commercial vendors. Hours of operation are commonly 24 hours per day, 7 days per week, and a toll-free line makes it easy for members to access the service. Nurses staffing advice lines typically have access to information about the member, including eligibility and claims history. When a member calls for advice about a medical issue, the nurse provides it by working through an algorithm containing common clinical scenarios and applicable advice. The nurses are not practicing medicine, but only providing medical advice, so they tend to be conservative and do not try to prevent a member from seeking care from a physician, clinic, or the emergency department. They also keep records of the call, and may record it (members are informed that the call may be recorded). All records are subject to the same privacy protections given to any type of protected health information (PHI) under the Health Insurance Portability and Accountability Act (HIPAA; see Chapter 29).

Nurse advice lines can also be proactive, not confined to answering calls from members. This is discussed further in the other sections covering demand management. Special market segments such as Medicare and Medicaid (see Chapters 24 and 25, respectively) benefit from dedicated programs, and some states require their use. Attention to the special problems and concerns of seniors will go a long way toward improving health status and can be a major contributor to the overall management of care in this population. Easy access to medical advice in the Medicaid population may allow these members to avoid a trip to the emergency department. However, Medicaid members are more likely than commercial members to not have a permanent telephone number, or even a telephone, although the appearance of pay-as-you-go cell phone plans has helped.

Self-Care and Self-Evaluation Programs

Self-care and self-evaluation simply means providing information to members that allows them to take care of minor medical problems, or to better evaluate whether or not they need to see a physician. With the increasing focus on making health care consumers more informed, payers have been creating or providing access to tools and information that has been expanding in scope and functionality. In most cases, payers outsource this or contract with a company that specializes in these services, and often add their own brand and logo to it. Self-care programs are now also eligible for accreditation or recognition by two accreditation organizations that most commonly accredit managed care plans, the National Committee for Quality Assurance (NCQA) and URAC,[†] as discussed in Chapter 15.

Self-care tools and information is almost always available through Internet member portals, but since members have different preferred communication channels, it is typically also available through other media such as mailings and hard-copy manuals. Nurse advice lines also provide self-care guidelines. Both the content and the way it is delivered may also vary for commercial, Medicare Advantage (MA), and Medicaid managed care plans. And though not specific to payers, the federal government has a portal that provides self-care and self-evaluation tools (www.healthfinder.gov/HealthTools/[‡]) and the ACA calls for additional investment. Online tools are passive, and payers sometimes take a more proactive approach for focused types of self-care communications, the preferred route typically by mail. For example, a payer may mail self-care material about back pain to members who have generated back pain-related claims. Self-care programs have been evaluated since the early 1980s. Typical results from the 1980s showed $2.50–3.50 saved for every $1 invested and/or reductions in office visits.[19, 20] A structured study in a staff model HMO in the 1990s reported that the targeted use of self-care manuals resulted in decreased outpatient visits and a 2:1 return on the cost of the program.[21]

---

[*]In a health plan, the use of the term *triage nurse* is not recommended if for no other reason than its military history. "Triage" is a term used in battlefield medicine that refers to the separation of casualties into three categories: immediate attention required, attention can be delayed, and casualty is beyond hope and only will be given palliative care. Use of the term *advice nurse* is more appropriate.

[†]URAC is no longer an acronym for anything.
[‡]Current as of July 9, 2011.

Preventive Services

Preventive services were the hallmark of the HMO industry from its earliest days. But over the past decade or more, almost all types of payers became interested in it, as well as large employer groups. The ACA made first-dollar coverage of prevention a requirement for all health plans shortly after its passage.[22] Prevention is covered in detail in Chapter 13, so only a brief mention of some of these activities is provided here.

Common preventive services include immunizations, mammograms, routine physical examinations, and counseling regarding behaviors that members can undertake to lower their risk of ill health. Counseling and education also may be directed toward specific clinical conditions or members who are at risk for complications. For example, a 2008 controlled randomized study compared the impact on at-risk members of mailing reminders to get an influenza vaccination, or both mailing a reminder and having an advice nurse directly call them, reported a return on investment (ROI) of $2.51 for mailings and $24.24 for mailing plus a nurse call.[23]

Prevention certainly has a positive impact on overall health, although mostly for individuals who actually change unhealthy behaviors. Many case studies report a positive financial ROI,[24] but some broad-based prevention programs do not. For example, a recent study of two employer-sponsored health management programs covering over 200,000 health plan members did not show any savings, although there was a slight decline in hospitalizations, and the lack of savings did not even count the cost of administering the program.[25]

Primary prevention has a positive impact on health and, generally speaking, on the overall cost of care. Prevention in chronic conditions such as high cholesterol, hypertension, and so forth also has a positive impact on health, but a recent analysis of prevention concluded that "Less than 20 percent of the preventive options (and a similar percentage for treatment) fall in the cost-saving category—80 percent add more to medical costs than they save."[26] This is not a secret. Even before the ACA mandated first-dollar coverage of prevention, health insurers and HMOs covered it not to save money, but because sometimes the right thing to do is the right thing to do.

Health Risk Appraisals*

The health risk appraisal (HRA)[†] is a tool designed to elicit information from a member regarding certain activities and behaviors that can influence health status. HRAs are administered in multiple formats, most commonly through an Internet member portal, but also using paper forms or even via telephone. Many employers support the use of HRAs and some offer incentives for employees and their dependents to complete them, for example, bonus dollars in flexible spending accounts, modest reductions in their payroll contribution toward the cost of coverage, or coupons for health-related services.

The objective of the HRA is to collect information and through analysis, create a member profile of an individual's health risks and needs for behavior modification that may improve a member's health outcomes. Ultimately, the health appraisal findings trigger applicable care management programs, including wellness and behavior modification programs focusing on common topics such as smoking cessation, stress reduction, or weight management. Disease-specific HRAs also exist and may be incorporated into a DM program. In all cases, HRA results are shared with the member and may be used by the payer's care management department. Results may also be shared with the member's physician, but that is inconsistent.

The value of HRAs is not easily assessed, but like prevention in general, it may actually increase costs in the short run. For example, a study comparing employees and dependents who were offered HRAs to those that were not found that women, healthier people, and people in CDHPs are more likely than others to complete an HRA; and among those who completed an HRA, use of office visits, prescription drugs, and cervical cancer screenings increased compared with those who are not offered an HRA.[27]

HRAs may be broadly classified into three categories:[28]

1. Risk-based HRA: It is the earliest type of HRA. It focuses on patient behavior and its effect on health risk.
2. Habit-based HRA: It is similar to the risk-based HRA. It not only looks at habits that create increased health risk, but also incorporates elements of health education and behavioral change.
3. Utilization-based HRA: A form of HRA that focuses on predictors of utilization. These are typically part of a DM program (Chapter 8).

Predictive modeling, which first came into heavy use in DM programs, has also been applied to HRAs that add questions about an individual's level of involvement in their health and in life in general. In this way, the HRAs both identify health risks and provide an indication of which at-risk members are more likely than others to respond to interventions or assistance. In plans that have a large Medicare enrollment, the plan may take extra steps in an initial assessment that go beyond the typical HRA. The most common extra step is an in-home assessment of the new MA member by a trained nurse or medical social worker. The assessment would include areas that injuries typically occur, such as the bathroom, and if the plan gives the new

---

*A payer may use the term "health appraisal" so as to eliminate any perceived negative connotations around the word "risk," but this is purely cosmetic.
†Not to be confused with the other meaning of the acronym HRA: health reimbursement account, discussed in Chapter 2.

MA enrollee a bath mat or shower chair, it will significantly reduce the risk of a hip fracture from falling in the bathtub. An inventory of the member's diet also may yield valuable information that will enable the new member's provider to improve health status by lowering sodium intake or the amount of dietary saturated fat.

Shared Decision-Making Programs

Shared decision making means having the member actively participate in choosing a course of care. While this general philosophy may be prevalent in the routine interactions between patients and physicians, shared decision programs are more focused, providing patients in-depth information on specific procedures. By doing so, patients gain a deeper understanding of not only the disease process, but also the treatment alternatives.

Shared decision making began to become popular in the 1980s when studies of surgical options for transurethral resection of the prostate and for mastectomies found that less invasive options were often as good as or better than invasive ones. In a few cases, HMOs would not even finalize authorization for certain elective procedures until the member completed a shared decision-making program. Some states even passed laws making it mandatory for surgeons to provide information on all surgical treatment options for mastectomies. Through the 1980s and into the 2000s, the value of shared decision-making programs was regularly documented.[29-32] However, in the case of mastectomies for breast cancer, shared decision making appears to actually increase the amount of more invasive surgery as patients chose more invasive types of mastectomies even when their surgeons recommended less invasive ones.[33, 34]

A number of commercial services produce these programs, some with innovative business model designs. Many use online tools, interactive DVDs, printed materials, or (in the past) CD-ROMs to provide information. A nurse or physician's assistant may also help a member go through the issues. Closed-panel HMOs sometimes have a private kiosk or workstation at a clinic that a member may use, as well as the ability to discuss the alternatives with the physician after the patient has reviewed the material. IDSs can easily adopt all of these approaches as well.

Personal Health Record and Personal Health Manager Tools

As health care in the United States continues to move to a more consumer-driven model where the member is expected to be more involved in the health care decision, a trend has evolved in the creation of personal health records (PHR). Personal health management involves activities like tracking and monitoring personal health measures (e.g., blood pressure, cholesterol), selecting health providers, managing health dollars (e.g., flexible spending, health spending, and health payment accounts), and understanding and influencing treatment.

It is important to note that a PHR is not the same as an electronic health record (EHR). Personal health management tools allow the data to be shared in multiple directions and business rules can drive key messages, actions, reminders, and content. The information is personalized, secure, and includes multiple data sources such as claims, authorizations, and results from an HRA. An initiative sponsored by the primary trade association for the health insurance industry, America's Health Insurance Plans (AHIP), in 2007 led to standardizing the core data elements of the PHR so as to improve interoperability between health plans.

■ CATEGORIES OF UTILIZATION MANAGEMENT

Before there was UM, there was utilization review (UR), and it still makes up the core of most UM programs, albeit in a far more sophisticated way than when it first appeared. The primary purpose of UR was, and still is, the first of the three main areas of focus for UM overall: to inform decisions about whether or not certain medical services or products will be covered under the benefits plan, and under what conditions. UR for benefits coverage determinations can occur at different points in time, so it is divided into three categories:

1. Prospective, meaning it takes place before medical services or products have been provided;
2. Concurrent, meaning it takes place while medical services are being provided, not before or after; or
3. Retrospective, meaning it takes place after medical services or products were provided.

The vehicle used to signal whether or not a medical service is covered, and under what circumstances, is the authorization system, so these same three categories also appear in the section on authorizations and precertification, but with several different variants. Although benefits determinations make up the majority of what takes place in UM, there are some activities that do not involve it, but even then there is a relationship. For example, case management, which is found in almost all types of managed health care plans and large IDSs, and is a central element in PCMHs and ACOs, may be triggered during all three types of UR. Other UM processes that focus on managing costs through the use of more cost-effective services, and on reducing practice variation through the promotion of evidence-based medical practices, may also take place because of UR and CM.

The purpose of identifying these categories here is to provide an overall framework for UM. Prospective and retrospective UM is applicable to all types of services, but concurrent UM is only applicable to inpatient or extended outpatient services. CM and the use of alternatives to inpatient services are applicable to most types of services as well, but differently than are the three main categories of UM. The focus on each category varies from payer to payer, both by plan type and by a plan's overall philosophical approach to managing utilization. This includes the specific activities within each category as well as the degree of assertiveness.

■ DETERMINATION OF COVERAGE, MEDICAL NECESSITY, AND EVIDENCE-BASED CLINICAL GUIDELINES

Most benefits coverage decisions are relatively straightforward and are typically described in a health plan's evidence of coverage (EOC) or schedule of benefits documents. For coverage determinations, most routine medical care requires little or no documentation other than what's required in the provider's claim for payment (see Chapter 18). Some care requires a small amount of additional documentation in order to determine coverage. For example, precertification of an elective admission is usually required by any type of health plan, and failure to comply can result in less or no coverage regardless of any clinical criteria (this is not the case for urgent or emergency care); in the case of in-network providers in HMOs and most PPOs, noncompliance results in less or no payment to the provider, but no member liability.

Coverage decisions can be based on administrative issues such as a member no longer being covered by the health plan or a particular service not being covered under the plan's schedule of benefits, regardless of whether a member or provider thinks it should be. For example, no commercial health insurers cover the cost of custodial care, and Medicare doesn't either. Only Medicaid covers it, and only for low-income or indigent individuals[*] (see Chapter 25). (Because the focus of this chapter is UM, purely administrative causes for benefits denial or reduction are discussed in Chapter 18, but not here.)

Coverage may also be denied or reduced due to failure to comply with certain requirements such as obtaining precertification, which is discussed in detail later. In this case, the impact on coverage or payment is intended to reinforce compliance with the UM program, not because of a service not being covered under any condition or because it's not considered medically necessary.

Coverage Decisions versus Medical Care Decisions

An important distinction must be drawn concerning the first of the three major areas of focus for UM: benefits coverage decisions. With the exception of closed-panel HMOs, managed health care plans *only* make coverage decisions. They

do not actually provide the care or prevent care from being provided. A statement like "My HMO wouldn't authorize my care," really means the HMO won't authorize coverage or payment for a particular medical service. A member can still get that service, but would have to pay for it out of pocket unless the provider agreed to render it without being paid. This distinction is an important one since managed health care plans are not practicing medicine.

Pointing out this distinction is not meant to pretend that coverage decisions can't influence whether or not a person gets a particular medical service. Obviously denial of coverage creates a substantial barrier to costly medical services, although not an absolute one. Some people do indeed go ahead and pay out of their own pockets. Also, a provider could forgo payment, but charity care is beyond the scope of this book.

When coverage is denied based on medical necessity, which is discussed next, it is rarely arbitrary and not necessarily immutable. Members have the right to appeal denial decisions, and initial coverage denials are often reversed when information is corrected or additional information is provided. If benefits coverage is still denied, members have the right to demand external physician review. The appeals and review processes are discussed in detail in Chapter 20 because they are typically managed by member services.

Medical Necessity

Part of the UM process is to ensure, as much as possible, that appropriate medical necessity criteria are met, that the benefits are being applied as they should be, and that they are being applied consistently to all members. A major portion of this is determining whether or not a service is "medically necessary" or meets the definition of "medical necessity." For example, a treating physician may be asked to provide clinical justification about why a very costly type of test is being requested when a less costly test will provide much the same information. Medical necessity may be a factor in benefits coverage decisions that occur at any point in the UM process, meaning it may be an element in prospective, concurrent, or retrospective UM. Medical necessity is discussed in Chapters 20 and 30 in the context of appeal rights created by the Employee Retirement Income Security Act (ERISA) and the ACA. The concepts are the same for purposes of this chapter, but the focus is on how payers typically apply it. Medical necessity is typically defined in the EOC, and also summarized in a new document defined in the ACA called a Summary of Coverage (SOC) beginning in 2012. The EOC also describes various rules such as compliance with UM, as well as various cost-sharing provisions or benefits limitations. These documents and the information within them are addressed in Chapters 20 and 30.

High-level definitions of medical necessity are not standardized and may differ some from one benefits plan to another, although there is general consistency in its overall

---

[*] Commercial long-term care insurance may cover it, but that is not health insurance.

application by payers. The ACA does not address either except as applicable to coverage of emergency care.[35] Medical necessity in commercial health benefits plans is typically defined beginning with items or services that may be justified as reasonable, necessary, and/or appropriate, based on evidence-based clinical standards of care. Definitions also typically describe what is excluded from coverage due to not being considered medically necessary; for example:

- Services that are primarily for the convenience of the patient or physician;
- Services that are more costly than an alternative service or sequence of services at least as likely to produce equivalent results;
- Custodial care or care that is essentially assistance with acts of daily living;
- Experimental or investigational care, except in defined circumstances; and
- Care not considered medically appropriate by generally accepted standards of medical practice.

Regardless of language in the benefits booklet, the terms "medical necessity" or "medically necessary" are sometimes difficult for those who are not involved in benefits determinations to understand. A provider or member may consider a medical service to be necessary, but that service still may not be considered medically necessary as applied to benefits coverage. This is because it still must meet the definitions, exclusions, and coverage requirements of the benefits plan, as noted earlier in the example of custodial care. Medical necessity may also be predicated on meeting certain clinical criteria or on demonstrating a lack of effectiveness of a less expensive option, which is the focus of this discussion.

Coverage decisions involving medical necessity are made with input from many possible sources, but the primary source is typically the treating physician. In the case of HMOs using PCP gatekeepers, which is described in detail later, authorization for coverage of specialty physician care is usually the sole responsibility of the PCP. But for all other types of UM, supporting information comes primarily from a member's treating physician. In some cases, however, UM managers and medical directors require additional information and/or opinions beyond that provided by the treating physician.

Variations in practice and inconsistent adherence to evidence-based medical practices are the main reasons a coverage determination might be required, but they are not the only reasons. Several studies published in reputable medical journals have confirmed that a sizable percentage of physicians are willing to deceive insurance companies or manipulate insurance coverage rules in order to obtain benefits for their patients.[36-40] Willingness to deceive an insurance company ranges from approximately one-third of physicians to over half when a patient has a serious condition. These studies do not mean that physicians are bad people. As discussed in the studies themselves, physicians see their primary duty as toward their patient, not an insurer, which should be no surprise since most people who go into medicine have a genuine desire to help people. Physician deception of health insurance companies is not condoned by clinical leaders,[41, 42] but it occurs nevertheless and is another reason why additional information may be required and why medical directors make independent coverage decisions.

Use of Evidence-Based Clinical Criteria and Guidelines

Benefits coverage decisions involving medical necessity are not arbitrary or based on the whim of a medical director, much less the apocryphal "bean counter" of the backlash days. Unsupportable decisions do not result in good service or good coverage decisions, and are ultimately harmful in the market and in court. The use of evidence-based clinical criteria and guidelines are just the opposite because they are based on formal medical studies and clinical trials that compare different approaches to care, with their results published in peer-reviewed medical journals.

Clinical criteria and guidelines are used in UM both for benefits determinations based on medical necessity and to assist the facilitation activities noted at the beginning of the chapter but not yet discussed. In the context of UM, benefits determinations may be a matter of covered or not covered under any circumstances, but just as often are also a matter of what is covered under what particular circumstances, and evidence-based clinical criteria and guidelines can be applicable to both. For example, an inpatient precertification request (described in detail shortly) may be evaluated based on criteria that support the need for hospitalization versus providing the care on an ambulatory basis. A case that does not meet those criteria may be subject to benefits denial or reduction for inpatient care, but would be fully covered if done as an outpatient; conversely, an individual may be so sick and frail that coverage of an inpatient meets criteria for medical necessity.

Criteria are also used for an initial assignment of a maximum length of stay that will be covered, and in the evaluation of whether or not continued inpatient days beyond that are medically justified and covered. Recalling the prohibition on balance billing in HMO provider contracts discussed in Chapters 4 and 6, a determination that additional days will not be covered usually results in facilitating the discharge since the hospital will not be paid for the excess days and may not bill the patient for them either.

It is important to bear in mind that guidelines are just that: guidelines. They are not intended to be absolute. Guidelines are used to inform the process and to facilitate consistency based on evidence-based practices. But there will always be cases that fall outside of the norm. For example, most inpatient procedures are done on the day of admission, but a frail elderly person with kidney and heart failure is likely to need to be properly hydrated or otherwise attended to so that already risky surgery is not made riskier.

In the early days, HMOs mostly created their own criteria by combining existing standards with internally generated ones. This could be a frustrating business since many clinical guidelines in the 1970s were not evidence-based, but rather were codifications of existing practices. That began to change in the early 1980s when InterQual® started publishing clinically grounded criteria for use in evaluating admissions, level of service, and discharges.[43] Payers began to adopt InterQual criteria, although the take-up rate was variable. Beginning in 1990, the actuarial firm Milliman (then called Milliman & Robertson) also began licensing evidence-based clinical criteria and guidelines,[44] and the use of both became widespread.

Currently, the Milliman Care Guidelines®[45] and guidelines created by InterQual,[46] now a division of McKesson, are widely used by payers for most routine and even complex benefits decisions, as well as supporting the other aspects of UM.* Hospitals and health systems as well as governmental agencies also frequently use them. There are multiple reasons for their widespread success: they are evidence-based, as already discussed; they are kept up to date, for current subscribers at least, which is not easy to do when there are so many criteria; they are available in many formats; and they are routinely automated and used in computerized decision-support systems.

When they first appeared, they were sold as two- or three-volume publications in three-ring binders (to make it easy to update a single guideline). The purchase price typically included a year's updates, and most payers subscribed every year. Paper-based versions are still available, for now at least, but it is much more typical for guidelines to be accessed electronically. Both Milliman and InterQual license them for a specified number of users for a specified period of time under multiple different platforms, including:

- Loaded into the care management decision-support application of a payer's core transactional processing systems;
- Loaded onto a third-party medical management decision-support software program that may be integrated with a payer's core systems or free-standing;
- Through a browser application that accesses a vendor's online support program;
- Installed on a payer's server and accessed through the payer's intranet;

- Installed on a PC; and
- Installed on a hand-held device such as a personal digital assistant (PDA) or smartphone.

Clinical criteria and guidelines are often separated into different categories, or areas of focus, although some may be combined under a single license. The most common categories are:

- Medical and surgical care
  - Inpatient care, together or separate from
  - Outpatient and ambulatory facility-based care;
- Behavioral health care;
- Imaging and other costly diagnostic services;
- Durable medical equipment, devices, and home care; and
- Long-term or chronic care.

Many payers modify these guidelines to some degree to conform to particular local conditions or to align with the focus of their UM priorities or business requirements. Payers may also supplement the guidelines with ones developed by their own clinical advisors or with other externally available guidelines for particular types of specialized care. There are thousands of evidence-based clinical guidelines for specific conditions, treatments, and procedures accessible through a federal clearinghouse† that can be very useful in determining medical necessity in complex cases and in the review of an appeal of a denial of benefits.

Both Milliman and InterQual market and license decision-support programs that will allow guidelines to be used more efficiently and effectively. Their criteria and guidelines are also used in systems provided by third-party vendors or incorporated into a payer's transactional processing system as seen in the platform examples above.

In most cases, guidelines used for precertification and medical benefits coverage determinations can be fully automated, converting decision support to decision making. When a potential denial of coverage is based on the use of fully automated guidelines, however, it typically is pended for review, not denied by the software program. Finally, some payers make the guidelines accessible on a self-service basis to all of their providers through a web portal.

The Benefits Determination Process in Complex Cases

The processes followed by UM for performing the initial determination of medical necessity in a complex case or the internal review of a denial of coverage appeal may take place on a prospective, concurrent, or retrospective basis, but the process is the same. The appeals process as described here serves to describe the process regardless of whether or not it is an initial determination or an internal review of an appeal, although timeframes may not be identical.

---

*Except for gratitude to the authors of Chapter 22 who are principals at Milliman, as well as knowing some individuals at both organizations simply from being in this industry since it was steam powered, the author has no relationship with either Milliman or InterQual.

---

† It is located at www.guideline.gov, current as of July 20, 2011.

The ACA requires all covered individuals to have the right to both an internal and external review of an appeal.[47] The administrative requirements of the formal appeals process is discussed in detail in Chapters 20 and 30, and only the basic clinical internal review process is described here; the external process is likewise described in Chapters 20 and 30. Timeliness requirements for internal review of urgent and nonurgent cases must conform to the following timeframes:

- An individual has at least 180 days to file an initial appeal;
- Urgent appeals must be reviewed in 72 hours or less;
- Preauthorization appeals must be reviewed within 30 days; and
- Postservice appeals must be reviewed within 60 days.

Case managers facilitate the internal processes, but final benefits determinations in cases of benefits limitations or denials are typically the responsibility of a medical director. It is a valid responsibility that is recognized by respected professional organizations including the American Medical Association (AMA)[48] and the American College of Physicians (ACP).[49] Medical directors are not providing care to the members for whom they are also making a coverage decision based on medical necessity. Charged with managing the finite resources of the benefits plan, their objective is to approach each benefits decision in an even and consistent fashion.

The processes used typically include:

- Use of computerized systems to track notes and information;
- Use of evidence-based clinical criteria and guidelines;
- Use of clinical data to support benefits determinations;
- Discussion of cases with the case management nurses as needed;
- Review of records and notes that pertain to the benefits issue or issues under consideration;
- Request for additional information as necessary;
- Communications with the member's provider and family as necessary;
- Use of benefits specialists to provide guidance on benefits language, when needed;
- Use of the specific benefits language in a plan to support the benefits determination; and
- The medical director(s), not nonphysicians, being responsible for making the benefits determination.

Finally, it is not typical for a case manager or medical director to personally examine a member. The member is not the patient of the medical director and the medical director does not provide or direct the provision of care; the medical director addresses only whether or not a service or product qualifies for coverage under the benefits plan.

■ AUTHORIZATION AND PRECERTIFICATION

One of the earliest elements to appear in managed health care was an authorization system, meaning certain types of medical services, sometimes only under certain conditions, required authorization before they would be covered; in other words, under defined circumstances, benefits are covered only if they are authorized, not simply provided. Authorizations may also take place on a prospective, concurrent, or retrospective basis. And, stating the obvious, authorization applies only for services that may be covered under the benefits plan.

While the term "authorization" can be used broadly, prospective authorizations are usually referred to as preauthorization or precertification.[*] These two terms are often used interchangeably, but within the managed health care industry the terms "authorization" or "preauthorization" often apply to a PCP's authorization for coverage of specialty physician services in an HMO, while "precertification" usually applies to coverage for facility-based services in any type of plan. However, there is considerable overlap in usage of both terms and breaking with the past, this chapter will not rigidly confine itself to only one use of either term.

As already discussed, authorizations and precertifications apply only to benefits coverage and/or claims payment; they do not prohibit the service itself, since the payer does not practice medicine. Also discussed earlier under the topic of benefit design, lack of authorization does not automatically mean zero coverage in all circumstances. In a pure HMO, lack of authorization for nonurgent or emergency care may well result in zero coverage, but non-HMO types of plans typically still provide coverage, although not as much. For example, an HMO with a POS plan may cover 60% of allowed charges for out-of-network or nonauthorized services.

In an HMO or a PPO, the penalty for failure to comply with UM requirements for authorizations typically falls solely on the contracted provider, who may not balance bill the member for the amount of the penalty. Failure to comply with authorization requirements when care is provided by noncontracted providers is the member's responsibility.

In some cases, a plan may authorize payment for only a portion of the claim. For example, if a patient is held over the weekend in the hospital because a clinical service was not available, the plan may not pay the charges related to the extra days even though the inpatient stay was authorized. This concept also applies to nonpayment for costs associated with "never events," discussed in Chapter 5.

---

[*] In common usage, they are often referred to as "preauth" and "precert," respectively.

Timing also can affect how authorizations are applied to claims payment if the claim arrives before the authorization. This is most likely to happen in a POS plan where PCPs must authorize full coverage of specialty physician services. If the plan receives the specialty physician's claim before the PCP transmits the authorization, the claims system will automatically process it as nonauthorized and pay only a portion of it. It must then be corrected after the fact, which is administratively costly and associated with member (and specialty physician) dissatisfaction. The advent of standardized electronic authorizations and authorization queries under HIPAA and the increase in connectivity has reduced, but not eliminated, this problem.

Authorization does not necessarily guarantee payment of a claim. One reason might be that a member is no longer covered by the plan at the time medical services are actually provided. Another reason authorization does not guarantee payment is because of retrospective loss of coverage. For example, a member may have appeared to be eligible for coverage at the time the authorization was issued because it occurred during the grace period allowed for reinstatement right after failure to pay a premium, but nonpayment ultimately results in a loss of coverage extending back to the last time coverage was paid for.

Finally, there are multiple additional reasons for authorization systems, including:

- To allow the medical management functions of the plan to review a case for medical necessity;
- To channel care to the most appropriate location (e.g., the outpatient setting or to a participating specialist rather than a nonparticipating one);
- To provide timely information to the concurrent utilization review and large case management (described later); and
- To provide finance with data to assist in accruing monthly for the cost of medical care already provided but for which a claim has not yet been received, referred to as incurred but not reported (IBNR) estimations (see Chapter 21).

Definition of Services Requiring Coverage Authorization or Precertification

One requirement in any authorization system is to define what will require authorization and what will not, and under what circumstances. There are no managed care systems that require authorization for primary care services, but authorization may be required for other types of services, which varies based on the type of plan and the benefits design. The source of the authorization is typically a payer's UM function except when it may come from a PCP in an HMO.

Most HMOs require members to choose a single PCP to coordinate care (except for so-called "open access"

HMOs that operate more like PPOs), and accessing the PCP never requires any form of authorization. As discussed in Chapter 4, most HMOs also covered direct access for obstetrics and gynecology (ob/gyn) even before it became required under the ACA.[50] HMOs typically require the PCP to authorize coverage for services from other types of specialty physicians, although some states have passed laws requiring HMOs to cover direct access to an even greater array of providers such as chiropractors. It is also common for HMOs to cover direct access to behavioral health providers, as discussed in Chapter 12, although such direct access may be limited to contracted behavioral health providers.

All types of payers typically require precertification for many or even most elective hospitalizations, as well as many ambulatory procedures. Emergency or urgent problems are not elective and not subject to precertification, but still may require some type of coverage authorization, which may take place during a hospitalization (concurrent review) or after discharge (retrospective review). Certain requirements may also be defined regarding the member's obligation in those circumstances (e.g., notification within 24 hours of the emergency). Such requirements do not allow for automatic authorization even if the plan is notified within 24 hours, but only for automatic review of the case to determine medical necessity. Such reviews use the "reasonable layperson's standard" required under many state and federal laws, including the ACA (see Chapter 30).

Not all admissions or ambulatory procedures require precertification or even authorization, although which one varies by payer. Even when precertification or authorization is not required, most payers still require a hospital to notify the plan within 24 hours of admission in order to capture the information. Childbirth is an example of a type of admission that typically only requires notification. Common low-cost ambulatory procedures such as a simple surgical biopsy are also less likely to require precertification. Other types of ambulatory procedures such as routine colonoscopy in adults over 50 years of age typically also do not require precertification.

Risk-based payment also can affect the definition of what requires authorization, especially capitation. For example, if an HMO has a contract with an IPA based on full professional risk, it is usually up to the IPA to determine the extent of authorization requirements. On a more focused basis, when a particular specialty or service is capitated—for example, endoscopy—precertification is usually not required.

Precertification is increasingly included as part of an overall focus on specific types of costly services that are highly variable in their use, and for which there are less costly alternatives, for example, expensive imaging such as positron emission tomography (PET) scans when less costly alternatives such as computerized tomography (CT) scans or even plain X-rays might suffice. This is discussed in more detail later in the chapter.

Definition of Who Can Authorize Coverage of Services

Authorization and precertification systems must also define who has the ability to authorize coverage for defined services, and to what extent. This may vary considerably depending on the type of plan and the degree to its medically managed. As just discussed, all types of payers typically require authorization and precertification of coverage for facility-based and nonprofessional services, and HMOs typically require PCP authorization of specialty physician services.

In the early days of HMOs, PCP would often have the responsibility for authorizing coverage of hospital admissions or any facility-based services, rather than the HMO performing that function, and some still work this way. Non-HMO payers and even most HMOs now place precertification within UM, not with the PCP. Precertification of routine services usually requires only minimal review, but in situations where the payer has negotiated a special arrangement for high-cost services, precertification not only serves to review the medical necessity of the service, but ensures that the care will be delivered at an institution that has contracted with the plan.

Review by a medical director, or a secondary or higher level review, may be required for coverage authorization in select cases, and in some cases the determination of coverage authorization is made. This is usually the case for expensive procedures such as transplants or bariatric surgery for morbid obesity, as well as for controversial procedures or treatments that may be considered experimental or of limited value except in particular circumstances.

Categories of Authorization

Authorizations may be classified into six types, the first three of which are familiar:

- Prospective
- Concurrent
- Retrospective
- Pended (for review)
- Denial (no authorization)
- Subauthorization

The value in categorizing authorization types is twofold: to understand how the system works and, for plan managers, to identify problem areas. For example, if all elective admissions are being classified as having prospective authorization but it turns out that most are actually being authorized either concurrently or, worse yet, retrospectively,

UM will be unable to function effectively in managing hospital cases due to not knowing about them. A brief description of the authorization categories follows.

Prospective

Prospective means the authorization is issued before any service is rendered. When carried out by the payer, it is synonymous with precertification. Precertification of elective inpatient care is the most common form of prospective authorization, followed by precertification of selected ambulatory procedures and diagnostic testing, and selected drugs and biologics. In its simplest form, precertification means evaluating whether or not an admission, procedure, or costly test meets clinical criteria.

Concurrent

A concurrent authorization is generated at the time the service is rendered. For example, a hospital calls the health plan to notify it that a member is in the process of being admitted. An authorization is then generated by UM. Concurrent authorization does not allow UM to have an effect on services before they're provided, so may result in care being inappropriately delivered or delivered in a setting that is not cost effective. But it does allow UM to facilitate a more cost-effective direction when necessary, even though care has already commenced. This is especially true in the case of large case management, as discussed later.

Retrospective

As the term indicates, retrospective authorizations take place after the fact. For example, a patient is admitted, has surgery, and is discharged, and only then does the plan find out. If the care was elective, payment is usually denied or reduced, but if it was urgent or an emergency, it is typically covered in part or in full, depending on the circumstances.

Inexperienced managers often believe not only that most authorizations are prospective but that, except for emergency cases, there are few retrospective authorizations. Unfortunately, some payers may generate a significant volume of retrospective authorizations if the participating providers fail to cooperate with the authorization system. This usually occurs when a payer does not enforce the contractual requirement to cooperate by not paying the claim. Most payers, however, do not pay claims that have not been prospectively or concurrently authorized, forcing the noncompliant providers to write off the expense. This is more likely to happen in an HMO than any other type of health plan. Refusal to pay will certainly get a provider's attention, but it comes at some cost in provider relations. Even so, sometimes it becomes necessary if discussions and education attempts fail.

If a payer's systems allow an authorization to be classified as prospective or concurrent regardless of when it is created relative to the delivery of the service, it is a sure thing that retrospective authorizations will occur, but many will be labeled concurrent, not retrospective. This can occur when individuals in UM do not want to "penalize" providers they know well, when very powerful hospitals ignore authorization requirements because they feel secure, or if the claims system allows a cold claim to be linked to another authorized claim.

When HMOs were relatively small, the ability to create a retrospective authorization was strictly limited to the medical director or UM department, but as they became large, the ability to manage this problem required a loosening of that policy. Even then, most tightly managed plans restrict the ability to create prospective authorizations once the service has actually been rendered, and concurrent authorizations cannot be created after 24 hours have passed since the service was rendered.

Pended (For Review)

Pended is a claims term that refers to a state of authorization purgatory. In this situation, it is not known whether an authorization will be issued, and the case has been pended for review. The treatment of pended claims is addressed in Chapter 18, but in brief, the main reasons a claim may be pended are:

- For medical review, which may be due to a diagnosis-procedure mismatch, a claim for a chest X-ray has a diagnosis for a broken leg, for example;
- For medical necessity review such as an emergency department claim;
- For medical policy review to determine if the service is covered under the schedule of benefits; or
- For administrative review such as coordination of benefits.

Denial

Denial refers to the certainty that there will be no authorization forthcoming. In an HMO, denial means no payment at all. In a POS, PPO, or CDHP, denial may mean no payment at all, but may also mean that payment will be made, but at a lesser level of coverage if the service is still considered medically necessary.

Subauthorization

This is a special category that allows one authorization to hitchhike on another. This is most common for hospital-based professional services. For example, a single authorization may be issued for a hospitalization, and that authorization is used to cover anesthesia, pathology, radiology, or even a surgeon's or consultant's fees.

In some HMOs, an authorization to a referral specialist may be used to authorize diagnostic and therapeutic services ordered by that specialist. For example, a referral to an orthopedist automatically allows for authorized payment for radiological services, a referral to a cardiologist allows for electrocardiograms, and so forth. Claims systems usually have algorithms in place to determine payment for real or imputed subauthorizations, with exceptions pended for manual review.

A particular issue in subauthorizations is self-referral. This means a physician owns or leases an expensive device or service, either alone or as one of a number of investors, and is also able to order its use. Self-referral is strongly associated with overutilization, so payers try to limit the ease with which subauthorizations for costly services can be created in self-referral situations. This is discussed later in the chapter.

Standardized Electronic Authorization Transactions

As noted earlier and as described in Chapter 18, HIPAA mandated standards for the electronic transmission of authorization data, among other types of electronic transactions. The American National Standards Institute (ANSI) X12 standard 278 is the Prior Authorization Request and Response Transaction. It is used both to request and to receive a response for referrals, certification, and authorization of the following:

- Health care services,
- Health care admission,
- Extend certification, and
- Certification appeal.

The field descriptions and data requirements of the 278 transaction standard are more complex than those found in older paper-based systems. Use of this electronic transaction occurs when many of those data fields are populated by the system itself such as a practice management support system or a hospital information system. The electronic standard is also used in Web-based portals where physicians and hospitals can request an authorization or query the payer to see if an authorization exists, and provide or obtain necessary nonclinical information.

Like so many of the standardized transactions required under HIPAA, there remained many areas of variation in implementation by commercial, state, and federal governmental payers. Examples of areas of variation included:

- Differences in data content
  - Some data fields are definable, and allow considerable flexibility;
  - Some data fields are defined based on the type and nature of data in other data fields;
  - Some data fields may be ignored based on contractual terms between trading partners if the data is not necessary to process the transaction;

- Payers could define specific types of data that must be provided or the transaction would not be completed;
- Differences in connectivity
  - Some required the use of a clearinghouse;
  - Some allowed direct connectivity;
  - Some allowed both;
  - Some allowed direct connectivity for some transactions but not others;
- Differences in transaction processing
  - Some processed only through batch mode on a nightly basis;
  - Some processed in real time; and
  - Some did both, but for different transactions.

Guides for the transaction data standards, including variations in implementation, are provided by each payer, and can be substantial in length. For example, the average size of the implementation guides for the ANSI 278 standard by five commercial payers, one federal payer, one state payer, and one municipal payer was 35 pages; the largest was 61 pages, and the smallest was 17.[51] Approximately one-quarter of each did not pertain directly to implementation standards, but that leaves a great deal of room for variances.

To address this, the ACA requires the Department of Health and Human Services (DHHS) to develop standard operating rules to reduce the amount of administrative variance that remained even after implementation of the standardized transactions under HIPAA.[52] At the time of publication, those rules had not yet been developed, and no implantation timeframe issued.

Nonelectronic Authorizations and Queries

The use of electronic transactions for authorizations continues to rise, but there are still some providers that rely on other means to transmit or inquire about authorizations. Secure web portals are a popular option, which is a kind of electronic transaction that requires no electronic capability by the provider other than having a browser.

Precertification is often done over the telephone with a live conversation between the payer's precertification personnel and the physician verifying the need. In some cases, it may be done by a physician's office staff finding out what the payer requires in documentation first. Telephone-based precertifications are typically then followed by a faxed form for the physician to sign, attesting to the information contained on the form. In other cases, a telephonic automated voice response system may be used, although this is more likely to be used to verify an authorization than to submit one.

Though archaic, many physicians still generate paper-based authorizations. It is usually a form, often with preprinted questions that may be answered by checking the appropriate boxes. Forms are then either mailed or, more commonly, faxed to the payer.

■ MANAGING UTILIZATION OF PHYSICIAN SERVICES

Managing physician services really refers to specialty services. There are very practical reasons why HMOs encourage or even require members to access PCPs for routine services, whether through the use of differential copays or through the use of a PCP "gatekeeper" model. The obvious reason in most managed health care plans is that the cost of specially care services is greater than the cost of primary care services, often between 1½ and 2 times as high. On top of that, there is also the cost of services ordered by specialists such as diagnostic studies, and the even more costly procedures that specialty physicians typically perform.

A third and equally important reason is that in many cases, a specialist only deals with the condition in which they specialize. There certainly are studies showing that a specialist is better at treating a specific condition than is a generalist,[53] and there are other examples of when a specialist will be better at managing the care of chronic and complex diseases such as severe diabetes,[54] chronic rheumatic and musculoskeletal diseases,[55] or debilitating congestive heart failure.[56] However, providing better care for a specific condition does not necessarily equate to providing better coordination of care when patients have multiple chronic conditions, as is discussed later.

Several studies in the late 1980s and early 1990s demonstrated the ability of PCP-model HMOs to lower costs and maintain quality.[57-62] The rapid growth of HMOs peaked at the end of the 1990s (see Chapter 1), but even then, studies continued to confirm that savings generated by managing specialty physician services were actually twice the amount generated from hospital UM (adjusted for severity and case mix),[63] including the use of specialty services in Medicare and Medicaid managed care plans.[64]

The peak of HMO growth was also accompanied by questions from patients about the PCP gatekeeper role and how the interaction between the PCP and the financial incentive system affected utilization.[65] Physician attitudes were also variable. For example, nearly one in four HMO PCPs in one large survey felt that the scope of care they were expected to provide was greater than it should be.[66] In another survey, physicians reported that the PCP gatekeeper model was effective in controlling costs and other aspects of care, but complained about the imposition of administrative requirements and access to specialists, testing, and other measures; however, overall, 72% still thought that the gatekeeper model was better than or comparable to traditional care arrangements.[67]

These types of sentiments have subsided to some degree as HMOs declined in enrollment. But most HMOs still require PCPs to authorize coverage of specialty care services. And even non-HMOs seek in some way to encourage the use of PCPs for routine services. The most common approach is to use differential copay requirements; for example, the benefits plan may require a $20.00 copay to see a PCP and a $40.00 copay to see a specialist, a differential used my most HMOs as well.

A PCP-oriented approach to care coordination is also incorporated into the PCMH model described in Chapter 2, but unlike the HMO gatekeeper model, there is no member or patient lock-in because they were designed for non-HMO plans such as FFS Medicare or a commercial PPO. In any case, unlike HMOs that focus on the sick and the healthy, the focus of these newer models is on patients with significant chronic medical problems, especially those with multiple chronic medical conditions.

PCMHs are a new concept at the time of publication, but the notion of better primary care coordination of chronically ill patients being associated with better outcomes and lower costs in a non-HMO setting has been examined. One study simply looked at PCP concentration in a community, and found that places with higher concentrations of PCPs did not show any real differences in overall costs compared to low-concentration communities.[68] A different study that looked a little deeper concluded that PCPs varied in their capabilities to effectively coordinate their patients' care, but those that were effective showed a greater commitment to interpersonal continuity of care through coordination, and office systems that supported it.[69] On a thoroughly positive note, a study in which primary care physician-nurse teams provided proactive, evidence-based comprehensive health care to patients with multiple chronic conditions demonstrated impressive improvements in reduced utilization and lower costs, even accounting for the additional costs associated with the enhanced support structure.[70] What the second and third studies have in common is that better coordination is associated with larger or more organized medical groups.

Unfortunately, the proportion of medical school graduates who enter into primary care specialties has been falling for over a decade, and in some communities there are not enough to meet even current demand. This is not surprising given the higher income associated with almost all non-primary-care specialties (excluding psychiatry), and with procedure-based specialties in particular.

The flip side of the positive studies noted previously is the serious problem of diminished coordination of care in the absence of an enhanced support structure. The effects of this on inpatient utilization, postdischarge transition, and the prevention of avoidable readmissions are looked at following the next section on facility-based UM. The related topic of managing complex chronic illnesses follows that.

■ MANAGING UTILIZATION OF FACILITY-BASED SERVICES

Hospitals and ambulatory facility-based services account for nearly half of all medical costs in the commercial sector (see Figure 7-1), and that does not even take into account

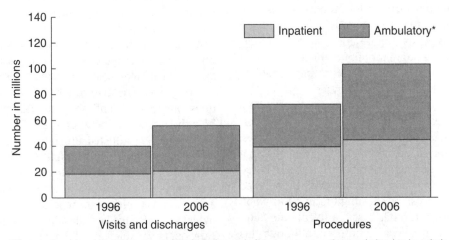

*The number of ambulatory surgery visits includes ambulatory surgery patients admitted to hospitals as inpatients for both 1996 and 2006. As a result, the data differ form those presented in the 1996 report (5).

FIGURE 7-4 Growth in Number of Ambulatory Procedures, 1996–2006

Source: Ambulatory Surgery in the United States, 2006, National Health Statistics Reports #11, January 28, 2009, www.cdc.gov/nchs/data/nhsr/nhsr011.pdf.

the cost of physician services associated with facility-based care. Chapter 5 looked at the high prices charged by hospitals and health systems and how they have been increasing for a decade, which accounts for a significant portion of the cost. But utilization is also a major factor, particularly in certain parts of the country, as seen in the earlier discussion about variation.

Inpatient care and ambulatory care are both facility based, but differ in major ways. UM processes addressing ambulatory procedures are also used for inpatient UM, but concurrent UM is only used for inpatient and certain rehabilitation services.

Ambulatory Procedures and High-Cost Imaging Services

Ambulatory procedures encompass a heterogeneous group of outpatient care. In the context of UM, it refers to outpatient procedures done in some type of specialized facility, unlike office visits or minor office-based procedures. Common examples applicable to this section include:

- Ambulatory surgical centers (ASCs),
- Endoscopy centers,
- Lithotripsy centers,
- Radiation oncology and chemotherapy centers, and
- High-cost diagnostics and imaging centers.

High-cost diagnostic and imaging centers are technically considered ancillary services rather than ambulatory procedure centers. But because they overlap with ASCs in some important ways applicable to UM, they are discussed here instead. For the same reason, physician-owned centers and physician-owned in-office ancillary services are also discussed in this section.

Managing utilization of ambulatory procedures has taken on increasing importance over the past 10 years. When HMOs and managed care first arrived, most facility-based care was done on an inpatient basis. Simply moving care to the ambulatory setting yielded immediate savings, as did reducing the ALOS and the admission rate. However, as addressed in Chapter 5, facilities quickly raised prices for ambulatory services, to the point where an inpatient day may be less expensive. In theory, admitting the patient would save money in such cases, but hospital policies and even contracts routinely preclude that.

Data from the National Center for Health Statistics showing growth in the absolute number of ambulatory procedures is found in **Figure 7-4**, and the shift to free-standing ASCs is seen in **Figure 7-5**.

Ambulatory scoping procedures make up a considerable portion of all procedures, and they too have shown an increased rate of growth. As **Figure 7-6** illustrates, the increase in ambulatory upper endoscopy has doubled in the 10 years between 1996 and 2006, and ambulatory colonoscopy has tripled.

Utilization of costly imaging services rose even faster than ambulatory procedures, especially MRI, magnetic resonance angiography (MRA), positron emission tomography

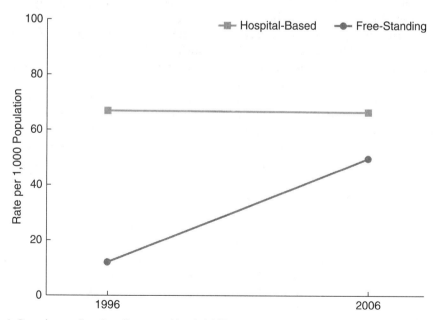

FIGURE 7-5 Growth Rate in Procedures at Free-Standing versus Hospital ASCs, 1996–2006

Source: Ambulatory Surgery in the United States, 2006, National Health Statistics Reports #11, January 28, 2009, www.cdc.gov/nchs/data/nhsr/nhsr011.pdf.

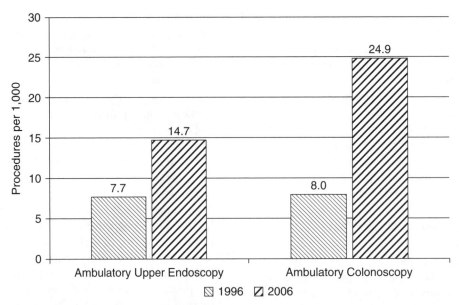

FIGURE 7-6 Ambulatory Gastrointestinal Scoping Procedures per 1,000 in the General Population, 1996–2006
Source: Created by author using data from the National Center for Health Statistics, National Ambulatory Medical Care Survey and National Hospital Ambulatory Medical Care Survey, 2009.

(PET) scans, nuclear stress testing, and CT. Looking at MRI and CT alone, utilization related to office visits has nearly tripled in the 10 years between 1996 and 2006, while that associated with emergency department (ED) visits has quadrupled, as seen in **Figure 7-7**.

Physician Ownership and Self-Referral

As has been discussed in Chapters 4 and 5 and at several points in this chapter, physician ownership of an expensive device or service is strongly associated with an increase in its use by the physician, resulting in overall cost increases. The term for this is "physician self-referral" and the concept is simple: the desire by some physicians to improve their own bottom lines, whether conscious or unconscious. By no means is self-referral condoned by all physicians. A great many actively oppose it, and leading medical journals have been in the forefront of publishing well-crafted studies showing the impact of self-referral on utilization and costs. That has not stopped it from growing.

This association between self-referral and higher utilization and costs has been known for decades now. For example, studies published in the late 1980s and early 1990s reported that physician ownership of radiology equipment was associated with a fourfold increase in imaging examinations and significant increases in charges compared to physicians who referred such studies to radiologists.[71] Similar results were reported for laboratory services[72] and a wide variety of ancillary services.[73]

Congress attempted to close the door, at least for Medicare and Medicaid, by prohibiting physicians from referring patients to facilities in which the physician has a financial interest.[74] However, it did not prohibit referring patients for ancillary services provided within the physician's office, which is known as an in-office ancillary services exception (IOASE). Because of that loophole, the problem has only grown worse, fueled by aggressive sales by manufacturers, including leasing arrangements and assistance with financing.

The following studies, representing only a sample of a much larger body of evidence, provide examples of higher utilization and costs being associated with self-referral:

- Physician-ownership in ambulatory surgical centers is linked to a doubling of surgical volume.[75]
- Comparisons of physician owner versus nonowner volume of orthopedic inpatient and outpatient surgical cases found that ownership correlates with a 54–129% increase for carpal tunnel repair, a 33–100% increase for rotator cuff repair, and a 27–78% increase for arthroscopy.[76]
- Highly compensated in-office (i.e., self-referral) myocardial perfusion imaging by cardiologists occurs six times more often than when the procedure is referred to a radiologist.[77]
- The number of MRI procedures orthopedists ordered within 30 days of a first visit increased by about 38% after they acquired their own MRI equipment, and not

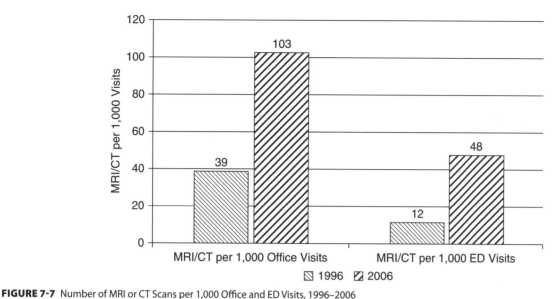

FIGURE 7-7 Number of MRI or CT Scans per 1,000 Office and ED Visits, 1996–2006

Source: Created by author using data from the National Center for Health Statistics, National Ambulatory Medical Care Survey and National Hospital Ambulatory Medical Care Survey, 2009.

only did MRI costs increase, but spending for other aspects of care rose as well.[78]

- A study looking at 20 common combinations of medical conditions and types of imaging found that self-referral was associated with significantly and substantially higher episode costs for most of them, and there was no decrease in the length of illness, except when doctors self-referred patients to receive X-rays for a few common conditions.[79]

- Despite arguments that physician-owned imaging devices provide "one-stop shopping" for patients, an analysis of 2006 and 2007 Medicare data showed that self-referral provided same-day imaging for 74% of straightforward X-rays, but for only 15% of more advanced procedures such as CT and MRI.[80]

Research on this topic is not uniformly dismal, however. In at least one study, for example, physician-owned cardiac hospitals had only a small increase in utilization and costs for cardiac procedures compared to non-physician-owned.[81] But even citing this single study misrepresents the relative volume of studies looking at self-referral and its association with utilization and cost increases.

Despite how well understood this problem is, the opportunity to address it through health reform was tepid at best, and even then only as it applies to care paid for by Medicare or Medicaid. The ACA froze development of new physician-owned specialty hospitals, but grandfathered existing ones, including those not yet completed. It also prohibited existing physician-owned hospitals from increasing their number of operating rooms, and requires them to report annually to CMS.[82] The ACA also now requires physicians who own or operate imaging services or devices to inform a patient in writing at the time of the referral with a written list of other imaging services in the area.[83]

Some commercial payers and many HMOs specifically added nonpayment for self-referral into their physician contracts. But even when it was in the contract, it was not always easy to enforce or even detect. The reality in the market is that many physicians will not sign a contract prohibiting them from billing for self-referred services. Nonparticipating physicians also often offer to waive any cost-sharing requirements associated with the use of an out-of-network facility and physician, which many consider fraud, as was noted in Chapter 5. When the benefits design cannot be used to effectively stop this, a personal member contact by a UM nurse or appropriately trained member services representative (see Chapter 20) often results in the member going in-network instead.

In addition to requiring precertification for selected expensive testing procedures, the best method for dealing with this issue is to contractually prohibit or markedly restrict the use of such services. When possible, a useful approach is a benefit design that has a very aggressive benefits difference, or eliminates coverage completely for certain costly elective services from noncontract providers. Most managed care plans contract with a limited number of vendors for such ancillary services and may limit referral to only those vendors, as discussed in Chapter 7.

Common Approaches to UM for Ambulatory Procedures and Imaging Services

Other than through payment terms described in Chapter 4, the primary approach to UM for ASCs and high-cost imaging services is precertification. Most require little documentation other than the physician's statement or request. HMOs with PCP gatekeepers may require the PCP to authorize it, but most payers work directly with the requesting physician or their office staff. Defining when precertification applies to ambulatory facility-based services overall was discussed earlier in the section "Definition of Services Requiring Coverage Authorization or Precertification."

Some costly procedures or diagnostic studies are done for medical conditions where there are less costly treatment alternatives, as already noted. Precertification may also determine that a more costly alternative meets medical necessity criteria after failure of the less costly alternative; for example, joint replacement because physical therapy has not brought sufficient relief to a patient, or a PET and CT combined scan because a CT or MRI scan was unable to detect a metastasis despite clinical signs and symptoms.

In some cases, the less costly alternative was not pursued, in which case the requesting physician is usually required to provide clinical information and/or having a telephone conversation with a UM nurse or physician to justify its use, which is then reviewed using evidence-based clinical guidelines appropriate to the medical condition. In other cases the review may be more complex and is done using the processes described earlier in the section "Medical Necessity and Determination of Benefits Coverage."

Routine precertification may sometimes be outsourced to companies that employ well-trained UM nurses. This serves to lower costs, which is increasingly important due to limits on administrative spending created by the ACA. It requires proper systems access and support, of course. When routine precertification is outsourced, a payer will still have local medical managers available as well.

Outsourcing Focused UM

Certain types of highly-cost ancillary services may be subject to a much more focused UM effort. It is used most often for costly imaging because of the substantial rise in utilization and costs, but it could apply to any costly type of service for which a payer finds a pattern of higher than expected utilization or a high inflation rate. Focused UM means that precertification based on review against criteria is required every time, and requests are not routinely approved. Focused UM may be carried out by the payer using specialized criteria and guidelines licensed from a third party but often it is outsourced to a company that specializes in managing utilization for that type of service. The precertification process is typically more detailed than for routine ambulatory procedures. For example, the UM company's radiologists may review copies of existing imaging studies, or speak directly with the requesting specialist. Focused UM is particularly useful where physician self-referral is a problem, and may even apply primarily to physicians who do it.

Hospital-Based ASCs

The shift from hospital-based ASCs to free-standing ones has had a negative impact on hospital margins, as discussed in Chapters 4 and 5. But one of the reasons for that is that patients at hospital-based ASCs are either generally sicker than those at free-standing facilities, or are having more complex procedures. This is evidenced by the longer periods of time patients spent in hospital-based ASCs, noted in a 2006 report by the CDC National Center for Health Statistics and shown in **Figure 7-8**.

The reason to note this disparity at all is because ambulatory procedures on sicker patients, and complex procedures, are more likely to have complications that may result in an admission. The admission might be for a short observation stay, or it could be due to significant medical problems. This doesn't change how UM is applied prospectively, but policies and procedures must be in place to ensure that admissions from the ASC are quickly brought into the concurrent process to be described shortly.

Emergency Department

The ED, which used to be called the emergency room (ER[*]), refers to emergency services provided by hospitals, not to urgent care centers. According to the Centers for Disease Control and Prevention, the ED visit rate for the general population in 2008 (meaning insured, uninsured, Medicare, and Medicaid combined) was approximately 410 visits per thousand people per year.[84] This is about twice the typical rate in a commercial payer, and approximately the same rate as a commercial MA plan. In a related report on the use of the ED in the general population in 2007, the distribution of how ED personnel rated the immediacy with which patients should be seen (in order from most severe to least severe) was as follows:

- Immediate: 4.5%
- Emergent: 11.3%
- Urgent: 38.5%
- Semi-urgent: 21.0%
- Nonurgent: 7.9%
- No triage or unknown: 16.0%[85]

---

[*]The term was so common that in 1994, when Michael Crichton created a new television show set in the ED, he named it *ER*, even though the term was going out of use in the medical community.

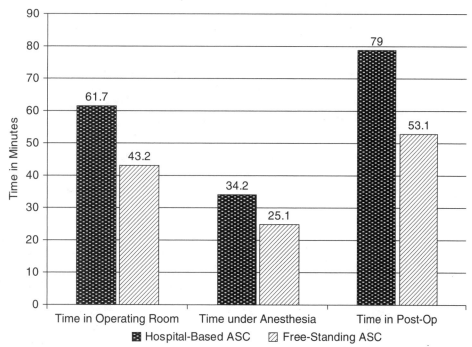

FIGURE 7-8 Comparison of Procedure Times, in Minutes, between Hospital-Based and Free-Standing ASCs, 2006

Source: Created by author using data from the National Center for Health Statistics, National Ambulatory Medical Care Survey and National Hospital Ambulatory Medical Care Survey, 2009.

In the distant past, some HMOs required a member to obtain precertification of coverage before going to the ED, except for serious emergencies. During the same time period, hospitals might actually turn a patient away if the patient had no insurance, or would wait until the HMO precertified the visit before providing care, also excepting serious emergencies. But in 1986, the federal government passed the Emergency Medical Treatment and Active Labor Act (EMTALA) to prevent transfer or "dumping" of uninsured patients by private hospitals.[86] It requires that all patients presenting to any hospital ED must have a medical screening exam performed by qualified personnel, usually the emergency physician. The medical screening exam cannot be delayed for insurance reasons, either to obtain insurance information or to obtain preauthorization for examination.

While theoretically the HMO could deny payment even though the ED was required by law to provide services, hospitals rightly refused to agree to those terms. Increasing numbers of lawsuits also demonstrated the higher liabilities associated with ED precertification requirements. As a result of both of these changes, HMOs abandoned precertification for basic ED services. The entire issue of precertification for ED became moot in any event under provisions of the ACA requiring health benefits plans to cover all emergency services based on the in-network level of benefits, and prohibiting a precertification requirement.[87]

In place of precertification, payers, including HMOs, increased the levels of cost-sharing for basic ED services. As discussed in the section on benefits design, the cost-sharing is supposed to cause the member to think twice about whether or not to go to the ED. The change was supported by a 1985 study on the effects of cost-sharing that concluded that cost-sharing decreased inappropriate use of the ED without having a negative impact on appropriate use.[88] This was affirmed in studies in 1989, 1996, and 1997.[89-91] The ACA may require coverage of emergency services at the in-network level, but it does not prohibit different cost-sharing for ED than for routine medical care, even on an in-network basis.

Patients show up in the ED in several ways. They may self-refer based on their perceived need to receive care (e.g., they may be having chest or abdominal pains, or may have cut themselves), they may be transported there by emergency services (e.g., after a motor vehicle accident), or they may be directed there by their physician on a payer's nurse advice line (e.g., after calling to find out what to do about chest pain). One recent study reported that 13.7–27.1% of all ED visits was for care that could have been provided at an urgent care center or a retail clinic that provides services for routine and noncomplex problems (see Chapter 4).[92] For that reason, some HMOs have their own urgent care centers or contract with existing ones, and many payers also have contracts with retail clinics.

The ED is both a source of utilization and expense in its own right, and a gateway to inpatient admission. At the time of publication, the most recent data on a national basis for the population as a whole is from 2008. Those data showed 15.53% of all ED visits led to an inpatient admission; the age distribution for patients admitted through the ED was:

- <1 year of age: 7.71%
- 1–17: 3.83%
- 18–44: 7.86%
- 45–64: 20.31%
- 65–84: 39.22%
- 85+: 49.02%
- Age data missing: 19.67%[93]

In the case of trauma or other obvious significant medical conditions, the role of UM is the same as for any other type of inpatient case. For many other common medical conditions, most EDs have created standardized protocols that improve efficiency and outcomes. But because of concerns about legal liability, many EDs have established chest pain protocols that result either in an admission to the cardiac care unit or in an observation stay, regardless of how serious the patient's condition appears to be or whether or not there is diagnostic data to support the existence of a serious and acute heart problem. This is costly to the plan and to the member too, depending on the degree of cost-sharing.

Some plans have addressed this problem by negotiating special rates for such admissions when there is no subsequent evidence of a heart attack. Other plans actually contract with specialty management companies to assume responsibility for the evaluation and disposition of these cases at each hospital's ED, as noted in Chapter 4.

Inpatient Acute Care UM

Inpatient care is almost the only type of service in which every type of UM is used: prospective, concurrent, and retrospective. Alternatives of acute care hospitals (discussed later) and some noninpatient services such as physical rehabilitation may also use all three to some degree, but not with the level of effort used for inpatient care. The reason for the attention to acute-care hospital admissions is cost. As seen in Figure 7-1 at the beginning of the chapter, physician cost may be slightly higher in aggregate than hospital cost is, but it takes a lot of office visits and surgical fees to add up to a single day in a hospital.

HMOs typically have the lowest levels of inpatient utilization, reflecting their strong focus on UM and care coordination. In the last decade, inpatient utilization for both HMOs and PPOs had fallen to relatively low levels, possibly caused by reduced capacity at hospitals with few empty beds. Hospitals have been expanding capacity, building new facilities and expanding existing ones, so the pressure to move patients out has been replaced with the pressure to keep the census up. Whether that is a coincidence or not, inpatient utilization has been climbing steadily since 2005, as seen in **Figure 7-9** showing HMO and PPO bed-days per thousand for non-Medicare members.

As is the case for ambulatory care, procedures make up a considerable portion of overall inpatient-related costs and, with a few exceptions, have also been rising in absolute frequency. The same federal report used to create Figures 7-7 and 7-8 also looked at selected types of procedures, including those that used a costly implant. As shown in **Figure 7-10**, for the U.S. population overall, between 1996 and 2006 the rate per 1,000 for total hip replacement rose by 26%, for partial hip replacement it rose by 58%, and for total knee replacement it rose by 66%.

Not surprisingly, costs also rose. The Healthcare Cost and Utilization Project (HCUP) by the federal Agency for Healthcare Research and Quality (AHRQ) looked at data on six selected procedures, comparing changes in overall cost between 1999 and 2006. For five of the six, costs rose between 147% and 289%; the exception was coronary artery bypass grafting, which declined by 3% from lower utilization due to the use of stents. These data are shown in **Figure 7-11**. The rising costs shown in Figure 7-11 are made up of three, not two, components. The two obvious ones are hospital price increases, as discussed in Chapter 5, and an increase in the total number of procedures per 1,000 people, as already shown. But the third component for the cases in Figure 7-11 is the astonishingly high costs of the implants themselves, which may account for half the total cost, as has been shown in Table 6-9 in the previous chapter.

Precertification

The basic precertification process has already been described, so is not repeated here. Avoiding unnecessary admissions and directing care to the most appropriate location is as applicable to inpatient stays as to any other service subject to precertification. In the case of inpatient care, however, it serves several additional functions depending on the situation. For example, precertifications and authorizations capture data for financial accruals. It won't capture every case, but typically does capture around 90-95%. By knowing the number and nature of hospital cases as well as potential or existing catastrophic cases, the plan may more accurately accrue for expenses rather than have to wait for claims to come in. It allows financial managers to take action early so as to avoid nasty financial surprises. (Accrual methodology is discussed in Chapter 21.)

Routine Cases

Routine or uncomplicated cases are typically precertified on the spot. Requests by telephone or secure fax typically are

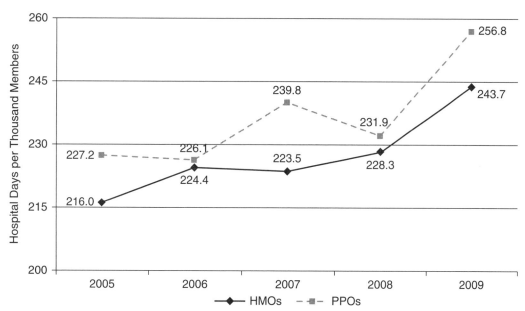

FIGURE 7-9 HMO and PPO Hospital Bed-Days per Thousand Non-Medicare Members, 2005–2009

Source: SDI © 2010 in The Sanofi-Aventis Managed Care Digest Series®/HMO-PPO Digest 2010. www.managedcaredigest.com. Used with permission.

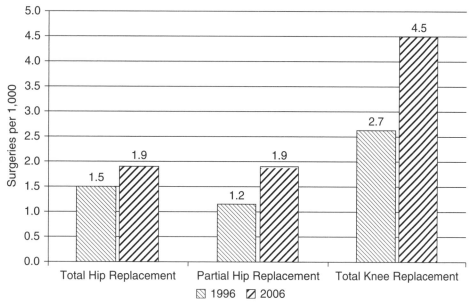

FIGURE 7-10 Inpatient Admits per 1,000 for Total Hip, Partial Hip, and Total Knee Replacement, U.S. Population, 1996–2006

Source: Data from the National Center for Health Statistics, National Ambulatory Medical Care Survey and National Hospital Ambulatory Medical Care Survey, 2009.

routed to UM reviewers who quickly determine if all necessary information is present, and review it against criteria for admission. The use of standardized electronic transactions, discussed earlier, is increasing, which improves efficiency for payers and for providers. Electronic input also supports a higher level of automation, pending only on cases where an admission clearly meets criteria.

Some types of inpatient stays that are routine and uncomplicated may not be precertified at all, or the precertification may be created at the time of diagnosis. The most common example is labor and delivery. When the expectant mother is admitted, the hospital simply notifies UM to allow capture of the information. UM typically does little in routine obstetrical admissions, but may become quite

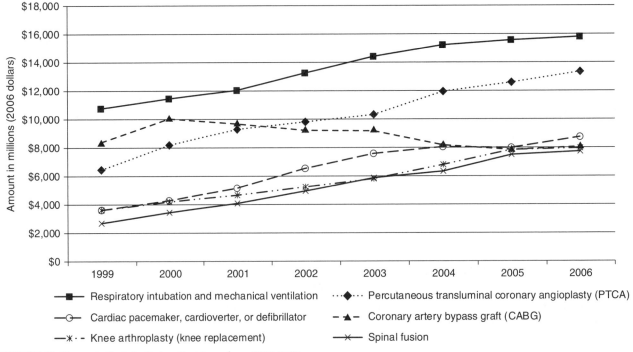

FIGURE 7-11 Change in Costs for Six Inpatient Procedures, 1999–2006

Source: Data from the Agency for Healthcare Research and Quality, Healthcare Cost and Utilization Project, Nationwide Inpatient Sample, Health, United States, 2009.

involved in the event of a fragile or significantly premature neonate. In other cases, closed-panel HMOs for example, precertification may simply consist of notification to case managers who facilitate patient expectations and discharge planning.

Authorization of an Urgent or Emergency Admission

Authorizations taking place after an urgent or emergency admission are not, by definition, prospective. But the first step in any inpatient UM is creating a record of the admission and beginning the process of determining whether or not it will be covered, which most closely resembles precertification. Urgent or emergency admissions are typically authorized, although participating hospitals may be paid a reduced amount or nothing if it fails to comply with timely notification of an admission. On occasion, an elective inpatient stay is not precertified and there is no clinical reason it was not, in which case coverage is typically denied.

This initial authorization of an urgent or emergency admission is particularly valuable for early identification of cases that may become very costly. Such cases are often called catastrophic cases, and are the same as what the actuaries call "shock claims." In UM, identification of a catastrophic case will trigger case management, which is discussed later.

Assignment of Length of Stay

A very important element of precertification or postadmission authorization is an assignment of LOS, meaning the maximum number of inpatient days that will be covered in the absence of medical justification for additional days. As expected, this is done through the use of clinical guidelines and criteria, as discussed earlier. It is typically automated for most cases. Multiple medical conditions or comorbidities are typically factored into the initial LOS assignment, although comorbidities do not automatically lead to a longer initial LOS assignment. The assigned LOS applies only to coverage, and UM does not have any ability to actually discharge a patient, nor provide care during an admission. As is addressed shortly under concurrent UM, an initial LOS assignment may be changed during the course of an admission. The exceptions to the use of evidence-based clinical guidelines for the initial assignment of LOS are state and federal laws mandating a minimum LOS. During the managed care backlash (see Chapter 1), for example, a federal law was passed that mandated a 48-hour minimum LOS for a routine delivery and 96 hours for a delivery by caesarean section.[94] That requirement still stands, even though subsequent studies demonstrated no significant effect on the health outcomes of newborns brought about by this policy.[95] It even prohibits a plan from encouraging a shorter LOS. From a clinical standpoint, a 1-day LOS for obstetrics is still acceptable if the patient wants to go and the obstetrician agrees, but 2 days is the minimum that can be assigned.

Input to Concurrent UM

The first basic element of concurrent UM for elective admissions is not concurrent at all, it is prospective, but is an integral part of the process. Precertification of elective inpatient care notifies concurrent review that a case will be occurring, and enables UM to prepare discharge planning ahead of time when appropriate; for example, an admission that will result in a recovery stay at a nonacute facility. It also provides time for UM nurses to help set expectations with the patient and the patient's family; for example, knowing what a typical length of stay is for that type of case, or how best to plan for the patient's return home.

If there are particular challenges or issues with a specific facility, precertification also allows UM to take whatever step to help address those challenges. As is discussed shortly, for example, primary care physicians no longer admit as many patients as they once did, or even admit patients at all in some hospitals. Specialists or hospitalists (see Chapter 4) provide the inpatient care, but do not always communicate properly with a patient's regular physician. UM may then take measures to improve communications prior to and after discharge.

Centers of Excellence for High-Cost and/or High-Complexity Cases

As discussed in Chapter 4, payers often contract with one or more "centers of excellence," which are facilities that provide care for very costly and/or complex elective care. Common examples include bariatric surgery for morbid obesity, transplants, and cardiac surgery. A favorable rate is typically not the only criteria used, and data about outcomes and experience also come into play. Precertification requests for procedures for which there is a center of excellence are approved at the preferred rate of member cost-sharing only when the centers are used. Depending on the type of plan, use of a facility other than a center is subject to greater cost-sharing or no coverage at all.

Under typical center of excellence contract terms, case rates or other payment models are used, and the payer's UM process is only peripherally involved during the inpatient stay until the time of discharge approaches. At that point, case management is used in a similar way to what is described later.

Preadmission Testing and Same-Day Surgery for Routine Elective Cases

Decades ago, patients were admitted for an elective procedure the day before to get any necessary preoperative lab work or X-rays. Beginning with HMOs, precertification made it clear that coverage would only apply to elective preadmission testing if done as an outpatient prior to admission, and coverage of the inpatient stay would only begin the day of the surgery or procedure. Initially resisted by hospitals, physicians, and patients, it is now a routine coverage requirement in all types of health plans, commercial or governmental. Indeed, most hospitals would refuse to admit a patient the day before a procedure in most cases. Exceptions are typically confined to complex cases such as a transplant in an immune-compromised individual.

Mandatory Outpatient Surgery

During the same period of time that patients were admitted for preoperative testing, most surgical procedures were done on an inpatient basis. Once again it was HMOs that led in moving cases from being performed on an inpatient basis to outpatient. As with preoperative testing, there was resistance, followed by its routine use. As discussed earlier in this chapter and in depth in Chapter 5, this produced substantial savings when the shift began, but that is no longer the case due to very high prices, made worse by charge-based payment terms. In any case, inpatient surgery and procedures continue to migrate to the outpatient setting.

Inpatient Attending Physicians: Specialists and Hospitalists

Prior to describing the roles and processes involved with concurrent UM on inpatient cases, it's worth looking at who the physicians are that are actually attending those cases. As admission rates have dropped and more care is provided in ambulatory facilities, patients that are admitted tend to be sicker or require more intense services or major surgery. This has been accompanied by the near disappearance of PCPs managing inpatient cases. Only a few years into the new century, PCP's management of inpatients had fallen from 40% of their time to just 10%.[96]

Specialty physicians now manage the majority of inpatient cases, but that too is shifting, at least for nonsurgical care. As discussed in Chapter 4, many hospitals have two types of relationships with their physicians: privately practicing physicians who admit to the hospital, and hospital-employed physicians. And within those two categories, each has seen the appearance of hospitalist physicians, which is addressed shortly. Recall from Chapter 4 that hospital employment of physicians has extended to all types of specialties, surgical and medical. But even then, many, if not most, of these employed physicians will practice in sites other than the main hospital and may not provide inpatient care.

The term "hospitalist" was coined in the mid-1990s by Wachter and Goldman in an article in the *New England Journal of Medicine* in which they described a "new breed of physicians we call 'hospitalists'—specialists in inpatient medicine—who will be responsible for managing the care of hospitalized patients in the same way that primary care physicians are responsible for managing the care of outpatients."[97] The primary feature of this model is that the physician providing care in the outpatient setting relinquishes responsibility for the admission, and the hospitalist assumes it. In 2009, the Society of Hospital Medicine (SHM), the professional organization for hospitalists, defined a hospitalist as "a physician who specializes in the practice of hospital medicine."[98]

According to the SHM, as of 2010:

- There are more than 30,000 hospitalists practicing in 3,300 hospitals, including over 80% of hospitals with more than 200 beds;
- Approximately 84% of hospitalists are trained in internal medicine;
- They are employed through multiple models as follows:
  - 40% are employed by hospitals or hospital corporations,
  - 18% are employed by academic hospital medicine programs,
  - 14.5% are employed by a local hospitalist-only medical group practice,
  - 14.5% are employed by a multispecialty or primary care medical group practice,* and
  - 13% are employed by a multistate hospitalist-only medical group.[99]

A related approach used in the past and still used in some groups is a designated admitting physician or rounding physician, in which a medical group practice designates one physician to care for all of the group's admissions to a given hospital or hospital service. Unlike a hospitalist model, the designated admitting physician model is rotated amongst the members of the medical group, meaning the physicians still see patients in the office.

Hospitalists are often supported by a team of nonphysician providers (see Chapter 6). The most common types of team members are physician's assistants, clinical or advanced nurse practitioners, dedicated rounding nurses, clinical pharmacists, and medical social workers. These types of teams are most suited for medical groups or hospitals that provide care for a high number of patients with serious and complex conditions, and are also commonly found in teaching hospitals, regardless of payer considerations.

The reasoning behind the hospitalist model is that a dedicated, on-site physician will be closer to the care that the patient is receiving, is in a better position to coordinate needed services, and is able to monitor care for quality and appropriateness. A dedicated hospitalist is also better able to obtain diagnostic study reports, consultations, and so forth in a timely manner. A hospitalist is available all day, though not necessarily 24 hours per day on-site, rather than once or twice per day, which is the norm when private practice physicians care for inpatients. Of course, there will be many clinical conditions where the hospitalist is not at all in a primary caregiver situation, for example, during chemotherapy, for obstetrics, for surgical procedures, and so forth. In that case, the hospitalist may still monitor inpatient cases, or simply be available for consultation or assistance as the need arises.

Payers are generally supportive of the hospitalist role, but have become a bit more cautious for two primary reasons. The first is the impact of the increasing trend in hospital physician employment on utilization. As noted in Chapter 5, hospital-employed physicians providing office-based care are typically directed to use the hospital's ancillary and imaging services rather than lower-cost alternatives, likewise for ambulatory procedures or any services the health system provides.

The second reason is the increasing disconnection between inpatient care and office-based care associated with hospitalists. As a result, a recent study found that the reduced hospital costs associated with hospitalists was more than offset by higher medical utilization and costs after discharge.[100] That topic is covered in in the section on managing the postdischarge transition.

Concurrent Review and Management

Concurrent UM is at the core of managing inpatient utilization. As noted earlier, it takes place during a hospital stay, and this is almost the only type of medical service in which it is used. The other services that use concurrent review are extended types of care such as rehabilitation, physical therapy, or similar care that can reach a point where it is no longer beneficial or meets the demands of medical necessity.†

There is substantial variability between payers in the degree of effort or the types of concurrent UM activities they undertake. Loosely managed plans such as CDHPs and some PPOs may not aggressively manage inpatient utilization once the member is in the hospital, becoming involved only if a case becomes very costly, but otherwise depend on hospitals' own internal UR to manage any cases. PPOs with strong hospital contracts may simply depend

---

*This includes hospitalists in closed-panel HMOs.

†It also may be used on occasion for treatment with costly drugs or biological agents, as described in Chapter 11.

on retrospective review, which is discussed later in the chapter, to identify cases where some or all of the charges will be denied.

Some believe that concurrent UM has run its course, and that practice patterns have changed to the point where it is unnecessary. That is not the case. For example, the senior officer in charge of the UM function at a major national payer reported that internal analyses of concurrent UM data found that even in 2011, 5–6% of inpatient days are being categorized as medically inappropriate.[101]

Payers that rely on fixed or semi-fixed payment methods such as diagnosis-related groups (DRGs), Medicare-Severity adjusted DRGs (MS-DRGs), bundled payments or case rates, and capitation may also be less aggressive with concurrent UM under the belief that once the patient is admitted, the hospital will manage the case since payment to the hospital is fixed. That may have been the case 10 or 15 years ago, but as discussed at length in Chapter 5, chargemaster-defined outliers now make up such a substantial percentage of inpatient cases that this belief is no longer warranted. HMOs that use any charge- or volume-based payment method such as per diems or discounted charges are most likely to have aggressively concurrent UM.

UM Nurse and Concurrent Review

The one individual who is most important to the success of a UM program is the UM nurse. It is the UM nurse who is the eyes and ears of the health plan's medical management department, who is able to apply clinical knowledge to cases, who will coordinate the discharge planning, and who will facilitate all the activities of utilization management.

UM Nurse Staffing

Staffing levels for UM nurses and others involved in UM overall varies depending on the size of the geographic area, the number of hospitals, the size of the plan, and the intensity with which UM will be performed. Automated clinical decision-support applications, either as part of a payer's main IT system or as an integrated free-standing set of applications, allow a UM nurse to access not only the clinical criteria and guidelines previously discussed, but also patient demographics, eligibility, claims history (including pharmacy claims), stored information from prior hospitalizations, associated physicians, and other relevant information. Access to these support systems is not confined to central locations, but accessible through secure wireless connections from anywhere.

Though concurrent UM takes place during a hospital stay, the range of specific UM nurse activities is broad. In some plans, the role simply involves telephone information-gathering. In other plans, there will be a more proactive role, including active hospital rounding; frequent communication with attending physicians, the medical director, the hospitals, and the hospitalized members and their families; and discharge planning and facilitation. Some of these activities are briefly described below.

UM nurse staffing ratios vary accordingly. These ratios were once widely available in published studies, but have since become proprietary to the organizations that collect such benchmarking data, with a few exceptions such as reports on new models of care, which is discussed a bit later. However, the ranges in **Table 7-4** are based on the author's personal experience with HMOs and PPOs with strong medical management.

UM Nurse Concurrent Review Rounding

The one fundamental function of the UM nurse is information-gathering. Information about hospital cases must be obtained in an accurate and timely fashion. It falls to the UM nurse to be the focal point of this information collection effort and to ensure that it is obtained and communicated to the necessary individuals in medical management. Depending on circumstances, this might be a medical director, a case manager, a DM nurse, or other clinical department.

Notification of urgent or emergency admissions are typically done by the hospital, but the UM nurse may discover a case in the normal course of work. Cases for which notification was provided still require confirmation and usually more information, depending on what was provided by the hospital. Necessary information includes admission date and diagnosis, the type of hospital service to which the patient was admitted (e.g., medical, surgical, maternity), the admitting physician, specialists, planned procedures by type and timing, expected discharge date, needed discharge planning, and any other pertinent information the plan managers may need.

Information gathered by the UM nurse or by any other individuals in the UM department are typically entered into the medical management decision support systems noted earlier. Because of the breadth of information available through those systems, the UM nurse may be able to

TABLE 7-4	Approximate UM Nurse Staffing Ratio Ranges per 100,000 Commercial Members
Role	**Approximate Staffing Ratio**
All UM functions	6–13 UM nurses per 100,000 members
Precertification and concurrent UM	2–8 UM nurses per 100,000 members
Case management	2–5 UM nurses per 100,000 members

provide clinical information from the payer's claims system that was not available in an urgent admission; for example, payers often have the only really complete record of all the medications a patient has had filled and when they were filled, as well as prior reasons for admissions or procedures.

Criteria Review for LOS Extensions

The topic of using evidence-based clinical criteria and guidelines has been thoroughly explored by this point. As applied to concurrent UM, the most important aspect is its use in any coverage authorization extension of an inpatients stay. In many cases it is straightforward and even automated. When it is not clear-cut, the criteria and guidelines assist in a more focused review.

Telephone Rounding

In some plans, information-gathering is done strictly by telephone, also referred to as telephone rounding. Although network hospitals are typically required to notify a payer of an unplanned admission, compliance is highly variable. Therefore, the first call is to the admitting office to see if plan members were admitted. The next call is to the hospital's UM department to obtain information about all unplanned admissions and any routine admissions that are near or past the authorized LOS.

HMOs are the least likely to rely primarily on telephone rounding, and often use it only in locations where there is too much geographic area to cover and the plan cannot yet justify adding more UM nurses. It also may be done in those rare instances where a hospital refuses to give the HMO's UM nurse rounding privileges on hospitalized plan members.

Non-HMOs are the most likely to use telephone rounding, if they do concurrent UM at all. The greater the pressure on administrative costs, the more likely telephone rounding will be the only type of rounding, and even then only to identify clear outliers. Also, where once nearly all HMOs used telephone rounding as their least preferred approach, there are now many that use it almost exclusively. As is discussed at the end of the chapter, pressures on administrative costs by the ACA may increase the use of telephone rounding compared to more labor-intensive approaches.

Hospital Rounding

For effective UM, rounding in person is far superior to telephone rounding, but is more labor intensive and therefore more costly. HMOs are the most likely type of payer to have UN nurses do hospital rounding.

The most intense type of concurrent UM is daily rounding by a UM nurse on every hospitalized member. This ensures that the medical director will obtain the most accurate and timely information, including information

that might not otherwise be obtainable. For example, in a good-quality management program (see Chapter 14), the rounding UM nurse can watch for quality problems or significant events that would trigger a QM review, or even a peer review. The rounding nurse is also in the best position to identify "never events," which are events that should never happen in a hospital (e.g., a serious medication error leading to complications). As discussed in Chapter 5, payers typically do not pay a hospital for costs associated with "never events."

A rounding nurse can pick up information about a patient's condition that may affect discharge planning—information that the attending physician may have failed to communicate such as home durable medical equipment that must be ordered. The UM nurse also can detect practice behavior that increases utilization simply for the convenience of the physician or the hospital. For example, a patient may be ready for discharge but the physician may have missed making rounds that morning and will not be back until the next day, or the hospital may have rescheduled surgery for its own reasons and the patient will have to stay an extra, unnecessary day. In situations such as these, the UM nurse must not be put into an adversarial position, but rather should refer such matters to the medical director.

Occasionally hospitals will refuse to grant rounding privileges to a UM nurse, the typical excuse being that the hospital already has a UM department. The hospital UM department may be inadequate for the needs of an HMO that truly manages care, however. Another frequent excuse is the need to protect the confidentiality of patients. That excuse does not hold if the plan's UM nurse is only rounding on plan members and is properly performing utilization and quality management; even the privacy requirements under HIPAA (see Chapter 29) recognize UM as a legitimate function and allow access to protected medical information to qualified personnel. Regrettably, the most likely reason a hospital will refuse an HMO UM nurse to round is that it has enough market power to demand it. Fortunately, hospitals and HMOs are usually able to come to agreement around on-site rounding.

Medical Director Responsibilities

In addition to monitoring the elements discussed in this chapter, there are a few specific functions that medical directors working in UM should perform. The first of these is communications. UM nurses typically handle routine types of communications as part of the precertification and concurrent UM process. But a medical director is usually involved in the most difficult cases. The difficulty may not necessarily be medical, but rather may be a problem with a physician, a hospital, a member, or a member's family. When it is medical, reliance on evidence-based medicine and industry standards is the norm.

Sometimes medical directors are in direct communication with the attending physician in complex cases where there may be alternatives available or when the UM nurse is unable to obtain adequate information. This is especially important when it comes to managing the growing problem of outlier cases discussed in Chapter 5. In some payers, medical directors are involved in most instances of direct communications with other physicians. In most cases in which there is a disagreement or dispute with an attending or consulting physician that involves UM, including coverage issues based on the member's specific benefits plan, it is appropriate for a medical director to be involved, not the UM nurse.

The most aggressive type of concurrent UM is typically found in HMOs or in medical groups or IDSs under global capitation, which does not mean that all HMOs or capitated providers use it. In an aggressive UM program, a medical director reviews the full list of hospitalized members every day. This task may seem onerous—and it can be—but it is the only way a medical director can consistently spot problems in time to do something about them. There are obviously limits to what a single medical director can review, so even in an aggressive UM program, the UM nurses will identify the cases they believe the medical director needs to focus on. Nevertheless, the most aggressive UM involves medical director review each day, even if prioritized. Furthermore, plans with aggressive UM will not try to stretch the medical director too thin, but will have more than one physician involved as appropriate.

As a practical matter, in most payer UM programs, review of active inpatient cases is done by exception, focusing only on those cases where the UM nurse wishes the medical director to become involved or at least offer advice or an opinion.

Discharge Planning

Discharge planning is an ongoing effort beginning with admission or preadmission screening, and is part of concurrent UM. Discharge planning includes an estimate of how long the patient will be in the hospital, what the expected outcome will be, and any special requirements on discharge. But what sets it apart from concurrent review is facilitating the provision of those special requirements. Clinical guidelines may still be used, although it is not always necessary, but in this case it is to help arrange for things, not solely to make benefits determinations.

For example, if a patient was admitted with a fractured hip or a hip replacement, it is known from the outset that many weeks of rehabilitation will be necessary. It is therefore helpful to contact the rehabilitation facility prior to discharge to ensure that a bed will be available at the time of transfer. If it is known that a patient will need durable medical equipment, the equipment should be ordered early

so that the patient does not spend extra days in the hospital waiting for it to arrive.

As noted earlier, an often overlooked aspect of discharge planning is informing and assisting the patient and family well in advance of actual discharge. Otherwise they may be upset when the physician tells them that the patient is being discharged since they may have different expectations. Informing the patient and family from the start about when they can expect discharge, how the patient will be feeling, what they might need to prepare for at home, and how follow-up will occur will help to smooth things considerably. Finally, discharge planning in relation to preventing avoidable readmission to the hospital is addressed following a review of common alternatives to acute-care hospitalization.

Alternatives to Acute-Care Hospitalization

There are many instances where patients are ill or disabled but not to the extent that they need to be in an acute-care hospital, yet that is where they are. In some cases, the patient initially needed acute-care services, surgery for example, but recovery requires far fewer resources. In other cases, there is simply no place for the patient to go; for example, a patient is recovering from a broken femur but lives alone and has no support system. When care is still required but at a lower intensity, UM may promote the use of acute-care hospital alternatives. This may occur as part of concurrent UM for an inpatient or prospectively, in which case no acute-care stay is involved.

Subacute Care

One alternative to acute care hospitalization is a subacute care facility. This is most suited for prolonged convalescence or recovery cases. There are several types of subacute care facilities, including:

- Skilled nursing;
- Intermediate nursing;
- Physical rehabilitation;
- Surgical recovery and rehabilitation, including
  - General,
  - Specialty-specific such as orthopedic or cardiac, and
- Condition-specific such as trauma recovery.

To illustrate, if a patient with a broken femur requires more traction than can be provided safely at home and requires many months to recover, the cost for a bed-day in a subacute facility will be much less than in an acute-care hospital. The same goes for rehabilitation cases such as stroke or trauma to the brain when the damage is too extensive for the patient to go home immediately.

Over the past several years, the subacute-care industry has focused on making their facilities a practical alternative to an acute-care hospital for a larger variety of medical cases. For example, some subacute-care facilities provide a cost-effective location for the administration of chemotherapy that requires close supervision. In some cases, the treatment of certain medical conditions such as acute pneumonia or osteomyelitis when a patient is too sick to be cared for at home may be done in a subacute facility. In other cases, a patient may be able to be cared for at home, but it is still more cost-effective to deliver the therapy in the subacute facility through economies of scale.

Skilled or intermediate nursing facilities typically offer subacute-care services, but the patient or the family may object to the use of a "nursing home," particularly in the case of young patients. There is a stigma attached to nursing homes, even if they are renamed subacute facilities, that triggers some people to associate them with warehouses for the infirm elderly. To overcome this stigma, a proactive approach is required. For example, the facility might ensure that the plan's members are given a private room or are placed in a room with a patient with a similar functional status. Subacute care should also be provided in a separate wing or floor than is used for permanent residents.

When discussing this alternative with the patient and the family, it is best done well in advance of the actual move. Nothing is as distressing as suddenly finding out that you will be shipped out in the morning to a nursing home. If possible, have the family visit the subacute facility to meet the staff and see the environment before the patient is transferred.

When a member is in subacute facilities for any extended period of time, concurrent review should be done on a periodic basis. Continued coverage is typically based on continuing improvement. If an individual is no longer showing progress but is still unable to go home and be cared for by family, then the stay is for custodial care, meaning assistance with the acts of daily living. And, as noted earlier, neither commercial health plans nor Medicare (or MA) cover custodial care.

Facing the end of benefits coverage can be an emotionally wrenching experience both for the member's family and for the medical managers involved. The problem of who will pay for long-term custodial care is a national dilemma, but it becomes profoundly personal when a family is faced with high costs because the benefits the plan provides do not continue indefinitely. If it is possible or likely that benefits will end, it is wise to inform the family early on. Referring them to community resources may also help.

Step-Down Units

A step-down unit is a ward or section of a ward in an acute-care hospital that is used in much the same way as a skilled nursing facility. A patient who requires less care and monitoring, such as someone recovering from a hip replacement (after all the drains have been removed), may need only bed rest, traction, and minimal nursing care. In recognition of the lesser resource needs, the charge per day is less.

The step-down unit has the advantage of being convenient for the physician and UM nurse and is more acceptable to the patient and the family. It also does not require transfer outside the facility. Although the cost per day is sometimes slightly higher than that of a subacute facility, the difference may be worth it in terms of member acceptability.

Hospice Care

Hospice care is care given to terminally ill patients. It tends to be care that is supportive to the patient and the family. Much hospice care is outpatient or home-care based, but inpatient forms of hospice are also available and are used most often when such care cannot be given in the home. Statistically speaking, most hospice patients are covered under Medicare. In commercial managed care, it is now a routine benefit, although it once was not. In fact, many payers will not cover acute-care hospitalization for purely palliative care for terminally ill patients, requiring the use of hospice for such care. Care of the terminally ill patient has not been a focus of most medical management programs, even though it should be considered a form of case management.

Home Health Care

Home health care is a frequent alternative to acute inpatient or subacute facility care. Services that are particularly amenable to home health care include nursing care for routine reasons (e.g., checking on a newborn, changing dressings, and the like), home intravenous treatment (e.g., for osteomyelitis, certain forms of chemotherapy, or home intravenous nutrition), home physical therapy, respiratory therapy, and rehabilitation care. Most payers have contracts in each community with one or more licensed home health providers since the scope of services may not be the same for each.

Concurrent review should be performed on home health. Because the physician and UM nurse seldom visit the patient receiving home health care, it often defaults to the home health nurse to determine how often and how long the patient should receive services, and this practice can lead to some surprising costs. It is advisable to have a firm policy regarding the number of home health visits covered under a single authorization and a requirement for physician review for continued authorization.

Case Management

Traditional case management (CM), sometimes called large case management (LCM), refers to identifying and managing high-cost inpatient cases. CM of complex chronic conditions is discussed later in this chapter and in Chapter 8.

Upon identification of a case that is appropriate to a CM program, an assessment is completed that identifies problems, goals, and applicable interventions for the case. The hallmark of CM is longitudinal management of the case by a single UM nurse or department. CM spans hospital care, rehabilitation, outpatient care, professional services, home health care, ancillary services, and so forth. As an aside, rehabilitation is not just physical rehabilitation following trauma or surgery; it includes cardiac, pulmonary, and neurological rehabilitation as well. It is in the active coordination of care that both quality and cost-effectiveness are maintained. One important element is to facilitate the transfer of information from the inpatient treating physicians to the patient's physician since this is a common point of breakdown, as discussed shortly.

In addition to the standard methods of managing utilization, CM often involves two other approaches. First is the use of community resources. Some catastrophic cases require support structures to help the member function or even return home. Examples of such support include family members, social service agencies, churches, special foundations, and so forth. Another approach is to go beyond the contractual benefits to better manage the case, logically referred to as extra-contractual benefits. For example, if the benefits structure of the group has only limited coverage for durable medical equipment, it may still be in the plan's financial interest as well as the member's to cover such expenses to get the patient home and out of the hospital. In self-funded groups, the group administrator may actually be willing to fund extra-contractual benefits simply as a benefit for an employee or dependent that is experiencing a terrible medical problem. Prenatal care is a specialized form of CM because active coordination occurs before the newborn is delivered. Prenatal CM involves identification of high-risk pregnancies early enough to intervene to improve the chances of a good outcome. With the staggering costs of neonatal intensive care, it only takes a few improved outcomes to yield dramatic savings. Methods for identifying cases include sending out information about pregnancy to all members, reviewing the claims system for pregnancy-related claims, asking (or requiring) PCPs and obstetricians to notify the plan when a delivery is expected, and so forth. After the UM department is informed of the case, the member may be proactively contacted, and an assessment undertaken to identify risk factors (e.g., very young maternal age, diabetes, smoking, alcohol or drug use, other medical problems, poor nutrition). If risk factors are noted, then the plan can coordinate prenatal care in a very proactive manner. Although it is impossible to force a member to seek care and to follow up on problems, it is possible to increase the amount and quality of prenatal care that is delivered. When the pregnant patient is also abusing drugs or alcohol, close coordination with the substance abuse program must then occur.

The degree to which the plan can become involved in CM is in part a function of the benefits structure. In a tightly run managed health care plan, it is common for the UM department to be proactive in CM; in simple PPOs, CM is often voluntary on the part of the member (in other words, if the member chooses not to cooperate, there is little impact on benefits). Even in situations requiring strictly voluntary cooperation by the members and physicians, CM is still highly effective.

Self-funded plans and payers with reinsurance must comply with one critically important element of CM or, more appropriately, LCM. As described in Chapter 2, reinsurance is fundamentally different from health insurance, including how and when the reinsurer has any liabilities for reinsurance claims. While there is a form of reinsurance called "Occurrence" that does not necessarily require timely notification, it is uncommon. The two common forms, called "claims made" and "claims paid," do require it. Any failure to notify the reinsurer according to the policy's requirements means no reinsurance recovery. And most policies also require active CM to manage the case as well.

The biggest challenge to medical managers charged with oversight of CM is in knowing when to stop. It is not uncommon for CM nurses to continue to provide support or maintain contact with members long after there is any real demonstrable return or impact. This is not to minimize the value of emotional support, but at some point decisions must be made about the appropriate use of resources. The most direct way to address this is by regularly reviewing cases against criteria to determine if continued CM intervention will have enough impact to warrant the use of resources.

The Postdischarge Transition

Upon discharge, most members will convalesce or recover at home and have few difficulties. But when a member has multiple chronic conditions or is otherwise frail or at risk, however, the transition from inpatient care to home can present a special challenge. Some individuals may not have the resources to self-manage their care according to a printed sheet of instructions, have poor medication compliance, or simply may not be seen in follow-up by their physician. In many cases, their PCP may not have received any information from the stay, or even have known about the admission. In other words, there is insufficient or absent coordination of their care, leaving them especially vulnerable following discharge. A number of them will be readmitted shortly after discharge for either the same condition or for medical conditions related to the first admission, either of which was preventable. Recall from Figure 7-2 the high concentration of costs in a small percentage of individuals—multiple hospital admissions make up a major portion of those costs.

Avoidable Readmissions

Preventing avoidable readmissions is an aspect of discharge planning that has received renewed attention, although it is not a new problem. Adverse events occur frequently in the immediate postdischarge period, and many can potentially be prevented by using simple strategies.[102] Despite long-standing awareness of the problem of avoidable readmissions, the extent of it was surprising to many, or at least many of those not involved with aggressive UM programs. It was brought into focus with the 2009 publication of a study analyzing traditional FFS Medicare claims data from 2003–2004 that found for all Medicare beneficiaries who were discharged from the hospital:

- Just under 20% were readmitted within 30 days;
- 34% were readmitted within 90 days;
- 50% of the patients who had initially been discharged with medical conditions and who were readmitted within 30 days had not seen a physician postdischarge; and
- 70% of the patients who had initially been discharged following surgery and who were readmitted within 30 days were readmitted with medical conditions.[103]

One reaction to this report was a push by CMS to include it in hospital payment reform. Congress agreed and included provisions in the ACA to require CMS to reduce overall payments to hospitals it classifies as having excess avoidable readmissions starting in 2013, as described in Chapter 5. This has had the effect of sharply increasing hospitals' attention, which is very helpful to health plans.

Several studies compared readmission rates between traditional FFS Medicare and MA plans. A 2009 Johns Hopkins study commissioned by the Alliance of Community Health Plans found that the readmission rate for their MA plans was 27% lower compared to traditional FFS Medicare.[104] This is similar to findings of a study commissioned by America's Health Insurance Plans (AHIP), the trade organization representing insurers and managed health care plans.[105] Why MA plans should show lower readmission rates than traditional FFS Medicare is most likely attributable to better care coordination, as is discussed next, but the studies only looked at rates, not root causes.

The Communications Challenge in Inpatient to Outpatient Continuity of Care

If hospital-employed physicians provide most of a member's care, including office-based primary care, then coordination and continuity of care can be maintained, much like a closed-panel HMO. Except in that situation, there has been an increasing lack of connection between community PCPs and the specialty physicians or hospitalists who provide and manage inpatient care, with some exceptions to be described shortly. For example, a survey of PCPs and specialty physicians about communications reported that 69.3% of primary care physicians reported "always" or "most of the time" sending notification of a patient's history and reason for consultation to specialists, but only 34.8% of specialists said they "always" or "most of the time" received such notification. Both PCPs and specialty physicians said lack of communication threatened quality.[106]

The rise of hospitalists has exacerbated the problem in many places. A 2008 survey of physicians in various communities reported a lack of coordination and accountability for the quality of care postdischarge, although companies and multispecialty medical groups that employed hospitalists were more likely than others to establish routines for ensuring coordinated transitions upon hospital admission and discharge.[107] This fits with the finding in the 2009 study cited earlier that 50% of avoidable readmissions had not seen a physician between the first discharge and readmission.

Studies in the late 1990s and early 2000s found that implementation of hospitalist programs was associated with significant reductions in resource use, usually measured as hospital costs (average decrease, 13.4%) or average length of stay (average decrease, 16.6%).[108] Other studies around that same time concluded that the benefits of using a hospitalist only became significant in the second year of use.[109, 110] Some recent studies show a continuing positive impact on quality, but more modest in scope.[111]

Of far more concern are studies associating hospitalist care with higher utilization and cost levels after discharge compared to patients cared for by community physicians. For example, a 2011 study demonstrated that for Medicare inpatients receiving hospitalist care, hospital charges were $282 lower, but Medicare costs in the 30-day postdischarge period were $332 higher, and hospitalists' inpatients were less likely to be discharged to the home.[112] Over time, EMRs should attenuate, though not eliminate this problem, as will better hospitalist training and communications. But those solutions have been, and remain, a long time in coming.

Transitional Case Management

The core of transitional case management (TCM) is a program to call members shortly after discharge. Many HMOs or other managed health care plans incorporate a simple "welcome home" type of call to make sure things are going well, answer any questions, or see if assistance is required. Hospitals also typically make such calls. Outbound calling may be automated, and TCM nurses typically use software systems that provide decision support, access to guidelines, electronic record-keeping, and tracking.

The call should at a minimum have a checklist to ensure that all major elements are covered. It also allows the nurse to educate, coach, and confirm with the member/caregiver that the treatment plan for post-acute care is clear and being followed. A focused postdischarge call is useful even when a member is in a health plan's DM program (see Chapter 8) because it is designed specifically to address preventable readmissions. For example, looking at MA members who were in their chronic DM program and who were hospitalized in 2008, those who received a call within 14 days of discharge had a 23% lower 30-day readmission rate compared to similar members who did not receive such a call.[113]

A more intense focus may be applied for those who are at the highest risk of readmission based on their underlying illness, length of stay, or clinical complexity. If the TCM nurse does not reach the individual or a caregiver within a few days of discharge, they typically will persist with multiple attempts at contact. The checklist is usually more extensive too. Examples of topics covered include:

- Assessing medication adherence;
- Screening for polypharmacy, drug duplication, or potentially adverse drug interactions;
- Encouraging or assisting with scheduling a physician office appointment in a timely way;
- Identifying and helping to resolve barriers to receiving medical care such as transportation;
- Getting necessary follow-up lab work or other types of diagnostic studies;
- Assessing diet and nutrition;
- Doing a depression screening;
- Performing a safety risk assessment;
- Screening and support of caregivers;
- Assessing level of functioning;
- Educating the individual and his or her caregiver about the clinical condition;
- Providing or reinforcing instructions and self-care or caregiving such as dressing changes, monitoring blood glucose levels, and so forth; and
- Performing condition-specific clinical assessments.

TCM nurses also usually have easy access to a physician advisor or medical director to provide support or guidance. In cases where medication compliance is the key to preventing readmission, a clinical pharmacist can make the call; for example, a follow-up phone call by a pharmacist involved in the hospital care of patients was associated with increased patient satisfaction, resolution of medication-related problems, and fewer return visits to the emergency department.[114] When focused on those most at risk, the impact is striking. In one study, for example, there was a fourfold reduction in the risk of readmission for those

who participated in TCM compared to those that did not, and there was also an association with how timely contact was made.[115]

Even more intense programs may be used. One example is the Care Transitions Program,[SM*] a highly structured 4-week program. The topic of individuals at high risk for readmission provides a segue into the next topic, which is the overall management of complex chronic conditions.

■ MANAGEMENT OF COMPLEX CHRONIC CONDITIONS

The small percentage of individuals responsible for the high percentage of costs has been brought up many times in this chapter in relation to specific UM topics. This section provides a very brief overview of the overall approach to managing cost and quality in members with multiple complex chronic conditions.

The current system of paying providers does not reward providers for managing the care of complex cases, it rewards procedures. And since it does not reward for managing complex care, time spent doing it is time not billing for something else; in essence, it may even cost them money. But it is also at the heart of newer IDS models such as PCMHs and ACOs (see Chapter 2). At the time of publication, however, PCMHs were still in the pilot stage and CMS had not finalized any payment models. Insurers and MA plans at risk for medical costs do realize the savings that comes from better managing these cases, just as they realize the savings from UM or DM overall, and have been piloting initiatives in several parts of the country.

Managing the care of individuals with complex chronic conditions is essentially a matter of coordination and continuity, and the practice of evidence-based medicine. As became clear in the preceding discussion, simply making sure that medications are taken properly, follow-up appointments are made and kept, and other basic measures can have a positive impact immediately following discharge. This can be beneficial in managing complex chronic conditions. Predictive modeling software, as described in Chapter 8, is also routinely employed. A more aggressive approach uses a support infrastructure involving multidisciplinary clinical teams, co-location of a care manager and physician, expanded use of home telemonitoring and remote sensing, and higher levels of patient interaction. The most intense approach uses "high-risk clinics" instead of primary care, having specially trained physicians and advanced nurse practitioners focusing on a small panel of patients.

Unfortunately, studies documenting savings show mixed results when postdischarge transition is not included; in

---

*www.caretransitions.org, current as of July 26, 2011.

other words, TCM demonstrates consistent savings, but savings that do not involve readmissions are less clear. It is also not clear what combination of techniques and in what settings produce the best results.[116]

■ RETROSPECTIVE REVIEW

Retrospective review is exactly what it sounds like—reviewing utilization and costs after care has been provided and paid for. There are two primary types: claims review and pattern review.

Claims Review

Claims review is the examination of individual claims for improprieties or mistakes. All payers use software to screen for and identify claims that are incorrect, misleading, or falsified. The most common problems are the result of coding errors by providers, such as diagnosis-procedure mismatch. Other common problems include "upcoding" (i.e., submitting a claim using the code for a procedure or diagnosis that is more complex than what was actually the case, but will result in higher payment) and "unbundling" (i.e., submitting multiple claims by separating out various components and charging for each).

Some payers have taken this process one step further and use software to automatically change claims that are determined to be problematic, for example, rebundling unbundled claims and paying only the appropriate payment. A more forceful step is to use the software to automatically downcode claims based on statistical norms; in other words, reduce the payment by reducing the type of code, based on how often those types of codes appear under normal circumstances. This last activity has resulted in legal class action by physicians, with some major health plans settling out of court while others continue to defend the practice. While still used by many payers, using automated systems to adjust claims downward is now less broadly applied, or used as part of retrospective pattern review.

It is routine for plans to review large claims to verify whether services were actually delivered, or whether mistakes were made in collating the claims data. In such large cases, the plan may actually send a representative on-site to the hospital to review the medical record against the claims record. In most cases, this results in some level of payment reduction when information supporting the charges cannot be found.

Specific claims will also take place when fraud or abuse is detected, usually through pattern review, as discussed next. Fraud refers to deliberate criminal activity to submit fraudulent claims, while abuse refers to billing practices that, while not specifically fraudulent, represent attempts to obtain payment far above what is appropriate. When detected, a claims examiner specializing in the identification of fraud or abuse conduct detailed reviews of submitted claims and supporting documentation (or lack thereof). If suspicion appears warranted, the payer typically exercises its contractual right to conduct on-site reviews (see Chapter 6), and does so unannounced. If fraud or abuse is confirmed, the payer usually attempts to recover the money either through direct payment or through offsets to future payment. In some cases, review takes place before the claims are actually paid. Law enforcement is also brought in when appropriate and reporting fraud and abuse to the federal government for Medicare and Medicaid services is required by law. (Fraud and billing abuse are discussed in Chapter 19.)

Pattern Review

Payers often examine patterns of utilization to determine where action must be taken. This is used not only to detect claims errors or falsifications, as discussed above, but also refers to detecting patterns of services and utilization that may allow for improvements in cost or quality of care. For example, if three hospitals in the area perform coronary artery bypass surgery, the plan may look to see which one has the best clinical outcomes, the shortest lengths of stay, and the lowest charges. The plan may then preferentially send all such cases to that hospital. Pattern review also allows the plan to focus UM efforts primarily on those areas needing greater attention (i.e., Sutton's Law: Go where the money is!).

The payer must first decide what it wants to look at since computer systems do not recognize patterns without being programmed to do so. Said another way, managers must choose what to look for because no computer system can analyze every type of event for every member, every PCP, every specialist, every hospital, every pharmacy, every ambulatory care facility, every home care agency, and so forth. In some cases, the focus of pattern analysis is on utilization, for example:

- Referral rates in an HMO that relies of FFS to reimburse specialists, or
- Hospital inpatient utilization rates and costs.

Recent examples in the industry applicable to outcomes include:

- Increasing the percentage of people who are prescribed beta blockers after a heart attack by analyzing pharmacy claims data, and
- Using physician claims data to increase compliance with prevention by reminding diabetics (and their physicians) about the need to get regular retinal exams.

The identification of patterns using claims data faces some challenges that can limit what it may be able to find.

In even selecting what to look for, the following aspects come into play:

- Sample size—there must be sufficient events that a typical statistical analytics system will be able to identify when the frequency of an event is significantly above or below expectations;
- Frequency of an event—the flip side of the sample size issue, the events being measured must occur with sufficiently high frequency to actually mean something:
  - This is the reason that DM programs and typical HMO pattern analyses focus on common chronic conditions, affecting a sizable number of members and occurring with sufficient frequency to capture meaningful data;
  - It is also therefore not typical for a payer to program its system to look for rare events unless it is tied to payment policies;
- Selection of a condition for which great variations exist in clinical practices, that is, there must be a reason for choosing what to look at; for example:
  - If physicians vary in their adherence to evidence-based medical practice, by not always prescribing beta blockers following an acute heart attack for instance, then pattern analysis can provide useful information for feedback to noncompliant physicians, including a reevaluation 6 months after such feedback was provided;
  - If providers typically adhere to accepted evidence-based medical practice for a particular condition, the ongoing pattern analysis may not be worth the effort.

Problems may exist with consistency and integrity of data, particularly when providers do not code properly or even capture all relevant data on the claims form. Capitated providers will have little or no incentive to submit detailed claims or encounter data. Providers paid by FFS are incented to submit claims, but are paid based on what they do, not on the diagnoses, so they typically are careful to code the type of visit or procedure, but are less careful about coding the diagnosis. Even similar providers do not necessarily provide the same array of services; for example, some cardiologists do invasive procedures such as placing pacemakers and stents, while other cardiologists are more limited in the procedures they perform.

Association does not equate to causality either, meaning that events or results may appear to be related, but it is not clear if one actually caused the other or that there is even a causal relationship at all. For example, if a physician appears to have much higher total member medical costs than his or her peers, this could reflect any or all of the following:

- Insufficient attention to cost-effective practice,
- Having a substantially sicker panel of patients, or
- Reflect care provided by or ordered by other physicians.

Because of complexities involved with retrospective pattern detection and review, it is addressed in more depth in Chapter 10 along with other uses of data in medical management. One other use of pattern review is to provide feedback to providers. Although not as powerful as active UM by the plan's own department, feedback sometimes can have an effect in and of itself. When combined with other management functions and financial incentives, meaningful and actionable feedback to providers is a useful management tool. (This topic is explored in Chapter 9.)

ROUTINE ANCILLARY SERVICES

High-cost imaging and diagnostic and therapeutic ancillary services were addressed earlier in the discussion about facility-based ambulatory services. The more traditional types of ancillary services such as laboratory, routine X-ray, ultrasound, and so forth typically do not present a major challenge in UM, and utilization has been relatively steady. If the overall costs for ancillary services is higher than expected, analyzing claims data usually identifies the specific ones causing the increase, and it is managed similarly to high-cost imaging.

Duplicate testing secondary to the absence of an EMR shared by all providers is regularly touted in support of EMR adoption, but substantial EMR-related savings from reduced testing have yet to be proven. The biggest problem caused by routine ancillary testing is from false positives that may set off a costly pursuit of a diagnosis that doesn't exist.

The ability to manage utilization of ancillary services will be directly related to the ability to capture accurate and timely data. If there is no way to capture data regarding ancillary services, there will be difficulty controlling utilization. Lack of data will also make contracting problematic because no vendor will be willing to contract aggressively without having some idea of projected utilization (at least not on terms that will be beneficial to the plan or medical group responsible for the cost).

Ancillary services utilization may be incorporated into payment methodologies, including pay-for-performance (Chapter 5). Physician self-referral for routine ancillary services also can be a problem, even though not as costly as for imaging, it is addressed the same way.

In older studies, simple feedback about test ordering led to modest reductions in use,[117, 118] and somewhat greater decreases have been seen when feedback was combined with other written guidelines or peer review.[119] (See Chapter 9 for additional discussion of physician behavior.)

THE POTENTIAL IMPACT OF THE ACA ON UTILIZATION MANAGEMENT

The ACA has been referenced many times already, but there are some remaining elements of the law that have the potential for a significant impact on UM. The ACA requires health insurers, but not self-funded health plans, to have a medical loss ratio (MLR) of no less than 85% of premiums for each insured large group account, and 80% in the individual and small group markets. This means that the combination of sales, governance, administration, and profit* may not exceed 15% or 20% of the premium, respectively. Insurers and HMOs must rebate the difference to their customers if the MLR is lower, but absorb the extra costs if it is higher (other restrictions also apply, as described in Chapter 30).

Health plan activities related to improving quality and patient safety may be counted as medical expenses, but UM activities are counted as administrative expenses, along with all costs associated with managing the provider network, claims processing, member services, sales and marketing, and so forth. Because of MLR limitations, payers are looking closely at all costs, including costs to do UM. In other words, the ACA effectively reduces the value of lowering medical costs while limiting how much can be spent on administration, including the contracting and medical management functions that address costs most directly.

At the time of publication, health insurers and HMOs have issued rebates in many cases, but have not yet substantially cut back on any medical management functions. However, that could change, and payers have several options. One option is not to change, which is certainly viable if they are currently able to do so, but it is also possible that they will make changes so at the very least, administrative dollars can be used elsewhere. Another option is to do less UM, which will typically result in higher medical costs, raising the MLR, which also indirectly raises the amount available for administration. A third option is to outsource some medical management functions, just like they sometimes do for network management, as discussed in Chapter 4, which some payers are exploring.

A fourth and increasingly attractive option is almost a return to the past, which is to move the responsibility for UM to the providers themselves, and pay them for it. This is what closed-panel and (to a lesser degree) IPA HMOs do, which accounts for why their MLRs may be 90% or higher, since UM, network management, case management, and so forth are counted as medical costs. It is also what is envisioned for PCMHs and ACOs. Many provider organizations are able to do this, but as discussed in Chapters 1 and 2, most cannot, at least not yet. In any case, moving UM to the providers without properly aligning the financial incentives is unlikely to end well, as discussed in Chapters 1 and 5.

▓ CONCLUSION

Basic medical-surgical UM involves a broad continuum. UM focuses primarily on the use of precertification and

authorization for coverage of services based on evidence-based clinical criteria and guidelines; UM does not actually provide or forbid the use of medical care, though coverage obviously can have a significant impact. UM uses the techniques of managing basic demand, referral and specialty services, and ambulatory and inpatient facility-based services, and often increases its focus on areas with excessive utilization such as that associated with physician self-referral. The tools and technology utilized by health plans to perform these types of UM services have evolved to support multiple channels and provide a more sophisticated level of analytics and business rules to improve efficiency and effectiveness of the programs, as well as acknowledging the longitudinal member record that includes key information regarding health risks, wellness programs, and condition management program participation.

The management of hospital or institutional utilization is one of the most important aspects of managing overall health care costs. The methods used to manage hospital utilization vary from relatively weak and mechanical to tightly managed, longitudinally integrated, and highly labor-intensive. Special attention is now being given to the prevention of avoidable readmissions and to individuals with complex chronic conditions. How this will evolve under the ACA and changes in the provider landscape is, at the time of publication, open to speculation at best.

Endnotes

1 Robinson JC, Yegian JM. Medical management after managed care. *Health Affairs.* May 2004;Suppl Web Exclusives:W4–269–280.

2 Anderson G. *Chronic care: Making the case for ongoing care.* Princeton, NJ: Robert Wood Johnson Foundation, 2010. Available at: www.rwjf.org/pr/product.jsp?id=50968. Accessed July 16, 2011.

3 The Patient Protection and Affordable Care Act (P.L. 111-148) as amended by the Health Care and Education Reconciliation Act of 2010 (P.L. 111-152), which was signed into law on March 30, 2010. For purposes of this chapter, the Affordable Care Act (ACA) includes both laws.

4 Van Horn RL, Burns LR, Wholey DR. The impact of physician involvement in managed care on efficient use of hospital resources. *Med Care.* 1997;35(9):873–889.

5 Wennberg JE, Gittlesohn A. Variations in medical care among small areas. *Sci Am.* 1982;246(4):120–134.

6 Wennberg J, Caper P. Medical practice: Why does it vary so much? *Hospitals.* 1985;59(5):89.

7 Wennberg JE, Fisher ES, Stukel TA, Shart SM. Use of Medicare claims data to monitor provider-specific performance among patients with severe chronic illness. *Health Affairs.* October 2004;Suppl Variation:VAR5–VAR18. Available at: http://content

---

*Occasionally called the administrative loss ratio or ALR, but the term is not used nearly as often as MLR is.

.healthaffairs.org/cgi/content/full/hlthaff.var.5/DC3. Accessed August 1, 2006.

8   Fisher ES, Wennberg DE, Stukel TA, Gottliev DJ. Variations in the longitudinal efficiency of academic medical centers. *Health Affairs.* October 2004;Suppl Variation:VAR19-VAR32. Available at: http://content.healthaffairs.org/cgi/content/full/hlthaff.var.19/DC3. Accessed August 1, 2006.

9   Sutherland, JM, Fisher ES, Skinner JS. Getting past denial—The high cost of health care in the United States. *N Engl J Med.* 2009;361(13):1227–1230.

10 Zuckerman S. Clarifying sources of geographic differences in Medicare spending. *N Engl J Med.* 2010; 363(1):54–62.

11 Medicare Payment Advisory Commission (MedPAC). Report to the Congress: Regional variation in Medicare service use. Washington, DC: MedPac, January 2011.

12 Chernew ME, Sabik LM, Chandra A, et al. Geographic correlation between large-firm commercial spending and Medicare spending. *Am J Manag Care.* 2010;16(2): 131–138.

13 ACA Section 1302 42 U.S.C. § 18022 (d).

14 Brook RH, Ware JE, Rogers WH, et al. *The effect of coinsurance on the health of adults: Results from the Rand Health Insurance Experiment.* Santa Monica, CA: Rand Corporation, December 1984.

15 Beeuwkes Buntin M, Damberg C, Haviland A, et al. Consumer-directed health care: Early evidence about effects on cost and quality. *Health Affairs.* 2006;25(6): w516–w530.

16 Beeuwkes Buntin M, Haviland A, McDevitt R, Sood N. Healthcare spending and preventive care in high-deductible and consumer-directed health plans. *Am J Manag Care.* 2011;17(3):222–230.

17 Lo Sasso AT, Shah M, Frogner BK. Health savings accounts and health care spending. *Health Serv Res.* 2010;45(4):1041–1060.

18 Swartz K. Cost-sharing: Effects on spending and outcomes. Research Synthesis Report No. 20. Princeton, NJ: Robert Wood Johnson Foundation, December 2010.

19 Vickery DM, Kalmer H, Lowry D. Effect of a self-care education program on medical visits. *JAMA.* 1983; 250(21):2952–2956.

20 Robinson JS, Schwartz ML, Magwene KS, et al. The impact of fever health education on clinic utilization. *Am J Dis Child.* 1989;143(6):698–704.

21 Elsenhans VD, Marquardt C, Bledsoe T. Use of self-care manual shifts utilization pattern. *HMO Pract.* June 1995; 9(2):88–90.

22 ACA Section 2717 42 U.S.C. §300gg-17 (b).

23 Berg GD, Silverstein SS, Thomas E, Korn AM. Cost and utilization avoidance with mail prompts: A randomized controlled trial. *Am J Manag Care.* 2008;14(11): 748–754.

24 For example, see Pronk N, ed. *The ACSM's worksite health handbook: A guide to building healthy and productive companies.* 2nd ed. Champaign, IL: Human Kinetics; 2009. Available at: www.humankinetics.com/products/all-products/acsm%27s-worksite-health-handbook—2nd-edition. Accessed July 9, 2011.

25 Mattke S, Serxner SA, Zakowske SL, et al. Impact of 2 employer-sponsored population health management programs on medical care cost and utilization. *Am J Manag Care.* 2009;15(2):113–120.

26 Russell LB. Preventing chronic disease: An important investment, but don't count on cost savings. *Health Affairs.* 2009;28(1):42–45.

27 Huskamp HA, Rosenthal MB. Health risk appraisals: How much do they influence employees' health behavior? *Health Affairs.* 2009;28(5):1532–1540.

28 Elias WS. Introduction to health risk appraisals. In: Kongstvedt PK, Plocher DW, eds. *Best practices in medical management.* Gaithersburg, MD: Aspen Publishers; 1998.

29 O'Connor AM, Llewellyn-Thomas HA, Flood AB. Modifying unwarranted variations in health care: Shared decision making using patient decision aids. *Health Affairs.* 2004;Suppl Variation:VAR63–VAR72.

30 Sepucha KR, Fowler FJ Jr, Mulley AG Jr. Policy support for patient-centered care: The need for measurable improvements in decision quality. *Health Affairs.* 2004;Suppl Variation:VAR54–VAR62.

31 Weinstein JN, Bronner KK, Morgan TS, Wennberg JE. Trends and geographic variations in major surgery for degenerative diseases of the hip, knee, and spine. *Health Affairs.* 2004;Suppl Variation:VAR81–VAR89.

32 O'Connor AM, Stacey D, Rovner D, et al. Decision aids for people facing health treatment or screening decisions. *Cochrane Database Syst Rev.* 2009, Issue 3. Art. No.: CD001431. DOI: 10.1002/14651858.CD001431.pub2.

33 Katz SJ, Lantz PM, Janz NK, et al. Patient involvement in surgery treatment decisions for breast cancer. *J Clin Oncol.* 2005;23(24):5526–5533.

34 Katz SJ, Lantz PM, Janz NK, et al. Patterns and correlates of local therapy for women with ductal carcinoma-in-situ. *J Clin Oncol.* 2005;23(13):3001–3007.

35 ACA Section 2719A 42 U.S.C. §300gg-19a (b)(2)(A).

36 Sade RM. Ethics in cardiothoracic surgery: Deceiving insurance companies: new expression of an ancient tradition. *Ann Thorac Surg.* 2001;72(5):1449–1453.

37 Freeman VG, Rathore SS, Weinfurt KP, Schulman KA, Sulmasy DP. Lying for patients: Physician deception of third-party payers. *Arch Intern Med.* 1999;159(19): 2263–2270.

38 VanGeest JB, Wynia MK, Cummins DS, Wilson IB. Measuring deception: Test-retest reliability of physicians' self-reported manipulation of reimbursement rules for patients. *Med Care Res Rev.* 2002;59(2): 184–196.

39 Novack DH, Detering BJ, Arnold R, et al. Physicians' attitudes toward using deception to resolve difficult ethical problems. *JAMA*. 1989;261(20):2980–2985.

40 VanGeest J, Weiner S, Johnson T, Cummins D. Impact of managed care on physicians' decisions to manipulate reimbursement rules: An explanatory model. *J Health Serv Res Policy*. 2007;12(3):147–152.

41 Wynia MK, Cummins DS, VanGeest JB, Wilson IB. Physician manipulation of reimbursement rules for patients: Between a rock and a hard place. *JAMA*. 2000; 283(14):1858–1865.

42 Morreim EH. Gaming the system. Dodging the rules, ruling the dodgers. *Arch Intern Med*. 1991;151(3): 443–447.

43 Mitus JA. The birth of InterQual: Evidence-based decision support criteria that helped change healthcare, professional case management. *Prof Case Manag*. 2008;13(4):228–233.

44 Milliman Care Guidelines. Available at: www.careguidelines.com/company/qna/methodology.shtml. Accessed July 20, 2011.

45 www.careguidelines.com, accessed July 20, 2011.

46 www.mckesson.com/en_us/McKesson.com/For%2BPayors/Private%2BSector/Private%2BSector.html. Accessed July 20, 2011.

47 ACA Section 2719 42 U.S.C. §300gg-19 (a) and (b).

48 American Medical Association. *CEJA Report 3 – A-99: Ethical Obligations of Medical Directors*. 1999. Available at: www.ama-assn.org/ama1/pub/upload/mm/369/ceja_3a99.pdf. Accessed September 26, 2008.

49 Povar GJ, Blumen H, Daniel J, et al. Ethics in practice: Managed care and the changing health care environment. *Ann Intern Med*. 2004;141(2):131–136.

50 ACA Section 2719A 42 U.S.C. §300gg-19a (d).

51 Scan conducted by author on July 12, 2011, by entering the phrase "X12 278 implementation guide" into Google, and selecting eight guides from the first page of results. The selections were not random in order to have at least one federal, one state, and one municipal guide; commercial payer guides were selected in the order they appeared on the search results page.

52 ACA Section 1104 42 U.S.C. §1320d note.

53 Cram P, Ettinger WH. Generalists or specialists—Who does it better? *Physician Exec*. 1998;24(1):40–45.

54 Quickel KE. Managed care and diabetes, with special attention to the issue of who should provide care. *Trans Am Clin Climatol Assoc*. 1997;108:184–199.

55 Committee of the American College of Rheumatology Council on Health Care Research. Role of specialty care for chronic diseases: A report from an ad hoc committee of the American College of Rheumatology. *Mayo Clin Proc*. 1996;71(12):1179–1181.

56 Bello D, Shah NG, Edep ME, et al. Self-reported differences between cardiologists and heart failure

specialists in the management of chronic heart failure. *Am Heart J*. 1999;138(1, Pt. 1):100–107.

57 Ware JE, Brook RH, Rogers WH, et al. Comparison of health outcomes at a health maintenance organization with those of fee-for-service care. *Lancet*. 1986;1(8488): 1017–1022.

58 Udvarhelyi IS, Jennison K, Phillips RS. Comparison of the quality of ambulatory care for fee-for-service and prepaid patients. *Ann Intern Med*. 1991;115:394–400.

59 Sloss EM, Keeler EB, Brook RH, et al. Effect of a health maintenance organization on physiologic health. *Ann Intern Med*. 1987;106(1):130–138.

60 Clancy CM, Hillner BE. Physicians as gatekeepers—The impact of financial incentives. *Arch Intern Med*. 1989;149(4):917–920.

61 Martin DP, Diehr P, Price KF, Richardson WC. Effect of a gatekeeper plan on health services use and charges: A randomized trial. *Am J Public Health*. 1989;79(12):1628–1632.

62 Hurley RE, Freund DA, Gage BJ, et al. Gatekeeper effects of patterns of physician use. *J Fam Pract*. 1991; 32(2):167–174.

63 Flood AB, Fremont AM, Jin KB, et al. How do HMOs achieve savings? The effectiveness of one organization's strategies. *Health Serv Res*. 1998;33(1):79–99.

64 Forrest CB, Reid RJ. Passing the baton: HMOs' influence on referrals to specialty care. *Health Affairs*. 1997;16(6):157–162.

65 Gallagher TH, St. Peter RF, Chesney M, Lo B. Patients' attitudes toward cost containment bonuses for managed care physicians. *Health Affairs*. 2001;20(2): 186–192.

66 St. Peter RF, Reed MC, Kemper P, Blumenthal D. Changes in the scope of care provided by primary care physicians. *N Engl J Med*. 1999;341(26):1980–1985.

67 Halm EA, Causine N, Blumenthal D. Is gatekeeping better than traditional care? *JAMA*. 1997;278(20): 1677–1681.

68 Chernew ME, Sabik L, Chandra A, Newhouse JP. Would having more primary care doctors cut health spending growth? *Health Affairs*. 2009;28(5):1327–1335.

69 O'Malley AS, Tynan A, Cohen G, et al. Coordination of care by primary care practices: Strategies, lessons and implications. *Center for Studying Health System Change Research*. April 2009; Research Brief No. 12.

70 Leff B, Reider L, Frick KD, et al. Guided care and the cost of complex healthcare: A preliminary report. *Am J Manag Care*. 2009;15(8):555–559.

71 Hillman BJ, Joseph CA, Mabry MR, et al. Frequency and costs of diagnostic imaging in office practice—A comparison of self-referring and radiologist-referring physicians. *N Engl J Med*. 1990;323(23):1604–1608.

72 Office of the Inspector General. *Financial Arrangements between Physicians and Health Care*

Businesses: Report to Congress. Washington, DC: U.S. Department of Health and Human Services; 1989. U.S. Department of Health and Human Services publication OAI-12-88-01410.

73 State of Florida Health Care Cost Containment Board. *Joint Ventures among Health Care Providers in Florida.* Tallahassee, FL: State of Florida; 1991;2.

74 The Ethics in Patient Referrals Act—Omnibus Budget Reconciliation Act of 1989.

75 Hollingsworth JM, Ye Z, Strope SA, et al. Physician-ownership of ambulatory surgical centers linked to higher volume of surgeries. *Health Affairs.* 2010;29(4): 683–689.

76 Mitchell JM. Effect of physician ownership of specialty hospitals and ambulatory surgery centers on frequency of use of outpatient orthopedic surgery. *Arch Surg.* 2010;145(8):732–738.

77 Levin DC, Rao VM, Parker L, Frangos AJ, Intenzo CM. Recent payment and utilization trends in radionuclide myocardial perfusion imaging: Comparison between self-referral and referral to radiologists. *J Am Coll Radiol.* 2009;6(6):437–41.

78 Baker LC. Acquisition of MRI equipment by doctors drives up imaging use and spending. *Health Affairs.* 2010;29(12):2252–2259.

79 Hughes DR, Bhargavan M, Sunshine JH. Imaging self-referral associated with higher costs and limited impact on duration of illness. *Health Affairs.* 2010;29(12): 2244–2251.

80 Sunshine J, Bhargavan M. The practice of imaging self-referral doesn't produce much one-stop service. *Health Affairs.* 2010;29(12):2237–2243.

81 Stensland J, Winter A. Do physician-owned cardiac hospitals increase utilization? *Health Affairs.* 2006; 25(1):119–129.

82 ACA Section 6001 42 U.S.C. §1395nn (a)(i)(1)(B) and (E), and (a)(i)(1)(C), (D), and (G).

83 ACA Section 6003 42 U.S.C. §1395nn(b)(2) (a).

84 Centers for Disease Control and Prevention. National Hospital Ambulatory Medical Care Survey: 2008 Emergency Department Summary Tables. Available at: www.cdc.gov/nchs/data/ahcd/nhamcs_emergency/nhamcsed2008.pdf. Accessed July 14, 2011.

85 Niska R, Bhuiya F, and Xu J. National Hospital Ambulatory Medical Care Survey: 2007 Emergency Department Summary. National Health Statistics Reports; no. 26. Hyattsville, MD: National Center for Health Statistics. 2010.

86 42, U.S.C 1395 dd (1986) Pub. L. No. 99–272.

87 ACA Section 2719A 42 U.S.C. §300gg-19a (b)(1) and (2).

88 Grady KF, Mannng WG, Newhouse JP, Brook RH. The impact of cost sharing on emergency department use. *N Engl J Med.* 1985;313(8):484–490.

89 Shapiro MF, Hayward RA, Freeman HE, Sudman S, Corey CR. Out-of-pocket payments and use of care for serious and minor symptoms. *Arch Intern Med.* 1989;149(7):1645–1648.

90 Selby JV, Fireman BH, Swain BE. Effect of a copayment on use of the emergency department in a health maintenance organization. *N Engl J Med.* 1996;334(10):635–641.

91 Magid DJ, Koepsell TD, Every NT, et al. Absence of association between insurance copayments and delays in seeking emergency care among patients with myocardial infarction. *N Engl J Med.* 1997;336(24): 1722–1729.

92 Weinick RM, Burns RM, Mehrotra A. Many emergency department visits could be managed at urgent care centers and retail clinics. *Health Affairs.* 2010;29(9):1630–1636.

93 Interactive data portal of the Healthcare Cost and Utilization Project (HCUP) at the U.S. Agency for Healthcare Research and Quality. Available at: http://hcupnet.ahrq.gov/HCUPnet.jsp. Accessed July 15, 2011.

94 The Newborns' and Mothers' Health Protection Act of 1996 (PL 104-204).

95 Madden JM, Soumerai SB, Lieu TA, et al. Effects of a law against early postpartum discharge on newborn follow-up, adverse events, and HMO expenditures. *N Engl J Med.* 2002;347(25):2031–2039.

96 Wachter RM. Hospitalists in the United States— Mission accomplished or work in progress? *N Engl J Med.* 2004;350(19):1935–1936.

97 Wachter RM, Goldman L. The emerging role of "hospitalists" in the American health care system. *N Engl J Med.* 1996;335(7):514–517.

98 Society of Hospital Medicine. Available at: www.hospitalmedicine.org. Accessed July 25, 2011.

99 Society of Hospital Medicine. SHM fact sheet: About hospital medicine. Updated July 12, 2010. Available at: www.hospitalmedicine.org/AM/Template.cfm? Section = Media_Kit&Template = /CM/ContentDisplay.cfm&ContentID = 26269. Accessed July 25, 2011.

100 Kuo Y-F, Goodwin JS. Association of hospitalist care with medical utilization after discharge: Evidence of Cost Shift from a Cohort Study. *Ann Intern Med.* 2011; 155:152–159.

101 Personal communication with author in 2011. For appropriate business reasons, the identity of the individual and the payer organization are confidential.

102 Forster AJ, Murff HJ, Peterson JF, et al. The incidence and severity of adverse events affecting patients after discharge from the hospital. *Ann Intern Med.* 2003; 138(3):161–167.

103 Jencks SF, Williams MV, Coleman EA. Rehospitalizations among patients in the Medicare fee-for-service program. *N Engl J Med.* 2009;360(14):1418–1428.

104 Anderson G. The benefits of care coordination: A comparison of Medicare fee-for-service and Medicare Advantage. Report prepared for the Alliance of Community Health Plans. September 1, 2009. Available at: www.google.com/url?sa = t&source = web&cd = 1&ved = 0CBgQFjAA&url = http%3A%2F%2Fwww .achp.org%2Ffiles.php%3Fforce%26file%3Dfront%2 FJohnsHopkinsStudy-FinalReport.pdf&ei = aWEsTsLr Danz0gG0uLjkDg&usg = AFQjCNGfkEYpwzNJYUCxh GtOl1XkBbsXyA&sig2 = tR7er6x_9pKqqu_oWhaQMQ. Accessed July 24, 2011.

105 America's Health Insurance Plans. Working paper: Using state hospital discharge data to compare readmission rates in Medicare Advantage and Medicare's traditional fee-for-service program. May, 2010. Available at: www.ahipresearch.org/pdfs/9State-Readmits.pdf. Accessed July 24, 2011.

106 O'Malley AS, Reschovsky JD. Referral and consultation communication between primary care and specialist physicians. *Arch Intern Med.* 2011;171(1):56–65.

107 Pham HH, Grossman JM, Cohen G, Bodenheimer T. Hospitalists and care transitions: The divorce of inpatient and outpatient care. *Health Affairs.* 2008; 27(5):1315–1327.

108 Wachter RM, Goldman L. The hospitalist movement 5 years later. *JAMA.* 2002;287(4):487–494.

109 Auerbach AD, Wachter RM, Katz P, et al. Implementation of a voluntary hospitalist service at a community teaching hospital: Improved clinical efficiency and patient outcomes. *Ann Intern Med.* 2002;137(11): 859–865.

110 Meltzer D, Manning WG, Morrison J, et al. Effects of physician experience on costs and outcomes on an academic general medicine service: Results of a trial of hospitalists. *Ann Intern Med.* 2002;137(11): 866–874.

111 Vasilevskis EE, Knebel J, Dudley RA, et al. Cross-sectional analysis of hospitalist prevalence and quality of care in California. *J Hosp Med.* 2010;5(4):200–207.

112 Kou Y-F and Goodwin JS. Association of hospitalist care with medical utilization after discharge: Evidence of cost shift from a cohort study. *Ann Internal Med.* 2011;155(3):152–159.

113 Harrison PL, Hara PA, Pope JE, et al. The impact of post-discharge telephonic follow-up on hospital readmissions. *Popul Health Manag.* 2011;14(1):27–32.

114 Dudas V, Bookwalter T, Kerr KM, Pantilat SZ. The impact of follow-up telephone calls to patients after hospitalization. *Am J Med.* 2001;111(9B):26S–30S.

115 Ahmed OI, Rak DJ. Hospital readmission among participants in a transitional case management program. *Am J Manag Care.* 2010;16(10):778–783.

116 Bodenheimer T, Berry-Millett R. Care management of patients with complex health care needs. Research Synthesis Report No. 19. Princeton, NJ: Robert Wood Johnson Foundation, December 2009.

117 Berwick DM, Coltin KL. Feedback reduces test use in a health maintenance organization. *JAMA.* 1986; 255(11):1450–1454.

118 Marton KI, Tul V, Sox HC. Modifying test-ordering behavior in the outpatient medical clinic. *Arch Intern Med.* 1985;145(5):816–821.

119 Martin AR, Wolf MA, Thibodeau LA, et al. A trial of two strategies to modify the test-ordering behavior of medical residents. *N Engl J Med.* 1980;303(23): 1330–1336.

Fundamentals and Core Competencies of Disease Management

David W. Plocher

STUDY OBJECTIVES

- Understand the meaning of disease management (DM) and be able to explain what is unique about the term
- Understand how conventional case management differs from disease management
- Understand the most important characteristics of a disease that make it appropriate for this model
- Understand where DM operates
- Understand the pros and cons of building versus outsourcing DM
- Understand difficulties in measuring DM return on investment

DISCUSSION TOPICS

1. Discuss what is unique about disease management.
2. Discuss the key differences between conventional case management and disease management.
3. Describe some characteristics of a disease that would make it appropriate for this model.
4. Discuss how information technology can make disease management programs more successful.

■ INTRODUCTION

This chapter highlights current and anticipated developments in disease management (DM). There is a specialized form of DM, behavioral health and substance abuse services, that is discussed fully in Chapter 12 and is not the subject of this chapter. Related in many ways to DM and with some overlap, case management (CM) is briefly discussed in Chapter 7 and is noted in this chapter only as it relates to DM activities. Finally, some of the main elements found in DM overlap with those found in basic utilization management (UM), which was also described in Chapter 7.

■ CHRONIC CONDITIONS

As discussed in Chapter 7 and illustrated in Figure 7-2, health care costs are highly concentrated, with 1% of the population accounting for 20% of total costs, 10% of the population accounting for 64% of total costs, and 20% of the population accounting for 80% of total costs. Recall as well from that chapter that a report on Medicare costs by the Johns Hopkins Bloomberg School of Public Health on behalf of the Robert Wood Johnson Foundation showed the relationship between the number of chronic medical conditions and costs, which is summarized as follows:

- 0 chronic conditions – 1% of Medicare expenditures,
- 1 chronic condition – 3%,
- 2 chronic conditions – 6%,
- 3 chronic conditions –10%,
- 4 chronic conditions – 9%, and
- 5 chronic conditions – 79%.[1]

Those conditions are primarily heart disease, diabetes, glaucoma, asthma, chronic obstructive pulmonary disease, and cancer.[2] Just below the senior threshold are baby boomers, who by 2020 will raise the level to 25% of Americans having multiple chronic conditions, and the associated care costs are projected to total $1.07 trillion.

Attempts by individual physicians to influence the course of chronic illness have been hampered by payment methods primarily rewarding treatment of acute illness and performance of procedures. Physicians are financially dissuaded from investing time and effort in preventing illness or preventing complications. Unfortunately, it is more remunerative for them to treat complications.

During the 1980s and early 1990s, experiments with full risk capitation of large medical groups intended to remedy this disconnect (see Chapters 2 and 5). However, the labor shortages of the 1990s and associated managed care backlash (see Chapter 1) all but extinguished such efforts. Furthermore, the office visit with a primary care physician is becoming uncomfortably similar to a 5-minute speed bump. Busy physicians, according to Rand research, use the best evidence-based guidelines for care only about half the time.[3] Compounding this problem, patients adhere to their prescription regimens at roughly the same rate.[4]

DM vendors appeared in the market to address these problems. Affordable at a scale that can only be accomplished using staffing ratios achievable at large regional call centers, these companies check in on patients *between* physician visits. They review the treatment plan for evidence-based medicine concordance, and if the ordering physician appears to have overlooked something, he or she is contacted. More often, the patients are coached and counseled on adherence to their complex medical regimens. A lot can happen—or not happen—during that 3- to 4-month interval between routine physician visits.

■ DEFINITION OF DISEASE MANAGEMENT

According to the Disease Management Association of America (DMAA; recently renamed the Care Continuum Alliance),[5] DM is a system of coordinated health care interventions and communications for populations with conditions in which patient self-care efforts are significant. Disease management:

- Supports the physician or practitioner–patient relationship and plan of care;
- Emphasizes prevention of exacerbations and complications utilizing evidence-based practice guidelines and patient empowerment strategies; and
- Evaluates clinical, humanistic, and economic outcomes on an ongoing basis with the goal of improving overall health.

DM components include the following:[*]

- Population identification processes:
- Evidence-based practice guidelines;[†]
- Collaborative practice models to include physician and support-service providers
- Patient self-management education (may include primary prevention, behavior modification programs, and compliance/surveillance);
- Process and outcomes measurement, evaluation, and management; and
- Routine reporting/feedback loop (may include communication with patient, physician, health plan and ancillary providers, and practice profiling).

■ DISEASE MANAGEMENT COMPANIES

The typical DM company, whether publicly traded or privately held, is primarily call center based, especially for the commercial sector. For the upper age bands in the commercial sector and more commonly with seniors, home-monitoring technology is added for transmission of weight and multiple vital signs, usually over the Internet to the call centers. This remote monitoring technology has recently evolved rapidly, promising to improve quality and cost of care for patients with chronic illnesses.

The Medicaid market (Chapter 25) requires other layers of intervention, including interaction with participants at community centers, with county public health nurses, with home care agencies (including a resurgence of house calls by physicians), as well as specialized programs such as free (restricted-use) cell phones for convenient call center contact and pushing reminders to participants, and even training neighborhood peers to serve as coaches. Individual companies vary by preferred purchaser. The majority contract with a health plan. Fewer have the inclination to bypass the health plan and contract directly with the large,

---

[*]Full-service DM programs must include all six components. Programs consisting of fewer components are DM support services.
[†]Guidelines are updated at least annually as the peer-reviewed medical literature evolves.

self-insured employer (potentially risky because neither partner is replete with health plan infrastructure). Similarly, few have invested in the specialized programs required for the Medicaid population, which is the domain of managed Medicaid plans (Chapter 25). Regardless of customer focus, there is less variation in the end-user focus for these companies: the majority are member-centered. Very few companies have developed a physician-centered program.

COMPONENTS COMMON TO MOST PROGRAMS

There are a number of components typically found in most DM programs. They are described as follows.

Condition Selection and Prioritization

The analysis of a payer's claims data forms the basis for condition selection and prioritization, and this begins with understanding which major diagnostic categories are the largest drivers of claim trend (see also Chapter 10). Within these, study of disease prevalence versus benchmarks will advance the cause. Then, comparison of the disease per member per month (PMPM) claim cost or annual episode claim cost versus benchmarks will complete the calculation of the financial priority and opportunity.

Next is the feasibility analysis. The foundation for treatment decisions should be widely agreed-upon evidence-based guidelines. The patients themselves should be symptomatic, motivating them to change behaviors. Preferably, the circumstances will allow incentives to be applied to both patients and physicians. The health plan has a responsibility in such motivation, for example, financial rewards for enrollment or waiving copays on generic drugs

and supplies used to treat these conditions (discussed later in this chapter).

In aggregate, the condition selected must have a resource-consumption course that can be modified using the DM arsenal, beginning with the call center. That is, one must ask if this patient and this condition could show behavior change and resource consumption change if only prompted by a phone call from a nurse, perhaps not for the socially isolated, sickest seniors, or most socioeconomically challenged Medicaid members. This modification must be accomplished at an acceptable overhead cost, or the program evaluation will show an unfavorable cost-benefit ratio.

Participant Identification

Most DM companies apply algorithms (with condition-definition rules) to the payer's claims data. This is usually a straightforward diagnosis-finding method. In addition, DM companies apply predictive modeling tools that are beyond diagnosis code dependency. They scan claims experience (sometimes using artificial intelligence and neural net modeling, or simply clinical rules, which is generally a speedier method) to discover candidates projected to become high in cost. The resulting candidates are screened by CM or DM intake specialists to determine whether CM, DM, or another program is applicable. **Figure 8-1** summarizes these case-finding techniques.

Once a candidate for DM is found, the next layer of predictive modeling or stratification becomes condition-specific to plan for intensity of outreach resources. In some settings, the most morbid DM participants may require at least temporary management by CM for stabilization and benefits modeling.

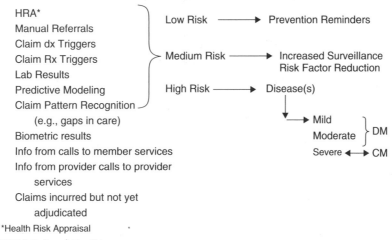

Population Triage

Case Finding Data Supplied to a Single Call Center

HRA*
Manual Referrals
Claim dx Triggers
Claim Rx Triggers
Lab Results
Predictive Modeling
Claim Pattern Recognition
   (e.g., gaps in care)
Biometric results
Info from calls to member services
Info from provider calls to provider
   services
Claims incurred but not yet
   adjudicated
*Health Risk Appraisal

Low Risk → Prevention Reminders

Medium Risk → Increased Surveillance / Risk Factor Reduction

High Risk → Disease(s)
   → Mild
   Moderate } DM
   Severe ↔ CM

FIGURE 8-1 Population Triage

Source: Adapted from *Best Practices in Medical Management.* Gaithersburg, MD: Aspen Publishing, 1998.

During the past few years, a further layer of data-mining has evolved. Claim pattern recognition software is applied to scan for gaps in care. Beyond conventional drug interaction software, these few vendors can determine whether a patient with a key diagnosis is not on recommended prescriptions, not refilling necessary prescriptions, not seeing the physician at a minimum frequency, not being immunized, or not having a recommended screening test, and so forth. Such services have evolved, in part, in response to the requirement that claims analysis and reporting must produce information that is *actionable*. Typical actions, beyond equipping the call center nurse with the care gap information, will include outreach by mail or phone to the patient, patient's physician, or the patient's pharmacist, depending on the type and urgency of the care gap. Recall from Chapter 7 that these are the very problems associated with avoidable readmissions.

Recruitment and Engagement

Historic attempts using the opt-in model, whereby the candidate must initiate an enrollment process, have yielded, at most, 30% participation rates. The opt-out method, in which the candidate is automatically enrolled based on passing tests in the rule-based, case-finding algorithm, averages 70% participation rates. The 30% nonparticipation is the sum of true opting out (10%), bad phone numbers (18%), and

false-positives (2%).[*] There is rapid evolution in the industry around these activities, to be discussed later in this chapter.

Interaction and Management

Here resides the most important activity of the disease manager. The call center nurse is dynamically interviewing the patients, motivating them to adhere to their complex medical regimens. This is not simply traditional CM, and **Table 8-1** summarizes the key activity differences between DM and CS.

Ten years ago, patients with asthma received much of the attention. Adolescents relying on albuterol for rescue and failing to use steroid inhalers for prevention were vigorously prompted to reverse course. The next most dramatic improvements were made for patients with chronic congestive heart failure, who were offered guidance on low-sodium diets, weight change parameters, diuretic dose adjustments, initiation of angiotensin-converting enzyme inhibitors (or, more recently, angiotensin receptor blockers) followed by more recent institution of beta blockers.

Subsequently, the majority of attention was given to patients with diabetes for blood sugar control, in concert with patients with coronary artery disease, both groups

---

[*]Data from author's experience.

TABLE 8-1	Differences between Case Management and Disease Management
Traditional/catastrophic case management	**Disease management**
Emphasis is on single patient	Emphasis is on population with a chronic illness
Early identification of people with acute catastrophic conditions (known high cost or known diagnoses that lead to high cost in the near term)	Early identification of all people with targeted chronic diseases (20–40) whether mild, moderate, or severe
Acuity level of catastrophic cases is high; acuity level of traditional cases is high to moderate	Acuity level is moderate
Applies to 0.5–1% of commercial membership	Applies to 15–25% of commercial membership
Value relies heavily on price negotiations and benefit flexing	Value is result of member and provider behavior change that results in improved health status
Requires plan design manipulation (e.g., adding more home care visits)	Requires plan design changes that reward enrollment in DM and shrink drug copays
Primary objective is to arrange for care using the least restrictive, clinically appropriate alternatives	Primary objective is to avoid hospitalization *and* modify risk factors, lifestyle, and medication adherence to improve health status
Episode is 60–90 days	Intervention is 365 days for most conditions
Site of interaction primarily hospital, hospice, subacute facility, or HHC	Site of interaction includes work, school, home, and MD office
Driven by need for arrangement of support services, community resources, transportation	Driven by nonadherence to medical regimens
Outcome metrics are single-admit LOS and cost per case	Outcome metrics are annual cost per diseased member and disease-specific functional status and gaps in care

Note: HHC, home health care; LOS, length of stay.

requiring reinforcement of blood pressure and cholesterol management.

Outbound Calls to Participant

Following are descriptions of the primary activities applied in the commercial sector by call centers.

Initial welcome call:
- Orientation to program;
- Administration of health risk appraisal (general) or condition-specific risk assessment;
- Determination of readiness to change;
- Establishing participant's baseline understanding of condition;
- Agreement on preferred language and mode of subsequent communications such as
  - Phone with desired time of day;
  - Mail;
  - Internet;
  - Interactive voice response (IVR);
  - Review of care plan;
  - Discussion of methods for closing gaps in care; and
  - Referral to ancillary programs such as smoking cessation.

Subsequent care calls:
- Establish progress toward achieving care plan goals and optimal regimen adherence;
- Measure improvement in participant's understanding of condition; and
- Coaching on questions to ask during next physician visit.

Reminder calls: Incidental prompts regarding necessary modalities; for example, flu shots.

Mailings

The following are typically sent by U.S. mail.

Welcome packet:
- Complete documentation of program,
- Education about condition, and
- A symptom checklist (when to call for help).

Periodic updates:
- Reminders about periodic services needed for condition, and
- Updates in educational materials based on medical advances.

Inbound Calls from Participants

Any participant can access the call center to discuss changes in symptoms or other questions about the condition or care plan.

Outbound Calls to Physician

These are rarely needed, unless the member has contacted the call center with a particularly urgent problem, or the claim pattern recognition software has discovered a gap in care, requiring prompt attention.

Mailings to Physician

The following are typically sent to physicians by U.S. mail.

Program orientation: These are informational for the physician, containing confirmation that the program is simply an adjunct to his or her care.

- Baseline set of practice guidelines pertinent to participant's condition
- List of patients in physician panel who have the index condition

Periodic guideline updates: As the literature advances over time, certain contents of evidence-based guidelines may change.

Periodic participant update: When timing is ideal, these occur just before an electively scheduled office visit. They contain information on the participant's

- Recent contacts with the call center,
- Recent emergency department (ED) visits, and
- Any necessary reminders about tests due or other gaps in care.

Inbound Calls from Physicians

These are very rare and usually consist of questions to aid understanding of the program.

Home Telemonitoring

Participants in the highest risk group with chronic heart failure, chronic obstructive pulmonary disease, and so forth, are equipped with home devices connected (usually) to the Internet so that call centers can monitor real-time results. The most common biometrics transmitted are weight, respiratory rate, blood pressure, heart rate, and oxygen saturation.

Medication Adherence Technology

Several vendors have deployed technology to provide prompts and reminders for participants on complex medication regimens. These take the form of electronic pill boxes, beepers, and specially equipped cell phones.

Documentation

On intake, each new participant's risk stratification is documented. This is usually done informally by each DM company, although the criteria to establish each stratification level, such as 1 through 4 (low severity to high severity), are objective. Alternatively, there is early use of specialized predictive modeling software designed to be used *not* for the entire population but only for a cohort of participants with a particular condition, again ranking them by levels of severity. The practical purpose is for establishing necessary outbound call frequencies. Similarly, it is essential to document all baseline inventory obtained during the welcome call, such as scoring and risk stratifying a completed health risk appraisal, readiness to change, and participants' comprehension of their condition. Periodic care call content is also documented, as are occurrences of preventive care reminder calls and mailings.

Information Technology Support

Leading DM companies have invested multiple millions of dollars in the technology providing decision support, automated connections with other programs, and reports. Information technology (IT) is discussed more broadly and at greater length in Chapter 23. Also, some of these practices overlap in technique with those described for Member Services in Chapter 20.

Examples of a few leading practices in the application of IT to DM include the following:

- Automated creation of care plans;
- Automated routing of a new participant's care plan to the correct disease manager;
- Auto dialers facilitating the DM nurse capacity to complete calls;
- Disease manager's ability to view past 12–18 months of claim history of the participant; and
- Disease manager's ability to view the participant's electronic medical record (EMR) at primary care clinic (most advanced practice).

Reporting

Later in this chapter, clinical and economic reporting is addressed. However, for the highest volume of reporting, DM companies produce fulfillment reports. These contain the following information:

- Call frequencies, in- and outbound;
- Mailing frequencies;
- Participants by condition by stratification level;
- Participants receiving mail-only versus calls;
- Opt-outs;
- Bad phone numbers;
- False-positives;
- Complaints and satisfaction survey results for participants and physicians.

■   MEASURING EFFECTIVENESS

Methods and metrics used for DM program evaluation were summarized several years ago.[6] This continues to be a source of evolution in this industry.

The most common method uses the pre- and poststudy. Because many metrics are similar or even identical to the Healthcare Effectiveness Data Information Set (HEDIS®; see Chapter 15), reflecting guidelines used for process measures based on testing required in a year, a requirement of 12 months' continuous enrollment is common. Examples of typical metrics include:

- Percentage of diabetes participants with a hemoglobin A_1C (HbA$_1$C) test or low-density lipoprotein (LDL) cholesterol test per year,
- Percentage of coronary artery disease (CAD) participants with LDL cholesterol test per year,
- Percentage of heart failure participants on an angiotensin converting enzyme inhibitor (ACEI), and
- Percentage of CAD (or post–myocardial infarction) participants on a beta blocker.

The preceding process measures have clear advantages over outcome measures because of the following reasons:

- Severity adjustment is not needed;
- Sample sizes can be much smaller than those used in outcome data; and
- Physicians see process measures as reflecting activity within their more immediate control, whereas there are many other contributors to an unfavorable outcome.

Measures of process or outcome can also be organized from a pre- and poststudy, although customers are often interested in using a concurrent control group. This method needs to find a cohort of participants using the same condition—finding algorithms but not being managed by the call center of a DM company. The most difficult challenge associated with this method is assurance that the two cohorts are actually comparable. Adjustments needed to make them comparable usually include:

- Geography,
- Demographics,
- Age,
- Gender,
- Illness burden,
- Provider networks,
- Provider contracts,
- Plan design, and
- Rigor of other medical management programs.

Trusting that such adjustments can be made, the outcome metrics of greatest interest have been as follows:

- Financial:
- PMPM cost;
- Annual episode of care cost;
- Utilization
  - Acute hospital admits and days per 1,000 and
  - ED visits per 1,000.

Return on Investment

Return on investment (ROI) has been the single largest controversy in the DM industry. The traditional method establishes baseline participant PMPM cost and projects the following year's expected cost using various trend assumptions such as the nondisease trend, disease trend, and overall trend. Such analysis typically excludes outliers, using definitions conventionally above 2 or 3 standard deviations beyond the mean. There are other total exclusions, such as acquired immune deficiency syndrome (AIDS), cancer, transplants, trauma, burns, and others. The actual observed following year's cost is then compared with the cost that had been projected. Trusting that the observed cost is less than projected, the difference is gross savings, from which program administrative/overhead costs are subtracted to produce net savings. This benefit-to-cost ratio, or ROI, is sometimes modestly positive and varies by condition.

There are certainly weaknesses in this method. For example, there is little agreement on which trend assumption to use. The largest objection is that this pre- and post-method is influenced by regression to the mean. Hence, there are several new methods in development at the time of publication that attempt to mitigate the error introduced by disease migration, which is the natural progression and regression of various disease care costs over time. Early indications suggest that these methods can produce a positive ROI, but less positive than the traditional method. Note that nearly all of the work to date on DM ROI has been done within the population-oriented opt-out engagement model. For those using the opt-in model, methodology revision will be needed.

For a current review on DM ROI, Motheral[7] has created a balanced review. There are nonfinancial reasons to deliver DM, but the financial summary in her detailed analysis seems to suggest chronic heart failure management holds some promise for the CFO, while other diseases do not.

■ CHALLENGES USING CURRENT ENGAGEMENT MODEL

Several valuable lessons have recently been learned after years of operating with the current opt-out engagement model.

Privacy

The Health Insurance Portability and Accountability Act (HIPAA; Chapter 29) has influenced DM companies with regard to protected health information (PHI). This risk occurs in the setting of the opt-out engagement model. That is, on its surface, one at least can question HIPAA compliance when PHI is being exchanged around a patient who may not even be aware of his or her automatic enrollment in the DM program and, if aware, might object. The wording of the final rule around PHI does appear to provide for the use of the opt-out model, but if there is any question, a health plan should rely on proper legal counsel.

Meaningful Engagement

Other recruitment and engagement approaches may be considered. Although the opt-in model has inherent weakness regarding recruitment success, perhaps the opt-out model is the other extreme. For example, opt-out participants might only be receiving but not reading their mail, may not be aware of their participation status, or have other potential barriers to higher success for the DM program. The near future will likely see a new recruitment model that consolidates the participants into a subset who are confirmed to be engaged.

Physician Integration

As discussed earlier, most DM activity is member-centered. As community physicians find out more about DM, there is understandable resentment based on the notion that "Treating diseases is why I went to medical school." Because of this, over the past few years there have been further efforts to involve physicians. Community physicians have become progressively more vocal about their resentment over being bypassed, or worse, suggesting that the DM company interferes with the doctor–patient relationship. Ironically, it was originally the intent of most DM companies to "not bother" busy physicians. Resolving such a dilemma may require a series of compromises. However, in the end it remains likely that in most cases, community physicians will not exert a direct role in DM as defined here, nor will they likely obtain a revenue stream from DM. The main reasons are as follows.

As the industry learned during the decade of integrated delivery system (IDS) development (see Chapters 1 and 2), the owner of DM has to be the owner of full financial risk. Today, that owner is the health plan (commercial, Medicare Advantage, or Managed Medicaid), the employer, Centers for Medicare and Medicaid Services, or the state Medicaid department. The physician owns only the office visit component of treatment delivery on a fee-for-service (FFS) basis and, in some cases, the professional component of an ER visit and/or hospitalization. Therefore, the success of DM, which reduces most of these categories of utilization, would reduce the physician's FFS revenue.

However, today, new delivery system models, such as patient-centered medical homes (PCMHs) and accountable care organizations (ACOs) as discussed in Chapters 2, 5, and 30, are attempting to recreate what IDSs of the 1990s tried in the name of shouldering some or all of the financial risk. With regard to success at DM, these new models need to undergo radical change to incorporate the former DM infrastructure of the health plan or DM vendor. As discussed in Chapter 7, the typical practicing office-based community physician is unaware of what the chronically ill patient is experiencing between office visits. The risk-sharing/risk-bearing PCMH or ACO will need to perform (or license from the health plan) identification and stratification of members in order to prioritize outreach and prevent hospitalizations and ED visits.

Next, the PCMH or ACO needs to decide where the medical call center will reside. Though the largest delivery systems may wish to host their own, those who have attempted cannot operate at the affordability scale of the DM companies' large call centers. That is, for health plans to yield and create separate payment schemes for individual medical offices to telephone patients between visits would be grossly inefficient in an environment characterized by enormous pressure on health plans to reduce overhead. Mature call centers can staff at the level of one nurse for every 1,000 coronary artery disease members—a ratio not conceivable by a typical provider system.

■ HEALTH PLAN DECISION TO BUILD VERSUS BUY

Large payer organizations will either build and operate their own DM capability, or buy it by contracting with a DM company. The debate on having an in-house versus outsourced program is summarized in **Table 8-2**.

Recent developments find the outsourced mode under pressure. When DM began over 15 years ago, health plans had little expertise for delivery. Today, after climbing the learning curve, health plans are taking a hard look at vendor fees and new integration demands. The nursing shortage notwithstanding, there are multiple experiments with in-house programs today.

■ OUTSOURCING CONTRACT FINANCIAL RISKS

The early years featured risk-sharing terms based on a variety of required milestones around service, satisfaction, and achievement of various process and outcome results,

including ROI. The ROI terms are the most rapidly evolving. For example, there is controversy on how to measure in years 3–5 of the program: to use original baseline or update the baseline year. Other controversies arise over what happens to people continuously enrolled over 3–5 years. If ROI results become more conservative over time, although proof of concept seems no longer in doubt, it seems logical to waive formal financial ROI risk and related reconciliation overhead. In fact, selected self-insured employers have begun to elect that option, usually in exchange for a reduced program fee and consideration to substitute nonfinancial items, such as adherence to evidence-based process of care measures.

■ LINKS TO OTHER HEALTH CARE PROGRAMS

In addition to current, conventional hand-offs to and from the health plan's other medical management programs as discussed in Chapters 7 and 12, new linkages are developing for the following types of programs.

Consumer-Directed Health Plans

Consumer-directed health plans (CDHPs; see Chapter 2), now in their sixth to eighth year, demonstrated the importance of first-dollar coverage for preventive services. Under the Patient Protection and Affordable Care Act (ACA), all health plans must now provide first-dollar coverage for prevention.

Recent experience suggests CDHP enrollees, at least those that enroll in a CDHP on a voluntary basis (i.e., they can choose between a CDHP and a more traditional type of health plan such as a PPO or HMO), are healthier than

TABLE 8-2	**Outsourcing Debate Summary**	
Build	**Buy**
Medical management is our core competency.	Lack of internal skills and time to manage rare or complex diseases.
Large organization with existing IT and managerial skills to perform DM.	Speed to market—would take more than 18 months to build.
Tried outsourcing—disagreed on metrics to determine risk-based fee refund.	Revised metrics and contract terms to place vendor at risk.
Tried outsourcing—vendor failed to affect claim cost or advertised ROI is "too good to be true."	After years of reliable service, transitioned to FFS contract to reduce overhead—no need for risk contract.
Tried outsourcing—vendor used nonclinicians in call center.	Local region has too few RNs with right capabilities to staff call center.
Need control and flexibility.	Require vendor to test guidelines with providers.
Too few dollars at stake for prenatal care and asthma.	Use broad, multicondition DM program.
Tried outsourcing—our members with multiple comorbidities received multiple calls from DM, CM, and UM.	Use single vendor for horizontal contact center.
Integration costs are more than the savings from an outsourced vendor.	Require vendor to use plan identity during communications.

Source: Multiple health plan chief medical officer interviews conducted by author.

non-CDHP enrollees are.* CDHPs with members who have chronic illnesses should consider benefits designs to lower or waive copays for medicines (at least generics) and supplies used for these conditions. Risk-adjusted contribution to health savings accounts may also be an option to accommodate those with chronic illnesses.

Participant Incentives

Several experiments have been a way to motivate enrollees, such as immediate reward of cash or gift certificates for agreeing to enroll in DM, or additional cash awards for completion of a health risk assessment. Similarly, copays for generic medications that manage chronic illnesses have been waived, and brand name drug copays have been reduced.

Physician Incentives

Recent initiatives around pay-for-performance (P4P; see Chapter 5) have linked metrics described earlier to bonus calculations for physicians. Beyond such clinical measures, other P4P experiments are adding to the bonus calculation the agreement by the physician to adopt an electronic medical record (EMR) and participate in e-prescribing. The interfaces between EMR and DM are multiple, such as electronically checking lab test results, medication lists, and so forth. This capability, under the industry term "disease registry," is also key for the PCMH or ACO, whereby, for example, the physician can obtain a list of panel diabetics, specifying who has not had a visit in 6 months or who had an elevated HbA_1C at last visit.

Personal Health Records, Regional Health Information Organizations, and Health Information Exchanges

The newest adjuncts to DM in technology are still to be proven. Personal health records (PHRs), which are populated primarily with data from health plans, may enable more real-time entry and retrieval of participants' health status information. Whether participants will agree on the data entry physicians will retrieve is being tested. Similarly, regional health information organizations (RHIOs) and state- or federal-sponsored health information exchanges (HIE) have the promise in DM of assisting with the capture of longitudinal episodes of care (gathering data from all sites of care) as well as transmission of EMR content from provider to provider. As with PHR, both funding and adoption are being tested. (PHRs, EMRs, RHIOs, and HIEs are discussed in Chapter 23.)

■ INTERNATIONAL DISEASE MANAGEMENT

United States–based DM companies have expanded into other countries. Most of the early adopters—primarily

Germany, followed by Japan, the United Kingdom, Australia, and South America—have presented the implementation challenges of a socialized system. These environments feature largely unregulated physicians and, in some cases, far more use of complementary and alternative medicine modalities, anecdotally already associated with baseline care costs much lower than in the United States. International application of managed health care is discussed further in Chapter 27.

■ POTENTIAL FUTURE APPLICATIONS OF DISEASE MANAGEMENT

DM programs continue to be market-driven, and are rapidly evolving. Some older approaches have failed, while others evolve and new ones emerge. Integration of multiple types of programs and activities has also become more common.

New Approaches

An area for intervention that is currently addressed primarily only by prevention and wellness programs (see Chapter 13) is the premorbid population. In the conventional approach to DM, the occurrence of a discharge from the hospital for a myocardial infarction might be the main trigger for enrollment in a coronary artery disease (CAD) DM program. Can a DM program move upstream and still make it affordable?

Using the findings of asymptomatic hypertension and cholesterol elevation as examples, various experiments are under way to improve upon the older versions of step therapy and the conventional DM call center programs. This draws upon two observations from health care ecology:

- The most frequent health care professional interaction for a patient is with the pharmacist.
- Nonphysician practitioners appear to be "a better buy" for certain routine services (compared to physicians).

Anticipate PCMH and ACO deployment of pharmacists and nurse practitioners into the care of individuals whose cases are not extremely complex but who have major risk factors. This should allow tolerance for the multiyear window needed to find impact from risk-factor reduction.[8, 9]

Failed Diseases and Failed Approaches

To use resources most effectively, each DM company or program must exert rigorous program evaluation techniques upon each disease in its roster. In the spirit of continuous improvement, the mix should change over time as the low-yield conditions are retired. In addition, greater sophistication will occur as to what interventions fade in effectiveness over time and under what circumstances interventions should be reduced or eliminated, not just changed.

---

*Author's analysis.

Integration

Medical management strategists have recently proposed a single point of contact for the member, allowing convenient triage to specialized services. The member is to be treated to customized "push" messages at correct intervals. Lavish coaching and counsel that assist the member in navigating the health care system to achieve optimal value are required. This appears to be an outgrowth of the current leading approach to addressing patients with multiple chronic conditions in which a single point of contact is used for managing all conditions.

■ CONCLUSION

DM is a continually evolving but effective approach to managing both the cost and quality of care for those members with the most expensive chronic conditions. Predicated on preventing avoidable complications leading to expensive care in the hospital setting, DM is a necessary component of any high-performing care management program.

Endnotes

1   Anderson G. *Chronic Care: Making the case for ongoing care.* Princeton, NJ: Robert Wood Johnson Foundation, 2010. Available at: www.rwjf.org/pr/product.jsp?id = 50968. Accessed July 16, 2011.

2   Landro L. Eliminating conflicts in medical treatment. *Wall Street Journal.* February 8, 2006:D5.

3   McGlynn EA, Asch SM, Adams J, et al. The quality of healthcare delivered to adults in the United States. *N Eng J Med.* 2003;348(26):2635–2645.

4   Oterberg L, Blaschke T. Adherence to medication. *N Eng J Med.* 2005;353(5):487–497.

5   Disease Management Association of America. DMAA definition of disease management. Available at: www .dmaa.org/definition.html. Accessed September 18, 2006.

6   Fitzner K, Sidorov J, Fetterolf D, et al. Principles for assessing disease management outcomes. *Dis Management.* 2004;7(3):191–201.

7   Motheral B. Telephone-based disease management: Why it does not save money. *Am J Manag Care.* 2011;17(1): e10–e16.

8   DiTusa L, Luzier A, Brady G, Reinhardt M, Snyder B. A pharmacy-based approach to cholesterol management. *Am J Manage Care.* 2001;7(10):973–979.

9   Menerich J, Lousberg T, Brennan S, Calonge N. Optimizing treatment for dyslipidemia in patients with coronary artery disease in the managed-care environment (The Rocky Mountain Kaiser Permanente experience). *Am J Cardiol.* 2000;85(3A):36A–42A.

Physician Practice Behavior and Managed Health Care

JAY WANT AND PETER R. KONGSTVEDT

STUDY OBJECTIVES

- Understand the inherent difficulties in modifying physician behavior
- Understand the role financial incentives and disincentives can play
- Understand how physician practice behavior issues have changed over the years
- Understand general approaches to modifying physician behavior
- Understand programmatic and specific approaches to modifying physician behavior, and the strengths and weaknesses of these approaches
- Understand discipline and sanctioning as applied to physicians

STUDY QUESTIONS

1. Describe the routine actions a payer should take to positively influence provider behavior.
2. What behavior on the part of a payer would likely engender negative provider behavior?
3. Develop policies and procedures for a physician sanction program to deal with unacceptable physician behavior.
4. Describe common physician perceptions, both negative and positive, of managed care. What steps might a health maintenance organization take in regard to those perceptions?
5. How might an organized provider system approach physician behavior change in contrast to a payer?

■ INTRODUCTION

The vast majority of medical expenditures originate with a physician's pen, or increasingly, with a physician's keyboard. Irrespective of the type of organization—traditional health plan, physician-hospital organization (PHO; see Chapter 2), medical group or independent practice association (IPA; see Chapter 2)—the key to producing excellent clinical and financial results is engaging physician behavior toward these shared goals. One of the bitter lessons of the last round of managed care in the 1980s and 1990s (see Chapter 1) was that imposing rules on physicians against their will to produce results that they didn't believe benefited them or their patients was a difficult and unhappy process.

In this chapter, we discuss three general areas: (1) the underlying issues and social norms that must be considered in working with physicians; (2) the methods by which these issues might be addressed and norms changed; and (3) those measures that must be undertaken when physician behavior puts the greater enterprise at risk.

While extrinsic motivators such as financial incentives are clearly helpful in this regard, they are not the subject of this chapter. As a rule, extrinsic motivators can be useful in getting physicians' attention initially, but their effects tend to be limited in duration, as is true of most extrinsic motivation. Many medical management practitioners have seen providers change practice patterns commensurate with particular financial rewards, only to see those practice patterns revert to baseline once the rewards are withdrawn. In essence, physicians "study for the test" as well as other people, and forget the underlying material just as readily. (For more detail on physician payment, including pay-for-performance and similar measures, please see Chapter 5.)

What we discuss here is the more fundamental problem of tapping physicians' *intrinsic* motivations by understanding their underlying predispositions, and hopefully aligning the goals of the organization and those motivators.

■ GENERAL ASPECTS OF PHYSICIAN PRACTICE BEHAVIOR

Physicians are selected for medical school because of certain characteristics. Among these are analytic thinking, competitiveness, independence, and verbal facility. In many ways, physician selection and training have not much changed the type of individual selected into the profession during the last half-century. The selection and training also creates practitioners who are driven by a sense of personal excellence, responsibility, and oftentimes guilt. We should not be surprised by this. At mid-century, an era largely devoid of measures and data by which to judge physician performance, professional pride and guilt were the predominant mechanisms available for regulating physician behavior.

Following selection, these characteristics are reinforced during education and training, leading many physicians to believe, consciously or subconsciously, that they are superior to other humans in many ways. Medical training delivers many messages. Some are positive, such as the value of a well-honed sense of genuine caring. But some of the implicit messages are less so. Through long work hours, hierarchical training, and exercises that imply error is rooted in lack of character (e.g., "morbidity and mortality conference"), many implicit messages are sent:

- Medicine is too complex to be understood by normal people. Therefore, normal people are unqualified to judge your performance as a physician.
- The task of medical practice is so difficult that wide latitude should be afforded you in your practice to compensate for the extreme difficulty of the task.
- Your financial compensation is only partial compensation for the burden you carry, and insufficient at that.
- Given such wide latitude to operate, errors are moral failings as they often do harm to people who give

us their trust, and therefore are not to be discussed, much less analyzed.
- Error is minimized by repetition of known algorithms imparted by experts.

These messages naturally make several functions in medical management difficult when they inhibit physician cooperation. Among these functions are utilization management (UM), practice reengineering, guideline development, and budget management. All of these activities run counter to the preceding messages, and strike many physicians on the surface as violations of the social contract they agreed to when they entered the profession. They were promised broad autonomy and minimal oversight of their practices in return for regulating themselves and each other through "oneupsmanship," guilt, and blame. Even physicians new to practice have been exposed to these messages, and regardless of whether or not a physician consciously agrees with any of them, they have been absorbed nevertheless. But these messages are anachronisms and a continuing source of cognitive dissonance that exacts a terrible toll on physicians' psyches over time.

Environmental Factors

Several forces have increasingly pressured the traditional small, independent physician practice model over the past two decades. First, the seminal articles from the Institute of Medicine, "To Err Is Human" and "Crossing the Quality Chasm,"[1, 2] have directly challenged the quality and effectiveness produced by the old model, charging the profession with almost 100,000 preventable deaths in the United States every year. Published a decade ago, more recent articles have contended that we are not doing much better today.[3] Elizabeth McGlynn's study of recommended care found that in a wide variety of settings, generally accepted best-practice was only delivered 55% of the time.[4]

Second, the retreat of managed care after the tight controls of the mid-1990s described in Chapter 1 turned out to be simply that, a retreat and not a defeat. The appetite for tighter medical management has increased as purchasers of all stripes have found the cost of health care benefits increasingly unaffordable relative to other private and public goods. The willingness to pay for choice and freedom to use services in an unregulated way correlates with the public's self-perception of wealth. The recessions in both the early and late 2000s have eroded that perception and willingness.

Third, there are paradigms in many areas of quality today that have demonstrated that it is possible to lower cost, raise quality, and thereby provide greater value, if an enterprise has sufficient infrastructure and appropriately aligned goals and incentives; for example, the Geisinger Clinic's ProvenCare model[5] demonstrates that it is possible to "give a warranty" on medical work, and prosper financially and clinically doing so. While many legitimate explanations have been offered as to why such systems are "not like my setting" among physicians, it has been hard to contend that everyone else is operating at optimal effectiveness and efficiency. For example, Peter Provonost's work with surgical checklists[6] has demonstrated that in some areas it is possible to reduce error to near zero. These and many other examples challenge the comforting delusion that physicians live in Garrison Keillor's "Lake Wobegon,"[7] where everyone is above average.

Fourth, like other goods and services, the local market for physician services is becoming increasingly national, and sometimes global. Where once practitioners could rely on geographic isolation or blind loyalty from patients based on prior emotional experiences, the explosive growth of information enabled by the Internet has and will empower purchasers to shop for value beyond traditional geographic boundaries. Medical tourism in which major elective procedures are outsourced to foreign hospitals of superior value is a growing trend and is beginning to be embraced by major payers.[8] While this trend has not yet been demonstrated to shift the individual patient's purchasing behavior, many will argue that this is because patients are still relatively shielded from the economic consequences of their clinical preferences. Many are betting that this will change as the economic burden of their care is increasingly shifted from purchasers and insurers to individual responsibility.

Finally, we can no longer afford as a nation to devote an ever increasing portion of our gross domestic product to health care. As this is published, we are staring at 17% of GDP, or more than $2.5 trillion annually, devoted to American health care. Pundits are making the connection between health care as a very expensive means of production for American companies and America's growing difficulty in producing goods and services that are globally competitive. Economic stresses are already eroding our nation's position in the global marketplace. If we risk losing our preeminence as a nation because the added burden of medical inflation remains unchecked, it is quite likely that we will see creative solutions that limit American medicine's top line. It is probable that the existing model of diffuse or nonexistent accountability for health care outcomes is ending, and the next model or models will have much more physician accountability for outcomes. Among the infrastructure it is necessary to assume that accountability will be an effective mechanism to change physician practice patterns.

■ HOW PHYSICIANS ARE RESPONDING TO THESE FACTORS

Psychologically, the preceding is a set-up for physicians to feel a loss of respect, autonomy, and community status. Instead of the traditional quid pro quo where they are afforded respect and wide practicing latitude in exchange for long hours and decision-making pressure, the emerging "give and get" is providing correct diagnosis and/or treatment relative to a national standard, for a cost that purchasers consider reasonable.* This gets closer to commoditizing their work, which is the exact opposite of the traditional value proposition, where physicians are prized for their uniqueness and individual judgment. The unsurprising result is that many physicians initially choose to resist any medical management as an infringement on their professional value proposition.

What we should all learn from this is that authoritarian approaches to medical management are quite likely to fail because they reinforce physicians' fears of loss of respect, position, and autonomy, and enhance the likelihood of experiencing guilt for "not having done the right thing." It is relatively easy in the physician's mind to equate attempts to change his or her professional decisions with "the greedy (insert loathed authority here—health plan, hospital, employer, medical group) putting profit above patient welfare." This aligns the physician's interest in not being questioned with the patient's health interests in the physician's mind, and therefore gives him or her a "moral" justification for fighting with the medical manager. It can in extreme examples become a morality play, as we have seen in some high-profile cases in the press.[9] This greatly contributed to the first retreat from managed care described in Chapter 1, and into the medically unmanaged open-access models of the early 2000s.

■ WHAT WE SHOULD DO INSTEAD: SEVERAL PRINCIPLES

There are four principles that are important to bear in mind when dealing with changing physician practice behavior in managed health care:

1. Relationships matter;
2. Let the data speak for itself;
3. Peers are a powerful influencer of physician practice patterns; and
4. Peer leaders must understand and communicate the big picture.

Principle One: Relationships Matter

It is much easier to demonize people we don't know. It is very important that physicians doing UM, quality improvement, or any other activity that involves persuading the physician to change his or her mind get to know their practicing peers. While in most situations it is impossible to have a one-on-one conversation with each network physician, it is important when the medical manager has occasion to have such conversations that he or she approach the conversation as a respectful colleague, and not as a

---

* It may plausibly be argued that we passed "reasonable" long, long ago.

punishing authority. Often the inquiry is best couched in terms of lack of understanding. "Hello, Dr. Kelly. I'm sorry to bother you, but I think I must be missing something in your referral to our orthopedist on Ms. Jones for low back pain. The referral shows no focal findings and no trial of physical therapy. Could she benefit from a course of PT, since most patients improve with that? I almost never get a complete picture from here. Can you help me understand?"

It is important for the medical manager to be present for social occasions and other informal meetings with the physicians so they might get to know that person outside the context of medical management, and as a peer. Unless the medical manager communicates her values continuously and proactively, she will have values assigned to her that fit the physicians' hypothesis about her motives. This assignment of values and motives is almost always negative and incorrect.

Principle Two: Let the Data Speak for Itself

Inevitably in the course of examining performance data on cost, quality, and value, differences between practitioners come to light. It is often tempting to leap to the conclusion that one practitioner is just a worse clinician than another, more risk adverse, less well-read, and so on. This then colors one's judgment on how to handle the variation. We not infrequently conclude that education is the answer, which at best is often ignored by physicians, and at worst is taken as condescension. It is just as important for medical managers not to assign values to medical practitioners as the converse.

Instead, it is usually much more effective to view the performance differences as a starting point for investigation. Is the data acuity adjusted? Perhaps Dr. B is dealing with a sicker population than Dr. A. Is one practicing with a different demographic than another? One practitioner in a network one of the authors managed at one time had extraordinarily low utilization, so much so that he worried about underutilization. It turned out that the practitioner was dealing with a Southeast Asian immigrant population, who had a distrust of Western medicine and extensive use of traditional Chinese medicine. His utilization was appropriate for the population he was serving.

However, oftentimes after investigating such factors, differences persist. When that happens, simply presenting the data to clinicians, unblinded and with peer comparison, will help generate hypotheses than can then be tested by analysts to explain variation. If the analysts cannot validate the hypotheses, then it sets up peers to have the conversation with the physician with the unusual practice pattern. This leads to the next principle.

Principle Three: Peers Are a Powerful Influencer of Physician Practice Patterns

Early on in his medical management career, one of the authors was fortunate enough to work with a doctorate-level pharmacologist. She would do presentation after presentation about different drug classes, trying to increase the use of generics over brand drugs. This is a technique called academic detailing,[10] described by Dr. Jerry Avorn.

She was puzzled, however, that the effect of her talks on practice pattern was very small. Reading Dr. Avorn's literature, she realized that they were approaching the learning process incorrectly if the goal was to change behavior. Many people can become *educated* by listening to a lecture, but few will actually *change their prescribing behavior* based on a unidirectional communication format, the traditional lecture. She subsequently changed to a discussion format, and began using physician *peers* to deliver the same message, with much greater effect.

The peer family doctor down the street* has several advantages over the doctorate-level pharmacologist in such discussions. First, the family doctor is doing exactly the same thing as the audience is, in a similar setting, so has immediate acceptance as "someone like me." Second, she can answer objections raised by the audience from her own experience, either confirming that they should have concern X, or refuting it. Third, having a peer conversation fits into the regulatory mechanism embedded in the physicians' training and minds, that physicians should modify each others' behaviors, and not have it done by nonphysicians. Objectively, the pharmacologist knew 10 times what any clinician knew about any particular drug; she just didn't know how it felt to prescribe it in the exam room, and for clinicians that was a critical difference. Did patients have trouble with nausea with that drug? She could cite the statistics from studies, but could never say, "Yes, my patients complain of that, too, and I always have them take it on a full stomach as a result."

Principle Four: Peer Leaders Must Understand and Communicate the Big Picture

It is a truism that successful organizations are able to connect their members with their overall mission in a direct and personal way. Never is this more true and necessary than in changing physician behavior. One can construct rules to compel certain behaviors in a small way, but inevitably such rules are limited, and easily circumvented by smart people who do not agree with their intent. This was often the case in 1990s managed care.

If not by rules, then how does one accomplish the organization's goals in dealing with the network? What likely will be necessary in this round of managed care is an alignment of incentives and goals beyond the basic capitation in use for decades now. In the end, a cadre of professionals who understand and agree with what an organization is trying to accomplish is usually able to defeat a similar cadre operating off of a set of orders or rules drawn up at

---

*The term is used metaphorically, since, as discussed in Chapter 4, the trend in many parts of the country is for physicians to become employees of hospitals or larger groups. In such cases, substitute the words "down the hall" for "down the street."

headquarters, but lacking buy-in by the troops. Similarly, a set of guidelines or referral rules handed down from a health care organization's headquarters is likely to fail to achieve desired goals by being disregarded or circumvented by the network. Modern organizations have applied this principle in other industries, including the U.S. Army in their war games simulations.[11] Therefore, it is important that every medical manager be able to speak to the organization's *intent* when dealing with other physicians in the network. This is a question every medical manager should be able to answer on the spot: Why is your organization trying to manage physicians in the first place? For the benefit of patients through great application of evidence-based medicine? To make care affordable for everyone in their community? To make the organization more profitable, thereby preserving jobs? To generate return on investment for shareholders of the organization? All of these are perfectly valid motivations are from different perspectives, and should be understood by medical managers as well as all other staff. However, they may generate different reactions from physicians depending on whether they identify with the organization or not.

Inherently medical management is about making choices with limited resources to optimize an outcome. But to what is the resulting efficiency purposed? Being able to say, for example, "to preserve a critical resource in short supply in our community, access to primary care" makes a big difference in how providers receive the message of limits. While these might seem to be lofty and ethereal issues, they are not. The question of whether a physician changes an order or a referral request depends greatly on what answers she receives to these questions. These principles can be summed up in the following equation:

Trust + Clean Data + Committed Peers => Physician Change

This is not intended to imply that physician change happens every time you assemble the three elements on the left-hand side of the arrow. Instead, it is intended to state that without all three elements, chances of affecting physician practice patterns in a sustainable way are not good.

◼ TOOLS FOR CHANGING PHYSICIAN BEHAVIOR

Tools for changing physician behavior refer to the techniques or supporting elements a leader should use for support. Like the principles discussed above, it is up to each leader to determine what will be most useful in any given situation, but their use should not be ignored or bypassed.

Communicate, Communicate, Communicate; Repeat

Ongoing communication with physicians and their office managers is at the core of changing physician behavior. This can take many forms. Electronic or paper newsletters, updates, and network notifications are the least labor-intensive and the most scalable. Unfortunately, they also have the worst penetration rates, in that they are usually opened and read by a small percentage of those to whom they are sent. Almost all of us have the experience daily of deleting e-mails that we find repetitive or irrelevant to us, often reading only the subject line. Busy physicians and their staffs are no different.

Group meetings with physicians, office managers, or both give people a chance to meet and evaluate the organization personally. Often these can be coupled with some kind of continuing medical education, giving physicians an additional incentive to attend. This gives everyone a chance to understand one another better, to voice concerns, and to get questions answered. This interaction cannot be emphasized enough. It is actually the act of *receiving feedback* as an organization, not giving it, that builds trust. Done with respect and humility, it sends the message, "We're not perfect, and we care about you and the effect our work has on yours. Please help us do better."

It can be difficult for some medical managers to embrace this model. They, too, can be caught up in the negative attributions about their role, thinking they are somehow there to "prevent physicians from abusing the system." Often they are subjected to abuse by angry physicians who view interacting with medical managers as a needless irritation or, worse, as an affront. But the more humility or empathy is demonstrated, the more likely the practicing physician is to view the medical manager as an ally and not as an enemy. It takes character and patience not to return fire with fire, and it is absolutely critical that medical managers not engage in such reciprocity.

An additional communication medium currently evolving is social networking. The use of Twitter, Facebook, blogging, and similar tools is only beginning for many health care organizations, but their use serves the same purposes as it does in other industries. The ability to create understanding, connection, and loyalty among a widely dispersed network will likely be very important going forward, particularly with younger physicians who have grown up using these media and not traditional paper-based communications. What these tools do is create the opportunity to get to know the organization and its personality by increasing the number of brief contacts it offers physicians. Just as with the live interactions, it gives physicians a basis to form a more nuanced understanding of the organization, its motives, and ethics beyond the interactions that the normal course of medical management might entail. Social media has limitations, of course, and chief among them from the standpoint of medical management is a lack of privacy and security, and is therefore suited to communications that contain no protected health information.

Data: Information or Knowledge?

For most of the managed care era, the challenge has been to get enough information to be able to take action. This is still a significant challenge, with the antiquated systems often still in use in many organizations or, worse, in the absence of data management systems at all. The details of a data infrastructure necessary to manage a network are covered in Chapter 10, and are beyond the scope of this discussion. But suffice it to say, the availability of current data to change utilization patterns is fundamental to the tasks of medical management. There is a saying from W.E. Deming, one of the pioneers in modern process improvement: "Information is not knowledge. The world is drowning in information but is slow in acquisition of knowledge. There is no substitute for knowledge."[12]

More and more, the challenge for American physicians (as well as most other Americans) will not be getting information, but knowing which information can be translated into knowledge that will be useful to them. For example, it is one thing to know that one doctor's dermatology costs are twice what another's is. It is quite another to understand that this variation arises because the dermatologist the first refers to most often does Mohs surgery on everything, whereas the second only does that procedure on faces.[*] Knowing a doctor's costs are higher is information. Knowing why is knowledge, knowledge that may potentially affect a physician's referral choices going forward.

One of the biases inherent in physician training is that we are taught to believe in data and objective conclusion. The roots of this go back all the way to the Flexner report[13] around the turn of the last century, when it urged medical schools to become much more data-driven to raise the respectability of the profession. Using credible data aligns with this training bias, and creates cognitive dissonance when these data say one's performance as a clinician is worse than peers'. Physicians are relatively adept at relieving this type of cognitive dissonance. The first avenue to do this is usually to attack the credibility of the data. By finding some error in the spreadsheet, the logic goes like this: "If this cell is wrong, every other cell on this spreadsheet is suspect. Therefore, I can dismiss this report until someone proves its validity to me. I don't need to change because I could potentially be changing in the wrong ways due to faulty data. That could harm my patients, and that violates my highest values. I am therefore morally justified in ignoring your recommendations."

The obvious conclusion is that one's data presented to physicians must be checked and rechecked for accuracy, and be squeaky clean on presentation. If a suspected error is raised, it should be investigated and fed back to the physician promptly and honestly, even if it was in fact an analysis error. The important issue here is trust and credibility. One tries to present data of impeccable quality, and whenever one fails to do so (as will inevitably happen in any human process some percentage of the time), it should be admitted promptly and transparently to preserve the integrity of the reporter, if not the report.

Other frequently used techniques to relieve cognitive dissonance generally involve claiming differences in populations (my patients are sicker, richer, poorer, more demanding, more passive, etc.). Every attempt should be made to either confirm or disprove these differences, and to correct the analysis for these effects where possible.

Should information from analysis be disseminated widely within an organization, or only to the physician in question privately? For example, should the percentage completion of dilated retinal exams in diabetics for every physician in the network be shown at a group meeting, with physician names associated with the numbers? This is a controversial subject, depending on organizational norms. As previously stated, any perceptions of authoritarian criticism are to be avoided. The goal is to communicate that such revelation is not intended to shame, but to point out that there are commonly areas in which each participant can help the organization achieve its goals. Credit and respect for good intent should always be given, as it is almost uniformly present.

No one wakes up in the morning and goes to work intending to do a mediocre job. However, there is data to suggest that wider dissemination of such information results in greater behavior change. Judith Hibbard published a study looking at quality improvement activity among Wisconsin hospitals, separated into two groups. In the first, the quality scores were given to each hospital in private. In the second group, the hospitals were given the results and told that they would be publicly disseminated in the press a few months later. The result was that there was twice as much quality improvement effort engendered in the public reporting group as in the private reporting group.[14]

And, with disclosure to peers within the group, a wonderful thing often happens. Frequently the physicians with the lowest performance will seek out those with the best performance to understand how they did it. It is a wonderful demonstration of the value of collective intelligence, and how it gets magnified and released in a community of trust. But it will not happen in communities where physicians see each other more strongly as competitors than collaborators. Individual discretion is advised in assessing whether the community is "safe" enough for this kind of disclosure.

Mission Clarity: What Are We Trying To Do?

As stated previously, a widespread understanding of what the organization is trying to accomplish is extremely valuable in changing behavior. Success in changing physician behavior is likely better correlated with the number of physicians in a network that understand and embrace the goals of the organization, rather than the depth of understanding for a few individuals, no matter how influential.

---

[*]Mohs surgery costs 10 times as much as wide excision, and is intended to produce a better cosmetic result.

Unfortunately, most often because of the costly and labor-intensive nature of imparting such understanding, many organizations default to deep understanding among leadership, and relative ignorance within the network.

Citing Deming again, in order to change an organization, one doesn't need to have everyone onboard, but one does need the square root of n, where n is the total number of individuals.[15] For example, if you need to change a 100-person organization, you need a minimum of 10 individuals to understand and champion the change. Deming estimated that once that number is recruited, the change can be reasonably self-sustaining. The ability of individuals on the front lines to be able to articulate and endorse the change is a critical variable in the change process.

■ FINANCIAL INCENTIVES

Financial incentives are a programmatic approach to changing behavior, intended or not. Because it is discussed at great length in Chapter 5, it is only touched upon here. As demonstrated amply in Chapter 5, how physicians are paid has been and still is a major factor in utilization and pricing. To believe otherwise is irrational. But unlike other cases in which payment has a direct impact on behavior, factory piecework, for example, the impact on physicians is likely to be buried. Few physicians would say they make any practice decisions based on pay, and only make them based on "what's best for the patient." Sadly, the evidence is just the opposite, and the reader is urged to read the section in Chapter 7 on physician self-referral to see a depressing example of it.

On the bright side, while physicians show consistent differences in their use of discretionary care based on payment methodology, they show no differences in the use of life-saving care.[16] This also affirms why capitation has not been shown to lead to poorer outcomes, as discussed and referenced in Chapter 5. Even relatively modest changes may be associated with behavior change. In a 2009 study most applicable to medical groups, closed-panel health maintenance organizations (HMOs), and health systems with employed physicians, changing physicians from a basic salaried compensation model to a lower base salary with additional piece rates for encounters and select procedures produced an 11-61% increase in the combination of total encounters, number of procedures performed, and time worked, despite no change in the patient population.[17]

The blend of malleability of discretionary behavior based on compensation and the lack of malleability of life-saving or nondiscretionary care is certainly comforting, and allows medical managers to consider how to best apply financial incentives as a part of an overall approach to changing physician behavior. This is particularly the case when using evidence-based clinical guidelines, as discussed later in the next section.

■ PROGRAMMATIC APPROACHES TO CHANGING PHYSICIAN BEHAVIOR

Programmatic approaches refer to specific types of methods for addressing physician behavior change. They are not equally effective. In fact, a review of various combinations of approaches found that there was no unifying theory of physician behavior change, and attempts to affect individual physicians' performance often failed or demonstrated mixed results; multiple interventions did yield somewhat better results, however.[18] On the other hand, there are some that if applied properly, do have a capacity to at least promote changes in practice behavior.

Formal Continuing Medical Education

Formal continuing medical education (CME) is the provision of additional clinical training or medically oriented information through seminars, conferences, home-study, and so forth. The hallmark of CME is that it provides CME credits by virtue of the accreditation of the sponsoring body. This method of information dissemination, while traditionally the most prevalent, is relatively ineffective when it comes to changing behavior. Review studies of the medical literature have found little evidence that traditional CME changed patient outcomes or changed behavior.[19-23] There is some evidence that changes in behavior will occur when the curriculum is *designed* to change specific types of behavior, for example, by creating in the CME program a strong focus on change.[24] Other useful adjuncts to CME include academic detailing (as in the pharmacist example above), reminders (i.e., specific reminders at the time of a patient visit), and the influence of opinion leaders.[25] The addition of more intensive and personalized interventions such as the ability to practice new skills (an intervention more useful for learning procedures than for changing practice behavior) or a high level of individual interactivity may also affect some level of change in the setting of a CME program.[25]

Based on this evidence, formal CME may be a useful tool for disseminating clinical information, and may be a useful adjunct to other approaches to changing physician behavior in general. However, formal didactic CME alone is not a useful tool for changing physician practice behavior when compared to other available methodologies. As above, they can serve as an attractant for physician meetings/relationship building, and as an excuse for face-to-face interactions between medical managers and practitioners. In and of themselves, however, they are a poor method to change behavior.

Data and Feedback

As has been mentioned in the beginning of this chapter and in other chapters, data regarding quality, utilization, and cost are an integral part of a managed care plan. For purposes of medical management, the value of data should predominantly be measured by the amount of practice change it generates in the network. Thus, data that stays with medical managers and is never shared with practitioners is of limited value. In the extreme, if the only data physicians get are letters at the end of the year informing them that all of their withheld funds are used up, they can credibly argue that they were blindsided, because in fact they were. Providing regular and accurate data about an individual physician's performance, from a quality, utilization, and (for risk/bonus models) an economic standpoint, is important for changing behavior. Most physicians will want to perform well, but can only do so when they can judge their own performance against that of their peers and/or against expectations.

The research literature is actually mixed in its support for feedback alone as a means of changing behavior, although a small majority of the research data is positive. There are studies reporting significant reductions in utilization and costs in response to feedback about individual physician behavior.[26-34] There are, however, other studies that report no effect from information feedback, report that feedback has little lasting effect unless continuously reinforced, or are at best ambiguous regarding the role of feedback.[35-41] As stated above, data is only one required element in effecting physician change, and variability in the other elements may account for the variability in outcomes of these studies.

When reviewing the possible reasons for feedback being shown to be effective or ineffective (at least over the long term), it is possible to conjecture on some other factors that improve the effectiveness of feedback. These conjectures, while not studied in the research literature, are valid from the standpoint of industry experience.

- Physicians must believe that their behavior needs to change, whether for clinical reasons, economic reasons, or simply in order to remain part of the participating panel in the plan; if physicians do not believe that they need to change, then feedback provides little value. (Goal alignment)
- Feedback must be credible; in other words, the data must be seen as taking into account such things as differences in acuity and demographics for patient-related practice profiling. (Clean data)
- Feedback must be consistent and usable; in other words, a physician must clearly understand the data in the report and be able to use that information in a concrete way and be able to keep using it to measure his or her own performance. (Knowledge vs. uninterpreted information)
- Feedback needs to be closely related to what a physician is doing at the time; in other words, feedback about behavior that is remote in time or infrequent is less likely to be acted upon. (Timeliness)

- Feedback must be regular in order to sustain changed behavior; feedback that is sporadic or unsustained will result in behavior changes returning to the condition before the feedback caused any change to begin with, assuming that any change took place at all. (Reinforced)
- Lastly, feedback that is linked to economic performance may be more likely to produce substantial change than feedback that is not so linked; in other words, feedback about utilization or nonutilization measures that are tied to compensation has more potential for use by the physician than data that does not have such a linkage. (Extrinsic motivation)

Practice Guidelines and Clinical Protocols

Practice guidelines and clinical protocols refer to codified approaches to medical care using evidence-based medical care; in other words, they rely on research published in peer-reviewed medical journals. Guidelines may be for both diagnostic and therapeutic modalities, and they may be used to guide physicians in the care of patients with defined diseases or symptoms, or as surveillance tools to monitor practice on a retrospective basis. (Guidelines and criteria, as they are implemented today, are discussed at length in Chapter 7 in the context of UM, as is the related concept of "medical necessity," and the reader is urged to review that section if those concepts remain hazy at this point.)

In the past, published guidelines were often inconsistent or did not conform to other published guidelines.[42] Physicians at the time often had an initial negative reaction, feeling that guidelines made for cookbook medicine. [43, 44] In the most recent decade, guidelines and clinical criteria have become much more consistent and have a much stronger basis in evidence-based practices. As hospitals and physician offices adopt electronic medical records and clinical support systems, they are increasingly licensing the same third-part guidelines and criteria payers use. Payers also frequently provide access to those guidelines on their systems for any participating physician to use, not only for medical care but to assist in understanding coverage issues. Attempting to put comprehensive practice guidelines into place is a daunting task if applied to too many guidelines at once. There is some evidence that simple publication of practice guidelines alone may predispose physicians to consider changing their behavior, but that publication alone is unlikely to create rapid change.[45, 46] When such protocols are accompanied by direct presentations by opinion leaders, so-called academic detailing, then changes are more sustained.[47]

What has also been found effective over the past 10 years is to focus on a small number of very specific guidelines and provide regular and systematized feedback to physicians. The earliest success story is around prescribing beta blockers to patients upon admission for a heart attack, and then upon discharge; early dismal rates of compliance noted in the "To Err is Human" report cited at the beginning of the chapter has shown a remarkable improvement through a combination of continual feedback from payers (based on pharmacy claims data), pay for performance (both by payers and by Medicare), and hospital protocol development. Other common conditions such as congestive heart failure and chronic obstructive pulmonary disease have followed.

The lesson from all this is that in contrast to past decades, evidence-based medical guidelines are now demonstrating increasing effectiveness as a component of physician practice behavior change. But the use of evidence-based medical guidelines to achieve change is best done through combining several attributes:

- Efforts must be focused; in other words, rolling out 20 new guidelines at once is likely to fail, but choosing one or two at a time and waiting until those have taken hold before implementing new ones has a higher success rate;
- Guidelines should focus on those conditions or practices that occur frequently, and for which there is a lot of practice variation;
- Implementation of guidelines must be accompanied by regular feedback on a consistent basis, preferably at each occurrence rather than a summarized report issued on a periodic basis (see prior section); and
- Financial rewards such as pay for performance or other approaches help to sharpen focus and facilitate change.*

Small Group Programs

There is good evidence that educating physicians in a highly interactive, small group setting can produce positive changes in behavior, including improved outcomes and lower utilization. Several authors of studies about interactive, small group physician education believe that the effectiveness is explained by theories of self-regulation.[48–50] These small group seminars or educational sessions are frequently focused on specific clinical conditions; for example, asthma,[50] hypertension,[51] hysterectomy,[52] pelvic pain and/or abnormal uterine bleeding,[53] sciatica,[54] and spinal stenosis.[55] The same approach has been studied in physician practice behavior for chronic conditions in general (including the creation of physician-patient "partnerships")[56] and for test ordering behavior.[57]

Well-regarded academic or community physicians are most appropriate for conducting these types of highly interactive small group seminars or educational sessions. Due to potential concerns of conflict of interest, medical managers from the organization are not in a good position to conduct such seminars unless the program is based on data and feedback that only the sponsoring organization has. The investment required to conduct these programs is potentially sizable, so it is important for an organization to leverage its resources to improve the likelihood of a positive outcome. One approach is for an organization to provide educational supporting grants to an academic center or tertiary health system to conduct the program. Supporting grants may be restricted to seminars focusing on improving quality and utilization, although ethically the organization should not attempt to dictate the educational content. Though only superficially related to formal CME, such a session should still provide for CME credit.

As hospitals increase the number of physicians they employ (see Chapter 4), as well as the creation of new ACOs and PCMHs, these types of small group meetings will become very important, and much easier to make happen. For provider organizations, often speakers can be drawn from members of the group and/or affiliated physicians. This may have ancillary benefits by improving rapport between referring and consulting physicians. This effect can be powerful enough that some attention may be necessary to giving equal opportunities to speak between physicians in the same specialty. The same cautions apply in terms of not dictating content and providing CME credit.

■ ADDRESSING NONCOMPLIANCE BY INDIVIDUAL PHYSICIANS

There are no programmatic approaches to changing practice behavior that will have a positive impact on every single physician in the network. Many variables such as geographic location, local practice attitudes, the training a physician has received, economic or financial conditions, availability and acceptability of data and information, personality, and so forth will have effects on the degree of success medical managers will achieve. The benefit design that the organization is administering in the marketplace will also have an effect, with those plans that are more restrictive (e.g., a "pure" HMO) having greater need and ability to address practice behavior change as compared to relatively loosely managed plans (e.g., a PPO). But in all events, there will be variability in the degrees or amount of positive changes that each individual physician makes. In some cases, there will be so little positive change that medical managers must undertake an approach focused on an individual physician.

The amount of investment in medical management an organization makes is directly related to the types of

---

*At the risk of being repetitious, the reader can find additional discussion in Chapter 5 about how factors such as time lag between an event and payments, the use of specific events versus aggregate results, and so forth affects the impact of any approach to physician payment and incentives.

approaches that are possible to use for changing behavior. Those organizations that make little investment in medical management will rely more on data dissemination and rules, while organizations that make heavier investments in medical management will use the broader array of available options discussed previously. Loosely managed networks may choose to not deal with individual physician behavior at all, whereas organizations at risk are far more likely to do so. Organizations with very large networks will need to focus on those physicians that are significantly out of conformance, while those with smaller networks can take the approach of working with a higher percentage of individual physicians. Medical groups, closed-panel HMOs, and health systems with a large panel of employed physicians are the most likely to focus resources here. Of course, the degree to which medical managers are able to focus on individual physicians will at least in part be dependent on available resources such as personnel (especially medical directors), valid data, and time.

Positive feedback is a powerful long-term approach.[*] As noted earlier in the chapter, it is an effective tool for change that most managers fail to use to any great degree. Positive feedback does not refer to mindless or misleading praise, but to letting a physician know when things are done well. Most managers get so involved in firefighting that they tend to neglect sending positive messages to those providers who are managing well. In the absence of such messages, providers have to figure out for themselves what they are doing right, although the plan will usually tell them what they are doing wrong. This is certainly a missed opportunity. The prior example in this chapter of disseminating performance statistics for well-performing physicians on measures as well as poor-performing ones is one in which a medical manager can take some time and attention with the network to highlight exemplary performers, and perhaps some of the mechanisms those physicians used to achieve such a high level. Most often, those performers cite office systems above individual effort as the cause of the superior performance.

Stepwise Approach to Changing Behavior in Individual Physicians

Changing behavior in individual providers requires a stepwise approach. The first and most common step is *collegial discussion*. Discussing cases and utilization patterns in a nonthreatening way, colleague to colleague, is generally an effective method of bringing about change. In most cases, this is adequate and no further steps are necessary. In a

fair number of cases, there are circumstances unknown to the reviewing and/or reviewed physician prior to the conversation that allow for a collaborative solution to be co-generated.

Persuasion is also commonly used. Somewhat stronger than collegial discussion, persuasion refers to plan managers persuading providers to act in ways that the providers may not initially choose themselves. For example, if a patient requires intravenous antibiotics for a chronic infection but is generally doing well, that patient is a candidate for home intravenous therapy. Some physicians will resist discharging the patient to home therapy because it is inconvenient to follow the case; keeping the patient in the hospital is a lot easier in terms of rounding. The physician must then be persuaded to discharge the patient because of the cost effectiveness of home therapy. Again, reminding the physician of the group aims the organization is attempting to achieve may be helpful because it gives a common basis for evaluating courses of action that aren't "yours" or "mine," but "ours."

Firm direction of plan policies, procedures, and requirements (i.e., the "rules and regulations") is the next step after persuasion. If a physician refuses to cooperate with the plan to deliver care cost-effectively and discussions and persuasion have failed, a medical director may be required to give a physician firm direction, reminding him or her of the underlying commitment to cooperate with organizational policies and procedures. In difficult cases, it may be necessary to invoke legal and contractual obligations. Behind firm direction is the implied threat of nonpayment and/or group sanctions, up to and including termination of contract or group participation. It is clearly a display of power and should not be done with a heavy hand, or without due contemplation of consequences for both the provider and the organization.

When giving firm direction, it is best to not be drawn into repetitive and unresolvable arguments. This is sometimes called a "broken record" type of response because it is often apparent that the medical director is giving the same response, irrespective of changes in the circumstances. Medical managers should reserve the firm direction approach to behavior change for those instances when the approaches discussed earlier are ineffective. Inexperienced managers, or managers who are overwhelmed with work and have little time or resources, may use this as a first step. In the short term, that may be effective, but it will come at the cost of lost trust, relationship, and future ability to use softer measures to change behavior. Medical managers are often not aware that they carry their organization's brand in every interaction they have with their network. The brand can be thought of as the repository of future trust and cooperation engendered by past actions, and should be managed extremely carefully. Ignoring its importance is a very expensive oversight in the long run.

---

[*] The use of the term "positive feedback" here is different than when using the term "feedback" regarding data. While both forms of feedback provide information to the provider regarding performance, data feedback is objective, while positive feedback in the context of this section refers to subjective information from plan managers.

One last thought in this section: Avoid global responses to individual problems. When managers are uncomfortable confronting individual physicians about problems in behavior, a dysfunctional response is to make a global change in policy or procedure because of the actions of one or two physicians. That type of response frequently has the effect of alienating all the other physicians who have been working positively within the group or the network, while failing to change the behavior of the problem providers. If a policy change is required, make it. But if the problem is really just with one or two individuals, deal with them and do not harass the rest of the physicians.

Discipline and Sanctions

This section discusses the most serious form of behavior modification. Sanctions or threats of sanctions are only applied when the problem is so serious that action must be taken and the provider fails to cooperate to improve the situation.* Any disciplinary action, especially one that leads to termination or even the threat of termination, should only be undertaken because the other approaches have failed. In addition to the significant emotional trauma and potential financial consequences to the provider, the sanctioning process has legal overtones that must be kept in mind.

In some situations, managed care organizations may initiate disciplinary actions short of a formal sanction process. In most cases, such discipline is also helpful in creating documentation of chronic problems or failure to cooperate. Discipline may involve verbal warnings or letters; in either case, the thrust of the action is to document the offensive behavior and to describe the consequences of failure to cooperate.

One example of verbal discipline is sometimes called "ticketing," so called because it is similar to getting a ticket from a traffic cop. This is a verbal reprimand about a specific behavior; the behavior and corrective action are described, as are the consequences of failure to carry out the corrective action. Much like the firm direction described above, the medical director refuses to get into an argument at that time and requires the offending physician to make an appointment at a future date to discuss the issue (similar to a court date). This allows tempers to cool off a bit and ensures that the disciplinary message does not get muddied up with other issues. When a medical director issues a ticket, there should be a document placed in a file that describes what transpired. Ticketing is a viable approach when significant time and energy have already been expended to no effect, and should not be used unless the more collegial approaches have been exhausted.

A more formal approach is an actual disciplinary letter. Like a ticket, the letter describes the offending behavior and the required corrective action and invites the provider to make an appointment to discuss the issue. In the case of a verbal ticket or a disciplinary letter, the consequence of failure to change errant ways is initiation of the formal sanctioning process. This is typically not done unless the peer review committee (see Chapter 3) is in agreement.

Formal sanctioning has potentially serious legal overtones. Due process, or a policy regarding rights and responsibilities of both parties, is a requirement for an effective sanctioning procedure, at least when one is sanctioning for reasons of quality. The Healthcare Quality Improvement Act of 1986 (HCQIA) has formalized due process in the sanctioning procedure as it relates to quality and a health system or plan must adhered to the prescribed steps, actions, and physician rights in order to maintain protection from antitrust action. Although this act was primarily aimed at hospital peer review activities, HMOs are specifically mentioned, and other forms of managed care are potentially subject to it as well.[58] Note that this is applicable when dealing with network models and independent practitioners; in an employment situation, there are bodies of employment law that are applicable to this subject that are beyond the scope of this chapter. It is important in those situations to be familiar with both sets of requirements, and to use the mechanisms applicable to the circumstance. For example, disciplining a provider for violating terms of their employment agreement by limiting hospital privileges may confuse the behaviors being sanctioned and may give the physician grounds for claiming unfair treatment.

Following the requirements of the HCQIA regarding due process is cumbersome and is obviously the final step before removing a physician from the panel for reasons of poor-quality care. Termination of a provider for reasons of quality is a serious charge and has a very negative impact on a physician. Because it is such a drastic step, compliance with the HCQIA, including the reporting requirements, is the best protection the organization has against a legal action. Again, in an employment situation, applicable employment law also needs to be taken into consideration and consultation with human resources and/or counsel specializing in these issues is strongly advised.

It should be emphasized that the HCQIA, in regard to peer review activities, promotes actions against physicians for quality problems. If a physician fails to cooperate with contractually agreed-to plan policies and procedures, the organization may have reason to terminate the contract with the physician "for cause," as discussed in Chapter 6 on legal issues in contracting. Even in that case, it may be wise to have a due process and peer review policy that allows for formal steps to be taken in the event that the plan contemplates termination, although it may not be required. Presentation of facts to a medical advisory committee made up of physicians who are not in direct economic competition with

---

*In some cases the provider may be willing to cooperate, but the offense is so serious that sanctions must be taken anyway, for example, a documented serious problem in quality of care.

the involved physician provides a back-up to plan management. Such a committee may be able to effect changes by the physician where the medical director may not. A decision by the peer review committee underscores that severe sanctions are not arbitrary, but are the result of failure on the part of the physician, not plan management.

There may arise situations where a physician's utilization performance is such that there is a clear mismatch with managed care practice philosophy. The quality of the physician's medical care may be adequate, and there even may have been no gross lack of cooperation with plan policies and procedures, but the physician simply practices medicine in such a style that medical resources are heavily and inappropriately overutilized. In such cases, the medical director must assess whether the physician can change his or her behavior. Assuming that the medical director concludes that the provider in question cannot change (or change sufficiently) or has failed to change despite warnings and feedback, the organization may choose to terminate the relationship solely on the basis of contractual terms that allow either party to terminate without cause when adequate notice is given (see Chapter 6).

When the organization deselects a physician in this way, it is not always subject to a due process type of review. The reason is that the separation is based on practice style and fit, not accusations of rule-breaking or poor quality. Terminating physicians in this manner has the potential for creating adverse relations in the network if there is the perception that the organization is acting arbitrarily and without reason. In effect, such terminations have cultural consequences for the network or group, in addition to other types of consequences for the individual in question. Even without the need for a due process approach in these situations, such steps are drastic and should not be done frequently or lightly.

Finally, many states as well as Medicare have laws and regulations about physician termination from health plans, including due process and appeal rights. Chapters 6, 28, and 29 provide an overview, but readers will themselves need to obtain current information applicable to their own needs and not rely on this book.

■ CONCLUSION

Changing physician behavior is central to the success of any health care organization managing cost and outcomes. Physicians are chosen and acculturated to respond to several influences: people/organizations they know and trust; clean, timely, accurate, and actionable data; peers they believe understand their circumstances and pressures; and shared missions that they have endorsed. Medical managers can exacerbate the difficulties in changing physician behavior by failing to establish or maintain positive relationships, failing to provide accurate and timely information to facilitate change, failing to provide positive feedback, failing to address specific problems with providers early, and failing to take a stepwise approach to managing change.

Systematic approaches to changing physician behavior can be successfully used for many aspects of practice. Continuing education, small group seminars, creation and dissemination of practice protocols, and data feedback are all potentially useful techniques. A focused approach to increasing the adoption of evidence-based clinical guidelines, when accompanied by regular and specific feedback and financial incentives, is of particular value.

When reasonable efforts to obtain necessary and important physician practice behavior change are unsuccessful, discipline and sanctions may be required. Due process must be followed before termination for poor quality, and it may be useful in other settings as well. In the final analysis, it is the plan's responsibility to make the effort to effect changes in provider behavior that will benefit all the parties concerned, and it is the plan's responsibility to take action when necessary.

Endnotes

1 Committee on Quality of Health Care in America, Institute of Medicine. *To err is human: Building a safer health system.* Washington, DC: National Academy Press, November 1, 1999. Available at: www.nap.edu/books/0309068371/html. Accessed April 2011.

2 Committee on Quality of Health Care in America, Institute of Medicine. *Crossing the quality chasm: A new health system for the 21st century.* Washington, DC: National Academy Press, March 1, 2001. Available at: www.nap.edu/html/quality_chasm/reportbrief.pdf. Accessed April 2011.

3 Dentzer S. Still crossing the quality chasm—or suspended over it? *Health Affairs.* 2011;30(4):554–555.

4 McGlynn EA, Asch SM, Adams J, et al. The quality of health care delivered to adults in the United States. *N Engl J Med.* 2003;348(26):2635–2645.

5 Geisinger Health System. *About proven care.* July 27, 2010. Available at: www.geisinger.org/provencare/. Accessed April 2011.

6 Provonost P, Needham D, Berenholtz S, et al. An intervention to decrease catheter-related bloodstream infections in the ICU. *N Engl J Med.* 2006;355(26):2725–2732.

7 Wikipedia. *The Lake Wobegon effect.* April 19, 2011. Available at: http://en.wikipedia.org/wiki/Lake_Wobegon. Accessed April 2011.

8 Kantor A. *Medical tourism takes off.* June, 2008. Available at: www.ahip.org/content/default.aspx?bc=31%7C130%7C136%7C23417%7C23420. Accessed April 2011.

9   Peeno L. *The confession of a managed care medical director.* May 2006. Available at: www.cchfreedom. org/issues/peeno596test.php3. Accessed April 2011.

10 Avorn J, Soumerai SB. Improving drug-therapy decisions through educational outreach – A randomized controlled trial of academically based detailing. *N Engl J Med.* 1983;308(24):1457–1463.

11 Pascale P, Millemann M, Gioja L. Changing the way we change. *Harvard Bus Rev.* 1997;75(6):126–139.

12 Deming WE. *The new economics: For industry, government, education.* Cambridge, MA: MIT Press; 1993.

13 Beck AH. The Flexner report and the standardization of American medical education. *JAMA.* 2004;291(17): 2139–2140.

14 Hibbard JH, Stockard J, Tusler M. Hospital performance reports: Impact on quality, market share, and reputation. *Health Affairs.* 2005;24(4):1150–1160.

15 Wachter R. *In conversation with...Brent James, MD, MStat.* February 2011. Available at: www.webmm.ahrq. gov/perspective.aspx?perspectiveID = 97. Accessed April 2011.

16 Shen J, Andersen R, Brook R, et al. The effects of payment method on clinical decision-making: physician responses to clinical scenarios. *Med Care.* 2004;42: 297–302.

17 Helmchen LA and Lo Sasso AT. How sensitive is physician performance to alternative compensation schedules? Evidence from a large network of primary care clinics. *Health Econ.* 2010;19:1300–1317.

18 Smith WR. Evidence for the effectiveness of techniques to change physician behavior. *Chest.* 2000;118:8S–17S.

19 Heale J, Davis DA, Norman GR, et al. A randomized controlled trial assessing the impact of problem-based versus didactic teaching methods in CME. *Proc Annu Conf Res Med Educ.* 1988;27:72–77.

20 Browner WS, Baron RB, Solkowitz S, et al. Physician management of hypercholesterolemia: A randomized trial of continuing medical education. *West J Med.* 1994;161(6):572–578.

21 Boissel JP, Collet JP, Alborini A, et al. Education program for general practitioners on breast and cervical cancer screening: A randomized trial. *Rev Epidemiol Sante Publique.* 1995;43(6):541–547.

22 Davis DA, Thomson MA, Oxman AD, Haynes RB. Evidence for the effectiveness of CME: A review of 50 randomized controlled trials. *JAMA.* 1992;268(9): 1111–1117.

23 Davis D, O'Brien MA, Freemantle N, et al. Impact of formal continuing medical education: Do conferences, workshops, rounds, and other traditional continuing education activities change physician behavior or health care outcomes? *JAMA.* 1999;282(9): 867–874.

24 White CW, Albanese MA, Brown DD, Caplan RM. The effectiveness of continuing medical education in changing the behavior of physicians caring for patients with acute myocardial infarction: A controlled randomized trial. *Ann Intern Med.* 1985;102(5): 686–692.

25 Davis DA, Thomson MA, Oxman AD, Haynes RB. Changing physician performance: A systematic review of the effect of continuing medical education strategies. *JAMA.* 1995;274(9):700–706.

26 Myers SA, Gleicher N. A successful program to lower cesarean section rates. *N Engl J Med.* 1989;319(23): 1511–1516.

27 Wennberg JE, Blowers L, Parker R, Gittelsohn AM. Changes in tonsillectomy rates associated with feedback and review. *Pediatrics.* 1977;59(6):821–826.

28 Frazier LM, Brown JT, Divine GW, et al. Academia and clinic: Can physician education lower the cost of prescription drugs? A prospective, controlled trial. *Ann Intern Med.* 1991;115(2):116–121.

29 Marton KI, Tul V, Sox HC. Modifying test-ordering behavior in the outpatient medical clinic. *Arch Intern Med.* 1985;145(5):816–821.

30 Berwick DM, Coltin KL. Feedback reduces test use in a health maintenance organization. *JAMA.* 1986;255(11): 1450–1454.

31 Billi JE, Hejna GF, Wolf FM, et al. The effects of a cost-education program on hospital charges. *J Gen Internal Med.* 1987;2(5):306–311.

32 Billi JE, Duran-Arenas L, Wise CE, et al. The effects of a low-cost intervention program on hospital costs. *J Gen Internal Med.* 1992;7(4):411–416.

33 Manheim LM, Feinglass J, Hughs R, et al. Training house officers to be cost conscious: Effects of an educational intervention on charges and length of stay. *Med Care.* 1990; 28:29–42.

34 Zablocki E. *Sharing data with physicians, in changing physician practice patterns: Strategies for success in a capitated health care system.* Gaithersburg, MD: Aspen Executive Reports, Aspen Publishers; 1995.

35 Dyck FJ, Murphy FA, Murphy JK, et al. Effect of surveillance on the number of hysterectomies in the province of Saskatchewan. *N Engl J Med.* 1977;296(23):1326–1328.

36 Lomas J, Enkin M, Anderson GM, et al. Opinion leaders vs. audits and feedback to implement practice guidelines: Delivery after previous cesarean section. *JAMA.* 1991;265(17):2202–2207.

37 Lee TH, Pearson SD, Johnson PA, et al. Failure of information as an intervention to modify clinical management: A time-series trial in patients with acute chest pain. *Ann Intern Med.* 1995;122(6):434–437.

38 Axt-Adam P, van der Wouden JC, van der Does E. Influencing behavior of physicians ordering laboratory tests: A literature study. *Med Care.* 1993;31(9):784–794.

39 Parrino TA. The nonvalue of retrospective peer comparison feedback in containing hospital antibiotic costs. *Am J Med.* 1989;86(4):442–448.

40 Soumerai SB, McLaughlin TJ, Avorn J. Improving drug prescribing in primary care: A critical analysis of the experimental literature. *Milbank Q.* 1989;67(2):268–317.

41 Martin AR, Wolf MA, Thibodeau LA, et al. A trial of two strategies to modify the test-ordering behavior of medical residents. *N Engl J Med.* 1980;303(23):1330–1336.

42 Shanayfelt TM, Mayo-Smith MF, Rothwangl J. Are guidelines following guidelines? The methodological quality of clinical practice guidelines in the peer-reviewed medical literature. *JAMA.* 1999;281(20):1900–1905.

43 Costantini O, Papp KK, Como J, et al. Attitudes of faculty, housestaff, and medical students toward clinical practice guidelines. *Acad Med.* 1999;74(10):1138–1143.

44 Woolf SH. Practice guidelines: A new reality in medicine-III: Impact on patient care. *Arch Intern Med.* 1993;153(23):2646–2655.

45 Kosecoff J, Kanouse DE, Rogers WH, et al. Effects of the National Institutes of Health Consensus Development Program on physician practice. *JAMA.* 1987;258(19):2708–2713.

46 Lomas J, Anderson GM, Domnik-Pierre K, et al. Do practice guidelines guide practice? The effect of a consensus statement on the practice of physicians. *N Engl J Med.* 1989;321(19):1306–1311.

47 Soumersai SB, Avorn J. Principles of educational outreach ("academic detailing") to improve clinical decision making. *JAMA.* 1990;263:549–556.

48 Bandura A. *Social Foundations of Thought and Action.* Englewood Cliffs, NJ: Prentice Hall; 1986.

49 Clark N, Zimmerman BJ. A social cognitive view of self-regulated learning about health. *Health Educ Res.* 1990;5(3):371–379.

50 Clark NM, Gong M, Schork A, et al. Impact of education for physicians on patient outcomes. *Pediatrics.* 1998;101(5):831–836.

51 Inui TS, Yourtee EL, Williamson JW. Improving outcomes in hypertension after physician tutorials. *Ann Intern Med.* 1976;84(6):646–651.

52 Carlson KJ, Miller BA, Fowler FJ Jr. The Maine Women's Health Study I: Outcomes of hysterectomy. *Obstet Gynecol.* 1994;83(4):556–565.

53 Carlson KJ, Miller BA, Fowler FJ Jr. The Maine Women's Health Study II: Outcomes of non-surgical management of leiomyomas, abnormal bleeding, and chronic pelvic pain. *Obstet Gynecol.* 1994;83(4):566–572.

54 Atlas SJ, Deyo RA, Keller RB, *et al.* The Maine Lumbar Spine Study II: One year outcomes of surgical and non-surgical treatment of sciatica. *Spine.* 1996;21(15):1777–1786.

55 Atlas SJ et al. The Maine Lumbar Spine Study II: One year outcomes of surgical and non-surgical treatment of lumbar spinal stenosis. *Spine.* 1996;21(15):1787–1795.

56 Clark NM, Nothwehr F, Gong M, et al. Physician-patient partnership in managing chronic illness. *Acad Med.* 1995;70(11):957–959.

57 Spiegal JS, Shapiro MF, Berman B, Greenfield S. Changing physician test ordering in a university hospital: An intervention of physician participation, explicit criteria, and feedback. *Arch Intern Med.* 1989;149(3):549–553.

58 Healthcare Quality Improvement Act of 1986. 45 US Code §11101–11152. Sec 412, Standards for Professional Review Actions. http://www.nejm.org/toc/nejm/308/24/.

CHAPTER 10

Data Analysis and Provider Profiling in Health Plans

DAVID W. PLOCHER AND NANCY GARRETT

STUDY OBJECTIVES

- Understand general requirements for using data in medical management
- Understand basic report format requirements
- Understand basic types of reports and data for inpatient, outpatient, and ambulatory utilization
- Understand basic concepts of profiling, and the problems of profiling and approaches to dealing with those problems
- Understand the uses of data, and the strengths and weaknesses of different approaches to using data to manage medical care
- Understand the general advantages and pitfalls of case-mix/risk adjustment systems
- Understand the trends in profiling and medical informatics

DISCUSSION TOPICS

1. Discuss the principles of using data to manage health care delivery systems.
2. List and discuss the most important utilization and cost reports a medical director would need by model type, and describe the key elements in those reports.
3. Discuss the most common technical, clinical, and organizational problems medical directors face in using data to manage utilization, and what steps might be taken to deal with those problems.
4. Discuss the most important principles in provider profiling.
5. Discuss the most common problems with profiling and how a plan might address those problems.
6. Identify and discuss common sources of data accessed in producing data for medical management, and how problems with each of these data sources cause problems with the others.
7. Discuss the types of case mix measures available for each type of health care encounter, and the strengths and weaknesses of each type.
8. Discuss legal requirements regarding privacy and protected health information.
9. Discuss the challenges of public versus confidential disclosure of provider information
10. Discuss some of the questions to consider when considering a case-mix/risk adjustment system and/or profiling vendor.

■ INTRODUCTION

Employers, the main purchasers of commercial health services, are under increased pressure to price their products and services more competitively in a global economy. The highest priority for employers has become health care affordability. Large self-funded employers (Chapter 2) are increasingly turning to analysis of financial and clinical data for insights into the unique drivers of their health care cost excesses and demanding solutions. In response, health plans are putting more resources into development of reporting and analyses that will help plans provide these insights and solutions. Additionally, large employers often work with third-party consulting firms that specialize in data analysis and who are able to provide summarized data from many employers for comparison, rather than rely on the perspective of a single health plan.

In addition to large employer groups, other users of health plan measures include government programs such as Medicare Advantage (MA) and Medicare/Medicaid managed care plans, medical managers in health plans, providers, consumers, and the community. However, all health plan analytic activities can ultimately be linked to their use in providing service to health plans' customers: employers and members. Even as health plans continue to collaborate more with providers, as is discussed later in this chapter, the friendly reminder in all of these initiatives reverts to: "What do the people whose money you're spending think about you?" By necessity, the focus of these analytics is on administrative claims data. Claims are a type of universal language in the health plan business. Because of government standardization in the way health plan claims are submitted[*] and increasing sophistication by health plans, consulting firms, and health services researchers in applying uniform rules and definitions to claims data, measures based on administrative data can be compared across employer groups, plans, and regions of the country. Using claims data for analysis is affordable because the data are already collected for the purposes of claims payment and is based on common rules and definitions. Although use of administrative data has many limits and nuances, which are discussed further, it forms the backbone of health plans' analytic services.

The latter part of this chapter focuses on a specific analytic activity: provider profiling. *Profiling* means the identification, collection, collation, and analysis of data to develop provider-specific characterization of their performance. As used in this chapter, providers can be any type of provider of health services, including physicians, clinics, and hospitals. Provider profiling represents an important

application of analytics to efforts to improve quality and reduce costs for employer groups.

■ DATA SOURCES

In recent years data sources collected and used by health plans for data analysis have expanded beyond administrative claims data. They include lab test results, biometric information such as blood pressure or body mass index, feeds from electronic health records at clinics or hospitals, patient satisfaction with care received, and operational information on health management programs run by plans or vendors.

However, administrative claims data are still the backbone of most reporting and analysis efforts across plans. Because health plans pay the providers of care through claims, including hospitals, pharmacies, group physician practices, and individual physicians, this data is widely available and provides a complete view of how employers' health care dollars are being spent. Before it is useful for reporting and analysis, however, the data must be standardized and stored in a data warehouse.

Data Warehousing

The setting in which a health service takes place helps to determine the kind of claims that are submitted to the health plan. For example, electronic claims from a health care facility are submitted using a standard, the American National Standards Institute (ANSI) X12N 837 (required under the Health Insurance Portability and Accountability Act [HIPAA] for electronic claims submissions; see Chapters 18 and 23). Pharmacy claims are submitted in a different format maintained by the National Council for Prescription Drug Programs (NCPDP), often through a pharmacy benefit manager (PBM), a company that specializes in processing pharmacy claims, as discussed in Chapter 11.

Other types of administrative data used for health plan payment include membership information, demographic information about the health plan members and the benefits they have; and provider information, demographic and practice information about providers. Because the sources of the data are unique, plans often have separate software systems to process each type of data for claims payment.

To capture and integrate these diverse data sources for clinical reporting and analysis, plans have developed data warehouses. A *data warehouse* is a collection of a broad set of data spanning a significant period of time, as well as a repository of information derived from those data. Standard rules and definitions are applied to reduce data errors and make the data as consistent as possible. This process of applying uniform rules is challenging, given the many different systems that can exist within the same health plan and the differences in how individual providers of care code similar events.

---

[*]The mandate for standardization of electronic claims and other administrative transactions is a result of the Health Insurance Portability and Accountability Act, as discussed in Chapter 23.

Building a data warehouse also requires agreement within a plan on how business rules apply to various data sources. For example, one business unit such as underwriting may use a different definition of what makes up a managed care product compared to another unit, such as marketing. Therefore, creating a useful warehouse requires the collaboration of people throughout an organization.

Data warehouses are also built to maximize efficiency in reporting so that queries can be quickly returned even when accessing files with millions of claim lines. As the speed of the servers that store data and the software that queries against it improves, plans will be able to devote less time to pull data out of the warehouse and more time to analyze what it means. As an example of the types of data that would be available for analysis in a data warehouse, for provider profiling purposes the following data elements are generally necessary:

- Unique patient identifier (scrambled for patient confidentiality)
- Diagnostic information—typically provided using codes from the *International Classification of Diseases, Ninth Edition, Clinical Modification* (ICD-9-CM). The ICD-9 system will be replaced with the ICD-10 code set maintained by the World Health Organization in the United States on October 1, 2013.
- Procedural information—derived from Volume III of ICD-9-CM (which will be replaced with the ICD-10 Procedure Coding System in 2013), current procedure terminology (CPT), and HCFA Common Procedure Coding System (HCPCS) codes. In addition, identifying information relative to the name of the pharmaceutical used is often present.
- Level of service information—such as that provided by evaluation and management CPT codes.
- Paid dollar amounts from services ordered by the physician or health care facility. It is important to also know the total allowed amount for each service, decomposed into the amount the member and provider pays. This represents the total cost to society of health services, which is increasingly important as the share of member liability increases.[1]
- Unique provider identifier. A unique National Provider Identifier (NPI) is issued to health care providers by the Centers for Medicare and Medicaid Services (CMS), as discussed in Chapter 4.

Data warehouses are also being built across multiple health plans by national data consolidators. These consolidators, often private consulting and actuarial firms, specialize in cleansing data and applying uniform rules so that use of health care services can be analyzed for large populations. The consolidators use the national data warehouses for several purposes, including providing data comparing health plans on cost and utilization to large employers; calculating benchmarks of use and cost of health care services that plans can use to compare their performance to others; and conducting studies of postmarket drug reactions. The work of the consolidators in helping large employers interpret and compare their health care patterns is putting pressure on individual health plans to provide more analytical services to their clients. Also known as data cooperatives, these multipayer or, rarely, all-payer clearinghouses are especially valuable when a single payer has too little market share in the service area of interest. It provides more statistical power in comparative analytics by region because of larger sample sizes. And providers appreciate the convenience of mining data in only one source, versus each local payer's separate database.

Because creating a central data warehouse is very costly, another model being used to allow analytics across many payers is a distributed data warehouse. In this design, each plan keeps its data warehouse onsite, and common algorithms are applied to each set of data to produce consistent results. An example of this approach is the FDA's Sentinel Initiative, which is building a system for monitoring the postmarket safety of drugs and medical products using separate data warehouses from health insurance providers, health care systems, and the government.[2]

■ VALIDITY AND RELIABILITY

One issue in using claims data for reporting and analysis is validity, or the extent to which they actually mean what you think they mean. Even when there is great attention to diagnostic coding, the reason for a visit may or may not be related to everything that gets done (e.g., a patient is seen with the diagnosis of hypertension but also gets a hearing test) or the diagnostic code may not be the same as the underlying disease (e.g., a patient is seen for an upper respiratory infection, but the relevant diagnosis is emphysema). In addition to coding validity, it is important to validate data against other potential sources of the same data. The measures built using claims data must also be meaningful. It is of no value to measure things that have no real impact on the plan's ability to manage the system or a physician's ability to practice effectively. So the true test is whether the information obtained from the analytic report is actionable.

Another important consideration is the reliability of claims data, or the extent to which data are consistent and mean the same thing from provider to provider. For example, one provider may code differently from other providers for the same procedures, and a hospital may code an event differently from the attending physician. Diagnostic coding is particularly problematic when analyzing data from physician outpatient reports. Because diagnostic coding is not as important as procedural information in determining what a physician is paid, there is a great deal of laxity in diagnostic coding for office visits. Procedure coding tends to be more accurate because there is a direct relationship between what a provider codes as having been performed and what the provider gets paid.

Accuracy, however, does not rule out creative coding, coding abuse, or even fraud, resulting in deliberate coding inconsistencies, as discussed in Chapter 19. For example, one surgeon may bill for a total hysterectomy, whereas another surgeon performing the same procedure may bill for an exploratory laparotomy, removal of the uterus, removal of the ovaries, and lysis of adhesions, all of which generate a fee. The need for consistency may mean having to change or otherwise modify data to force conformance of meaning in the construction of a data warehouse.

Another challenge for health plans is the existence of different systems for claims processing for different products. It is common, for example, for the same plan to use one claims system to process commercial claims and a different system to process claims for its government programs such as Medicaid. The data coming from each source system must be standardized for a data warehouse to produce reliable data. Data standards mandated by HIPAA may have made this a bit easier, but it did not eliminate it as a challenge.

USE OF CLAIMS DATA FOR ANALYSIS AND REPORTING

Despite the challenges with reliability and validity of administrative claims data, they are the closest type of information we have to a universal language in the health plan business. Because there is no need for additional data collection efforts such as clinical chart abstraction, using claims data is relatively cost-effective. However, with recently increased adoption of electronic health records (EHRs), rich additions to reporting information are gradually being integrated with claims data into reports. Though it is beyond the scope of this chapter to expand beyond the use of claims data, there is great interest in adding information derived from EHRs, lab test results, health risk appraisals, patient satisfaction, patient self-reported health status, patient demographics/socioeconomic status/ethnicity, and so on. These additional data sources hold the promise of tracking measures of outcomes of care, such as whether a person's blood pressure level is controlled. At this time for most health plans, however, clinical data is incomplete and not yet fully integrated with administrative claims data.

Claims data are used to produce reports that monitor the utilization patterns and cost of health care, often on a per member per month (PMPM) basis, so that health plan actuaries can monitor changes in the population-wide cost of specific services. Reports provide a picture of utilization patterns from a clinical perspective, showing the types of treatment that members receive. By tracking the services

used by members with particular conditions, plans can produce process measures of the quality of care delivered. Claims also provide a basis for ad hoc investigation into specific clinical questions.

Although still sometimes criticized, claims-based data have been widely used for quality improvement purposes.[3] For example, the Maine Medical Assessment Project has extensively utilized inpatient claims data for the purpose of developing physician-specific profiles.[4] These profiles are then released directly to the physician. This project has had a significant impact on medical practice, not only because of the rigorous scientific nature of data elements used within the physician profiles, but, just as important, the release process of the profiles. That is, the physician profiles are not only released for internal purposes, but senior physicians have provided extensive follow-up to the physicians involved in this profile effort.

Controversy still exists with respect to the validity of using claims-based data for quality improvement purposes. Recently published literature has begun to address this controversy. Chen and colleagues at Yale University determined that at least one methodology—that used in the creation of the *U.S. News and World Report* Quality Ranking—correlated with outcomes and processes of care for the one condition examined, acute myocardial infarction (AMI, or "heart attack").[5] On the other hand, Iezzoni and colleagues determined that complication rates derived from claims data do not correlate with quality of care information abstracted from the medical record.[6] Health plans should be cognizant of the limitations of quality measures that rely only on claims data.

Visit-based ambulatory care claims data can also be used to provide comparative information pertaining to utilization of services across providers (provided that procedures are not a significant part of the case-mix adjustment that is used to account for differences in illness severity of the patient).[7] So long as the objective is clearly specified, profiling can also provide information pertaining to quality of care provided to enrollees. Thus, the following types of information obtained from visit-based ambulatory claims data are useful for physician profiles for quality monitoring purposes:

- Absence of a particular procedure, often referred to as a "gap in care" (such as vaccination or mammogram for preventive services or a retinal examination for a diabetic patient). Some HEDIS rates measure gaps in care, and many health management vendors develop and maintain sets of gaps in care measures that health plans can purchase. These vendors use complex algorithms to mine data for patterns indicating that patients have not received services important to managing their conditions. They also search for gaps in pharmacy use for patients who have been prescribed drugs for chronic disease management, calculating medication possession ratios (the day's supply of medication divided by the days between refills).

- Inappropriate use of health care services that do not follow practice guidelines and may unnecessarily increase health care costs. Examples include an MRI during a first office visit for uncomplicated low back pain, antibiotics used for viral upper respiratory infections, and brand name antibiotics used when a generic exists.

As summarized in a review of claims data used for physician report cards published in 1998: "Despite the imperfections, claims data can be extremely useful probes to improve utilization, target continuing medical education, help manage complex patients, identify underserved patients and detect misprescribing, as well as fraud and abuse."[8]

■ THE NEED TO ADJUST FOR RISK

When comparing populations on outcomes related to the quality or cost of care, an important step is to adjust for differences in the illness burden between them. A useful definition of risk adjustment is: "Risk adjustment (RA) consists of a series of techniques that account for the health status of patients when predicting or explaining costs of health care for defined populations or for evaluating retrospectively the performance of providers who care for them."[9] Without rigorous risk adjustment techniques, comparisons of outcomes between populations may be a result of the demographic and health characteristics of each group rather than the care provided.

The terms *risk adjustment*, *severity adjustment*, and *case-mix adjustment* are often used interchangeably. Sometimes, however, *case-mix adjustment* is used specifically to adjust inpatient hospital episodes, as opposed to a population-wide approach to controlling for differences in health status across patients. Until the industry arrives at more standardization of this terminology, it is therefore important to be clear about the definitions used in any particular situation.

Because risk adjustment techniques aim to separate the effect of treatment from characteristics inherent to the members, they need to be based on diagnosis rather than procedure codes. For example, a diagnosis code of diabetes indicates that a person is in a higher risk category for health care utilization compared to someone without diabetes. However, two people with the diagnosis of diabetes may have very different treatment patterns, and these treatment patterns should not influence the risk category because they are part of the outcome of interest. Traditionally, age and sex served as a proxy for severity and case-mix adjustments, as was discussed in Chapter 5 regarding capitation payments to physicians. The basic and valid argument is that utilization is predictable based on age and sex, using actuarial tables. However, age and sex account for only a portion

of risk, and more sophisticated models take into account population morbidity or other factors as well. Risk adjustment systems typically explain about 30% of the variance in outcomes. Other unmeasured population differences that influence health include socioeconomic status and psychosocial characteristics.

Risk adjustment requires different tools and approaches depending on the focus of analysis. Approaches for ambulatory visits, inpatient episodes, diagnosis-based risk adjustment, and nursing home care are discussed later.

Ambulatory Visits

Two classification systems were developed and are used in the profiling of individual ambulatory visits or encounters: ambulatory patient groups (APGs) and ambulatory payment classifications (APCs). APGs were developed as a forerunner and are quite similar to APCs. Both are in the public domain. The APCs are used by CMS for outpatient prospective payment in hospital outpatient departments and ambulatory surgery centers for Medicare patients as discussed in Chapter 5. APGs are also used by a variety of payers (e.g., Medicaid and many Blue Cross and Blue Shield plans). A number of companies produce software to implement these classification systems.

Inpatient Episodes

A number of case-mix classification systems are available for profiling of inpatient care. Two such examples are as follows:

- Medicare severity diagnosis-related groups (MS-DRGs) are used by CMS for prospective payment under Medicare. They include severity adjustment, often in three categories: without complications/comorbidities, with complications/comorbidities, and with major complications/comorbidities.
- All Patient Refined Diagnosis Related Groups (APR-DRGs; 3M/HIS Inc.) are proprietary, use claims data, and are commonly used for inpatient severity adjustment.

A number of intermediary vendors aggregate severity-adjusted data from either their own customers or from public use data to produce comparative data. These include not-for-profit alliances and proprietary companies. A practical issue the user needs to decide is whether to mold and manipulate the data in-house and thus have greater flexibility in creating one's own reports or to send the data to a third party and receive reports from that intermediary. Thus, for example, with respect to the APR-DRGs, users can license a workstation that provides both standard and ad hoc reports, but they still must load in their data, or they can work with a third-party vendor that processes the data and provides canned or, at a higher price, tailored reports. This choice is made based on economic issues, internal capabilities, and the need to manipulate data on a frequent basis.

A health plan or large provider system should understand several theoretical issues. One of the most contentious is the inclusion of complications versus comorbidities in the logic of the risk adjustment. For example, with specific respect to AMI, many secondary diagnoses present on admission after an AMI likely represent comorbidities or sequelae of the AMI. For example, if a patient develops complete atrioventricular blockage (a complication resulting in the heart's inability to beat properly) on the second day of admission, it is likely that this secondary diagnosis represents a comorbidity of the AMI and not an *avoidable* complication of an AMI. One could extend this analysis to a large number of other secondary diagnoses with specific respect to AMI, though not all, and the same issue occurs with many other acute illnesses.

Medicare has taken a step toward identifying avoidable complications in inpatient stays by determining whether a particular diagnosis is a hospital-acquired condition. Each diagnosis code is designated as either present on admission (POA), or not. If the diagnosis is present at the time of admission it is not considered a hospital-acquired condition. If it is not present at the time of admission, it may be categorized as a hospital-acquired condition if it meets certain criteria. Hospital-acquired conditions do not count as complications and may reduce the payment for a given inpatient MS-DRG. (Avoidable readmissions are discussed in some detail in Chapter 7.) That is, cases that contain hospital acquired conditions are paid as though the condition was not present, hence no added payment for secondary diagnoses categorized as hospital acquired conditions.

Diagnosis-Based Risk Adjustment

Several systems have been developed that adjust for risk based on combined inpatient, ambulatory, and pharmacy data. These systems involve algorithms that look for patterns of diagnosis codes that are associated with higher population morbidity and resource consumption. They allow for comparison of utilization between populations while holding the overall illness burden constant. Thus, they have been used to determine payments to health plans and providers, as well as for clinical analysis. Three major systems in this category are adjusted clinical groups (ACGs),[10] episode resource groups (ERGs), and diagnostic cost groups (DCGs).[11]

Nursing Home, Rehabilitation Facilities, and Home Care

The numerous proposals and enacted federal legislation to pay for these services on a prospective basis have heightened the importance of case-mix measures. Health plans will increasingly need to become familiar with these case-mix measures as disease management programs begin to use these types of facilities more frequently. Commonly used case-mix measures are as follows.

Resource utilization groups (RUGs) have the least severity adjustment built into the system. They are currently used in the prospective payment for nursing homes.[12] Functional independence measure (FIM) and the Patient Evaluation and Conference System (PECS) are used primarily for rehabilitation facilities. Both have excellent severity adjustment measures built into the system. Recently, function resource groups (FRGs) were developed, using the FIM, for prospective payment. The Outcome and Assessment Information Set (OASIS) has been developed as both a quality of care and payment tool for home care services.

■ PATIENT DATA CONFIDENTIALITY

There have always been requirements on providers and health plans to protect the confidentiality of patient information. Those requirements have been variable from state to state to some degree. That changed with HIPAA's stringent minimum set of privacy and security standards, although states remain free to impose even greater stringency (see Chapters 28 and 29). In addition to privacy and security standards, as noted earlier the implementing regulations for electronic business transactions also include detailed technical specifications based on ANSI X.12N transaction data standards for both the data fields contained in a transaction and for the electronic format for transmitting a transaction, and also mandates the use of standard procedure and diagnostic codes (discussed in Chapters 18 and 23). The Patient Protection and Affordable Care Act of 2010 (ACA) further strengthened HIPAA's privacy requirements.

HIPAA focuses on requirements to maintain the physical security of health information. The legislation applies to any person or organization that maintains or transmits electronic health information. HIPAA outlines standards for maintaining reasonable and appropriate administrative, technical, and physical safeguards. The safeguards aim to protect the physical security and integrity of personal health information from threats, hazards, or unauthorized uses. HIPAA prohibits wrongful disclosures of individually identifiable health information and prescribes penalties for violations.

HIPAA allows data to be used for medical management, including managing utilization and quality. It also allows for the use of "blinded" data—aggregate data for purposes of producing population-level reports—as long as there is no way for someone to use those data to trace back to an individual patient. Special protections are provided for mental health records. There are also situations where specific permission to use the data must be obtained from the patient (e.g., providing that information to an employer or to anyone who is not involved in the provision or direct management of the patient's medical care). HIPAA expressly prohibits the sale of patient-identifiable data for any marketing or sales purpose. The specific elements are described in Chapters 23 and 29 and the complete text of the HIPAA regulation is available at the CMS website.[13]

Based on the preceding, it is clear that the use of data for analytic purposes requires a high degree of attention to policy and procedure to protect member confidentiality. Methods to produce reports must take these confidentiality requirements into account. Nevertheless, these confidentiality requirements, while creating high standards, do not prevent health plans from using data.

■ EMPLOYER REPORTING AND ANALYSIS

The purchaser of health coverage is primarily interested in the data analyst's ability to identify cost drivers, that is, the main causes of claim trend escalation. Such discoveries are expected to lead to focused or customized solutions for reducing health care costs. The goal is trend mitigation, and employers would like to see their claim trend approximate the consumer price index.

The Fundamentals

Each employer wishes to see how its paid claims trend compares to competing employers in the same industry. Next, the portion of employee liability is also of interest. That is, has the employer been too paternalistic in taking on the vast majority of health care costs—or, conversely, has the option to cost shift been maximized to the point of contributing to workforce turnover?

For each type of service, the employer wants to see the health plan's accounting of exactly where excesses occur. For acute inpatient hospital services, is it unit cost (payment per confinement) or unit frequency (admits per thousand)? Such analysis continues for outpatient/ambulatory services. In addition, a repricing analysis may be performed in which unit cost is held constant in order to determine sources of excess utilization.

These excesses must be justified using credible benchmarks. As stated earlier, benchmarks should match the industry. There should also be adjustment by region of the country, product type such as health maintenance organization (HMO) versus preferred provider organization (PPO), demographic (commercial vs. MA vs. managed Medicaid), and illness burden (adjustment for severity of illness of the employer's workforce and dependants).

Clinical analyses of where an employer's health care dollars are being spent are often constructed using a Pareto chart of clinical categories of care, such as the major diagnostic categories recommended by the Agency for Health Care Research and Quality (AHRQ).[14] For the commercial employed population, the top three categories are often oncology, musculoskeletal, and cardiovascular. As excesses are explored, micro-contributors need to be addressed.

For example, high levels of emergency department services or of diagnostic imaging may represent overutilization that should be addressed.

Reports are often produced quarterly from the beginning of the year, with each quarter added on cumulatively so that the fourth quarter report represents the entire year of experience. This allows an employer to compare cost and utilization for a given set of quarters to the same period in the previous year and assess the impact of benefit design changes that usually occur on January 1.

Another important concept in analytics is claims run-out. Run-out refers to time that elapses after a reporting period to allow claims incurred during that period to be submitted by providers and processed by the plan. A typical employer report displays claims incurred during a reporting period with a 3-month run-out that allows for the most complete picture of utilization that occurred during that period. The employer is usually most concerned with the amount it pays toward the health care services, but it is also important to include the total allowed amount with member liability so the employer can assess the total cost of care and the cost burden on employees.

Increasingly, plans are delivering reports to employers through interactive websites. These sites allow employers to download prepopulated reports, produce reports by selecting variables like a timeframe or subpopulation, or create their own custom reports with report-building tools. Many vendors build these interactive reports for plans, while some plans use their internal information technology departments to build the reports. However, many employers don't have analysts on staff that can take full advantage of sophisticated reporting tools and may still rely on health plan analysts or third-party consultants to create and interpret reports.

Program Evaluation

Especially when the health plan charges an added fee for a particular medical management program, the plan analyst is required to show, using rigorous methods and metrics, the benefits-to-cost ratio for each program. Program evaluation involves both process and outcomes measures. For most employers the ultimate goal of health improvement programs is to save money by improving health, so analysts must determine return on investment (ROI) of each program. This is usually expressed as the ratio of dollars saved for each dollar invested (e.g., a 2:1 ROI). For the most controversial programs, shared payment of such reconciliation by an independent third party may be required.

For disease management programs, recently used methodologies include either a pre- and post-study measuring results with trended projections, as described in Chapter 8, or a controlled study, sometimes randomized, in which the two cohorts undergo adjustments to ensure comparability.

The Care Continuum Alliance has developed guidelines for measuring disease management programs to try to standardize methods and allow for comparison of programs.* To evaluate utilization management programs, an analyst first compares the service units per 1,000 for services that undergo a prior authorization process and compares the results to industry benchmarks (recall that various common utilization metrics were defined in Chapter 7). If utilization exceeds the benchmarks, the analyst creates a model to determine, for example, whether the added administrative costs of the prior authorization process are offset by savings associated with reducing the number of services.

Historic program evaluation techniques are centered on changes in direct claim costs, usually driven by utilization improvements. Today's analysts must add estimates of the indirect cost gains for the employer caused by improvements in productivity and "presenteeism." These indirect costs are harder to measure, but are necessary to provide a complete picture of the benefits of health improvement programs. An emerging body of research is helping to provide more tools to make this possible.[15]

Applied Research Studies

Health plans may also conduct applied health services research studies of topics of interest to employers. For example, a health plan could use its administrative claims data and analytical expertise to conduct a study of the effectiveness of consumer-directed health plans (CDHPs; see Chapter 2) in reducing utilization and cost. These studies help plans provide consultations to employers about effective medical management and motivational plan designs.[16, 17]

■ PROVIDER PROFILING

The purpose and uses of provider profiling span a wide range of provider strategies. Among those are payer–provider collaboration initiatives involving academic detailing, whereby a plan physician visits with provider groups to present their data and explain how they compare to the average of their specialty-matched peers. The discussions are collegial, and usually include options for performance improvement. Payers also use such data to determine which provider groups may be exempted from prior authorization requirements, due to the absence of excess utilization and internal capabilities. Profiling data is used to equip pay for performance programs (P4P; see Chapter 5) with metrics used for bonus calculation. Most metrics have been based on quality, although

sometimes metrics include efficiency or cost-effectiveness, such as the generic prescribing rate.

The natural extension of such detailed quality and cost data is to use it on a network level to divide, for example, the PPO into two tiers; the preferred tier with better quality and cost results have lower member cost-sharing, as described in Chapter 4. Or the same information can be used to form an exclusive provider organization (EPO; see Chapter 2) whereby the payer positions the most expensive providers who show no quality advantage to be out of network. A related application of similar data forms the basis for expanding a payer's centers of excellence network beyond solid organ and bone marrow transplants to, for example, bariatric surgery. Finally, in the pursuit of arrangements more conducive to enlightened payment reform and the ACA, performance data may be used as the basis for patient-centered medical homes and accountable care organizations (PCMHs and ACOs, respectively; see Chapter 2). Providers are increasingly as interested as payers in their big-picture comparative performance and how well their current practice patterns will serve them as they consider bundled payment contracts, gain- or risk-sharing terms, and global capitation.

When designing provider profiling reports, the following principles should be kept in mind:

- Identify high-volume and costly clinical areas to profile.
- Involve appropriate internal and external customers in the development and implementation of the profile.
- Involve the providers in the development and implementation of the profile.
- Compare results with published performance (external vs. internal norms).
- Report performance using a uniform clinical data set.
- When possible, employ an external data source for independent validation of the provider's data.
- Consider onsite verification of data from the provider's information system.
- Present comparative performance using clinically relevant risk stratification.
- Require measures of statistical significance for comparisons and establish thresholds for minimum sample size.
- Revise performance measurements using formal severity adjustment instruments.

Customers and Users of Provider Profiles

There are many customers or users of provider profiles. Identification of these customers and paying attention to their needs when developing and implementing the profile are important to success. Profiles are not inexpensive in both time and money. Profile customers include the following:

---

*Located at www.carecontinuum.org/OGR5_user_agreement.asp, current as of March 12, 2011.

- **Health plans:** All levels (provider relations, medical directors, etc.).
- **Consumers:** Although consumers are a key customer, we are still in the process of developing profiles and approaches to the effective dissemination to health plan members.[18]
- **Employers:** With notable exceptions, most employers are still less interested in quality than they are in cost control. Thus, to get employers interested in quality one must use tools and approaches that integrate cost control with quality.
- **Providers:** Most providers are interested in change if methods to measure performance are well grounded in scientific evidence or professional consensus.[19]

Public versus Internal Disclosure of Provider Profiles

A key flashpoint of debate is internal versus external disclosure of provider profiles. By way of example, there are nearly 20 states that produce publicly available profiles of hospital services. Health plans are beginning to use this information in their feedback loop to hospitals. The report format itself is an important aspect of the development process. For example, the state of Florida, which has released hospital-specific mortality and severity of illness rates for several years, has established wide confidence intervals and designed a format that places great emphasis on information and deliberately underemphasizes identification of poor or excellent performers. This approach improves the acceptance and utility of the report, while lowering the potential for sensationalism. The Commonwealth of Pennsylvania has undertaken similar efforts in producing reports on hospitals, taking into account severity adjustments, for years.

The National Committee for Quality Assurance (NCQA) uses the Healthcare Effectiveness Data Information Set (HEDIS®) to evaluate health plans and make this information available through its *Quality Compass* publication; see Chapter 15 for further discussion about NCQA, HEDIS, and health plan accreditation. The Integrated Healthcare Association in California as well as the Pacific Business Group on Health have used the HEDIS data set to evaluate medical groups and hospitals that contract with health plans. Minnesota Community Measurement is another example of an effort to pool data across health plans to provide quality measures to purchasers and consumers, and increasingly uses clinical data reported directly from providers to supplement claims data.[20] There are also several commercial Internet websites that provide rankings of health plans, hospitals, and/or physicians.

More recently, some health plans and employers have produced and released physician practice quality and service profiles to their members or employees and have reported a shifting in enrollment into practices that were reported as "best practices."[21] This is a significant step forward in the development of physician profiles for external or public release. Its importance derives from the fact that many physicians, particularly on the West Coast, are not solo practitioners or members of small medical groups; they are members of large medical groups that contract with health plans for the entire risk and are the key providers of medical care. Counterbalancing this concept, organized medicine in many states have successfully sued health plans to prevent disclosing physician-specific profiles.

■ DESIRED CHARACTERISTICS OF PROVIDER PROFILES

Provider profiles should share certain characteristics. They should:

- Accurately identify the provider in the profile;
- Accurately identify the specialty of the provider;
- Help to improve the process and outcome of care, both dollar and quality outcomes;
- Have a firm basis in scientific literature and professional consensus;
- Meet certain statistical thresholds of validity and reliability;
- Compare the provider to a norm;
- Cost the minimum amount possible to produce; and
- Respect patient confidentiality and, if obtaining information from the medical record or using patient-derived information, obtain patient consent.

Accurate Identification of the Provider

Methods to attribute health care services to a provider are critically important in producing provider profiles that are useful and acceptable to all parties. In a fragmented health care system where plans are increasingly set up on an open access model, attribution is not an easy problem to solve. To illustrate, some examples of methods considered in a provider profiling effort led by the state of Minnesota in 2010 include:

1. Plurality-minimum—All care is attributed to the one clinic with the greatest number of evaluation and management visits
2. Multiple-proportional—Care is attributed to clinics in proportion to the percent of evaluation and management visits so that one clinical episode of care could be assigned to multiple providers

Each of these methods has advantages and disadvantages. For example, in the multiple-proportional method, complex patients are attributed to each provider that works with them, which is easier to understand and may provide a stronger incentive for providers to coordinate care. However, this method may discourage a primary care physician from acting as the main manager of a complex patient's care.[22]

The level of analysis is also important to consider in provider profiling. Profiling at the individual physician level is often not possible because the number of episodes for each physician is too small. The resulting statistical instability introduces too much error to lead to robust comparative conclusions, as also noted in Chapter 5 in the discussion about P4P. Instead, profiling is often done at the clinic/group level. This also has the advantage of taking into account the fact that care is delivered by teams of providers, particularly for complex and chronic diseases; however, it is not without controversy as one study found that group results were not accurate predictors of individual physician performance within the group.[23]

There are increased efforts to link hospital and physician payment for services provided in the hospital because these data are usually not coming from the same sources. In other words, physician claims or encounters are entered into the system via both claims and medical management, whereas hospital data are likewise entered, but independently from the physician data. And none of these sets of data are automatically linked in most information systems. New models of payment under consideration for traditional Medicare such as bundled pricing and value-based payment (discussed in Chapter 5), all depend on some degree to being able to provide these linkages. More dramatic approaches, both those underway before passage of the ACA such as PCMHs and new models incorporated into the ACA such as ACOs depend very heavily on the ability to properly attribute costs of care to providers.

A final problem concerns the ability to detect linkages between practices and ancillary services. Examples include orthopedists who own physical therapy practices or neurologists who have a proprietary interest in a magnetic resonance imaging center. (This topic was explored in Chapter 7 in the section on physician self-referral.)

Accurate Identification of the Specialty Type

The specialty of the physician is not always clear. Most health plans have provider files that indicate what specialty type a physician has self-indicated, but it is surprising how often that information does not match up with specialty indicators in the claims file. Of course, health plans that perform comprehensive verification of board specialty status as part of the credentialing process (see Chapter 4) will have more accurate data than health plans that depend on self-reporting by physicians.

The problem of provider specialty definition is particularly acute when looking at primary care physicians (PCPs). As discussed in Chapter 4, many board-certified medical specialists actually spend a considerable amount of time performing primary care, whereas others spend the majority of their time practicing true specialty medicine. This has great implications for how a health plan will evaluate performance of specialists as well as PCPs when comparisons to peers are used (a common practice). Even within a single specialty there are differences in how specialized a specialist is. For example, a specialist may have a majority of primary care patients or may not care for patients in the intensive care unit (ICU). Therefore, the health plan will want to look at the degree to which a physician is truly a specialist in his or her mix of routine and complex cases.

Even when the issue of specialty definition is resolved, there remains the problem that no two practices are exactly alike. As an example, some general internists perform flexible sigmoidoscopies and some do not. If one looks only at charge patterns, the internist who performs the procedure will look more expensive compared to the internist who does not, but that analysis will fail to pick up the fact that the internist who does not perform flexible sigmoidoscopies instead refers them all to a gastroenterologist who charges more than the first internist (in addition, the first internist could be overutilizing the procedure or the second internist could be failing to provide this common preventive care activity, but those are separate types of analysis). The same problem arises outside of primary care medicine. For example, when neurosurgeons are assumed to be a homogeneous group, accurate profiling cannot be done when one neurosurgeon works only on arteriovenous malformations, another on brain tumors, and so on. This problem extends to related procedures, such as whether neurosurgeons or vascular surgeons perform carotid endarterectomies or whether neurosurgeons or orthopedists perform various types of spine fusions.

Improve Processes and Outcomes Using Scientific Criteria

Using data and profiling is also carried out by comparing performance against evidence-based clinical guidelines. Generally speaking, this can be done in one of four ways:

1. Accrediting organizations, such as NCQA, have increasingly put their screening items through a rigorous evaluation process.
2. Several proprietary software packages from reputable developers include guidelines or quality of care criteria.
3. Most will use professional literature, including peer-reviewed journals or trusted locations on the Internet, such as the website hosted by the Agency for Health Care Policy and Research, www.guideline.gov.
4. Self-development is always an option, but development of reliable and valid quality of care criteria always takes more time than one expects.

(Evidence-based clinical guidelines, including those provided by commercial vendors, are discussed at some length in Chapter 7.)

Need for Statistics

Appropriate statistical techniques are required for both care quality and efficiency criteria. Without their use, one can easily be misled by noise into arriving at a mistaken conclusion. Most stand-alone software packages have statistical tests embedded. If one is obtaining reports from the information technology department, it is important to ask for the addition of statistical tests, especially when faced with decisions pertaining to network determination. Reports should include basic measures of confidence, such as standard deviations or P values.

From a design point of view, it is likely that there will be enough data over time to profile a provider using statistical process control (SPC). "SPC consists of a set of powerful techniques to ensure the continued stability of any process and to detect the presence of sources of instability."[24] One can develop control charts or simpler reports if one is not able to use SPC for a wide variety of independent variables using claims data such as the following:

- Daily hospital census
- Length of stay
- Cost of care (by type of cost; claims forms are divided into approximately 20 departmental categories ranging from pharmaceutical to medical supply to intensive care units)

Compare the Provider to a Norm

Practice profiles are of no use unless the results are compared to some type of standard. Certain problems are inherent with comparisons in provider profiling, as already discussed. All these problems are resolvable, but medical managers need to be aware of them before embarking on profiling. Comparison against norms is necessary, but it is fraught with potential difficulties, chief of which is *defining* the norm. There are, broadly speaking, two types of norms: internal norms (i.e., one's own norms if one has enough members or patients) and comparative norms (using external data).

The usual way of comparing profiling results is to provide data for each individual practice in comparison to one or more of the following internal norms discussed earlier:

- **Total health plan average result**. This standard is simply the average for the entire health plan and is the crudest method of comparison.
- **Independent practice association (IPA) or preferred provider organization (PPO)**. A variation of health plan average, this compares the practice only to other practices within a set of providers smaller than the entire network. This approach may be combined with multiple other approaches when a health plan contracts through organized provider systems. Another variation on this is geography, even in the absence of organized provider groups.

- **Specialty specific or peer groups**. This compares each practice only to its own specialty (e.g., internists are only compared to other internists).
- **Peer group, adjusted for age, sex, and case mix/ severity of illness**. This is the most complicated approach, as noted earlier, but provides the most meaningful comparative data.
- **Budget**. This compares the profile to budgeted utilization and cost, a necessary activity when providers are accepting full or substantial risk for medical expenses.
- **Advanced and statistically based comparisons**. This is coupled with confidence intervals so that a provider will know whether the difference versus the peer group is statistically significant. Examples of comparative norms include the following:
  - Hospital charges or costs
  - Mortality
  - Group practice charges
  - Certain outcomes, such as hospital admission rates
  - Parameters of greatest interest to health plans, such as utilization rates (e.g., prescribing behavior), immunization, mammography, or other HEDIS rates

Some of these norms, such as hospital charges and mortality, may be augmented through public use state data files. Occasionally, state data repositories, such as those in Florida, California, Pennsylvania, and Texas, are adjusted using a reputable severity adjustment tool. More often than not, the state data repository is either not available or, if it is, no risk adjustment is performed. Normative data sets may be internally generated if the health plan is large or part of an alliance that pools similar data. Data sets tailored to the needs of a specific organization are also available for purchase from reputable commercial organizations.

Episodes of Care

As touched on earlier, grouping claims data into episodes of care is increasingly becoming a standard approach to efficiency analysis across providers. It provides a complete picture of care delivered across the health care continuum.

Episodes of care are defined as time-related intervals that have meaning to the behavior requiring measurement. Episodes may vary considerably both by clinical condition and by provider type. In the case of obstetrics, obvious measures, such as Caesarian section rate, are important but will not reveal the full picture. Looking at the entire prenatal and postnatal episode may reveal significant differences in the use of ultrasound and other diagnostics, differences in early detection and prevention of complications, or perhaps a great deal of unbundled claims during the prenatal period.

Furthermore, it is possible for patients with multiple medical conditions to have overlapping episodes of care, making it more difficult to sort out which resources are being used for which episode. Several of the proprietary software programs attempt to deal with this issue by, for example, identifying patients with both congestive heart failure (CHF) and diabetes and separating this group of patients from those who only have CHF.

Related to the issue of episode construction is the problem of identifying which provider is actually responsible for the patient's care at any one time. As an example, an internist or an endocrinologist may be responsible for the care of a diabetic but may have little responsibility for managing that patient's broken leg, other than to refer the patient to an orthopedist. Identification of the responsible physician is especially difficult for hospitalized patients; it is not uncommon for the admitting physician not to be the attending physician, especially when surgery is involved. The rapid increase in hospitalists providing much of the inpatient care further muddies the waters.

The hallmark of episode definition is the ability to link all the health resources into a defined event. This may mean diagnostic services (e.g., laboratory or imaging), therapeutic services (e.g., physical therapy), drugs, consultations, outpatient visits, and inpatient visits. In other words, it must be a patient-based analysis rather than a provider-based one; the analysis of the behavior of providers is a product of examining what happens to their patients. Several vendors have constructed proprietary episode grouping systems, such as Episode Treatment Groups (ETG)[25] and the Medical Episode Grouper (MEG).[26] However, episodes of care may contain heterogeneous levels of severity and thus require further risk adjustment to use them to compare utilization across populations.

■ LOCATION OF PROFILING ACTIVITY

Plans increasingly have capabilities to perform provider profiling on cost and quality in-house, using their data warehouse, analytic expertise, and purchased capabilities such as episode grouping and risk adjustment software and gaps in care or quality measurement algorithms. Another option is to outsource this activity to a third-party vendor, which can have the advantage of appearing more neutral to provider groups who are interested in as objective an analysis as possible of their performance.

■ IMPACT OF ICD-10

The complete planning for the impact of *International Classification of Disease, 10th Revision* (ICD-10) on the measurement activities discussed in this chapter would surpass space available in this book. In general, the huge redefinition of code values to ICD-10—scheduled for October 1, 2013—will likely require a transitional period of dual use.

An example is the potential impact on PCMH, ACO, and disease management program processes for the identification and stratification of members for outreach,

due to the deeper levels of information detail (assuming it is properly implemented in the first place). This is in concert with improved risk adjustment due to increased diagnosis code granularity, which will help target health management. It is important to note that as of today, we haven't quantified the improvement in predictive validity.

Provider performance measurement and monitoring will become more robust on several fronts. Medical necessity of device deployment will be much more precise, since the device coding will be enhanced. Fraud detection will be similarly improved. The increased density of diagnosis codes and procedure codes will improve the evaluation of provider effectiveness, since accuracy will improve for both cost and quality information. Cost information will be specifically enhanced when such coding improves payment accuracy, especially for risk adjusted payments. End results will include more meaningful pay for performance programs and public report cards. Furthermore, all benchmarking databases will have to be upgraded, and for the first time we will make more accurate international comparisons, for so many locations already on ICD-10.

Training and retraining for professionals involved in performance measurement will be considerable, with anecdotal estimates of at least 50 hours for each coder to learn ICD-10. On the plus side, ICD-10 may mean a much lower volume of physician office submission of supplemental information, since the richness of the new codes will more often suffice; however, ICD-10 does not replace the Current Procedural Terminology, 4th Revision (CPT-4) used by most physicians for billing, so the overall impact is hard to determine.

ICD-10 will have a major impact on MA Star ratings (Chapter 24) and HEDIS measures because the expanded diagnosis codes are in the denominators. HEDIS will begin to phase out of ICD-9 in 2015 (for the 2014 measurement year), codes will be removed from a measure when the look-back period for the measure, plus one additional year, has been exhausted, and there will be an overlap period.[*]

■ CONCLUSION

The primary future use of health plan data and analysis will reside under the umbrella term "transparency." For consumers, data will be accessed through the Internet to allow easily comprehended comparisons in cost and quality among providers. This will prompt more consumers to "vote with their feet," although the magnitude of market share shifts remains to be seen.

For providers, data and analysis provided by health plans, particularly when data are aggregated, allow them to see a more complete picture of the care they provide. Bolstered by seeing their contributions to longitudinal episodes

---

[*]Details are available at www.ncqa.org/tabid/1260/Default.aspx; current as of August 9, 2011.

and seeing their performance within their specialty, compared to matched peers, regional national averages, and gold standards, they will have customized information on which to produce quality/performance improvement programs. ACOs will likely accelerate this.

The secondary future use of these data is the same as it is today, which is for original health services research. By having access to national inventories of claims data, investigators will be in a unique position more quickly to find out "what works." For example, postmarket surveillance of Food and Drug Administration–approved drugs is often a poorly funded ad hoc process. Increasingly, one can use claims data for this purpose, avoiding the expense and time of conducting clinical studies. By isolating a drug code, initiating a downstream search for specific complications (ICD-10 diagnosis coded), and comparing the results with those who did not use that particular drug, postmarket drug surveillance can be expanded and improved. Similar analysis can be conducted looking for the unintended consequences of deployment of new medical devices.

It will represent a major step up from the still-to-be-admired data analyses and reports of the Agency for Healthcare Research and Quality through its Medical Expenditure Panel Survey.[*] Furthermore, research will be accelerated for discovering what kinds of behaviors are prompted by various innovations in benefit design. Ultimately, there will be better answers about the relationship between cost and quality in the delivery of health care services.

Endnotes

1 Claxton G, DiJulio B, Whitmore H, Pickreign JD, McHugh M, Osei-Anto A, Finder B. Health benefits in 2010: Premiums rise modestly, workers pay more toward coverage. *Health Affairs.* 2010;29(10):1942–1950.

2 U.S. Department of Health and Human Services, U.S. Food and Drug Administration, Center for Drug Evaluation and Research, Office of Medical Policy, The Sentinal Initiative: Access to Healthcare Data for More Than 25 Million Lives. July 2010. www.fda.gov/downloads/Safety/FDAsSentinelInitiative/UCM233360.pdf. Accessed March 24, 2011.

3 Goldfield N. *Physician Profiling and Risk Adjustment.* 2nd ed. Gaithersburg, MD: Aspen Publishers; 1999.

4 Schneiter EJ, Keller RB, Wennberg D. Physician partnering in Maine: An update from the Maine Medical Assessment Foundation. *Jt Comm J Qual Improv.* 1998;24(10):579–584.

5 Chen J, Radford MJ, Wang Y, Marciniak TA, Krumholz HM. Do "America's best hospitals" perform better for acute myocardial infarction? *N Engl J Med.* 1999;340(4):286–292.

6 Iezzoni LI, Davis RB, Palmer RH, et al. Does the Complications Screening Program flag cases with process of care problems? Using explicit criteria to judge processes. *Int J Qual Health Care.* 1999;11(2):107–118.

7 Goldfield N. A quality improvement process for ambulatory prospective payment. *J Ambul Care Manage.* 1993;16(2):50–60.

8 Dans PE. Caveat doctor: How to analyze claims-based report cards. *Jt Comm J Qual Improv.* 1998;24(1):21–30.

9 Blumenthal D, Weissman JS, Wachterman M, et al. The who, what, and why of risk adjustment: A technology on the cusp of adoption. *J Health Polit Policy Law.* 2005;30(3):453–473.

10 Starfield B, Weiner J, Mumford L, Steinwachs D. Ambulatory care groups: A categorization of diagnoses for research and management. *Health Serv Res.* 1991;26(1):53–74.

11 Ash A, Porell F, Gruenberg L, Sawitz E, Beiser A. Adjusting Medicare capitation payments using prior hospitalization data. *Health Care Financ Rev.* 1989;10(4):17–29.

12 MedPAC suggests modifications to SNF PPS system, new RUG III group may be an option. *Natl Rep Subacute Care.* March 10, 1999;7(5):3–5.

13 U.S. Department of Health and Human Services. Centers for Medicare and Medicaid Services: HIPPA Overview. www.cms.gov/HIPAAGenInfo/. Accessed March 25, 2011.

14 U.S. Department of Health and Human Services. Agency for Healthcare Research and Quality. www.ahrq.gov. Accessed May 19, 2006.

15 Goetzel RZ, Long SR, Ozminkowski RJ, et al. Health, absence, disability, and presenteeism cost estimates of certain physical and mental health conditions affecting U.S. employers. *J Occup Environ Med.* 2004;46(4):398–412.

16 Wilson AR, Rodin H, Garrett NA, Bargman EP, Harris LA, Pederson MK, Plocher DW. Comparing quality of care between a consumer-directed health plan and a traditional plan: An analysis of HEDIS measures related to management of chronic diseases. *Popul Health Manag.* 2009 Apr;12(2):61–67.

17 Wilson AR, Bargman EP, Pederson D, Wilson A, Garrett NA, Plocher DW, Ailiff PL Jr. More preventive care, and fewer emergency room visits and prescription drugs: Health care utilization in a consumer-driven health plan. *Benefits Q.* 2008;24(1):46–54.

18 Goldfield N, Larson C, Roblin D, *et al.* The content of report cards: Do primary care physicians and managed care medical directors know what health plan members think is important? *Jt Comm J Qual Improv.* 1999;25(8):422–433.

---

[*]www.meps.ahrq.gov/mepsweb/; current as of August 9, 2011.

19 Stason WB, Auerbach B, Bloomberg M, et al. *Principles for Profiling Physician Performance.* Walton: Massachusetts Medical Society; 1999.

20 Minnesota Community Measurement. 2010 Health Care Quality Report. Available at: http://www.mncm.org/site/. Accessed March 25, 2011.

21 Larkin H. Doctors starting to feel report cards' impact. *Am Med News.* July 26, 1999.

22 Brown R. "Provider Peer Grouping: Methodological Issues." Presentation at October 15, 2010, MN Community Measurement Forum, St. Paul, MN.

23 Mehrotra1 A, Adams JL, Thomas JT, McGlynn EA. Cost profiles: Should the focus be on individual physicians or physician groups? *Health Affairs.* 2010;29(8): 1532–1538.

24 Goldfield N. *Physician Profiling and Risk Adjustment.* 2nd ed. Gaithersburg, MD: Aspen Publishers; 1999.

25 Symmetry Health Data Systems. Episode Treatment Groups: An Illness Classification and Episode Building System. 2004. Available at: www.symmetry-health.com/ETGTut_Desc1.htm. Accessed March 30, 2006.

26 Thompson Medstat. Medical Episode Grouper. Available at: http://thomsonreuters.com/products_services/healthcare/healthcare_products/a-z/med_episode_grouper_health_plans/. Accessed March 25, 2011.

CHAPTER 11

Prescription Drug Benefits in Managed Care*

ROBERT P. NAVARRO, CRAIG S. STERN, AND RUSTY HAILEY

STUDY OBJECTIVES

- Understand why health plans began to manage pharmacy program costs in the early 1980s
- Understand the factors that contribute to pharmacy program costs
- Understand trends in pharmacy program costs and utilization rates
- Understand the metrics commonly used to measure and compare pharmacy program performance
- Understand the basic components of a pharmacy benefit management (PBM) information system
- Understand the advantages and disadvantages of using a PBM for pharmacy program management
- Understand how the Certificate of Coverage affects pharmacy benefit design
- Understand the basis components of a pharmacy benefit management program
- Understand factors involved in the legal basis of pharmacy benefit management
- Understand the components in a managed care pharmacy distribution network
- Understand the essential elements of a pharmacy provider contract, including the administrative requirements surrounding the dispensing process
- Understand the role of the drug formulary in pharmacy benefit management
- Understand the potential impact of drug formularies on drug access and utilization
- Understand the influence of prescription drug patient copayments on program costs, drug access, and utilization

DISCUSSION TOPICS

1. Discuss the market forces, trends, and changes in the drug benefit over the past 15 years.
2. Discuss the essential elements of a managed care pharmacy benefit management program.
3. Identify the components of pharmacy program costs and discuss the implications of each.

---

*Note: Company names in the chapter are current at the time of publication, but subsequent merger or acquisition with a resulting name change is always possible.

4. Discuss the advantages and disadvantages for a managed care plan in using a PBM to managed its pharmacy services.

5. Discuss the impact of prescription copayments, cost-sharing, and formulary tiering on pharmacy program costs, drug access, and utilization.

■ INTRODUCTION

Prescription drug benefits are a vital component of a comprehensive health care benefit. Appropriately prescribed and used pharmaceuticals are valuable medical resources to prevent or delay disease progression and reduce the use of expensive, higher-risk, medical interventions for many high-cost and high-prevalence diseases. Some of the medical conditions for which drugs commonly provide clinical, economic, or quality of life benefits include arthritis, asthma, numerous infections, many cancers, chronic obstructive pulmonary disease, dyslipidemia, depression, diabetes, gastroesophogeal reflux disease, heart failure, hypertension, migraine, multiple sclerosis, and many others.

Over 99% of employed workers, all state Medicaid beneficiaries, and, as of 2006, all Medicare Parts A- or B-eligible recipients, are eligible for Part D, outpatient prescription drug benefits.[1] Prescription drugs are a highly utilized health benefit. Persons in the age range of 19 to 64 years on average consume 11.3 retail prescriptions per year. Medicare age persons (65 years and older) obtain an average of 31.2 retail prescriptions per year.[2]

■ PRESCRIPTION DRUG COST AND UTILIZATION TRENDS

Prescription drug benefits represent a significant component of health care resource expenditures, and require continuous cost and quality management. Thirty years ago, health plan pharmacy benefits represented approximately 5% of total direct medical expenditures. Several important pharmaceutical market and benefit trends are occurring that will challenge prescription drug benefit management. Today, prescription drugs represent 10% of total U.S. health care expenditures,[3] although the pharmacy budget component of managed care organizations is closer to 20% and inpatient and outpatient medical costs are both just over 30%. Over 93% of all outpatient prescriptions dispensed are covered by a managed prescription drug program. The Medicare drug spend represented 19.8%, Medicaid was 8.5%, and other third parties represented 62.9% of the total spend. Cash represented only 8.8% of the retail prescription sales, down from 14% in 2005.[3]

The U.S. pharmaceutical market exceeded $300 billion for the first time in 2009. After historically low growth of 1.8% in 2008, the 2009 sales trend was 5.1%, with a 2.1% growth in prescriptions. Oncology drugs, the specialty

category, and generics each grew by almost 11%. At the same time, total prescription utilization growth was only 2.1%. Brand name drugs have shown a negative utilization trend, and generics now represent almost two-thirds of total prescription volume (although only 10% of sales).[4]

These data represent the entire U.S. market, including retail sales into commercial, Medicaid, and Medicare plans, with highly variable levels of prescription drug program management. In contrast, Express Scripts, a large pharmacy benefit manager (PBM), experienced in managing pharmacy program costs and utilization, reported their 2010 overall drug cost trend increased 3.0% (including prevalence, cost per unit, units per prescription, patent expirations, and new drug entries), although the traditional drug trend was 1.2% and the specialty trend was 16.4%.[5]

In 2010, pharmaceutical sales grew only 2%, while prescription volume grew just over 1%. Brand name drugs exhibited a slightly negative sales growth in 2010, with over a 10% reduction in total prescription volume. Generic sales grew by 22% and generic prescription volume grew by almost 6%.[6] Continued low-growth pharmacy program costs are expected due to almost $90 billion of important brand name drugs losing their patent over the next several years.[7] **Figure 11-1** summarizes the historical growth in U.S. pharmaceutical sales.

The management of prescription drug benefits continues to evolve to meet the dynamic and complex changes

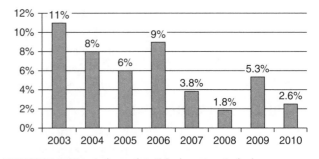

Prescription drug average annual sales increase

FIGURE 11-1 Historical growth in U.S. pharmaceutical sales.

Source: RP Navarro, 2011, based on data from the Kaiser Family Foundation Prescription Drug Trends 2010. Available at: www.kff.org/rxdrugs/upload/3057-08.pdf. Accessed April 8, 2011; IMS Health 2009 U.S. Pharmaceutical Market Trends: A Picture of Increasing Trends. Available at: www.imshealth.com/portal/site/imshealth/menuitem.a46c6d4df3db4b3d88f611019418c22a/?vgnextoid=b52325 7373a96210VgnVCM100000ed152ca2RCRD&vgnextfmt=default. Accessed April 8, 2011; D Long. IMS Health National Prescription Audit, November 2010, presented at the PCMA Managed Markets Educational Forum, Miami, FL, February 8, 2010.

occurring in private and public health care delivery and financing. The 2006 introduction of the Medicare Part D outpatient prescription drug benefit was a significant development that had a direct influence on commercial pharmacy benefit programs and formularies, as well as pharmacy costs. Within 5 years, the Centers for Medicare and Medicaid Services (CMS), through Medicare Part D, and, to a lesser degree, Medicaid program policies and regulations, has become as important as commercial plan sponsors in influencing outpatient prescription drug coverage and management. Within 10 years, the CMS programs will become the dominant force in the outpatient prescription market.

FUTURE TRENDS AFFECTING PHARMACY PROGRAM MANAGEMENT

The gradual implementation of the 2010 Patient Protection and Affordable Care Act (ACA) will have a dramatic, yet unknown, impact on total health care costs and outcomes due to the sweeping benefit coverage changes, the influx of previously uninsured patients, and the vague potential impact of various litigations that may challenge the legitimacy and implementation of portions of the Act.

Important trends will influence access and cost of prescription drug programs, as well as the outcomes expected from the appropriate use of cost-effective pharmaceuticals:

- The patent loss of approximately $90 billion of brand name drugs, resulting in sustained, low-cost trends in traditional, nonspecialty pharmaceuticals, largely a generic and more easily managed drug benefit.
- Simultaneously, there will be an increase in the number of specialty drugs approved by the Food and Drug Administration (FDA). Almost one-half of the approvals will be for self-injectable subcutaneous specialty drugs that will be covered under the prescription drug benefit with a coinsurance.
- As a result of the preceding trend, health plans will integrate some portion of the management of specialty drugs currently under the medical benefit (usually infused in physician offices or infusion centers) with their pharmacy benefits. The average cost of specialty prescriptions often exceeds $1,000 per month, and even a modest patient coinsurance of 20% or 30% may exceed the ability to pay for many patients. Lack of adherence leading to potential clinical failure may be an unintended consequence, and may lead to consumption of other more expensive medical resources, such as hospitalization.
- By 2019, CMS projects the number of beneficiaries in Medicare and Medicaid to grow by approximately 30%, while the number of members in private health insurance plans will remain fairly stable. There may also be 30 million individuals receiving health insurance through an insurance exchange, as a result of the ACA.[8]

- The ACA and CMS policy support the development of several initiatives to measure and promote practice patterns and risk-sharing contracts that improve outcomes and the quality of care. Comparative effective research (CER) offers the promise of providing data that allow greater consideration of outcomes in drug formulary decisions and future benefit design. Accountable care organizations and patient-centered medical homes (ACOs and PCMHs, respectively; see Chapter 2) present an opportunity for health plans and medical groups to expand risk-sharing that may include the cost of prescriptions for participating physicians. If drug cost and outcomes are included into risk-sharing contracts and pay-for-performance contracts, in theory outcomes-based contracting with pharmaceutical manufacturers could also occur.
- ACOs and PCMHs would be difficult without integrated health information technology (HIT) and intelligent decision support systems. Electronic prescribing is an important component that may reduce drug interactions and adverse effects (and possibly reduced hospitalizations secondary to adverse drug events), as well as improve formulary conformance and enhance drug adherence by alerting physicians when patients are delinquent in refilling prescriptions.
- Finally, as the focus on cost containment increases, health plans and PBM will likely implement greater restrictions on their formularies, and we may see a revival of closed formularies popular in the past. As more drugs are launched into specialty categories, these drugs will also be subject to similar cost and utilization management strategies that have been successfully applied to manage prescription drug programs for four decades.

These and other nonpharmacy trends, such as the growing epidemic of obesity (contributing to diabetes and cardiovascular disease) and the expanding over-65 age cohort (with increasing drug use subsequent to the medical vicissitudes of age), will present impossible challenges to U.S. health care policymakers and administrators of prescription drug programs.

BUSINESS RELATIONSHIPS AND THE FLOW OF MONEY

Prescription drug benefits are developed and managed within health plans or by PBMs, or both. A PBM may be unnecessary for health plans with an adequate pharmacy department staff capable of operating a complete pharmacy program without using an external PBM. However, PBMs offer a variety of services in a cost-efficient manner, and most health plans use PBMs for some services. Even large health plans and insurers may use an external PBM for some services, such as for claims processing or a pharmacy network.

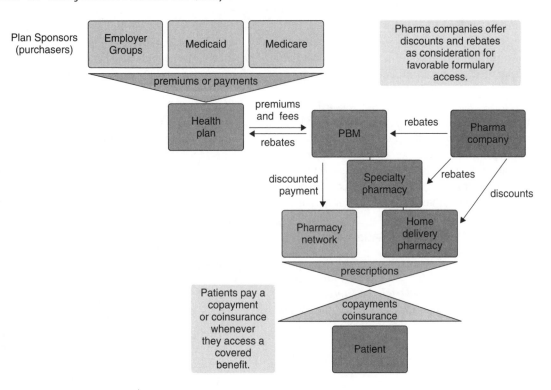

FIGURE 11-2 Role of a PBM when providing prescription drug benefits through a health plan.
Source: Navarro (2011).

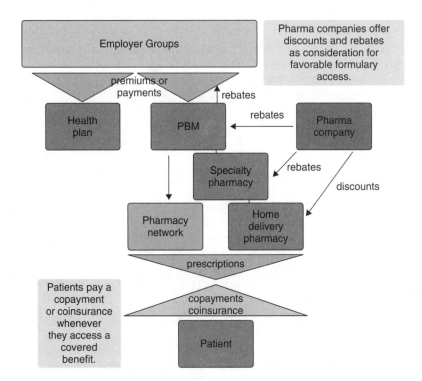

FIGURE 11-3 Role of a PBM when providing carve-out prescription drug benefits directly to plan sponsors.
Source: Navarro (2011).

In **Figure 11-2** and **Figure 11-3**, the PBM is shown to have internal mail service and specialty pharmacies, but contracts with community retail pharmacies to provide the majority of outpatient prescription drugs paid to members. The pharmacy department within a large insurer is often termed a "captive PBM," as they offer all PBM services, and may offer their services to plan sponsors outside of the parent health plan. CIGNA Pharmacy Management and Humana Pharmacy Solutions may be considered examples of captive PBMs. As discussed later, PBMs often contract directly with pharmaceutical manufacturers to obtain discounts and rebates on contracted products in exchange for improved formulary access, and health plans obtain access to discounted pharmaceuticals under PBM contracts. Large health plans may contract directly with pharmaceutical companies and not through a PBM (but usually not directly *and* through a PBM without specific written notification).

Plan sponsors are purchasers of health or pharmacy benefits. Plan sponsors include private corporations (commercial plans), State Medicaid programs, CMS Medicare plans, and other purchasers. Figure 11-2 illustrates the business relationships when plan sponsors contract with a health plan for medical and pharmacy benefits and the health plan subcontracts with a PBM to provide all or some of the components of a prescription drug benefit, including contracting with pharmaceutical manufacturers.

Plan sponsors may also contract directly with PBMs to purchase carve-out prescription drug benefits, as illustrated in Figure 11-3. PBMs and Medicare Advantage plans may also offer Medicare Part D prescription drug benefits directly to individual Medicare recipients, independent of health plan benefits (not shown in figure).

Health plans also contract directly with pharmaceutical manufacturers, bypassing the PBM from the flow of rebate dollars (not shown in figure).

▪ PHARMACY BENEFIT MANAGERS

PBMs are companies that specialize in developing and managing prescription drug benefits for a variety of private and public plan sponsors.[9] The largest three PBMs at the time of publication—CVS Caremark, Medco Health,[*] and Express Scripts—provide prescription drug benefits to over 200 million Americans through commercial, managed Medicaid, and Medicare Part D programs. CVS Caremark had net revenue of approximately $98 billion in 2010, providing prescription benefits for 67 million members.[10] Medco 2010 net revenue was $66 billion and processed over 740 million prescriptions (3.6 million were e-prescriptions), including almost 110 million prescriptions dispensed through their own mail service pharmacy.[11] In 2010, Express Scripts

processed 753 million prescriptions, and had 2010 revenue of $44 billion, almost double the 2009 revenue.[12] Obviously, PBMs, as well as others, are dominant forces in prescription drug benefit programs and management.

The economies of scale allow PBMs to provide comprehensive prescription drug benefits or various pharmacy benefit management components to augment internal health plan prescription drug benefits.[†] For example, a large, sophisticated health plan with an internal pharmacy benefit may only use the PBM for claims processing, and develop and manage all other aspects of a prescription drug benefit internally. In contrast, smaller health plans may maintain the responsibility for formulary decisions, but use the PBM for all other pharmacy benefit requirements (e.g., claims processing, drug contracting, pharmacy network development, and pharmacy program experience reports). A large employer group does not have the internal knowledge or resources to develop and manage a prescription drug program and will obtain this benefit through their medical provider plan or contract directly with a PBM.

PBMs generally do not accept a fiduciary responsibility for the customers, and rarely accept the risk of the prescription drug benefits they administer.[13] Instead, most PBM contracts with plan sponsors are administrative services only (ASO) contracts through which the PBM passes discounted paid claims, plus an administrative fee, to the plan sponsor for payment. Several analyses have shown that PBMs have been controlling the cost of prescription drug program operations. As early as 2003, the U.S. General Accounting Office reported PBMs obtained substantial pharmacy program savings for the Federal Employee Health Benefit Program.[14]

Pharmacy benefit management is a highly competitive business, and PBMs must understand and satisfy the diverse and dynamic cost and quality management objectives of their plan sponsors. Not wishing to compete on price alone, PBMs have developed an array of related management, patient care, and clinical services to improve adherence, appropriate use, and drug-related outcomes. PBMs had been criticized for a lack of transparency in passing on the value of pharmaceutical manufacturer rebate contracts to their plan sponsor customers. Private and government litigations[15, 16] over the past two decades have improved rebate accountability. In response, many PBMs claim transparency in pharmaceutical contracting, although the contracts remain confidential; some PBMs claim to be "100% transparent."[17]

Although PBMs are responsible for prescription drug benefit costs and not medical benefit costs, it would be incorrect to assume PBMs are unconcerned with clinical and economic outcomes. PBMs attempt to act in the best long-term interests of plan sponsors and offer a clinically

---

[*] At the time of publication, Medco Health announced it was being acquired by Express Scripts, but the acquisition had not yet been completed.

[†] A directory of PBMs is available from the Pharmacy Benefit Management Institute (www.pbmi.com/pbmdir.asp).

balanced drug formulary at the lowest possible cost without jeopardizing patient care. PBMs provide a variety of management services, either as a comprehensive pharmacy benefit or as à la carte components to supplement the internal pharmacy programs of large health plans that manage their pharmacy benefit with an internal pharmacy department.

Typical services offered by a PBM, customized for the need of plan sponsors and health plan customers, are:

- Claims processing and management reports
- Community retail pharmacy provider network
- Home delivery prescriptions (mail service pharmacy option)
- Specialty pharmacy distribution services
- Drug formulary development and management
- Pharmaceutical manufacturer contracting
- Customized pharmacy benefit design development and administration
- Clinical pharmacy programs, including drug utilization review and medication therapy management (MTM) programs
- Other customized services requested by plan sponsor.

Future PBM Services

PBMs will embellish their core services with greater focus on patient services, improved adherence interventions, behavior modification to encourage healthy lifestyles and appropriate drug utilization, and genomics testing (see later) to be prepared to develop personalized pharmacotherapy solutions when the market develops to the point of broad commercialization. Express Scripts has a separate website that addresses behavioral modification to improve patients' effectiveness in making lifestyle and health care access and utilization decisions.[18] PBMs are well positioned to increase their membership and structure novel benefit designs to accommodate the coming changes emerging from implementation of the ACA.

■ PRESCRIPTION DRUG PROGRAM MANAGEMENT COMPONENTS

Aggressively managed prescription drug programs are able to reduce pharmacy expenses by 25% or more, depending on the prior benefit design and the willingness of the plan sponsor to implement strident management strategies, as discussed later. However, today it is unlikely to find an employer group naive to managed prescription drug programs, and significant incremental pharmacy program cost reductions are difficult to achieve, except with greater cost-shifting to patients and aggressive use of generic drugs. The PBM CVS Caremark claims an ability to achieve a 20% reduction in pharmacy benefit costs by implementing specific strategies presumably in a relatively unmanaged plan sponsor.[19]

Managed prescription drug programs share the same general components that have been used for over 30 years, but are highly variable in project objectives, benefit design emphasis, and component execution intensity. The most striking evolution is the advance in health information technology that has allowed health plans and PBMs to implement their programs more effectively and accurately with greater customer flexibility, and obtain actionable data for timely decisions. Prescription drug benefit program management strategies are designed to manage the supply cost and utilization demand to best meet, or exceed, the business and quality objectives of plan sponsors. The general approach used for over three decades have included the following:

- Certificate or evidence of coverage—legal enforcement of the benefit design
- Pharmacy benefit design—plan sponsor-specific benefit management strategies
- Drug formulary—dynamic list of covered drugs and access rules
- Pharmacy provider network—drug distribution channels to provide member access to covered drugs
- Information technology—claims processing and decision support systems to optimize program performance
- Drug Utilization Review (DUR), MTM, and clinical programs—resources to support patients and maximize outcomes

■ PHARMACY BENEFIT DESIGN

The benefit design is a summation of covered benefits and access rules the health plan or PBM develops in concert with the plan sponsor purchasing the pharmacy benefit. The provider and customer, often with the counsel of an external benefit consultant, discusses and negotiates the specific coverage options, additional services, access rules, and patient cost-sharing strategies that will best satisfy the plan sponsor's goals of providing pharmacy benefits for employees or beneficiaries. All parties must not forget that drugs generally represent a cost-beneficial health care expenditure if they are able to prevent or delay the consumption of more expensive medical resources, such as an inpatient stay or ER visit.

The art and science of designing and managing a benefit that balances cost and quality of care is a challenge. Cost management should consider near-term pharmacy budget expenses, of course, but must also consider long-term total direct medical costs and the potential contribution of drug use on both short- and long-term medical outcomes and costs. This potential value of pharmacy benefits is often lost on plan sponsors that are desperate to reduce near-term costs and implements significantly higher cost-sharing onto employees. The unintended consequences resulting from drug nonadherence may be more costly than the avoided drug costs. Rather than severely restricting or eliminating pharmacy benefits, MCOs and PBMs attempt to counsel their plan sponsor customers to purchase a balanced and clinically responsive benefit design than allows affordable access to necessary drugs, while providing incentives for patients to ask their physicians to prescribe generic or preferred brand name drugs whenever possible and necessary. Many high-cost and popular traditional (nonspecialty) brand name drugs will lose their patent over the next decade and as generic drug use increases, there will be a mitigation of the pharmacy cost trend. Additionally, a growing percent of pipeline drugs are specialty drugs, and the cost contribution will grow in importance and replace the current concern on brand name nonspecialty drugs. As we discuss later, health plans are moving specialty medications now covered under the medical benefit to the pharmacy benefit, or are applying pharmacy benefit management strategies to injectables that remain under the medical benefit. This will result in greater patient cost-sharing and coinsurance that may threaten adherence based on the patient's inability to pay. These issues will require innovative approaches to benefit design that consider the prescription drug benefit not as an isolated cost center, but a potential value center. This may especially challenge some PBMs that are measured primarily on pharmacy budget cost trends and patient satisfaction. Clearly, plan sponsors must take an integrated approach to designing their medical and pharmacy benefit designs.

Approximately a decade ago the concept of a value-based insurance design (VBID) was introduced to reduce copayment barriers for high-value pharmaceuticals. Some employer groups and health plans have lowered the member cost-share burden on selected "high-value" drugs with the intended consequence of lowering the cost-share burden to the patient. The literature reports some positive experiences with VBID adherence.[20-22] However, an extensive review of the VBID literature revealed equivocal if not disappointing outcomes of VBID.[23] Clearly, additional research is required, especially as we move to an era of greater accountability and emphasis on quality outcomes.

■ EVIDENCE OF COVERAGE

Managed prescription drug programs are governed by state and federal laws and regulations, as described in Chapters 2, 20, 28, and 29. In addition, state Boards of Pharmacy govern the practice of pharmacy, and variable state pharmacy laws may influence drug coverage, generic substitution and therapeutic interchange, "any willing provider" pharmacy provider contracting and payment, mail service pharmacy delivery, specialty drug handling, and other issues.

Prescription drug benefits are also subject to the contract between the benefit purchaser (plan sponsor) and the insurer, health plan, or PBM providing pharmacy benefits. This contract, often named the evidence of coverage (EOC), certificate of coverage, or other similar term, defines the pharmacy benefit inclusions, exclusions, specific riders to include specific drug categories (e.g., oral contraceptives, smoking cessation, sexual dysfunction, infertility drugs), drug access rules (e.g., drug formulary, member cost-sharing [copayments or coinsurance], and member deductibles, out-of-pocket maximums, and many other benefit coverage stipulations).[24] The EOC is discussed further in Chapter 20.

Health plans (or PBMs) execute contracts with the pharmacy providers within their network to dispense covered prescription benefits to covered members according the *Pharmacy Provider Policy and Procedure Manual.* The drug formularies are dynamic and continuously updated as new drugs are launched, and new safety and efficacy data are published. Therefore, the plan sponsor and pharmacy provider contracts could not identify covered drugs by name. Rather, the contracts specify that covered benefits include those drugs listed in the plan or PBM drug formulary, and the specific drugs covered "will change from time to time." However, the EOC and the pharmacy provider contracts summarize covered benefits and access rules, and usually specify the general types or categories of drugs that are excluded from coverage:

- Experimental or investigational drugs (drugs not approved by the FDA for commercial sale within the United States).
- FDA-approved drugs when prescribed for unapproved indications ("off-label" use).
- Drugs used for cosmetic purposes (e.g., botulinum toxin) or specific purposes (e.g., erectile dysfunction, smoking cessation, infertility, others). These drugs may be specifically covered through a plan sponsor contract rider, but may incur higher premium and/or patient cost-sharing requirements.
- Drugs available without a prescription (over-the-counter [OTC] drugs). Insulin is a nonprescription drug in many states but generally is covered by health plan and PBM prescription drug programs.
- Most EOCs have riders that specifically address plan sponsor coverage decisions. For example, the documents often include language that excludes coverage for "unproven" uses, even of FDA-approved drugs. This refers to the plan or PBM having full discretion to not cover a drug for an unlabeled, off-label use. This is generally unenforceable for prescriptions not requiring prior approval before dispensing (i.e., most nonspecialty prescriptions dispensed through a community or mail service pharmacy). This does not indicate plans or PBMs will avoid covering all off-label coverage, if

possible. In fact, they will specifically cover off-label use if it is justified or necessary and supported by specialty opinions, guidelines, compendia, published literature, or other evidence-based information.

Neither the plan, the PBM, nor the EOC regulate what a physician may *prescribe* for a health plan or PBM member, but it does govern what the plan or PBM will *pay*. Members may confuse this point, and may not understand why an FDA-approved, prescribed drug is not covered. It is also important to note that health plans and PBMs allow for coverage of an otherwise noncovered drug with a medical exception, if requested by the member's physician and if approved by the health plan or PBM. Additionally, patients may pay cash for any noncovered prescription.

■ HEALTH INFORMATION SYSTEMS AND CLAIMS PROCESSING[25]

Effective prescription drug benefit management is highly dependent upon accurate claims adjudication systems and internal information-processing systems. Organizations that are best equipped to collect, analyze, and manage information will improve decision making and compete more effectively in the highly competitive health care marketplace. Participating pharmacy providers rely upon point-of-service access to accurate eligibility information to quickly and accurately process millions of third-party claims every day. The amount of demographic, financial, and clinical information that pharmacists need to acquire and manage their patients is staggering and growing in complexity. Online, real-time pharmacy claims processing has followed a universal data processing standard maintained by the National Council for Prescription Drug Programs (NCPDP). The NCPDP standard has allowed pharmacies the unique capability to process over 96% of pharmacy claims interactively in real time with hundreds of third-party payers. This has offered the pharmacy an unparalleled position in electronic commerce that other segments of the health care industry are still striving to achieve, even after almost three decades.

Medical and pharmacy benefit designs are becoming increasingly numerous, dynamic, and complex. Insurers must manage a variety of products such as:

- Commercial insured products;
- Self-funded employer benefits plans;
- Managed Medicaid for several states;
- Medicare Part D benefits;
- Different benefit designs such as
  - HMOs,
  - PPOs, and
  - Point of service (POS) plans, hybrids;
- Plans associated with various savings options such as
  - High-deductible health plans (HDHPs),

- Consumer-directed health plans (CDHPs) with
  - A health savings account (HSA) or
  - A health reimbursement account (HRA); and
- Flexible spending accounts (FSAs).

All of these plans, designs, and accounts, which are described in Chapter 2, potentially have different formularies and cost-sharing and tier structures. Data from these and other files must be converted into actionable information accessible by a variety of individuals for disparate applications throughout the business day. Drug claim files may be merged with medical claim files to generate an integrated database suitable to support clinical management decisions and clinical research.

■ ELECTRONIC PRESCRIBING

Electronic prescribing (e-prescribing) establishes an electronic communications network among a prescribing physician, a dispensing pharmacy, and a claims adjudicator. A switching company is usually involved that develops and maintains the electronic system. Hospitals, especially Veterans Administration hospitals, have used computerized physician order entry (CPOE) and electronic medical records for several years as a method of reducing ordering errors, providing health care professionals more complete and timely patient information at the point of care, and improving order and delivery efficiency. Outpatient e-prescribing pilot programs began over a decade ago, and today deployment is slowly expanding by several e-prescribing solution companies.

A physician or a designated health care professional engages in e-prescribing at or near the point of care using a computer or a hand-held device. The e-prescribing device provides the physician with the drug formulary options for a specific patient, a copayment amount, and a complete history of prescription drug claims for the patient that have been captured by the system, even if written by other physicians. The system will not include a cash prescription transaction not processed through the claims system. The physician can renew or prescribe a new drug for a specific patient that conforms with the patient's drug formulary, and ideally the system will guide the physician in avoiding drug interactions, redundant medications (based on the provided drug history), dosing errors, or other prescription problems, and will send the prescription to the participating pharmacy of the patient's choice. Prescriptions are considered "clean" if it clears the various edits. However, studies have shown physicians using e-prescribing continue to make input errors, and transmitted electronic prescriptions are not 100% error-free. Some existing systems are ponderously slow, with the patient arriving at the pharmacy before the electronic prescription.

The Surescripts 2009 National Progress Report on E-Prescribing indicates 81 million prescriptions were transmitted electronically in 2009 to 53,000 community pharmacies (85% of all retail pharmacies).[26] (Surescripts is a health information technology company that offers an e-prescribing solution.) Approximately 25% of all prescribers have access to an e-prescribing portal. However, the cost of deployment and the acceptance by many physicians remains a barrier to rapid deployment, and e-prescribing should benefit by the Health Information Technology for Economic and Clinical Health (HITECH) Act component of the American Recovery and Reinvestment Act dedicated toward health information technology, funded at $19 billion.[27] Experience will prove if e-prescribing fulfills the promise of improved patient safety, reduced drug interaction, lower costs, and improved adherence. Surescripts reports that 20% of paper prescriptions are never brought to the pharmacy, and e-prescribing has increased the number of prescriptions filled by 11%.[28]

The development of ACOs and PCMHs (see later) will depend on a sophisticated health information technology system; e-prescribing is a logical requirement to ensure physicians have the necessary drug history and prescribing information at the point of prescribing. Medco Health accepted over 10% of processed claims through e-prescribing in 2009.[29]

■ PHARMACY DISTRIBUTION NETWORK

Efficient and accurate drug distribution completes the journey of the drug product from the pharmaceutical company to the patient. The three primary channels of distribution include retail pharmacy, mail service (also called "home delivery"), and specialty pharmacies for specialty

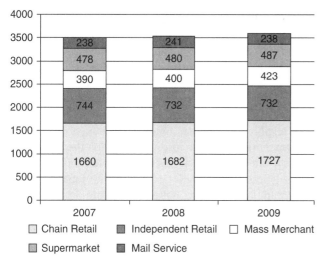

FIGURE 11-4 Trends in prescription volume in retail, mail, and specialty pharmacy. (*Y*-axis is in millions of prescriptions.)
Source: Navarro (2011). Adapted from data found at NACDS Community Pharmacy Results. Available at www.nacds.org/wmspage.cfm?parm1=6538. Accessed April 6, 2011.

pharmaceuticals. Retail remains the most important distribution channel. Approximately 14% of nonspecialty prescriptions are dispensed through mail delivery. **Figure 11-4** illustrates the retail prescription volume dispensed by store type.

■ DEVELOPING AN OUTPATIENT PHARMACY PROVIDER NETWORK[30]

Health plans and PBMs develop pharmacy distribution channels that balance pharmacy benefit access and cost management for their plan sponsors' members. Closed-panel health plans such as staff or group model HMOs (see Chapter 2) may operate their own outpatient pharmacies within their medical clinics for greater cost management and formulary control. If their membership is distributed through a large service area, they may supplement their internal network with community pharmacies and mail service. Open-model plans and national insurers use a community retail pharmacy network supplemented with mail service pharmacy. Plans may develop their own pharmacy network; most use their PBM's network.

Outpatient pharmacy network geographic coverage is based on the location of health plan medical facilities and plan sponsor members. Health plan and PBM contracts with plan sponsors may require a pharmacy provider be within a defined distance from members' homes or workplaces (e.g., 5 miles or less). There is an inverse relationship between pharmacy outpatient network size and cost; that is, a small number of contracted pharmacies (usually chains) will accept a lower prescription payment in exchange for having access to a larger number of members. Large national pharmacy networks may contain approximately 60,000 retail pharmacies. A restricted network may contain 5,000 pharmacies or less for a plan sponsor or health plan with a limited service area. Restricted networks generally include one or two national pharmacy chains and mail service to accommodate members visiting other states.

■ PHARMACY PROVIDER CONTRACTS AND CLAIMS ADJUDICATION

All contracted pharmacies are bound by a provider agreement that stipulates they will dispense prescriptions to eligible members in accordance with drug benefit and coverage policies, as explained in the *Participating Pharmacy Policy and Procedure Manual*, updated from time to time by the health plan or PBM. Participating pharmacies must use an online, real-time point-of-dispensing claims adjudication system to verify member, provider, and drug eligibility, and to determine drug coverage status, member copayment, and verify payments. Participating pharmacies also agree to participate in onsite audits by a representative of contracting health plans and PBMs.

Retail pharmacy payment is currently based on a discounted average wholesale price (AWP), such as AWP −15% to −17% for brand name drugs, and AWP −20% to −25% for multisource generic drugs not subject to a maximum allowable cost (MAC). The AWP basis for payment is likely to change as a result of recent litigation, although the replacement pricing benchmark has not been established.

AWP is a calculated price and not reflective of a real drug cost and is universally known by retail pharmacists and pharmacies managing health plan or PBM prescription drug benefit programs. For over 30 years, health plans and PBMs have used a discounted AWP payment for retail prescriptions to approximate the actual acquisition cost by pharmacies and to allow a small profit. The wholesaler acquisition cost (WAC) is a reasonable benchmark (and WAC-plus pricing is a potential AWP alternative). It is impossible for a pharmacist to report the actual acquisition cost of every tablet, capsule, gram, or milliliter of a drug product, as a prescription may be dispensed using bulk drug containers purchased at different times and at different costs. Also, pharmacies may retroactively receive purchase time–payment discounts, volume purchase discounts, or seasonal special promotions, all of which may result in a different product cost. Therefore, managed care organizations began using a discounted AWP in the early 1980s to pay for brand name drugs.

Generic drugs are known to also have an actual acquisition cost (AAC), which is different than a published WAC. Generic manufacturers offer retail pharmacies significant price discounts based on volume and other special deals through wholesalers that can result in significantly discounted AACs, which remain confidential.

Some of the major mass merchandizers such as Walmart or Target also offer a cash discount price on selected generic products, such as up to a month for $4 and up to 90 days for $10. If cash transactions are not captured by health plans or PBMs, the prescriptions will not appear in patient medication histories and may not contribute to satisfaction of out-of-pocket front-end deductibles. Additionally, prescriptions not processed through a third-party claims adjudication system will not be included in an e-prescribing patient drug history.

■ PHARMACEUTICAL CONTRACTING

Health plans and PBMs contract with pharmaceutical manufacturers to obtain price concessions to reduce the net cost of contracted drugs. The lower net price improves the drug value, which will result in the contracted drug being placed in a preferred formulary position (e.g., tier two in a three-tier formulary structure).[31] Pharmaceutical manufacturer discounts and rebates reduce pharmacy expenses in two ways:

- Drugs subject to rebates and discounts have a lower net cost, and these costs result in lower plan sponsor premiums.
- Discounted and rebated brand name drugs are placed in preferred formulary positions with lower member copayments, and members save money when they are prescribed a contracted product.

Closed-panel plans that operate their own pharmacies and PBMs that operate mail service pharmacies take possession of drugs they dispense, and participate in wholesale chargebacks to obtain significant discounts on drugs under contract with generic and brand name drug manufacturers. Open health plans and PBMs using a contracted community pharmacy network use rebate contracts with pharmaceutical manufacturers to reduce net drug cost. Rebates are offered on brand name drugs but not generics drugs. Discounts on generic products are offered through wholesaler chargebacks to pharmacies that take possession of drug products (e.g., mail service pharmacies, staff or group model plans with owned pharmacies).

Rebate contracts often consist of two components: a flat access rebate that is paid if the contracted drug is given a preferred formulary position, and an additive performance component based upon an increase in the utilization rate or market share of the contracted product. The specific performance criteria vary by contract and manufacturer. In open drug formularies that include most drugs available on one of generally three tiers, rebates are usually offered for the tier two preferred position. As open formularies, by definition, generally pay for most drugs, the worst formulary position is tier three. Therefore, most pharmaceutical manufacturers will not offer a rebate for tier three in an open formulary, unless a rebate is offered to "contract away" a dispensing limitation, as a step-edit or prior authorization.

In contrast, closed formularies, such as those often used by group or staff model health plans, and many Medicare Part D plans, by definition do not cover all drugs. Therefore, there is a worse position than having a high copayment on tier three: not covered and not paid. Consequently, pharmaceutical manufacturers may offer a contract for tier three to be eligible for payment and avoid being "not covered." Pharmaceutical manufacturers will offer the minimum necessary to achieve their desired formulary position, and that will result in a positive return on the rebate amount paid. Manufacturers may not offer a rebate on an innovative drug that must be covered by plans and PBMs due to its unique clinical value. Minimally differentiated products in crowded therapeutic classes often have very high rebates (e.g., 30% or higher). Medicaid Best Price is the minimum Medicaid rebate pharmaceutical manufacturers must offer Medicaid programs if they are included in a Medicaid formulary (although this may vary by state).

Pharmaceutical manufacturers often used Medicaid Best Price as an artificial commercial rebate ceiling, although many manufacturers offered higher contracts. Medicaid Best Price is increasing to 23.1% (up from 15.1%).

Most plans operate under PBM contracts due to the ability of PBMs to negotiate deeper discounts from pharmaceutical manufacturers by aggregating membership of their customers. PBMs pass the rebate share to customers based on their utilization of contracted products; however, customers of PBMs are never certain they are obtaining total rebate value. Today, all PBMs claim to be transparent regarding contracting, although the rebate contracts with pharmaceutical manufacturers are kept confidential. This is discussed further in the section on PBMs.

■ DRUG FORMULARY MANAGEMENT

The drug formulary is the linchpin of the pharmacy benefit, for it describes and defines the benefit design and pharmacy program richness or limitations.[32] A drug formulary is not a static list of drugs, but reflects a therapeutic methodology of satisfying the clinical and economic needs of plan sponsors and their member patients. Certainly health plans and PBMs develop and support different formularies for various customers, but absent some specific drug categories (e.g., drugs for erectile dysfunction, oral contraceptives), drug formularies meet therapeutic needs, although perhaps with a different number of drugs within comparative therapeutic categories, within different tier structures, and available at different copayment amounts.

Managed care has borrowed the concepts of drug formularies and the Pharmacy & Therapeutics (P&T) Committee from hospitals. The Academy of Managed Care Pharmacy (AMCP) defines a drug formulary thusly:

> A drug formulary, or preferred drug list, is a continually updated list of medications and related products supported by current evidence-based medicine, judgment of physicians, pharmacists and other experts in the diagnosis and treatment of disease and preservation of health. The primary purpose of the formulary is to encourage the use of safe, effective and most affordable medications.[33]

The formulary system organizes drugs in a specific rational format and hierarchy selected by the parent organization. A common high-level organization is by organ systems, and subcategorized by disease or medical conditions under which appear drug classes, pharmacological categories, and finally specific drugs covered by generic and brand name. Each drug entry also displays any coverage limitation or restriction, such as a step-edit (e.g., a generic must be used before a brand is covered) or a prior authorization (the physician or pharmacist must request coverage approval for a specific patient for a defined reason, and for a limited period of time). Some drugs are not eligible for coverage and payment for various defined reasons.

Drug formularies are accessible online via an intranet or Internet system or an e-prescribing system for the physician, and through the pharmacy point-of-dispensing prescription claims adjudication system for the pharmacist. Many health plans also publish their drug formulary and recent changes online for members or the public to view. Several private companies (e.g., Fingertip Formulary, Epocrates) provide electronic access to a compilation of drug formularies and covered drugs by health plan and PBM, and often by state.

Impact of Generic Drugs

The use of generic drugs is an important cost management component in managed care prescription drug program formularies. Generic drugs typically have a published WAC of approximately 40–60% less than their brand name drug equivalents, and with mandatory generic substitution, the actual net cost of a generic drug may be 70–90% less than its brand name equivalent. On average, the retail price impact of a generic drug is 75% lower than the brand name drug.[34]

Closed-panel plans with owned pharmacies have greater control of their formulary and degree of generic substitution and dispense 80% or more of total prescriptions as generic drugs (termed the generic dispensing ratio). Open-model health plans with open formularies using community pharmacy networks have somewhat less control, but with a strong generic substitution policy they may achieve a generic dispensing ratio of 60–70%. One study found that every 1 percent increase in generic dispensing ratio is associated with a drop of 2.5% in gross pharmacy expenditures (one-half of the savings from brand-to-generic conversions; one-half from reduced brand name drug utilization).[35] The percent of prescriptions dispensed with generic drugs will increase substantially over the next decade, as many important brand name drugs will lose their patent protection.

Generic drug acceptance is influenced by copayment differential between tier one (generic drugs) and brand name drug copayments (tier two and higher tiers). A financial incentive of $15 or more generally influences patient demand for a lower-tier drug. Also, most plans and PBMs have a mandatory generic substitution program for most commonly available multisource generic drugs. Generic drugs available from three or more generic manufacturers experience price competition and generally have an actual acquisition cost (AAC) of 70–90% less than the published list price after aggressive discounts from drug wholesalers. For such generic drugs, health plans and PBMs are assigned a maximum allowable cost (MAC), an estimate of the AAC, and the upper level of payment for drugs subject to a MAC.

Types of Drug Formularies

Drug formularies were developed to support specific insurance products. The drug formulary for a commercial product will be different in structure and covered drugs than for a Medicaid or Medicare Part D formulary. The drugs included are selected to meet the clinical needs of the age range of covered members, thus commercial and Medicaid formularies would include pediatric medications and a Medicare Part D formulary would not.

Drug formularies are often classified as "open" or "closed." An open formulary generally covers most drugs within a tiered system (discussed in the next section). Even though most drugs may be covered, some may be subject to dispensing limitations (e.g., prior authorization, step-edits, quantity or duration limits). Some drug classes such as those for cosmetic use or over-the-counter drugs may be excluded from open formulary coverage according to the EOC. A closed formulary is more restrictive, not covering as many drugs as an open formulary, and also using tiers and dispensing limitations. Drugs not included in the formulary are not eligible for payment except by an approved medical exception. Members always have the option of paying cash for a noncovered prescribed drug. Closed formularies may be more common in staff or group model plans. Large insurers often offer plan sponsors a variety of formulary options, including closed, open, and Medicare Part D, with various tier options.

Drug Formulary Tier Structure

Drugs on most commercial and Medicare Part D formularies are assigned to a formulary tier, which is reflective of the plan benefit design, the drug patent status (e.g., generic or brand), and the relative net cost to the parent organization. Many commercial and Medicare Part D formularies use a three-tier formulary for nonspecialty drugs. A traditional three-tier formulary includes generic drugs on tier one, preferred brand name drugs on tier two, and nonpreferred drugs on tier three. Thus, generics drugs on tier one are expected to have an overall lower net cost to the plan. Preferred drugs on tier two are considered preferred brand name drugs. Drugs are preferred for one or more reasons: they may be clinically superior, have a lower list price, or have a lower net price to the plan as a result of a rebate or discount contract with a pharmaceutical manufacturer. Tier three drugs are nonpreferred because they do not meet the clinical and net cost attributes of brand name drugs on tier two, and they are generally not subject to a pharmaceutical manufacturer contract. (Exceptions exist; tier three products on Medicare Part D formularies are often subject to a pharmaceutical manufacturer contract.)

Each tier is associated with a dollar copayment the member must pay as a form of financial cost-sharing when a covered drug is dispensed. Tier one drugs have the lowest copayment to encourage the use of a generic drug whenever

clinically appropriate. If a brand name drug is required, members are incentivized to obtain a tier two brand name drug, which has a copayment higher than tier one, but lower than tier three. Finally, nonpreferred, often noncontracted brand name drugs in tier three generally have a higher net cost, and have the highest copayment in a three-tier formulary structure. A minority of commercial plans also offer a fourth tier, often used for self-injectable specialty drugs, available at a percentage coinsurance. **Table 11-1** illustrates a typical three-tier open formulary structure for a commercial payer.

In 2010, 65% of commercial plans offered a three-tier formulary and 13% of commercial plans offered a four-tier formulary. The remaining plans had flat or two-tier formularies.[36] **Table 11-2** illustrates the structure of copayments and coinsurance in a four-tier commercial drug formulary structure. Employer groups are asking plans and PBMs to shift more costs to utilizing members. **Figure 11-5** shows the increase in retail commercial pharmacy benefit copayments over the past decade.

In addition to flat (fixed) dollar copayments, plans and PBMs may use percentage coinsurance as a form of member cost-sharing. Percent coinsurance levels are often used for expensive medications on tier three (or a higher tier some plans or PBMs). Percentage coinsurance is often used with self-injectable specialty medications. Self-injectable specialty drugs are often on tier four, if it exists. Exceptions exist to the three-tier formulary structure. Some insurers offer five or more tier formularies, including tier one for preferred/lower-cost generics, tier two for nonpreferred/higher-cost generics, tier three for preferred brand name drugs, and so on.

TABLE 11-1	Example of an Antidepressant Class in a Commercial Three-Tier Open Drug Formulary		
Serotonin—norepinephrine reuptake inhibitor antidepressant class drugs	Tier	Quantity limit	Step-edit
CYMBALTA®	2	√	√
EFFEXOR®	3	√	√
EFFEXOR XR®	3	√	√
PRISTIQ®	2	√	√
Venlafaxine*	1	√	
Venlafaxine ER (cap)	1	√	
VENLAFAXINE ER® (TAB)	3	√	√
Venlafaxine SR (tab)	1	√	

* Generic equivalent of Effexor.
Note: Uppercase, brand name drug; lowercase, generic drug.
Source: RP Navarro, 2011. Adapted from an Aetna three-tier open drug formulary. Available at www.aetna.com/FSE/planType.do. Accessed April 8, 2011.

TABLE 11-2	Example of Copayments in a Four-Tier Commercial Drug Formulary Structure			
Product	Tier one generic	Tier two preferred brand	Tier three nonpreferred brand	Tier four self-injectables
Commercial	$10	$25	$50	50% coinsurance ($500 per month MOOP)

Note: MOOP, maximum out-of-pocket (per month; plan pays 100% after MOOP is satisfied each month)
Source: Navarro (2011).

Medicare Part D pharmacy benefit formularies are similar in tier structure, but are highly variable. Aetna offers several Medicare Part D options, including a five-tier drug formulary.[37] Medicaid usually has zero-dollar or low-dollar flat copayments, and all drugs on a single tier. Each state may have specific restrictions, such as a maximum number available for coverage per month or prior authorization on all brand name drugs.

■ MAIL SERVICE PHARMACY

Members in some health plans and PBMs have the option of receiving prescriptions sent to them via the U.S. Postal Service or a private carrier. Mail service delivery, also termed home delivery, is offered by most major chain pharmacies and large PBMs, some of which own mail service pharmacies. Mail delivery is growing slowly. Medco Health reports 14% of outpatient managed care prescriptions are dispensed through a mail service pharmacy in 2009.[38] Some employer groups provide financial incentives (e.g., discounted copayments) for members to use mail delivery for chronic medications, especially when a generic substitute is available. The largest PBMs—Medco Health, CVS Caremark, Express Scripts, and others—own mail service pharmacies, and as a result of heavy promotion and financial incentives for members, some PBM employer group customers may have 20% or more of their prescriptions dispensed through mail service.

Source of Mail Service Costs Savings

Mail service prescriptions can offer cost savings of approximately 10% to plan sponsors.[39] Members also save money by paying lower and fewer copayments if they access mail service, especially for generic drugs. Mail service traditionally offers two cost advantages over retail pharmacy prescriptions as well as one potential disadvantage. Mail service pharmacies take possession of drugs, and due to the deep volume discounts and highly efficient dispensing automation, the cost of dispensing is less than a retail prescription. Mail service pharmacies promote generics heavily. Medco Health claims 71% of mail prescriptions were dispensed with generic drugs, a 3.5% increase from 2009.

Generic drugs are the primary source of profit and cost savings of mail service pharmacies. The prescription costs PBMs guarantee to their plan sponsors of brand name drug expenses are approximately 8% less than through retail (e.g., AWP −25% through mail; −17% through retail), and guarantee a generic prescription discount of AWP −40% or more, or the MAC amount. Of course, the actual net acquisition cost of generic drugs is often AWP −70% to −90% for some highly competitive generics.

Most plan sponsors use financial incentives to encourage members to use mail delivery prescription services. Members may obtain a 60- or 90-day supply of a chronic maintenance medication for one copayment, rather than paying one copayment per 30-day supply through a retail pharmacy. To compete with mail service pharmacies, many retail pharmacies, especially chains, will also offer to dispense a 60- or 90-day supply of medication for one

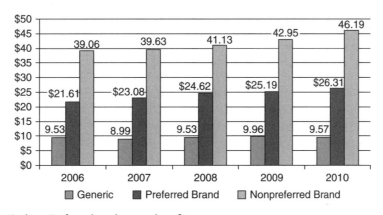

FIGURE 11-5 Retail copayment in three-tier formulary pharmacy benefits.
Source: Navarro (2011). Adapted from data found at NACDS Community Pharmacy Results. Available at www.nacds.org/wmspage.cfm?parm1=6538. Accessed April 6, 2011.

copayment. This depends on the benefit design and the willingness of the pharmacy provider.

Employers should know PBMs often use more than one MAC list: one list to pay network pharmacies and another, higher MAC to guarantee generic prices to plan sponsors.[40, 41] The difference between what is paid out to pharmacies and what is guaranteed to plan sponsors is the "spread," often retained by the PBM as profit. This practice is common and acceptable unless prohibited by the contract the PBM has with its plan sponsors. PBMs defend this practice by stating this is their source of profit and, as long as they meet or exceed the guaranteed drug costs specified in their contract with the plan sponsor, there should be no claim on these profits by plan sponsors. Conversely, the plan sponsor contract often requires that PBMs pay a financial penalty if the guaranteed prices are exceeded. Finally, PBMs do not consider themselves fiduciaries, and this is often specified in the contract.

Patient Interaction Satisfaction

A potential disadvantage of mail service pharmacy is the lack of face-to-face interaction with the dispensing pharmacy when a prescription is dispensed at a retail pharmacy. Regular personal interaction provides opportunities for more personal patient counseling and medication therapy management (MTM) interventions. Pharmacists are available by telephone or e-mail at mail service pharmacies, and some members, especially those with limited mobility, may prefer the convenience. The JD Power 2010 Pharmacy Satisfaction Survey shows mixed patient satisfaction ratings of retail and mail service pharmacies. The Veterans Administration and Kaiser-Permanente received the highest mail service ratings ("among the best"), with Express Scripts and Humana mail services being rated as "better than most."[42–44]

■ SPECIALTY PHARMACY DISTRIBUTION

Specialty pharmaceuticals represent a critical challenge for cost and quality management for health care managers and plan sponsors. Specialty drugs can provide life-altering treatment for patients with chronic and complex diseases including multiple sclerosis, blood deficiencies, HIV/AIDS, hepatitis C, cancer, hemophilia, growth deficiencies, pulmonary arterial hypertension, rheumatoid arthritis and other types of arthritis, Crohn's disease, and others. Specialty pharmaceuticals often have complex delivery methods or dosing schedules and may require special handling and patient monitoring. Many specialty dugs are administered by subcutaneous injection, intramuscular injection, or intravenous infusion. However, specialty products are becoming available in oral dosage forms, but retain a specialty pharmacy profile due to special handling, the need for patient monitoring, and high cost.

The PBM Express Scripts reported the cost trend of traditional pharmaceuticals (nonspecialty drugs) was 1.2% while specialty drugs had a 19.6% cost trend.[45] Part of the specialty trend growth is fueled by a high utilization trend. In 2009, PBMs and specialty pharmacy providers reported a utilization trend of 15%; one-fifth experienced a 20% growth in utilization.[46]

Infused (IV) injectable products are generally covered under the medical benefit, which may contribute up to 11.2% of total medical benefit costs.[47] Subcutaneous injection and oral products are usually covered under the pharmacy benefit. While 40% of the costs in the specialty segment are spent on self-injected specialty pharmaceuticals, 60% under the medical benefit is largely unmanaged, and specialty drugs under the medical benefit are 2–30% more expensive than drugs under the pharmacy benefit.[48] As a result, many plans are moving medical benefit specialty products to the pharmacy benefit, or integrating management of specialty pharmaceuticals under the medical and pharmacy benefits.[40]

Approximately 75% of commercial plan members were subject to some type of specialty cost-sharing mechanism.[49] Twenty-eight percent of health plans have specialty products in a specialty formulary tier (often tier four or tier five), and apply a percentage coinsurance cost-share, possibly with a front-end deductible, a member out-of-pocket maximum, and a benefit cap.[40]

As the number of specialty drugs subject to pharmacy benefit management increases, many members may not have the ability or willingness to pay the cost-sharing portion of expensive pharmaceuticals. Nonadherence may jeopardize outcomes and concerned physicians may hospitalize patients to administer specialty products, an unintended consequence of increasing member cost-sharing and reduced physician outpatient specialty drug payment.

Specialty Pharmacy Distribution[50]

The unique distribution and storage of injectables has caused the development of specialty pharmacies that may send injectables directly to a physician's office or infusion center specifically for a patient appointment, or mail specialty drugs directly to a member's home. Volume purchasing introduces cost efficiencies into the system that are passed on to payers and members. Specialty pharmacies also contract with pharmaceutical manufacturers for rebates, provide formulary-style product steerage, collect copayments and coinsurance, and bill for drugs covered under the pharmacy benefit.

Health plans also may use specialty pharmacies to buy and store inventory on behalf of physicians, which prevents physicians from stocking and storing expensive medications and removes them from the flow of dollars. In this scheme, the specialty pharmacy bills the health plan and/or member directly, and the physician is paid an infusion and/or administration fee by the health plan. Traditional discounted payment of injectable products in a Part B Medicare Benefit will be altered through the use of a CMS average selling price (ASP) plus 6% method. Many plans are adopting this Medicare-style cost plus payment for injectables in their commercial plans as well.

Managing Specialty Pharmaceuticals

Specialty pharmacies apply the standard pharmacy management strategies used to manage traditional drugs, as described in previous sections of this chapter, including specialty formulary management, patient cost-sharing, pharmaceutical contracting, and patient care services. One large specialty pharmacy reported 75% of health plan clients were subject to formulary management.[51] **Figure 11-6** illustrates the most commonly managed therapeutic classes, as well as those classes most commonly associated with rebate contracts.

Specialty Pharmaceuticals in the Future

Specialty pharmacy management presents unique cost and quality of care management challenges. The average member cost-share is 17% of the drug cost in 2010, and this will increase,[52] threatening adherence and outcomes. The ACA provides for pathways to facilitate approval of "biosimilars," also termed "follow-on biologics," as less expensive products that are "highly similar" to reference products. The approval process for biosimilars is under consideration to prepare for the anticipated arrival of several products. The price of biosimilars should be less than that of the reference products, and may assist in specialty pharmacy cost-containment efforts. Biosimilars are expected in the following therapeutic categories: human growth hormones, recombinant insulins, epoetin alfa, drugs for neutropenia, rheumatoid arthritis, interferon-alfa, and others.[53] Specialty

pharmacies are uniquely positioned and equipped to address these concerns, and their role will continue to grow as specialty pharmaceuticals dominate managed care PBM programs.

■ CLINICAL PHARMACY PROGRAMS

The clinical elements in pharmacy programs are typically categorized as those applicable to the general membership such as drug utilization review (DUR); those applicable to focused care management such as disease management (DM), including adherence management; and medication treatment management (MTM) under Medicare Part D as discussed in that section. The other elements are discussed as follows.

Drug Utilization Review Programs[54]

DUR programs are designed to identify and correct inappropriate or unsafe drug utilization or patterns. DUR programs have been implemented in most health plans and PBMs are part of their commitment to pursue cost and quality management on behalf of their plan sponsor customers and their members. In addition to improving clinical outcomes, DUR programs identify opportunities for cost reduction, such as reversing excessive use of prescriptions written as "dispense as written" (DAW) that may prevent generic conversion opportunities, pharmacies that fail to cause a brand-to-generic conversion, excessive quantity and duration, and patients abuse controlled drugs by accessing similar prescriptions from multiple physicians and pharmacies. DUR programs generally use only pharmacy claims data, although when a drug-use pattern of concern is discovered, pharmacists conducting the review will often integrate medical claims data, if available, to gain a complete understanding of a patient's clinical situation. Perhaps the medical data, such as a

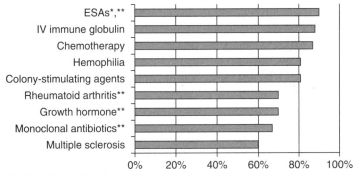

*Erythropoiesis-stimulating agents

** Therapeutic classes in which more than 69% of ICORE specialty pharmacy health plan lives are receiving pharmaceutical rebates.

FIGURE 11-6 Commonly managed specialty drug therapeutic classes.

Source: Navarro (2011). Adapted from ICORE Trend Report 2010, pp. 9, 10. Available at www.icorehealthcare.com/trends.aspx. Accessed April 7, 2011.

diagnosis of cancer, may explain high opioid doses for a prolonged period of time. DUR program reports may identify drug abuse and diversion, such as multiple prescriptions of opioids prescribed by two or more physicians and filled at multiple pharmacies. If a drug-abuse pattern is discovered, plan pharmacists generally contact the physicians involved and restrict the patient to one physician and one pharmacy.

DUR programs can be prospective, concurrent, and retrospective. Health plans and PBMs generally perform all three types of DUR activities on a periodic basis. Many organizations schedule preprogrammed DUR reports be automatically run on a monthly or quarterly basis. DUR programs identify medication nonadherence and identify Medicare D recipients that meet the MTM inclusion criteria, and to follow up on the results of an MTM intervention.

Prospective, Concurrent, and Retrospective DUR Programs

A prospective review occurs before the patient has received the medication. The primary advantage of this type of analysis is that problems are identified and resolved before medication is dispensed. Prospective DUR serves as an excellent member-teaching opportunity for pharmacists. Concurrent DUR programs are performed at the point-of-prescribing in the dispensing pharmacy. While performing the claims adjudication process, pharmacists are provided clinical and benefit design edits that provide an alert for potential clinical conflict that should be evaluated before the product is dispensed. Retrospective DUR is performed after the prescription is dispensed. **Table 11-3** summarizes and compares drug-use exceptions commonly identified through the three types of DUR screening programs.

The Role of Pharmacy Programs in Disease Management

Disease prevention and management are core principles of managed health care and remain key objectives in health care plans today. In addition to developing clinically balanced drug formularies, health plan pharmacists are involved in disease management programs, DUR programs, and Medicare Part D MTM programs to monitor and optimize drug use.

Health plans often provide active case management and care coordination for specific high-risk and high-cost, comorbid patients who typically are taking many medications. These coordinated care programs, often termed DM, include the pharmacy department if the diseases managed include pharmaceuticals. Diseases commonly included in DM programs include asthma, chronic obstructive pulmonary disease (COPD), congestive heart failure, diabetes, and hypertension. Pharmacists may be

TABLE 11-3	Type of Drug Use Exception Identified by Prospective, Concurrent, and Retrospective DURs		
DUR elements	**Prospective DUR exceptions identified**	**Concurrent DUR exceptions identified**	**Retrospective DUR exceptions identified**
Adherence (low or high)	√	√	√
Drug–disease contraindications	√	√	√
Drug–disease contraindications	√	√	√
Drug–drug interactions	√	√	√
Drug formulary conformance	√	√	√
Drug–gender conflicts		√	√
Drug–pregnancy precautions		√	
High-cost outliers			√
Incorrect dosage	√	√	√
Misuse and abuse patterns	√		√
Therapeutic redundancy	√		√

Source: RP Navarro, 2011. Adapted from tables found in Peterson AM, Chan V, and Wilson MD. Drug utilization review strategies. In: Navarro RP (ed.). *Managed Care Pharmacy Practice.* Sudbury, MA: Jones and Bartlett; 2009.

involved in DM programs to monitor and counsel patients on drug adherence, appropriate utilization, and drug information.

Health plans may offer disease-specific management programs to augment health care services provided by plan physicians that may include general disease education, diagnostic screening events, and case management.

Health plan pharmacy departments and PBMs often play a supportive role in health plan and employer DM programs. Pharmacy program drug utilization data are often used to identify patients with poorly controlled medical conditions (identified by the number and type of medications used) or have drug adherence problems (through inconsistent prescription refill records). Pharmacy departments may obtain resource support from pharmaceutical manufacturers that often provide unbranded DM resources (e.g., physician or patient education materials or educational grants) to supplement health plan efforts. DM offered from pharmaceutical manufacturers will not influence formulary decisions, and in fact the reverse influence exists. That is, health plans and MCOs may seek clinical program support from manufacturers whose drugs have been previously selected for preferred formulary positions.

Adherence Programs

Adherence to prescribed medications has long been a challenge. Retail pharmacies may offer adherence services that include an auto-refill if members forget to call in a refill order for a chronic medication. Some pharmacies will call members if they fail to refill a chronic medication to determine if the patient is experiencing an adverse effect or if the physician changed the prescription order.

In addition to not ordering a refill drug, approximately 11% of patients do not return to the pharmacy to pick up their prescription. This behavior, termed "prescription abandonment," occurs in almost 7% of brand name prescriptions and over 4% of generic prescriptions.[55] PBMs also claim mail service prescriptions that provide for a 60- or 90-day supply, especially with an auto-refill option, improves adherence. Express Scripts reports a medication possession ratio (MPR) of approximately 80%, which is considered relatively high for most therapeutic categories (notably, asthma was under 70%).[56] CVS Caremark also offers an adherence improvement program, and claims a 15% improvement in adherence and 35% of patients who discontinued therapy restarted their medications after an intervention.[57]

■ MEDICARE AND MEDICAID PHARMACY BENEFITS

Medicaid is a health program for eligible individuals and families with low incomes and resources; Medicare is a federal program for older adults that covers hospital, physician, drug benefits, and related services. CMS directly administers Medicare, while states administer Medicaid. Medicare has a managed care component (Part C), and many states now manage their Medicaid programs. With the advent of Medicare Part D in 2006, an outpatient prescription drug benefit was introduced for eligible Medicare and Medicaid patients. By 2008, Medicare Part D retail prescriptions accounted for nearly 20% of total prescriptions in the United States.[58]

The Medicare Prescription Drug, Improvement, and Modernization Act of 2003 (MMA; Pub. L. No. 108-173) was signed into law on December 8, 2003. It created a new Medicare Part D, which established a voluntary outpatient prescription drug benefit for seniors and qualified disabled persons. Prior to Part D, there was an interim drug discount card program that started on June 1, 2004, and ended on May 15, 2006. The full prescription drug benefit began on January 1, 2006.

Medicare is a federal program that has four components:

- Part A—covers inpatient care (e.g., hospital, skilled nursing facility care, home health care, hospice)
- Part B—covers outpatient care (e.g., medical visits, durable medical equipment [DME], a few prescription drugs)
- Part C—covers managed care (enacted as Medicare+Choice in 1997 and now known as Medicare Advantage)
- Part D—covers voluntary prescription drug benefit

By 2010, Medicare enrollment was 47 million, including 8 million individuals with disabilities (under age 65) and 39 million older adults (age 65 and older).[59] In 2011, approximately 38 million Medicare recipients participated in Part D.[60] Part D plans include prescription drug plans (PDPs)—private, stand-alone plans that offer drug-only coverage and Medicare Advantage prescription drug (MA-PDs) plans—that offer both prescription drug and health coverage. These plans exist in every state except Alaska and Vermont. Residents of Puerto Rico and other territories are not eligible for Part D subsidies. Other insurers, for which benefits must be coordinated with Part D payments, provide competing or alternative insurance coverage.

Of the almost 47 million Medicare members in 2010, 38% (17.7 million) obtained t heir drug coverage through a stand-alone PDP, 21% (9.9 million) obtained drug coverage through their Medicare Advantage drug plan, 10% (4.7 million) had elected to receive no drug coverage, and 31% (14.1 million) obtained their drug coverage through a retiree drug benefit or had some other drug coverage.[61]

PDPs and MA-PDs are established in geographical regions of the United States. Regions are established based on the following key factors: eligibility of the population, the capacity of health care systems for service delivery, beneficiary considerations, and limited variation in prescription drug spending. Using these criteria, CMS established 34 PDP and 26 MA-PD regions across the country.

Part D prescription drug plans must offer a basic drug benefit called the "standard benefit," may offer supplemental benefits called "enhanced benefits," can be flexible in benefit design, and must follow marketing guidelines. Certain beneficiaries will have the greatest benefit from Part D. These are patients with no current drug insurance, those who qualify for limited income assistance, those in Medicare Advantage plans with no drug coverage, and those who spend more than $800 per year on prescription drugs.

Enrollment

Each individual entitled to Medicare Part A or enrolled in Part B qualifies for Part D coverage. Individuals enrolled in traditional Medicare will receive their benefits through a stand-alone PDP. Individuals enrolled in a Medicare

Advantage plan will have coverage through an MA-PD plan. Most eligible Part D beneficiaries were able to choose a Part D plan. Two special groups were identified for consideration:

- *Dual eligible.* Nearly 9 million Medicaid beneficiaries are "dual eligible": low-income seniors and younger persons with disabilities enrolled in both the Medicare and Medicaid programs. They are among the sickest and poorest individuals covered by either programs, and must navigate both Medicare and Medicaid to access services. Medicaid pays Medicare premiums and covers critical benefits Medicare does not cover, such as long-term care.
- *Limited-income beneficiaries.* These individuals were eligible for a limited income subsidy (LIS). A LIS enrollee is auto-assigned through the bid process, and not by the beneficiary, plan, or employer.

Retirees must follow their employers' plan coverage rules to remain eligible for their retirement coverage. However, if retirees decide to leave their employer coverage midyear, they may enroll in a Medicare Part D plan only during the Medicare open-enrollment period. For example, if a retiree left the employer's Part D plan in July, he or she would have to wait until the November open-enrollment period for coverage for the following year. Exceptions are allowed for the following special circumstances:

- Beneficiaries who permanently move out of the plan service area
- Individuals entering, residing in, or leaving a long-term care facility
- Involuntary loss, reduction, or non-notification of creditable coverage
- Other exceptional circumstances

Standard and Low Income Benefits

The standard benefit design entails a monthly premium of approximately $37 that varies by PDP and MA-PD region. The annual deductible is $310 in 2010 and 2011, and is indexed annually. The primary coverage after the deductible requires the beneficiary to be responsible for approximately 25% of drug costs until he or she reaches $2,830 in 2010 in drug spending (not including monthly premiums). After spending $2,840 (not including monthly premiums) in 2011 (compared to $2,830 in 2010), the beneficiary is responsible for 100% of drug costs until he or she reaches $4,550 in 2011 (vs. $4,550 in 2010) in true out-of-pocket costs. This is referred to as the "coverage gap." This responsibility corresponds to more than $6,000 of total prescription drug spending (more if a person has a wraparound plan). After $6,447.50 of total prescription drug spending in 2011 (vs. $6,440 in 2010), the beneficiary receives catastrophic coverage. For this coverage the beneficiary is responsible for about 5% of drug costs.

Under provisions of the ACA, the coverage gap will decline over time. In 2011, beneficiaries received a 50% discount from manufacturers as well as a modest federal subsidy for generic drugs. Beginning in 2013, Medicare will provide additional subsidies for brand name drugs and generics so that by 2020 the coinsurance rate in the coverage gap will be 25%.

The "true out-of-pocket cost" (TrOOP) is the beneficiary cost-sharing for Medicare Part D benefits before catastrophic coverage begins. TrOOP includes all covered medication costs except drugs purchased outside of the United States, OTC drugs, drugs not on the plan's formulary, and drugs not covered by law.

State Medicaid drug benefits are now available or coordinated with Part D for state employees, retirees, and dependents, many of whom may be Medicare beneficiaries; Medicaid coverage provided to low-income beneficiaries, many of whom may be Medicare dual eligible who will now receive most drug coverage from Medicare Part D; and supplemental drug coverage offered to seniors through state pharmaceutical assistance programs (SPAPs). In light of the rollover of Medicaid benefits to Part D, all benefits must be coordinated with other employee benefits. The fundamental guiding principle for coordination of benefits (COB) is that MMA requires coordination between CMS, state agencies, insurers, and employers to ensure that the benefits provided to Part D beneficiaries are maximized. States have special coordination concerns because of their dual status as employers and insurers. Coordination with SPAPs is a high priority for CMS. As a rule, Part D usually pays first, except for group health plans and workers' compensation.

Pharmacy Network Contracting and Medicare Part D

Part D pharmacy network contracts require specific expectations for the plan sponsors. Sponsors expect these plans to meet specific criteria including work plans that must be included in the application, performance and service criteria that must be included in pharmacy contracts, contracts must contain any willing providers, and contracts must have convenient access requirements for patients who routinely receive benefits through the network.

Initially, Part D plans had to establish pharmacy networks by August 1, 2005. These networks had to obey standards that could be no less than the TRICARE Retail Pharmacy access standards. These requirements are based on state, not PDP or MA-PD region. MMA contains an "any willing provider" provision such that any pharmacy that wishes to participate in a Medicare plan can participate if they accept the standard terms and conditions of the participating pharmacy agreement. This requirement pertains only to initial networking and did not extend past August 1,

2005. After this time, health plans could close the pharmacy networks if they chose.

There is a so-called level playing field requirement that no mandatory mail service is allowed. In addition, PDP sponsors may not include only mail service pharmacies in their network. This requirement is not completely exclusive. For example, if retail pharmacies refuse the 90-day option, then a PDP can still offer a 90-day mail option. Adequate retail emergency access for enrollees is also necessary. However, the patient is responsible for any higher cost-sharing that applies at a retail pharmacy; for example, the patient may pay the normal copay plus the difference between the mail and retail 90-day rates. The implications of this requirement are that if a Part D plan offers a 90-day supply by mail, then it must offer a 90-day supply option at retail; the plan is not required to offer a 90-day supply option at retail if it does not have a 90-day mail option.

Plans can offer benefits with preferred pharmacies. These discounts apply to standard benefits but not to dual-eligible or low-income beneficiaries. Plans with preferred pharmacies can provide lower payment to participating pharmacies and, in turn, provide more advantageous copays and co-insurances to beneficiaries. However, plans must maintain actuarial equivalence of 25% patient responsibility, meaning that the preferred pharmacy benefits still must obey the standard benefit package.

Congress did not set a minimum or maximum requirement for pharmacy payment rates. The plan—that is, the market—determines payment based on its network contracting. Dispensing fees do have some limitations. They are limited only to those costs associated with the transfer and possession of a drug. These costs include checking for coverage information, performing quality assurance (QA) activities as mandated by the state, filling the container and providing to the customer, delivery at the point of sale, and overhead. Also, dispensing fees do not include any activities beyond the point of sale (e.g., pharmacy follow-up telephone calls or medication therapy management).

Formularies and Medicare Part D

Formularies are encouraged for PDP and MA-PD plans. While each plan may develop its own formulary, there are several rules governing the design of these formularies. CMS contracted with the United States Pharmacopoeia (USP) to develop formulary guidelines. USP identified 146 therapeutic categories that must be included in all Part D formularies. In addition, if a generic is available, it must be included in the formulary. If the pharmacy dispenses a brand name drug, they must inform the Part D patient of any differential between the price of the brand name drug and the price of the lowest-priced generic version of that drug available at that pharmacy. This disclosure is mandatory, and plans must ensure compliance with this provision on the retail level.

Also, if preferred drugs are defined, the rebates collected must go to the payer to decrease the cost of the program.

Part D formularies must also comply with the following requirements:

- They must include at least two drugs in each therapeutic category and class of covered Part D drugs also known as "key drug types," or FKDTs. The FKDTs are part of the "outlier" test for formulary review.
- They must include prior authorizations, step therapy, generic drug requirements, and preferred brand name drugs.
- They must include all or substantially all drugs in the following classes: antidepressants, antipsychotics, anticonvulsants, anticancer, immunosuppressants, and HIV/AIDS medications.

Part D allows for preferred drug levels defined by formulary tiers. The first tier (tier 1) is the lowest level of cost-sharing for the beneficiary. Subsequent tiers have higher cost sharing in ascending order. CMS reviews all plan formulary submissions to identify drug categories that may discourage enrollment of certain beneficiaries with Medicare by placing drugs in nonpreferred tiers. These plans must have exception procedures for these tiered formularies.

Medication Therapy Management[62]

MTM includes a distinct service or group of services that optimize therapeutic outcomes for individual patients. MTM services are independent of, but can occur in conjunction with, prescription dispensing. MTM services may be provided by a qualified health care professional other than a pharmacist. However, the CMS reports that pharmacists provided 99.9% of MTM programs in 2010.[63]

The MMA requires Part D sponsors implement programs to control cost and quality improvement in prescription drug programs that may be performed by a pharmacist. The programs, defined as MTM, were established to ensure that medications covered and used by Medicare recipients are "appropriately used to optimize therapeutic outcomes through improved medication use, and to reduce the risk of adverse events, including adverse drug interactions."[64]

These services include but are not limited to the following, according to the individual needs of the patient:[65]

- Performing or obtaining necessary assessments of the patient's health status.
- Formulating a medication treatment plan.
- Selecting, initiating, modifying, or administering medication therapy.
- Monitoring and evaluating the patient's response to therapy, including safety and effectiveness.
- Performing a comprehensive medication review to identify, resolve, and prevent medication-related problems, including adverse drug events.

- Documenting the care delivered and communicating essential information to the patient's other primary care providers.
- Providing verbal education and training designed to enhance patient understanding and appropriate use of his or her medications.
- Providing information, support services, and resources designed to enhance patient adherence with his or her therapeutic regimens.
- Coordinating and integrating medication therapy management services within the broader health care-management services being provided to the patient.

The ACA expands the role and responsibilities of MTM programs for Medicare beneficiaries. Part D sponsors may determine how MTM services are provided, and many pay dispensing pharmacies if the services are documented. University colleges of pharmacy are also MTM providers for Medicare Part D plans.[66] The CMS will not dictate how much sponsors should offer pharmacies in MTM compensation; however, sponsors must explain their fee structure. MTM program requirements were significantly expanded for the 2010 contract year to increase the number of beneficiaries eligible for MTM services and the intensity of interventions, and to provide for the collection of more robust plan-reported data for outcomes analysis.[67]

Targeted beneficiaries for the MTM program are enrollees in Part D plans "who have multiple chronic diseases, are taking multiple Part D drugs, and are likely to incur annual costs for covered Part D drugs that exceed a predetermined level as specified by the Secretary." The cost threshold was lowered to $3,000 for 2010. Sponsors are required to target beneficiaries with multiple chronic diseases, and they define the minimum threshold for eligibility into their MTM program. Regardless of contract type, approximately 72% of 2010 MTM programs require a minimum of three chronic diseases to be eligible for enrollment. Ninety-five percent of health plans are targeting beneficiaries with specific chronic diseases, the most frequent in 2010 being diabetes (96.8% of plans), heart failure (93.7%), hypertension (79.1%), and dyslipidemia (76.3%). Almost 60% of programs are broadly targeting beneficiaries with "cardiovascular" diseases.[47]

Plans also use the number of drugs as a criterion for MTM enrollment. For 2010, CMS also established both a ceiling and a floor in the minimum number of drugs that may be required (two to eight). In 2009, almost 90% of MTM programs were already targeting beneficiaries with a minimum threshold of eight or fewer Part D drugs.[47] The average age of members reached by the call center is 65 years. The individuals take an average of 15 medications and have an average of 10 chronic disease states.[46]

Sponsors must target beneficiaries for enrollment in the MTM at least quarterly during each plan year. Over two-thirds (68.0%) of 2010 MTM programs identify targeted beneficiaries quarterly and 26.5% of programs identify beneficiaries monthly. Sponsors must enroll targeted beneficiaries using an opt-out method of enrollment only.[68]

The American Pharmacists Association, in concert with several other professional pharmacy organizations, have provided MTM training and resources for pharmacists and have conducted research on MTM programs. As in previous years, providers reported a variety of fee structures for MTM services. Eleven percent use capitation, 43% use fee-for-service, and 47% use a flat rate per service.[48]

An integrated health care system in Minnesota has provided clinical pharmacy services, quite similar to what are now described as MTM, for over a decade. From 1998 to 2008, the integrated system documented 38,631 drug therapy problems during 33,706 encounters with 9,068 patients. The most frequent problems encountered were the need for additional drug therapy ($n = 10,870$, 28.1%) and subtherapeutic dosages ($n = 10,100$, 26.1%). The clinical status of 55% of the 4,849 patients not at goal when they enrolled in the program improved, 23% of patients were unchanged, and 22% worsened during the course of MTM services. Pharmacists estimated the ROI of the MTM program over 10 years was $1.29 per $1 spent on MTM administrative costs. In the patient satisfaction survey, 95.3% of respondents agreed or strongly agreed that their overall health and well-being had improved because of MTM.[69]

DM, DUR programs, and MTM services provide opportunities for clinical pharmacists in Medicare Part D programs and participating community pharmacists to participate in clinical pharmacy services to help ensure cost management and quality of care is enhanced for participating members and beneficiaries.

Skilled Nursing Facility/Nursing Facility Impact

There are approximately 1.6 million Medicare/Medicaid-certified skilled nursing facilities (SNFs) and nursing facilities (NFs), with even more assisted-living facilities. Nearly 3 million of the 40 million Medicare beneficiaries will reside in one of these long-term care (LTC) facilities for some period of time in any given year. These patients will be generally 75 years and older, 70% female, may suffer from cognitive disorders, require assistance with activities of daily living, and utilize approximately 9–10 medications at any given time.

In order to comply with Part D, plans must offer standard contracting terms, contract with any willing LTC pharmacy, and ensure convenient access to LTC pharmacies. To participate, LTC pharmacies must enter into network agreements with PDPs. While the PDPs manage formularies, a Part D plan may require that an LTC pharmacy must offer a portfolio of services including drug packaging (e.g., blister packs), labeling, delivery (including emergencies around the clock), prescription ordering, access to urgent medications, pharmacist on-call services, emergency boxes and log systems, drug disposition for controlled and noncontrolled drugs, IV medications, compounding, and medication administration records (MARs). However, pharmacies may negotiate with PDPs for additional payment for services.

Of particular concern are utilization management requirements for psychotherapeutic medications and the impact of copay tiers on specialty pharmaceuticals that commonly exceed limits of $500 in monthly costs. Ultimately, the NF is responsible for all aspects of care for residents, including drugs. The facility is responsible, not the LTC pharmacy, if Part D does not cover drug therapy.

Quality Measures

Quality variations are much higher in health care than in other national industries. Nominal quality differences are reported in other industries such as airlines, banking, and manufacturing; however, the quality "gap" may be as high as 20% on existing measures within health care.

Quality measures fall under three broad categories in pharmacy programs:

1. Administrative measures—this is the basis of the Joint Commission Accreditation of Healthcare Organizations (JCAHO) measures that focus on inpatient pharmacy operations.
2. Operational measures—these are typical of PBM contracts that focus on computer-generated information and customer service requests.
3. Integrated health quality measures—these are typical of Health Plan Employer Data and Information Set (HEDIS®) measures that focus on patient care from a medical perspective and include pharmacy measures for specific diseases.
4. In addition to the aforementioned quality rating systems, CMS publishes a "Medicare 5 Star Ratings System" for Medicare Advantage Plans. The goal is to help consumers to choose plans that meet their personal needs and requirements. Consumers should consider the 5 Star Rating and also review plans who target and achieve optimal outcomes in medication adherence, MTM, and medication oversight. The goal of any quality program or rating system should be to ensure that the plan is helping the consumer achieve therapeutic goals. (See Chapter 24, Health Plans and Medicare)

Specific language for PDPs is contained within Part D—PDPs must have "quality assurance measures and systems to reduce medication errors and adverse drug interactions and improve medication use." Part D requires that medication measures be developed that demonstrate the quality of drug use for areas determined by CMS. The measures must be based on clinically supported research and evaluated by a technical expert panel. The measures must consider the technical and data limitations of PDPs. CMS draft guidance for developing these measures occurred in spring 2006.

The ideal measures for quality must be based on the Institute of Medicine (IOM) domains of safety, effectiveness, patient-centeredness, timeliness, efficiency, and equitability. They must be based on scientific evidence, and there must be consistency within the guidelines. They must be applicable to one or more purposes: quality improvement; patient safety; evaluating and monitoring clinical and economic impacts; and oversight for the purposes of controlling fraud, abuse, and waste. Finally, there must be public reporting of the measures. A list of metrics published in 2006 included such things as enrollment and disenrollment, claim reversals, MTM beneficiary eligibility and enrollment, generic dispensing rate, grievances, prior authorization, step-edit and exceptions, appeals, call center measures, overpayment, rebates, discounts and price concessions, and financial and solvency statistics.

When deficiencies in compliance are identified, the plan can issue a corrective action plan (CAP). CAPs provide an opportunity to identify risk areas within an organization. The CAP text on the CMS website can provide insight into what CMS considers inadequate and what improvements should be made by the organization. Areas commonly emphasized by CMS are grievances, coverage determination, and appeals; marketing materials; and formulary, transition process, and P&T.

In addition to compliance reviews of plan reports and materials, Medicare collects data for every paid claim. This is the Medicare Part D prescription drug events (PDEs) that are data from prescription claims that are reported to CMS by PDPs and MA-PDs. The PDE data is used by CMS for reporting to Congress and the public on the overall statistics associated with the Medicare prescription drug benefit, reconciliation of payments by plan sponsors, evaluations of the program, making legislative proposals, and conducting demonstration projects. Because plans are paid by CMS prospectively, the PDE dataflow ensures that plans report all eligible beneficiaries and data for payment reconciliation. Errors in submissions will result in underpayments to the plans or CMS chargebacks of payments from the plans.

Management of Medicare and Medicaid Drug Benefits in the Future

As Medicaid programs transition to Medicare, there is also discussion to shift Medicaid programs to private managed care programs with similar elements to the Part D programs. The argument is that the states do not wish to be dependent on the federal government for benefits and costly subsidies. While Medicare will continue to expand services, many of the state Medicaid programs will probably shift to managed care programs, either public or private in order to decrease cost. It is important to realize that this is one grand experiment where the public funds the cost, but the results are unknown for 5–10 years.

■ MEASURING FINANCIAL PERFORMANCE

The competitive managed care environment requires that health plans and PBMs effectively manage their pharmacy programs to achieve desired clinical and economic objectives for their plan sponsors and members. Health plans manage medical and pharmacy benefits and should integrate the management of both benefits. This may encourage consideration of the outcomes value of pharmaceuticals, as opposed to only managing pharmacy budget expenses independent of the medical budget. PBMs only manage pharmacy programs and are criticized for focusing on drug cost minimization rather than considering the potential for medical budget cost offsets.

Pharmacy directors monitor specific metrics on a regular basis to compare with actual versus forecasted performance, including the following:

- Various cost parameters (e.g., program expenses; high-cost therapeutic categories and high-cost drugs within categories; billed and paid claims; copayment deductions; and others). Costs may be reported as total, monthly per-member-per-month (PMPM), by product, benefit design, or a variety of other breakdowns
- Prescription utilization (PMPM and per member per year [PMPY]) and trends, through a variety of reports as indicated above
- Administrative and claims processing fees (overall, per prescription, trends)
- Prescription discount or rebate (total amount, per prescription, PMPM, and PMPY, etc.)
- Generic dispensing and conversion rate (overall, by pharmacy, by group, by therapeutic class, and by physician) and missed generic substitution opportunities
- Drug formulary conformance rate (overall, by physician, and by pharmacy)
- Patient satisfaction and member complaints related to the pharmacy program
- Number of drug formulary prior authorization exception requests and approvals and review of authorization trend
- NCQA HEDIS measure scores related to pharmacy (e.g., percent of post-myocardial infarction patients receiving a beta blocker)
- Drug utilization review exception reports

There are many more performance measurements that pharmacy directors routinely monitor, especially with more sophisticated programs that may include drug formulary conversion, compliance, and persistence activities. However, with the preceding basic performance measurements, pharmacy directors can evaluate the effectiveness of prescription drug management strategies.

■ PHARMACY BENEFIT QUALITY MEASURES AND PATIENT SATISFACTION

Health plans and PBMs respond to intensive market competition by designing and offering a variety of benefit designs to meet the varied demands of an array of customers, including health and welfare trusts, self-funded employers, health plans (for PBMs), and third-party administrators. Some may also offer Medicaid, Medicare, and other government programs. According to the WilsonRx Health Insurance Satisfaction Survey, plan sponsors generally offer two or more coverage options.[70] Generally, members of major health plans indicated they were satisfied with their health care selection. Prescription benefit coverage was ranked in the middle of the "ten most important health care issues," with "quality of medical care received" as the top issue.[71] The availability of drugs, the copayment level, and the coverage of generics were some of the top quality concerns specifically related to prescription drug benefits. These issues were ranked higher than was coverage of brand name drugs, indicating members are not only comfortable with generics but prefer them over brand name drugs due to cost savings.[72]

MCOs attempt to design and administer high-quality health care benefits that provide for covered clinical and economic objectives of plan sponsors and their members. Quality initiatives have a long history in managed care, and preventive care and quality of care were objectives of early HMOs. A complete review on quality in managed health care is provided in Chapter 14. This chapter provides information on quality initiates that are specific to prescription drug program outcomes only.

The National Committee on Quality Assurance (NCQA; see Chapter 15) has provided quality assurance tools since 1991, and offers a health plan accreditation for organizations offering comprehensive health care benefits that have delivered high-quality outcomes.[73] NCQA publishes annual updates to its Healthcare Effectiveness Data and Information Set (see also Chapter 15) measures used to measure quality of care in health plans. Some measures are process oriented, more are becoming outcomes oriented. Some specifically or implicitly refer to effective drug therapy to contribute to the HEDIS measure outcome.[74] The increasing number of pharmacotherapy-related HEDIS measures indicates an awareness of the important role the appropriate use of pharmaceuticals may have in achieving high-quality outcomes. URAC (see Chapter 15), another organization that accredits various types of health care organizations, also accredits PBM, drug therapy management, specialty pharmacy, and mail service pharmacy.[75] URAC evaluates PBMs; NCQA does not. The Pharmacy Quality Alliance (PQA) is a collaborative initiative of organizations interested in improving quality of care. The PQA sponsors a number of initiatives that promotes and measures quality outcomes in pharmacy benefit programs. (The JD Power U.S. National Pharmacy patient satisfaction reports are discussed in the section on PBMs.)

■ PHARMACOGENOMICS

The concept of personalized medicine integrates individual genetic characteristics and drug pharmacokinetics and pharmacodynamics to achieve better clinical outcomes, greater safety, and efficacy in drug design and development. Individualized medicine is particularly important in oncology, whereby most clinically used anti-cancer drugs have a narrow therapeutic window and exhibit large interindividual pharmacokinetic and pharmacodynamic variability. The three largest PBMs are exploring the role of pharmacogenomics to improve dosage precision, increase the probability of a desired therapeutic response, minimize adverse effects, reduce waste, and manage costs.[76, 77] The FDA is exploring how to include pharmacogenomics data in new drug application (NDA) submissions, and has issued a guidance document.[78] Such data are not required now, but the FDA encourages such data be included in investigational new drug (IND) applications.[79]

The use of pharmacogenomics to individualize drug therapy brings ethical considerations. Genotyping of large patient populations in the entire nation raises privacy issues. A pharmaceutical company may elect not to develop a drug for an orphan disease, or a poor country unable to afford a specialty drug, if the identified genotype group does not represent a viable business opportunity.[80]

■ CONCLUSION

Prescription drug benefits are a critical, high-value health care delivery component. Near-term trends will change the management priorities of pharmacy program directors. As many high-cost brands of traditional drugs lose their patent protection over the next decade, generic drug use will dominate the outpatient retail prescription market and costs should be easily contained. Specialty pharmaceuticals will replace traditional pharmaceuticals as the focus of cost and quality of care management. The Medicare Part D and Medicaid drug benefits will double, and mandated benefits will increase cost containment pressure on plans and PBMs. Policymakers, plan sponsors, and plan leaders must take caution to focus on the value of pharmaceuticals when the proper drug is used appropriately, and avoid the expediency of myopically focusing on cost minimization alone.

Recommended Reading

Navarro RP, ed. *Managed Care Pharmacy Practice.* Sudbury, MA: Jones and Bartlett; 2009.

Endnotes

1 Kaiser/HRET Employer Health Benefits 2010 Annual Survey. Available at: http://ehbs.kff.org/. Accessed March 15, 2011.

2 Kaiser Family Foundation. Retail prescription drugs filled pharmacies (Annual per capita by age), 2009. State Health Facts. Available at: www.statehealthfacts .org/comparetable.jsp?ind = 268&cat = 5. Accessed March 15, 2011.

3 Kaiser Family Foundation. Prescription drug trends 2010. May 2010. Available at: www.kff.org/rxdrugs/ upload/3057-08.pdf. Accessed April 8, 2011.

4 Long D. U.S. Pharmaceutical market trends: A picture of increasing trends. *IMS Health.* Spring 2010. Available at: www.imshealth.com/portal/site/imshealth/menuitem. a46c6d4df3db4b3d88f611019418c22a/?vgnextoid = b52 3257373a96210VgnVCM100000ed152ca2RCRD&vgnext fmt = default. Accessed April 9, 2011.

5 *Express Scripts Drug Trend Report 2010.* Available at: www.express-scripts.com/. Accessed April 11, 2011.

6 Long D. IMS Health National Prescription Audit, November 2010. Presented at: PCMA Managed Markets Educational Forum; February 8, 2010, Miami, FL.

7 IMS Health 2009 US Pharmaceutical Market Trends: A Picture of Increasing Trends. Available at www .imshealth.com/portal/site/imshealth/menuitem.a46c6 d4df3db4b3d88f611019418c22a/?vgnextoid = b52325737 3a96210VgnVCM100000ed152ca2RCRD&vgnextfmt = de fault. Accessed April 7, 2011.

8 Centers for Medicare and Medicaid Services. National health expenditure projections 2009–2019. September 2010. Available at: www.cms.gov/NationalHealthExpendData/ downloads/NHEProjections2009to2019.pdf. Accessed April 9, 2011.

9 Navarro RP, Becker Aw, Francis W, et al. Pharmacy benefit management companies. In: Navarro RP, ed. *Managed Care Pharmacy Practice.* 2nd ed. Sudbury, MA: Jones and Bartlett; 2009:95–114.

10 *CVS Caremark 2010 Annual Report.* Available at: http://thomson.mobular.net/thomson/7/3169/4424/ document_0/Annual%20Report%202010%20Final.pdf. Accessed April 9, 2011.

11 *Medco Health 2010 Annual Report.* Available at: http:// phx.corporate-ir.net/External.File?item = UGFyZW50SU Q9ODY0MTV8Q2hpbGRJRD0tMXxUeXBlPTM = &t = 1. Accessed April 9, 2011.

12 *Express Scripts 2010 Annual Report.* Available at: http:// phx.corporate-ir.net/External.File?item = UGFyZW50SU Q9ODY0MTV8Q2hpbGRJRD0tMXxUeXBlPTM = &t = 1. Accessed April 9, 2011.

13 Goliath Press webpage. *Fiduciary concerns spur new PBM models.* Available at: http://goliath.ecnext.com/ coms2/gi_0198–161376/Fiduciary-concerns-spur-new-PBM.html. Accessed April 10, 2011.

14 Government Accounting Office. *Effects of using pharmacy benefit managers on health plans, enrollees, and pharmacies.* Available at: http://www.gao.gov/ new.items/d03196.pdf. Accessed April 8, 2011.

15 National Community Pharmacist Association website. *Federal cases (PBMs).* Available at: www.ncpanet .org/index.php/legal-proceedings/federal-cases-pbms. Accessed April 10, 2011.

16 Pharmacy Times website. *National PBM settles federal claims of fraud, kickbacks.* Available at: www .pharmacytimes.com/publications/issue/2007/2007-06/2007-06-6588. Accessed April 11, 2011.

17 MedImpact website. *MedImpact markets itself as "the transparent PBM" with "complete transparency."* Available at: www.medimpact.com. Accessed April 8, 2011.

18 Express Scripts Consumerology website. Available at: www.consumerology.com. Accessed April 7, 2011.

19 CVS Caremark website. Available at: http://info .cvscaremark.com/sites/cvsca. Accessed April 8, 2011.

20 Matthew L, Maciejewski ML, Parker J, Wansink D. Copayment reductions generate greater medication adherence in targeted patients. *Health Affairs.* Available at: http://content.healthaffairs.org/content/29/11/2002 .full?ijkey = quBxP9SBsXsYs&keytype = ref&siteid = healt haff. Accessed April 9, 2011.

21 Mahoney JJ. Reducing patient drug acquisition costs can lower diabetes. *Am J Manag Care.* 2005;11(5 Suppl): S170–S176.

22 Fendrick AM, Chernow AE. Value based insurance design: Maintaining a focus on health in an era of cost containment. *American Journal of Managed Care.* 2009; 15(10 Suppl):S277–S283.

23 Fairman KA, Curtiss FR. What do we really know about VBID? Quality of the evidence and ethical considerations for health plan sponsors. *J Manag Care Pharm.* 2011;17(2):156–174.

24 Jones J. Pharmacy benefit design, marketing, and customer contracting. In: Navarro RP, ed. *Managed Care Pharmacy Practice.* 2nd ed. Sudbury, MA: Jones and Bartlett; 2009:54–58.

25 Black GE, Romza JH. Managed care pharmacy information systems. In: Navarro RP, ed. *Managed Care Pharmacy Practice.* 2nd ed. Sudbury, MA: Jones and Bartlett; 2009: 183–214.

26 Surescripts. Surescripts 2009 National Report on E-Prescribing. 2010. Available at: www.surescripts .com/about-e-prescribing/progress-reports/national-progress-reports.aspx. Accessed April 7, 2011.

27 USDHHS website. *HITECH Act enforcement interim rule.* Available at: www.hhs.gov/ocr/privacy/hipaa/ administrative/enforcementrule/hitechenforcementifr .html. Accessed April 11, 2011.

28 Surescripts website. *Benefits of e-prescribing to pharmacists.* Available at: www.surescripts.com/about-e-prescribing/benefits-of-e-prescribing_for-pharmacies .aspx. Accessed April 11, 2011.

29 Medco Health Solutions, Inc. *Medco Health 2010 Annual Report.* Available at: www.sendd.com/~webdrop/ EZHTML/201103/C27IuV67ybckD6ehYOcc/pdf/ MedcoHealthSolutions_BMK.pdf. Accessed April 8, 2011.

30 Sterler LT, Stephens D. Pharmacy distribution systems and network management. In: Navarro RP, ed. *Managed Care Pharmacy Practice.* 2nd ed. Sudbury, MA: Jones and Bartlett; 2009:115–121.

31 Navarro RP, Kenney JT, Haily R, Kramer D, Urick PN. Managed care contracts with pharmaceutical manufacturers. In: Navarro RP, ed. *Managed Care Pharmacy Practice.* 2nd ed. Sudbury, MA: Jones and Bartlett; 2009: 361–383.

32 Navarro RP, Dillon MJ, Grzegorczyk J. Role of drug formularies in managed care organizations. In: Navarro RP, ed. *Managed Care Pharmacy Practice.* 2nd ed. Sudbury, MA: Jones and Bartlett; 2009:233–252.

33 Academy of Managed Care Pharmacy website. Available at: http://amcp.org/Sec.aspx?id = 5399. Accessed August 15, 2011.

34 Congressional Budget Office. *Effects of using generic drugs on Medicare's prescription drug spnding.* Washington, DC: Congressional Budget Office; 2010. Publication 4043. Available at: www.cbo.gov/ftpdocs/ 118xx/doc11838/09-15-PrescriptionDrugs.pdf. Accessed April 11, 2011.

35 Liberman JN, Roebuck C. Prescription drug costs and the generic dispensing ratio. *Manag Care Pharm.* 2010; 16(7):502–506.

36 Kaiser/HRET. Employer Health Benefits 2010 Annual Survey. Available at: http://ehbs.kff.org. Accessed April 8, 2011.

37 Aetna. Aetna Medicare 2011 formulary (List of covered drugs). August 16, 2010. Available at: www.aetnamedicare .com/documents/individual/2011/formularies/2011_ medicare_preferred_drug_list.pdf. Accessed April 14, 2011.

38 Medco Health website. Available at: http://phx .corporate-ir.net/phoenix.zhtml?c = 131268&p = irol-homeProfile. Accessed April 9, 2011.

39 The Lewin Group. Mail-service pharmacy savings and the cost of proposed limitations in medicare and the commercial sector. Available at: www.lewin.com/ content/publications/3480.pdf. Accessed August 15, 2011.

40 Managed Care website. *Don't get caught by PBM's MAC mousetraps.* Available at: www.managedcaremag.com/ archives/0809/0809.maxallowable.html. Accessed April 7, 2011.

41 American Journal of Health Benefits website. Comparing pharmacy benefit managers: Moving well beyond the simple spreadsheet analysis. Available at: www .ahdbonline.com/feature/comparing-pharmacy-benefit-managers-moving-well-beyond-simple-spreadsheet-analysis. Accessed April 5, 2011.

42 JD Power website. 2010 Pharmacy satisfaction study: Pharmacy ratings (Mail order). Available at: www .jdpower.com/Healthcare/ratings/pharmacy-ratings-(mail-order)/. Accessed April 7, 2011.

43 JD Power website. 2010 Pharmacy satisfaction study: Pharmacy ratings (Brick and mortar): Chain. Available at:

www.jdpower.com/healthcare/ratings/pharmacy-ratings-(brick-and-mortar)/chain/. Accessed April 6, 2011.

44 JD Power website. 2010 Pharmacy satisfaction study. Pharmacy ratings (Brick and mortar): Mass merchandiser. Available at: www.jdpower.com/healthcare/ratings/pharmacy-ratings-(brick-and-mortar)/mass-merchandiser/. Accessed April 6, 2011.

45 Express Scripts Drug Cost Trend 2010. Ibid., p. 26.

46 *Biotechnology Monitor & Survey.* 2010. Plainsboro, NJ: Bristol-Myers Squibb; 2010:6.

47 Ibid., pp. 18–19.

48 Johnson KJ, Siegel MJ. Specialty Pharmaceuticals. In: Navarro RP, ed. *Managed Care Pharmacy Practice.* 2nd ed. Sudbury, MA: Jones and Bartlett; 2009:165–179.

49 ICORE. The 2010 medical injectibles and oncology trend report. 2010:14. Available at: www.icorehealthcare.com/trends.aspx. Accessed April 7, 2011.

50 Johnson KA, Siegel JM. Specialty pharmaceuticals. In: Navarro RP, ed. *Managed Care Pharmacy Practice.* 2nd ed. Sudbury, MA: Jones and Bartlett; 2009:151–163.

51 Ibid., p. 9.

52 Ibid., p. 6.

53 BiotechBlog website. *Biosimilar drugs to gain greater priority as decade progresses.* Available at: www.biotechblog.com/2010/06/21/biosimilar-drugs-to-gain-greater-priority-as-decade-progresses/. Accessed April 14, 2011.

54 Peterson AM, Chan V, Wilson MD. Drug utilization review strategies. In: Navarro RP, ed. *Managed Care Pharmacy Practice.* 2nd ed. Sudbury, MA: Jones and Bartlett; 2009:215–232.

55 Pharmaceutical Executive website. *Prescription abandonment rates on the rise.* Available at: http://pharmexec.findpharma.com/pharmexec/article/articleDetail.jsp?id = 590840. Accessed April 8, 2011.

56 Express Scripts Drug Trend Report 2010, p. 33. Available at: www.express-scripts.com/research/studies/drugtrendreport/. Accessed April 11, 2011.

57 CVS Caremark Annual Report 2010. Available at: http://info.cvscaremark.com/sites/cvscaremark.com/files/TrendsRx_2009.pdf. Accessed April 8, 2011.

58 Cain P. Medicare D–Nearly 20% of prescriptions. *IMS Health.* July 2009. Available at: www.imshealth.com/portal/site/imshealth/menuitem.a46c6d4df3db4b3d88f611019418c22a/?vgnextoid = 3c87c71e81a32210VgnVCM100000ed152ca2RCRD&vgnextfmt = default. Accessed April 7, 2011.

59 Kaiser Family Foundation. Medicare enrollment, 1966–2010. Available at: http://facts.kff.org/chart.aspx?ch = 1714. Accessed April 10, 2011

60 Hoadley J, Cubanski J, Hargrave E, Summer L, Neuman T. Medicare Part D spotlight: Part D plan availability in 2011 and key changes since 2006. Kaiser Family Foundation.

Available at: www.kff.org/medicare/upload/8107.pdf. Accessed April 7, 2011.

61 Kaiser Family Foundation. Medicare enrollment, 1966–2010. Available at: http://facts.kff.org/chart.aspx?ch = 1714. Accessed April 9, 2011.

62 Kehoe D. Medication therapy management. In: Navarro RP, ed. *Managed Care Pharmacy Practice.* 2nd ed. Sudbury, MA: Jones and Bartlett; 2009:491–513.

63 Centers for Medicare and Medicaid. 2010 Medicare Part D medication therapy management (MTM) programs. Available at: www.cms.gov/PrescriptionDrugCovContra/Downloads/MTMFactSheet.pdf. Accessed April 8, 2011.

64 Schumock GT, Butler MG, Meek PD, et al. Evidence of the economic benefit of clinical pharmacy services. *Pharmacotherapy.* 2003;23(1):113–132.

65 Bluml BM. Definition of medication therapy management development of profession-wide consensus. *J Am Pharm Assoc.* 2005;45(5):566–572.

66 Erickson AK. Changing lives one phone call at a time. *Am Pharm.* 2011 (Feb.):42–44.

67 Centers for Medicare and Medicaid. 2010 Medicare Part D medication therapy management (MTM) programs. Available at: www.cms.gov/PrescriptionDrugCovContra/Downloads/MTMFactSheet.pdf. Accessed April 8, 2011.

68 American Pharmacist Association. Tracking the expansion of MTM in 2010. Exploring the consumer of perspective. *Medication Therapy Management Digest.* March 2011. Available at: www.pharmacist.com/AM/Template.cfm?Section = MTM&TEMPLATE = /CM/ContentDisplay.cfm&CONTENTID = 25712. Accessed April 8, 2011.

69 Ramalho de Oliveira D, Brummel AR, Miller DB. Medication therapy management: 10 years of experience in a large integrated health care system. *J Manag Care Pharm.* 2010;16(3):185–195.

70 Wilson JM. Member satisfaction strategies. In: Navarro RP, ed. *Managed Care Pharmacy Practice.* 2nd ed. Sudbury, MA: Jones and Bartlett; 2009:253–261.

71 Ibid., p. 258.

72 Ibid., p. 269.

73 NCQA website. Available at: www.ncqa.org/Home.aspx. Accessed April 8, 2011.

74 NCQA website. Available at: www.ncqa.org/tabid/1223/Default.aspx. Accessed April 8, 2011.

75 URAC website. Available at: www.urac.org/pqm/dtm.asp. Accessed April 8, 2011.

76 Dovepress website. *Pharmacogenomics and personalized medicine.* Available at: www.dovepress.com/aims-and-scope-pharmacogenomics-and-personalized-medicine-d30-j38. Accessed March 25, 2011.

77 Medco Health website. Available at: www.medcohealth.com/medco/corporate/home.jsp?ltSess = y&articleID = CorpPM_PersonalizedMedicine. Accessed April 16, 2011.

78 U.S. Department of Health and Human Services Food and Drug Administration. Guidance for industry: Pharmacogenomic data submissions. March 2005. Available at: www.fda.gov/downloads/RegulatoryInformation/Guidances/ucm126957.pdf. Accessed April 14, 2011.

79 Innovaro pharmalicensing website. *Pharmacogenomics in drug development*. Available at: http://pharmalicensing. com/public/articles/view/1090249172_40fbe1d4c4ef9/pharmacogenomics-in-drug-development. Accessed April 14, 2011.

80 Bartfai T. Pharmacogenomics in drug development: Societal and technical aspects. *Pharmacogenomics J.* 2004; 4:226–232. Available at: www.nature.com/tpj/journal/v4/n4/full/6500249a.html. Accessed April 14, 2011.

Introduction to Managed Behavioral Health Care Organizations

Joann Albright, Deborah Heggie, Anthony M. Kotin, Connie Salgy, Wanda Sullivan, and Fred Waxenberg

STUDY OBJECTIVES

- Understand the differences between behavioral health managed care and medical-surgical managed care
- Understand the impact of federal legislation on the management of behavioral health care
- Understand the different forms of managed care treatment in behavioral health managed care
- Understand how behavioral health managed care is integrated into the larger health system
- Understand the different approaches a behavioral health management organization might take for different types of health plans

DISCUSSION TOPICS

1. Discuss the unique factors that present special challenges to behavioral health management as compared to medical-surgical management.
2. Discuss which types of behavioral health treatment methods form the backbone of managed care service.
3. Discuss the advantages and disadvantages of a managed care plan using an external behavioral health vendor versus an internal behavioral health department.

■ INTRODUCTION: THE NATURE AND UNIQUENESS OF BEHAVIORAL HEALTH

Although generally misunderstood, there is increasing acknowledgment that mental health is not a minor issue—as a singular issue affecting the health and productivity of the population but also as an amplifier of the impact of chronic illness, both in quality of life and cost of care. For example, as **Table 12-1** shows, depressive and anxiety disorders affect large numbers of people.

Despite their widespread occurrence, psychiatric conditions remain poorly understood by the general public and incompletely understood by most clinicians who practice outside the field of psychiatry. This issue extends to the treatment of substance-related disorders. Franklin et al note that "stigma associated with the term *alcoholism*

frequently inhibits physicians and patients from exploring the connection between [substance] abuse and biopsychosocial consequences."[1] They further note that "psychiatrists participating in a hospital survey positively identified alcohol abuse two-thirds of the time, whereas physicians treating gynecology patients diagnosed the disorder only 10 percent of the time."[1, 2]

As understanding of brain chemistry has evolved, there has been a concomitant and significant impact on the treatment of behavioral health conditions. Schatzberg et al. summarize this view when they argue that over the past 30 years, psychiatry's "move from a largely psychoanalytic orientation toward a more biological stance radically changed not only its basic approaches to patients but also the professional identities of psychiatrists."[3]

TABLE 12-1	Prevalence of Depressive and Anxiety Disorders in Adults	
Disorder	**Estimated prevalence**	
Dysthymic disorder	10,800,000	
Major depressive disorder	9,900,000	
Posttraumatic stress disorder	5,500,000	
Social phobia	5,300,000	
Generalized anxiety disorder	4,100,000	
Obsessive-compulsive disorder	3,300,000	
Agoraphobia	3,000,000	
Panic disorder	2,500,000	
Bipolar disorder	2,300,000	

Source: National Institutes of Mental Health (2007).

At its core, behavioral health attempts to interpret neurophysiology as manifested by behavior. This is by no means a simple task and proves daunting for even the most talented professionals. Behavior can reasonably be interpreted as the consequence of activities in the mind, and the mind as a state of being both influenced by and influencing brain chemistry. Yet psychiatric nosology (i.e., the systematic classification of diseases) partly ignores this paradigm by its shift from imputed motivation in certain conditions to a phenomenological approach that relies solely on the observation of behavior or a patient's self-report.

Nothing, for example, in the American Psychiatric Association's (APA) description of a major depressive episode implies a psychological antecedent to depression.[4] The description relies solely on the patient's report and/or observation by the clinician or others of a depressed mood, markedly diminished interest in or pleasure from activities, significant weight loss or decreased or increased appetite, insomnia or hypersomnia, psychomotor agitation or retardation, fatigue or loss of energy, feelings of worthlessness or excessive/inappropriate guilt, diminished ability to think or concentrate, and recurrent thoughts of death or suicidal ideation.

Given the plethora of theories and schools of thought about the psychology of human beings, the emphasis on observation of behavior and patient self-report is necessary for the creation of an empirical system that is manageable and easily validated. While such a system serves the health care industry well, it is necessarily circumscribed and unable to match the complexity of the human condition, especially in regard to an individual's motivation, which may be a key to effecting therapeutic change.

While the APA's catalog of symptoms, as just presented, makes the diagnosis of depression a relatively straightforward task for a psychiatrist or behavioral health clinician, even such a basic task is complicated by differential diagnosis. For example, the symptoms of a major depressive episode occur within the context of major depressive disorder, or they may constitute the depressive phase of bipolar disorder, depression secondary to a medical condition, depression as related to substance use or withdrawal, depression as manifested in premenstrual dysphoric disorder, depression as related to bereavement or complicated bereavement, or depression as associated with cyclothymic disorder.

It is small wonder, then, that the diagnosis of behavioral health disorders poses many challenges to clinicians and patients alike. Thus, it becomes obvious that expecting acute care, general medical clinicians to understand the nuances of behavioral diagnosis under the structural and process pressures inherent in general practice settings is unrealistic or in the public interest.

Another emerging facet of the field of behavioral health is the growing evidence for and understanding of the connection between the body and the mind. Psychosomatic medicine, which is rooted in consultation-liaison psychiatry and has grown from modest beginnings in American medicine in the 1930s, remains a valuable subspecialty. With an emphasis on the mind-body connection, psychosomatic medicine remains a vital force in opposition to the split—predominantly an artifact of systemic versus clinical factors—that too readily occurs between physical and mental approaches to diagnosis and treatment. Mainstream psychiatry acknowledges the mind-body connection by its elimination of "functional" (being emotional or psychological in nature) and "organic" (being physiological or anatomical in nature) concepts and terms in recent editions of the *Diagnostic and Statistical Manual of Mental Disorders*.

Proper diagnosis is, of course, of paramount importance in any medical specialty. It is no less so in behavioral health. Treatment plans can be effective only if based on proper diagnosis because the diagnosis determines not only the treatments offered (e.g., medication and/or psychotherapy), but also risk factors and prognosis. Yet, as the example of depression demonstrates, a clear diagnosis is not always evident to even the most skilled clinician, especially upon initial evaluation.

Accuracy of diagnosis and appropriateness of treatment planning have ramifications for an individual's morbidity, productivity, and sense of well-being, as well as for the cost of effective treatment. Furthermore, since many behavioral health disorders are chronic, and chronicity may become evident only after adequate time in treatment, incorrect diagnosis and inappropriate treatment planning can foster noncompliance and relapse and result in excessive costs for treatment. Risk of inaccurate diagnosis and resulting inappropriate or ineffective treatment is not as pronounced for general medical conditions (e.g., hypertension, hyperlipidemia, or diabetes) where laboratory or physical tests to identify and monitor these conditions are readily available.

In response to these challenges, managed behavioral health care organizations (MBHOs) have gone beyond the traditional gatekeeper function of utilization management. Prevention and disease management programs identify members at risk because of behavioral health and/or medical conditions, and provide education and outreach to reduce morbidity and enhance well-being. Intensive care management programs meet the needs of members with more serious or long-term care needs. Alongside these initiatives are outcome measurement protocols that measure effectiveness in terms of reduction in morbidity and increase in productivity—key issues for the health plans and employers that typically cover the costs of care.

Furthering the impetus for care collaboration is the promotion of the concept of the patient-centered medical home—now finding favor with most managed care organizations (MCOs). In this context, behavioral health is a key element in terms of screening and management of its impact on physical health conditions. The Patient Protection and Affordable Care Act (ACA) has taken this integration concept further with the establishment of integrated health homes, which specifically include the management of individuals with serious mental illness as one of the sentinel conditions.

The health care delivery system is now better poised to more holistically address the mind-body continuum. It will remain to be seen if the models that have been put forth can and will be put into practice.

■ LEGISLATION AFFECTING MANAGEMENT OF BEHAVIORAL HEALTH CARE

The Mental Health Parity and Addiction Equity Act and the ACA have a profound impact on the management of mental health benefits, essentially redefining the marketplace. Interim final regulations for the application of mental health parity, a law that was heavily supported by the managed behavioral health industry, were distinctly adverse to behavioral health management.

The ACA, assuming its provisions do not change significantly, will greatly expand the industry's management of the government sector by virtue of creating new coverage for a population that is anticipated to have significant behavioral health conditions. It will also create new opportunities and challenges for the industry as state-run health exchanges come to fruition. The creation of the CMS offices for Innovation and Duals will also force the creation of new models of care that will affect the industry.

Parity

The Mental Health Parity and Addiction Equity Act passed in October 2008 was a watershed event for those suffering from mental health conditions. Its original intent was to ensure that coverage for behavioral health conditions would be on par with coverage for physical health maladies. The regulations

that ensued not only embraced this intent but went further by equilibrating the management of behavioral health conditions to that of physical health. This was done through a new and unanticipated concept of "nonquantitative treatment limits." The thought was that not only should there be benefit equivalence in terms of days in treatment or restrictions in site of service, but there should be parity in the manner in which care is managed. While logical in a simplistic sense, the practical reality is that much of the provision of behavioral health services occurs in an ambulatory environment. Physical health utilization management is primarily focused on procedures and inpatient management. Thus, trying to equilibrate what is allowed under parity in this light clearly strains the ability for MBHOs to provide the historical degree of utilization management services and protections to clients and members.

Health Care Reform

One result of the sweeping impact of ACA will be the expansion of coverage in 2014 to approximately 14 million recipients who are believed to have a significant degree of mental health issues. Typically, these are low-income, single males for whom substance use disorders are felt to be prominent. This expansion of covered lives will greatly define the strategy for the industry in terms of competing for government-funded business.

In addition to this expansion, the new law creates a number of opportunities to pilot new programs that are designed to promote a truly integrated approach to clinical management. One particular section of the bill, 2703, creates the opportunity for states to implement "integrated health homes." The section specifically allows for these homes to accommodate the seriously mentally ill (SMI) as their primary source of care. Add to this the concerted effort to rationalize funding for the aged, blind, and disabled (ABD) and dually eligible (individuals funded by both Medicaid and Medicare) through the newly created CMS offices of Innovation and Duals, and it becomes easy to see how transformative the legislation will be.

Why is there such an impact on the managed behavioral health industry? Nearly 30% of the ABD population and almost 50% of the dual-eligible population carry a diagnosis of SMI. Historically, these population cohorts have been predominantly covered in a fee-for-service environment. With coordinated funding and the opportunity to have payment models that allow for risk assumption, the market will dramatically change.

Enhancing this impact is the fact that as opposed to simply believing that there needs to be more integration around the management of behavioral health and physical health in the comorbid population, the ACA is now providing a significant impetus to make it happen. How this plays out in the government sector and how it will influence the commercial sector will largely determine the face of the managed behavioral health industry of the future.

THE PUBLIC SECTOR

If individuals with mental health and substance use disorders pose special challenges for health care systems, individuals who receive care through Medicaid benefits present additional, complex problems. (Medicaid managed care is also discussed in Chapter 25.)

Medicaid populations have a much higher incidence of debilitating psychiatric illness, such as schizophrenia and bipolar disorder, than the general population. Medicaid beneficiaries by definition lack resources to easily access the private health care system, and the serious and persistent nature of their behavioral disorders makes them less likely to comply with treatment or maintain routine follow-up care. Reduced or absent access to routine and preventive care, cultural and linguistic factors, lack of family and social supports, and lack of community resources conspire to make effective participation in behavioral health treatment much less likely. MBHOs have been able to address the unique needs of Medicaid populations through innovative, evidence-based programs that provide solutions to the complex, myriad barriers that reduce participation in behavioral health care.

NETWORKS

As discussed in Chapters 2 and 4, one of the defining features of managed care in general, and managed behavioral health care in particular, is the establishment and use of a credentialed clinical network. The philosophy of behavioral health network management has changed over the past few decades. Originally, MBHOs developed small, contained networks, contracting with facilities and providers at discounted rates in return for increased referral streams to these preferred providers. The modest size of these networks allowed behavioral health care companies to track utilization and quality indicators and helped control the cost of care.

As the managed care industry matured, consumers opted for less restrictive products with more choice of providers than in traditional health maintenance organizations (HMOs). MBHOs responded by expanding their networks to include a larger selection of providers to allow greater consumer choice and clinical specialization. Companies created mechanisms to decrease barriers to access and enabled members to search for providers using Internet and telephone technologies. The downside to the development of broader and larger networks was reduced opportunity to collect and interpret meaningful quality data on credentialed providers. Recently, MBHOs have responded to this challenge by implementing new strategies designed to collect outcomes and/or quality data regardless of network size and composition.

PAYMENT MECHANISMS

In the last two decades, behavioral health care payment strategies mirrored to a large extent those developed in the medical arena, as discussed in Chapter 5. As HMOs developed and matured, there was a movement to share financial risk with large provider groups and delivery systems through capitation contracts. Subcapitated groups were paid set rates regardless of the number of patients served. Contracts varied as to the levels of care and services covered. By the year 2000, however, the popularity of capitation as a risk-sharing strategy ebbed due to the well-publicized collapse of a number of large provider groups, as described in Chapter 1.

More recently, different financing strategies have developed based on whether a mental health and substance abuse provider operates at the inpatient or outpatient level. Outpatient providers have been contracted with and paid using fee-for-service (FFS) with varying specific, negotiated fee schedules. FFS rate schedules depend on provider type (psychiatrist, psychologist, social worker, etc.), Current Procedural Terminology (CPT) codes, and state(s) in which services are rendered.

Facility-based providers more recently have been paid using per diem schedules specific to the type of service and program (e.g., hospital inpatient, intermediate care, residential treatment, partial hospitalization, day treatment, and intensive outpatient). The rates depend on a number of variables, including the facility's retail rates, location, availability of comparable services in the same area, and prevailing market rates.

NEW TYPES OF SERVICE DELIVERY SYSTEMS

New federal regulations, including the ACA, are encouraging an overarching improvement to health care. As a result, federal and state governments are exploring new types of service delivery systems, such as accountable care organizations and patient-centered medical homes (ACOs and PCMHs, respectively; see Chapters 2 and 30). Both care delivery systems actively engage the patients and the right participants to improve the experience of care, improve the health of populations, and reduce per capita costs of health care.

Medical and health organizations have tried organizing such operations before. However, because of the new regulations and new funding available, insurers are stepping up their role to take part. Health plans, medical groups, behavioral health groups, and hospitals are creating ACOs, and are offering financial incentives and alternative payment strategies in an attempt to change the care delivery system.

By definition, an ACO typically consists of medical physicians, behavioral health physicians, hospitals, and a health plan or governmental payer. There is a 3-year commitment to belong to an ACO, and the ACO is responsible for the care delivered to its members. The main objectives of the ACO are to improve quality of care, lower medical costs, and improve patient satisfaction. The ACO builds in accountability by rewarding the providers for results through a shared-savings model (Chapter 5).

Key success factors of an ACO include:

- Ability to identify the population to manage
- Ability to understand and manage cost
- Ability to manage quality
- Ability to integrate care

A medical home is not a place but a type of clinical practice. Focusing primarily on patients with serious mental illness and/or chronic comorbid conditions, it is a practice in which a doctor—either a behavioral health doctor or medical doctor—coordinates primary care for patients. In addition, through technology, the treating providers and the patient become more connected to the care and treatment. Often, an ACO is the organization that supports the clinical model, but it is not a prerequisite. Other medical or provider organizations may have a medical home clinical model, but they may not be a part of an ACO.

Common members of a medical home team include a physician, medical assistant (MA), registered nurse (RN)/ coach, behavioral health team member, and a health plan case manager. Through health information exchange technology, electronic medical records, and e-solutions, the practice team shares information and integrates both physical and behavioral health care for the patients. This is depicted graphically in **Figure 12-1**.

Key success factors of a medical home include:

- Improved quality of care
- Improved status of comorbid conditions
- Increased satisfaction of patients
- Reduction of avoidable comorbid hospitalizations
- Reduction of acute occurrences
- Reduction of inpatient admissions
- Reduction of long-term care admissions

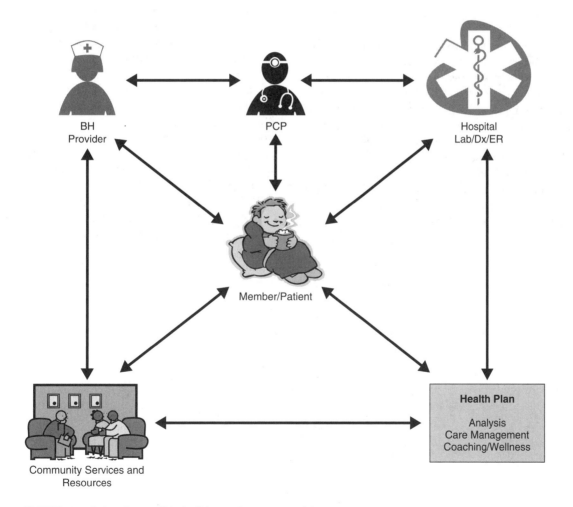

FIGURE 12-1 Patient-Centered Medical Home—Integration and Communication

■ BEHAVIORAL HEALTH CARE PROFESSIONAL PROVIDERS

Behavioral health as a discipline is served by a variety of licensed professionals, including psychiatrists, psychologists, social workers, licensed professional counselors, marriage and family therapists, and clinical nurse specialists. MBHOs create their own requirements for acceptance of these provider classes because states vary greatly on their requirements for licensure and the degree of professional autonomy associated with specific licenses.

Some of the more commonly recognized subspecialties are:

- Child/adolescent
- Substance use disorders
- Eating disorders
- Anxiety disorders
- Gay/lesbian/transgender issues
- HIV/AIDS
- Faith-based counseling
- Workplace/career issues

Access and Density Standards

As MBHOs grew national in scope, they began to review their clinical networks using access and density standards. Such review was necessary because of variation in the number and availability of mental health and substance use providers across regions and in rural versus urban settings.

A number of factors are considered in reviewing access and density. Access is defined as the availability of a provider within a certain geographical distance of the population. Access standards vary depending on whether an area is considered urban, suburban, or rural as determined by U.S. Census data in conjunction with the latest U.S. Postal Service zip code updates.

- Urban = population of 3,000 or more per square mile
- Suburban = population of 1,000–2,999 per square mile
- Rural = population of less than 1,000 per square mile

Table 12-2 illustrates access standards for urban, suburban, and rural areas.

Density refers to the type and number of professionals per a defined number of covered members. Psychiatrists are

TABLE 12-2	Network Provider Access Standards			
MHSA	**Urban areas**	**Suburban areas**	**Rural areas**
One psychiatrist and one other behavioral professional	90% within 10 miles	90% within 25 miles	90% within 40 miles
One organizational provider (facility)	90% within 25 miles	90% within 40 miles	90% within 60 miles

TABLE 12-3	Network Provider Density Standards			
Psychiatrist	**Nonpsychiatris**	**Total**	**Number of covered lives**
2	8	10	10,000

broken out from the other classes of therapists due to the specialized services they provide. **Table 12-3** illustrates density standards for psychiatrists and nonpsychiatrists. Behavioral health care organizations typically use commercially developed computer programs to determine the adequacy of their networks in relation to the characteristics of the population they are serving.

Credentialing*

Providers undergo a standard credentialing and contracting process before they are included in a network. National accrediting bodies such as the National Committee for Quality Assurance (NCQA), The Joint Commission (TJC), and URAC[†] have established standards for the types of information that must be collected and verified in the credentialing process. External accreditation is discussed in detail in Chapter 15.

Use of standardized credentialing applications, such as that supported by the Council on Affordable Quality Healthcare (CAQH), Universal Provider Datasource, or state-mandated forms, has increased in recent years to reduce the administrative burden for providers credentialed across a number of health plans. Verification processes performed by MBHOs include review of providers' credentials, such as licensure, board certification, education and training, Medicaid and Medicare sanctions, and work history.

Primary source verification of credentials has increased in efficiency as such data are now commonly provided online by the various states and federal and professional certification agencies. Credentialing also incorporates review of supplemental information indicated by the provider, such as clinical specialties, languages spoken, experience with special populations, and ethnicity. This information supports improved member self-referral activity, as well as care manager facilitated referrals.

A review of credentials and other provider practice information is performed by a clinical credentialing committee once the administrative aspects of the credentialing process are completed. The clinical reviewers make the final decision as to whether to credential the provider for network participation.

* The authors express their appreciation to Mary Shorter-Fahimi, LCSW, who provided content for the credentialing section.
† URAC was once an acronym, but it no longer is.

MBHOs perform ongoing monitoring of its network providers for the occurrence of disciplinary actions on licenses and sanctions imposed by Medicaid or Medicare, including exclusion from participation in those programs. Discovery of such actions may affect the provider's network participation status.

Network providers are fully recredentialed every 3 years, at which time information is reverified to ensure currency and updated with any new credentials obtained since the previous credentialing activity. Licensure, board certification, presence of any Medicaid/Medicare or license sanctions, and new professional liability claims are again primary source verified, and providers queried for any updated clinical specialty information. Once administrative verifications are complete, the clinical credentialing committee again reviews the provider's credentials, supplements this with relevant quality information—such as member satisfaction, clinical practice guidelines studies, treatment record review results, and outcome trends—and renders a decision about the provider's ongoing network participation.

■ TYPES OF SERVICES DELIVERED BY BEHAVIORAL NETWORKS

Behavioral health care networks allow for the provision of an extensive array of services and levels of care. The typical commercial delivery system classification includes:

Inpatient Services Inpatient services are the highest level of skilled psychiatric and substance abuse services and are usually provided in a hospital facility involving 24-hour medical and nursing care, such as a free-standing psychiatric facility, a general hospital, or a detoxification unit in a hospital.

Residential Treatment Residential treatment services are rendered in a facility that offers 24-hour care and provides patients with severe mental disorders or substance-related disorders a continuum of therapeutic services. Licensure requirements vary by state, but settings that are eligible for this level of care are licensed at the residential intermediate level or as an intermediate care facility.

Partial Hospitalization Partial hospitalization programs provide structured mental health or substance abuse therapeutic services for at least 4 hours per day and at least 3 days per week. Services are delivered by a multidisciplinary team.

Intensive Outpatient Program Intensive outpatient programs provide structured therapeutic services for at least 2 hours per day and at least 3 days per week. Services are comprised of coordinated and integrated multidisciplinary services, such as individual, family, or multifamily group therapy; psychoeducational services; and medical monitoring.

Outpatient Treatment Traditional outpatient therapy includes individual, family, or group treatment rendered by a licensed professional for a specified duration of time. This includes medication evaluation and monitoring by a professional licensed to provide that service (typically psychiatrists or clinical nurse specialists).

Employment Assistance Programs (EAPs) EAP professionals deliver short-term, problem-focused services for employees and their families. Services are delivered in an outpatient setting and focus on finding solutions for work and personal problems. Services are free to the user and delivered within a three-, five-, or seven-session model.

■ NETWORKS IN THE PUBLIC SECTOR

Public sector networks frequently encompass a greater range of services and delivery systems due to myriad services needed by the public sector population. Consequently, these networks often include nontraditional provider and organization types, such as those listed below, which usually are provided under the supervision of a community mental health center.

Supervised Living Supervised living includes community-based residential detoxification programs, community-based residential rehabilitation in halfway or quarter-way houses, specialized foster care homes, and group homes. Services include a combination of outpatient therapy and assistance in managing basic day-to-day living activities.

Programs for Assertive Community Treatment (PACT/ACT Teams) In PACT/ACT units, multidisciplinary teams deliver services directly in the community to members who demonstrate a pattern of recidivism and symptom chronicity and severity. The structure of the teams and delivery system are highly standardized.

Peer Support In peer support programs, consumers who have attained a high level of recovery work under the supervision of a behavioral health provider that assists patients in building confidence and in improving life skills.

Continuous Treatment Teams (CTT) Continuous treatment teams are multidisciplinary and provide a range of intensive integrated case management, treatment, and rehabilitative services in an effort to prevent a child's removal from the home to a more restrictive level of care. The team uses a community-based family strengths model and philosophy.

Community Case Management Community case management workers coordinate care and social services delivered within the community. They collaborate with the systems and providers rendering the care.

■ QUALITY MANAGEMENT OF NETWORKS

MBHOs monitor the safety and quality of care for members and the services delivered by their network providers and facilities through a variety of means. This includes self-reported outcomes by treated members, treatment record audits, experience of care/satisfaction data, and the tracking of complaints, adverse incidents, and quality of care concerns.

With the movement to use externally validated measures and reportable patient outcomes, MBHOs also review within their contracted networks the use of evidence-based practices and performance on nationally reported data sets such as NCQA's Healthcare Effectiveness Data and Information Set (HEDIS®). Four behavioral health measures within HEDIS are of specific emphasis in reviewing provider practices: timely ambulatory follow-up after an inpatient hospitalization, antidepressant medication management, follow-up care for children prescribed medication for attention-deficit/hyperactivity disorder, and initiation and engagement of alcohol and other drug dependence treatment.

Providers treating members in the public sector are monitored based on measures such as the National Outcomes Measures (NOMS) established by the Substance Abuse and Mental Health Services Administration (SAMHSA). **Table 12-4** provides the NOMS categories for measures.

In the 2011 report, the National Strategy for Quality Improvement, to Congress from the Secretary of the Department of Health and Human Services, it is recommended that payment arrangements in health care should offer incentives that foster better health and promote quality improvement and greater value while creating an environment that fosters innovation. Two practices related to quality management

TABLE 12-4	National Outcomes Measures Categories	
Reduced Morbidity	Access/Capacity
Employment/Education	Retention
Crime and Criminal Justice	Perception of Care
Stability in Housing	Cost Effectiveness
Social Connectedness	Use of Evidence-Based Practices

of networks that reflect this direction are provider/facility profiles based on clinical, outcomes, and utilization data, and pay for performance (P4P) initiatives.[5-7] These have received mixed reviews due to lack of clarity in the purpose, questionable evidence that outcomes measurement improves a patient's participation in treatment, lack of risk adjustment systems, and excessive administrative burden for providers.

One of the major challenges in implementation of provider profiling and P4P systems in behavioral health care is that, unlike medical-surgical care, easily identified and accepted tests that indicate improvement in a patient's mental health and well-being are not available. The stigma associated with mental health diagnoses may be another factor in the slow adoption of these practices.[8] Despite these challenges, MBHOs are implementing pilot programs for provider profiling and P4P. [6, 7]

Successful P4P initiatives, as described in Chapter 5, are characterized by involvement of the provider community in the program design, adoption of nationally recognized and reliable measurements that are viewed as clinically relevant, a financial incentive that is of a size and structure that is meaningful to the provider, and a compensation methodology that is easy to understand and calculate.[9, 10] Under the direction and leadership of the Centers for Medicare and Medicaid Services (CMS), the public sector has been one of the leaders in the adoption and rollout of P4P initiatives. A summary document prepared by the Center for Health Care Strategies summarizes the different P4P initiatives that are being tracked across states. Several of the initiatives relate specifically to behavioral health populations[11] including adolescent readmissions to residential facilities, ambulatory follow-up visits within 30 days post-discharge, and community tenure.

Another large measurement program is the System for Tracking Audit and Payment (STAR), developed by CMS as a quality profiling demonstration program. The program applies to Medicare Advantage plans, private FFS, and medical savings accounts and special needs plans. The program is comprised of five categories, which include 36 measures. Health plans are ranked on their overall performance in the five categories and are awarded stars for performance, which are publicly reported. Plan members can review ratings of the health plans. While the health plan is responsible for reporting these measures, behavioral health plans support them in reporting on select measures and providers' performance is tracked as they contribute to successful achievement of the measures.

■ USE OF STANDARDIZED ASSESSMENT TOOLS

In recent years, the managed behavioral health care industry has begun using standardized assessment tools in day-to-day clinical operations. This represents a major shift in the industry. The major focus of behavioral health managed care in the 1970s and 1980s was cost containment achieved through the determination of what was medically necessary and what was not, and managing benefits accordingly. Increasingly, employers, health care purchasers, and government agencies are requiring clinical outcomes in addition to cost containment for purposes of comparison and health care transparency. Health care transparency and health care accountability are critical aspects of health care reform. Quality improvement and performance measurement are essential for achievement of both.

Through the management of care, behavioral health companies have found that just as in medical-surgical care, the majority of the costs are associated with a minority of chronic patients who require repeated interventions over time. The reason is that once a condition becomes full-blown, it often requires very intensive and high-cost services to manage, often with limited success. To conserve resources and achieve optimal return with an ever-growing demand for services, MBHOs are increasing their focus on identification and management of individuals with complex care needs. The goal is to proactively intervene in early phases of illness and to manage the care throughout the course of the chronic condition. MBHOs are demonstrating that accurate behavioral diagnosis and attention to medical, neurological, and substance abuse issues reduces repeat hospitalizations and excessive ambulatory visits, with reductions in attendant costs of care and burden of illness.

A growing aspect of the trend toward proactive identification and intervention is an emphasis on high-prevalence mental disorders, such as depressive and anxiety disorders, that frequently coexist with medical disorders, such as heart disease, diabetes, and cancer. This emphasis is based on the belief that medical costs can be significantly lowered if coexisting mental disorders are aggressively managed, such that patients are more engaged in and compliant with medical treatment. This belief is borne out by a growing body of data suggesting that the course and prognosis for at least some medical conditions are affected or mediated by mental disorders. For example, the link between recovery after a coronary event and the presence or absence of depression is now well established.

MBHOs have become more directly involved with general medical patients in activities that provide added value to the efforts of medical providers to reduce impact, course, and severity of medical disorders. MBHOs are increasingly working with their health plan customers in the development of both medical homes and integrated health homes, where patient-centered care and care coordination is emphasized.

MBHOs have developed disease management programs to address chronic conditions, and a variety of coordinated models have been developed in concert with health plans, including having mental health care managers co-located with medical care managers. Disease management programs (see also Chapter 8) are designed to meet two objectives: (1) to help patients successfully manage chronic behavioral disorders and (2) to identify and mitigate the effects of mental disorders that may reduce treatment effectiveness and increase costs of care for physical illnesses, such as diabetes.

In the service of motivating medical patients to engage in self-care and treatments that address their coexisting mental disorders, MBHOs have embraced the technique of motivational coaching. Coaching is offered to patients directly by the MBHO, providing education, encouragement, and other assistance to enhance motivation for and engagement in treatment, assist in the coordination of care with multiple providers, and support the patient during the therapeutic process.

Disease management and coaching activities are indications of a major paradigm shift in which MBHOs work directly with patients and not solely with providers. Since these are new and innovative approaches, their clinical and financial effectiveness has not been proven. To demonstrate the return on investment, MBHOs have embedded ongoing outcomes measurement, using standard assessment instruments to establish baseline status and improvement during treatment, into program design.

At present, most MBHOs are using internally developed health risk assessments, which assess a range of behavioral and physical conditions to target areas for assistance. Other widely used general assessment tools include QualityMetric, Incorporated's SF-36™ and SF-12™, and the Consumer Health Inventory (CHI). Other standardized assessment tools targeted to assess a specific condition such as depression, anxiety, or substance abuse include the PHQ-9 and Beck Depression Inventory for depression, and the CAGE and AUDIT for substance use disorders.

Some MBHOs offer trainings for providers and practitioners in the use of standard assessment tools for patients and, in some cases, provide the tools for contracted providers. With the expansion of medical and integrated health homes, it is likely that use of assessment tools for measurement of patient outcomes and for the promotion of health care transparency will continue to grow.

■ UTILIZATION MANAGEMENT

For most managed care companies, utilization management is conducted telephonically by licensed mental health professionals, referred to as care managers, who review cases with the provider, facility, or program personnel. Reviews also may be conducted with other members of the treatment team as needed. The care managers use evidence-based medical necessity criteria addressing intensity of services and severity of need to determine the most appropriate level of care. The care managers have access to licensed clinical supervisors, board-certified psychiatrists, and addictionologists to assist in clinical decision making.

Utilization review occurs when treatment is requested and is reviewed at intervals thereafter to assess treatment issues, screen for potential quality of care issues, and arrange for discharge and aftercare planning.

■ OUTPATIENT MANAGEMENT

Trends in MBHOs' management of outpatient services have varied during the past few decades. Initially, MBHOs used precertification and concurrent review to manage outpatient care. Typically, 3–10 sessions were authorized at the start of treatment. If the clinician required additional sessions, he or she submitted a request that included clinical information on which a clinical reviewer could determine case severity, progress to date, and necessity of additional treatment.

Over time, MBHOs reduced the amount of information needed for reviewing care and introduced technologies, such as telephonic and Web-enabled forms, to reduce the administrative burden for clinicians. Currently, MBHOs serving commercial populations vary in the use of precertification and concurrent review for the management of outpatient care. These activities increasingly are being combined with data-driven strategies tailored to members' specific, identified health care needs.

As a result of the parity legislation and ACA, the management of behavioral health and substance abuse conditions, particularly on the outpatient level where most of this treatment occurs, is undergoing a major paradigm shift based on the elimination of defined outpatient benefit limits separate and apart from medical benefits. Because in most cases there will be no limit to the number of sessions allowed, the management of care is now moving to models where patients and providers are being encouraged by managed care to adopt the concepts of recovery and resiliency as goals for treatment.

■ MANAGEMENT OF INPATIENT AND INTERMEDIATE LEVELS OF CARE

Initially, inpatient and intermediate level of care management efforts focused on containment strategies, such as primary care gatekeepers, benefit limitations, discounted provider fees, and restrictions on coverage of certain types of conditions. When MBHOs arrived on the scene, the focus shifted to promoting the delivery of clinically effective specialty care and services in the least restrictive setting that was safe and effective for a given patient.

As MBHOs evolved, utilization management strategies have begun to emphasize:

- Addressing the psychosocial precipitants to admission to high levels of care in order to get early treatment response and avert the need for admission.
- Increasing ambulatory follow-up to help prevent unnecessary readmission to high levels of care.

- Reducing readmission through intensive interventions for at-risk patients.
- Measuring and tracking clinical performance with a focus on outcomes and efficiency.
- Reducing relapse through effective aftercare planning and use of community and social supports.
- Coordinating services among multiple agencies and providers.
- Emphasizing the quality of services provided through supervision, clinical rounds, live call and documentation audits, analysis of complaints, patient and provider satisfaction surveying, in-service staff training, and outcomes tracking.

Two other factors have had a role in utilization management of inpatient and other high levels of care. Employee assistance programs have reduced utilization because EAP counselors assist people in handling social, vocational, and behavioral issues and problems before they reach crisis levels that may require higher levels of care. The use of networks with specialty care clinicians also has reduced high-level utilization, through accurate matching of patients with providers who specialize in the presenting issues. Such matching can increase the likelihood that behavioral health needs will be addressed adequately and will not escalate such that higher levels of care will be needed.

■ RECENT TRENDS IN UTILIZATION MANAGEMENT

The absolute cost of behavioral health services relative to medical costs has historically been, and remains, a relatively small proportion. Thus, the intensity of management resource applied to a large number of members must be carefully managed as the savings opportunity per each contact is far less than for members with a medical condition.

This has resulted in a shift of focus from case by case to targeted, data-driven efforts and increased partnerships with providers. For example:

- Through the management of patient and provider data gathered over many years, MBHOs have developed national and regional norms, by diagnosis, for higher levels of care. Routine decisions can be based on these norms, with review resources used for complicated cases at high risk for readmission based on past history.
- Reviews increasingly focus on how providers can improve the quality and/or efficiency of treatment and how the MBHO can assist through specialized services, such as intensive care management.
- Field care management programs, in which MBHO staff members work with patients in the community, have been found effective in maintaining patient stability while reducing use of higher levels of care.

- Provider education and communication, based on outcomes monitoring, have become the norm.
- Partnerships between MBHOs and facilities or programs with similar values have reduced front-end utilization management and increased joint management by outcomes.

While utilization management will remain a basic function of MBHOs, current trends suggest that utilization increasingly will be addressed through cooperative efforts with providers on how to increase the quality and efficiency of care and boost provider self-management through education and data management. Continued innovative efforts, such as field care management aimed at the chronic high-risk population, also will be an ongoing focus.

■ RECOVERY AND RESILIENCY

Recovery and resiliency are concepts originally developed within the public sector. The ideas that patients are dependent on their providers for all their care and that curing the condition is the goal of treatment are no longer the norm, particularly for serious mental illness conditions. A new emerging philosophy of care promotes the idea that the expectation of curing these conditions, particularly serious mental illness conditions, may be unrealistic. A more reasonable and practical goal is for patients to learn how to take responsibility (with the encouragement and help of their providers and other "nonprovider" resources) to pursue their life goals, while accepting and managing their conditions as independently as possible in the process.

The premise is that the more patients work toward fulfilling their potential to the greatest extent possible, the more they become empowered and motivated to manage their conditions rather than focusing on being victims of and disabled by their conditions, dependent on their providers with limited hopes for the future.

As a result of this paradigm shift, MBHOs have taken two new directions:

1. In discussion with providers on patient care, there is a new focus on patient strengths and empowerment, patient-determined goals (aside from symptom relief) and progress, and addressing barriers to progress.
2. There are increasing types of direct interaction between managed care professionals and consumers. Programs such as intensive care management, disease management, field care management, and coaching are all focused on promoting patient empowerment, where patients successfully learn how to assume greater responsibility for their health and well-being, as well as focus on progress toward their life goals.

■ SPECIALIZED SERVICES

MBHOs increasingly are using health risk assessment questionnaires, claims, and pharmacy data to link members proactively to services appropriate to the severity of their condition. Members are assigned to a defined risk level based on their questionnaire responses, diagnosis, and historical utilization pattern. Care management services are then provided based on the associated risk level. This continuum typically ranges from prevention and psychoeducational interventions to intensive care management (ICM) involving direct contact with both members and providers.

The recent parity legislation closely focuses on the goal of integration of care. It is well known that the combination of mental health and substance abuse conditions are quite common and that each can exacerbate the other, making these patients more vulnerable to decompensation. It is also well known that either of these singly or in combination can adversely affect medical conditions (or vice versa). In response to these issues, MBHOs are engaging in new initiatives.

With respect to substance abuse conditions, there is greater focus on identifying co-occurring diagnosis situations (mental health and substance abuse) to better co-jointly manage these cases. Additionally, there is a movement to increase the use of ambulatory detoxification for alcohol and opioid conditions to allow more patients to receive treatment without disrupting or impacting their home or work environments (if conditions are appropriate to do so).

There has been an increased focus in research on substance use and neurobiology, which has resulted in the identification of a number of medications that can reduce cravings and enhance relapse prevention. Most recently, research is focusing on targeting the use of certain types of medications with certain types of patients. The use of these medications has been addressed by respected government and accreditation and substance abuse organizations such as SAMSHA, APA, and NCQA as desired practices in the industry. Efforts are underway for MCOs to work collaboratively with the provider community to increase the use of these medications when appropriate through media communications, direct education, and individual case discussions with providers.

With regard to integration of behavioral health and medical treatment, new models of care such as the integrated medical home are being initiated, where all care is coordinated and overseen by one caregiver who is responsible for a consumer's total health needs. New initiatives have also begun in which behavioral health experts are training medical personnel in techniques designed to promote increased patient motivation for change in the interest of their health and well-being, and to improve consumer buy-in with adherence to their treatment and medications.

As can be seen in these changes in treatment focus and new initiatives, there is real movement taking place to manage care by improving the quality of care through treatment integration as well as by the promotion of the philosophy of care toward patient empowerment.

■ TELEMENTAL HEALTH SERVICES

Telepsychiatry or telemental health is becoming more widespread and less costly, and new applications are emerging. According to the American Psychiatric Association, telepsychiatry is a specifically defined form of videoconferencing that can provide psychiatric services to patients living in remote locations or otherwise underserved areas. It can connect patients, psychiatrists, physicians, and other health care professionals through the use of cameras and microphones.

Telemental health currently provides an array of services, including but not limited to diagnosis and assessment, medication management, and individual and group therapy. It also provides an opportunity for consultative services between psychiatrists, primary care physicians, and other health care providers. Telepsychiatry also is being used to provide patients with second opinions in areas where only one psychiatrist is available.[12]

Overall, telepsychiatry provides increased access to services and has helped enhance the provision of services to families with children and other patients who are homebound. Patients participating in telepsychiatry say they are satisfied with the care they are receiving and that they feel telepsychiatry is a reliable form of practice. Various delivery mechanisms are available and include:

- **Hub-and-spoke networks:** These integrated networks link large tertiary centers with outlying clinics.
- **Health provider-home connections:** This links primary care providers, specialists, and home health nurses with patients over single-line phone-video systems for interactive consults. These services can also be extended to residential care centers such as nursing homes.
- **Web-based e-health patient service sites:** These links provide direct consumer outreach and services over the Internet.[13]

Telehealth poses some significant challenges for behavioral health provider organizations, including technology infrastructure, cost, regulatory issues, and payment.

Technology Infrastructure

The universe of technologies available for use in telehealth is constantly expanding. In behavioral health, the most common application is the substitution of face-to-face evaluation and therapy with videoconferencing, using computer-based video systems.

Cost

The capital investment required for telehealth infrastructure can be prohibitive for some organizations, as well as for communities aiming to bring services to remote areas. The federal government has addressed the cost concern through various initiatives, including the following:

- In November 2007, the Federal Communications Commission made awards totaling $417 million to 42 states and three U.S. territories to construct 69 statewide or regional broadband telehealth networks.
- The Rural Health Care Pilot Program received 81 applications representing 6,800 health care facilities; 69 applicants were selected based on their ability to support innovative telehealth and, in particular, telemedicine services.
- In 2007, the Health Research and Services Administration (HRSA) awarded $56 million in grants to advance health IT and telemedicine in 35 states and the District of Columbia.

State Licensing and Regulation

In addition to cost and infrastructure issues, provider organizations must be aware of licensing and regulation requirements, which vary from state to state. Many states require providers using telemedicine technology across state lines to hold a valid state license in the state where the consumer is located.

Currently, professionals who want to practice in more than one state must apply for a separate license or certification in each state. However, the Federation of State Medical Boards has drafted a model state law that creates reciprocal agreements among states and allows professionals licensed in any participating state to practice in all other participating states. According to the Center for Telehealth and E-Health Law, 10 states have enacted the statute so far: Alabama, California, Minnesota, Montana, Nevada, New Mexico, Ohio, Oregon, Tennessee, and Texas. HRSA's grant program for telehealth includes assistance for state Licensure Portability Grant Programs.

Payment

In the past year, a number of payer organizations have started covering telehealth and "Web visits" for their members. Provider payment levels vary according to the health care provider's contract and by market.[14]

■ INTENSIVE CARE MANAGEMENT

ICM services have a long history in the public behavioral health delivery system. These services emerged out of utilization research showing that a small percent of patients repeatedly used costly inpatient services. In the late 1970s

Stein and Test implemented an ICM program in Wisconsin characterized by assertive outreach to individuals with frequent psychiatric hospitalization, "hands-on" ICM by care managers, and ongoing involvement with patients across service setting.[15] Consistently, such hands-on ICM services have been found effective in reducing inpatient services in the public sector.[16-18]

By the early 2000s, many commercial behavioral health organizations had implemented telephonically based ICM services for their members. Like their public sector counterparts, internal studies by these MBHOs found that a small percent of members utilized a disproportional amount of treatment services. This research found that age, diagnosis, and comorbidity of diagnoses were factors that contributed to a higher risk of readmission or greater overall cost. Not only was this costly to the MBHOs, but the quality of care was considered less optimal as best illustrated by the pain and disruption in the members' and families' lives that resulted from repeated psychiatric admissions. One large MBHO found that of those members who utilized behavioral health services, 5% accounted for 53% of total costs, as illustrated in **Figure 12-2**.

In companies with such programs, ICM candidates are typically identified by either claims data, notification of an inpatient admission, or by care managers from the managed behavioral health care entity or the health plan partner. Once identified, ICM care managers contact members to explain the program and obtain consent to participate. The ICM care managers then work directly with the members to develop personalized treatment plans that address their clinical needs, and then coordinate care delivery with the members and their behavioral health providers across service settings.

Additional activities may also include integration of behavioral health services with general medical care to address critical areas such as timely communication with primary care practitioners/providers, collaboration with medical practitioners to increase appropriate use of psychotropic medications, and evaluation of access, continuity, coordination, and follow-up to medically necessary care within the behavioral health and general medical communities.

Over the past few years the philosophy of ICM programs has expanded to include components of the chronic care model, such as the promotion of self-management skills and integration with evidence-based decision support tools. These concepts associated with the management of chronic illnesses have been adopted by the behavioral health community to address the severity and chronicity of certain mental illnesses such as bipolar disorder, schizophrenia, major depression, and substance abuse. Self-management support involves patient education, problem solving, and collaborative decision making.[19] Care managers use these strategies to support the goals of self-efficacy and behavior change. This requires ICM care managers to use different skill sets—such as motivational interviewing, promotion of recovery-based concepts, and resiliency—as they work collaboratively with members and providers during the delivery of care.

MBHOs have begun to use clinical outcomes and return on investment (ROI) measures to evaluate the efficacy and impact of their ICM programs.[20] One such program resulted in decreases in admissions, lengths of stay, and overall care costs. These results are promising, although yet to be confirmed by other studies.

■ QUALITY OF CARE

Quality of care, as defined by the Institute of Medicine, is "the degree to which health services for individuals and populations increase the likelihood of desired health outcomes and are consistent with current professional knowledge."[21] Six aims for high-quality care were identified in the IOM's seminal reports, *Crossing the Quality Chasm: A New Health System for the 21st Century*[19] and *Improving the Quality of Health Care for Mental and Substance-Use Conditions.*[22] These aims define care that is:

- **Safe:** Avoiding injuries to patients from the care that is intended to help them.
- **Effective:** Providing services based on scientific knowledge to all who could benefit and refraining from providing services to those not likely to benefit (avoiding underuse and overuse, respectively).
- **Patient-centered:** Providing care that is respectful of and responsive to individual patient preferences, needs, and values and ensuring that patient values guide all clinical decisions.
- **Timely:** Reducing waits and sometimes harmful delays for both those who receive and those who give care.

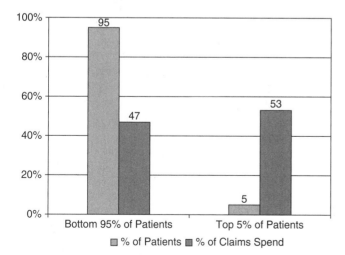

Figure 12-2 Proportion of High-Cost Patients
Source: Magellan Health Services; used with permission.

- **Efficient:** Reducing waste, including waste of equipment, supplies, ideas, and energy.
- **Equitable:** Providing care that does not vary in quality because of personal characteristics such as gender, ethnicity, geographical location, and socioeconomic status.

The ACA required the Secretary of the Department of Health and Human Services to establish a National Strategy for Quality Improvement in Health Care. In a 2011 report to Congress, six priorities were set forth:

- Making care safer by reducing harm caused in the delivery of care.
- Ensuring that each person and family are engaged as partners in their care.
- Promoting effective communication and coordination of care.
- Promoting the most effective prevention and treatment practices for the leading causes of mortality.
- Working with communities to promote wide use of best practices to enable healthy living.
- Making quality care more affordable for individuals, families, employers, and governments by developing and spreading new health care delivery models.

Quality management programs within behavioral health care set priorities similar to those listed above using program descriptions, annual work plans, and selected performance measures with established targets and national benchmarks.

Quality Management

Since 2003, the Agency for Healthcare Research and Quality (AHRQ) with various partners has published annual National Healthcare Quality and Disparities Reports.* Overall, these reports find that while health care quality is improving, the pace of that improvement is slow. With increased attention on patient safety, use of evidence-based practices, demonstrated accountability, optimal transparency, measured and reportable outcomes, strong clinical interventions, and use of stakeholder input, quality management has a central role within behavioral health care management. Patel and colleagues stated that "developing quality improvement resources is fundamental to improving mental health care."[5]

Quality management as a term encompasses practices such as quality control and auditing, quality assurance, quality improvement, and process improvement. Early origins of quality management in behavioral health care can be traced to the American College of Surgeons who, in the interest of understanding the variability of patient outcomes, published in 1913 the first set of quality standards for hospitals.[23] In

the 1980s and 1990s, the health care industry and behavioral health care began applying principles of total quality management (TQM) and continuous quality improvement (CQI) built on the theories of Walter Shewhart, W. Edwards Deming, Joseph M. Juran, Philip Crosby, and Donald Berwick. These systems and processes were designed to measure process variability and methods for reducing variability to acceptable levels. A universal model used for the continuous process of quality control/improvement within health care is plan, do, check, act (PDCA):[24]

- **Plan:** Identify opportunity for improvement
- **Do:** Implement interventions
- **Check:** Measure affect of interventions
- **Act:** Adjust interventions/change interventions

Another standard model for continuous quality improvement, taken from Lean Six Sigma,[25-27] also referred to as an operations roadmap, is the DMAIC process consisting of the following steps:

- **Define:** Identify the scope of the problem and estimated benefits of the solution
- **Measure:** Measure the current variation of the performance data included in the problem
- **Analyze:** Find potential sources of variation of the performance data
- **Improve:** Verify, control, and optimize the sources of variation of the performance data
- **Control:** Establish a system of controls to mange the gains of the solution

In its 2001 report, *Crossing the Quality Chasm: A New Health System for the 21st Century,* the Institute of Medicine's Committee on Quality of Health Care wrote, "The performance of the health care system varies considerably."[19] Quality management programs within behavioral health care, therefore, focus on the variation challenges of system-wide data with limited connectivity, multiple treatment methods and practices, and treatment for diverse populations delivered by a wide array of providers in different disciplines. Examples of variations in quality of care and services are found in the practices of providers in their use of risk assessment protocols, screening for substance abuse, application of evidence-based practices, adoption of electronic treatment records, diagnostic coding procedures, and utilization review procedures.

Components of Quality Management Programs

Quality management program components frequently are grouped into structures, processes, and outcomes, based on a framework proposed by Donabedian.[28] *Structures* are the components of behavioral health care's quality improvement program. *Processes* represent the behavioral health services provided to, or on behalf of, a patient. *Outcomes*

---

*www.ahrq.gov/qual/measurix.htm#quality.

are the results of the services and care provided to patients. The quality of behavioral health care is measured, monitored, and improved over time using performance measures.

Quality programs in MBHOs vary in size and scope based on the complexity of the organization, the type of products provided, the size of the provider network, and the characteristics of the population served or managed. Another factor affecting the complexity of an MBHO's quality program is its participation in programs that accredit or certify quality processes, such as those of NCQA, URAC, or the Joint Commission.

Most MBHO quality programs have a quality committee with subcommittees and workgroups as the structural elements of the program. In addition, an extensive set of policies and procedures outline the standards and practices that govern operations and quality reviews. Performance measures with established targets and benchmarks are used as markers of progress and program achievement. When goals are not met and/or opportunities for improvement are identified, a formal system of review using PDCA or DAMIC steps is implemented to identify undue variation in quality or utilization, barriers, and root causes, and to initiate interventions for improvement. Formal systems for assessing quality improvement initiatives have been developed. For example, NCQA has developed standards for quality improvement activities (QIAs), and URAC has developed standards for quality improvement projects (QIPs).

Comprehensive quality improvement programs rely on feedback and cooperation from multiple stakeholders. Within the public sector, open forums and consumer-oriented meetings are conducted on the quality of care and services provided. One model used by an MBHO involves consumers and providers participating on a governing board for review of quality program components. Stakeholder input (consumers, providers, family members, advocates, customers) is gathered through multiple activities including surveys, websites, and participation on quality committees and workgroups.

Quality programs depend heavily on the use of analytics, data, and fact-based decision making. With large data sets available to MBHOs, accurate reporting of data is essential for strong quality programs. Equally important is the use of advanced analytics for explanatory and predictive purposes. Thomas Davenport advocates for smart use of analytics as a key business strategy.[29] Skilled use of analytics within a quality program supports not only continuous quality improvement, but guides fact-based decision making related to quality care and services for patients.

Performance Measurement and Outcomes

"Policy makers, purchasers, and other stakeholders have a strong interest in the measurement of quality of care and increased attention has been lent to the development of reliable and valid measures."[30] Multiple reasons exist for performance measurement: transparency and accountability, quality improvement, education and engagement of consumers, patient safety, and research. [31, 32]

Performance measurement program components can be categorized similarly to quality program components. *Structural* measures are features of a behavioral health care organization relevant to its capacity to provide services and care. *Process* measures are usually expressed as a rate and assess a health care service. *Outcome* measures are the "effects of interventions (or lack of interventions) on primary and secondary consumers."[33] Outcomes-based measures of quality reflect the cumulative impact of multiple processes of care.[34]

Valid and reliable measures are the cornerstone of monitoring quality improvement efforts. There is a growing emphasis on use of nationally endorsed measures to provide information that is timely, actionable, and meaningful to both providers and patients. The National Quality Measures Clearinghouse (NQMC), operated by the Agency for Healthcare Research and Quality, includes measures for mental health and substance abuse,[35] as does the National Inventory of Mental Health Quality Measures. Lists of performance indicators for use in measuring the quality of mental health and substance abuse treatment have been compiled and published.[30, 36] An example of sources on performance measures is provided in **Table 12-5**.

The challenge for behavioral health care is not a lack of measures, but difficulties arising from the quality and availability of data, the validity of measures, their applicability to the populations served, the administrative burden of data collection, and complexity in computation. A wide array of data sources is used to collect performance metrics in behavioral health care, as illustrated in **Figure 12-3**.

TABLE 12-5	Sources on Measures Applicable in Behavioral Health Care Quality Improvement
Developer	**Measurement set**
Child and Adolescent Residential Psychiatric Programs (CHARPP)	CHARPP Improvement Measurement Program
U.S. Department of Health and Human Services (HHS)	National Quality Measures Clearinghouse
The Joint Commission	Core Measure Sets
National Committee for Quality Assurance (NCQA)	Healthcare Effectiveness Data and Information Set (HEDIS)
National Quality Forum (NQF)	NQF-endorsed™ standards
Mental Health Statistics Improvement Program (MHSIP)	Process measures derived from MHSIP Consumer Survey items
The Washington Circle	Washington Circle Performance Measures

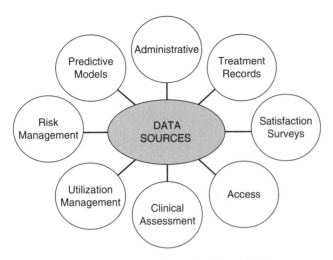

FIGURE 12-3 Data Sources for Behavioral Healthcare Quality Improvement

TABLE 12-6	Performance Measures Used for Quality Improvement	
Domain	Measure	Data source
Structure	QI and UM program descriptions	Quality data
	Medical necessity criteria	Clinical data
Process	Timeliness of telephone access	Administrative data
	Readmission rates	Utilization data
	Appeals overturn rate	Administrative data
	Intensive care management enrollment	Administrative data
	Adverse events	Clinical data
	Patient experience of care	Patient survey
Outcome	Symptom and function improvement of members	Patient self-report

These types of data are described as follows:

- *Administrative data* include claims, eligibility information, and various coding sets;
- *Treatment records* contain detailed clinical information;
- *Survey data* are obtained from providers and consumers and measure experiences and satisfaction with care and services;
- *Access data* are gathered from telephone systems and reviews of provider appointment availability;
- *Clinical assessments* involve consumer self-report and provider and caretaker observations related to functional health, symptoms, substance use, coping skills, strengths, and the nature of the provider relationship;
- *Utilization management data* include requests for care, nonauthorizations, and appeals;
- *Risk management data* include adverse events, medication errors, and rates of seclusion and restraints; and
- *Predictive modeling data* are derived from utilization data and population risk adjustment formulas.

Data challenges are significant within behavioral health care. Behavioral health is difficult to measure as there are few relevant laboratory tests for program monitoring. Use of self-report and provider observations result in wide variation and expensive capture mechanisms. Providers' use of electronic technology is limited for claims submission and treatment records. Code sets and definitions vary widely across the continuum of care, resulting in data interface issues. Calculation problems arise due to the many variations in data capture and coding systems.

Measurement Selection

Drawing on the available data sources, behavioral health care companies select performance measures based on internal and external needs, customer contracts, and state and federal regulations. The most widely used measurement set in health care is HEDIS, developed by NCQA. While HEDIS measures are reported by MCOs, as subcontractors to managed care organizations, MBHOs share in the collection of data. HEDIS includes behavioral health measures with established thresholds for utilization and effectiveness. Annually, NCQA publishes MCOs' HEDIS results; employers use the results to select among managed care plans and set benchmarks for performance. A sample of performance measures used for quality improvement and accountability by one behavioral health company is presented in **Table 12-6**.

Outcomes

Clinical outcomes measurement is a key function for MBHOs and serves multiple stakeholders. Purchasers of behavioral health care want demonstrated ROI and maximum clinical improvement for minimal premium dollars. At the patient or consumer level, outcomes allow for comparison with a standard and/or with consumers using similar services. At the aggregate level, population health and well-being can be assessed, as well as program effectiveness and efficacy. Another purpose, gaining momentum in health care, is that of linking outcome and performance measurement data with incentives to improve quality.[37–39] Health care reform offers initiatives and investments to push the health care system to exceed current performance.[32]

Most MBHOs use clinical assessment systems that monitor members' response to treatment and progress over time. The modalities used by MBHOs vary, with some requiring providers to complete assessments and others relying on member self-report. The focus of clinical assessment is broadening from solely behavioral health to incorporate physical health, recovery and resilience, and productivity, with the intent to equip consumers with data that empowers them to be active partners in treatment planning and to promote ownership of one's health and wellness.

Patients are increasingly recognized as valid judges of the quality of their health care experience.[40] With the shift to patient-centered care, clinical outcomes reported from the patient perspective are being used by patients and clinicians for treatment planning and monitoring. "Ultimately, the most important questions in assessing quality of care are whether symptoms remit, functioning and quality of life improve, adverse events are avoided and consumers are satisfied."[36]

Incentives to Drive Quality

An additional function of clinical outcomes data is in support of incentive programs. Provider profiles and scorecards increasingly are used to aid consumers in choice and selection of providers. P4P programs reward high performers for demonstrated quality through the use of financial incentives. Nonfinancial incentives include recognition programs, administrative burden reduction, and preferred provider status. Tying provider incentive payments to investment in technology and using variable co-payments to encourage consumers to choose providers with better-quality profiles have also been proposed.[41]

As noted in Chapter 5, it is unclear which incentive programs work best and how much they improve quality of care and access to services, if they are effective at all. The development of a set of principles to guide P4P systems by the Joint Commission and the IOM's charge for use and measurement of evidence-based practices suggest that incentives to improve quality will grow with greater use and scrutiny in the years to come. Groups such as Leapfrog, an employer-based group, and the NQF play a significant role in setting quality standards, use of performance measurement, and reviewing incentives to drive quality.

Evidence demonstrates that health plans play a meaningful role in improving health care quality.[42] With the movement to public reporting on quality for consumers to choose among plans and with health care reform resulting in higher standards for care and service delivery and efficiency, managed behavioral health plans will be expected to demonstrate innovative leadership in quality and performance measurement.

■ ACCREDITATION

The major accreditation organizations used by MBHOs are the Joint Commission, NCQA, and URAC (see Chapter 15). Applicable standards are continuously revised, requiring MBHOs with accreditation to modify procedures and measurement processes to meet changing standards. This is

a resource-intensive process, as accreditation entities expect a state of continuous readiness and will conduct impromptu visits to check on the quality status of operations. Preparation for such visits and formal surveys entails presentation of policies and procedures with extensive documentation supporting adherence to standards, with random utilization file audits to assess timeliness and clinical documentation.

Accreditation by these organizations is voluntary and designed to provide external validation of a behavioral health care company's quality program with assurance of quality for consumers and purchasers of services. Increasingly, states require MBHOs to meet accreditation requirements to obtain a utilization review license and/or to deliver services within their state.

In the absence of state-mandated accreditation, MBHOs historically have sought to distinguish themselves on the basis of accreditations. An important factor in voluntary accreditations is that medical MCOs that contract with MBHOs in a carve-out arrangement frequently require them to be externally accredited and set monetary guarantees and penalties based on accreditation performance. While accreditation standards for behavioral health care vary by agency, they include constructs such as those shown in **Table 12-7**.

MBHOs seeking accreditation must demonstrate that they have identified opportunities for improvement in service and clinical areas, with targeted interventions and measurement of the effectiveness of interventions. Examples of clinical improvement activities in behavioral health care include increasing the rate of members who attend an ambulatory follow-up visit in the 7 days following hospitalization, improving the rate of provider identification of comorbidities, strengthening coordination of care between behavioral and primary care clinicians, and use of medicated assisted treatment for substance abuse.

TABLE 12-7	Common Constructs in Behavioral Health Care Accreditation Standards	
Quality program and improvement activities	Patient safety
Enrollee and provider satisfaction	Performance measures and outcomes
Utilization review program components	Member rights and responsibilities
Medical necessity criteria	Preventive behavioral health
Appeals and complaints	Clinical practice guidelines
Credentialing of providers and organizations	Stakeholder input
Confidentiality and HIPAA compliance	Cultural diversity

With the maturation of MBHO quality programs and increasing numbers of companies obtaining accreditation, a shift is occurring from an emphasis on structures and processes to performance-based measurement and demonstrable outcomes.

■ IN-HOUSE VERSUS OUTSOURCED MANAGEMENT OF BEHAVIORAL HEALTH SERVICES

Although written from the perspective of a MBHO for reasons of consistency, much of the discussion in this chapter is applicable whether the management of behavioral health services is performed by an in-house department or by a MBHO under contract. It has and is done both ways.

As for the future, the managed behavioral health care industry is in flux and will likely remain so. Significant tension exists among MCOs regarding whether the behavioral management function should be in-house or outsourced. The illusion that the percentage of the medical spend allocated to behavioral health is now small relative to the overall medical spend may suggest that it does not merit a carve-out management approach. Added to this is the growing acknowledgment that there is a significant intersection between behavioral health issues and physical health, leading MCOs to the conclusion that coordinated management under one roof is the preferred way to proceed.

These arguments are counterbalanced with the reality that managing patients who are suffering from emotional distress requires a different set of skills, a broader network of provider types, and specialized claims processing standards. These dynamics will continue to play out with strong advocates on each side of the equation. Most of the large national carriers have built or bought the capability, but the regional and local players will continue to assess their strategic direction on a regular basis.

■ CONCLUSION

Mental and behavioral health care and substance abuse services are both related and integrated with traditional medical-surgical health care, but are also highly unique. Managing behavioral health care uses many of the same approaches used in traditional utilization management, but only as described at a high level. When looking at the specifics of how utilization and quality are managed in managed health care, substantial differences are instantly apparent. But even though behavioral health care makes up a small percentage of the overall cost of care, its indirect impact is very high, particularly for vulnerable individuals with multiple medical conditions. The impact of substance abuse on overall health care costs is equally high. Therefore, competent management of behavioral health care and substance abuse services is felt throughout a payer organization.

Endnotes

1 Franklin JE, Levenson JL, McCance-Katz EF. *Substance-related Disorders: Textbook of Psychosomatic Medicine.* Washington, DC: American Psychiatric Publishing; 2005.

2 Moore RD, Bone LR, Geller G., et al. Prevalence, detection and treatment of alcoholism in hospitalized patients. *JAMA.* 1989;261:403–407.

3 Schatzberg AF, Cole JO, DeBattista C. *Manual of Clinical Psychopharmacology.* 5th edition. Washington, DC: American Psychiatric Publishing; 2005.

4 American Psychiatric Association. *Diagnostic and Statistical Manual of Mental Disorders DSM-IV-TR.* Washington, DC: American Psychiatric Association; 2004.

5 Patel KK, Butler B, Wells, KB. What is necessary to transform the quality of mental health care. *Health Affairs.* 2006;25(3):681–693.

6 Bremmer RW, Scholle SH, Keyser D, Knox Houtsinger JV, Pincus HA. Pay for performance in behavioral health. *Psychiatr Serv.* 2008;59(12):1419–1429.

7 Liptzin B. Quality improvement, pay for performance, and "outcomes measurement": What makes sense? *Psychiatr Serv.* 2009;60(1):108–111.

8 Pomerantz JM. Drug Benefit Trends. 2005–17, 273–274.

9 Young G, White B, Burgess J, Berlowitz D, Meterko M, Guldin M, Bokhour B. Conceptual issues in the design and implementation of pay-for-quality programs. *Am J Med Qual.* 2005;20:144–150.

10 Endsley S, Kirkegaard M, Baker G, Murcko A. Getting rewards for your results: Pay-for-performance programs. Family Practice Management 2004;11(3):45–50.

11 Balit Health Purchasing. Performance incentive model options. Center for Health Care Strategies. 2005.

12 American Psychiatric Association. APA document on telepsychiatry via videoconferencing. 1998. Available at: www.psych.org/lib_archives/archives/199821.pdf. Accessed August 12, 2011.

13 American Telemedicine Association. About telemedicine. 2011. Available at: www.americantelemed.org/i4a/pages/index.cfm?pageid = 3331. Accessed August 12, 2011.

14 Marsh Cupino E. Telehealth and the behavioral health market: Adoption of new technologies will change service delivery forever. *OPEN MINDS, The Behavioral Health and Social Service Industry Analyst.* 2008;20(1):4–5.

15 Stein LI, Test MA. Alternative to mental hospital treatment, I: conceptual model, treatment program and clinical evaluation. *Arch Gen Psychiatr.* 1920;37:392–397.

16 Bond GR, Miller LD, Krumwied MHA, et al. Assertive case management in three CMHCs: A controlled study. *Hosp Community Psych.* 1988;39(4):411–417.

17 Tibbo P, Chue P, Wright E. Hospital outcome measures following assertive community treatment in Edmonton, Alberta. *Can J Psychiatr.* 1999;44:276–79.

18 Ziguras SJ, Stuart GW. (2000). A meta-analysis of the effectiveness of mental health case management over 20 years. *Psychiatr Serv.* 2000;51:1410–421.

19 Institute of Medicine. *Crossing the Quality Chasm: A New Health System for the 21st Century.* Washington, DC: National Academy Press; 2001.

20 Taylor EC, LoPiccolo CJ, Eisdorfer C, & Clemence C. Best Practices: Reducing rehospitalization with telephonic targeted care management in a managed health care plan. *Psychiatr Serv.* 2005;56(6):652–654.

21 Lohr KN (ed). (1990). *Medicare: A Strategy for Quality Assurance.* Washington, DC: National Academy Press Available at: www.nap.edu/catalog.php?record_id = 1547. Accessed August 12, 2011.

22 Institute of Medicine. *Improving the Quality of Health Care for Mental and Substance-Use Conditions.* Washington, DC: National Academy Press; 2006.

23 Ruetsch C, Wadell D, Dewan N. Improving quality and accountability through Information systems. In: Dewan NA, Lorenzi, NM, Riley RT (eds), *Behavioral Health Informatics.* New York: Springer-Verlag; 2001.

24 Brassard M, Ritter D. *The Memory Jogger II: A Pocket Guide of Tools for Continuous Improvement and Effective Planning.* Methuen, MA: GOAL/QPC; 1994.

25 George ML, Rowlands D, Price M, Maxey J. *Lean Six Sigma Pocket Toolbook.* New York, NY: McGraw-Hill. 2005.

26 Zinkgraf S. *Six Sigma: The first 90 days.* Upper Saddle River, NJ: Prentice Hall; 2006.

27 Smith C, Wood S, Bradly B. Thinking lean: Implementing DMAIC methods to improve efficiency within a cystic fibrosis clinic. *J Health Care Qual.* 2011;33(2):37–46.

28 Donabedian A. *Exploration in Quality Assessment and Monitoring: The Definition of Quality and Approaches to Its Assessment.* Ann Arbor, MI: Health Administration Press; 1980.

29 Davenport TH, Harris JG, Morison R. *Analytics at Work; Smarter Decision, Better Results.* Boston: Harvard Business Press; 2010.

30 Watkins K, Horvitz-Lennon M, Caldarone LB, et al. (2011).

31 Solberg LI, Mosser G, McDonald S. The three faces of performance measurement: Improvement, accountability, and research. *Jt Comm J Qual Improv.* 1997;23(3):135–47.

32 National Committee for Quality Assurance. The State of Health Care Quality. Reform, the Quality Agenda and Resource Use. 2010. Retrieved from www.ncqa.org. Accessed April 5, 2010.

33 Decision Support 2000+ Outcomes Measurement Process, Project Overview and Deliberation of Steering Committee; 2003.

34 AcademyHealth. Health Outcomes Core Library Project. Washington, DC: National Information Center on Health Services Research and Health Care Technology, National Library of Medicine; 2004.

35 Agency for Healthcare Research and Quality. National Quality Measures Clearinghouse. 2004. Available at: www.qualitymeasures.ahrq.gov/resources/measure_use.aspx#attributes. Accessed September 20, 2004.

36 Hermann RC. *Improving Mental Healthcare: A Guide to Measurement-Based Quality Improvement.* Washington, DC: American Psychiatric Publishing; 2005.

37 Dudley R, Frolish A, Robinowitz D, Talavera JA, Broadhead P, Luft HS. Strategies to support quality-based purchasing: A review of the evidence. Summary, Technical Review No. 10. 2004. Agency for Healthcare Research and Quality. Available at: www.ahrq.gov/clinic/epcsums/qpurchsum.htm. Accessed November 8, 2006.

38 Rosenthal MB, Fernandopulle HRS, Landon B. Paying for quality: Provider incentives for quality improvement. *Health Aff (Millwood).* 2004;23(2):127–141.

39 Bachman J. "Pay for performance" in the behavioral healthcare arena. 2004. Available at: www.wpic.pitt.edu/dppc/journalwatch_2004_11.htm. Accessed September 20, 2004.

40 Iezzoni, L. (1997). Assessing quality using administrative data. *Ann Intern Med. 127*:666–674.

41 Steinberg EP. Improving the quality of care—can we practice what we preach? *N Engl J Med.* 2003;348(26):2681–2683.

42 Baker L, Hopkins D. The contributions of health plans and provider organizations to variations in measured plan quality. *Int J Qual Health C.* 2010;22(3):210–218.

CHAPTER

13

Disease Prevention in Managed Health Care Plans

MARC MANLEY

STUDY OBJECTIVES

- Understand the role of health plans in prevention
- Understand the different approaches a managed care plan can use in preventing disease
- Understand the economic value of prevention

DISCUSSION TOPICS

1. Discuss the value of disease prevention; use concrete examples and measures.
2. Discuss how a health plan might implement, monitor, and modify a prevention program.
3. Discuss the potential impact of health care reform on disease prevention programs in health plans.

■ INTRODUCTION

The prevention of disease has always been an integral component of the practice of medicine. Hippocrates, the most famous physician of the ancient Greeks, proclaimed, "The function of protecting and developing health must rank even above that of restoring it when it is impaired." Disease prevention strategies have produced major improvements in human longevity, the quality of our lives, and the capability of entire societies. Safe drinking water, polio vaccination, and screening for breast cancer are but three examples of the powerful impact prevention can have on a community's health.

Yet in the 21st century, the role of prevention in U.S. health care is far from prominent. Less than 2% of the nation's expenditure on health care is spent on population-based prevention.[1] In contrast, about 70% of the nation's health care expenditures are devoted to treating people with chronic diseases;[2] almost all of these diseases are preventable.

Prevention has often been regarded as an essential element of managed care. Indeed, the expansion of health maintenance organizations (HMOs) and other managed care organizations (MCOs) in the 1970s and 1980s was expected to result in a greater emphasis on prevention and therefore improved health and control of health care costs, as described in Chapter 1. This chapter presents the rationale behind prevention and then reviews the current practices health plans use to prevent illness, including benefit selection, member services, provider contracting, and influencing public policy. The discussion focuses largely on the prevention of common chronic diseases in adults.

In the context of health and health care, prevention can be defined as "action taken to decrease the chance of getting a disease or condition."[3] Three levels of prevention are commonly recognized.

- *Primary prevention* is the prevention of disease before it starts. For example, individuals who smoke can help avoid lung cancer by quitting smoking before any neoplasm has begun.

- *Secondary prevention* is the detection of disease before it becomes symptomatic, which allows for earlier and more successful treatment. Mammography is an example of secondary prevention, in which breast cancer is detected before a patient is aware of its existence and the cancer is treated before it has metastasized.
- *Tertiary prevention* is the prevention of complications of a chronic disease after diagnosis.

Health plans address tertiary prevention through case management and (very specifically) disease management programs, as discussed in Chapters 7 and 8, respectively. The focus of this chapter, therefore, is on the need for and practice of primary and secondary prevention strategies.

■ THE CASE FOR PREVENTION: A COST-EFFECTIVE SOLUTION FOR SAVING LIVES

In the early 21st century, noninfectious diseases have replaced infectious diseases as the leading causes of death, illness, and health care costs. Heart disease and cancer lead this list, together causing an estimated 1,178,942 deaths each year.[4] Chronic diseases cause about 70% of all U.S. deaths each year,[5] and five chronic diseases—heart disease, cancer, stroke, chronic obstructive pulmonary disease, and diabetes—are responsible for most of these deaths.[6] Health care costs are a growing burden on our economy. Heart disease, cancer, and stroke—the top three causes of death in the United States[7]—cost an estimated $402.8 billion each year in direct medical costs.[8]

These statistics convey the toll—in human and economic terms—of chronic diseases. But they do not convey one fundamental fact: most chronic diseases (and thus, the associated mortality and health care costs) are partially or even entirely preventable. At least one-third of all deaths in the United States can be attributed to three very modifiable behaviors: tobacco use, lack of physical activity, and poor eating habits.[9]

Similarly, the costs associated with these avoidable causes of chronic disease are immense. Tobacco use alone is responsible for $96 billion in annual health care costs, with an additional $97 billion per year in lost productivity.[10] Obesity is estimated to cost the nation's health care system $147 billion annually, with up to an additional $66 billion per year in lost productivity.[11]

Numerous studies have shown the remarkable results that preventive measures can achieve:

- Patients at risk for diabetes could reduce their risk by 58% simply by walking an average of 30 minutes a day, 5 days a week, and by lowering their intake of fat and calories.[12]

- Cervical cancer screening programs can reduce cervical cancer mortality rates by 20–60%.[13]
- Treatment for high blood pressure can reduce heart attacks by 21% and strokes by 37%.[14]

By using existing technologies and evidence-based practices known today, we have the potential to reduce chronic disease to nearly the same extent that immunization reduced infectious disease in the 19th and 20th centuries.

Return on Investment

For a society, the health and financial benefits of preventing disease are obvious. Full implementation of disease prevention programs could produce major reductions in morbidity and mortality caused by chronic disease. Prevention has the potential to produce financial savings for individuals, employers, health plans, governments, and entire societies. Several factors impair the willingness or ability of health plans to implement successful primary prevention efforts.

- The time it takes to realize financial gains from prevention is highly variable, depending on the disease that is being prevented, the type of prevention program employed, and the point of view of the return on investment (ROI) calculation.
- The benefits of member-focused interventions may not be realized by the health plan or employer. The people who start exercising and lose weight now, employees of Company A and members of Health Plan B, may avoid heart disease and diabetes 10 years from now, but at that point they may well work for a different employer and be covered by a different health plan.
- For purchasers and even some health plans, the benefits of primary prevention tend to be abstract and distant, whereas the up-front costs are tangible and immediate; they must come out of this year's already-tight budget.

Adding to the complexity, the financial benefits of different prevention programs and services have been calculated and described in many different ways. Thus, it has not always been easy to associate programs with clear, short-term financial ROI. However, well-designed studies have documented a positive ROI for many health improvement programs. One literature review found an average return of $3.48 for each dollar invested in these programs.[15] A review of worksite health promotion and disease prevention programs found that for every dollar companies spend, the median benefit-to-cost ratio is $3.14.[16] Programs to reduce smoking have been studied frequently and found to produce positive returns. One study that examined the relationship between modifiable health risks and short-term health care charges in a health plan population aged 40 years and older found that current tobacco use was related to 18% higher health care charges over an 18-month period.[17] Such results provide evidence that reducing these health risks may offer health plans relatively short-term ROI for persons in this age group.

Another analysis, based on a worksite simulation analysis, suggests that for a health plan with a 10% annual turnover rate, a smoking cessation program would more than pay for itself based exclusively on savings in health care costs.[18] A related article suggests that such a program would reach the break-even point for a firm implementing it in just over 3 years. The worksite simulation included not just medical care costs but also related costs such as productivity, absenteeism, and life insurance.[19]

A COMPLETE PREVENTION PROGRAM

Organized and strategic interventions are required to achieve the successful implementation and maintenance of preventive strategies. Health plans have a variety of prevention tools at their disposal. To have the maximum impact on health and health care costs, health plans need to use the entire set of prevention tools available to them. Health plans need to offer the right member benefits, provide the right services for members, contract effectively with providers, and—perhaps most important—support and implement the right public policies. **Table 13-1** shows examples of each of these four basic strategies. Each is described in more detail in the following subsections.

TABLE 13-1	Components of a Strong Health Plan Prevention Program
Component	**Examples**
Member benefits	• Immunization and screening included in benefit sets
	• No copayments for preventive services or products
	• Coverage for nicotine-cessation medications and weight-loss drugs
	• Coverage for provider visits for tobacco use and weight management
Services for members	• Health risk assessments
	• Behavior change programs
	• Membership discounts at fitness centers or weight-loss programs
Contracts with providers	• Pay-for-performance programs
	• Performance feedback
	• Increases in taxes on tobacco products
	• Clean indoor air laws
Public policies	• Complete Streets policies

MEMBER BENEFITS

Health plans typically offer three general types of clinical preventive services: immunizations, screening services, and counseling services. Immunizations, once a routine part of pediatric care only, are now used for the prevention of disease in adults as well. The role of immunizations in adult preventive care is likely to increase. In June 2006, the Food and Drug Administration approved a vaccine for girls and women ages 9–26 for the prevention of cervical cancer.[20] Immunizations that prevent cancer in other sites may be used in the future. Screening services are most often performed to prevent cancer and heart disease in adults, but also include screening of newborns and children for a variety of illnesses. Screening may be accomplished through laboratory tests (e.g., cholesterol levels), imaging studies (e.g., mammography), or a clinical examination (e.g., a skin exam to detect cancer). Counseling helps people change their behavior to avoid disease. Counseling to help people quit smoking or lose weight results in the prevention of cancer and heart disease.

One challenge for all health plans is choosing the correct list of preventive services to provide as benefits for their members. Plan leaders understand the importance of providing benefits for services that are proven to prevent disease, but the science of prevention does not always provide complete information.

Most health plans choose to adopt the recommendations of a single organization, relying on the expertise of this body for these difficult judgments. Since the U.S. Preventive Services Task Force (USPSTF) first published the *Guide to Clinical Preventive Services* in 1989, it has become the primary resource for many health plans as they design their health maintenance programs and benefit packages. **Table 13-2** presents the USPSTF's recommendations as they stand in 2010.

A report issued by the National Commission on Prevention Priorities—a panel of key representatives from health plans, employer groups, academia, clinical practice, and governmental health agencies—ranked preventive services according to two measures: the clinically preventable burden of disease and the cost-effectiveness of the service.[21] The combined score of these two measures provides a rough measure of the value of each service. Each service received a score of 1–5 on each of the two measures, for a total score possible of 10. **Table 13-3** shows the ranking.

Of all preventive services with evidence of effectiveness, the three that ranked highest were aspirin use in high-risk adults, childhood immunization series, and tobacco use screening and brief intervention. This same study ranked the preventive services that would provide the most health benefits if 90% of patients received the service. Tobacco use screening and brief intervention, colorectal cancer

TABLE 13-2 **Preventive Services Recommended by the U.S. Preventive Services Task Force, 2010**

Recommendations	Adult men	Adult women	Pregnant women	Children
Abdominal aortic aneurysm, screening	X			
Alcohol misuse, screening and behavioral counseling interventions	X	X	X	
Aspirin for the prevention of cardiovascular disease	X	X		
Asymptomatic bacteriuria in adults, screening			X	
Breast cancer, screening		X		
Breast and ovarian cancer susceptibility, genetic risk assessment and BRCA mutation testing		X		
Breast-feeding, primary care interventions		X	X	
Cervical cancer, screening		X		
Chlamydial infection, screening		X	X	
Colorectal cancer, screening	X	X		
Congenital hypothyroidism, screening				X
Depression (adults), screening	X	X		
Folic acid supplementation		X		
Gonorrhea, screening		X		
Gonorrhea, prophylactic medication				X
Hearing loss in newborns, screening				X
Hepatitis B virus infection, screening			X	
High blood pressure, screening	X	X		
HIV, screening	X	X	X	X
Iron-deficiency anemia, prevention				X
Iron-deficiency anemia, screening			X	
Lipid disorders in adults, screening	X	X		
Major depressive disorder in children and adolescents, screening				X
Obesity in adults, screening	X	X		
Obesity in children and adolescents, screening				X
Osteoporosis, screening		X		
Phenylketonuria, screening				X
Rh (D) incompatibility, screening			X	
Sexually transmitted infections, counseling	X	X		X
Sickle cell disease, screening				X
Syphilis infection, screening	X	X	X	
Tobacco use and tobacco-caused disease, counseling and interventions	X	X	X	
Type 2 diabetes mellitus in adults, screening	X	X		
Visual impairment in children younger than age 5 years, screening				X

Note: This table does not include recommendations for immunizations, which are revised frequently.
Source: U.S. Department of Health and Human Services, Agency for Healthcare Research and Quality. "The guide to clinical preventive services 2010–2011: Recommendations of the U.S. Preventive Services Task Force". Available at: www.ahrq.gov/clinic/pocketgd1011/pocketgd1011.pdf. Accessed April 14, 2011.

TABLE 13-3	Priorities Among Effective Clinical Preventive Services		
Clinical preventive services	**Score for clinically preventable burden**	**Score for cost-effectiveness**	**Total score**
Aspirin chemoprophylaxis	5	5	10
Childhood immunization series	5	5	10
Tobacco use screening and brief intervention	5	5	10
Colorectal cancer screening	4	4	8
Hypertension screening	5	3	8
Influenza immunization	4	4	8
Pneumococcal immunization	3	5	8
Problem drinking screening and brief counseling	4	4	8
Vision screening—adults	3	5	8
Cervical cancer screening	4	3	7
Cholesterol screening	5	2	7
Breast cancer screening	4	2	6
Chlamydia screening	2	4	6
Calcium chemoprophylaxis	3	3	6
Vision screening—children	2	4	6
Folic acid chemoprophylaxis	2	3	5
Obesity screening	3	2	5
Depression screening	3	1	4
Hearing screening	2	2	4
Injury prevention counseling	1	3	4
Osteoporosis screening	2	2	4
Cholesterol screening, high risk	1	1	2
Diabetes screening	1	1	2
Diet counseling	1	1	2
Tetanus-diphtheria booster	1	1	2

Source: Reprinted from Maciosek MV, Coffield AB, Edwards NM, et al. Priorities among effective preventive services: Results of a systematic review and analysis. *Am J Prev Med.* July 2006;31(1):52–61. Used with permission from Elsevier.

screening, and influenza vaccine for adults were the three highest-ranking services.[22]

Based on evidence that reducing patients' out-of-pocket costs increases the number of smokers who use smoking cessation interventions, as well as the number of smokers who subsequently quit, the Task Force on Community Preventive Services (TFCPS) recommends coverage or payment to patients for expenses incurred for proven smoking cessation interventions.[23] Increasingly, health plans provide coverage for first-line pharmacotherapies and telephone counseling to help smokers quit successfully.[24]

In addition to scientific evidence and expert opinion, other forces may affect the selection of preventive services. Some benefits may be required by regulators or accreditors, mandated by state laws, or requested by customers. The National Committee for Quality Assurance (NCQA) assesses the prevention efforts of health plans, including whether the plan has guidelines for doctors about the need to provide immunizations and screening tests to plan members. NCQA evaluates how the plans educate providers and patients about preventive measures and assesses the percentage of eligible patients who receive appropriate services. Accreditation, including examples of these types of measures, is discussed fully in Chapter 15. Coverage for cancer screening in particular has become a political issue in several states. Many states have mandated some form of cancer screening, but what screening services are covered varies from state to state. As of 2010, most states required health insurers to provide coverage for mammograms.[25] Many states also require coverage for cervical and colorectal cancer screenings. Twenty-eight states have passed legislation requiring health insurers to cover the full range of colon cancer screening tests. Only four of those use USPSTF guidelines.[26]

Health plans define the copayments, deductibles, and other incentives or disincentives applied to these benefits. Because cost-sharing by members decreases the use of at least some preventive services, some health plans eliminated copayments for appropriate preventive services, often those recommended by a trusted national or state organization, such as the USPSTF or the Institute for Clinical Systems Improvement. Early experience with consumer-driven health plans (CDHPs; see Chapter 2) found that CDHP plan members were significantly more likely than members of traditional health plans to participate in health-promoting and preventive behaviors, including joining a wellness program and receiving regular checkups from a physician.[27]

Since 2010, the Patient Protection and Affordable Care Act of 2010 (ACA) has required all health plans and self-insured group health benefits plans to provide coverage without cost-sharing for all preventive services recommended by the USPSTF. This provision took effect in 2010 and applied to all Task Force recommendations with an A or B level of evidence (the strongest evidence) and to all immunizations approved by the Centers for Disease Control and Prevention's Advisory Committee on Immunization Practices. Similar changes were made to Medicare and Medicaid. Other provisions of this Act are discussed later in this chapter.

■ SERVICES FOR MEMBERS

In addition to defined benefits, health plans can provide a wide variety of other services to help members stay healthy and improve their health. Health plans typically offer some or all of four types of prevention-oriented services: information, assessments of members' health risks, programs to change behaviors, and financial incentives to improve health.

Information

Health plans have been providing prevention information to patients for decades. Printed materials such as brochures and newsletters contain screening recommendations, encouragement for healthy behaviors, and reminders about the use of appropriate immunizations. Many regulators and accreditors expect or require these communications. There is very little evidence that these materials alone change knowledge or behavior.[28]

Health plans have increasingly turned to the Internet to supply prevention information to their members. Health plans have developed or purchased voluminous web-based information on prevention and other health issues. The impact of this information on the health behaviors of health plan members is not well documented. It is known that the Internet is a popular resource for health information for the U.S. public: 74% of American adults use the Internet[29] and of these, 80% have searched for health-related information.[30]

Assessment of Members' Health Risks

A major challenge of supplying useful information to patients is the need to tailor information to each person. A nonsmoker, for example, may get no benefit from a brochure promoting a smoking-cessation program. Health risk assessments (HRAs) were developed, in part, to address this issue. HRAs are questionnaires about an individual's health behaviors, health status, screening, and immunization history. Algorithms allow the individual's responses to trigger a tailored plan that addresses the specific risks and needs of that individual. Pencil-and-paper HRAs still exist, but HRAs are more commonly administered and scored electronically. HRAs are also an effective tool for collecting information about a population. That cumulative information can then drive decisions about appropriate interventions. In large populations, the most significant challenge can be encouraging or requiring people to complete the HRA. Employers and some health plans have increased use of HRAs by offering financial or other incentives to individuals who complete them.

Programs to Change Behaviors

HRAs require follow-up. When a person is identified with a risk factor for disease (such as smoking or obesity), services should be offered to address that issue. Such services can be delivered through e-mail or the Internet, through mailed materials, by telephone, and through face-to-face counseling. Many health plans offer or sell these services to their members. Most commonly, health plans offer members different "modules" to help them with a particular health issue that is identified by the individual's HRA results. Often the modules are Internet-based programs that provide information and e-mail reminders. Common modules cover diet, physical activity, tobacco use, and stress.

HRAs may also be used to direct members to formal counseling programs that help individuals change behavior. Because tobacco use and obesity are the first and second causes of premature death, programs to address these issues are commonly provided to members.[31,32] Tobacco cessation counseling over the telephone is effective and widely available through vendors, state health departments, and health plans. Of all counseling methods, telephone counseling is the most widely covered by health plans.[33] The TFCPS found ample evidence to strongly recommend telephone cessation counseling, especially when used in conjunction with other cessation methods, such as tobacco cessation medications.[34] Several other studies have found telephone counseling to be highly effective in helping patients to modify behaviors and improve health.[35, 36, 37]

There is less evidence that Internet programs help smokers quit successfully. A recent review found that Internet-based interventions can help smokers quit if they are tailored to the users and include frequent contacts with the users.[38] Smoking cessation programs delivered through mobile telephones have also been tested, but their long-term impact is not clear.[39] Group and individual face-to-face counseling is effective, but those methods are utilized by a very small fraction of people trying to quit. A study conducted on the cost-effectiveness of counseling intervention options found group intensive counseling to be the most cost-effective, yet only 5% of smokers were interested in participating in this intervention option.[40]

Programs to treat obesity come in many different formats. There are promising Internet- and telephone-based programs, but their effectiveness is not firmly established. An overview of studies on Internet-based programs found that participants acquired wider knowledge and understanding of chronic conditions and achieved greater health-promoting behavioral modifications.[41] Several studies have found that Internet-based weight-loss programs are more effective when they are tailored or include an interactive behavioral counseling component, such as personalized e-mail feedback from trained weight-loss counselors.[42, 43] A study on the effectiveness of telephone counseling for treating obesity found that patients who received individualized, telephone-based behavioral counseling from trained professionals achieved weight loss comparable to patients who attend face-to-face behavioral programs.[44] At least one group support program (Weight Watchers®) has been shown to help people lose weight.[45] There are also more intensive group and individualized programs, some requiring medical management of severe caloric restrictions.

Financial Incentives to Improve Health

Health plans also promote prevention by providing discounted prices for specific services. For example, discounts may be offered for participation in fitness centers. Such discounts frequently are paid only when a member uses the fitness center a minimum number of times per month (e.g., 12 times per month). Discounts may also be offered for weight management programs, such as Weight Watchers. Here again, an incentive program may pay the discount only for those members who attend the program regularly. It is important to select programs that can reach large numbers of people, can expect to affect their health, have been

studied adequately, and can be reasonably expected to provide a ROI. Some incentive programs reward health outcomes, not program participation. For example, members may receive a financial incentive for achieving a healthy weight, blood pressure, or cholesterol level, or by being a nonsmoker. These programs typically require the individual to be screened by a clinician to document their achievement of these health outcomes.

■ CONTRACTING WITH HEALTH CARE PROVIDERS

MCOs can also use the power of the purse to influence physicians and their delivery of preventive services. Health plans' contracts with provider organizations are potentially important tools for promoting good preventive care. For many years, health plans paid clinics to institute quality improvement programs that were designed to make "systems changes" in the care of patients. Payment was often tied to completing the quality improvement project, not necessarily to improving actual care. In recent years, pay-for-performance programs have attempted to provide financial incentives for providers to deliver documented improvement in patient outcomes. Many of these programs have strengthened the delivery of preventive services, such as cancer screening or tobacco counseling. As noted in Chapter 5, rigorous studies have not yet confirmed the effectiveness of pay-for-performance programs,[46, 47, 48] but many plans are using this technique, which is discussed in Chapter 5.

In recent years, health plans and provider organizations have developed new models of care and payment. Patient-centered medical homes and accountable care organizations (PCMHs and ACOs, respectively), discussed in Chapter 2 and 4, are two concepts that have generated these new models. Health plans are beginning to develop new ways of contracting with provider organizations that provide financial rewards if certain preventive services are performed.

Another approach to promote the delivery of appropriate preventive services is the use of performance feedback for health care providers. Using administrative claims data, health plans have provided information to provider groups and individual practitioners about their patients' use of preventive and other services. Information about an individual provider's performance improves the delivery of preventive services.[49,50] Information that compares a practitioner's or provider's performance to other peers can be particularly compelling.

In addition to performance feedback, health plans have also provided reminders to providers about specific patients' needs for services. Using administrative data, health plans have notified clinics about patients who may be overdue for specific screening tests or immunizations. The use of provider reminders to promote screening and immunization has been shown to be effective as a way to increase rates of both immunization and screenings. Electronic medical record systems that create computer-generated reminders have been found to increase the frequency of follow-up visits,[51] to increase the likelihood that practitioners provide preventive care,[52] and to allow clinics to easily provide individualized outreach and services to patients.[53] The work of prevention requires information that isn't commonly found in a health plan's administrative claims data sets, such as tobacco use, body mass index, and dates of immunizations. It also requires information that isn't commonly found in a patient's medical record, such as benefits coverage and HRA results. In the future, HRA results may augment health plans' data sets and provide information that can guide programs and monitor progress. Similarly, as electronic medical records become more common, we should expect major improvements in the ability of health plans and health care providers to use their collective information for tailored interventions.

■ PUBLIC POLICIES

Health plans have both financial and ethical reasons to prevent disease and promote health. Their traditional sphere of influence lies within their membership, their benefits and services, and their provider contracts. Recent decades have seen some notable public health improvements (e.g., in immunization rates and smoking rates), but these improvements have not been accomplished through clinical interventions alone. Major improvements in public health come about through multifaceted intervention programs that may include clinical tactics but rely most heavily on public policy. Public policies influence people every day and can provide encouragement, incentives, and (at times) requirements to change behavior in a positive way.

Childhood immunizations provide a good example of the effects of public policy. Vaccination is a clinical intervention, but high rates of childhood immunization were not achieved by clinical means alone. The most powerful intervention for increasing immunization rates has been the public policy that requires children to be vaccinated before they can attend school. All 50 states now require proof of current immunization to enter school, although the specific immunization requirements vary from state to state.[54] This "no shots, no school" policy has made immunization almost universal among school-age children. A review of immunization interventions concluded that the enforcement of immunization laws requiring proof of vaccination for school attendance resulted in more than 95% of school-age children receiving the proper vaccinations.[55] Although most states allow exemptions for medical, religious, or philosophical reasons, only 1–3% of school-age children are exempted.[56]

Adult immunizations are not as widely utilized as childhood immunizations. Vaccines to prevent influenza and pneumococcal pneumonia are both effective and cost-effective, but no public policies require their use. Instead, health departments and health plans invest in programs to encourage voluntary vaccination, and achieve much lower immunization rates. Immunization has the potential to save thousands of adults who die each year from diseases that can be prevented, including influenza and hepatitis B. Yet in recent years, only 40% of U.S. adults were vaccinated against influenza.[57]

Tobacco use is also affected by public policy. There are effective clinical treatments for nicotine addiction, but large-scale reductions in the prevalence of tobacco use require a multifaceted approach that goes far beyond clinical interventions. Changes in public policy have much larger impact on smoking rates. Two public policies make a big difference: (1) increases in the excise tax (and therefore the price) on tobacco and (2) strong clean indoor air laws that prohibit smoking in all public workplaces, including restaurants and bars. States that have enacted a comprehensive tobacco control program, including public policy and a variety of options to help smokers quit, have seen notable decreases in smoking rates.[58]

Changes in public policies are far more cost-effective methods for improving health than any clinical intervention. A study that compared the cost-effectiveness of cigarette tax increases, nicotine replacement therapies, and "nonprice interventions," including smoking bans, bans on advertising, and public education campaigns, found that tax increases are both the most effective and the most cost-effective intervention. All of the interventions were shown to be cost-effective when compared with the cost in lives and preventable medical expenses, but policy interventions are more cost-efficient because they incur only administrative and enforcement costs as opposed to nicotine replacement therapies, which have the added cost of the pharmacological product.[59] Health plans that lead or contribute to lobbying efforts for effective primary and secondary prevention strategies demonstrate visible public leadership and active concern for their members' health. Public policy advocacy is a relatively new role for health plans but one that may gain traction as health plans, purchasers, and other community leaders realize the cost-effectiveness of this approach.

■ PREVENTION AND HEALTH CARE REFORM

In 2010, Congress passed the ACA, which required a series of changes in health insurance and other aspects of health care over a period of several years. As noted earlier in the context of member cost-sharing, included in the ACA were many major initiatives and policies related to prevention.[60] The entire law is discussed in more detail in Chapter 30.

The ACA addressed clinical preventive services in several ways. A provision that went into effect in 2010 required health plans and self-insured employers to eliminate coinsurance or copays for all effective clinical preventive services when obtained through in-network providers. These are the services identified as effective by the USPSTF, with an A or B rating of the strength of evidence for effectiveness. This list of preventive services included cancer screening (such as mammography and colonoscopy), vaccinations, and a variety of counseling interventions. The law also required Medicare and Medicaid to remove the same deductibles for effective clinical preventive services and required Medicare to provide coverage for an annual wellness visit.

In addition to clinical preventive services, the health care reform law also addressed prevention programs at the workplace, in the community and at the state level. Several provisions addressed prevention at the workplace. The law provided funding to support effective worksite wellness programs in small businesses (100 or fewer employees). Small businesses often don't have worksite wellness programs. The ACA also made it possible for all employers to offer larger financial rewards to employees who participate in wellness programs offered at work. These can be rewards for participation in a program (such as a weight-loss program) or rewards for achieving a certain prevention goal (such as a healthy body mass index). The ACA appropriated significant funding for prevention programs in states and communities. Most of these programs are intended to reduce the major risk factors for chronic disease, such as tobacco use and obesity. The Department of Health and Human Services (DHHS) was directed to spend up to $2 billion per year to support state and local programs. In addition, DHHS will provide grants to states to support incentives for Medicaid members to participate in prevention programs. DHHS was further instructed to conduct a national outreach and education campaign to promote the prevention of major diseases.

Also included in the health care reform law was a significant policy unrelated to health care delivery but important for prevention of disease. It was a policy requiring chain restaurants to include calorie counts for items on their menus. It also required them to provide more complete nutritional information for customers who want it. This menu-labeling provision was based on similar laws in several states and cities. The information on calorie counts is meant to inform consumers who are trying to manage their weight. Unfortunately, the law preempted state and local governments from enacting stronger laws, such as requiring fat or sodium content on menus.

The 28 prevention provisions in the ACA together constitute a strong and comprehensive national prevention program to address major chronic diseases. These preventive provisions addressed the issue of cost containment in health care. As discussed earlier in this chapter, chronic diseases cause the majority of health care spending, and most of them are preventable. A multiyear commitment to a comprehensive prevention program could produce a significant improvement in health and reduction in health care costs.

■ CONCLUSION

Prevention saves lives and improves health. It is an effective and often cost-effective strategy. In fact, the health and financial case for prevention has never been stronger as concerns about rising health care costs grow. Health plans have a wide array of tools to promote primary and secondary prevention, including member benefits, member services, provider contracts, and the promotion of public policies. Health plans should work to educate both purchasers and members about effective prevention methods. The policy arena clearly holds the most promise for major future gains. Health plans can expand their roles by becoming catalysts for collaborative efforts among other health plans, purchasers, and other community stakeholders.

Endnotes

1 Satcher D. Perspective: The prevention challenge and opportunity. *Health Affairs.* 2006;25(4):1009–1011. Available at: http://content.healthaffairs.org/content/25/4/1009.full#R3. Accessed April 14, 2011.

2 Agency for Healthcare Research and Quality (AHRQ). Health care costs fact sheet. Available at: www.ahrq.gov/news/costsfact.htm. Accessed April 12, 2011.

3 National Cancer Institute and U.S. National Institutes of Health. Dictionary of cancer terms. Available at: www.nci.nih.gov/dictionary/. Accessed March 10, 2011.

4 Jiaquan X, Kochanek KD, Xu J, Murphy SL, Tejada-Vera B. Deaths: Final data for 2007. *Natl Vital Stat Rep.* 2010:58(19):1–135. Available at: www.cdc.gov/nchs/data/nvsr/nvsr58/nvsr58_19.pdf. Accessed April 7, 2011.

5 U.S. Centers for Disease Control and Prevention (CDC). The power of prevention: Chronic disease . . . the public health challenge of the 21st century. Atlanta, GA: U.S. Department of Health and Human Services, 2009. Available at: www.cdc.gov/chronicdisease/pdf/2009-Power-of-Prevention.pdf. Accessed March 31, 2011.

6 Jiaquan X, Kochanek KD, Xu J, Murphy SL, Tejada-Vera B. Deaths: Final data for 2007. *Natl Vital Stat Rep.* 2010:58(19):1–135. Available at: www.cdc.gov/nchs/data/nvsr/nvsr58/nvsr58_19.pdf. Accessed April 7, 2011.

7 Jiaquan X, Kochanek KD, Xu J, Murphy SL, Tejada-Vera B. Deaths: Final data for 2007. *Natl Vital Stat Rep.* 2010:58(19):1–135. Available at: www.cdc.gov/nchs/data/nvsr/nvsr58/nvsr58_19.pdf. Accessed April 7, 2011.

8   U.S. Centers for Disease Control and Prevention (CDC). The power of prevention: Chronic disease . . . the public health challenge of the 21st century. Atlanta, GA: U.S. Department of Health and Human Services, 2009. Available at: www.cdc.gov/chronicdisease/pdf/2009-Power-of-Prevention.pdf. Accessed March 10, 2011.

9   Mokdad AH, Marks JS, Stroup DF, et al. Actual causes of death in the United States, 2000. *JAMA*. 2004;291(10): 1238–1245.

10   U.S. Centers for Disease Control and Prevention (CDC). Smoking-attributable mortality, years of potential life lost, and productivity losses—United States, 2000–2004. *MMWR Weekly*. November 14, 2008;57(45):1226–1228. Available at: www.cdc.gov/mmwr/preview/mmwrhtml/mm5745a3.htm. Accessed March 31, 2011.

11   Hammond RA, Levine R. The economic impact of obesity in the United States. *Diabetes Metab Syndr Obes*. 2010;3:285–295. Available at: www.brookings.edu/~/media/Files/rc/articles/2010/0914_obesity_cost_hammond_levine/0914_obesity_cost_hammond_levine.pdf. Accessed April 5, 2011.

12   Diabetes Prevention Program Research Group. Reduction in the incidence of type 2 diabetes with lifestyle interventions or metformin. *N Engl J Med*. 2002;346:393–403.

13   U.S. Preventive Services Task Force. *Guide to clinical preventive services*. 2nd ed. Washington, DC: U.S. Department of Health and Human Services, Office of Disease Prevention and Health Promotion; 1996. Available at: http://odphp.osophs.dhhs.gov/pubs/guidecps/PDF/CH09.PDF. Accessed March 31, 2011.

14   U.S. Centers for Disease Control and Prevention (CDC). Heart disease and stroke prevention: Addressing the nation's leading killers. At a glance 2010. Available at: www.cdc.gov/chronicdisease/resources/publications/aag/pdf/2010/dhdsp.pdf. Accessed March 31, 2011.

15   Aldana SG. Financial impact of health promotion programs: A comprehensive review of the literature. *Am J Health Prom*. 2001;15(5):296–320.

16   U.S. Department of Health and Human Services. Prevention makes common "cents." September 2003. Available at: http://aspe.hhs.gov/health/prevention. Accessed April 6, 2011.

17   Pronk NP, Goodman MJ, O'Connor PJ, Martinson BC. Relationship between modifiable health risks and short-term health care charges. *JAMA*. 1999;282(23): 2235–2239.

18   Warner KE. Smoking out the incentives for tobacco control in managed care settings. *Tobac Contr*. 1998;7(Suppl): S50–S54. Available at: http://tc.bmjjournals.com/cgi/content/full/7/suppl_1/S50. Accessed March 31, 2011.

19   Warner KE, Smith RJ, Smith DG, Fries BE. Health and economic implications of a work-site smoking cessation program: A simulation analysis. *J Occ Envir Med*. 1996;38(10):981–992.

20   U.S. Food and Drug Administration. FDA licenses new vaccine for prevention of cervical cancer and other diseases in females caused by human papillomavirus. *FDA News*. June 8, 2006. Available at: www.fda.gov/NewsEvents/Newsroom/PressAnnouncements/2006/ucm108666.htm. Accessed March 31, 2011.

21   Maciosek MV, Coffield AB, Edwards NM, Flottenmesch TJ, Goodman MJ, Solberg LI. Priorities among effective preventive services: Results of a systematic review and analysis. *Am J Prev Med*. 2006;31(1):52–61.

22   Maciosek MV, Coffield AB, Edwards NM, Flottenmesch TJ, Goodman MJ, Solberg LI. Priorities among effective preventive services: Results of a systematic review and analysis. *Am J Prev Med*. 2006;31(1):52–61.

23   Task Force on Community Preventive Services. Recommendations regarding interventions to reduce tobacco use and exposure to environmental tobacco use. *Am J Prev Med*. 2001;20(2S):10–15. Available at: www.thecommunityguide.org/tobacco/tobac-AJPM-recs.pdf. Accessed April 12, 2011.

24   McPhillips-Tangum C, Bocchino C, Carreon R, Erceg C, Rehm B. Addressing tobacco in managed care: Results of the 2002 survey. *Prev Chron Dis*. October 2004;1(4):A04.

25   National Cancer Institute, State Legislative Database Program. Fact sheet: Breast cancer. Bethesda, MD: National Cancer Institute, 2006. Available at: www.scld-nci.net/linkdocs/products/factsheets14.pdf. Accessed April 6, 2011.

26   American Cancer Society Cancer Action Network. Internal analysis of 2010 and 2011 data. 2011.

27   Agrawal V, Ehrbeck T, Packard KO, Mango P. Consumer-directed health plan report—early evidence is promising: Insights from primary consumer research. Pittsburgh, PA: McKinsey & Company; 2005. Available at: www.mckinsey.com/clientservice/payorprovider/Health_Plan_Report.pdf. Accessed March 31, 2011.

28   Lancaster T, Stead LF. Self-help interventions for smoking cessation. Cochrane Database of Systematic Reviews. 2005;3. Art. No. CD001118. doi: 10.1002/14651858.CD001118.pub2.

29   The Pew Research Center's Internet & American Life Project. Report: Internet, broadband, and cell phone statistics. January 5, 2010. Available at: www.pewinternet.org/Reports/2010/Internet-broadband-and-cell-phone-statistics/Report.aspx. Accessed March 31, 2011.

30   Pew Research Center. Generations 2010. December 16, 2010. Available at: www.pewinternet.org/Reports/2010/Generations-2010.aspx. Accessed April 6, 2011.

31   McPhillips-Tangum C, Bocchino C, Carreon R, Erceg C, Rehm B. Addressing tobacco in managed care: Results of the 2002 survey. *Prev Chron Dis*. October 2004;1(4): A04.

32 National Institute for Health Care Management. Health plans emerging as pragmatic partners in fight against obesity. April 2005. Available at: http://nihcm.org/pdf/ObesityReport.pdf. Accessed April 12, 2011.

33 McPhillips-Tangum C, Rehm B, Carreon R, Erceg C, Rehm B, Bocchino C. Addressing tobacco in managed care: Results of the 2003 survey. *Prev Chron Dis.* July 2006:3(3). Available at: www.cdc.gov/PCD/issues/2006/jul/pdf/05_0173.pdf. Accessed April 7, 2011.

34 Task Force on Community Preventive Services. Recommendations regarding interventions to reduce tobacco use and exposure to environmental tobacco use. *Am J Prev Med.* 2001;20(2S):10–15.

35 Zhu SH, Anderson CM, Tedeschi GJ, et al. Evidence of real-world effectiveness of a telephone quitline for smokers. *N Engl J Med.* 2002;347(14):1087–1093.

36 Lichtenstein E, Glasgow RE, Lando HA, Ossip-Klein DJ, Boles SM. Telephone counseling for smoking cessation: Rationales and meta-analytic review of evidence. *Health Ed Res.* 1996;11(2):243–257.

37 Boucher JL, Schaumann JD, Pronk NP, Priest B, Ett T, Gray CM. The effectiveness of telephone-based counseling for weight management. Diabetes Spectrum. 1999:12(2):121–123.

38 Civljak M, Sheikh A, Stead LF, Car J. Internet-based interventions for smoking cessation. U.S. National Library of Medicine, National Institutes of Health, Pub Med. 2010. Available at: www.pewinternet.org/Press-Releases/2011/Health-Topics.aspx. Accessed March 31, 2011.

39 Whittaker R, Borland R, Bullen C, Lin RB, McRobbie H, Rodgers A. Mobile phone-based interventions for smoking cessation. U.S. National Library of Medicine, National Institutes of Health, PubMed. 2010. Available at: www.ncbi.nlm.nih.gov/pubmed/19821377. Accessed March 31, 2011.

40 Cromwell J, Bartosch WJ, Fiore MC, Hasselblad V, Baker T. Cost-effectiveness of the clinical practice recommendations in the AHCPR guideline for smoking cessation. Agency for Health Care Policy and Research. *JAMA.* 1997;278(21):1759–1766. Available at: http://jama.ama-assn.org/content/278/21/1759.full.pdf+html. Accessed April 12, 2011.

41 Wantland DJ, Portillo CJ, Holzemer WL, Slaughter R, McGhee EM. The effectiveness of Web-based vs. non-Web-based interventions: A meta-analysis of behavioral change outcomes. *J Med Internet Res.* 2004;6(4). Available at: www.jmir.org/2004/4/e40/. Accessed March 31, 2011.

42 Rothert K, Strecher VJ, Doyle LA, et al. Web-based weight management programs in an integrated health care setting: A randomized, controlled trial. *Obesity.* 2006;14(2):266–272.

43 Tate DF, Jackvony EH, Wing RR. Effects of Internet behavioral counseling on weight loss in adults at risk for type 2 diabetes: A randomized trial. *JAMA.* 2003;289(14):1833–1836.

44 Boucher JL, Schaumann JD, Pronk NP, Priest B, Ett T, Gray CM. The effectiveness of telephone-based counseling for weight management. *Diabetes Spectrum.* 1999;12(2):121–123. Available at: http://journal.diabetes.org/diabetesspectrum/99v12n2/pg121.htm. Accessed March 31, 2011.

45 Tsai AG, Wadden TA. Systematic review: An evaluation of major commercial weight loss programs in the United States. *Ann Intern Med.* 2005;142(1):56–66.

46 Dudley RA. Pay-for-performance research: How to learn what clinicians and policy makers need to know. *JAMA.* 2005;294(14):1821–1823.

47 Rosenthal MB, Frank RG. What is the empirical basis for paying for quality in health care? *Med Care Res Rev.* 2006;63(2):135–157.

48 Rosenthal MB, Frank RG, Li Z, Epstein AM. Early experience with pay-for-performance: From concept to practice. *JAMA.* 2005;294(14):1788–1793.

49 Bordley WC, Chelminski A, Margolis PA, Kraus R, Szilagyi PG, Vann JJ. The effect of audit and feedback on immunization delivery. *Am J Prev Med.* 2000;18(4):343–350.

50 Kiefe CI, Allison JJ, Williams OD, Person SD, Weaver MT, Weissman NW. Improving quality improvement using achievable benchmarks for physician feedback. *JAMA.* 2001;285(22):2871–2879.

51 Barnett GO, Winickoff RN, Morgan MM, Zielstorff RD. A computer-based monitoring system for follow-up of elevated blood pressure. *Med Care.* April 1983;21(4):400–409.

52 McDonald CJ, Hui SL, Smith DM, et al. Reminders to physicians from an introspective computer medical record: A two-year randomized trial. *Ann Intern Med.* 1984;100(1):130–138.

53 Kleschen MZ, Holbrook J, Rothbaum AK, Stringer RA, McInerney MJ, Helgerson SD. Improving the pneumococcal immunization rate for patients with diabetes in a managed care population: A simple intervention with a rapid effect. *Joint Commission J Qual Patient Safety.* 2000;26(9):538–546.

54 National Network for Immunization Information. Exemptions from immunization laws. Updated April 5, 2011. Available at: www.immunizationinfo.org/issues/immunization-policy/exemptions-immunization-laws#footnote1_g9eyr0h. Accessed April 14, 2011.

55 Briss PA, Rodewald LE, Hinman AR, et al. Reviews of evidence regarding interventions to improve vaccination coverage in children, adolescents, and adults. *Am J Prev Med.* 2000;18(Suppl 1):97–140.

56 The Council of State Governments' Healthy States Initiative. Exemptions from school immunization requirements – policy brief. 2007. Available at: www.healthystates.csg.org/NR/rdonlyres/7B29EF52-6408-4D67-904D-CFBE28AF35CA/0/ExemptionsLPB.pdf. Accessed April 12, 2011.

57 Centers for Disease Control and Prevention. Final estimates of 2009-10 influenza vaccination coverage—United States, Behavioral Risk Factor Surveillance System and national 2009 H1N1 flu survey, May 2010. Available at: www.cdc.gov/flu/professionals/vaccination/reporti0910/reportII0910/. Accessed April 12, 2011.

58 Centers for Disease Control and Prevention (CDC). Tobacco use: Targeting the nation's leading killer. At a glance 2011. Available at: www.cdc.gov/chronicdisease/resources/publications/AAG/osh.htm. Accessed April 12, 2011.

59 Ranson K, Jha P, Chaloupka FJ, Nguyen S. The effectiveness and cost-effectiveness of price increases and other tobacco control policies. In: Jha P, Chaloupka FJ, eds. *Tobacco Control in Developing Countries*. New York: Oxford University Press; 2000:427–447. Available at: http://tigger.uic.edu/ ~ fjc/Presentations/Scans/Final%20PDFs/tc427to448.pdf. Accessed March 31, 2011.

60 Compilation of Patient Protection and Affordable Care Act [as amended through May 1, 2010] including Patient Protection and Affordable Care Act health-related portions of the Health Care and Education Reconciliation Act of 2010. Prepared by the Office of the Legislative Counsel for the U.S. House of Representatives, May 2010. Available at: http://docs.house.gov/energycommerce/ACAcon.pdf. Accessed March 31, 2011.

Quality Management in Managed Health Care

Pamela B. Siren

STUDY OBJECTIVES

- Understand the components of a traditional quality assurance program
- Understand the differences between traditional quality assurance and quality management
- Identify customers of managed care
- Understand managed care processes and outcomes and how they meet customer need
- Understand the key measures used to assess performance of managed care processes

DISCUSSION TOPICS

1. Describe and discuss the three criteria Donabedian developed to assess quality and identify circumstances in which they can be applied.
2. Discuss the key components of a quality management program and what features distinguish a quality management program from traditional quality assurance.
3. Discuss how the quality management model can be applied to the development of a new program in preventions such as one to reduce teen smoking.
4. Describe and discuss the strategies a managed care organization can use to involve physicians in managed care processes.

▪ INTRODUCTION

The Patient Protection and Affordable Care Act (ACA) was signed into law by President Barack Obama on March 23, 2010. Health care reform has been based on the foundation of double-digit health insurance premium increases and the disproportionate share that health services consume of the gross national product without corresponding performance in key health indicators.

Three significant publications from the Institute of Medicine (IOM) examined the quality in our health care system including *To Err is Human: Building a Safer Health System* (1999)[1] and *Crossing the Quality Chasm* (2001),[2] and *Unequal Treatment; Confronting Racial and Ethnic Disparities in Healthcare* (2003).[3] Adding to this rich and fertile foundation is one of many pivotal perspectives for national health care reform from Donald Berwick, the former president and CEO of the Institute for Healthcare Improvement and, at the time of publication, the director of the Centers for Medicare and Medicaid Services (CMS). Dr. Berwick suggests that the "Triple Aim" requires the simultaneous pursuit of three aims to improve the U.S. health care system: improving patient experience of care, improving the health of populations, and reducing per capita cost of health care.[4]

A fundamental premise of the Triple Aim is the existence of an organization (an integrator) that accepts responsibility for all three aims for a population. This "organization" must build relationships with individuals and families, redesign the way primary care is delivered, provide population health management and financial management, and work within an integrated system of health. The organization may be a multispecialty group practice, an integrated delivery system, an accountable care organization (ACO), or a managed care organization (MCO).

■ FOUNDATIONS OF REFORM: PREMISE FOR QUALITY MANAGEMENT

The foundational arguments were based on the work of the Committee on Quality of Health Care in America that was formed in June 1998 and was charged with developing a strategy that would result in substantial improvement in the quality of health care over the ensuing 10 years. Their first work addressed an urgent quality problem: patient safety. *To Err is Human: Building a Safer Health Care System* concluded that tens of thousands of Americans die each year from medical errors and hundreds of thousands suffer nonfatal injuries that a high-quality health care system would be able to prevent. In 2003, the Committee proposed six aims for improvement in our health care system:

- **Safe:** Avoiding injuries to patients from the care that is intended to help them.
- **Effective:** Provision of services on basic scientific knowledge to all who could benefit and refraining from providing services to those not likely to benefit (avoiding overuse and underuse, respectively).
- **Patient-centered:** Providing care that is respectful of and responsive to patient preferences, needs, values, and ensuring patient values guide clinical decisions.
- **Timely:** Reducing waits and sometimes harmful delays for both those who receive and those who give care.
- **Efficient:** Avoiding waste, including waste of equipment, supplies, ideas, and energy, with the desired outcome of cost efficiency.
- **Equitable:** Providing care that does not vary in quality because of personal characteristics such as gender, ethnicity, geographic location, and socioeconomic status. Disparities in health care delivery and outcomes are described in IOM's report "Unequal Treatment." State governments, health delivery systems and purchasers are becoming increasingly aware that health inequities exist.

Many MCOs have worked to incorporate these goals into their quality management programs. However, it must be noted that the IOM's six goals are provider oriented. In other words, the primary focus of both the report and the goals is on how providers deliver health care, for example, reducing medication errors (particularly in the inpatient setting) or providing appropriate care more quickly to a patient having a heart attack. Because of this, payers typically work to incorporate these six goals on a population basis, not a patient-by-patient basis, with the exception of cases in which a specific quality concern is brought to the attention of the plan's medical managers. Except for closed-panel health maintenance organizations (HMOs), MCOs have little ability to directly measure and manage these six goals on a day-to-day basis. What they can do is refuse to pay providers for the cost of care associated with a "never event," as discussed in Chapter 5. (Never events are the same as serious reportable events, which are discussed later in the chapter.)

Finally, on a historical note, quality assurance and management programs were initially focused more on HMOs than on other types of payer organizations. As discussed in Chapter 1, this was an element of the HMO Act of 1973, and was put in place because HMO members were limited to using providers who were in the HMO. Quality programs have expanded to other types of plans, but remain the most robust in HMOs even today. While this chapter refers to MCOs by using that generic acronym, the material reflects the HMO experience.

■ HISTORICAL PERSPECTIVE: THE EVOLUTION

In prior editions of *The Essentials of Managed Health Care*, this chapter provided a primer for the development of a managed care quality management program. Considering the changes in the marketplace, those core concepts are still important today and are repeated, but the concepts also employ the principles of measurement, customer focus, and statistically based decision making and are enhanced to address the issues of day.

■ TRADITIONAL QUALITY ASSURANCE

Advocacy for performance assessment in health care can be traced to E. A. Codman, a surgeon who practiced at Massachusetts General Hospital in the early 1900s. He was among the first advocates of systematic performance assessment in health care. His efforts included evaluation of the care provided to his own patients.

In the 1960s and 1970s, the introduction of computers and large administrative data sets (used initially to support Medicare claims processing) permitted investigators to use powerful epidemiological methods in their analyses of practice variations and related phenomena. In this period, Avedias Donabedian developed three criteria for the assessment of quality that are still used today: structure, process, and outcome. His approach to quality assessment of care has stood the test of time and remains useful in managed care settings.

Structure Criteria

Structural measures of health care performance focus on the context in which care and services are provided. These measures provide inferences about the MCO's capability to provide the services it proposes to offer. Examples of structural measures include board certification of physicians, licensure of facilities, compliance with safety codes, medical record-keeping, and physician network appointments. Many such requirements are delineated in federal, state, and local regulations that govern licensing or accreditation (Chapters 15 and 28) and mandate periodic review and reporting mechanisms.

Accreditation and regulatory bodies have historically emphasized structural criteria because of their ease of documentation and requisite requirement upon which a quality program is built. Purchasers support this tradition by requesting such information in their contract negotiations with MCOs. The role of the MCO's leadership in improving performance is increasing and is evaluated by accrediting agencies through assessment of core processes and the outcomes the processes produce. MCO leadership, executive and governance, need a complete understanding of the role and the responsibility they have in ensuring quality of care and service.

Integrated delivery systems' criteria for structural quality are more complex. The regulations and standards that may govern MCOs, such as those of the National Committee for Quality Assurance (NCQA; see Chapter 15), may be different from the standards to which member hospitals are held accountable, such as those of The Joint Commission (TJC) or to those public health licensing requirements for which the primary care practice sites are held responsible. Reconciliation of at least the minimal and widely accepted standards within the MCO and across an integrated delivery system is the first step to developing structural measures and evaluating structural performance and its impact on the quality and cost of health care delivery.

Structural measures generally do not offer adequate specificity to differentiate the capabilities of providers or organizations beyond meeting minimum standards. In addition, the relationship between structure and other measures of performance, such as outcomes, must be evaluated to ensure that enforcing structural standards leads to better quality results. In an era of increasing demand by consumers and increasing costs, MCOs must manage their structural resources strategically while being mindful of the IOM aims for improvement. For example, some states, in collaboration with MCOs, are streamlining the provider credentialing process through centralization using an intermediary. In Massachusetts, for example, MCOs purchase provider credentialing information for a subscription fee. The efficiency achieved is twofold: Providers have a single application to complete for all of the state's MCOs, and MCOs can reduce resources associated with their credentialing function without compromising the integrity of the process. From a quality perspective, required credentialing criteria can be consistently met in a timely fashion with a minimum of variation and error. (This approach is discussed further in Chapter 4.)

Process Criteria

The second traditional criterion for health care quality assessment is process. Langley and Nolan describe a process as a set of causes and conditions that repeatedly come together in a series of steps to transfer inputs into outcomes.[5] Processes of care measures evaluate the way in which care is provided. The IOM aims for improvement in process measures' focus on safe, effective, timely, patient-centered, efficient, and equitable health care. Examples of process measures for MCOs include the number of referrals made out-of-network, preventive health screening rates (e.g., mammography and cholesterol screening), follow-up rates for abnormal diagnostic results, and assessment of adherence to clinical guidelines for different health conditions. Such measures are frequently evaluated against national criteria or benchmarks. Process of service measures are also frequently used, for example, appointment waiting times and membership application processing times. As with structural measures, it is important to link process measures to outcomes. Although the field of outcomes research continues to grow, the link between many health care processes and key outcomes has not always been clearly defined.

Freedom of choice and ease of access to specialty care are often common themes in patient-centered approaches to process measurement. For example, a number of HMOs have been experimenting with referral-less or open access specialty networks. They are doing so because if processing a referral is not embraced as an opportunity for care management, there may be little value and added administrative expense for requiring one. Evaluation of both the cost and clinical value for specialty referrals as well as designing networks with some flexibility of choice should therefore be considered. The ACA emphasizes the delivery of patient-centered care in patient-centered medical homes and health homes.

Outcome Criteria

The third traditional category of quality assessment is the outcome of care or service. Examples of traditional outcomes measurements include infection rates, morbidity, and mortality. Relatively poor outcomes performance generally mandates careful review. Unfortunately, although outcomes measures are purported to reflect the performance of the entire system of care and service processes, they often offer little insight into the causes of poor performance.

Despite the limitations of current outcomes assessment, MCOs have systems in place to assess for adverse events. These screening criteria are often evaluated during the utilization review process to detect sentinel events. Some of these same measures are being applied to the peer review process within the MCO.

Peer Review and Appropriateness Evaluation

In addition to Donabedian's three quality criteria, peer review and appropriateness review have been key components of the traditional quality assurance model. Peer review and appropriateness of care are central to the managed care debate, and they are discussed here.

Peer Review

Peer review, which is also discussed in Chapter 5, involves a comparison of an individual provider's practice either by the provider's peers or against an acceptable standard of care. These standards, or practice guidelines, may be developed within the MCO, be described by national professional associations (eg, the American Academy of Pediatrics), or be created or compiled by a regulatory or legislative agency (e.g., the Agency for Healthcare Research and Quality). (Practice guidelines are discussed further in a later section of this chapter as well as in Chapter 7.)

Cases for peer review are identified either as outliers to specific indicators, perceived deviations from a norm, or through audits of medical records. Peer review has traditionally been used as an informal yet effective educational tool. It is typified by morbidity and mortality conferences currently in existence within medical groups. Within an MCO, peer review frequently occurs following a sentinel or "never event" such as a member suicide during the course of receiving behavioral health treatment or the wrong body part being operated on. These never events are called that because they should never occur. In 2006, the National Quality Forum (NQF) built on the committee's work and identified 28 evidence-based adverse events that are serious, largely preventable, and of concern to health care providers, consumers, and all stakeholders for public reporting. CMS and a number of states have taken this a step further and have implemented policies of nonpayment for serious reportable events to incent the delivery system to improve processes that result in such events, as described in Chapter 5. The scope of Reportable Events has been limited to inpatient acute care, and are listed in **Table 14-1**. The NQF is seeking to expand that to ambulatory surgical centers, skilled nursing facilities, and physician office practices.

Peer review has its limitations. Opportunities for improvement may be missed by a paradigm that rests on conformance with standards. W. Edwards Deming, a statistician and early adopter of statistical process control in industry, emphasized that merely meeting specifications does not result in constant improvement, but rather ensures the status quo. Peer review

is limited by the scope of the indicators or processes under review and is traditionally driven by sentinel events.

In today's MCO, more emphasis is being placed on the what, the how, and the who of making clinical decisions to approve or deny coverage. An integral component of a modern quality management program is the evaluation of consistency of decision making by both MCO physicians and case managers. Interrater reliability audits are useful tools to be added to an MCO's internal peer review process to monitor consistency of decision making and application of criteria.

Appropriateness Evaluation

Appropriateness evaluation reviews the extent to which the MCO provides timely and necessary care at the right level of service to those who are likely to benefit. Appropriateness evaluation is closely aligned with the IOM's aims of effective and timely care delivery. This type of review frequently occurs before an elective clinical event (admission or procedure) or as part of a precertification process, as discussed in Chapter 7. Procedures or admissions most frequently selected for appropriateness review include those for which there is a wide variation of opinion as to their usefulness or effectiveness and those that have been notably expensive. Examples of procedures frequently selected for appropriateness review include hysterectomy, coronary artery bypass surgery, and laminectomy.

The proposed indication for the event is compared with a list of approved evidence-based indications developed by a professional society (e.g., American College of Radiology), a specialty vendor, or commercial source or designed by the MCO itself through their technology assessment process. The two most commonly used commercial vendors of evidence-based clinical criteria and guidelines are described in Chapter 7. Appropriateness review is intended to identify and minimize areas of overutilization. Optimal care management systems apply appropriateness criteria to assess the potential for underutilization of needed services.

■ BUILDING ON TRADITION: ADDITIONAL COMPONENTS

Donabedian's three criteria for quality assessment provide the essential tools to design a quality management program. The traditional quality assurance model can be improved, however, with an infusion of systems thinking, customer focus, and knowledge for improvement.

Systems Thinking

Systems thinking recognizes that processes are interrelated and offers a method for structural design, assessment, and management of performance with a clear aim and shared purpose. A shared aim permits payers and providers to form

TABLE 14-1	**Serious Reportable Events in Health Care**

1. Surgical events
   a. Surgery performed on the wrong body part
   b. Surgery performed on the wrong patient
   c. Wrong surgical procedure performed on a patient
   d. Unintended retention of a foreign object in a patient after surgery or other procedure
   e. Intraoperative or immediately postoperative death in an ASA Class I patient

2. Product or device events
   a. Patient death or serious disability associated with the use of contaminated drugs, devices, or biologics provided by the health care facility
   b. Patient death or serious disability associated with the use or function of a device in patient care in which the device is used or functions other than as intended
   c. Patient death or serious disability associated with intravascular air embolism that occurs while being cared for in a health care facility

3. Patient protection events
   a. Infant discharged to the wrong person
   b. Patient death or serious disability associated with patient elopement (disappearance)
   c. Patient suicide, or attempted suicide, resulting in serious disability while being cared for in a health care facility

4. Care management events
   a. Patient death or serious disability associated with a medication error (e.g., errors involving the wrong drug wrong dose, wrong patient, wrong time, wrong rate, wrong preparation, or wrong route of administration)
   b. Patient death or serious disability associated with a hemolytic reaction due to the administration of ABO/HLA-incompatible blood or blood products
   c. Maternal death or serious disability associated with labor or delivery in a low-risk pregnancy while being cared for in a health care facility
   d. Patient death or serious disability associated with hypoglycemia, the onset of which occurs while the patient is being cared for in a health care facility
   e. Death or serious disability (kernicterus) associated with failure to identify and treat hyperbilirubinemia in neonates
   f. Stage 3 or 4 pressure ulcers acquired after admission to a health care facility
   g. Patient death or serious disability due to spinal manipulative therapy
   h. Artificial insemination with the wrong donor sperm or wrong egg

5. Environmental events
   a. Patient death or serious disability associated with an electric shock while being cared for in a health care facility
   b. Any incident in which a line designated for oxygen or other gas to be delivered to a patient contains the wrong gas or is contaminated by toxic substances
   c. Patient death or serious disability associated with a burn incurred from any source while being cared for in a health care facility
   d. Patient death or serious disability associated with a fall while being cared for in a health care facility
   e. Patient death or serious disability associated with the use of restraints or bedrails while being cared for in a health care facility

6. Criminal events
   a. Any instance of care ordered by or provided by someone impersonating a physician, nurse, pharmacist, or other licensed health care provider
   b. Abduction of a patient of any age
   c. Sexual assault on a patient within or on the grounds of a health care facility
   d. Death or significant injury of a patient or staff member resulting from a physical assault (i.e., battery) that occurs within or on the grounds of a health care facility

a connected, efficient network. Generally, a disconnected network will eventually engage in contradictory, inefficient behaviors and potentially duplicative harmful behaviors such as prescribing medication that may be contraindicated with current medication. Organizational goals are achieved by identifying customer needs of an organization, unify-ing that purpose within the organization, and expanding the shared purpose across the integrated delivery system. Shared purpose and a shared financial risk between MCO and provider groups offers the potential to promote the quality of care delivered through the reduction of inappropriate care/service denials and improved coordination of care.

Customer Focus

Customer focus is the cornerstone of all quality management programs in health care and in industry overall. An organization that embraces this philosophy as part of its strategic vision is well suited to address the needs associated with increasing consumerism. A robust quality management program identifies key customers, anticipates customer needs, measures how effectively customer needs are met, and improves processes to meet those needs.

Knowledge for Improvement

Finally, an enhancement of the traditional quality assurance model is knowledge for improvement. Improvement involves the methods of measurement and change management. As illustrated in **Figure 14-1**, three fundamental questions are used to guide for improvement efforts:

1. What are you trying to accomplish? Information gained from understanding customer needs, the current process and outcome performance, and expected performance will assist the MCO in answering this question.
2. How will you know that a change is an improvement? Establishing performance expectations in comparison with the current level of performance before implementing an improvement activity assists the MCO in understanding whether a change is necessary and if there is an improvement.
3. What changes can be made that will result in an improvement?

To develop tests and implement changes, the plan–do–study–act (PDSA) cycle is used as a framework for an efficient trial and learning model. The term "study" is used in the third cycle to emphasize this phase's primary purpose: to gain knowledge. Increased knowledge leads to a better prediction of whether a change in a given process will result in an improvement.

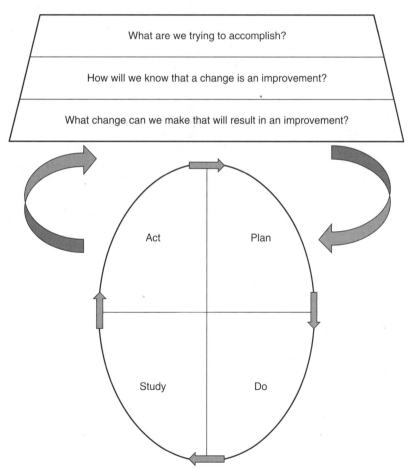

FIGURE 14-1 The Model for Improvement

Adapted from Langley et al. (2009). Reproduced with permission of John Wiley & Sons, Inc.

To be considered a PDSA cycle, the following aspects of the activity should be identifiable. First, the activity must be planned, including a strategy to collect data. Second, the plan must be attempted. Third, time must be set aside to analyze the data and study the results. Finally, action must be rationally based on what was learned. For example, an MCO experimenting with the most effective means to ensure an adequate response rate on a member self-reported health risk assessment (see Chapters 7 and 13) might deploy two strategies. One strategy includes a telephone call to the member; in the other strategy, a written survey is mailed. Response rates are collected for both methods to determine which yields the most favorable rates. If findings identify that telephone calls yield a higher response rate, then this is the strategy to be deployed. In all events, improvement strategies do not necessarily have to be broad, sweeping changes. Rather, small, incremental improvements offer sustainability over time.

■ CONTINUOUS IMPROVEMENT PROCESS MODEL

The remainder of this chapter discusses the key steps in developing a modern quality management program that is based on the fundamentals of quality assurance, incorporates the improvement aims of the Institute of Medicine, and is responsive to the changing marketplace. **Figure 14-2** illustrates the components of this model.

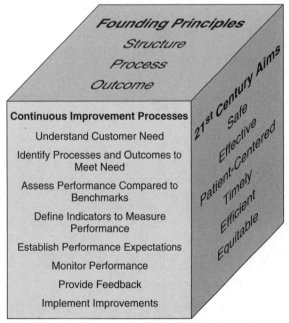

FIGURE 14-2 Quality Management in Three Dimensions
Source: Developed by Neighborhood Health Plan, Inc. ©2006. Used with permission.

Understand Customer Need

Understanding customer need is the basis of all quality management programs. Customers are anyone who is affected by a product or process. Three categories of customers are external customers, internal customers, and suppliers. External customers of an MCO include members or beneficiaries, providers, and purchasers, either employers or state/federal purchasers. Internal customers include the departments and services within the MCO, such as claims processing and member education, as well as the MCO's health care professionals themselves. Negotiating and balancing the needs of these diverse and sometimes conflicting customer groups represent a challenge for MCOs, as they do for any organization.

Methods to understand customer need are as diverse as the customer groups. Reactive understanding of customer needs usually comes in the form of complaints. Customer complaints are a usual signal of a quality problem. Low levels of complaints, however, do not necessarily mean high satisfaction. Frequently, dissatisfied customers will purchase services elsewhere without ever registering a complaint. Most MCOs have a formal process to systematically survey their membership for satisfaction with care or services, as discussed in Chapter 20. Member surveys often use a common format, as described in Chapter 15 on accreditation.

MCOs need to carefully examine their internal policies and processes that have a direct impact on members. Evaluation of front-end member services to assess the ease of access to care and services and responsiveness to meet member needs is essential. Medical management operations must evaluate the appropriateness and consistency of care decisions, particularly denials, and the degree to which care is coordinated. Analysis of member appeals should focus on the reason for the care denial but also should inform the process of negotiating; balancing the diverse groups of customer needs can represent a challenge. It is important to recognize that some customers are more important than others. It is typical that 80% of the total sales volume comes from about 20% of the customers; these are the vital few customers who command priority. Within these key customer groups, there is a distribution of individual customers that may also have a hierarchy of importance, such as a government agency, a gold card employer account, or an academic teaching center. Explicit understanding of the needs of all the MCO customer groups will minimize situations in which one customer's needs are met to the exclusion of another's. MCOs also have the ability to influence and direct their membership to high-quality hospitals or centers of excellence, as discussed in Chapters 4 and 7. The customer need for patient safety is also being expressed by purchasers and employer groups who are diligently working to inform their constituents. An example is the Leapfrog Group, an organization of purchasers that asks hospitals if they adhere to three quality and safety practices because significant scientific evidence shows that these practices reduce unnecessary deaths and injuries:

1. Computerized physician order entry
2. Intensive care unit (ICU) staffing with health care providers who have special training in critical care
3. High-risk treatments—the process of selecting a hospital with extensive experience and results for specific procedures, surgeries, or conditions is known as evidence-based hospital referral[6]

Equitable health care means providing care that does not vary in quality because of personal characteristics such as gender, ethnicity, geographic location, and socioeconomic status; and it is a growing customer need. In *Unequal Treatment*, the Institute of Medicine found that racial and ethnic groups receive lower quality of care and needed services than nonminorities do even when factors related to access to care are controlled. MCOs are uniquely positioned to study health equity given their substantial data warehouses of health services information. For example, an MCO in Massachusetts found that their African American female members were less likely to have had a screening mammogram than their white or Latina counterparts. This same MCO found that their members of Dominican Republican descent with diabetes demonstrated better comprehensive management of their disease than their Puerto Rican counterparts[7] MCOs must focus on health equity as they design their improvement strategies.

Identify Processes and Outcomes That Meet Customer Need

Identification of processes and outcomes that meet customer need is the next step of the continuous improvement process. How do customers view the MCO's quality? To begin with, they want to know whether the MCO meets their expectations. MCOs are expected to treat members who are ill and to maintain the health and functional capabilities of those who are not. To treat sick patients, MCOs first have to make it easy for them to access services, and second must provide them with appropriate care. Purchasers value assessments of disease screening activities and service quality and encounter outcomes to the extent that they support or embellish information about access and appropriateness. Similarly, purchasers know that to maintain health and functional capacity, MCOs must support prevention of illness and management of health status. (These types of activities are discussed further in the other chapters in Part III of this book.)

Assess Performance Compared with Professional or "Best-of-Class" Standards

The third step of the continuous improvement process is assessing the MCO's performance compared with a professional or "best-of-class" standard. This concept of comparison was discussed earlier. Performance can be assessed through appropriateness and peer review, benchmarking, and outcomes assessment.

Appropriateness Review

As discussed for the traditional quality assurance model, appropriateness indicators evaluate the extent to which the MCO provides necessary care and does not provide unnecessary care in the service location best suited for quality and cost efficiencies. Purchasers understand that they cannot obtain good value from an MCO unless it provides appropriate services, so that these indicators are as important as those for accessibility. Unfortunately, in some cases at least, improving the assessment of appropriateness has been dogged by methodological problems, such as adjusting the data for case mix (discussed later) and the surprising lack of data from controlled trials that would define appropriate care in the first place. This issue affects the evaluation of both overutilization and underutilization of services.

In response to these challenges, the MCO can do two things. First, the MCO can identify minimum performance standards for high-cost diagnoses and use them to select processes having excess utilization. Second, the MCO can demonstrate evidence of consistent success and/or an improvement trend in clinical appropriateness indicators. If these two approaches are employed, purchasers seem inclined to offer MCOs some flexibility in the short run even if some isolated indicators suggest that there may be quality problems.

Peer Review

As discussed previously, peer review involves a comparison of an individual provider's practice against an accepted standard of care. A key difference between peer review in a traditional quality assurance model and that in a modern quality management model is the topic of comparison.

Benchmarking

A third method of assessing and comparing an MCO's performance is benchmarking or comparing the MCO's performance to the 90th percentile national performance or the MCO's toughest competitor. Two types of benchmarking may be used by MCOs. First, internal benchmarking identifies internal functions to serve as pilot sites for comparison for other internal functions. An example of internal benchmarking is the percentage of calls answered in 20 seconds in the Member Services department compared to the percentage of calls answered in 20 seconds in the Prior Authorization unit. This type of benchmarking is particularly useful in the second step of the Model for Improvement, *How will I know if a change is an improvement?* (see Figure 14-1). The second type of benchmarking is external or competitive benchmarking. Competitive benchmarking is the comparison of work processes with those of the best-in-class competitor. The benchmarking process can be applied to service and clinical processes for knowledge of current performance.

Outcomes Assessment

An MCO assesses performance through outcomes assessment. An outcomes assessment may be performed on the MCO's 10 high-volume or high-cost diagnoses or procedure groups, for example. An outcomes assessment permits the MCO to assess its own performance over time and to identify variation within the MCO. Outcomes assessments include measurement, monitoring, and management. Measures are observations at a point in time. Monitoring for outcomes measurements occur serially or over multiple points of time to assess a trend either in a favorable or unfavorable direction. And, like the Model for Improvement in Figure 14-1, the results of outcomes monitoring feeds back into the PDSA continuous improvement cycle.

Define Indicators to Measure Performance

Defining indicators to measure performance is the fourth step of the continuous improvement process. The MCO may apply the quality criteria (structure, process, and outcome) as discussed for the traditional quality assurance model. In addition, it is useful for MCOs to evaluate their process and outcomes by populations of customers served. A key issue faced by MCOs in indicator definition and analysis is case-mix adjustment. Case-mix adjustment is a statistical process to control for variations in illness or wellness in patient populations. It takes into account specific attributes of a patient population (e.g., age, gender, severity of illness, chronic health status, race and ethnicity) that are beyond the control of the MCO or health provider. This adjustment is particularly important in comparative analyses between providers or among MCOs. Case-mix adjustment permits fair comparisons among same-population groups because it accounts for preexisting phenomena that may affect the outcome of care.

Issues of case mix affect the analysis of both inpatient and outpatient care. The problem, however, is more serious for some performance measures than for others. Case mix is important for clinically oriented indicators such as appropriateness and outcomes. It also has a significant impact on assessments of health status, resource use, and member satisfaction. Case mix is not nearly as important for measures of access and prevention, and thus these measures should be considered more appropriate for physician profiles and report cards. The topic of case-mix adjustment exceeds the scope of this chapter. Chapter 10 provides further discussion of this topic.

NCQA has been a leader in indicator development for managed care. The indicator set developed by NCQA, the Healthcare Effectiveness Data and Information Set (HEDIS®; see Chapter 15), had its origins in preventive health screenings and procedures such as pediatric immunizations and cancer screenings. With recognition that the population of persons living with chronic conditions and the science of measurement have improved, new HEDIS measures have increasingly focused on care of chronic conditions and proper use of medications. NCQA is moving away from creating new measures that require review of medical records and is advancing toward more retrieval of health information from electronic medical records. For example, chronic disease treatment measures now include chronic obstructive pulmonary disease and rheumatoid arthritis. Medication monitoring measures a number of treatment domains, including antibiotics, psychoactive medications (for depression and attention-deficit/hyperactivity disorder), and persistent-use medications for chronic conditions such as asthma and hypercholesterolemia. Rates for the new measures are calculated using a combination of claims and pharmacy data.

Establish Performance Expectations

Establishing performance expectations is the fifth step of the continuous improvement process. Performance expectations are defined by understanding customer needs (step 1), evaluating the performance of the processes and outcomes designed to meet those needs (step 2), and comparing performance against "best-of-class" standards either internal or external to the MCO (step 3). Many MCOs submit the results of their indicators to NCQA's Quality Compass® each year. Quality Compass is a valuable source for MCOs from which to benchmark from and establish stretch goals for performance improvement.

Monitor Performance and Compare with Expectations

Following established expectations, the sixth step is the actual monitoring of performance and comparison with expectations. The frequency of monitoring is determined by the indicators the MCO has selected to measure performance. An MCO can compare its performance against its own over time and against other MCOs if the same indicator definitions are used.

Provide Feedback to Providers and Customers

The seventh step of the continuous improvement process is providing feedback. Two methods of feedback are discussed here: profiling, which assesses the performance of individual providers, and report cards, which assess overall MCO performance.

Profiling

Profiling focuses on the utilization patterns of an individual provider or group of providers rather than that provider's specific clinical decisions. As described by the Triple Aim, this is an assessment of population health. The population represents all the members assigned to a specific provider or group of providers. Performance is expressed as a rate of utilization divided by the population served (or population eligible for the service). An example of population profiling is the rate in which body mass index is assessed for the entire panel (population) of patients. Another example is the percentage of eligible women between the ages of 40 and 64 who have had a screening mammogram in the prior 24 months. The resulting profile can then be compared against a peer group of providers (external benchmarking) or a standard (Quality Compass).

MCOs are using profiling to measure provider performance, to guide quality improvement efforts, and to select providers for managed care networks. Other examples of measures used in provider profiling include average wait time to schedule a routine physical, number of hospital admissions, number of referrals out-of-network, number of emergency department visits, member satisfaction, percentage compliance with the MCO's clinical practice guidelines, and, if applicable, the percentage of children receiving appropriate immunizations and the Cesarean section rate. Chapter 10 discusses the approach to and uses of profiling in more detail.

Report Cards

Report cards have become a popular method of conveying performance within an individual MCO with multiple geographic sites or across many diverse MCOs. The purpose of a report card is to provide customers (purchasers and consumers) with comparable quality and cost information in a common language for the purpose of selecting a health plan. In 2010, NCQA partnered with Consumer Reports© to rank America's health plans on quality. The reports and the rankings are calculated from an MCO's NCQA accreditation status and their HEDIS and member satisfaction performance. The benefits of the report card movement (sometimes referred to as data transparency) include the stimulus for MCOs to build the capacity to produce performance information and strengthen data quality. Public disclosure of performance information also lends itself to plan, provider, and hospital accountability. Such public report cards should aim to include the issues of patient safety and equity.

A limitation of the report card movement continues to be measurement. Although the NCQA and HEDIS have made moves to standardize measurement, there continues to be variation in measurement, coding, and clinical classification. Additionally, there is variation in the administrative source data sets that plans use to obtain their measurements. Risk adjustment and a broader clinical focus are opportunities for improvement. Finally, no conclusion can be drawn about processes or outcomes that are not assessed by the report card measurements.

Implement Improvements

The eighth step of the continuous improvement process is implementation of improvements. The PDSA cycle described earlier is a vehicle for learning and acting. PDSA can be used to build knowledge about a process, to test a change, or to implement a change. Current strategies employed by MCOs as tools to improve health care delivery processes and outcomes are practice guidelines, improvement teams, and consumer education.

Practice Guidelines

Clinical practice guidelines are systematically developed statements to assist practitioners and patients in making decisions about appropriate health care for specific clinical circumstances, as described in Chapter 7. Clinical guidelines may inform a disease management program (see Chapter 8) or be applied separately. Clinical guidelines for selected, high-impact conditions are also incorporated into P4P programs, as discussed in Chapter 5.

Guidelines offer an opportunity to improve health care delivery processes by reducing unwanted variation and can also be viewed as restrictive when applied to care or service denials. An appointed committee of the Institute of Medicine recommended the following attributes of guideline design:

- Validity: Practice guidelines are deemed valid if they lead to the health and cost outcomes projected for them.
- *Reliability/reproducibility:* If given the same evidence and development methods, another set of experts would come up with the same recommendations, and the guidelines are interpreted and applied consistently across providers.
- *Clinical applicability:* Guidelines should apply to a clearly defined patient population.
- *Clinical flexibility:* Guidelines should recognize the generally anticipated exceptions to the recommendations proposed.

- *Multidisciplinary process:* Representatives of key disciplines involved in the process of care should participate in the guideline development process.
- *Scheduled review:* Guideline evaluation should be planned in advance and occur at a frequency that reflects the evolution of clinical evidence for the guideline topic.
- *Documentation:* Detailed summaries of the guideline development process that reflect the procedures followed, the participants involved, the evidence and analytical methods employed, and the assumptions and rationales accepted should be maintained.

For successful implementation of clinical practice guidelines, the MCO needs to examine its customers' needs, in this case the providers, and identify any driving or restraining forces that may impede guideline implementation. Thus, an MCO may want to convene a group of local content experts along with its own medical leadership to initiate guideline planning and adoption. An effective implementation team strengthens the driving forces for the guideline and weakens the restraining forces for a given clinical practice change. To implement guidelines as an improvement strategy, performance must be measured on two levels. First, the gap between prior and optimal practice is measured to assess the degree of implementation. Providers need to be informed about their performance either through profiling or report cards.

Consumer Education

The effectiveness of consumer education must also be a part of an MCO's quality plan. Consumer education is targeted at beneficiaries so that they can become effective health care consumers and participate in meeting the aforementioned needs of treating disease and managing health. Examples of consumer education utilized by MCOs include telephone resource lines, health risk appraisals, worksite-based consumer education programs, and consumer health education materials. Many MCOs have developed and provide members with self-care guidelines for preventing illness and treating common complaints at the time of enrollment. (These topics are also discussed briefly in Chapters 7 and 13.)

Setting the Improvement Agenda

Finally, the MCO must evaluate whether improvements actually made a change and met customer need. If not, the cycle begins again with step 1. If improvements did occur and customer need was met, the cycle can begin again for new or unaddressed customer needs.

How can an MCO design such a cycle? MCOs have limited resources with which to assess and improve performance, and strategic decisions must be made to target

resources effectively. An MCO's leadership group may begin the cycle of improvement by applying the following criteria:

1. Identify which customer need is being addressed by the proposed project.
2. Evaluate the strength of the evidence for the need to improve.
3. Assess the probability that there will be a measurable impact.
4. Determine the likelihood of success.
5. Identify the immediacy of impact in meeting the customer's need.

◼ VALUE-BASED PURCHASING

For skeptics who may underestimate the role of quality and performance in the health reform word, the reader is urged to consider the following. CMS has proposed a strategy for value-based purchasing for inpatient care of Medicare beneficiaries that has some similarities to pay-for-performance programs as described in Chapter 5. The purchasing (or payment) proposal is based on:

- Process measures (e.g., prescribing aspirin to a heart attack patient at discharge)
- Eight hospital-acquired conditions (HACs) (e.g., development of decubitus ulcers or retained surgical sponge)
- Thirty-day mortality rate
- Patient experience (e.g., member satisfaction)
- Efficiency measures (e.g., hospital spending per admission)

The Kaiser Family Foundation reports that 17% of all Americans are currently covered by Medicaid, the state/federal shared program for the poor and 46,589, or 12%, are covered by Medicare; in other words, almost 30% of all U.S. citizens are covered by government-sponsored insurance.[8] Those statistics illustrate the considerable purchasing power the states and the federal government have around health coverage and the government's responsibility to employ value-based purchasing.

◼ CONCLUSION

Health reform and persistent double-digit rate inflation annually for health care premiums, in an environment of excessive medical errors, and concerns that minorities are not receiving equal care and treatment suggests an opportunity for MCO quality managers to design effective and comprehensive quality programs. Tools to affect such a program are the foundations of quality assurance from Donabedian, addressing the IOM improvement aims for the 21st century, and using a planned and deliberate process improvement method based on data.

Recommended Readings

Institute of Medicine. *To Err Is Human: Building a Safer Health Care System*. Washington, DC: National Academy Press; 2000.

Institute of Medicine. *Crossing the Quality Chasm: A New Health System for the 21st Century*. Washington, DC: National Academy Press; 2001.

Institute of Medicine. *Unequal Treatment: Confronting Racial and Ethnic Disparities in Healthcare*. Washington, DC: National Academy Press; 2003.

Juran JM, Gryna FM. *Quality Planning and Analysis*. New York: McGraw-Hill; 1993.

Langley GJ, Moen RD, Nolan KM, et al. *The Improvement Guide: A Practical Approach to Enhancing Organizational Performance*. 2nd edition. San Francisco: Jossey-Bass; 2009.

Senge P. *The Fifth Discipline: The Art and Practice of the Learning Organization*. New York: Currency Doubleday; 1993.

Walton M. *The Deming Management Method*. New York: Putnam; 1986.

Endnotes

1 Institute of Medicine. *To Err Is Human: Building a Safer Health Care System*. Washington, DC: National Academy Press; 2000.

2 Institute of Medicine. *Crossing the Quality Chasm: A New Health System for the 21st Century*. Washington, DC: National Academy Press; 2001.

3 Institute of Medicine. *Unequal Treatment: Confronting Racial and Ethnic Disparities in Healthcare*. Washington, DC: National Academy Press; 2003.

4 Berwick DM, Nolan TW, and Whittington J. The triple aim: Care, health, and cost; *Health Affairs*. 2008;27(3): 759–769.

5 Langley GJ, Moen RD, Nolan KM, et al. *The Improvement Guide: A Practical Approach to Enhancing Organizational Performance*. 2nd edition. San Francisco: Jossey-Bass, 2009.

6 www.leapfroggroup.org/for_consumers/hospitals_asked_what. Accessed August 13, 2011.

7 Author's experience, Neighborhood Health Plan, 2010.

8 http://facts.kff.org/chart.aspx?ch=477. Accessed August 13, 2011.

Accreditation and Performance Measurement Programs in Managed Health Care

MARGARET E. O'KANE

STUDY OBJECTIVES

- Understand the rationale for accrediting health care organizations and the intended uses for the information provided by different accreditation/certification programs
- Give examples of the impact of accreditation and performance measurement programs on the health care system
- Understand the differences in approach and intent between the nation's three primary accreditors of managed care organizations
- Explain the difference between accreditation and performance measurement
- List at least four of the main elements of a typical health plan accreditation program
- List at least four of the main elements of the most commonly used performance measurement tool

DISCUSSION TOPICS

1. Discuss the main elements of the accreditation process, and the importance of each.
2. Discuss how different entities are accredited; for example, HMOs, PPOs, utilization review organizations, and credentialing verification organizations.
3. Discuss how accreditation information is currently used and how such use might evolve in the future.
4. Discuss the difference between accreditation and certification.
5. Discuss why a health plan may or may not participate in a voluntary accreditation program.
6. Discuss how accreditation differs from state or federal licensure.

■ INTRODUCTION

Since 1991, measurement, transparency, and accountability in accreditation and performance measurement have become enduring features in the managed care landscape. Information systems and key administrative and management functions have been refined or built from the ground up to promote quality improvement and satisfy the demands of external oversight. Driven by mandates from employers, state and federal government, consumers, and a desire by health plans to demonstrate quality objectively as market distinction, a majority of the nation's health maintenance organizations (HMOs) and point-of-service (POS) health plans—and many preferred provider organizations (PPOs)—now participate in some form of accreditation. Plan types are described in Chapter 2.

During this same period, the oversight process has evolved from its initial exclusive focus on HMOs to include accreditation, certification, recognition, and performance measurement programs that cover the full spectrum of affiliated health care organizations—managed behavioral health care organizations (MBHOs), credentials verification organizations (CVOs), PPOs, disease management programs, and provider groups. In addition, oversight programs have become more sophisticated and targeted, and are now able, using current information technology, to focus on specific population subsets and disease states.

Accreditation has grown through state and federal legislation. States have steadily added the requirement or recognition of accreditation (through deeming) in state insurance department and Medicaid programs. The 2010 Patient Protection and Accountable Care Act (ACA) calls for all health plans operating in the new health insurance exchanges to be accredited. In the meantime, employer evaluation programs incorporate accreditation results in the rating of health plans.

Despite the trend, it is notable that accreditation and performance measurement in managed care remain largely voluntary. Federal legislation requires Medicare health plans to submit performance data (see also Chapter 24), and the Office of Personnel Management has added a requirement for fee-for-service plans contracting with PPOs. At the state level, selected states require health plans to be accredited, provide performance measures, or both; sometimes this is a condition of licensure, in other instances it is to gain entry into the state employee market. In place of legislative mandates, however, the market has developed its own mandate. Dozens of the nation's leading corporations will not do business with a health plan that has not earned some form of external accreditation—in particular by the National Committee for Quality Assurance (NCQA). An even larger number of employers require their health plan partners to report on their performance, a prerequisite to assessing value.

Three organizations, each of which approaches its oversight role from a different perspective and each of which specializes in a different sector of the market, have developed managed care oversight programs of note: NCQA, URAC,* and the Accreditation Association for Ambulatory Health Care, also known as the Accreditation Association or AAAHC. Each of these accredits managed care organizations (MCOs) and offers related accreditation or certification programs. These organizations and the various oversight programs they offer are described later in this chapter. In addition, NCQA manages and implements the predominant performance measurement tool that evaluates managed care plans—the Healthcare Effectiveness Data and Information Set (HEDIS®)—used by more than 90% of all health plans and referred to in several other chapters in this book.

The Joint Commission (formerly the Joint Commission on Accreditation of Healthcare Organizations), a major organization for facility-based accreditation and certification, discontinued its network accreditation program for integrated delivery systems, MCOs, MBHOs, and PPOs effective January 1, 2006. However, the Joint Commission provides support services and oversight to organizations accredited under this program through the end of each organization's respective accreditation award period.

There are differences among the accreditation programs offered by each organization. These differences reflect the accreditors' varied histories and perspectives for which their programs were designed. While each of these organizations are discussed in detail later in this chapter, a brief description follows.

For **NCQA**, the major emphasis is on improving the quality of health care through measurement, transparency, and accountability and providing the market—consumers and employers—with information that allows for direct comparisons between the organizations on the basis of quality. NCQA's focus on quality is underscored by the fact that effectiveness of care and member experience performance make up 46% of the accreditation score. Using the objective, evidence-based HEDIS measures, NCQA puts emphasis on those mechanisms that the organization has established for continuous improvement in quality. Historically, NCQA focused on evaluating HMO and POS plans, but its agenda has expanded considerably in recent years and now includes MBHOs, PPOs, CVOs, provider groups, and other health care entities. NCQA believes that by providing the market with this information, it rewards those health plans that are providing excellent care and service, thus giving all health plans a strong incentive to focus on quality.

URAC was formed in 1990 with the backing of a broad range of consumers, employers, regulators, providers, and industry representatives to provide an efficient and effective method for evaluating utilization review (UR) processes. The organization has since branched out beyond UR oversight and into the evaluation of health plans and PPOs, CVOs, disease management programs, health websites, and other health care entities. The stated mission of URAC is "to promote continuous improvement in the quality and efficiency of health care management through processes of accreditation and education." Originally, URAC was incorporated under the name Utilization Review Accreditation Commission. That name was shortened to the acronym URAC in 1996, when URAC began accrediting other types of organizations such as health plans and PPOs. In addition, URAC sometimes uses a second corporate name or "DBA," which is the "American Accreditation HealthCare Commission, Inc."

AAAHC was formed in 1979 to assist ambulatory health care organizations to improve the quality of care provided to patients. AAAHC accredits more than 2,700 health care

---

* "URAC" was once an acronym, but it is now the official name of the organization.

organizations, including endoscopy centers, ambulatory surgery centers, office-based surgery centers, student health centers, and large medical and dental group practices. The AAAHC also surveys and accredits MCOs and independent physician associations (IPAs). The organization's managed care standards are developed with active industry input and include the evaluation of enrollee communications systems; enrollee complaint and grievance resolution systems; utilization management, including enrollee appeal procedures; quality management and improvement; and provider credentialing and recredentialing systems.

■ OVERSIGHT BY TYPE OF ORGANIZATION

Managed care is a loosely defined term that can be applied to a number of different types of health care organizations, including HMOs, POS plans, PPOs, IPAs, UR firms, and other derivative organizational models discussed in Chapter 2. Accreditation and performance measurement have not weighed equally on the various systems of care. Historically, only the most tightly managed delivery systems—HMO and POS plans—have been impelled to seek external accreditation. The reasons for the focus on HMO and POS plans were primarily due to responsible employers and leading health plans seeking market distinction volunteering to come forward. No

doubt, the movement was supported by the extensive media coverage of HMO "horror stories" described in Chapter 1, and the public's general reluctance in the 1990s to accept change in the health care system.

HMOs' participation in accreditation and performance measurement programs over the years has paid an important dividend: improved quality. For example, participating HMO and POS plans went from treating just 62% of heart attack patients with beta-blockers in 1996 to treating 96% by 2004, an improvement that continues to save thousands of lives every year. Furthermore, HEDIS scores for accredited plans outperform their nonaccredited counterparts, evidence that accredited health plans are providing superior care.

Figure 15-1 illustrates accredited and nonaccredited plans' improvement in several clinically important HEDIS measures over a decade.

By contrast, there have been few accreditation mechanisms for PPOs and little information available about what proportion of PPOs have quality-assurance programs or how effective those programs are. Until recently, most PPOs have not pursued external accreditation by any oversight organization because few purchasers have required it. NCQA's PPO and HMO accreditation evaluations are essentially the same, and minor differences in HEDIS reporting will phase out in 2012.

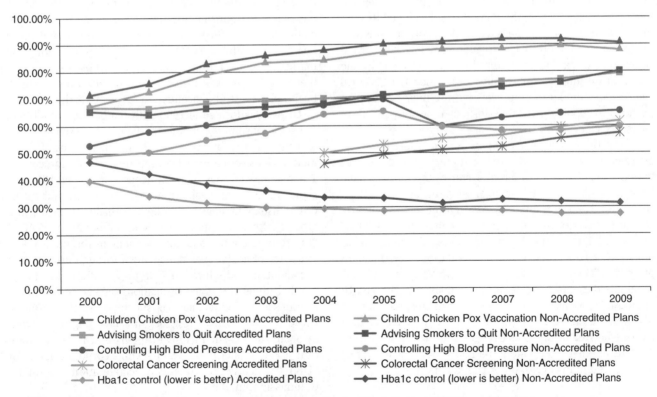

FIGURE 15-1 Changes in Select HEDIS Measures of Accredited and Nonaccredited Plans: National HMO Means, 2000–2009.

Source: National Committee for Quality Assurance, http://www.ncqa.org/.

Accreditation and performance measurement tools have become more sophisticated and versatile to adapt to changes in the health care delivery system. Several important organizations have challenged the health care industry to provide better and safer care and performance measurement, and more are focusing on individual physicians and patients with specific chronic diseases. In fact, a growing number of states are making data about hospitals' quality available online. Consumers—armed with this information, health education materials from the Internet, and health plan report cards from accreditation organizations—are making more informed choices.

As indicated previously, the accreditation programs offered by the three accreditation organizations discussed in this chapter have some similarities, but for the most part are unique, as are the organizations themselves. These differences are reflected in the focus of their review process, in the governance of the organizations, and in the actual accreditation process. A review of each of them follows.

■ NATIONAL COMMITTEE FOR QUALITY ASSURANCE

NCQA is a private, nonprofit organization dedicated to improving health care quality. NCQA accredits and certifies a wide range of health care organizations, including managed care plans (HMOs, POS products, PPOs), MBHOs, clinician organizations, and credentials verification organizations. NCQA implements and manages the evolution of HEDIS, a performance measurement tool used by more than 90% of the nation's health plans. NCQA is committed to providing health care quality information through the Web and the media in order to help consumers, employers, and others make more informed health care choices.

NCQA is governed by a board of directors of independent experts representing key stakeholders in health quality such as employers, consumers, labor representatives, health plans, quality experts, policymakers, and representatives from organized medicine. Copies of NCQA's accreditation standards, HEDIS specifications, application materials, and current accreditation status of health plans can be obtained by contacting NCQA by:

- Writing to NCQA at 1100 13th Street NW, Suite 1000, Washington, D.C. 20005;
- Calling NCQA at (888) 275-7585; or
- On the Internet at www.ncqa.org.

History

NCQA was established in 1979 by the Group Health Association of America and the American Managed Care Review Association, the trade associations at that time for HMOs and IPAs.[*] Original NCQA governance was by the HMO industry. In 1987 HMO industry leaders, believing that NCQA provided a good base for external quality review, studied a broader role for NCQA and began a process to separate it from the trade associations and make it independent, a recognized prerequisite for its credibility. As part of that process, the board was restructured to empower purchasers and other users.

In 1988, the Robert Wood Johnson Foundation funded a series of meetings to explore interest in the purchaser community in NCQA's potential as an independent external review organization. The group of purchaser representatives, benefits managers from Fortune 500 companies who were at the leading edge of external quality assessment, gave a resounding mandate for NCQA to go forward. In late 1989, the foundation awarded NCQA a grant to support its development as an independent entity. As evidence of industry support, the grant required that matching monies be raised from the managed care industry. Industry contributions demonstrated support and NCQA was officially launched in March 1990.

NCQA conducted the first health plan accreditation survey in 1991. Since then, the organization has conducted thousands of reviews of participating health plans and other health care entities. During the 1990s, NCQA took responsibility for the management and further development of what was initially called the Health Plan Employer Data and Information Set before being renamed the Healthcare Effectiveness Data Information Set (HEDIS), and introduced accreditation or certification programs for CVOs, MBHOs, physician organizations, and PPOs.

In 2001, NCQA began accreditation and certification of disease management programs and assumed management of the Diabetes Provider Recognition Program. In 2004, NCQA introduced *Quality Plus*, an initiative that recognizes health plans that take innovative approaches to ensuring that their members receive high-quality care.

In 2010, NCQA also introduced its Multicultural Health Care Distinction program, which evaluates health care plans' cultural competency in delivering health care in order to reduce health care disparities. The Multicultural Health Care Distinction evaluates organizations, such as health plans, wellness, disease management, and MBHOs through use of an evidence-based set of requirements. These standards create a roadmap for improving and refining initiatives.

---

[*]These trade associations eventually merged to become the American Association of Health Plans (AAHP), which then later merged with the Health Insurance Association of America (HIAA) to become America's Health Insurance Plans (AHIP). AHIP is the trade association that now represents the managed care and health insurance industries in the United States.

In the latter part of 2011, NCQA launched its Accountable Care Organization Accreditation. Accountable care organizations (ACOs; see Chapter 2) are provider-based organizations that take responsibility for meeting the health care needs of a defined population with the goal of simultaneously improving health, improving patient experience, and reducing per capita costs.

Areas of Health Plan Review

The content of NCQA's accreditation programs is determined by NCQA's Standards Committee, a 15- to 20-member group that represents employers, consumers, health plans, and policymakers. NCQA also actively solicits input on all its programs through public review and comment periods.

A health plan's overall accreditation status is based on its performance in three areas: clinical performance using HEDIS measures, member satisfaction using the Consumer Assessment of Health Providers and Systems (CAHPS®) survey, and a review of key structures and processes using NCQA Standards and Guidelines. HEDIS and CAHPS together account for about 45% of a health plan's accreditation results, with performance against standards accounting for the remainder. Using these methods, NCQA evaluates and reports to the public the following:

- **Access and service:** NCQA evaluates how well a health plan provides its members with access to needed care and with good customer service.
- **Qualified providers:** NCQA evaluates how a health plan ensures that each provider is licensed and appropriately trained to practice, and that members are satisfied with their doctors.
- **Staying healthy:** NCQA evaluates health plan activities that help people maintain good health and avoid illness.
- **Getting better:** NCQA evaluates health plan activities that help people recover from illness.
- **Living with illness:** NCQA evaluates health plan activities that help people manage chronic illness.

Compliance with NCQA Standards and Guidelines

Of a health plan's accreditation results, 54.14% are based on compliance with NCQA's Standards and Guidelines, including the scope and function of key operations:

- Quality improvement
- Utilization management
- Credentialing and network development
- Members' rights and responsibilities
- Member connections

Quality Improvement

The first and most rigorous area of NCQA review is a health plan's own internal quality control systems (see Chapter 14).

To meet NCQA standards, an organization must have a well-organized, comprehensive quality improvement (QI) program accountable to the governing body of the organization. The QI program must include a written description of the QI program, which is updated annually and overseen by a QI committee that meets regularly.

The QI program's scope must be comprehensive, covering the full spectrum of services included in the organization's benefit design. The QI program must focus on important aspects of care and services and address clinical issues with major impact on the health status of the enrolled population. These should include:

- Accessibility of health care services,
- Assistance for people with chronic health conditions and complex conditions,
- Continuity and coordination of care, and
- Coordination between medical and behavioral health care.
- Documentation of clinical quality improvement

To ensure practitioner participation in QI activities, contracts with physicians and other health care providers must be explicit about the requirement to cooperate with the health plan's QI program. In addition, the health plan must ensure access to care by creating a provider network that considers the needs of its members. The health plan must also develop and distribute clinical practice guidelines and policies for medical record documentation to its provider network.

If the health plan delegates QI activities to another organization, it must work with the delegated party to develop a mutually agreed-upon document that outlines responsibilities, delegated activities, and monitoring processes.

Most important, a health plan must document program effectiveness in improving its quality of care and service. Quality improvement can also be documented comparing successive years' HEDIS results in the areas where the health plan has chosen to focus (immunization rates, eye exams for diabetics, etc.).

NCQA establishes compliance with its standards through an onsite review and electronic surveys of a health plan's QI program, quality improvement studies, projects and monitoring activities, QI committee and governing body minutes, interviews with key staff, issue tracking, and documented evidence of quality improvement.

Processes for Reviewing and Authorizing Medical Care

Utilization management (UM; see Chapter 7), one of the foundations of effective managed care, is an important determinant of both the cost and quality of an MCO. To earn NCQA accreditation, a health plan must meet rigorous UM standards designed to ensure that this key function promotes good health care rather than acting as an arbitrary barrier to accessing appropriate services.

NCQA requires that review decisions be made by qualified medical professionals and that the organization have a written description of its program for managing care, which includes clearly documented criteria and procedures for approving and denying care. The UM plan must also address triage and referral for behavioral health care, procedures for drug coverage, access to emergency services without precertification, and the evaluation and coverage of new technology.

NCQA UM standards specify that qualified health professionals oversee all review decisions and that an appropriate practitioner reviews any denial of care based on medical necessity. These standards ensure that if a medical specialist appeals a decision to deny a requested treatment, another similarly trained practitioner will rule on the appeal. This issue is especially critical in appeals dealing with complex medical questions where simply referring to preexisting medical guidelines may not adequately account for a specific patient's situation.

Health plans must have written policies and procedures for the resolution of member UM appeals. To make sure that UM decisions and appeals are processed in a timely manner, NCQA sets explicit "turnaround time" requirements that specify the maximum allowable time between appeal and determination by the health plan.

While consumers and others are typically most concerned about overaggressive UM, insufficient UM can be problematic as well, leading to unnecessary care and expense. Thus, NCQA requires that a health plan's UM system monitor for over- as well as underutilization.

Compliance with UM standards is determined during a thorough onsite review and electronic surveys of a health plan's written UM program description and related policies and procedures, review determinations, appeals process and determinations, interviews with key staff, tracking of issues uncovered by the UM system, and documented evidence of appropriate oversight.

Delegation

Delegation occurs when the organization gives another entity the authority to carry out a function that it would otherwise perform to meet requirements within NCQA standards. This authority includes the right to decide what to do and how to do it, within the parameters agreed on by the organization and the other entity. When delegation exists, NCQA requires the presence of a mutual agreement between the delegating organization and its delegate that is performing specific functions related to NCQA standards. Although the organization does not directly perform delegated functions, it must oversee them to ensure that the delegate is performing the functions properly. The organization may reclaim the right to carry out its delegated functions at any time.

Subdelegation occurs when the organization's delegate gives a third entity the authority to carry out a delegated function. Subdelegation is acceptable if either the delegate or the organization oversees the work performed by the subdelegate to ensure that it meets NCQA standards. If the delegate oversees the subdelegate, it must report to the organization regarding the subdelegate's performance. NCQA holds the organization ultimately accountable for all NCQA-related activities performed by both the delegate and subdelegate on the organization's behalf.

Quality of Provider Network

To ensure the quality of the health plan's provider network, NCQA's accreditation process includes a thorough review of an organization's credentialing system (see Chapter 4). In addition to a credentialing process for primary care physicians and medical specialists, the health plan must also confirm that hospitals, home health care agencies, skilled nursing facilities, nursing homes, and behavioral health facilities in its network are in good standing with state and federal agencies and accrediting organizations.

NCQA requires that health plans have a process to identify which types of practitioners must be credentialed, clearly defined and documented procedures for assessing its practitioners' qualifications and practice history, and policies that define practitioner rights to review and correct credentialing information.

Prior to allowing network participation, health plans must verify practitioners' credentials, including a valid license to practice medicine, education and training, malpractice history, and work history. Before making a decision on a practitioner's qualifications, the health plan must receive and review information from third parties, such as information about any disciplinary actions. In addition, the health plan must verify through an onsite visit that primary care practitioners, obstetricians/gynecologists, and high-volume behavioral health care practitioners' offices meet the organization's standards.

An important part of ensuring delivery system integrity is periodic recertification of providers and NCQA requires that the health plan reevaluate practitioners' qualifications every 36 months. Before reevaluating a practitioner's qualifications, the health plan must receive information from third parties, such as information about disciplinary actions. Between recredentialing cycles, the organization must monitor practitioner member complaints and satisfaction and information from quality improvement activities. NCQA standards require the health plan to monitor sanctions, complaints, and quality issues on a regular basis and take appropriate action when issues are identified.

If the health plan delegates to a third party decisions on evaluating or reevaluating a provider's qualifications, the decision-making process—including the responsibilities of the plan and delegated party—must be clearly documented and the plan must evaluate and approve the delegated party's credentialing process on a regular basis. In 1995 NCQA released standards to certify CVOs, thus eliminating the need for health plans to conduct an annual review of those organizations. This program is described in more detail later in this chapter as well as in Chapter 4.

Compliance with credentialing standards is ascertained by reviewing an organization's credentialing policies and procedures, sampling individual provider files, conducting interviews with relevant staff, reviewing credentialing committee minutes, and tracking issues identified through the complaint system or quality improvement findings.

Member Rights and Responsibilities

To meet NCQA standards, a health plan must have written policies that state its commitment to treating members in a manner that respects their rights as well as delineate the plan's expectations of members' responsibilities. These policies must be distributed to members and participating practitioners.

NCQA requires a health plan to have a system for the timely resolution of member complaints and appeals, to aggregate and analyze complaint appeal data, and to use the information for quality improvement. This activity, often undertaken by the health plan's member services function, is also discussed in Chapter 20.

NCQA standards require written communication to members of certain types of information about how the health plan works, including benefits and charges for which members are responsible, as well as co-payments; how to obtain care; how to file a complaint or appeal; and how to choose a new provider when members' practitioners leave the plan's network.

The standards require that member information be written in readable prose and be available in the languages of the major population groups served. Health plans must also have mechanisms ensuring confidentiality and take steps to protect the privacy of members' information and records.

In 2008, NCQA introduced Physician and Hospital Quality Certification standards, which replaced the Distinction program. The revised standards represent a more comprehensive review of organizations' programs to measure and report quality and cost of care from physicians and hospitals. The standards also reflect changes in physician measurement since 2006. As a result, the updated program is Certification instead of Distinction.

A health plan's marketing materials must describe its procedures for approving or denying coverage; covered benefits, including pharmacy benefits; noncovered services; availability of practitioners and providers; and any applicable restrictions. In addition, the health plan must monitor new members' understanding of its procedures and update its marketing materials accordingly.

Compliance with member rights and responsibility standards is determined by reviewing an organization's written policies and procedures and marketing materials, conducting interviews with relevant staff, and tracking issues identified through the complaint and appeals system.

NCQA Member Connections standards are designed to measure how well health plans connect their members with important information such as their health status, the resources provided by their health plan, their care options, and the costs of different services and prescription drugs. Member Connections standards have been included in the NCQA HMO and PPO Accreditation standards since 2007 and Health Plan Accreditation since 2008. Some plans voluntarily achieved distinction in this area prior to its inclusion in accreditation.

HEDIS

As noted earlier, HEDIS is a performance measurement tool used by more than 90% of the nation's MCOs. It is a robust set of standardized measures that specifies how health plans collect, audit, and report on their performance in important areas such as delivery of preventive health services, member satisfaction with care, utilization of services, and treatment efficacy for various illnesses. Measures are reviewed annually, updated, revised, and even retired through a broad-based process that includes public comment on each proposed new measure or change.

By specifying not only what to measure but also how to measure it, HEDIS allows true "apples-to-apples" comparisons between health plans. HEDIS allows health plans to manage and improve quality and purchasers of health care to make informed choices. Every year, dozens of national news magazines, newspapers, employers, and others use HEDIS data to generate health plan "report cards" during open enrollment. All HEDIS data are independently audited and verified.

HEDIS consists of more than 70 measures (not including the CAHPS survey, which includes dozens of individual questions) that fall into eight broad categories or domains:

- Effectiveness of Care,
- Access/Availability of Care,
- Satisfaction with the Experience,
- Use of Services,
- Cost of Care,
- Health Plan Descriptive Information,
- Health Plan Stability, and
- Informed Health Care Choices.

The full 2011 HEDIS measure set is listed in **Table 15-1**.

Effectiveness of Care: Measures in this domain provide information about clinical care quality provided by the organization. The measures consider how well the organization incorporates widely accepted preventive practices and recommended screening for common diseases. This domain has been expanded to include some overuse and patient safety measures listed.

TABLE 15-1	2011 HEDIS® Measures

Effectiveness of care measures
(listed separately)

Prevention and screening

- Adult BMI assessment
- Weight assessment and counseling for nutrition and physical activity for children/adolescents
- Childhood immunization status
- Immunizations for adolescents
- Lead screening in children
- Breast cancer screening
- Cervical cancer screening
- Colorectal cancer screening
- Chlamydia screening in women
- Glaucoma screening in older adults
- Care for older adults

Respiratory conditions

- Appropriate testing for children with pharyngitis
- Appropriate treatment for children with upper respiratory infection
- Avoidance of antibiotic treatment in adults with acute bronchitis
- Use of spirometry testing in the assessment and diagnosis of COPD
- Pharmacotherapy management of COPD exacerbation
- Use of appropriate medications for people with asthma

Cardiovascular conditions

- Cholesterol management for patients with cardiovascular conditions
- Controlling high blood pressure
- Persistence of beta-blocker treatment after a heart attack

Diabetes

- Comprehensive diabetes care

Musculoskeletal conditions

- Disease-modifying antirheumatic drug therapy for rheumatoid arthritis
- Osteoporosis management in women who had a fracture
- Use of imaging studies for low back pain

Behavioral health care

- Antidepressant medication management
- Follow-up care for children prescribed with ADHA medication
- Follow-up after hospitalization for mental illness

Access/availability of care measures

- Adults' access to preventive/ambulatory health services
- Children and adolescents' access to primary care practitioners
- Annual dental visit
- Initiation and engagement of alcohol and other drug dependence treatment
- Prenatal and postpartum care
- Call abandonment
- Call answer timeliness

Satisfaction with the experience of care measures

- CAHPS Health Plan Survey 4.0h, Adult Version
- CAHPS Health Plan Survey 4.0h, Child Version
- Children with chronic conditions

Use of services measures

- Frequency of ongoing prenatal care
- Well-child visits in the first 15 months of life
- Well-child visits in the third, fourth, fifth, and sixth years of life
- Adolescent well-care visits
- Frequency of selected procedures

- Ambulatory care
- Inpatient utilization—general hospital/acute care
- Identification of alcohol and other drug services
- Mental health utilization
- Antibiotic utilization
- Plan all-cause readmissions *(new measure)*

Cost of care measures

- Relative resource use for people with diabetes
- Relative resource use for people with asthma
- Relative resource use for people with acute low back pain
- Relative resource use for people with cardiovascular conditions
- Relative resource use for people with uncomplicated hypertension
- Relative resource use for people with COPD

Health plan descriptive information measures

- Board certification
- Enrollment by product line
- Enrollment by state
- Language diversity of membership
- Race/ethnicity diversity of membership
- Weeks of pregnancy at time of enrollment

Health plan stability measure

- Total membership

Informed Health Care Choices Measure

- *Currently there are no measures in this domain.*

Access/Availability of Care: Measures in this category assess whether care is available to those who need it. Among others, important measures in this category include adults' access to preventive health care, children and adolescents' access to primary care, and women's access to prenatal and postpartum care.

Cost of Care: These measures provide information about how efficiently and effectively the organization uses available health services and available resources. Because potentially preventable hospital readmissions contributes to waste, overtreatment, and high cost, NCQA introduced a measure of hospital readmissions in 2010. Relative

| TABLE 15-2 | HEDIS Effectiveness of Care Measures for Accreditation | | | | | |

Measure	Commercial		Medicare		Medicaid	
	HMO/POS	PPO	HMO/POS	PPO	HMO/POS	PPO
Annual monitoring for patients on persistent medications (total rate)			√	√	HMO/POS	
Antidepressant medication management (both rates)	√	√	√	√	√	√
Appropriate testing for children with pharyngitis	√	√			√	√
Appropriate treatment for children with upper respiratory infection	√	√			√	√
Avoidance of antibiotic treatment in adults with acute bronchitis	√	√			√	√
Breast cancer screening	√	√	√	√	√	√
Cervical cancer screening	√	√			√	√
Childhood immunization status (combination 2)	√				√	
Chlamydia screening in women (total rate)	√	√			√	√
Cholesterol management for patients with cardiovascular conditions (LDL-C screening only)	√	√	√	√	√	√
Colorectal cancer screening	√	√	√	√		
Comprehensive diabetes care (eye exam, LDL-C screening, HbA1c testing, medical attention for nephropathy)	√	√	√	√	√	√
Comprehensive diabetes care	√	√	√	√	√	√
HbA1c poor control (> 9.0%)						
Controlling high blood pressure	√	√	√	√	√	√
Flu shots for adults (ages 50–64)	√	√				
Flu shots for older adults			√	√		
Follow-up after hospitalization for mental illness (7-day rate only)	√	√	√	√	√	√
Follow-up for children prescribed with ADHD medication (both rates)						
Glaucoma screening in older adults			√	√		
Medical assistance with smoking and tobacco use cessation (advising smokers and tobacco users to quit only)	√	√	√	√	√	√
Osteoporosis management in women who had a fracture			√	√		
Persistence of beta-blocker treatment after a heart attack	√	√	√	√		
Pneumonia vaccination status for older adults			√	√		
Prenatal and postpartum care (both rates)	√	√			√	√
Use of appropriate medications for people with asthma (total rate)	√	√			√	√
Use of high-risk medications in the elderly (both rates)			√	√		
Use of imaging studies for low back pain	√	√			√	√
Use of spirometry testing in the assessment and diagnosis of COPD	√	√	√	√	√	√

Source: NCQA.

resource use (RRU) measures indicate how intensively health plans use health care resources (such as physician visits and hospital stays), compared with other plans in the same region, serving similar members. Given the definition of value as the intersection of health plans' spending (resource use) and quality results, RRU reveals the value that competing plans offer. RRU analysis shows that more care is not always linked to better results, confirming that the saying "you get what you pay for" does not apply to health care.

Health Plan Descriptive Information: Measures in this domain provide information about the organization's staff (how many physicians leave the organization) and stability (including years in business).

Health Plan Stability: These measures—practitioner turnover, years in business, and total membership—provide information about the soundness and dependability of a health plan. They consider the organization's structure and type and number of participating physicians.

Informed Health Care Choices: There are currently no measures in this domain.

Satisfaction with the Experience of Care: These measures provide information on members' experiences with their health care organization and give a general indication of how well the organization meets their expectations.

Use of Services: These measures provide information about how the organization manages and expends resources. Measures in this category permit members and other users to understand patterns of service utilization across different health plans.

Significantly, HEDIS is applicable to public and private sector plans. The same measurement standards are applied to care provided to Medicaid beneficiaries, commercial health plan enrollees, and Medicare populations opting for managed care plans. This not only increases the efficiency of measurement but also allows for performance comparisons across populations and health plan types.

Measures included in HEDIS typically undergo exhaustive testing and review prior to inclusion and must possess three key attributes:

1. *Relevance:* Measures must address health issues of significant concern, and performance on measures should be at least partially controllable by the health plan. Also, information produced by a given measure should be useful to consumers and employers.
2. *Scientific soundness:* Measures must focus on processes of care that are evidence-based. They must generate reproducible, valid, and accurate results. Measures also must be sensitive enough to detect meaningful differences in performance between health plans.
3. *Feasibility:* It should be possible to collect the data required for a measure at a reasonable cost and effort.

As part of the NCQA accreditation process, health plans are required to report on their performance on HEDIS measures, including a subset from the effectiveness of care category and a subset derived from the CAHPS Health Plan surveys. To ensure that quality and performance are maintained between onsite surveys (which occur at least every 36 months), NCQA requires health plans to submit independently audited HEDIS results annually. Should these results, or other factors such as regulatory action, suggest a lapse in quality, NCQA may elect to resurvey the health plan sooner. Accreditation status can change as well.

CAHPS Health Plan Survey

Member satisfaction surveys have long been a popular way to assess health plan performance, and such a survey has been featured in HEDIS since 1996. Previously, information about member satisfaction was gathered using a variety of surveys and instruments developed by the health plans for use with their enrolled population. Because no standardized survey was in broad use, what little member satisfaction data were available could not be used to compare plans since the survey instruments and survey methodology varied from plan to plan.

At the insistence of various constituencies—including health plans, which were often required by their clients to field dozens of different satisfaction surveys annually—satisfaction survey data are now collected in a more rational, efficient manner using a standard tool, the CAHPS Health Plan Survey. This survey was jointly developed by NCQA and the federal Agency for Health Research and Quality (AHRQ).

CAHPS Health Plan surveys are similar to patient satisfaction surveys and include ratings of providers and health plans. But they go beyond this type of question by asking health plan members to report on their experiences with health care services. Reports about care are regarded as more specific, actionable, understandable, and objective than general ratings alone.

Since 1999, NCQA has required CAHPS Health Plan survey results from health plans seeking accreditation and/or submitting data as part of HEDIS. CAHPS, like HEDIS, is designed to be applicable to all health plans regardless of the population they serve: Medicare, Medicaid, or commercial. CAHPS consists of several surveys: one for the adult population, another designed to assess parents' impressions of their children's health care, and a third for Medicare and Medicaid populations. To ensure that CAHPS data are collected using only the approved, standardized methodology, health plans are required to contract with an NCQA-certified third-party vendor to administer the survey. The overarching goal of the CAHPS survey is to effectively and efficiently obtain standardized information about members' experiences with their health care organization.

While each CAHPS Health Plan survey consists of dozens of questions, the questions are grouped in "composites" to make comparisons between plans easier. The composites provide information on plan performance in the following areas:

- Getting needed care,
- Getting care quickly,
- How well doctors communicate,
- Courteous and helpful office staff,
- Customer service,
- Claims processing, and
- Overall rating of health plan.

HEDIS and CAHPS in Accreditation

HEDIS and CAHPS data are an integral part of NCQA Accreditation. As noted earlier, together these data comprise 45% of the total Accreditation score. This reflects an emphasis on quality performance and customer (member) satisfaction.

Today's competitive health care environment has generated an unprecedented demand for standardized information regarding consumer experiences with health plans. The HEDIS 2011 CAHPS Health Plan Survey reflects state-of-the-art consumer research that considers:

- Key components of health care quality
- Eliciting a broad range of consumer experience with these components
- Reporting information to the public in a meaningful way

NCQA publicly reports HEDIS and CAHPS scores on its website, in the annual NCQA Health Insurance Plan Rankings and the annual State of Health Care Quality report.

The HEDIS Compliance Audit™

An integral part of HEDIS assessment is validating data that organizations collect and report. Despite the clear specifications defined in HEDIS, data collection and calculation methods employed by organizations may vary, and other errors may taint the results, diminishing the usefulness of HEDIS data for comparison. NCQA's analysis of HEDIS data collected as part of a national report card and experience with numerous state and local projects confirm that these are justifiable concerns.

NCQA developed a precise, standardized methodology for verifying the integrity of HEDIS collection and calculation processes: the HEDIS Compliance Audit™. The audit ensures that HEDIS specifications are met and results are consistent and comparable. Audits by NCQA-authorized personnel help purchasers make more reliable "apples-to-apples" comparisons between organizations.

The NCQA HEDIS Compliance Audit indicates whether an organization has adequate and sound capabilities for processing medical, member, and provider information as a foundation for accurate and automated performance measurement, including HEDIS reporting. The audit standards were designed to complement other verification activities that already occur within organizations. As a result, the standards do not address information audited by other organizations (e.g., financial/accounting firms or state regulatory agencies), or information based on narrative descriptions of programs that are addressed in the NCQA Accreditation Standards, which are reviewed during accreditation survey visits.

The certified auditor evaluates a core set of measures across all applicable domains in HEDIS, and then extrapolates the findings from the core set to all measures reported by the organization. If problems areas are identified, the certified auditor may expand the core set measures. Following a completion of an audit, the organization can use NCQA's audit seal to market itself as having undergone an NCQA HEDIS Compliance Audit.

Certification of individual auditors and licensing of qualified organizations helps to ensure that standard auditing methodologies are used during all NCQA HEDIS Compliance Audits. NCQA has developed a qualifying exam with a division of the Educational Testing Service that individuals must pass before being designated NCQA-Certified HEDIS Compliance Auditors. The exam consists, in part, of an audit of a hypothetical organization's HEDIS processes against NCQA's standards. In order to maintain certification, auditors must participate in two audits per year, obtain 12 hours of preapproved continuing education credits, and attend the Auditor Update Conference annually. Recertification is required every 2 years.

NCQA also licenses organizations to conduct HEDIS Compliance Audits. Individuals taking the Certification Exam must be employed by or contract with an NCQA-Licensed Organization. NCQA also monitors the quality of an auditor's work through ongoing assessments of audit performances by individual auditors and licensed organizations.

A list of the licensed organizations and certified auditors can be found on NCQA's website at www.ncqa.org.

Physician and Hospital Quality Certification

NCQA's Physician and Hospital Quality (PHQ) Certification program evaluates how well health plans measure and report the quality and cost of physician and hospital services. PHQ Certification represents an impartial third-party certification of provider measurement programs. It also provides assurance that such efforts use valid, transparent methodologies and measure on quality—not cost alone. This program is open to any organization conducting functions evaluated by the standards, whether a health plan, a measurement collaborative, a provider network, or an information provider such as a website.

More than 60 health plans have achieved Distinction in Physician and Hospital Quality through the 2006 version of the program. In 2008, NCQA released a PHQ Certification program reflecting changes in the provider measurement field and demand from purchasers and regulators. Four key principles serve as the foundation of PHQ Certification:

1. **Standardization and sound methodology:** This allows results to be compared across organizations.
2. **Transparency:** Organizations should offer physicians the opportunity to provide input on measurement programs. Organizations should also provide clear, understandable information about how the results will be used.

3. **Collaboration:** Where possible, organizations should pool their data on standardized measures to produce results with greater statistical reliability.
4. **Action on quality and cost:** Organizations should not sacrifice quality for cost reduction. Organizations must not use results of cost measurement alone.

NCQA Accreditation Review Process

NCQA uses an Internet-based survey tool for health plan accreditation. The Interactive Survey System (ISS) allows an organization to perform a readiness evaluation at its own pace before submitting data to NCQA. A health plan can assess its programs and operations and estimate its performance against NCQA standards.

The NCQA review process begins with the submission of the survey tool and ends with an onsite survey. When a health plan applies for NCQA accreditation review, a date is set for the electronic submission of the survey tool and a subsequent onsite survey. The review process is separated into two stages:

- The offsite review of a health plan's electronically submitted materials and readiness evaluation.
- The onsite survey of an organization's credentialing, denial, and appeal files, as well as a review of the organization's delegation oversight.

The onsite survey occurs approximately 8 weeks after the submission of the survey tool. This part of the review process, which typically takes 2 days, consists of a brief opening/introduction, a review of the elements indicated for onsite review, completion of the review of previously submitted documentation, an interview with key personnel, and a closing conference.

During the onsite visit, members of the survey team complete an extensive review of health plan documentation, such as minutes of quality improvement committee and board meetings; policies and procedures relating to various areas of the standards; provider contracts; quality improvement studies, reports, and case files; utilization management review criteria, reports, and files; credentialing files; complaint and grievance files; and member satisfaction and disenrollment surveys.

The survey team also interviews the health plan's chief executive officer; medical director; directors of quality improvement, utilization management, provider relations, and member services; members of the quality improvement committee; a member of the board of directors; and participating physicians.

The survey team checks for evidence of compliance with each of the NCQA standards and presents a summary of its findings at the end of the site visit. A member of the review team prepares a report that is submitted to NCQA. An independent oversight committee analyzes the teams' findings and the organization's clinical performance and then assigns an overall accreditation outcome.

Reviewers

NCQA survey teams typically consist of one or two administrative reviewers and two or three physician reviewers. Administrative reviewers are nonphysician clinicians or quality management experts with extensive experience in quality improvement in MCOs. Physician reviewers are medical directors, associate medical directors, or directors of quality management from noncompeting health plans.

Accreditation Decisions and Information

Following an onsite survey, NCQA assigns the health plan one of five possible accreditation levels based on the plan's performance:

- **Excellent.** NCQA's highest accreditation outcome is granted only to those plans that demonstrate levels of service and clinical quality that meet or exceed NCQA's rigorous requirements for consumer protection and quality improvement. Plans earning this accreditation level must also achieve HEDIS results that are in the highest range of national or regional performance.
- **Commendable.** This accreditation outcome is awarded to plans that demonstrate levels of service and clinical quality that meet or exceed NCQA's rigorous requirements for consumer protection and quality improvement.
- **Accredited.** Health plans that earn the Accredited outcome must meet most of NCQA's basic requirements for consumer protection and quality improvement.
- **Provisional.** Provisional accreditation indicates that a health plan's service and clinical quality meet some, but not all, of NCQA's basic requirements for consumer protection and quality improvement.
- **Denied.** Denied is an indication that a health plan did not meet NCQA's requirements during its review.

Accreditation of New Health Plans

NCQA maintains an accreditation program designed for MCOs that otherwise would not be eligible to participate in NCQA accreditation: the Accreditation of New Health Plans Program. The program is designed especially for organizations and health plans less than 3 years old, using a core set of standards derived from the *Standards for the Accreditation of Managed Care Organizations (MCOs)*, making the program distinct and different from NCQA's Accreditation of MCO Program. This program for new health plans (NHPs) is fundamentally similar to NCQA's regular MCO accreditation program, except for three key differences:

- The NHP program contains no requirement that a plan demonstrate improvement over time (an unrealistic expectation given the short history of the plan),

- Results are on a pass-fail basis (to distinguish it from NCQA's main MCO accreditation program), and
- NHPs are not required to submit HEDIS or CAHPS data.

NHP Accreditation evaluates how well a plan that has been in operation less than 3 years manages its clinical and administrative systems in order to continuously improve health care for its members. The accreditation survey results are essentially on a pass-fail basis with plans receiving either NHP Accreditation or a Denial. Plans may apply for new health plan accreditation only once, and the accreditation period for plans that receive a "pass" designation is 3 years.

NCQA's standards for quality NHPs fall into six categories:

1. **Quality Management and Improvement:** The NHP must have the appropriate organizational structures and processes in place to monitor and improve the quality of care and service provided to its members and must fully examine the quality of care given to its members.
2. **Credentialing and Recredentialing:** The NHP must meet the specific NCQA requirements for investigating the training and experience of all practitioners in its network and assess practitioner qualifications and practice history. The NHP must identify which types of practitioners must be credentialed and have policies in place that define practitioner rights to review and correct credentialing information.
3. **Members' Rights and Responsibilities:** The NHP must clearly inform members about how to access health services, how to choose a practitioner or change practitioners, and how to make a complaint.
4. **Preventive Health Services:** The NHP must encourage members to use its preventive health programs and encourage its practitioners to deliver preventive services for its covered population.
5. **Utilization Management:** The NHP must use a reasonable and consistent process when deciding what health services are appropriate for individuals' needs, and when the NHP denies payment for services, it must respond appropriately to member and practitioner appeals.
6. **Medicaid Benefits and Services:** The NHP must provide Medicaid benefits that include direct access to women's health services, provide second opinion from in-network provider and cover out-of-network services when the NHP cannot provide services in a timely fashion.

Other NCQA Accreditation Programs

The managed health care era has given rise to a diverse array of managed systems of care beyond HMOs and POS plans—physician-hospital organizations, MBHOs, and many others—about which quality information historically had been scarce. To help address the need for information about these organizations and to facilitate NCQA's core MCO accreditation program by reducing the oversight burden for health plans, NCQA has implemented a number of other accreditation and certification programs. Taken together, these programs point to one of the trends for the future of quality oversight: targeted accreditation and certification programs suited to particular types of health care delivery systems.

Disease Management Accreditation and Certification

NCQA offers a flexible evaluation program, including Accreditation for organizations that offer comprehensive disease management (DM) programs with services to patients, practitioners, or both; and Certification for organizations that provide specific DM functions. Because they evaluate functions rather than specific types of organizations, NCQA's DM accreditation and certification programs are available to a wide variety of organizations, including DM organizations, health plans (HMOs and PPOs), pharmaceutical companies, provider organizations, pharmacy benefit management companies, medical groups, and nurse call centers.

NCQA offers four DM evaluation options.

Accreditation Options:

1. Patient- and practitioner-oriented accreditation—comprehensive accreditation that includes all standards and is for organizations that work with both patients and practitioners. It conveys the most automatic credit to health plans and MBHOs that contract with an accredited DM program.
2. Patient-oriented accreditation—comprehensive patient-focused accreditation that includes all standards that address all interventions toward patients and do not have regular contact with practitioners.

Certification Options:

3. Program design certification—specialized certification for organizations that develop the content for DM programs according to clinical guidelines. It does not include implementation.
4. Systems certification—specialized certification for organizations for the design of clinical information systems to support DM. It does not include implementation.

Disease Management Standards

NCQA DM standards address seven key areas that an organization is required to address for the implementation of disease management:

- **Patient services** standards include the provision of program information, patient participation, interventions, feedback to the patient, encouraging patient and practitioner communication, and patients' rights and responsibilities.

- **Practitioner services** standards include the provision of program information, practitioners' rights, and decision-support services such as interventions to the practitioner and feedback.
- **Measurement and quality improvement** addresses the selection, methodology, analysis, reporting, and action related to the organization's clinical quality measures, patient and practitioner feedback, and the evaluation of QI initiatives.
- **Program operations** of DM include access and service issues, marketing and advertising, staff training, qualifications, and credentialing.
- **Performance measurement** assesses its performance against a standardized, evidence-based set of measures. Organizations that meet this standard receive the designation of *Accredited with Performance Reporting*.
- **Evidence-based measurement** addresses whether the organization uses the best clinical evidence to develop program content.
- **Care coordination** standards include information about patients' care plans that are accessible to patients and practitioners.

Managed Behavioral Healthcare Organization Accreditation

NCQA's MBHO accreditation program was launched in 1996 to provide employers and the more than 140 million Americans enrolled in MBHOs with information about the quality of those organizations. Since then, NCQA's health plan and MBHO accreditation programs have become closely aligned, with nearly identical sets of standards applying to both types of organizations. Both accreditation programs seek to promote access to behavioral health care and coordination between medical and behavioral health professionals, a prerequisite to good quality care.

The NCQA MBHO standards were developed by the consensus of a task force representing employers, public purchasers, consumers, MCOs, MBHOs, and mental health and substance abuse experts. The standards emphasize the importance of access to care and services, coordination of behavioral health services with medical care, and preservation of patient confidentiality.

The MBHO review process consists of both on- and off-site evaluations conducted by teams of behavioral health clinicians (which may include psychologists, psychiatrists, and/or clinical social workers) and managed care experts. A national oversight committee analyzes the team's findings and assigns an accreditation level based on the MBHO's compliance with NCQA's standards.

The standards against which NCQA measures MBHOs are organized into five categories:

1. **Quality Management and Improvement:** The MBHO has systems in place to ensure that care and service improve over time.
2. **Utilization Management:** The MBHO is required to make decisions about approving or denying care in a fair, informed, and timely manner with a staff of qualified decision makers.
3. **Credentialing and Recredentialing:** NCQA reviews how thoroughly the MBHO checks the credentials of its providers.
4. **Members' Rights and Responsibilities:** The MBHO must do a good job of communicating with members and there needs to be evidence that member handbooks and customer service staff are accessible, and that members understand their rights and how the system works.
5. **Preventive Health Programs:** The organization is required to take proactive steps to keep members healthy.

Based on their compliance with NCQA's requirements, MBHOs can earn the following NCQA Accreditation status levels:

- **Full Accreditation** is granted for a period of 3 years to MBHOs that have excellent programs for continuous quality improvement and meet NCQA's standards.
- **One-Year Accreditation** is granted to MBHOs that have well-established quality improvement programs and meet most NCQA standards. NCQA provides these MBHOs with a specific list of recommendations, and reviews the MBHOs again after 1 year to determine if they have progressed enough to merit Full Accreditation.
- **Provisional Accreditation** is granted for 1 year to MBHOs that have adequate quality improvement programs and meet some of NCQA standards.
- **Denial of Accreditation** is given to MBHOs when NCQA's assessment reveals serious flaws in systems for consumer protection and quality improvement.

Other NCQA Certification Programs

NCQA also has several other certification programs, which are briefly described here.

Credentials Verification Organization (CVO) Certification Program

NCQA's CVO Certification is a quality assessment program designed to assist MCOs in evaluating CVOs and other organizations that verify the credentials of physicians (see Chapter 4). Certified CVOs have provided the protections required by NCQA's standards, that they have developed a sound management structure, and that they monitor, and are continually improving, the quality of the services they deliver.

The NCQA CVO survey is a rigorous on- and offsite evaluation conducted by a survey team that includes at least one certification surveyor and one administrative surveyor. A review oversight committee (ROC) of physicians analyzes the team's findings and assigns a certification status based on the CVO's performance against core standards and the requirements within applicable certification options.

The CVO standards were developed and are updated with the assistance of representatives from the credentials verification industry, as well as input from MCOs. Certified CVOs must meet these standards, as well as all applicable Credentialing Standards from NCQA's Standards for the Accreditation of Managed Care Organizations.

For MCOs seeking to be accredited by NCQA, CVO Certification takes the place of health plan review of a CVO's structure and performance in verifying provider credentials. Accordingly, health plans that contract for credentials verification with an organization that has been certified by NCQA are exempt from some due-diligence oversight requirements specified in NCQA Credentialing Standards.

There are two major components to the CVO Certification Survey:

1. Determination of compliance with the CVO Standards, which includes a review of an organization's:
   - Policies and procedures for credentials verification
   - Mechanisms for maintaining credentials data integrity and confidentiality
   - Capabilities for ongoing data collection
   - Internal quality assurance processes
   - Physician application components
   - Reporting of physician disciplinary actions
2. An audit of completed credentials files to determine compliance with NCQA's MCO Credentialing Standards.

Certification is awarded to participating organizations on an individual credentials element basis (e.g., verification of license to practice, DEA registration, etc.). CVOs may be certified for all, some, or none of the 10 credentials elements addressed in the NCQA Standards. These elements are:

1. License to Practice
2. Drug Enforcement Agency (DEA) Registration
3. Education and Training
4. Work History
5. Malpractice Claims History
6. Medical Board Sanctions
7. Medicare/Medicaid Sanctions
8. Practitioner Application Processing
9. CVO Application and Attestation Content
10. Ongoing Monitoring

There is one level of CVO certification and it is not considered all-inclusive. Status for all participating CVOs is maintained on an individual credentials element basis and pertains only to those elements reviewed as part of NCQA's CVO certification process.

Physician Organization Certification (POC)

Physician organizations (POs) such as medical groups and similar organizations play an important role as delegated providers of administrative and clinical services for HMOs and other health plans. The three standard categories for certification review are Quality Management and Improvement (QI), Utilization Management (UM), and Credentialing and Recredentialing (CR). This program focuses on the POs' role as a delegate or agent performing a function on behalf of health plans.

NCQA's PO Certification evaluates how well a physician organization manages its clinical and administrative systems in order to continuously improve health care for its members. Certification focuses on the PO's role as a delegate or agent performing a function on behalf of health plans. The survey process for physician organizations is fundamentally similar to that of health plans.

NCQA's Physician Organization Certification is a modular program. Unlike health plans, which must be reviewed on all sections of standards, POs vary in the services they provide relative to standards.

Utilization Management/Credentialing Certification

NCQA's Organization Certification (OC) program is available to organizations that perform CR and/or UM for health plans and other types of organizations eligible for NCQA accreditation or certification. Specialty plans such as chiropractic, dental, vision, and indemnity plans are eligible to apply for the OC program.

NCQA's certification review includes a rigorous on- and offsite evaluation conducted by a team of physicians and managed care experts. A review oversight committee of physicians analyzes the team's findings and assigns a certification status based on the organization's performance against standards within applicable certification options.

NCQA Clinician Recognition Programs

In collaboration with leading experts and consumer-related health care organizations, NCQA has implemented several clinician recognition programs. Consumers are able to identify physicians in their area using a search tool available on the NCQA website.

Diabetes Recognition Program: Honors physicians who demonstrate that they provide high-quality care to patients with diabetes. The program assesses key measures that were carefully defined and tested for their relationship to improved care for people with diabetes.

Heart/Stroke Recognition Program: Honors physicians who demonstrate that they provide high-quality care to patients with cardiac conditions or who have had a stroke.

Physician Practice Connections: Developed by NCQA in collaboration with Bridges to Excellence, a group of large employers, awards recognition to physician practices that use up-to-date information and systems to enhance patient care.

Patient-Centered Medical Home (PCMH): A method of organizing the provision of primary care that emphasizes care coordination and communication to transform care into "what patients want it to be." Research shows that medical homes can lead to higher quality and lower costs, and improve patients' and providers' reported experiences of care. Building on the joint principles developed by the primary care specialty societies, the program is a roadmap practices can follow to orient care to patients' needs and priorities, and then coordinate and track care over time.

The NCQA PCMH program is the most widely used medical home program in the country. Some MCOs have also incorporated these recognition programs into their pay-for-performance programs, as discussed in Chapter 5.

NCQA Report Cards

Since 1994, NCQA has made the results of all its accreditation and certification surveys available to the public through a set of Health Plan Report Card and Status Lists. These reports are all available online at NCQA's website, and they are searched or downloaded by thousands of visitors each month.

The most frequently used reports are:

- **Health Plan Report Card:** NCQA's Health Plan Report Card compares the performance of NCQA-accredited health plans across the country. This tool equips consumers with information about the quality of health plans (including HMOs, POS plans, and PPOs) based on their performance in five key areas—access and service, qualified providers, staying healthy, getting better, and living with illness—and overall accreditation. Consumers can compare the ratings of various health plans and get detailed information on individual plans.
- **Recognition Directory:** The Recognized Clinician Directory helps individuals find doctors who have demonstrated meeting NCQA's Recognition standards of care.
- **Health Insurance Plan Rankings:** NCQA issues its rankings each fall, which is the open enrollment period when many consumers choose their health plans.
- **The State of Health Care Quality:** This report is NCQA's main annual survey of aggregate trends in health care quality.

NCQA's other report cards are:

- **Credentialing and Utilization Management:** This lists specialty plans such as chiropractic, dental, vision, and indemnity plans that meet NCQA credentialing and UM requirements.
- **Credentials Verification Organizations:** This list comprises organizations that conduct credentials verification, report the credentialing information to clients, and have systems in place to protect the confidentiality and integrity of the information.
- **Disease Management:** This list contains DM-certified organizations that provide specific DM functions.
- **Health Information Products:** This is a list of organizations that provide services to health plans related to NCQA standards addressing member connections, care management, and health improvement standards addressing wellness and provider directories.
- **Quality Dividend Calculator:** This free on-line tool uses HEDIS plan data and employer demographics to calculate increased productivity and revenues when selecting accredited plans.
- **Managed Behavioral Healthcare Organizations:** MBHO Report Card is an interactive tool that makes quality information about MBHOs more accessible to employers, health plans, and consumers.
- **Managed Care Organizations:** This is a list of plans that have MCO status.
- **Multicultural Health Care Distinction:** NCQA's Multicultural Health Care (MHC) lists organizations that meet the NCQA standards to improve culturally and linguistically appropriate services and reduce health care disparities.
- **New Health Plan Accreditation:** The NHP Accreditation Status List catalogs all NHPs that have an accreditation status with NCQA, all NHPs with pending accreditation decisions, and all NHPs scheduled to be surveyed.
- **Physician and Hospital Quality:** The Physician and Hospital Quality (PHQ) list contains NCQA PHQ certified organizations that meet valid and transparent methods to evaluate quality, or quality and cost together, of services.
- **Physician Organizations:** This updated list contains all POs that provide primary, multispecialty, or single-specialty health care services through the use of practitioners of appropriate disciplines and perform the functions required in the standard category (or categories) for which they seek NCQA certification.
- **Wellness and Health Promotion Accreditation:** This is a list of organizations that meet NCQA's Wellness and Health Promotion (WHP) Accreditation, which comprehensively assesses key areas of health promotion,

including how wellness programs are implemented in the workplace, how coaching services are provided to help participants develop healthy choices, and how individual health information is properly safeguarded.

■ URAC

URAC is another leading accreditation organization that, similar to NCQA, provides accreditation and recognition programs for managed health care plans and related organizations. Copies of URAC's accreditation standards, application materials, and current accreditation status of health plans can be obtained by contacting URAC by:

- Writing to URAC at 1220 L Street NW, Suite 400, Washington, DC 20005;
- Calling URAC at (202) 202-216-9010; or
- On the Internet at: http://www.urac.org.

History

URAC is an independent non-profit organization that was established in December 1990 by the American Managed Care and Review Association (AMCRA), the trade association at that time for UR firms, PPOs, and HMOs. AMCRA's goal was to address provider concerns about the diversity of UR procedures and the growing impact of UR on physicians and hospitals. In addition, at the time of URAC's inception, managed care advocates believed that a number of state legislative initiatives under consideration would severely limit the impact of UR in some instances and make it impossible to conduct UR in others. URAC developed its first set of standards, the Health Utilization Management Standards, as a response to these legislative initiatives. URAC was originally incorporated under the name "Utilization Review Accreditation Commission." That name was shortened to the acronym "URAC" in 1996 when URAC began accrediting other types of health care entities in addition to UR organizations.

Over the years, URAC has continued to create accreditation programs covering a range of healthcare processes and organizations. URAC currently offers 28 health care accreditation and certification programs, several of which are relevant for managed care organizations. New programs are continually under development.

URAC Accreditation Process

URAC accreditation entails a rigorous review occurring in four phases. The initial phase, "Building the Application," usually takes several months and consists of completing the application forms and supplying supporting documentation. The remaining three phases take approximately three to six months and include:

Desktop Review

One or more full-time URAC reviewers analyze the applicant's documentation in relation to the URAC standards. The applicant's documentation usually consists of, but is not limited to, formal policies and procedures, organizational charts, position descriptions, contracts, sample template letters, and program descriptions and plans for departments such as quality management and credentialing. After receiving a desktop review summary, the applicant usually must provide additional documentation clarifying any pending issues.

Onsite Review

The same team that performed the desktop review conducts an onsite review to verify compliance with the standards. Management is interviewed about the organization's programs and staff is observed performing its duties. In addition, audits are conducted and personnel and credentialing files analyzed. Education and quality management programs are reviewed and URAC personnel share "best practices" and provide other guidance.

Committee Review

The last phase in the accreditation process is a review by two URAC committees that include professionals from a variety of areas in health care as well as industry experts from or chosen by URAC's member organizations. The committee review begins with a written summary documenting the findings of the desktop and onsite reviews. This summary is submitted to URAC's Accreditation Committee for evaluation with discussion with the review team as needed. An accreditation recommendation is then forwarded to URAC's Executive Committee, which has the authority to grant accreditation. After reviewing the summary and considering the Accreditation Committee's recommendation, the Executive Committee makes a final accreditation determination.

Accreditation Status and Reaccreditation

Applicants that successfully meet all requirements are awarded a Full two-year accreditation. Conditional accreditations may be awarded to applicants that have appropriate documentation, but incomplete implementation of certain policies and procedures.

Provisional accreditation may also be awarded to companies determined to be "start-ups," e.g., those that have not yet implemented their program or have not had at least six months of operational experience at the time of the onsite review.

Organizations that are unable to meet URAC standards may be placed on corrective action status, denied accreditation, or choose to withdraw.

Follow-up activities for organizations receiving Conditional or Provisional status or corrective action may include submission of additional or revised documentation and another onsite review. When these follow-up activities are complete, a follow-up executive summary is submitted to URAC's committees for a possible change to Full accreditation.

Accreditation is granted for two years starting the first day of the month following URAC's Executive Committee approval. Accredited companies seeking reaccreditation must submit the reaccreditation application at least four months before the accreditation expiration date or six months prior to expiration if the accredited company is a network reapplying for Health Plan or Health Network accreditation.

Ongoing Compliance with the Standards

Accredited organizations must continue to remain in compliance with the applicable standards throughout the accreditation cycle. If an accredited company is unable to comply with URAC Standards, its accreditation will likely be rescinded.

Complaints against an Accredited Company

URAC has a grievance procedure for investigation of complaints about an accredited company. Complaints may originate from consumers, providers or regulators. After an investigation of each complaint, which may or may not include an onsite visit, URAC may sanction an accredited company. Sanctions may range from a letter of reprimand to revocation of accreditation, depending on the nature and frequency of the violations.

URAC Core Accreditation Standards

The Core Standards serve as a common foundation for all of URAC's accreditation programs. This means that URAC-accredited companies must meet the requirements of the Core Standards, as well as the function-specific requirements for a particular accreditation program.

URAC offers stand-alone accreditation under the Core Standards for any health care organization that does not qualify for another URAC accreditation program. URAC Core Accreditation provides a general set of quality requirements that can be applied in any health care organization setting.

The Core Standards address critical issues of structure and process, including organizational structure, personnel management, quality improvement, oversight of delegated responsibilities and consumer protection.

Highlights of the Core Standards are:

Organizational Structure

Organizations clearly define their organizational structures and oversight responsibilities. They also maintain policies and procedures that govern all aspects of the operation. Organizations must implement a regulatory compliance program to ensure they are conducting business in accordance with applicable federal and state laws. Confidentiality and conflict of interest policies must be developed and followed. Other requirements include a structured quality management program and processes to protect the safety and welfare of consumers.

Personnel

Organizations must ensure that written job descriptions for all staff clearly define: education, training, professional experience, expected professional competencies, appropriate licensure andcertification requirements, as well as the scope and role of responsibilities. The organization verifies credentials of licensed or certified personnel and implements any corrective action given adverse changes in licensure or certification status. Likewise, a clear orientation, training, and evaluation program must be maintained and staff should be given the necessary guidelines to do their job.

Operations/Process

The organization should establish communication methods across all departments and disciplines to promote collaboration coordinate internal activities and provide quality services. Systems and processes must be in place for information management, business relationships, clinical oversight, regulatory compliance, and incentive programs.

Quality Improvement

The organization must maintain a quality management program that promotes objective and systematic monitoring and evaluation of consumer and client service and health care services. URAC also provides flexibility for an organization to implement its own quality management program.

Delegation of Responsibilities

The organization maintains responsibility and oversight for any function it delegates to another entity. Oversight requirements are somewhat relaxed if the entity is accredited by URAC.

Consumer Satisfaction and Protection

Communications to consumers and clients clearly and accurately represent information about the organization's services and how to obtain these services. A complaint or grievance forum or inputmechanism must be in place. The organization must have a process to respond quickly in situations that create an immediate threat to the safety or welfare of consumers.

Health Utilization Management Standards

URAC's Health Utilization Management Standards address:

- Medical necessity criteria that is evidence-based and promotes consumer safety;
- Specialty matched clinical peers for medical necessity review;
- Requirements for consistency in maintaining the highest confidentiality in UM processes as a new age is rapidly approaching with electronic health records (EHR) and health information exchanges;

- The need for flexibility for stand-alone UM organizations and UM functions within health benefit programs such as indemnity insurance, health maintenance organizations (HMOs), preferred provider organizations (PPOs), Consumer-Directed Health Care plans, and third party administrators (TPAs);
- Specialty UM organizations, such as mental health, dentistry, physical medicine rehabilitation, genetic testing, and hospitals.

URAC's Health UM Standards apply to a variety of organizations, including stand-alone UM organizations and UM functions within health benefits programs, such as indemnity insurance, health maintenance organizations (HMOs) or preferred provider organizations (PPOs).

Key aspects of the standards include:

Personnel

The organization employs qualified utilization management staff that is supported by written clinical review criteria. Nonclinical staff may perform limited data collection, intake screening, and scripted clinical screening. At each stage of the utilization review process, the organization must appropriately use qualified clinical staff.

Utilization Management Process

The organization must use a three-step process to determine if a proposed medical treatment or service is medically necessary. Licensed health professionals, such as nurses, must perform the first step—initial clinical review. If initial clinical review results in a certification, then the utilization management process ends for that case.

If the proposed service cannot be approved during initial clinical review, then the case must be referred to step two of the process—peer clinical review. A physician who is qualified to render a clinical opinion about the proposed service generally must perform this review. However, if the treating provider is a nonphysician, then a similar provider may also perform the peer clinical review. A provider who performs peer clinical review must be available to discuss review determination with the treating provider.

If peer clinical review results in a noncertification, the patient or the treating provider hasthe right to access step three of the process—appeals consideration. For cases involving ongoing or imminent medical care, the organization provides for an expedited appeals consideration mechanism.

Throughout the utilization management process, the UMO utilizes explicit clinical review criteria based on sound clinical principles and processes, and are reviewed and revised on a periodic basis. Upon request, the UMO discloses to the patient or treating provider the criteria upon which a non-certification decision was based.

Confidentiality

The organization must have written policies and procedures in place that assure information obtained during the UM process is kept confidential in accordance with applicable laws. Information must be limited to only what is necessary for UM to performthe services under review, and be used solely for the purpose of UM, quality management, discharge planning and case management. If provider-specific data is released to the public, the organization must have policies and procedures for exercising due care in compiling and releasing such data.

Health Network Standards

The Health Network Standards encourage open-panel networks to become more integrated in their operations and emphasize quality assurance and improvement. The Health Network Standards cover three areas: network management, credentialing, and consumer protection.

Network Management

The organization maintains a formal strategy for incorporating the perspectives of participating providers. It submits a general description of the criteria for selection to new providers and includes a provider relations program. The organization must have a written agreement with all providers, which details the terms between the organization and the provider.

Agreements cannot include language that restricts providers from discussing healthcare matters with consumers or that stresses cost over quality. Upon requestwithin 45 calendar days, the organization discloses a list of all payers who have access to the organization's networkto a provider. If the organization contracts with another network for access to its providers, it must ensure consistency in the contract terms. The organization also implements a policy addressing alleged violations by participating providers and a mechanism for dispute resolution and appeals. Finally, the organization implements a mechanism to immediately suspenda provider who is under investigation for criminal activities or negligence.

Provider Credentialing

The organization develops and implements a written plan for credentialing that is approved by the organization's executive management. The plan requires that practitioners who are within the scope of the program submit a credentialing application that includes an attestation of truthfulness and accuracy signed and dated by the applicant. The plan also includes the types of credentialing information to be collected. For verification of licensure and certification, the organization must use primary sources (i.e., the issuing source of the credential).

The credentialing plan requires that the organization recredentials providers every three years. For credentialing functions it delegates to another entity, the organization retains authority to make the final determination regarding participation status, and at least every three years, conducts an on-site review of the entity.

Consumer Protection

The organization maintains a confidentiality policy for protected information. It also orients the staff annually on the policy and requires staff to sign a confidentiality agreement.

The organization has a means of informing consumers about which providers participate in the provider network, such as a directory or other such avenue of communication.

Health Plan Standards

The Health Plan Standards apply to integrated networks, such as health maintenance organizations (HMOs) and risk-assuming preferred provider organizations (PPOs). Organizations must meet standards related to:

- Network management
- Credentialing
- Consumer protection
- Utilization management
- Quality management

Highlights of the Health Plan Standards include:

Network Management

The organization maintains a formal process for incorporating the perspectives of participating providers and submits a general description of the criteria for selection to new providers. The organization also includes a provider relations program that maintains communications between the organization and the provider about network activities.

Provider agreements cannot include language that restricts providers from discussing healthcare matters with consumers or that stresses cost over quality. If the organization contracts with another network for access to its providers, it must ensure consistency in the contract terms. The organization implements a policy addressing alleged violations by participating providers and a vehicle for dispute resolution and appeals.

Credentialing

The organization implements a program to verify the professional qualifications of all participating providers and facilities that provide services to consumers, with the senior clinical staff person overseeing the clinical portion of the program. The credentialing program has a committee consisting of at least one practicing provider who has no other role in the organization. The committee will provide, among other things, guidance to the organization on credentialing matters and vote on applications for participation status.

For verification of licensure and certification, the organization uses primary sources. The organization implements a way of determining which applications need further investigation and what factors affect the quality of care and then conducts the investigation. Each provider is recredentialed every three years.

Utilization Management

Organizations seeking health plan accreditation must comply with URAC's Utilization Management Standards. In addition, the organization establishes a wayfor consumers to access an independent review process.

Consumer Protection

The organization maintains a confidentiality policy and requires staff to sign a confidentiality agreement.

The organization has means ofinforming consumers aboutproviders in the provider network. The organization implements a safeguard to ensure that marketing and sales activities do not misrepresent the organization's services. Information available to consumers should include cost-sharing features, medical management and administrative requirements, as well asdisenrollment statistics.

Consumers must be notified prior to any changes to their benefits plan. The communication plan also provides consumers with the latest provider network information and a means to access the organization via telephone to obtain answers regarding benefits, assistance with selecting providers, answering claims questions, and acceptance of complaints. The organization provides constant telephone access (and online access) to consumers for urgent health care issues. The organization implements a venue for consumers to provide suggestions for better service.

Quality Management

In addition to the two quality improvement projects required under the Core Standards, the organization maintains at least one additional project. At least two of the three quality improvement projects focus on clinical quality.

Disease Management Standards

By focusing the attention of resources on members with significant health risks and needs, disease management programs can help health plans improve health status and conserve resources. To reach its full potential, a disease management program should adopt a comprehensive approach to assessing and responding to the needs of health plan members.

Performance Measurement and Reporting

The organization develops a valid process forevaluating and reporting its performance and provides results specific to each health condition within the scope of the DM program. The performance measurement process also accounts for consumers' satisfaction with the DM program and seeks feedback from healthcare providers.

Population Management

The organization implements a standard process to identify consumers who will participate in the DM program, and to evaluate the health needs of each participant. The disease management organization involves consumers in the DM process by informing them how disease management works and what information they can expect to receive.

Program Design

The organization implements a process to assess the health condition of each participant, taking into account cases where more than one chronic health condition may be present. Such assessment is conducted according to a standard process. Based on the assessment results, the disease management organization implements interventions that are designed to respond to the specific health needs of the patient. Decision-support tools used during the DM process are evidence-based, and they are reviewed and updated at least annually.

Health Provider Credentialing Standards

URAC developed Health Provider Credentialing Standards to encourage the implementation of credentialing programs to certify participating providers in a wide array of managed care networks. Examples of this type of organization include preferred provider organizations (PPOs), health maintenance organizations (HMOs), physician hospital organizations (PHOs), and workers' compensation networks.

There are nine categories of standards in the Health Provider Credentialing Standards: credentialing program; structure, organization and staffing; credentialing plan; credentialing program requirements; credentialing records; credentialing process; initial credentialing verification; recredentialing verification; and credentialing verification.

Scope of Services

These standards apply to credentialing programs within managed care networks, such as HMOs and PPOs. The network determines the scope of its credentialing program—does it credential physicians only, does it credential all providers, or is it somewhere in between?

The organization implements a program to verify the professional qualifications of all participating providers and facilities that provide services to consumers, with the senior clinical staff person overseeing the clinical portion of the program. The credentialing program has a committee consisting of at least one practicing provider who has no other role in the organization. The committee provides, among other things, guidance to the organization on credentialing matters and votes on applications for participation status.

The organization maintains a detailed written plan for its credentialing program that the committee approves.

The organization requires all practitioners requesting participation status to submit a written credentialing application that provides information pertinent to verify the applicant's qualifications. The organization maintains the confidentiality of credentialing information, with limited access, for each provider going through the credentialing process. The organization implements mechanisms to ensure accuracy of information, to communicate with providers about their credentialing status and to accept additional information.

For verification of licensure and certification, the organization must use primary sources. The organization determines which applications need further investigation and what factors affect the quality of care, upon which time the investigation is conducted.

The organization requires that the credentialing committee review and approve the application prior to granting participation status. The organization should not submit any application that is older than one year or verification information that is older than six months to the credentialing committee. The organization notifies providers of their status within 60 calendar days of the determination. The organization monitors providers for compliance and implements mechanisms to respond to cases of noncompliance.

Each provider is recredentialed every three years. The re-credentialing process focuses on information that is subject to change and based upon the performance of the provider within the health plan. For credentialing functions it delegates to another entity, the organization retains authority to make the final determination regarding participation status, and at least every three years, conducts an onsite review of the entity.

Credentials Verification Organizations

CVOs typically verify the qualifications of doctors and other health care practitioners with whom an HMO, PPO, or other network contracts. The purpose of the CVO standards is to ensure that the managed care organization includes only properly qualified healthcare practitioners in its network.

The CVO program standards cover such topics as:

CVO Personnel

The CVO trains staff in the its policies and procedures for verification, as well as in other responsibilities, including relevant URAC standards.

The Credentialing Process

The CVO verifies current licensure through primary sources. The practitioner has the right to request reconsideration if such sources show errors in data collection. The CVO also must have written policies and procedures governing the reporting of findings to the client, attempts to retrieve information, and the status of the practitioner within the verification process.

If the CVO conducts reviews of practitioner offices, it must use healthcare practitioners to conduct the onsite review. The review of the office must look at patient access; public health policies; and procedures and safety standards for fire, emergency, and equipment maintenance.

Quality Improvement

The CVO must have a written quality improvement plan that includes evidence of routine inspections of data and databases; annual random sampling of staff activities; and improvements in areas of concern.

Delegation of Responsibilities

The CVO retains authority and maintains oversight of all subcontracted verification activities and performs a comprehensive review of the subcontractor's verification program. The subcontractor maintains compliance with URAC standards. The CVO also performs quarterly reviews of the subcontractor's work and uses annual reviews with random audits of the files.

Confidentiality

The CVO must have a written policy and procedures concerning the integrity of its databases and update all acquired databases at least annually. The CVO may make public information about the practitioner only with the consent of the practitioner. The CVO secures electronic data with changing passwords and a daily backup.

Grievances & Complaints

Providers who go through the credentialing process must be permitted to submit information to correct errors or inconsistencies. If the CVO conducts an onsite review, the provider has the opportunity for reconsideration.

Health Website

The purpose of the Health Web Site program is to help consumers and others identify health care Web sites that meet high standards of quality and accountability.

The standards apply to a variety of health-related websites, including health care financing organizations, health delivery organizations, health management organizations and application service providers.

Operations/Process

The standards cover diverse topics that include organizational policies and structures, disclosure, health content, external linking, privacy, security, and accountability.

A URAC-accredited website must disclose a variety of information that can help consumers evaluate the site. The website must have certain processes in place regarding health content, including an editorial policy that identifies the author and requires that information be evidence-based. Also, there must be a clear distinction between paid advertising and content.

If the website links to other sites, it must have a process for selecting the sites to which it links, as well as a process for periodically reviewing the links in order to ensure they are current and appropriate.

Quality Improvement

To ensure organizations remain compliant with URAC standards, URAC conducts periodic reviews of the accredited site and a full review annually.

In addition, the organization must have a Quality Oversight Committee in place to oversee the website's quality. The Quality Oversight Committee includes the health professional(s) responsible for the health content on the Web site and the individual responsible for the Web site's privacy practices. The Quality Oversight Committee reviews all changes to the website's policies and procedures. The Committee also sets performance goals for the site and checks progress in meeting the goals.

Privacy and Security

The URAC standards provide strong rules and restrictions regarding the use and protection of personal information consumers may provide to a health website. For example, the Web site may not collect personal health information without first asking for permission to do so. The site must notify users if their information is to be sold to third-party entities. In addition, the site must demonstrate that its security protocols are sufficient to maintain the privacy of information collected on the site.

Delegation of Responsibilities

The organization discloses the involvement of third-party entities if they have significant interests in the Web site. The organization also discloses significant relationships between commercial sponsors and health content, specifically the sponsor's involvement in the development of health information and/or any preferential treatment the site might receive through its sponsor (priority listings in search engine results, product listing, etc.).

In addition, URAC reviews the use of contracted services to ensure maximum privacy and security.

■ ACCREDITATION ASSOCIATION FOR AMBULATORY HEALTH CARE

The AAAHC is the third accreditation organization for managed health care plans, but its emphasis is primarily on ambulatory care, consistent with its historical roots. Copies of AAAHC's accreditation standards, application materials, and current accreditation status of health plans can be obtained by contacting AAAHC by:

- Writing to AAAHC at 5250 Old Orchard Road, Suite 200, Skokie, IL 60077;
- Calling AAAHC at (847) 853-6060; or
- On the Internet at www.aaahc.org.

History

The AAAHC, also known as the Accreditation Association, was created in 1979 to assist ambulatory health care organizations improve the quality of care provided to patients. The founding members of the association were the American College Health Association, the American Group Practice Association (now known as the American Group Medical Association), the Federated Ambulatory Surgery Association, the Group Health Association of America (the successor of which is AHIP), the Medical Group Management Association, and the National Association of Community Health Centers. Presently, the AAAHC includes 16 member organizations representing a broad spectrum of ambulatory health care.

The AAAHC currently accredits more than 4,600 health care organizations, including endoscopy centers, ambulatory surgery centers, office-based surgery centers, student health centers, and large medical and dental group practices. In addition, the Accreditation Association surveys and accredits MCOs, including HMOs, PPOs, and IPAs. At the time of publication, it accredited only 18 HMOs or managed health care plans, all but one of which are in Florida.[*]

The AAAHC's managed care standards have been developed with industry input and incorporate the evaluation of functional areas such as member communications systems; member complaint and grievance resolution systems; utilization management, including member appeal procedures; quality management and improvement; and provider credentialing and recredentialing systems. The association's Managed Care Program has received Medicare Advantage Deemed Status from the Centers for Medicare and Medicaid Services.

AAAHC Accreditation Process

An accreditation decision is based on an assessment of a health care organization's compliance with applicable standards and adherence to the policies and procedures of the Accreditation Association. Compliance is assessed by AAAHC through at least one of the following means: documented evidence, answers to detailed questions concerning implementation, or onsite observations and interviews by surveyors.

---

[*] www.aaahc.org/eweb/dynamicpage.aspx?site = aaahc_site&webcode = find_orgs, search on "Organization Type," "Managed Care Organization." Accessed April 22, 2011.

The Accreditation Association surveyors are physicians, dentists, nurses, and administrators who are selected, to the extent possible, on the basis of their knowledge of and experience with the range of services provided by the organization seeking an accreditation survey. At the close of an onsite survey, the reviewers schedule a summation conference during which they present their findings to representatives of the organization for discussion and clarification. Members of the health care organization's governing body, medical staff, and administration are encouraged to comment on the findings as well as express their perceptions of the survey.

After the onsite survey is completed, association staff members review the survey findings and recommendations, including the survey team's recommendation regarding accreditation, and make a recommendation regarding accreditation to the Accreditation Committee of the AAAHC. Accreditation is awarded to organizations that demonstrate substantial compliance with the AAAHC standards and adhere to the AAAHC accreditation policies. Possible terms of accreditation awarded by the Accreditation Committee, include 3-year, 1-year, 6-month and denial or revocation of accreditation.

AAAHC Accreditation Standards

The AAAHC Accreditation Standards are divided into a set of core standards that apply to all organizations seeking accreditation, and adjunct standards that apply to organizations based on the specific programs and services they provide.

AAAHC Core Standards that apply to all organizations include:

1. Rights of Patients
2. Governance
3. Administration
4. Quality of Care Provided
5. Quality Management and Improvement
6. Clinical Records and Health Information
7. Infection Prevention and Control and Safety
8. Facilities and Environment

AAAHC Adjunct Standards that may apply to health plans include:

- Managed Care Organizations
- Health Education and Wellness

■ CONCLUSION

This chapter has presented a summary of three organizations that currently accredit MCOs and related health care entities, as well as some details of the oversight programs they offer. Like the organizations they review, the three accreditation organizations vary in their goals and in their approach to external review. Although they vary considerably in their approach, all of these organizations hold the potential for rationalizing and consolidating current external review processes for employers, state, federal, and individual purchasers. These processes are sometimes duplicative or contradictory in their requirements and, in some cases, may have a detrimental impact on managed care programs. Ultimately, however, their effectiveness must be judged in terms of their ability to improve the quality of care and service that health care organizations provide to their customers. And, most important, there is no doubt that these organizations have had a positive impact on the quality of health care in this country.

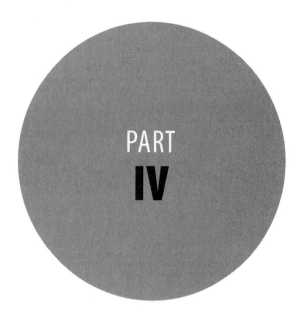

PART

IV

Sales, Finance, and Administration

"Being good in business is the most fascinating kind of art. Making money is art and working is art and good business is the best art."

Andy Warhol (1928–1987)
The Philosophy of Andy Warhol
(From A to B & Back Again)
[Harcourt Brace Jovanovich, 1975]

Marketing and Sales

Richard Birhanzel

STUDY OBJECTIVES

- Understand the basic activities of sales and marketing within a managed care organization
- Understand how marketing differs from sales
- Understand compensation of sales and marketing personnel
- Understand the different segments of the health care market
- Understand how sales and marketing differ depending on market segments
- Understand how metrics are used in the sales and marketing processes
- Understand the impact of the Patient Protection and Affordable Care Act on marketing and sales

DISCUSSION TOPICS

1. Discuss how each market segment is unique and how that affects sales and marketing.
2. Discuss how sales and marketing interact with other health plan functions.
3. Discuss how sales and marketing have evolved and how it may evolve in the future.
4. Discuss the different ways that sales and marketing success may be measured, and the strengths and weaknesses of each.
5. Discuss how a sales and marketing organizational structure may vary by health plan, by market segment, or by regulatory requirements.

▉ INTRODUCTION

Marketing and sales in health insurance and managed health care are on the verge of disruptive change, influenced by the convergence of reform-driven regulatory changes, economic challenges, and a marketplace increasingly expecting retail-caliber experiences. Anticipated disruptions range from transition away from medical underwriting, the basis for pricing health insurance for decades, to an expansion of sales channels to include an array of new and more direct selling approaches. This chapter defines

the fundamentals of health plan marketing and sales, focusing on the employer and individual market segments, not Medicare (see Chapter 24) or managed Medicaid (see Chapter 25). Marketing and sales for Medicare Advantage has a number of fundamental differences compared to the commercial sector, so it is addressed solely in Chapter 24 and not here; marketing and sales are not typically a feature of managed Medicaid plans.

Grounded in the foundation of the way things currently work, this chapter also looks to the future and shares perspective on how key marketing and sales capabilities are likely to change. The reader must bear in mind, however, that this book was published before most of the major provisions of the Patient Protection and Affordable Care Act (ACA) are to go into effect. The impact of some aspects of the ACA can only be estimated, and predicting anything in health care is always a difficult exercise. Furthermore, like all major legislation, the ACA will continually be subject to amendments, just like every single major law in the nation.

■ DEFINING THE MANAGED HEALTH CARE MARKETPLACE

In the commercial market, meaning employer group and individual health coverage but not Medicare or Medicaid, health plans organize around traditional segmentations of their customer base. These customer segments generally are based on membership size in the commercial space and include individual, small group (typically 2–50 member employers), mid-market (51 to approximately 5,000 members), and large case (more than 5,000 members).

Section 1304 [42 U.S.C. 18024] of the ACA has very concrete market definitions that are used in relation to state health insurance exchanges, medical loss ratio (MLR), limitations and underwriting requirements, all of which are discussed in Chapter 30 as well as in this chapter as appropriate. Those definitions are:

- **Individual**—meaning health insurance purchased individually, not through a group
- **Small Employer Group**—at least two or one[*] but not more than 100 employees on average but states can elect to define the small group market as up to 50
- **Large Employer Group**—more than 100 employees on average

Within the size-based market segments, health plans also typically apply some designation to reflect the risk arrangement, ranging from fully insured to self-funded administrative services only (ASO), as described in Chapter 2. Customers may also be differentiated by the product portfolio purchased, including medical, pharmaceutical, behavioral health, and other ancillary products. In considering health plan sales and marketing, it is important to understand the distinct characteristics and demands of the two broad means of accessing the market: employer-sponsored and individual markets.

The *employer-sponsored* channel is a business-to-business-to-consumer model characterized by heavy reliance on intermediary distribution channels, namely brokers and consultants. In this model, the relationship with the primary buyer, the employer, may be direct or indirect and the

relationship with the consumer is typically indirect. The aim of health plan sales and marketing in this model is primarily to influence employer buyers and distribution channel partners, with a secondary focus on consumers. In contrast, the *individual* channel is characterized by a closer relationship with the consumer. As such, health plan sales and marketing in this model is focused on influencing consumer buyers and the distribution channel partners that service them.

■ HEALTH PLAN MARKETING FUNDAMENTALS

Health plan marketing has historically been an area of relatively minimal focus when compared to other functions such as claims management or medical management. This changed in recent years as health plans focused more heavily on organic growth. Many health plans have recently invested in acquiring marketing talent from other industries in an effort to infuse cross-industry thinking. Furthermore, the onset of new products, particularly in the consumer-directed and Medicare spaces, has demanded a dramatic increase in marketing spend and improvement in marketing capabilities. Given this rather sudden shift toward a focus on marketing as a key differentiator, many health plans have struggled to advance their capability at a pace necessary to meet the growing demand of the marketplace.

Organizationally, health plans vary relative to a central marketing entity serving all market segments versus allocation of marketing resources to each market segment. In the employer-sponsored segments, sales and marketing are typically distinct organizations, whereas in the direct markets there is very little distinction between sales and the tactical component of marketing. Regardless of structure, most health plan marketing organizations perform a standard set of functions, described as follows.

Brand Management

The need to manage brand is a rather recent development in the managed care industry. The exception is Blue Cross and Blue Shield (BCBS) plans with a historic market presence, as described in Chapter 1. Marketplace longevity provided brand awareness, but the BCBS plans also have centralized brand management through the Blue Cross Blue Shield Association. This centralized brand management is limited in some ways since each individual plan is an independent entity, so the process described next applies to those individual plans. The brand management process begins with developing a view to the desired market positioning: how does the health plan want to be viewed in the eyes of employers, consumers, distribution partners, and providers? For example, is the health plan positioned as a high-touch, premium carrier? Or perhaps the health plan is positioned as a no-frills, low-cost carrier. Whatever the positioning, it is competitively important to clarify the desired market positioning and the key marketplace differentiators aligned

---

[*]For purposes of insurance, states typically define whether or not a single employee may be considered as a small group for coverage instead of only for individual coverage. As expensive as small group coverage is, it is usually less expensive than individual coverage and may also be more attainable.

with the positioning. Given the strategic importance of brand positioning, health plan C-suite executives are typically involved and health plans often seek assistance from advertising or strategy consulting firms in developing and managing their brand.

External Communications

Many health plan marketing organizations own public relations and external communications. This responsibility ranges from managing the content of external websites to providing counsel to spokespersons on public comments on specific issues. Marketing is also responsible for ensuring consistency of external communications with the aforementioned brand positioning.

Advertising

Like any other company, health plans utilize a variety of media to advertise their products and services, including television, radio, print, and the Internet. Health plans use advertising firms heavily in determining the mix of advertising channels and in executing broad-based and targeted advertising campaigns. The marketing organization is responsible for setting the overall advertising strategy and objectives, based on the brand positioning, and then providing oversight to the work of the advertising firms. As affinity relationships and go-to-market alliances become more prevalent, marketing organizations are also responsible for representing the health plan in shared branding and advertising.

Market Research

Marketing organizations execute basic market research in support of the health plan. Marketing's research scope typically includes marketplace trends, competitive intelligence, and surveying of health plan stakeholders, including employers, distribution partners, members, and providers. For specific needs, health plan marketing purchases specific research from niche vendors.

Lead Generation

As market research uncovers opportunities for new markets or customers, marketing provides leads to sales organizations in the various market segments. These leads may be as directional as market intelligence around the attractiveness of a particular industry or as specific as a list of prospective customers.

Sales Campaign Support

Marketing often provides guidance and support to the sales organizations in the planning and execution of campaigns, particularly around presentations and customer messaging. This support ranges from hands-on edits to proposals to employers to directional advice on key selling messages.

Increasingly, health plans' execution of campaigns involves marketing automation tools. These tools enable fast-paced and accurate setup and execution of new campaigns, tracking of campaign results, and management of marketing resources across multiple campaigns.

■ CHALLENGES TO EFFECTIVE HEALTH PLAN MARKETING

Health plan marketing organizations face several challenges in executing the fundamentals, particularly when compared to enablers commonly found in other industries. For example, marketing is severely limited by a lack of customer insight. Although the typical financial services or retail company is armed with advanced customer segmentation based on behaviors and preferences, health plan marketing organizations typically rely on anecdotal data or data that are not specific to the membership base they serve. This customer insight gap limits the ability to tailor marketing campaigns to influence employer or consumer behavior based on behaviors or preferences. Some health plans have mitigated this challenge in the direct markets by purchasing consumer insight from marketing database vendors. However, in the employer-sponsored market, meaningful customer insight around employers or employees has remained elusive.

Historically, health plans have limited investment in the marketing space. Although this has changed over the last few years, the impact of years of underinvestment is manifest in the gaps in human capital and technology assets that reside in many health plan marketing organizations. Only recently, health plans have looked to other industries for marketing talent and started to invest in modernizing supporting marketing technology, such as campaign automation tools. With limits on the MLR on insured business, as described in Chapters 21 and 30, the overall amount available to invest in marketing may be constrained, however. Targeted marketing in the employer-sponsored space can be very difficult because an employee's purchasing decision may be complex and has many potential influences, including employers, brokers, physicians, unions, other consumers, their own personal medical needs or those of a dependent, cultural issues, and media sources. This presents a challenge to health plan marketing organizations as they attempt to design and execute campaigns to establish brand position or promote a product or service.

■ HIGH PERFORMANCE IN HEALTH PLAN MARKETING PRACTICES

There is significant variability in health plans' execution of marketing fundamentals, and health plan marketing generally continues to lag other industries from a capability perspective. Nonetheless, some health plans have achieved marketplace differentiation in certain marketing practices in their pursuit of organic growth. Though not considered exceptional by cross-industry standards, examples of high-performance health plan marketing include the following.

Measuring Brand Value

Advanced health plan marketing organizations are able to measure the value of the brand they represent. Accomplished through quantitative surveys, this activity provides insight validating brand strategy, measuring the effectiveness of campaigns to adjust brand positioning, and quantifying the current value of the brand. Some are also developing an understanding of the brand and customer experience factors that drive conversion through the marketing funnel and yield increased sales and profitability.

Marketing Portfolio Optimization

Although limited by rudimentary capabilities to measure specific marketing return on investment (MROI), some health plans have started to apply a more scientific approach to the mix of marketing and advertising activities and investments. Health plan marketers currently rely on qualitative, survey-based information and third-party advice in adjusting the mix of their portfolios. Furthermore, they depend on basic information such as "cost per impression," rather than "cost per desired outcome" or quantitative ROI.

Consumer Segmentation

Beyond the traditional segmentation of members by age, gender, and claims experience, some health plans are adding qualitative, "life stage" information to their segments. This information is gathered through consumer surveys and clusters members based on the attitudes common to their life stage, a mix of demographics, socioeconomics, lifestyle, and views on health care issues. Some health plans are further advancing their consumer segmentation to include behavioral segmentation, as defined by utilization of health care services, call centers, and portals.

Targeted Marketing Campaigns

Leveraging advances in consumer segmentation, some health plans have effectively tailored marketing campaigns to support specific objectives, typically around the introduction of new products or services. Examples abound in the consumer-directed product space because health plans have developed intelligence on favorable consumer segments and key selling messages around these products. This intelligence has also been applied to drive advertising content and other marketing campaigns.

■ BENEFITS DESIGN

Benefits design is the creation of variations in benefits coverage, including defining what's covered and what's not, any benefits limitations, and the degree of cost-sharing.

For example, the consumer-directed health plans (CDHPs), described in Chapter 2, represent a benefits design with high levels of cost-sharing, combined with pretax savings options. The goal is to create products that are competitive and attractive in the marketplace.

For insured business, states typically mandate coverage of certain types of services, while self-funded plans are generally free to design their benefits plans as they see fit. But even self-funded plans must comply with certain benefits requirements under federal law such as mental health parity, meaning benefits for mental health services cannot differ from those for medical–surgical care. Benefits for prescription drugs are almost always included as a rider or secondary coverage, making them eligible for different types of cost-sharing. Annual and lifetime limits were also sometimes put in place.

Qualified Health Benefits under the ACA

The ACA has already changed some aspects of benefits design, and beginning in 2014 it will place very specific requirements on benefits coverage. These are referred to as essential health benefits, and qualified health plans or qualified health benefits plans will have to provide them. All health benefits plans, insured and self-funded, will have to meet these requirements or their health plans will not be considered "qualified." Exceptions for some, but not all, of these requirements are allowed for "grandfathered" plans, which are discussed shortly. Essential health benefits are listed in **Table 16-1**.

TABLE 16-1	Essential Health Benefits for Qualified Health Benefits Plans under the ACA	
Benefit	**Cost-sharing allowed**
Ambulatory patient service	Yes
Emergency services	Yes
Hospitalization	Yes
Maternity and newborn care	Yes
Pediatric services	Yes
Preventive and wellness services	No, first-dollar required
Prescription drugs	Yes, but type may differ from medical
Laboratory services	Yes
Mental health and substance use disorder services	Yes, and may not differ from medical
Chronic disease management	Yes
Rehabilitative and habilitative services and devices	Yes

Source: Copyright P.R. Kongstvedt Company, LLC. Used with permission.

TABLE 16-2	Cost-Sharing for Qualified Health Benefits Plans under the ACA
Benefit level	**Cost-sharing (actuarial value)***
Platinum	10%
Gold	20%
Silver	30%
Bronze	40%

*Does not include wellness and prevention, which have first-dollar coverage (excluding grandfathered plans).
Source: Copyright P.R. Kongstvedt Company, LLC. Used with permission.

TABLE 16-4	Provisions of the ACA In Effect for All Plans, Including Grandfathered Plans

- Prohibition on preexisting condition exclusion or discrimination based on health status for children under age 19
- Prohibition on rescissions after coverage begins except in the case of fraud or intentional misrepresentation
- No lifetime limits on coverage
- Extension of dependent coverage until age 26

Source: Copyright P.R. Kongstvedt Company, LLC. Used with permission.

The ACA also defines four different levels of allowable cost-sharing. Cost-sharing does not refer to coinsurance percentages but it refers to the actuarial value. For example, 20% cost-sharing means the total of all cost-sharing—deductibles, coinsurance, and copayments—must add up to 20% of total costs on average for the overall plan. Cost-sharing is applicable to in-network costs, so out-of-network cost-sharing could be higher except for emergency care, which must be provided as though it is in-network. Prevention and wellness must be covered without any cost-sharing, excluding grandfathered plans. The four levels of cost-sharing defined in the ACA are listed in **Table 16-2**. Already in effect, the ACA also prohibits lifetime limits on coverage, and annual limits are to be phased out through 2014.

Grandfathered Benefits Plans

Grandfathered health benefits plans refer to plans that were in effect on March 23, 2010, the date of enactment of the ACA. Grandfathered plans need not comply with many (but not all) of the ACA's requirements as long as they maintain

the grandfathered status. A grandfathered plan loses that status if one of a number of events occurs, as listed in **Table 16-3**.

Certain benefits requirements in the ACA apply to all health benefits plans, regardless of whether or not they are grandfathered. These are listed in **Table 16-4**.

■ SALES

Sales refers to the processes involved in actually selling the products and services that the health plan offers, regardless of the type of market. It is the concrete means of adding or retaining members. It differs between the employer-sponsored model and the individual model, and differences exist within the employer-sponsored model based on size and distribution channel. All are expected to face change under the ACA, but to differing degrees.

Sales Processes in the Employer-Sponsored Model

Employer-sponsored health plan sales are typically organized into two groups in each customer segment: (1) new sales and (2) account management for existing customers, focused on renewals. For both new and existing customers, sales activity is heavily reliant on well-established distribution channels, with more than 85% of employer-sponsored business involving an intermediary, typically a broker or consultant.

Brokers are typically focused on relatively smaller employers (2–1,000 members) and are compensated based on commissions paid by the health plan, meaning some percentage of the premiums paid by the employer to the health plan. Consultants are focused on larger employers and receive fee-based compensation paid by the employer. Health plans have no involvement with payment of fees to consultants.

Given the reliance on distribution partners in driving employer sales and renewals, it has become common among health plans to invest in capabilities that increase the effectiveness of these relationships, particularly the broker relationships. A majority of these investments are focused on driving broker loyalty and improving incentive compensation processes and tools. To drive broker loyalty, health plans have developed databases to gather insight

TABLE 16-3	Conditions under Which a Grandfathered Plan will Lose Grandfathered Status

- Benefits for a particular condition are eliminated or substantially reduced
- Co-insurance charges are increased
- Deductibles or out-of-pocket limits are significantly increased
- Office copay amounts are significantly increased
- Fixed-dollar deductibles are significantly raised
- Significantly lower employer contributions toward premiums
- Addition or lowering of annual limit
- Change in insurer
- Allowing new employees to join the plan will not cause a loss of grandfather status, but transferring employees to a new plan without different terms and without a bona-fide employment reason would cause loss of grandfather status

Source: Copyright P.R. Kongstvedt Company, LLC. Used with permission.

on broker attributes, including performance metrics such as productivity, volume, and profitability. Health plans leverage this insight to tailor relationships with brokers, including commissions and service strategies.

Considerable variation exists regarding commission amounts from plan to plan, and for new sales versus renewals. The execution of commission strategies has been significantly improved with the emergence of incentive compensation technology solutions that streamline and drive increased accuracy in commission payments, which have historically been a trouble spot for health plans. Conversely, many payers are decreasing commissions in response to MLR limits created by the ACA. In some cases, payers are paying flat commission rates. The commission structure for brokers will continue to face considerable pressure in coming years.

Completing the sales process quickly and accurately is a key differentiator from an employer's perspective. An important and increasingly common aid in effective selling is sales force automation (SFA). These applications and databases support the sales process from lead generation through the first sale and become the initial data set for account management to service an employer. SFA tools can also support the gathering of key sales performance metrics. Although specific measures may vary, most health plans evaluate sales based on membership, revenue, and, increasingly, profitability; these metrics serve as the basis for compensating sales resources and brokers.

Although these processes may vary by health plan, they typically follow several common steps, as depicted in **Figure 16-1**.

Lead Generation

The health plan sales process begins with the identification of "leads," prospective employer customers. Leads come from a variety of sources, including brokers and consultants, health plan marketing, and requests for proposals (RFPs) from employers. The basic information about a lead is typically logged in a database, establishing an initial record of the prospective customer.

Prospecting

The health plan salesperson is assigned a lead to qualify through research, initial conversations with the prospective customer, and collaboration with brokers and consultants. If the salesperson interacts directly with the employer, the interaction is likely with benefits coordinators, human resources executives, and potentially C-suite executives. In fact, the involvement of chief executive officers and chief financial officers in determining employee health benefits is rapidly increasing among larger employers because affordability of health insurance is a top priority for many businesses. Successful prospecting will yield enough additional information about a prospective customer to enable rating and underwriting and an initial price quote. This additional information is added to the prospective customer record.

Rating and Underwriting

Based on information gathered by brokers and aggregated and submitted by the salesperson, the underwriting organization will evaluate and score the risk to insure the employees of a prospective customer, which drives the initial pricing based on established margin targets. If the prospective customer is interested in ASO, the activity at this stage is focused on underwriting stop-loss insurance coverage and estimating administrative cost, yielding an initial price. Rating and underwriting is discussed more fully in Chapter 22.

Quoting

The next step is for the salesperson or distribution partner to communicate initial pricing to the prospective customer, based on several parameters, including the scope and design of employee benefits and network coverage. There may be several iterations to underwriting and price quoting as parameters are negotiated and adjusted.

First Sale—To the Employer

When the employer customer agrees to pricing, benefit design, products, network, and other contract parameters, the salesperson or broker finalizes the contract with the employer and completes the record of the sale in a database that will be used in setting up the customer on the health plan's information systems. In the small group segment, telesales (sometimes referred to as telemarketing) is increasing as an alternative to internal and broker-driven sales.

Case Installation

Upon the close of the "first sale," the customer's information, including the details of the services purchased,

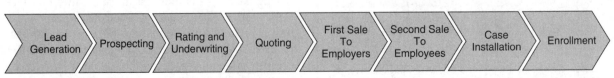

FIGURE 16-1 Employer-Sponsored Sales Process

is entered into the health plan's information systems. Although health plan sales is typically not directly involved in case installation, the quality and completeness of the customer information gathered by the salesperson influences the efficiency and quality of the case installation.

Second Sale—To the Employee

Although many employers offer insurance from only one health plan, some employers, particularly larger employers, often provide multiple health plan options to their employees. Health plans refer to this as "slice" business because any one insurer will likely service only a portion of the customer's employees. In these situations, there is an open enrollment period for employees to select a health plan. This is referred to as the "second sale," the sale to the employees. During the second sale, the health plan salesperson may be involved in promotions or campaigns to the employees in an effort to influence the selection of the health plan they represent.

Enrollment

When employee selection is complete, the enrolled employees (called subscribers) and dependants (called, along with the subscriber, members) are enrolled in the health plan's systems. Similar to case installation, the salesperson has a limited role in enrollment. However, the salesperson typically follows the status of enrollment to ensure timely completion of fulfillment (e.g., identification or ID cards to employees) by the employer's effective date. The duration from the first sale to employees' receipt of ID cards is viewed as an important end-to-end measure of a health plan's "front-end" operational efficiency. For small group customers, case installation and enrollment typically occur in one step because both the group and member information is loaded into health plan systems.

Account Management and Renewal in the Employer-Sponsored Model

Upon the conclusion of a successful sale, the employer relationship, or "account," is transitioned to an account manager. The account manager's primary responsibilities are to oversee the service provided to the employer and pursue the renewal of the health plan's contract with the employer. Depending on the products and services purchased by the employer, the account manager may interact with the employer on issues related to enrollment, claims, network, care management, and other ancillary services. In providing service to the employer, the account manager is expected to act as a quarterback, owning the customer relationship but able to quickly engage the appropriate health plan expert (e.g., care management or behavioral

health experts) as the issues and opportunities dictate. The volume and complexity of these service-related, transactional issues can diminish the time and focus available for the strategic component of the account manager's responsibilities: renewal and expansion of the customer relationship. Renewal of existing customer relationships has become a strategic focus because health plans generally view acquisition of new customers to be as much as four times as costly as the retention of existing customers.

The renewal process for small groups is often established as an auto-renewal. Essentially, in the weeks or months prior to the contract expiration, the small group receives a renewal letter that includes a description of services and pricing. If the expiration date is reached without any action by the small group, the renewal is automatically enacted. If the small group decides to consider changes to the current coverage, the process will resemble large group renewals. The large group renewal process begins with a look back at the results from the previous year, leveraging customer reporting that includes metrics demonstrating the service and value delivered. Based on the retrospective view and the anticipated future needs of the customer, the account manager, distribution partner, and employer discuss changes to benefits and other components of the contract. At times, the employer will issue an RFP to evaluate alternatives to the current health plan relationship. Regardless of whether there is an RFP or not, the consideration and negotiation of the renewal often requires multiple iterations. Similar to the sales process, changes to the specifics of the benefits, products, network, or other contract components typically require reconsideration by underwriting, as well as updated pricing. Upon the successful conclusion of the renewal, account management follows a process similar to sales, with oversight of updates to case installation, second sales, and updates to enrollment. Similar to sales, account management is evaluated based on membership, revenue, and profitability. However, account management is also evaluated based on employer satisfaction, employer retention, and member persistency, which is retention at the member level. Account managers and brokers are compensated, in part, on a composite view of these measures.

Seasonality in the Employer-Sponsored Model

Most employers purchase or renew health insurance on a calendar year, meaning the coverage period begins on January 1. As a result, both the first sale to the employer and the second sale to the employees have busy periods that resemble the peak volumes accountants face during tax season in the United States, as illustrated in **Figure 16-2.** In the case of the "second sale" peak that spans from September to December, health plans supplement the sales force with temporary resources to plan and participate in events such

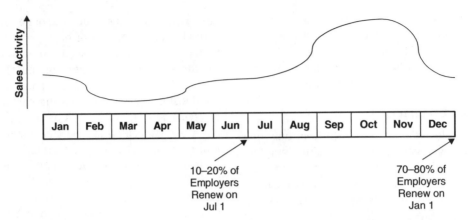

FIGURE 16-2 Seasonality of Sales Activity

as employee benefits fairs. The volume of activity and the inexperience of the team executing the second sale create a significant challenge.

Challenges to Effective Employer-Sponsored Sales

Amid the dynamics changing the employer-sponsored marketplace, health plans must also address more traditional challenges. As noted earlier when addressing marketing, valuable and usable insight around employers, brokers, and members is limited, by comparison to other industries. Driven by limitations in supporting technology, processes, and customer relationships, this gap in turn limits the ability of sales resources to identify solution needs proactively with targeted value propositions. The lack of customer insight also naturally limits the quality of the strategic account planning that is critical to growing customer relationships.

The products, networks, and services that health plans sell are becoming commoditized as employers see less differentiation as they consider health plan options. A significant driver of the commoditization is the lack of a demonstrated, quantifiable value story around services aimed at mitigating health care cost. A recent trend in some markets for narrower networks has the potential for reintroducing network-based market differentiation, but that is not yet the case. Just as is the case with targeted marketing, health plan sales and renewals are often complex, given the array of influences on employer buyers. These influences include their own health care needs or the needs of their dependants, other brokers, consultants, other employers, providers, employees, and governments. These entities often influence employers in divergent directions and there is a significant challenge for health plans to address the diverse employer concerns emanating from these influencers.

Anticipated Changes to Employer-Sponsored Sales

The traditional approach to employer-sponsored sales is changing. By the full enactment of ACA in 2014, assuming the relevant sections go into effect as written, several aspects of the current employer-sponsored sales model will look different. While ACA legislation and related regulatory activity is covered in full in Chapter 30, it is important to note several aspects of health insurance reform as a primary catalyst to anticipated changes to employer-sponsored sales.

State-Sponsored SHOP Insurance Exchanges

As noted earlier, by 2014 employers with 1–100 employees (or 1–50 for plan years beginning before 2016 if a state elects to define the market that way) will be able to purchase group coverage based on a qualified health benefits plan through their respective state's Small Business Health Options Program (SHOP) exchanges. In states that do not or are otherwise unable to create exchanges, the federal government will do so until the state takes it on. While the specifics of the operating models of these SHOP exchanges are still to be determined, the ACA creates a number of requirements around products and customer interactions. The main functions of insurance exchanges under the provisions of the ACA are listed in **Table 16-5**.

The ACA does not prohibit a market outside of SHOP exchanges, and does not require employers to use it. The law does state that any insurer offering coverage through a SHOP exchange must offer at least one Gold- and one Silver-level benefits plan for each product it offers. It is not required to offer Platinum or Bronze, although may elect to do so. An insurer must charge the same premium rates for the same product both inside and outside of an exchange.

The ACA does not require an insurer to offer through the exchange. Just the opposite—a state may prohibit an insurer from offering through the exchange based on several criteria. How this might affect the levels of risk for products sold through an exchange versus products sold exclusively outside of it is unknown. There is also an individual insurance exchange, and states have the option of merging the individual and small group exchanges. After 2017, states will have the option of opening up the exchange to

TABLE 16-5	Main Functions of an Insurance Exchange under the ACA

- Certifying, recertifying, and decertifying health plans offering coverage through the Exchange, called qualified health plans;
- Assigning ratings to each plan offered through the exchange on the basis of relative quality and price;
- Providing consumer information on qualified health plans in a standardized format;
- Creating an electronic calculator to allow consumers to assess the cost of coverage after application of any advance premium tax credits and cost-sharing reductions;
- Operating an Internet website and toll-free telephone hotline offering comparative information on qualified health plans and allowing consumers to apply for and purchase coverage if eligible;
- Determining eligibility for the Exchange, tax credits and cost-sharing reductions for private insurance, and other public health coverage programs, and facilitating enrollment of eligible individuals in those programs;
- Determining exemption from requirements on individuals to carry health insurance, granting approvals to individuals relating to hardship or other exemptions;
- Establishing a navigator program to assist consumers in making choices about their health care options and accessing their new health care coverage, including access to premium tax credits for some consumers; and
- Implementing outreach and education programs and complying with oversight and program integrity requirements.

Source: Adapted from Fact Sheets on Exchanges at HealthCare.gov. Available at: www.healthcare.gov/news/factsheets/exchanges07112011b.html. Accessed August 14, 2011.

businesses larger than 100 employees. Merging these different risk pools could also have a major impact on pricing and profitability for health plans offered through an exchange.

The ACA allows for brokers to sell through an exchange, but does not require it, so what role brokers play in exchanges is likely to vary from state to state as well as over time, and could even eliminate brokers as the primary distribution channel in the small group market. Indeed, SHOP exchanges will introduce an entirely new channel to a small group market segment that has been largely unchanged for decades.

Resegmentation of Markets

It is possible that market segments will be redefined based on exchanges and other provisions in the ACA. For example, the market for small groups could bifurcate into a market reliant on the exchange and one that is completely outside of it. Likewise, insurers that offer products to large and small groups alike might divide into those that serve the small group and individual markets, and those that serve the large and self-funded employer group markets. Only time will tell.

Reduction in the Use of Medical Underwriting

The way risk-based health insurance is priced will fundamentally change for the small group market. Health plans will no longer be able to differentiate rates based on the health status of the employees of prospective small employer group customers. While this may simplify the pricing steps of the sales process, it will introduce a challenge to health plans as leverage alternative methods, including improved analytics and community-based rating, to appropriately price their risk-based products in that market.

The law only requires a single annual open-enrollment period (not counting "life events" as described in Chapter 17), although states may elect to allow more. During periods without open enrollment, medical underwriting could be applicable, although without regulations it is not possible to know at the time of publication. Underwriting in support of risk-based experience premium rates are still allowable in the large group market since the community rating requirement is restricted to small groups and individuals.

Penalties for "Cadillac Plans"

By 2018, employers providing employee health benefits deemed too rich by regulators will be required to pay a material penalty. As a result, many larger employers are beginning a multiyear change to their employee benefit plans to ensure compliance by 2018. Health plans will be looked to as advisors and partners in helping employers successfully make this transition. In addition to these regulatory-driven impacts, there are a few market dynamics that also promise to cause change to employer-sponsored sales, described next.

Defined Contribution and Private Insurance Exchanges

A vast majority of employers provide a "defined health benefit" to employers, meaning the employer pays a portion of a benefit that is defined by the employer and, beginning in 2014, partially defined by the ACA. However, there is a shift occurring in the marketplace, a fast-growing shift toward "defined contribution" products. In the defined contribution model, the employer provides a lump-sum monetary contribution to the employee, who then chooses how to apply the contribution in selecting both medical and ancillary products. A prevalent approach to distribute defined contribution is a private insurance exchange, which is essentially a website that facilitates the employee shopping and buying experience. In some cases, employers directly engage private exchanges and offer employees options across health plans. In other cases, employers purchase from one health plan and employees engage the health plan's exchange to select from products offered by that health plan.

Continued Shift to Retail

As American consumers are exposed to improved experiences with retailers, banks, mobile phone companies, and others, the general expectation of the customer experience is rapidly changing. This trend is causing large employers to demand retail-like experiences for their employees as they engage with health plans. While this will affect member touch points in health-management and back-office functions, it also affects the execution of sales campaigns to employees, including the second sale during open enrollment.

Disruptive Change to Brokers and Agents

Given their uncertain role in the changing small group and individual markets, brokers and agents are reexamining their book of business, looking to diversify with a greater focus on product lines (e.g., ancillary) less affected by regulatory changes. Furthermore, these companies are exploring fee-based, consultative roles they could play in the small group market as commissions decline due to medical loss ratio limitations. Nevertheless, some will not survive this shift as there will be less business in this market. Health plans, heavily dependent on this distribution channel, will need to accelerate efforts to clarify and strengthen their most important broker and agent relationships, even as they mature their capabilities in the emerging direct channels.

Decomposition of the Small Group Market

Given economic challenges and newly established alternatives like the SHOP and individual exchanges, health plans are expecting a reduction in the traditional small group health insurance market by 2014. How much it will decline is the subject of much debate at the time of publication, however. If a state merges the individual and small group exchanges, it would likely accelerate that dynamic since any pricing advantage to remaining a small group would evaporate.* Health plans are focused on proactively converting small groups into defined contribution offerings or products in the expanding individual market.

Sales Processes in the Individual Model

In contrast to the employer-sponsored model, the individual markets generally employ a business-to-consumer "campaign" model in influencing consumers to purchase their respective products and services. The exclusion of the employer, however, does not indicate a purely direct consumer relationship. Brokers and other distribution partners remain relevant in this model as a connection to the consumers they serve. Another key distinction of individual markets

---

*In Massachusetts where exchanges similar to those in the ACA have been operative for several years, the individual market was more expensive than the small group market, and individuals came and went from the risk pool more often than did groups. When they merged the two markets, it increased the costs for small groups.

is that they tend to leverage marketing and customer insight more heavily than the employer-sponsored model does.

Individual market distribution strategies vary widely, due in large part to the vastly different characteristics of various individual consumer segments, ranging from uninsured to early retirees. As a result, health plans leverage a mix of individual market distribution channels, which are briefly described next.

Broker/Agent

The most prevalent distribution channel remains brokers and agents, who typically account for at least half of the individual product sold. Selling through this channel emulates the employer-sponsored selling model for small groups. It is likely to be under even more pressure than the broker and agent channel for small group business once state insurance exchanges are operational.

Web Sales

Online brokers act as Web-based clearinghouses for Web-savvy consumers seeking individual health insurance. In many cases, online brokers receive a commission for an online referral to the health plan's individual website, where the consumer can evaluate insurance options and, in most cases, purchase insurance. Across the health plans in individual markets, there is significant investment in Web sales capabilities, including the website and the functions it supports, such as underwriting and fulfillment. Some health plans intend to mimic the Web sales capabilities of retailers or auto insurers, in terms of the depth and breadth of on-line functionality. Depending on the targeted segment, Web sales tools may be provided directly to consumers or may be distributed to brokers to be used in selling to consumers.

Direct Mail

In the direct mail channel, the prospective members, or leads, are identified through health plan customer insight and segmentation, broker relationships, consumer purchasing organizations, or other sources. Typically, emerging products and services have characteristics that would suit certain consumers better than others. As health plans and their distribution partners apply criteria to prospects, they identify a list of targets for a specific campaign. This list is often delivered to print fulfillment vendors who subsequently distribute campaign materials to consumers.

Telesales

Growing significantly in the individual markets, telesales is similar to the direct mail model, with the exception at fulfillment. Instead of sending a list of targeted consumers to a print fulfillment vendor, the targets are delivered to an internal or external call center. Agents in these call centers contact target consumers telephonically, following a specific script intended to promote the sale of a product or service.

Retail Stores

An emerging individual market sales channel deployed by only a few health plans is the retail store. In this model, health plans set up stores that enable walk-in, in-person purchasing. Sales associates in the retail store consultatively engage the consumer and guide them through the purchase process. In many cases other channels (e.g., Web, mail) are leveraged to stimulate traffic to the retail store.

Challenges to Effective Individual Sales

Beyond the anticipated overhaul of individual markets discussed next, health plans will need to overcome challenges they face in the current model. For example, insight is also critical to direct markets aimed at consumers. Although customer insight is typically more advanced in the individual segments, these insight capabilities generally do not yet enable more advanced "retail" approaches, such as behavioral segmentation.

Although Web sales are viewed as important to the growing individual segments, health plan capabilities are generally immature in comparison to similar cross-industry capabilities such as automobile insurance or retail consumer products. As an example, health plans are not currently able to execute the "real-time" underwriting that is common among automobile insurers.

To a degree exceeding other consumer industries, health plans are burdened by non-ACA regulatory concerns in their pursuit of organic growth. Federal and state governments have various rules that restrict a pure "retail" model, such as the Health Insurance Portability and Accountability Act (HIPAA) regulations (see Chapter 29) that influence the aggregation and sharing of consumer data. These rules and regulations add an additional layer of complexity to health plan sales efforts in the direct markets. This dilemma is likely to only grow as much of the individual market converts to state-based insurance exchanges.

Anticipated Changes to Individual Sales

The individual markets will experience unprecedented growth and transformation by 2014, as this market will be most greatly affected by the ACA and associated regulatory activity. A few of the most important ones are described next.

State Insurance Exchanges

While the existing individual sales model will remain, reform creates the new and materially larger channel of the state-based insurance exchange, which will be the means of distributing health insurance to at least 30 million Americans.

There is still much to be decided by both federal agencies and states in terms of how this new channel will work specifically. The main functions of exchanges have already been provided in Table 16-5 earlier, but certain elements specific to the individual market include:

- *Citizenship validation:* Department of Homeland Security checks and verifies U.S. citizenship, a requirement to purchase insurance on the exchange.
- *Subsidy determination:* The Internal Revenue Service determines subsidy level based on income tax returns.
- *Shopping:* State citizens visit their respective insurance exchanges to begin the insurance purchasing process. On the exchange they are able to view and compare federally defined products offered by state-approved health plans.
- *Enrollment:* When citizens have made their selection, the exchange may direct them to the respective health plan's website for enrollment or the exchange may enable enrollment on the insurance exchange.
- *Navigators:* Exchanges will need to provide navigators to assist individuals in understanding their options and selecting the most appropriate choice. The federal government is also operating a web portal to provide similar information at HealthCare.gov.

Product Design and Implementation Challenges

Federal and state agencies will define and ultimately commoditize the products in this market, but effective health plans will need to have a capability to quickly assimilate to regulatory changes and get to market on time with product changes. Furthermore, designing products and services that are not dictated by regulation, including services like disease management and products such as vision and dental, will be critical to augmenting the revenue and profitability of this segment.

Analytics

Achieving consumer intimacy will surely be challenging in a market with so many unknowns. Yet, effective health plans will develop a consumer segmentation strategy that enables fast-paced dissemination of member data to drive the continuum of activities from retention strategies to disease management interventions to contact center approaches.

Channel Management

States will become a channel partner, in a sense. Health plans will need strong relationship management capabilities in qualifying with states to participate in the insurance exchange. Furthermore, if brokers and agents are allowed to engage as an intermediary for the individual insurance exchanges, health plans will continue to rely heavily on these companies as a primary driver of individual business.

■ CONCLUSION

Health plans face an inflection point as the mandates that will change the industry quickly approach. Which plans will successfully navigate the conversion of much of the profitable, risk-based group and individual marketplace to insurance exchanges? Which plans will deliver on the promise of a retail experience in the health insurance marketplace? Which plans will harness the potential of new, primarily online distribution channels? Which plans will abandon certain markets in order to focus on others? Health plan sales and marketing organizations will have a large role in answering these questions on behalf of their organizations. Whether they take up that challenge or not, the marketing and sales function, for the small group market at least, will undergo more dramatic change than any other operational function in a health plan.

Enrollment and Billing

KARL V. KOVACS, SCOTT McDANIEL, AND PETER R. KONGSTVEDT[*]

STUDY OBJECTIVES

- Understand the different ways in which an individual can be eligible for coverage under employer-sponsored group health plans
- Understand the concept of "life events" and their impact on eligibility in group health coverage
- Understand differences between employer-sponsored group health coverage and individual coverage, and how that will be affected by the Patient Protection and Affordable Care Act (ACA)
- Understand the basic commercial enrollment process
- Understand the basic commercial billing and payment process
- Understand the most basic levels of eligibility and enrollment for Medicare
- Understand the level of complexity involved with Medicaid eligibility

DISCUSSION TOPICS

1. Discuss possible scenarios in which a person's eligibility for group health coverage changes, and how that person should best act in those situations.
2. Discuss how errors can occur in the enrollment and billing process, and how those errors can affect an insurer.
3. Discuss the pros and cons of group health coverage versus individual coverage.
4. Discuss the interplay between commercial coverage, Medicare and Medicaid, and the potential impact of the ACA on that interplay.

◼ INTRODUCTION

Nothing can happen in any payer until it has members enrolled. The first step in that process is determining whether or not an individual is even eligible for coverage in the first place. The enrollment process itself simply means creating a record in the transactional processing system that an individual is eligible for benefits coverage, and links that record to a specific benefits schedule and a specific network of contracted providers. It is the basis for many of the

[*]Portions of this chapter were adapted from proprietary work products created and copyrighted by the P.R. Kongstvedt Company, LLC. It is used with permission and without further attribution. Additionally, information contained in Chapters 21 and 23 was drawn upon for use in sections of this chapter. Information from other chapters is noted as appropriate.

other transactions that take place in a payer organization, including claims processing, member services, and medical management. It is a dynamic process, occurring more than once a year in many cases.

Billing is how a payer organization is itself paid. For insured or at-risk commercial business, bills are generated for premiums. For self-funded or administrative services only (ASO) commercial accounts, bills are for administrative fees only.

Eligibility, enrollment, and billing differ for commercial group coverage, commercial individual coverage, Medicare Advantage, and managed Medicaid plans. All are addressed in this chapter in sequence, but additional detail about eligibility and enrollment rules and regulations are found in Chapter 24 for Medicare Advantage (MA) and Chapter 25 for managed Medicaid.

The Patient Protection and Affordable Care Act (ACA) created a new avenue for enrollment and billing through state-level health insurance exchanges for individuals and small employer groups. Exchanges will not become active until 2014, but when they do, they will add yet another unique approach to enrollment and billing.

This chapter is made up of three major sections: (1) the commercial market, (2) Medicare, and (3) Medicaid. Each addresses the three primary elements of enrollment and billing: (1) eligibility; (2) enrollment, including maintenance; and (3) billing.

■ THE COMMERCIAL MARKET SECTOR

The commercial market sector consists of employer groups and individuals who are not in Medicare or Medicaid. Employer sponsored coverage, which is the most common type of coverage, as discussed in Chapter 2, is typically either insured, meaning the health insurer or health maintenance organization (HMO) is at risk for medical costs, or is self-funded, meaning the employer is at risk for medical costs. Individual coverage is always fully insured, meaning the payer is at risk. Group coverage is discussed first, followed by issues specific to individual coverage.

Eligibility

Eligibility in the commercial market may be thought of in three categories: (1) eligibility in employer-sponsored group benefits plans, (2) eligibility changes based on life events, and (3) individual eligibility.

Eligibility in Employer-Sponsored Group Benefits Plans

Employers are not compelled to offer group health benefits, so employment by itself does not necessarily mean an employee will have coverage. The ACA will create incentives and penalties for some employers if they do not offer coverage, but that is subject to change. Regardless, almost all large employers offer coverage, while even

smaller employers offer coverage as well. If an employer does offer it, coverage cannot discriminate between people based on such things as income, position in the company or health status.

Employer-based coverage is made available to the employee, who can elect to be covered or choose to decline it. Most people elect to be covered, but those who decline it usually do so because they feel they cannot afford the payroll deduction and have no immediate health needs, or else they're covered under another plan such as their spouse's plan. Coverage is typically available for the employee's dependents as well, meaning a spouse and children. Under the ACA, a child can remain on the plan until age 26 if that child does not have any other group coverage available. Disabled adult children are also eligible to be enrolled.

Employers typically have an annual open-enrollment period if they offer more than one plan, which large employer groups almost always do. As noted in Chapter 16, this most often takes place in the fall for an effective date based on the calendar year, but can take place at other times as well. If an employer offers a new plan, it is typically introduced during the open-enrollment period. The annual open-enrollment period is the only time employees can change plans except in the case of life events, which are described shortly. If an employee does change plans, the enrollment process takes place during the open-enrollment period and (hopefully) prior to the effective date.

New employees must enroll within a specific time period after coming on board. In some cases there is a waiting period before a new employee is eligible to join the employer's plan. The length of time a new employee must wait to become eligible varies, but the ACA places a 90-day limit on any waiting periods beginning in 2014. During the period of time a new employee is eligible to enroll, which is typically a 30-day window, they must also enroll their dependents during that same time period if they want them covered too. If they fail to enroll themselves or their dependents during that period, they usually cannot enroll until the next open-enrollment period (discussed below). The exception is for life events, which are discussed next.

Eligibility Changes Based on Life Events

Eligibility may be affected by changes that occur in an employee's life, which is why they are referred to as "life events." It is important that the employee, employer, or agent transmits information related to a life event in a timely manner in order to make sure the benefits and billing are administered properly.

Life events are directly affected by several federal laws. State laws and regulations also affect eligibility and may provide greater protections than federal laws, but not less. These federal laws are discussed more fully in

Chapters 28, 29, and 30, but are listed here for convenience, and their pertinent provisions are noted as appropriate. These laws are:

- The Employee Retirement Income Security Act (ERISA),
- The Consolidated Omnibus Reconciliation Act (COBRA),
- The Health Insurance Portability and Accountability Act (HIPAA),
- The Newborns' and Mothers' Health Protection Act, and
- The ACA.

The U.S. Department of Labor (DOL) provides a resource for health care planning that links a life event with the applicable laws that protect the insured under a job-based health plan. **Table 17-1**, adapted from a fact sheet issued by the U.S. Department of Labor and supplemented by information in Chapter 29, lists the life events and their impact on employment-based health coverage.

Individual Eligibility

Except for individual eligibility associated with life events, individual eligibility varies a great deal from state to state, but only until 2014. Prior to 2014, individuals remain subject to medical underwriting in most cases, meaning they must

TABLE 17-1	Life Events' Impact on Health Benefits and Eligibility

Marriage

- HIPAA offers special enrollment rights for employees and spouses that allow them to enroll in a group health plan upon marriage and provides protections for individuals who have preexisting conditions or might suffer discrimination on the basis of health status when they switch plans.
- ERISA Disclosure Provisions provide individuals with rights to important information concerning benefits under their own or spouse's group health plan.

Birth or Adoption of a Child

- HIPAA prohibits preexisting condition exclusions from being applied to pregnancy, regardless of whether the mother had previous health coverage. In addition, HIPAA does not permit preexisting condition exclusions to be applied to newborns and adopted children who enroll within 30 days of birth or adoption.
- HIPAA also offers special enrollment rights for employees, spouses, and new dependents, allowing them to enroll in a group health plan upon birth, adoption, or placement for adoption.
- ERISA Claims Procedures help ensure timely and fair review of maternity and other claims under group health plans.
- The Newborns' and Mothers' Health Protection Act includes important new protections for mothers and their newborn children with regard to the lengths of hospital stays following the birth of a child.

Job Change or Loss

- COBRA generally requires that most group health plans of employers with at least 20 employees offer employees and their dependents the opportunity to continue their health plan coverage for limited periods of time when the employee loses his or her job or has a reduction in hours that would result in a loss of coverage. There is a 60-day window to accept coverage under COBRA. COBRA coverage is usually limited to 18 months, except for disabled individuals and people who've lost coverage due to divorce or death of their spouse, who may be covered for up to 36 months.
- HIPAA protects individuals who have preexisting conditions, helping them to keep coverage for those conditions or get coverage for them in no more than 12 or 18 months through limits on the length of preexisting condition exclusions. HIPAA also helps individuals who might suffer discrimination in health coverage on the basis of health status when they change jobs. Coverage under HIPAA is also available to people whose coverage under COBRA has run out, but only if they have had at least 18 months of continuous coverage.

Coverage for Family and Loved Ones

- ERISA permits a parent to obtain a court order to provide coverage for children under the noncustodial parent's health plan (called a qualified medical child support order).
- ERISA Disclosure Provisions help to ensure that individuals covered by group health plans receive clear information about their rights, benefits, and obligations under the plan, including information about COBRA continuation coverage, access to urgent or specialized care, and composition of physician and other provider networks.
- HIPAA includes protections for newborns and adopted children with preexisting conditions. Specifically, HIPAA does not permit a preexisting condition exclusion to be applied to a newborn or adopted child who enrolls within 30 days of birth or adoption.
- The ACA allows parents to continue their adult children on their medical plan up until age 26 if the adult child does not have access to group coverage through their employment.
- ERISA and the ACA's Claims Procedures help ensure timely and fair review of plan denials of claims.

continues

TABLE 17-1	(Continued)

Coverage Loss Due to Divorce or Death of a Spouse

- COBRA generally requires that group health plans of employers with at least 20 employees offer spouses and dependent children the opportunity to continue their health care coverage for limited periods of time in the event of the spouse's legal separation or divorce from or death of the employee covered by the plan. COBRA coverage in these situations may be extended for up to 36 months.
- HIPAA offers special enrollment rights, generally allowing employees and dependents who were covered under a spouse's plan to obtain coverage under the employee's plan upon legal separation, divorce, or death, if they are otherwise eligible.

Coverage in Later Years

- HIPAA offers protections for individuals who have preexisting conditions, helping them to keep coverage for those conditions or get coverage in no more than 12 or 18 months through limits on preexisting condition exclusions.
- HIPAA includes protections to help ensure individuals are not excluded from coverage under their group health plan or charged a higher premium based on health status.
- COBRA generally requires that group health plans of employers with at least 20 employees offer employees and their dependents the opportunity to continue their health plan coverage for limited periods of time when the employee loses his or her job due to retirement.
- ERISA Claims Procedures help ensure a fair and timely appeals process for covered individuals.
- ERISA Disclosure Provisions require that group health plan disclosure material furnished to plan participants and beneficiaries must contain information about specialists in the plan network and the plan's rules for accessing specialty care.
- ERISA Disclosure Provisions also require that plan disclosure material must describe the ability of the employer to reduce plan benefits or terminate the plan.

Source: Adapted from the United States Department of Labor, Employee Benefits Security Administration Fact Sheet on Life Events, www.dol.gov/ebsa/newsroom/fshealthy.html. and An Employer's Guide to Group Health Continuation Coverage Under COBRA, www.dol.gov/ebsa/publications/cobraemployer.html#WhoIsEntitledtoContinuationCoverage. Accessed July 29, 2011; and Chapter 29, "Federal Regulation of Health Insurance and Managed Health Care."

be free of any medical conditions. Individual applicants must fill out a medical questionnaire and agree to allow the insurer to obtain copies of their medical records. Sometimes an insurer will require an applicant to have a physical examination and some basic tests done as well.

Individuals who cannot obtain insurance because of medical underwriting may still have options, however. Thirty-four states have "high-risk pools" that provide limited coverage for individuals with significant health needs.[*] Also, some states require certain health insurers to have an annual open-enrollment period in which any applicant must be accepted, known as guaranteed issue. The majority of states do not require this, but of those that do, it may be confined to a state's nonprofit Blue Cross and Blue Shield plan(s) or nonprofit HMOs or may be required of all insurers.[†] Coverage under guaranteed issue may also be subject to children only, or as an "insurer of last resort," meaning the individual must have unsuccessfully sought coverage elsewhere.

As discussed in detail in Chapter 30 as well as in Chapter 16, the ACA will change individual eligibility rules and regulations effective January 2014. At that time,

guaranteed issue will be required of all insurers and HMOs, and individuals will be able to access coverage through new state health insurance exchanges. The ACA only requires states to have an annual open-enrollment period, so access may be confined to as brief a period as 30 days, but it could be longer if the state so chooses.

The Commercial Enrollment Process

Commercial enrollment applies to employer-sponsored group benefits plans and to individuals, so are addressed in that order.

Enrollment in Employer Sponsored Group Benefits Plans

As noted earlier here and discussed in detail in Chapter 16, large employers offering more than one plan hold annual open-enrollment periods, when employees can choose among the options. Smaller employers or any employer that offers only one plan may not have an annual open enrollment per se, but will still adjust benefits and rates on an annual basis. Open enrollment typically takes place in the months preceding the renewal or change of coverage. The majority of coverage renewals and changes occur on January 1, so the majority of employer open-enrollment periods occur in the fall. In the case of a new sale by a payer, enrollment takes place during that same open-enrollment period.

The first step in the enrollment process is modifying or setting up the account, which must be done prior to the employer's open-enrollment period. When an employer group is

---

[*] Kaiser Family Foundation, State Health Facts, www.statehealthfacts.org/comparetable.jsp?ind = 602&cat = 7&sub = 89. Accessed August 21, 2011.

[†] Kaiser Family Foundation, State Health Facts, www.statehealthfacts.org/comparetable.jsp?ind = 353&cat = 7. Accessed August 21, 2011.

a new account, this means entering all relevant information and creating the records for that account. For existing groups, only information that needs to be changed is modified, such as the benefits package and rates. In either case, it is typically carried out through a manual entry process.

Very high-level examples of account information include:

- All necessary contact information;
- Billing information, including
  - Contact name, address, and telephone number(s),
  - Type of billing,
  - Bank routing numbers if appropriate;
- Appropriate identifiers such as employer tax ID number(s);
- The employer group's industry code, using either the Standard Industrial Classification (SIC) Codes or the North American Industry Classification System (NAICS) Codes;
- The specific benefits plan and any modifications;
- Insured versus self-funded;
- If insured, premium rates by category, of which there may be many variations, including
  - Employee-only,
  - Employee plus spouse,
  - Employee plus child,
  - Employee plus children,
  - Family (employee, spouse, children, and dependents);
- If self-funded, recording various options, including
  - Specific services being administered,
  - Pricing,
  - Reinsurance information, and
  - Bank routing numbers;
- Effective dates of coverage.

Enrollment of employees creates a record for each employee, indicating that the individual is covered under their employer's benefits plan; covered dependents are also recorded in this record. In group coverage, the employee is the subscriber, while any covered dependents plus the employee are referred to as members. The subscriber record includes information such as:

- The employee's demographic information, including
  - Name;
  - Address;
  - Telephone number(s), including home, office, and mobile;
  - E-mail address(es);
  - Date of birth;
  - Gender;
  - Social Security number;
  - Contact information; and
  - Other identifiers;
- Any employment subgroup the employer uses, such as a specific subsidiary;

- The specific benefits plan applicable to the employee;
- The specific provider network associated with the employee's benefits plan;
- Effective date(s) of coverage;
- Dependent demographic information;
- Primary care physician selection in the case of some HMOs; and
- Any other coverage in place, such as coverage through their spouse's group benefits plan (to support Coordination of Benefits, discussed in Chapter 18).

The goal of the enrollment process is to create records for new employees or revise existing records before the coverage period starts or changes. However, it is inevitable that some information will arrive late, so any enrollment process must provide for retroactive enrollment. Retroactivity is often limited to a defined time period such as 3 months; however, it can make reconciliation of enrollment, claims payments, and coverage adjustments a real headache.

Enrollment was once heavily dependent on paper forms. In the past decade this has changed, and now electronic transactions are the norm, at least for large employers. In many cases, the enrollment information is recorded in the employer's system and transmitted to the payer electronically. This may be done through a secure line or Internet channel or on magnetic tape. Even smaller groups often enroll through a secure Internet portal, creating an electronic record on the spot.

As addressed in Chapter 23, covered entities such as payers are required to use certain standardized transactions as mandated under HIPAA's Administrative Simplification rules. Among these standard transactions are the American National Standards Institute (ANSI) X12 834, Benefit Enrollment and Maintenance Set. However, only covered entities are required to use the 834, not employers, so they often do not. The ACA requires new eligibility and enrollment transaction standards to supplement the 834, and also requires its use to be more widespread, so this will eventually truly become standard.

Paper enrollment forms are typically scanned into the system using optical character recognition software. The resulting electronic record is then reviewed manually to ensure its accuracy and correct any errors. Larger payers usually outsource this, often to an offshore company with low labor costs. The actual paper form remains with the payer, however, and the manual review is done using an image.

Errors in enrollment can cause significant problems for any payer. Examples of the kinds of problems encountered with enrollment errors include:

- Paying claims on somebody who is no longer covered or not yet eligible for coverage;
- Not paying claims on somebody who is supposed to be covered;

- Incorrect premium or administration payments to the payer, requiring later reconciliation;
- Improper calculation of capitation payments (Chapter 5); and
- The need to make after-the-fact adjustments with providers.

In all cases, correcting the errors and problems caused by enrollment errors is usually manual and costly. It also results in unhappy members and customers.

Enrollment in Individual Coverage

For individual enrollment, the process is more manual, at least for the subscriber. Individual coverage is almost always only for the subscriber, but under the ACA, individuals will be able to purchase family coverage beginning in 2014. Many insurers and HMOs provide a secure and user-friendly portal to individuals for entering the information. Paper enrollment forms are handled as described earlier.

Fulfillment

Fulfillment occurs after enrollment is completed. It refers to the creation of identification (ID) cards and distribution of material to members. Some large groups want to handle fulfillment on their own, through their own intranet, for example, while others have the payer do it. Payers always do it for individual coverage. Some or all of this may be outsourced.

The ID card is the most tangible connection between the member and the payer. In addition to demographic information, it contains information such as:

- Name
  - The member's name in many plans and all HMOs,
  - Only the subscriber's (employee's) name in some plans with older systems, or
  - The subscriber's name and all dependents' names;
- The group number;
- The policy number;
- Cost-sharing information, including
  - Copays,
  - Coinsurance, and
  - Deductibles;
- Pharmacy information, including
  - Name of the pharmacy benefits manager (PBM),
  - Pharmacy benefit numbers, and
  - Pharmacy-only cost-sharing and tiering;
- The provider network, if applicable;
- The name of the member's primary care physician in some HMOs;
- Plan contact information for customer service, and
- Additional telephone numbers as applicable, such as
  - Specialty services such as behavioral health, or
  - Nurse advice lines.

Member materials include such items as

- Member handbooks;
- Evidence (or certificate) of coverage (EOC); and
- The new Summary of Coverage (SOC) required under the ACA.

Distribution used to be entirely on paper, but electronic distribution is increasing in popularity. However, even if electronic distribution is the primary means of fulfillment, members have a right to paper copies upon demand.

The new health insurance exchanges under the ACA have fulfillment requirements, but at the time of publication it is not known how this will work or how it will apply to what any participating insurers or HMOs do.

Billing and Payment in Employer-Sponsored Groups

Billing and payment in employer-sponsored group coverage refers to the payer billing the employer, not the subscriber. It is applicable to billing for premiums and to billing for administrative fees for self-funded accounts. As discussed in Chapter 21, premiums account for the majority of money that comes in to a payer, far exceeding administrative fees that are a fraction of the cost of premiums. But in either case, it is the only way a payer is itself paid.

Billing takes place before the period of time it is applicable; in other words, bills are sent out for the coming month, and is typically highly automated. The premiums are developed as described in detail in Chapter 22, and, as already noted, that information is entered into the employer group record. The system pulls information from that employer record, and then from each employee's enrollment record, including the benefit package selected and spouse/dependent count. The information is summarized, listing the number of subscribers at each benefit level and its associated premium. A detailed list of names is also available to assist the employer in reconciling the bill. Premium billing also generates an accounts receivable record.

Premium bills can be distributed electronically with electronic funds transfer (EFT) to accept payment in a paperless fashion. Payment can be automatically posted to the system. The HIPAA-mandated standardized ANSI X12 for Payroll Deducted and other group Premium Payment for Insurance Products is the 820, and it can be used to make a premium payment for insurance products. Currently, employers are not required to use it, although payers must accept it and banks routinely accept it as well.

There are two broad ways billing takes place: self-billing and retroactive billing. Self-billing means the employer adjusts the billing invoice for changes in enrollment. It means the amount billed and recorded as receivable revenue will not be the same as what is actually paid by the employer group. This means the account must be adjusted each time. Advance notification by the employer can prevent the need to continually adjust the ledger. In any case, enrollment records under self-billing need to be modified as soon as the information is received. Some large employers do this themselves through direct access to the payer's enrollment module. Retroactive billing means that any adjustments are made on the next month's bill, even though changes in enrollment are recorded as soon as they are received.

Enrollment and billing must be regularly reconciled. Small errors can add up, and even when corrected it may not lead to proper billing. Many large employers require detailed information and perform their own reconciliations. Errors in billing are almost always directly associated with errors in enrollment, although there are other reasons they can occur. Employer systems also make errors. For that reason, payers and employers regularly reconcile enrollment records and billing and payment records.

Billing and Payment for Individual Coverage

Billing information is captured during the enrollment process for individual coverage. Insurers and HMOs often offer automated direct pay through EFT from the person's bank, or they may bill a credit card company. Electronic bills are typically offered, and paper bills are routinely offered as well. Many insurers require individuals to pay 3 months at a time, but the ACA may affect that.

Employer Group and Member Self-Service

Secure Internet portals for groups and individuals allow them to access such things as billing information, employee updates and changes, advice on creating a healthier workplace or personal environment, and benefit documentation. Various resources are provided, including Web-based training, administrative and instructional documents and forms, and URLs that link the employer group and member to various sites that provide provider network information, drug formularies, health promotion activities, and other insurer information.

Members have the ability to use the member portal to review various items that may include their benefit package, health promotion resources including health assessment options, eligibility, ordering additional ID cards, copayment or deductible balances, claims, and evidence of benefit statements. This functionality has become more important with the increase in consumer-directed and high-deductible benefits plans. In addition, the individual may call or visit customer service to deal with any issues or questions.

Health Insurance Exchanges

As discussed in Chapters 16 and 30, the ACA requires states to develop health insurance exchanges, but also gives them certain flexibility. On January 1, 2014, the exchanges are to be operational either through a state-operated exchange or a federal exchange if the state does not have an operational exchange. The ACA provides direction for the development of two exchanges: the individual

exchange and a Small Business Health Options Program (SHOP) exchange. Draft rules for exchanges have been promulgated and responses were due in September 2011, so are not available at the time of publication. Planning grants have been made available to the states to develop exchanges. At the time of this writing, legislatures in 13 states have passed legislation to establish exchanges and 26 have not.

In the individual exchange, individuals and families may be enrolled in a qualified health plan (QHP) that is approved by the exchange. Exchanges will be responsible for implementing tax credits and reduced cost-sharing options when appropriate. The states will have broad flexibility in the structure of the exchange. While needing to foster direct competition on price and quality, the exchange may implement either active or passive contracting with the QHPs. The exchange may utilize an "any willing and qualified" QHP approach; engage in selected contracting or have insurers bid for selection; or negotiate on a case-by-case basis. In addition, ACA requires coordination between the exchange and Medicaid.

The exchange will also provide grants to navigators who will conduct outreach and assist individuals and small groups in the enrollment process. While this discussion only presents a brief review of exchanges, there are aspects of the exchange that may impact the current individual and small group market and potentially the large group market in 2017. The exchange may provide a replacement for the individual portals currently available through insurers and agents. Agents may be replaced by the SHOP exchange and there may be a potential role change for agents in their relationship with large businesses.

■ MEDICARE

This section of the chapter focuses on enrollment for Medicare and its four parts in order to set the stage for Chapter 24's deeper look at the enrollment process for Medicare Advantage (MA) plans, also known as Medicare Part C. Medicare was addressed briefly in Chapter 1 and in depth in Chapter 24, and the reader is referred to those chapter for additional specifics about the Medicare program.

Enrollment: Stage One

In order to enroll in Medicare, the individual must first make application for Medicare to the Social Security Administration (SSA).[1] The SSA controls the enrollment for Social Security retirement benefits and enrollment for Medicare; however, the application for retirement benefits is not a requirement in applying for Medicare. The SSA has provided a website at www.socialsecurity.gov/info/isba/retirement/ to allow beneficiaries to enroll online. For those not wanting to apply over the Internet, the SSA provides 800 telephone access or the individual can apply at a local SSA office.

The Four Parts of Medicare

Title XVIII of the Social Security Act is Health Insurance for the Aged and Disabled and is made up of four parts.[2]

Part A: Hospital Insurance

Most citizens or permanent residents of the United States who are age 65 or older are eligible for premium-free Medicare hospital insurance known as Medicare Part A. Some are eligible if they meet requirements for time spent receiving Social Security disability benefits or are receiving a disability pension from the railroad retirement board. The regulations for Part A provide more specific information on who qualifies, including government workers, spouses, and children. There is also a regulation that allows a person to purchase Part A if the basic requirements for free Part A are not met. Part A coverage includes inpatient hospital care, skilled nursing facility care, hospice care, and home health care.

Part B: Supplementary Medical Insurance Benefits

If an individual is eligible for premium-free Medicare Part A hospital insurance, he or she can enroll in Medicare Part B medical insurance by paying a monthly premium.[3] Services covered under Part B include medically necessary services, physicians' services, and other medical services and supplies. The ACA also added the full array of preventive and wellness benefits to Medicare. If an individual is not eligible for premium-free Part A, he or she can buy Part B by paying a monthly premium if age and residency requirements are met.

Part C: Medicare Advantage*

The Balanced Budget Act of 1997 was passed in part to control the growth of Medicare spending and to offer Medicare beneficiaries choices for care through private health plans. Individuals eligible for Medicare Parts A and B were eligible to receive their health care services through the Medicare + Choice Program. With the passage of the Medicare Modernization Act in 2003, Medicare + Choice was renamed the MA Program. An MA plan must meet the regulatory requirements of the Centers for Medicare and Medicaid Services (CMS) to be eligible to enroll Part A and Part B beneficiaries.[4] Beneficiary choices include:

- Medicare HMO Plans,
- Medicare Preferred Provider Organization (PPO) Plans,
- Medicare Private Fee-for-Service (PFFS) Plans, and
- Medicare Special Needs Plans (SNPs).

---

*Formerly called Medicare + Choice.

Beneficiaries enrolled in an MA plan who decide to disenroll can enroll in original Medicare from January 1 until February 14.

Part D: Medicare Prescription Drug Plans

Individuals who have Medicare Parts A and B or are enrolled in a MA plan (Part C), are eligible to enroll in Part D for prescription drug coverage. The beneficiary may wait to enroll in Part D but the timing of enrollment and having other prescription coverage are important factors for the beneficiary to consider. Medicare extracts a penalty payment if the beneficiary does not enroll in the appropriate enrollment period.

Paying for Medicare

Medicare is not completely free to the beneficiary and is funded through a combination of sources. Part of the funding comes from a portion of the payroll taxes paid by workers and their employers; monthly premiums deducted from Social Security checks and premiums, coinsurance, and copays and deductibles paid by the Medicare beneficiary. The Federal Insurance Contributions Act (FICA) consists of two parts: the 6.2% Social Security Tax and the 1.45% Medicare tax. Both the employee and the employer must pay these taxes. The Social Security portion is based on the Social Security wage base and contributions are stopped when the employee meets that wage base. There is no wage base or limitation for the Medicare tax.

For Part A in 2011 the beneficiary's deductible is as follows:

- Days 1–60: $1,132 deductible
- Days 61–90: $283 coinsurance each day
- Days 91 and beyond: $566 coinsurance per each "lifetime reserve day" after day 90 for each benefit period (up to 60 days over your lifetime)
- Beyond lifetime reserve days: all costs
- Inpatient mental health care in a psychiatric hospital is limited to 190 days in a lifetime

In 2011 the beneficiary's annual deductible for Part B is $162. After the deductible is paid, the coinsurance for part B services is generally 20% and may be based on the billed amount, allowed amount, or a preset rate for service depending on the service type. In the case of outpatient mental health care, the beneficiary pays 20% of the Medicare-approved amount for services to diagnose or monitor the beneficiary's condition. The beneficiary pays 45% of the Medicare-approved amount for treatment services.

Dual Eligibles with Medicare and Medicaid

While some may confuse Medicare for Medicaid and vice versa, the two are very different programs that, however, intersect in some circumstances. Medicaid is the health program under Title XIX of the Social Security Act for low-income individuals and families. Chapter 25 provides a thorough review of Medicaid Managed Care. There are times when a Medicaid recipient also qualifies for Medicare. In this instance the individual may receive assistance in paying Medicare premiums, deductibles, co-insurance, and copays through the state's Medicare Savings Program. There are four Medicare Savings Programs for dual eligibles:

- Qualified Medicare Beneficiary (QMB)
- Specified Low-Income Medicare Beneficiary (SLMB)
- Qualifying Individual (QI)
- Qualified Disabled and Working Individual (QDWI)

In order to limit its liability for health care costs, the state Medicaid program may participate in the Medicare Buy-In program. In order to save state funds, it may "buy-in" for Medicare coverage for certain Medicaid eligibles. States may receive lists of Medicare eligibles from CMS and compare it to their list of Medicaid eligibles. The state may choose to buy either Part A and/or Part B for the Medicaid recipient. This is a cost-saving measure for the state because Medicare is the primary insurer in that it pays first on a claim. The state must have a claims payment system that adjudicates the claims with coordination of benefits, sometimes referred to in general as third-party liability. Coordination of benefits does not just occur for the "dual eligibles" with Medicaid and Medicare coverage but for other instances when a Medicare or Medicaid beneficiary has other insurance.

If the beneficiary has limited income and resources, they may qualify for assistance from Medicare for Part D. This is referred as low-income subsidy (LIS) by Medicare.

Medicare Information Technology: MARx

The information technology application that supports Parts C and D of Medicare as well as beneficiary payments is the Medicare Advantage and Prescription Drug system, referred to as MARx. In December 2010, CMS issued a letter to MA organizations, Medicare Prescription Drug Plans (PDPs), Programs for All Inclusive Care for the Elderly (PACE), and other health care organizations that use the MARx system, announcing the MARx System Redesign and Modernization software release in April 2011. Enclosed in the letter to the above organizations was the *MARx Redesign and Modernization Handbook.*[5]

The handbook represents the modifications and functionality added to the MARx application. The handbook provides insights into the MARx improvements, highlighting enrollment transaction codes, the transaction calendar, cancellation transactions, reply reports, residence reporting, and the plan user interface. The MARx user interface (UI) is the vehicle for information exchange between CMS and the MA plan using transaction type codes (TCs) and transaction reply codes (TRCs).

Eligibility for Medicare Advantage

An individual is eligible to enroll in an MA plan if they meet the following requirements:

- Entitled to Medicare Part A and enrolled in Part B and must be entitled to Medicare Part A and Part B benefits as of the effective date of coverage under the plan;
- Does not have end-stage renal disease (ESRD);
- Permanently resides in the service area of the MA plan;
- The individual or their legal representative completes an enrollment request;
- Agrees to abide by the rules of the MA plan;
- Makes a valid enrollment request during an enrollment period; and
- If requesting enrollment in a Special Needs Plan (SNP), the individual must meet the additional requirements for the SNP.

Medicare Advantage Enrollment

The application for enrolling in an MA plan is referred to as an "enrollment request." This enrollment request (ER) must be completed by the eligible individual or their legal representative. In addition, the ER must be provided to the MA plan within the required timeframes and during a valid enrollment period. There are other means of enrollment as well that include an optional employer/union enrollment request mechanism; passive enrollment by CMS; and group enrollment for employer- or union-sponsored plans.

MA organizations that offer MA plans to employers or unions may agree, but are not required, to accept voluntary enrollment requests from the employer or union without requiring a written enrollment request from the individual.

Passive enrollment occurs when CMS determines that continued enrollment in a certain MA plan would pose possible harm. In this instance, the beneficiary is changed to another MA plan and is considered to have made the enrollment request without taking action.

Group enrollment for employer- or union-sponsored group health plans is allowed by CMS. As long as there is advance notice to the employee/union member and CMS receives other insurance information for the population, the process is permissible.

Election Periods

The various election periods are described in Chapter 24, so are only noted here:[6]

- The annual election period (AEP),
- The initial coverage election period (ICEP),
- Open-enrollment period for institutionalized individuals (OEPI), and
- Special election period (SEP).

Enrollment Procedures

In order to make the enrollment process user-friendly and widely accessible, CMS requires that the MA plans accept enrollment requests in various formats. Enrollment requests can be made through face-to-face interviews, through the mail, by facsimile, or other methods defined by CMS. Enrollment may occur also by way of auto-facilitated enrollment, discussed later in this section. Within 10 calendar days of the receipt of the ER, the MA plan is required to acknowledge the request, request additional information if needed, or issue a denial of the ER.

Prior to the AEP, the MA plan is prohibited from soliciting or accepting ERs on paper, via telephone, or by way of the Internet. CMS expects that the MA plan, its brokers and agents, notify beneficiaries of this requirement. Recognizing that, regardless of the information provided by the MA plan, its brokers and agents, there will be enrollment requests submitted before the AEP. CMS has promulgated procedures on how MA plans are to process these enrollment requests using MARx. The MA plan must submit all transactions to the CMS systems (MARx) on the first day of the AEP with an "application date" of the same date.

The ER form must meet criteria stipulated by CMS and model forms have been developed by CMS for MA plans as well as a model short enrollment form. There is also a model plan selection mechanism for ERs in a beneficiary's enrollment in another plan offered by the same MA organization as well as a model EGHP enrollment mechanism. The enrollment mechanism must include the following acknowledgments by the applicant to:

- Continue to keep Parts A and B,
- Abide by the MA plan's rules,
- Consent to the disclosure and exchange of information necessary for the MA plan to operate,
- Participate in only one MA plan, and
- The right to appeal service and payment denials made by the MA plan.

Enrollment through the Internet

MA plans may offer enrollment through a secure Internet website. All CMS guidelines, including CMS' Internet security policies, must be followed for the enrollment process, website, and marketing materials. Applicants must be informed that they are participating in the online enrollment process and all CMS required information must be obtained. CMS provides another Internet method for enrolling. Beneficiaries can access the Medicare Online Enrollment Center (OEC) through the www.medicare.gov website.

Enrollment by Telephone

MA plans may allow telephonic enrollment, but the telephone call must originate with the beneficiary and no agent or representative must be present with the beneficiary during the call. The beneficiary must be advised that they are in the process of enrolling. The MA plan must inform the beneficiary that the telephone call is being recorded, obtain the beneficiaries consent and the beneficiary must attest to their intent to enroll. In addition, beneficiaries may contact the 1-800-MEDICARE call center.

Seamless Conversion and Auto-Facilitated Enrollment

For new MA eligibles, CMS allows MA plans to offer a seamless MA enrollment for individuals enrolled in the organization's commercial or Medicaid Health Plans at the time of the beneficiary's conversion to Medicare.

Auto-facilitated enrollment applies to MA plans that offer both MA-PD and MA-only plans. CMS requires that the plans have a process for auto-facilitated enrollment for LIS-eligible individuals who select a MA plan without Medicare prescription drug benefits. The LIS individual will be auto-facilitated enrolled into an MA-PD plan or into a PDP offered by the same organization. The individual has the right to decline enrollment.

Processing the Enrollment Request

During a face-to-face enrollment, the MA plan should use the person's Medicare card to verify critical data elements, including the health insurance claim number, entitlement dates, and so on. In the case of mailed or faxed ERs, the information should be verified either over the phone or by some other means or by having the beneficiary include a copy of their Medicare card with their application. Medicare provides a list of items required to consider an ER complete, such as permanent residence, entitlement information, effective date of coverage, attestations, and a signature and the date. CMS prohibits the MA plan from asking any health-related questions except for determining the ESRD status of the individual. MA personnel may not fill out the form on behalf of the beneficiary.

As part of ER processing, the MA plan must provide the individual with the option to (1) pay plan premiums by being billed directly by the plan or (2) have the premiums withheld from their SSA benefit check. The MA plan may offer other options such as monthly deductions from a bank savings account.

In the event that the ER is incomplete, the MA plan must notify the beneficiary of the needed information and maintain an audit trail explaining why the ER was deemed incomplete. Denial of an ER is required within 10 days of receipt of the ER. For those ERs that were determined incomplete, the denial must occur within 10 days of the expiration of the timeframe for the beneficiary to send the needed information.

In matters of ESRD, if the individual no longer requires regular dialysis or has had a kidney transplant, the individual should be instructed to send medical information to the MA plan as stipulated by CMS.

Transmitting Enrollments to CMS

The MA plan is required to send the enrollment information to CMS within 7 calendar days after receipt of the completed ER. The enrollment request receipt date is considered day zero. Enrollments are to be processed in chronological order of the day of receipt by the MA plan.

Information Sent to the Member

The MA plan is required to send certain information to the member before the effective date of coverage. However, there is certain information that can be sent after the member's effective date of coverage. Prior to the effective date of coverage the MA plan must send its rules, member's rights and responsibilities, and a copy of the paper enrollment request in the case of a paper ER or evidence that the Internet ER was received such as a confirmation number.

Within 10 days of the receipt of the ER, the MA plan must provide an acknowledgment of receipt of the ER with the effective day of coverage and proof of coverage. The proof of coverage may take the form of an identification card or a notice or letter to the member. The MA plan must inform the member of any cost for which they will be responsible such as premiums, co-pays, and fees; the disclosure authorization provided by the member; the "lock-in" to receive services through the MA plan; and the prospect of member financial responsibility for services received due to the member not meeting the requirement for Parts A and B entitlement.

After the effective date of coverage, the MA plan may send out all required information in instances where the enrollment request was received late in the month. The information must be transmitted within 10 days of the receipt of the ER. The MA plans are encouraged by CMS to contact these members by telephone within 1 to 3 days to provide the member with their effective date of coverage, MA plan rules, and information on how to access services.

Voluntary Disenrollment by the Member

Members may request disenrollment only during one of the election periods noted above and in Chapter 24. The member may disenroll by enrolling in another MA plan, by giving or faxing a written notice to the MA plan or through their employer or union, submitting the disenrollment via the Internet to the MA plan if the plan has that functionality, or by calling 1-800-MEDICARE. When the MA plan receives a verbal request to disenroll, the plan should direct the member to use one of the above mechanisms.

In the case of disenrollment requests sent via the Internet, the MA plan must have sufficient identification, authentication, and encryption protocols to ensure privacy. Written requests must contain the signature of the member or their legal representative. The MA plan is also responsible for determining the effective date of disenrollment and of notifying the member within 10 days of the receipt of the request and reminding the member that the lock-in provision remains in effect until the effective date of disenrollment.

MA plans that voluntarily offer employer/union MA plans the option to receive enrollment from the employer or union can also offer the option to disenroll through the employer, union, or their third party administrator. CMS also provides a process for group disenrollment from an employer- or union-sponsored MA plan.

Involuntary Disenrollment

There are instances when the MA plan must disenroll a member. These include:

- A change in residence, including incarceration, that makes the member no longer eligible to be served by the plan;
- Loss of entitlement to Parts A and B;
- In the case of a SNP, the member no longer meets the requirements for participation;
- Death of the member; or
- Termination of the MA plan's contract or a reduction in the MA plan's service area that makes the member no longer eligible.

Optional Involuntary Disenrollment

The MA plan may, but is not required, to disenroll members for the following reasons:

- Failure to pay premiums on a timely basis,
- Disruptive behavior, or
- Fraud committed as part of the enrollment request or allowing improper use of the identification card.

Processing Voluntary Disenrollments

The MA plan must have a system in place for receiving, processing, and tracking disenrollment requests according to CMS guidance. The MA plan is responsible for transmitting the disenrollment to CMS within 7 days of receipt of the completed disenrollment request.

Employer-/Union-Sponsored Disenrollments

This occurs when either the contract between the employer or union group and the MA plan are terminated or the member loses eligibility. In either instance the notification of disenrollment sent to the MA plan must be proactive and not retroactive.

Cancellations

Cancellations may be needed when a beneficiary mistakenly enrolls or disenrolls from the MA plan. CMS stipulates that a beneficiary may do this only prior to the effective date of the enrollment or disenrollment.

Reinstatements

If a disenrollment is not legally valid, reinstatement may be appropriate. The most common reasons for reinstatements are due to an erroneous death indicator, erroneous loss of Parts A and B, mistaken disenrollment, and plan error.

Retroactive Enrollments and Disenrollments

If the beneficiary has fulfilled the enrollment requirement, but the MA plan is not able to process the ER in a timely manner, CMS will process a retroactive enrollment. For enrollments that were not legally valid or were valid but not processed due to plan or system error, CMS may allow a retroactive disenrollment. Retroactive disenrollments may be submitted by the plan or the beneficiary.

In those instances where the MA plan has a contract with an employer/union group health plan (EGHP) and the EGHP processes enrollment, there may be a delay in the transmission of enrollment from the EGHP to the MA plan. CMS allows retroactive transactions for routine delays. For EGHP disenrollments, the MA plan must submit the disenrollment to CMS even if it has not received timely notice from the EGHP. Up to 90 days' payment adjustment is possible in this situation.

Storage of Enrollment and Disenrollment Record

Under the Code of Federal Regulations (42 CFR 422.60(c)(2)), MA plans must retain all enrollment and disenrollment records for the current year and for 10 prior years. CMS is flexible in terms of the storage medium as long as it allows access to signed forms and other enrollment requests.

■ MEDICAID

Medicaid is discussed in detail in Chapter 25. For purposes of completeness, this chapter summarizes only the highlights. Medicaid eligibility is more complicated than Medicare or Commercial eligibility. A joint federal and state program, Medicaid eligibility requirements vary from state to state. Most states include the Children's Health Insurance Program (CHIP, or sometimes S-CHIP) in their Medicaid benefits. Many states provide additional benefits through waivered programs. Some beneficiaries may have dual coverage under Medicaid and Medicare, as already noted. In most states, beneficiaries receive cash assistance from the Temporary Assistance for Needy Families (TANF) program, or from the federal Supplemental Security Income (SSI) program.

Eligibility Categories in Standard Medicaid

The eligibility requirements are complex and require coordination with other state agencies (public welfare agencies, department of health) as well as federal agencies (SSA and CMS). In standard Medicaid (not including CHIP or waivered programs), there are two general eligibility groups: the "categorically needy" and the "medically needy."

Mandatory Categorically Needy

The eligibility groups in mandatory "categorically needy" programs include the following:

- Limited-income families with children, as described in Section 1931 of the Social Security Act, who meet certain of the eligibility requirements in the state's Aid to Families with Dependent Children (AFDC) plan in effect on July 16, 1996;[*]
- SSI recipients, or in states using more restrictive criteria, aged, blind, and disabled individuals who meet criteria that are more restrictive than those of the SSI program and that were in place in the state's approved Medicaid plan as of January 1, 1972;
- Infants born to Medicaid-eligible pregnant women must remain Medicaid eligible throughout the first year of life so long as the infant remains in the mother's household and she remains eligible, or would be eligible if she were still pregnant;
- Children under age 6 and pregnant women whose family income is at or below 133% of the federal poverty level.
  - The minimum mandatory income level for pregnant women and infants in certain states may be higher than 133%; as of certain dates the state had established a higher percentage for covering those groups;
  - States are required to extend Medicaid eligibility until age 19 to all children born after September 30, 1983 (or such earlier date as the state may choose) in families with incomes at or below the federal poverty level;
  - Once eligibility is established, pregnant women remain eligible for Medicaid through the end of the calendar month in which the 60th day after the end of the pregnancy falls, regardless of any change in family income;
  - States are not required to have a resource test for these poverty-level related groups; however, any resource test imposed can be no more restrictive than that of the TANF program for infants and children and the SSI program for pregnant women;
- Recipients of adoption assistance and foster care under Title IV-E of the Social Security Act;
- Certain people with Medicare; and
- Special protected groups who may keep Medicaid for a period of time, for example,
  - People who lose SSI payments due to earnings from work or increased Social Security benefits; and

---

[*]The TANF program replaced the AFDC program in 1996 as part of an overall welfare reform initiative by the Clinton administration. Some people still refer to TANF as AFDC or welfare, but those terms are now archaic.

■ Families who are provided 6–12 months of Medicaid coverage following loss of eligibility under Section 1931 due to earnings, or 4 months of Medicaid coverage following loss of eligibility under Section 1931 due to an increase in child or spousal support.

Optional Categorically Needy

States also have the option to provide Medicaid coverage for other "categorically needy" groups. These optional groups share characteristics of the mandatory groups, but the eligibility criteria are somewhat more liberally defined. Examples of the optional groups that states may cover as categorically needy (and for which they will get federal matching funds) under the Medicaid program include the following:

- Infants up to age 1 and pregnant women not covered under the mandatory rules whose family income is below 185% of the federal poverty level (the percentage to be set by each state);
- Optional targeted low-income children;
- Certain aged, blind, or disabled adults who have incomes above those requiring mandatory coverage, but below the federal poverty level;
- Children under age 21 who meet income and resources requirements for the TANF program, but who otherwise are not eligible for TANF assistance;
- Institutionalized individuals with limited income and resources;
- Persons who would be eligible if institutionalized but are receiving care under home and community-based services waivers;
- Recipients of state supplementary payments;
- Tuberculosis-infected persons who would be financially eligible for Medicaid at the SSI level (only for TB-related ambulatory services and TB drugs); and
- Low-income, uninsured women screened and diagnosed through a Centers for Disease Control and Prevention (CDC) Breast and Cervical Cancer Early Detection Program (NBCCEDP) and determined to be in need of treatment for breast or cervical cancer.[*]

States may use more liberal income and resources methodologies to determine Medicaid eligibility for certain TANF-related and aged, blind, and disabled individuals under Sections 1902(r)(2) and 1931 of the Social Security Act. For some groups, the more liberal income methodologies cannot result in the individual's income exceeding the limits prescribed for federal matching.

Medically Needy

States can also offer medically needy programs. This allows the states to extend Medicaid eligibility to others who may have too much income or assets to qualify under the categorically needy programs in the preceding section. States have a number of methods to establish eligibility as medically needy.

Nutrition Assistance Program as the Basis for Medicaid and CHIP Eligibility

With the passage of the Affordable Care Act, additional changes to eligibility processes and business processes will have to be adopted. States will need to apply new rules to adjudicate eligibility for the program; enroll millions of newly eligible individuals through multiple channels; renew eligibility for existing beneficiaries and operate seamlessly with the health insurance exchanges; incorporate a streamlined application used to apply for multiple sources of coverage and health assistance; participate in a system to verify information from patients electronically; and produce notices and communications to applicants and beneficiaries concerning the process, outcomes, and their rights to dispute or appeal. Undoubtedly, there will be significantly more performance reporting requirements to both state and federal parties.

The Eligibility Determination Process

Part of Medicaid's complexity is that in order to determine eligibility for these different programs, information must be drawn from a wide variety of sources. The process to determine eligibility remains complex in comparison to any other form of health benefits eligibility, but just how complex and how the process works has varied over time.

Determination of Eligibility Prior to 1989

Most eligibility determinations were derived from the cash welfare assistance programs run by the states' public welfare agencies. State governments varied in the degree of automation of these tasks. In some states, the eligibility information was mostly gathered manually. It was not uncommon to have a 21-page questionnaire that required proof of residence, assets and income, birth, and other documents. Those eligible for cash assistance may stick it out to finish the application process. Many who were not eligible dropped out and remained uninsured.

Modernizing the Eligibility Determination Process

In 1989, a final rule was published excluding eligibility determination systems from the enhanced funding reasoning that the close interrelationship between cash assistance programs and Medicaid eligibility rendered such enhanced assistance redundant and unnecessary. Since the 1989 regulation, a series of statutory changes dramatically affected eligibility for Medicaid and how Medicaid eligibility is determined. Among other things, new eligibility coverage groups were created and expanded, and in 1996, Medicaid eligibility was "de-linked" from the receipt of

---

[*] Additional information may be found under "Downloads and Related Links Inside CMS."

cash assistance when the AFDC program was replaced by the TANF, as noted earlier in a footnote.

With the passage of the Balanced Budget Act of 1997, states were required to coordinate eligibility for and enrollment in Medicaid, with the new CHIP program to ensure enrollment of children in the appropriate program. With passage of the "Express Lane Eligibility" provisions of section 204 of the Children's Health Insurance Reauthorization Program Reauthorization Act of 2009, states were provided with the option, and are encouraged, to coordinate and expedite eligibility for children in Medicaid and CHIP by using findings regarding income and other eligibility criteria made by other agencies, such as the Supplemental Security Administration.

Retroactive Medicaid Eligibility

Retroactive Medicaid eligibility may be available to a Medicaid applicant who did not apply for assistance until after they received care, either because they were unaware of Medicaid or because the nature of their illness prevented the filing of an application. If an individual meets certain financial and need requirements before applying for Medicaid, eligibility for Medicaid is possible during all or part of a 3-month period before the date of the application (not the date eligibility was determined was valid). This period is called retroactive eligibility.

When a beneficiary has paid a provider for a service for which the beneficiary would be entitled to have payment made under Medicaid, the provider has the option to refund the payment to the beneficiary and bill Medicaid for the service if the beneficiary furnishes valid eligibility identification (a valid Medicaid identification card for the dates of services provided) during the timely filing requirements. Some services provided during the period of retroactive eligibility are special services that require prior authorization. The services cannot be denied because of failure to secure such prior authorization, but the authorization must be obtained before payment can be made.

Medicaid Information Technology Architecture and the Medicaid Business Process Model

In late 1972, a federal law was passed that provided for federal funding for states to design, develop, install, and operate claims processing and information retrieval systems approved by the Secretary of the U.S. Department of Health and Human Services (HHS). For Medicaid purposes, the mechanized claims processing and information retrieval system, which states are required to have unless this requirement is waived by the Secretary, is the Medicaid Management Information System (MMIS).

Since 2005, CMS developed and implemented the Medicaid Information Technology Architecture (MITA). MITA is intended to foster integrated business and IT transformation across the Medicaid enterprise to improve the administration of the Medicaid program. The MITA initiative began with the concept of moving the design and development of MMIS toward a more modern architecture. States vary in their adoption of the MITA framework and its architecture, however.

From a high level, the components of a Medicaid business process model includes the management of the member, the provider, contractors carrying out some part of the Medicaid program such as claims processing or data warehousing and reporting, operations, program, program integrity (fraud, abuse, waste), and other business relationships with state, federal, or other entities. The following models represent the typical Medicaid business process, using documents made available by CMS; the full set of MITA framework documents are available to the public at www.cms.gov/MedicaidInfoTechArch/.

The typical Medicaid business processes involve:

- Member management,
- Provider management,
- Contractor management,
- Operations management,
- Program management,
- Care management,
- Program integrity management, and
- Relationship management.

These are seen in **Figure 17-1**. Some of these will be delegated to other business partners or entities such as managed care organizations (MCOs). Following Figure 17-1, the remaining figures show the typical details of each of these processes.

The member management processes in a typical Medicaid program are depicted in **Figure 17-2**. Case workers in the state's human services division are frequently the ones who handle the enrollment. Hospitals often have staff specially trained to assist in the enrollment of uninsured individuals who qualify for Medicaid coverage. In some cases, some of these activities can be delegated to business partners; for example, enrollment brokers in some states will perform some or all of these activities to facilitate enrollment, including enrollment in a managed Medicaid plan.

Provider management, as shown in **Figure 17-3**, is another typical function of Medicaid in order to ensure the providers are qualified and in good standing, give direction on how to file claims and how to report adverse events, and file appeals and grievances on behalf of the member or for payment reasons. A managed Medicaid plan typically performs these processes. The state may retain certain services or eligibility groups and carry out these activities for those groups as well.

Figure 17-4 shows the contractor management processes that are performed by all Medicaid agencies. In addition to the contractors already noted, Medicaid typically contracts with an external quality review Organization to audit and review these contracts.

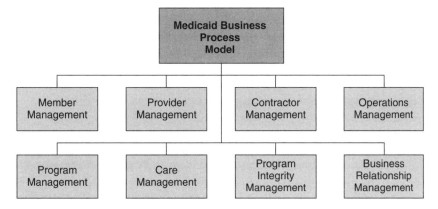

FIGURE 17-1 Medicaid Business Process

Source: Medicaid Information Technology Architecture (MITA), Centers for Medicare and Medicaid, www.cms
.gov/MedicaidInfoTechArch/. Accessed August 9, 2011.

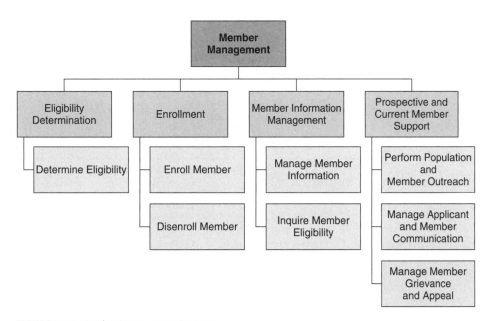

FIGURE 17-2 Member Management Processes

Source: Medicaid Information Technology Architecture (MITA), Centers for Medicare and Medicaid, www.cms.gov/
MedicaidInfoTechArch/. Accessed August 9, 2011.

Overall operations management is shown in **Figure 17-5**. This graphic gives an overview of the typical activities of a Medicaid program. If the agency pays claims, it performs the activities under the first two columns; if it contracts with a managed Medicaid plan, the third column is performed.

With all of the pressures to adopt MITA, the state also must implement the *International Classification of Diseases*, 10th Revision (ICD-10) just as commercial payers are, and must also integrate with the new health information exchanges when they are formed in 2013, prior to a 2014 "go live" date. This is a significant challenge under the best of circumstances. Some states are addressing this as they addressed basic Medicaid operational administration

already, by contracting with vendors to run the MMIS and provide the basic business processes such as maintaining databases, processing claims, and so forth. Other states chose to operate their own core systems.

MCOs receive their payments directly from the state. As outlined in the model above, the state will set its premium rates based on an actuarial analysis and recommendation. Some states provide extra ("bump") payments for services such as pregnancy or HIV/AIDS. Most states vary payments by region. Some states provide risk-based adjustments to protect MCOs against adverse risk selection.

All states have adopted standard HIPAA transaction sets to provide enrollment and premium information to

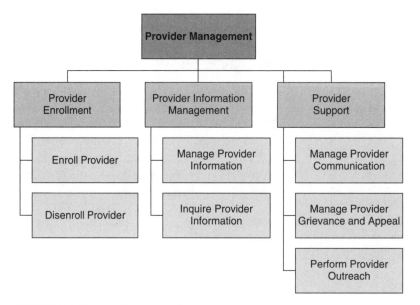

FIGURE 17-3 Provider Management Processes

Source: Medicaid Information Technology Architecture (MITA), Centers for Medicare and Medicaid, www.cms.gov/MedicaidInfoTechArch/. Accessed August 9, 2011.

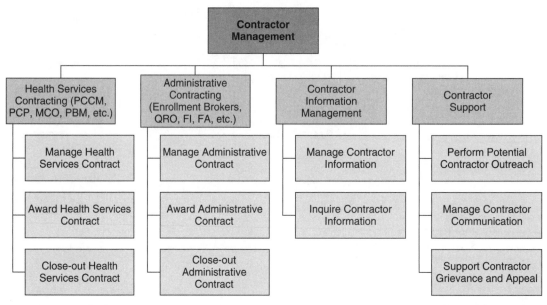

FIGURE 17-4 Contractor Management

Source: Medicaid Information Technology Architecture (MITA), Centers for Medicare and Medicaid, www.cms.gov/MedicaidInfoTechArch/. Accessed August 9, 2011.

the managed Medicaid plans. The ANSI X12 834 Benefit Enrollment format is used for enrollment, and the 820 Payment Order/Remittance Advice is used for premium payment. Even so, the information, in many cases, is supplemented through additional proprietary electronic formats and even on paper. The actual payment is typically directly transferred from the state's bank to the MCO's bank through EFT.

■ CONCLUSION

Enrollment is the first actual contact a new member has with a health plan. How well the enrollment process is handled, including timeliness and issuance of ID cards, has the outsized impact of all first impressions. The enrollment record is used by nearly all other transactional processes in a health plan, from utilization management to member

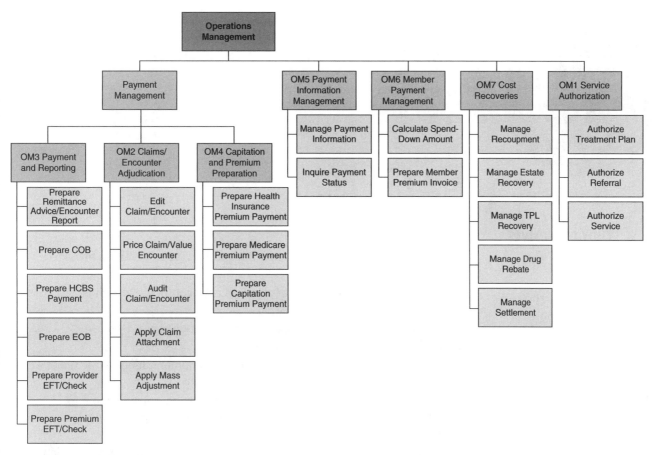

FIGURE 17-5 Operations Management

Source: Medicaid Information Technology Architecture (MITA), Centers for Medicare and Medicaid, www.cms.gov/MedicaidInfoTechArch/. Accessed August 9, 2011.

services. It is also the basis for how an insurer or HMO is paid the money to pay claims, for insured business, and pay for administering the benefits program for all lines of business. The commercial market has several variations, and Medicare and Medicaid vary even more.

The ACA will create yet new complexities and requirements around enrollment and billing, but will also flatten out some of the ways eligibility has been handled, eliminating many restrictions while it creates new requirements. But ACA or not, nothing can happen in any type of payer organization until members are actually enrolled in it.

Endnotes

1   Social Security website. *Medicare.* Available at: www.socialsecurity.gov/pubs/10043.html. Accessed July 29, 2011.

2   Official U.S. Government Site for Medicare. Available at: www.medicare.gov.

3   Medicare General Information, Eligibility, and Entitlement. *Chapter 3: Deductibles, Coinsurance Amounts, and Payment Limitations.* 2011. Available at: www.cms.gov/manuals/downloads/ge101c03.pdf. Accessed July 29, 2011.

4   Medicare Managed Care Manual Internet-Only Manuals (IOMs). *Chapter 2: Medicare Advantage Enrollment and Disenrollment.* Publication #100-16. Updated August 17, 2010. Available at: www.cms.gov/Manuals/IOM/itemdetail.asp?filterType = none&filterByDID = 99&sortByDID = 1&sortOrder = ascending&itemID = CMS019326&intNumPerPage = 10. Accessed July 29, 2011.

5   Centers for Medicare and Medicaid Services Memorandum. December 2, 2010. Announcement of the MARx System Redesign & Modernization Software Release in April 2011. Available at: www.cms.gov/MAPDHelpDesk/downloads/MARx_RM_HANDBOOK_Final_2010_12_16.pdf. Accessed July 29, 2011.

6   Centers for Medicare and Medicaid Services. Tip sheet: Understanding Medicare enrollment periods. CMS Product No. 11219. Available at: www.medicare.gov/Publications/Pubs/pdf/11219.pdf. Accessed July 29, 2011.

CHAPTER

18

Claims and Benefits Administration

DONALD L. FOWLER, JR. AND ELIZABETH A. PASCUZZI

STUDY OBJECTIVES

- Understand the purpose of the claims adjudication process within a managed care organization
- Understand the factors from other plan areas that contribute to, or hinder, accurate and timely claims processing
- Understand where claims and benefits administration play a key role in improving a plan's operations or market position
- Understand implications upon claims work flow of organizational structure of claims within an organization, and internal to claims
- Understand the major components of claims operational management to establish, monitor, and maintain efficient work flow, including pertinent measures for productivity and quality
- Understand standard accuracy measures, what they mean to an organization's sound fiscal, community relations, and market-competitive standing
- Understand the interrelationships between claims and other payer functions
- Understand how to identify common claims administration problems, their repercussions, and how to identify and rectify them

DISCUSSION TOPICS

1. Discuss the purpose of benefits administration and claims adjudication within a managed care organization.
2. Discuss the process and importance of inventory control.
3. Discuss what information reports support claims management.
4. Discuss the differences between "batch" and "online" adjudication, and the advantages or disadvantages of each.
5. Discuss productivity standards and turnaround times, including those factors that improve or hinder each.
6. Discuss the standard accuracy measures, and what reasonable levels of accuracy are within these measures.
7. Discuss the sources for definitive interpretation of benefits in order to determine plan liability when adjudicating a claim.
8. Discuss the factors that combine to contribute to the final claim payment amount.
9. Discuss the most common claims and benefits administration problems, their repercussions, and how to identify and rectify them.
10. Discuss the circumstances under which a plan would consider outsourcing their claims adjudication function.

INTRODUCTION

The modern claims capability, built on decades of evolving and competing demands, operates on a monumental scale. Nationally, today's claims capability facilitates nearly $2.5 trillion in claims payments annually (approximately 17.6% of the U.S. economy[1]), enough financing to fuel the largest sector of the American economy. As such it protects millions of citizens from catastrophic loss due to medical expenses through the health benefit programs it administers. In addition to processing claims, the modern claims capability:

- Supports disease management and specialized medical management programs for up to approximately 75 million Americans,
- Serves as the primary safeguard against fraud and abuse,
- Supports large social welfare programs (Medicare and Medicaid), and
- Plays a role in tracking national health trends and providing early warning signs for health pandemics and bioterrorism.

Closer to home, the modern claims capability is vital to the health and vitality of its payer organization, having a crucial impact on virtually all other departments and on the payer's bottom line. However, claims must rely on a number of other departments for faithful execution of their responsibilities in order to fulfill its mission: to serve customers, internal and external, via timely and accurate claims adjudication.

This chapter describes the evolution of the modern claims capability, defines the various functions within the claims capability, and examines management issues and core business steps. It concludes with a discussion of major risk areas. Several tables and figures are included to illustrate concepts or provide more detailed information.

EVOLUTION OF THE MODERN CLAIMS CAPABILITY

The modern claims capability has evolved over many decades of changes in health care delivery and insurance practices. Changes have been driven by expectations and demands of employer groups, individual policyholders, consumers, medical providers, legislators, and regulatory agencies. The Centers for Medicare and Medicaid Services (CMS),[*] which administers Medicare and Medicaid through various public-private business partnerships, has also influenced the modern claims capability in major ways.

Additionally, advances in medical technology on the provider side and in transactional processing systems on the payer side have driven claims operations managers to continually upgrade and redefine the role of the claims capability.

The roots of claims operations can be traced back to the 1940s when many employers began offering health care coverage as a method of attracting and retaining employees (see Chapter 1). Benefits initially focused on hospitalization, but as the labor force grew and large unions began negotiating improved benefit packages, coverage was extended to include the cost of doctors' fees, allied medical expenses, and prescription drugs. Union negotiated benefit plans influenced both product and benefit design and ultimately the benefit packages offered to salaried and other nonunion employees. This evolution in product and benefit design resulted in more and more variations of health insurance coverage, with some employer groups ultimately sponsoring dozens of benefit plans.

To finance and administer such programs, employer groups looked to multiline insurance companies with their in-house transaction capabilities and actuarial skills to price, underwrite, assume the financial risk, and process claims. Insurers were the first to introduce the idea of cost-sharing (deductibles, coinsurance, and stop-loss features) as well as underwriting principles to guard against adverse selection (the tendency of certain members of a defined population to utilize health care and file claims at a higher rate than the general population). At the same time that employer groups were developing programs with insurance carriers, medical providers were exploring other methods of providing and financing health care in the form of prepaid medical practices and health service plans.

While the financing and delivery of health care were evolving, provider billing practices also changed to reflect the ever increasing complexity in medical care. Initially, payment to providers (even in the form of barter) was expected from patients at the time medical services were rendered. Even if covered under an employer health plan, patients often paid for doctor visits or prescription drugs out of their own pockets. As health insurance covered more and more people and as benefits expanded to include physician visits, payers introduced the claim form as a way to organize the intake of medical bills to facilitate payment. Over time, hospitals and physicians began to file claims directly with third-party payers as a service to patients. When providers began filing claims, they began using more sophisticated methods of creating itemized bills. Itemized bills were submitted in a variety of formats and did not always contain all of the data required by the payer to determine coverage or payment.

It wasn't until 1966 that Common Procedure Terminology (CPT) codes were introduced by the American Medical Association to standardize itemized charges and provide

---

[*]CMS, initially known as the Health Care Financing Administration or HCFA, is part of the U.S. Department of Health and Human Services.

uniformity in billing practices. CPT codes were incorporated into the Healthcare Common Procedure Coding System (HCPCS) Level I, while Level II codes for ancillary medical services were introduced in 1983; revenue codes for hospital services were introduced in 1984. Even today, the medical community tries different submission techniques to streamline claims processing, improve claims turnaround time, and maximize payments.

The other major coding system, the *International Classification of Diseases* (ICD), grew from ongoing efforts by U.S. and European medical statisticians beginning in the early 20th century to classify causes of death. With substantial support by the United States, the effort was expanded considerably in mid-century and placed under the auspices of the World Health Organization (WHO). The 7th and 8th revisions in 1955 and 1965, respectively, were rapidly adopted by hospitals, and following the 9th revision in 1975, its use by hospitals became universal. Work on ICD-10 began in 1983, was completed by the WHO in 1992, and adopted shortly thereafter by almost every nation except the United States.

With the advent of government entitlement programs in 1965, the policies and procedures established for the administration of Medicare began to influence the health insurance industry. Medicare processing standards were ultimately adopted (and continue to be adopted) by most payers, even for non-Medicare benefits. Additionally, CMS, then called HCFA, pushed for uniformity in billing, and ultimately providers began to use standard claim forms, which, at that time, were referred to as the UB92 claim form for hospital services and HCFA 1500 claim forms for professional fees and ancillary services. Uniformity was still an issue in 1996 when the Health Insurance Portability and Accountability Act (HIPAA) mandated standardization of certain code sets and electronic transactions for more efficient communication among providers and payers.

On the heels of HIPAA, the United States began planning for the implementation of an updated accident and disease classification scheme that will provide more granular detail related to every patient's health condition. This updated classification scheme, based on the *International Classification of Diseases*, 10th Revision with Clinical Modification, advances society's interest in documenting and using health care information. Implementation of this new classification scheme will require several years to complete, but ICD-10-CM codes may be in use as early as October 1, 2013.

However, the most overarching change to American health care financing and delivery to occur in a generation came about with the signing into law of the Patient Protection and Affordable Care Act (ACA) on March 23, 2010. Some of the broad changes envisioned by this legislation include:

- Providing new health benefits for up to 75% of the nation's currently uninsured and underinsured (including some young adults),
- Reducing increases in Medicare payments to most health care providers,
- Introducing new payment methodologies in traditional Medicare,
- Creating more standardized wellness benefits for most Americans, and
- Increasing government focus on waste, fraud, and abuse within the health care delivery system.

At the time of this writing, expansion of family coverage to some young adults and reduced Medicare payments have already become reality. Full rule implementation related to the 2010 Act will require years to complete and ultimately have dramatic impacts on providers, payers, and Americans overall.

While standardization of coding helped to simplify claims adjudication during the late 1960s and 1970s, the provider practice of decomposing service codes, referred to as "unbundling," introduced a new element of complexity. Early unbundling largely related to hospital-based physician charges (i.e., ungrouped services that had been previously included within the hospital bill). As a result, a single hospital stay began to produce multiple paper claims including those for the hospital facility charges as well as those for professional fees (emergency room physicians, radiologists, surgeons, anesthesiologists, other specialists, ambulance, durable medical equipment, prescriptions, etc.). Later, unbundling was also carried out by physicians (including a practice known as upcoding) in order to maximize payments. This practice in turn led to the development of early programs to detect and prevent fraud and abuse, a topic further explored later in this chapter.

The growth of dual household incomes after 1970 increased the likelihood of dual health benefit coverage for all family members. As a result, coordination of benefits (COB) became another element of administrative complexity. Initially, primary coverage for dependent children was associated with the father's health plan. But as society changed, so did benefit determination rules, and the "birthday rule" (see Table 18-5 for definition) was established in 1984. Other party liability (OPL) rules associated with automobile insurance, workers' compensation, and subrogation also evolved. Insurers and government entitlement programs became increasingly focused on assigning financial responsibility and controlling claim payments.

The growth of health maintenance organizations (HMOs) in the 1970s and 1980s, spurred by the 1973 federal HMO Act, introduced two new elements to the developing claims capability: medical management and much broader use of provider payment agreements. In terms of medical management, claims adjudicators now had to determine if charges submitted by health care providers were preauthorized and/or met other medical management standards. In terms of provider payment agreements, claims adjudicators also had to ensure that the claims payment matched the appropriate fee schedule or even type of payment used for the particular type of service and benefit plan. In addition to fee schedules are other payment options for individual providers, including specific discounts and per diem rates, as described in detail in Chapter 6.

The evolving claims capability had to be adaptable, flexible, and forward-looking to keep pace with the growth in complexity (as shown in **Figure 18-1**) of benefit plans within multiple lines of business (commercial, Medicare, Medicaid, TRICARE, etc.); provider payment rules; increasingly sophisticated coding schemes such as ICD-10; unbundling practices; multifaceted referral/authorization rules; government mandates; other party liability rules; evolving cost-sharing features; and increasing vigilance in the detection of fraud. The claims capability had to be proactive and positioned to respond to changes in the health insurance marketplace, in the practice of medicine, in health care billing practices, and in the payer's own evolving information and technology needs. While the environment around it became increasingly complex, the claims operations continued to focus on its primary role of transaction processing to ensure the financial integrity of the payer.

As all of the variables shown in Figure 18-1 evolved over the course of the last century and as computer-based transaction processing matured, health insurance payers were required to make greater investment in technology and to continually upgrade both hardware and software. Payers also had to continue to invest in training and development to support evolving medical management practices. For this and a variety of other reasons, many of the multiline insurance carriers that together created the health insurance claims processing industry ultimately opted to divest their health insurance divisions. This divestiture created a new landscape that led to a new breed of organization that shifted the fundamental approach to the delivery and financing of health care from an actuarial point of view to a holistic care management point of view. This new breed of organization evolved during the 1980s and early 1990s into the payer organizations that dominate the health insurance market today. By the end of the last century mergers and acquisitions had become the norm, with some very large payers dominating the industry and subsequently moving the claims capability further along in its development.

■ 21ST-CENTURY DEVELOPMENTS

We touched on two significant developments affecting the health insurance and managed care industry in general and the claims capability in particular on the previous pages. One is the implementation of the updated scheme of diagnostic coding known as ICD-10. The other is the ACA.

ICD-10-CM

While ICD-10 was originally endorsed in the United States in 1992, it is only now being implemented with a currently mandated completion date of October 1, 2013. As part of the federal mandate, diagnoses will be described using the *International Classification of Diseases,* 10th Revision, Clinical Modification (ICD-10-CM) and inpatient procedures

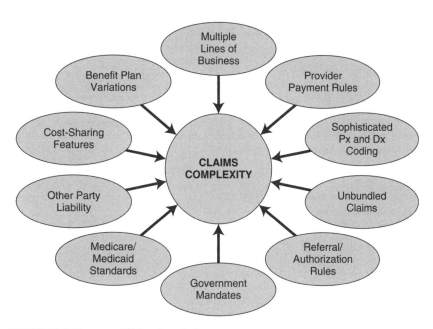

FIGURE 18-1 Elements of Claims Complexity

will be described using the *International Classification of Diseases*, 10th Revision, Procedure Classification System (ICD-10-PCS).[*]

Most health plans already have begun the transition from ICD-9 to ICD-10 in terms of system and business operation changes because ICD-10 applies to all entities covered under HIPAA. According to CMS, all outpatient claims with dates of service and all inpatient claims with dates of discharge on and after October 1, 2013, must include ICD-10 diagnostic codes or such claims must be rejected (denied) by managed care organizations (MCOs). However, in order to accommodate ICD-10, all health plans and providers dealing in electronic claims must have implemented the American National Standards Institute (ANSI) X12 version 50.10 standard for electronic health care transactions by January 1, 2012.

The transition of diagnosis coding from ICD-9 to ICD-10 directly affects the claims capability because diagnosis codes are a key element on all medical claims. ICD-9 codes were composed of four or five alpha-numeric characters, but ICD-10 codes are composed of seven alpha-numeric characters. The entire coding system has been reconfigured and will allow up to 16,000 different variations of clinical data. The files that control the automatic adjudication of claims must be updated to comply with ICD-10 diagnosis codes, and providers must bill with such codes by October 1, 2013, even if the 2012 mandatory compliance date is delayed. The claims capability must be proactive and available to adjudicate claims accurately even before the new diagnostic coding system goes into effect.

The Patient Protection and Affordable Care Act of 2010

The ACA represents significant regulation of the health care industry by the federal government, and is addressed in detail in Chapter 30. Some portions of the legislation became effective in 2010 and 2011 while others will not become effective until 2013 or 2014. The legislation expands access to health insurance to nearly all Americans. It also eliminates the preexisting condition provision for children (and later for adults) and extends coverage for dependents to age 26 under certain conditions. While there are numerous provisions in the ACA, specific provisions that affect the claims capability are those that define qualified health benefits plans.

As described in Chapter 16, the ACA allows for up to four different levels of coverage or tiers for covered services provided by in-network providers. These benefit tiers are labeled as Platinum (90% coverage), Gold (80% coverage), Silver (70% coverage), and Bronze (60% coverage). This standardized approach should enable consumers to comparison-shop among health plans, possibly even across state borders.

Comparisons will also be facilitated by a new Summary of Coverage (SOC) document described in Chapter 20.

Other ACA provisions affecting benefit plans include certain limitations on the application of deductibles, the elimination of lifetime limits in 2010 as well as annual limits by 2014, and the elimination of preexisting condition clauses in all benefit plans for all individuals by 2014. Another key provision is the prohibition of rescission, the practice of some health plans to cancel insurance coverage predicated on not having revealed a preexisting condition when a covered individual becomes ill; rescission is still allowable in cases of nonpayment or fraud on the part of the individual.

Just as with the implementation of ICD-10, the claims capability must be proactive to ensure that claims are accurately adjudicated as the new provisions of the ACA go into effect over the next several years. Similarly, it behooves the claims capability managers to stay abreast of developments as new regulations are published by the Department of Health and Human Services (HHS) and CMS, or as the ACA is amended by further congressional and/or judicial action.

■ DEFINING THE MODERN CLAIMS CAPABILITY

Simply stated, the modern claims capability is the set of operational functions within the payer organization that together process claims from receipt to issuance of payment and/or explanation of benefits (EOB). The set of operational functions (illustrated in **Figure 18-2**) includes:

- Receipt of electronically submitted claims through electronic data interchange (EDI)
- Receipt of paper claims
- Initial auto adjudication (first pass)
- Second-attempt auto adjudication following resolution of certain suspension edits

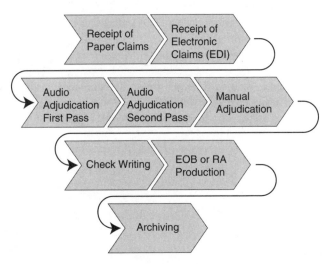

FIGURE 18-2 Claims Capability Operational Functions

---

[*]Work has already begun on ICD-11, but we are limiting our focus in this chapter to ICD-10.

- Manual processing for claims that cannot be auto-adjudicated
- Check-writing process
- Issuance of EOB and/or remittance advice (RA)
- Completing appropriate prepayment and postpayment analytics
- Archiving claim records and data

Most often, this collection of functions (described at length on the following pages) is referred to as "claims" by individuals both outside and inside of the payer organization. To those outside the payer organization, the claims process is often the "face" of the organization, particularly to the provider community. To payer business leaders, government agencies, and others within the health insurance industry, claims is the source of information that allows payers to gauge and improve its business performance and improve the health care of its members. As the modern claims capability continues to evolve, information management techniques will continue to create a place of greater prominence for the claims capability in the 21st century.

In studying the modern claims capability, one quickly concludes that four primary core competencies make up what many of us consider "claims." The core competencies include transactional processing, quality control, service delivery, and information management/analytics.

As shown in **Figure 18-3**, within each of these core competencies are three integrated components: proven business and communication processes, trained and motivated people,

and supporting tools and technology. Just as with a three-legged stool, weakness in any one integrated component will threaten the entire structure. Each of the core competencies and their integrated components are described in the next sections.

Core Competency 1: Transactional Processing

Transactional processing is a term that describes the handling and adjudication of health care claims. It is (and always has been) the primary competency of the claims capability. Failure to execute this competency has a profound impact on all of the other core competencies as well as on the payer organization as a whole. Successfully executing this competency requires an effective blend of proven business and communication processes, trained and motivated people, and supporting tools and technology.

Along with traditional "claims," many MCOs now process and/or track encounter information, which includes patient demographics, disease and treatment data, and other related information that helps health care professionals understand a particular patient's potential health outcomes. Encounter data is very important to MCOs because the reporting of complete encounter data can influence payment levels from government health programs. Such data can also help to complete a MCO's understanding of a member's health situation.

Business and communication processes should be detailed, transparent, thorough, and integrated. One process should lead to the next in a comprehensive course of events that allows for all contingencies. The initial business process actually begins with instructions to providers on how to file claims. Over the years, provider instructions have become much more complex yet very specific in terms of standardized claim forms and required data elements.

Two information elements that have undergone the most significant changes in recent years are the member and provider identification numbers. Following the passage of HIPAA, covered entities had to discontinue the use of Social Security numbers in favor of a payer-generated ID number. The original wording in HIPAA called for the creation of a national member ID. Concerned about privacy and security, Congress quickly permanently defunded any such efforts, so there will not be a national member ID in the foreseeable future. For provider ID numbers, covered entities had to convert to a national provider identifier (NPI). HIPAA also calls for a national health plan ID, but at the time of publication, CMS has not yet issued rules and regulations around that.

As for other required data elements, virtually all payers require the use of standardized place of service, diagnosis, and procedure codes (CPT, HCPCS, revenue, etc.) and have abandoned (for the most part) the use of so-called "home-grown" or local-use codes. Personnel outside of the claims capability (often the Provider Relations or Provider Contracting

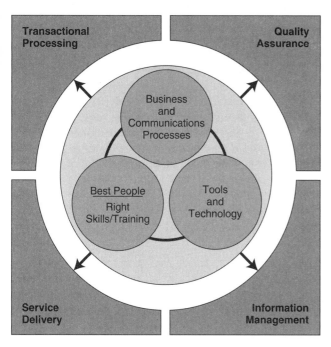

FIGURE 18-3 Claims Capability Core Competencies and Integrated Components

department; see Chapter 4) generally communicate instructions to providers regarding these and other data elements. However, the claims capability management team is responsible for reviewing and approving claims filing instructions periodically to ensure that new pertinent information is adequately and accurately included.

Within the payer organization, specific business processes govern more detailed policies and procedures for:

- Initially handling submitted claims (electronic or paper),
- Adjudicating claims for payment or denial,
- Resolving suspended claims,
- Limiting liability by administering other party liability programs, and
- Reopening processed claims due to errors or appeals.

These business processes are discussed in greater detail later in this chapter. Effective business processes must be well documented, tested, applied, revised, and reapplied in a quest for continuous process improvement. Business processes must also be coordinated with other payer departments to ensure that customer concerns are adequately addressed and that the payer delivers on its key commitments across constituencies.

The claims capability's business architecture (i.e., its business and communication processes) defines the tools needed to execute the transaction processing core competency. The key tool is the set of software applications that includes an integrated transactional processing system, a technically advanced software application designed to record data and adjudicate claims according to predetermined rules. This tool must be robust enough to accommodate existing business and membership levels, but flexible in its capacity (or scalable) to support membership growth and future complexity. Additional technology tools include scanning solutions for paper claims, applications that enable electronic claims submissions, and a host of special databases to support the management of products, benefit plans, provider contracts, regulatory requirements, and so on.

To optimize this complex set of tools:

- Functionality (including limitations) should be well understood and communicated,
- Capabilities should be fully exploited to deliver the greatest possible value, and
- Information files should be properly maintained and updated.

Optimizing the configuration and use of these tools is contingent upon integrating activities and communication within a variety of departments within the payer organization (often including functions and/or entities external to the organization).

When designing and developing products, benefit plans, provider payment terms, and business processes, the payer

should not allow a transactional processing system to dictate its business decisions. However, care should be taken to ensure that benefit plan features and/or provider payment methods are easily configured or programmable in the system and can be supported in such a manner as to avoid manual processing.

Historically, there has been a natural tension between the health insurers' and subsequent payers' desire to customize benefit plans and provider contracts in response to marketplace demands and the payer's internal constraints related to business processes and tools. To ensure this natural tension remains in balance, analysis of claims administration costs associated with nonstandard benefits or provider payment schemes is recommended before contracts are signed. In fact, some payer organizations pass the costs of nonstandard provisions onto the employer groups and providers who request them. Imbalance within this natural tension will ultimately lead to a decrease in profitable business either through unmanageable internal processes and related cost increases, or products that are too out of touch with the marketplace to retain membership.

Just as business processes and technology are important to transaction processing, so are trained and motivated people who perform the tasks required to process claims. It is the people who interact with each other, with other internal departments, and with customers that really put the "face" on the claims organization. Within the transaction-processing component of the modern claims capability, these people include:

- Technically proficient personnel who support electronic data interchange (EDI) transmissions,
- Clerical personnel who initially prep paper claims,
- Claims processors who adjudicate claims as well as make adjustments,
- Supervisors and managers who interpret policies and run daily operations,
- Specialized staff who support analytics, reporting, and continuous process improvements, and
- Directors and vice presidents who strategically manage investments in the claims capability as well as recruit and hire key talent and/or investigate other sourcing models.

Unfortunately, it is the technology component that is often the major focus of attention in many claims capability operations, with less and less emphasis placed on business process or personnel. Such an approach is shortsighted, especially while payers upgrade to new coding schemes, continue to receive paper claims, and suspensions of electronic claims remain common. Clerical personnel are still needed to open, date-stamp, sort, and stage paper claims. They also scan claims or key claims data into the transactional processing system. These front-end procedures are critical to an efficient and accurate process, since claims mishandled at this stage bog down the entire workflow and may lead to quality issues such as linking claims to the incorrect member and benefit plan or to the incorrect service provider and fee schedule.

Personnel are also needed to manage electronic claims submissions when claims are submitted via EDI or via the payer's provider portal. The EDI and portal process varies among payer organizations depending on the sophistication of their systems and the providers' EDI capabilities. The electronic process also depends on the efforts of the payer's personnel outside of the claims capability who are normally staffed in the information technology department and charged with establishing the electronic links with providers and other third-party invoicing organizations or billers. There must be strong two-way communication between the claims capability and those controlling the EDI and portal processes to ensure that all data is received according to established business processes.

The heart and soul of transaction processing is claims adjudication. According to research completed by America's Health Insurance Plans for 2009, transactional processing systems auto-adjudicated around 75%[2] of claims that are accepted into the processing system; claims that are not accepted into the processing system are considered "rejected" and never become part of the claims inventory within the payer organization. Some health plans report a higher auto-adjudication rate. For the remaining 25% or so of accepted claims, a suspension occurs during the adjudication process. Suspensions (sometimes called edits or pends) result in manual intervention. Well-trained and experienced claims adjudicators must review suspended claims and judge whether they should be paid or denied.

Adjudication not only depends on well-defined business and communication processes and technology and tools as previously described but also on the human element. Within the modern claims capability, it often takes 6 months or more to fully train a claims adjudicator. While initial training to on-board new employees is vital, ongoing training of tenured staff is also required to remain current in a rapidly changing environment. Claims adjudicators must also be properly motivated, accurately assessed, and suitably rewarded in terms of productivity and quality measures.

Core Competency 2: Quality Control

The second core competency of the modern claims capability is quality control. Quality control focuses on functions and processes from initial intake through preparation/staging and concludes with customer service, appeals, and ultimately renewal of the employer group or government contract. Claims adjudication is where the "rubber meets the road." It is the spot in the payer organization where its business processes and system files converge to produce an adjudicated outcome. As such, the claims capability is able to assess quality both "upstream" and "downstream."

"Upstream" refers to the processes and system files that govern and enable automatic and manual claims adjudication. Those areas and the individuals responsible for these files are usually outside of the traditional claims capability. Some upstream files contain high-level but fundamental information, including data about lines of business, group and subgroup structure, benefit plans, and other "control" data that apply across the board to all transactions. These files do not change much over time (with the exception of transitions such as ICD-10 diagnosis codes as described earlier). However, other upstream files are continually updated. These include member and provider records, provider payment terms and rates, referral and authorization decisions, and other party liability details as well as the files that define benefit coding and adjudication rules.

Errors in claims processing can often be traced back to errors in one or more upstream files or records. However, rather than identifying such errors only after claims have been erroneously processed (causing customer service issues), the modern claims capability is proactive in monitoring and testing upstream files before providers and members are negatively impacted. Just as a tenet of modern managed health care is preventive medicine, a tenet of the modern claims capability must be quality assessment through proactive testing, quality reviews, and preventive file maintenance on a prepayment basis. The people component of this core competency relies largely on communications with other departments that control upstream processes and files. Interdepartmental relationships must be established, maintained, and nurtured. Payer organizations without good governance models and open communication will never be as successful as those that encourage honest dialogue and collaboration.

"Downstream" refers primarily to the claims capability itself. The claims capability's primary goal is ensuring that claims processing error rates are kept as close to zero as possible while maintaining target production. Claims personnel are the primary focus in most downstream quality and process improvement efforts since downstream quality problems are often traced back to human error. Human error within the claims capability is generally due to carelessness, unclear policies or procedures, insufficient training, or less than attentive management practices. Preventive measures are also essential to downstream quality assessment in terms of routine claims adjudicator audits, ongoing policy and procedure review and updates, attention to training and retraining, and close daily supervision. Careful attention should also be paid to member and provider complaints and/or appeals as well as to returned checks and other voluntary refunds to discover the root causes of errors and subsequent design of corrective measures.

Other downstream factors that affect quality claims adjudication include medical management and many of the third-party programs such as pharmacy benefits management (PBM) and mental health care programs. Tort actions can also be a factor long after claims adjudication. For example, when the payer is notified by outside attorneys of accidents where automobile insurance, workers' compensation benefits, or subrogation is involved, the claims capability must review processed claims for potential adjustments. In addition to retrospective review of previously paid claims, measures must be taken to avoid future overpayments related to these situations. There have also been examples in recent years of provider class actions that require payers to retain records and payment documentation for longer periods than planned.

Whether errors are considered upstream or downstream, they have a negative impact on the "face" of the payer in terms of customer satisfaction. Continuous quality problems have a dampening effect on provider and member retention and could lead to the loss of business, negatively impacting the payer's bottom line. Even if such customer loss is avoided, quality problems still impact the bottom line in terms of costly rework. Devoting resources to preventing errors is far less expensive than the postadjudication analysis necessary to discover errors or the assets necessary to correct them. Costly rework can quickly change the financial assumptions underlying the payer organization's business plan.

Core Competency 3: Service Delivery

A third core competency of the modern claims capability is service delivery to both internal and external customers. Internal customers include those departments that directly interact with members and providers as well as finance, actuarial and underwriting, product development, sales and marketing, medical management, and internal audit. External customers, including employer groups, brokers, members, providers, and trading/business partners, are impacted by the claims capability and may have direct contact with the claims capability management team through periodic customer audits and site visits.

Service delivery focused on members or providers can be handled in two ways. One way is to house call centers that respond directly to member and provider claims concerns within the claims capability. The advantage to this approach is that claims adjudicators taking the calls may be able to immediately adjust errors or resolve suspended claims. The disadvantage to this approach is that the caller may have other concerns and must be transferred to a member or provider services representative for resolution. Another disadvantage is that constant interruptions with telephone calls severely impede claims adjudication productivity and quality if both tasks are assigned to the same person at the same time. Caution must be taken to segregate claims adjudication production tasks from call center tasks to ensure appropriate focus. Another issue to consider is whether claims adjudicators assigned to call center duty are trained in customer service skills. Excellent claims adjudicators may not be excellent customer service representatives.

The most common way to handle service delivery to members and providers is for the payer organization to have separate call center operations that responds to all member and/or provider inquiries, as described in Chapter 20 for member services. In this case, customer service representatives (CSR) must rely on the claims capability to promptly resolve claims problems. The advantage to a centralized call center is that the CSR is trained to respond to all sorts of issues, not just claims-related problems. A disadvantage is that additional extensive training on how claims are adjudicated may be needed to fully prepare CSRs to respond to claims inquiries. Another disadvantage is that adjustments will probably not be accomplished as quickly. To address this issue, the claims capability must establish and execute policies and procedures to promptly attend to problem claims identified by the CSRs.

As stated earlier, the claims capability uses technology and sundry tools to support service delivery. Transactional processing systems and other software applications facilitate communication among departments, provide data to research and uncover the root cause of errors, and support the execution of adjustments. Almost as important as the transactional processing system are the business and communication practices that enable an efficient and timely error resolution process. However, well-trained and motivated personnel are the key to delivering the service. The claims capability staff must be reminded that behind every claim is a patient who is ill or injured and is relying on the payer to deliver on its service commitments. If claims personnel understand the human component, they are more likely to understand their impact on customers and are less likely to think of themselves as just a traditional back-office support operation.

Core Competency 4: Information Management and Analysis

The fourth core competency of the modern claims capability is information management and analysis (i.e., the collection and management of data fundamental to the payer organization and its customers). Information management depends on good data stewardship and warehousing; information management enables appropriate security, standard and ad hoc analytics, care and disease management, fraud and abuse detection, other party liability administration, and financial functions such as forecasting and reporting. As previously noted, the claims capability is the source of much of the data that allows the payer to operate and improve its business. In short, it is claims data analysis that largely provides the customer insights that are critical to managing and growing the business. This fourth core competency relies on the previous three competencies, particularly transactional processing and quality control.

Technology, of course, is vital to information management. A robust transactional processing system and other technological tools allow the payer to categorize and house data. Personnel can then extract and manipulate key data elements to develop appropriate insights. In early processing systems, reporting was limited to so-called "canned" reports that were hard-coded into the software. Current systems are designed to make virtually all data elements "reportable" so that analysts can include any number of factors in business and health care improvement models.

During the past decade, robust analytics tool suites have helped shape a new informatics capability. Informatics is generally defined as "the collection, classification, storage, retrieval, and dissemination of recorded knowledge treated both as a pure and as an applied science."[3] The science of informatics has now grown from infancy to become a robust part of the payer organization's business and care delivery model. Moreover, newer and newer analysis tool suites provide the means of creating ever deeper insight.

As informatics has come of age, so have the parallel needs of developing and hiring more personnel with deep analytical skills. In order to optimize the resources and data collected, well-designed business processes are needed and must be fully coordinated with other operational departments. As such there is a need for two-way communication and understanding between claims personnel and other departments (and trading partners) to fully understand and realize the potential of all collected data. For example, administering a profitable COB and OPL program usually depends on data collected by personnel outside of the claims capability. If the Enrollment Department (or outside vendors) provides other health insurance information on members, it must be cognizant of the specific data elements needed in order for claims adjudicators to coordinate benefits successfully. Similarly, if utilization nurses identify other insurance potential due to accidental injury, they must be directed to record specific information that can be used to reduce the payer's liability in favor of automobile or workers' compensation insurance. Data collection, analysis, and management are ongoing processes that cannot be left unattended. Lags or gaps in maintaining data limits its usability and diminishes its value, robbing the payer of insights needed to run the business more effectively.

When claims-related information initially became more accessible through software and hardware designs and greater automation, it was mainly used for actuarial purposes to evaluate experience and set rates. Since the 1990s payers have developed more sophisticated means to retrieve data, thus exponentially expanding the use of the information they have collected. Information is now considered a vital asset not only to the payer but also to employer groups, members, providers, and external parties including state and federal governments.

For the payers, and for employer groups as well, claims experience helps to support product and benefit designs and expand the development of consumer-driven health plans/products. Members have more and more access to data that help them to determine and/or control costs and manage their own health care. Wellness initiatives and disease management programs continue to expand and benefit members, providers, and the payers in ways not imagined previously. Even the federal government is now realizing that payers are a unique aggregator of data that can identify early signs of global health threats or biological terrorism. Organizations such as regional health information organizations (RHIOs) are leveraging this growing information management and informatics experience.

Organization Considerations

The claims capability is typically managed as one consolidated department within a payer's operations division and reports to a chief operations officer or a chief financial officer. In large organizations, the claims capability may report to a senior vice president of operations. Within smaller payer organizations, the claims capability often reports to a director of operations. As shown in **Figure 18-4**, the claims capability is integral to managed care operations and depends on relationships with virtually all of the other departments.

Within the claims capability, the organization structure depends on the scope of responsibilities. A large payer organization with multiple lines of business may require a separate manager or director for each. An operation focused solely on commercial business may organize around major employer groups, especially if each employer group has nonstandard benefit plans that require a certain amount of manual adjudication. Payers with Medicare Advantage (MA) and/or managed Medicaid plans may organize based on the program guidelines for compliance. Within any of these models, further specialization could be assigned for pharmacy claims, behavioral health claims, durable medical equipment (DME) claims, claims involving other party liability (OPL), and so on.

Additional factors to consider involve the transactional processing system in use. Most transactional processing systems are structured by claim type (i.e., one set of processing screens and procedures for professional claims and another set of processing screens and procedures for institutional claims). This structure lends itself to organizing units of claims adjudicators by the types of claims they process. Some payers may have one or more legacy transactional processing systems that were developed for HMOs, preferred provider organizations (PPOs), or traditional indemnity plans. In some cases, this factor alone may dictate that the claims capability be organized around specific claims platforms.

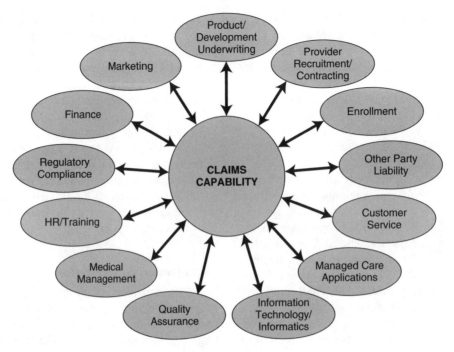

FIGURE 18-4 Claims Capability Relationships within the Payer

Figure 18-5 shows a claims capability organization chart for a large payer that incorporates many of these ideas. The organization chart shows several management levels that may or may not conform to specific payer strategies around organization design. This illustration also shows a claims organization that is rich in varied duties and levels, creating a career path vital for employee motivation and retention. Figure 18-5 is not a blueprint but rather an example that suggests options to consider when organizing personnel and business processes by line of business in relation to the available technology.

A single individual should be accountable for the claims capability, but whether the individual is a senior vice president, vice president, director, or manager depends on the size of the payer, the payer's human resources policies, the number of business lines, annual claims volume, and government protocols if the payer manages state or federal contracts. The organization chart shows only one supervisor under each manager. However, the number of supervisors (if any) depends on the number of adjudicators needed and the degree of processing specialization. Figure 18-5 also shows that quality assessment and training are often separate and shared services across the claims capability organization. These functions should report to the highest management level of the claims capability because they serve the entire claims operation. Placing these functions outside of the claims production environment is more likely to ensure (1) fair and equitable quality reviews, (2) an adequate focus on training and cross-training, and (3) the development of comprehensive training materials.

Another organizational issue relates to adjustments defined as those claims that must be corrected or adjusted due to a processing error or a decision reversed upon appeal. Adjustments due to errors include claims that are paid for the wrong patient, paid to the wrong provider, paid an incorrect amount (possibly off of the wrong fee schedule), paid for the wrong date of service, and paid at the wrong benefit level, as well as those denied erroneously. Adjustments also may be due to decisions reversed upon appeal, including claims denied for no eligibility, ineligible benefit, no authorization, or exhausted benefits. Claims may be reversed upon appeal by a first-time review within the appeals department (often located within claims capability), by medical management or other senior managers, or as the result of provider peer review or legal action. Although there may be some value in returning errors to the original adjudicator for correction, it is usually more efficient to have all adjustments handled by a special unit because the processing steps can be quite complicated. Choosing to staff each unit of the claims capability with adjustors who are familiar with the specific line of business, employer groups, government programs, provider contracts, and so on is a decision that must be made based on quality, productivity, and training challenges unique to the payer.

Over the last decade many large payers have developed an operations command center and made it part of the claims capability. The command center is typically responsible for analytics, workforce optimization and planning, and reporting. Such functions depend on claims data and ultimately help the payer improve its operational performance.

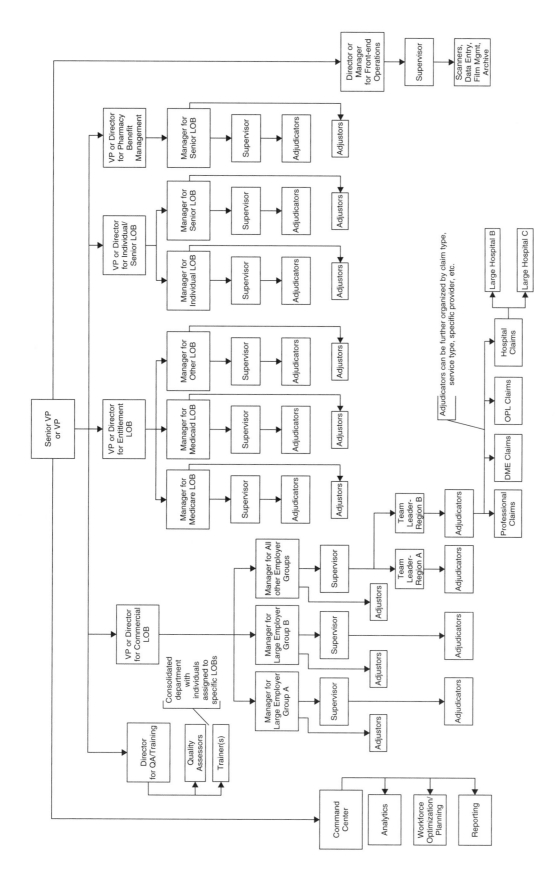

FIGURE 18-5 Claims Capability Organization Chart Options

TABLE 18-1   **Claims Capability Roles and Responsibilities Matrix**

	Sr VP	VP	Dir	Mgr	Sup	Team lead	Adjudicator	Adjustor	Clerical staff	Other
Overall responsibility for claims capability (depending on size of operation)	X	X	X	X						
Represents claims capability in management meetings	X	X	X	X						
Represents claims capability with providers and members	X	X	X	X						
Represents claims capability with ASO groups, government, trading partners, and external auditors	X	X	X	X						
Manages third party including sourcing	X	X	X	X						
Security	X	X	X	X						IT, compliance
Determines claims capability roles and responsibilities	X	X	X	X						
Determines individual management roles and responsibilities	X	X	X	X						
Determines individual non-management roles and responsibilities			X	X						
Establishes policies and procedures			X	X						
Enforces policies and procedures				X	X	X				
Coordinates policies and procedures with other departments			X	X	X	X				
Coordinates claims adjudication system rules			X	X						
Maintains claims adjudication system rules			X	X						IT
Responsible for training and development	X	X	X	X	X					Trainers
Manages workflow tools			X	X						IT
Manages work distribution at unit level			X	X						
Manages work distribution at individual level				X	X	X				
Quality assessment										Quality assessors, compliance

continues

TABLE 18-1	(Continued)									
	Sr VP	**VP**	**Dir**	**Mgr**	**Sup**	**Team lead**	**Adjudicator**	**Adjustor**	**Clerical staff**	**Other**
Inventory (backlog) management		X	X	X	X	X				
Continuous quality improvement		X	X							Cross-functional team
Analytics, workforce optimization/planning, and reporting										Command center
Hires, terminates, assesses performance	X	X	X	X	X					
Responds to problem resolution calls			X	X	X	X				
Special projects			X	X	X	X				
Resolves unadjudicated EDI claims							X			
Adjudicates paper claims							X			
Resolves suspended claims							X			
Adjusts claims due to processing errors or appeals								X		
Scans or keys claims data into system									X	
Archiving and purging									X	

Roles and responsibilities should be coordinated within the organizational model to drive outcomes related to the particular claims capability. **Table 18-1** displays a skills matrix that can help shape the various roles and responsibilities within the payer. Some responsibilities are marked for more than one managerial level and should be interpreted to apply to the highest level that exists in a particular payer. For example, "overall responsibility" is checked for a senior vice president, vice president, and director. However, if all three managerial levels exist, the responsibility resides with the senior vice president.

Claims capability managers often have questions about determining staffing ratios in terms of the number of claims adjudicators, supervisors, or managers needed to respond to the claims volume. There is very little in the way of industry standards to suggest the ideal staffing ratio because there are so many variables to consider. There are also variations in the way claims capability metrics are structured. Some claims osperations measure productivity by claims processed per hour; others measure by claims processed per day. The payer's historical experience can provide a starting point for creating productivity benchmarks if they are not already established. Productivity goals should be set, records kept and analyzed, and ultimately a claims per hour or claims per day (or claim line items per hour or day) quota should be established for staffing determinations as well as performance evaluations. Ultimately, the answer to staffing ratio questions depends on the number needed to meet volume demands, while maintaining quality standards and not relying on overtime hours as a permanent solution.

■ MANAGING THE CLAIMS CAPABILITY

Shared across the four claims capability core competencies as described previously are common, enterprisewide objectives, including:

- Enabling the payer to meet contractual obligations to employer groups, government agencies, members, and providers;
- Ensuring timely benefits administration for enrolled members including the accurate application of cost-sharing features, benefit limitations, maximums, and exclusions;
- Improving the health care of its members through the development and execution of care management plans;

- Administering medical management policies and medical necessity decisions;
- Providing prompt and accurate customer service to members, brokers, employer groups, and providers;
- Protecting financial liability by validating eligibility, avoiding duplicate and other inappropriate claims, ensuring accurate processing, administering other party liability programs, pursuing cost-containment activities related to known or specific financial leakage, and ensuring timely productivity to avoid processing penalties and interest payments; and
- Delivering on its corporate mission in a manner that contributes to effective and efficient use of the health care dollars it touches.

Each of these management priorities is discussed next in terms of achieving production and quality standards. Refer to **Figure 18-6** for a graphic representation of the process steps and functions described in this section.

Policies and Procedures

Although several references to policies and procedures have been made throughout this chapter, this topic deserves a section of its own in order to underscore its importance. Indeed, one cannot overstate the value of thorough, well-written, cross-functional, current, and accessible policies and procedures. They are used to explain the "why" (policy) and the "how" (procedure) of every operational task within the claims capability. Unfortunately, the policies and procedures responsibility is often an orphan. The task to develop and maintain such documentation is either specifically unassigned or it is listed as a responsibility for an overworked supervisor or manager who has neither the time nor resources necessary for proper execution. Ideally, the responsibilities for creating and maintaining policies and procedures should be specifically assigned to one or more persons who have claims knowledge and experience as well as analytic and written communication skills.

In a large organization, the policies and procedures responsibility can be part of the audit, quality assurance, or training function to ensure consistency across the claims capability in style and substance. In a smaller organization, the policies and procedures responsibility may have to be combined with other duties, but care should be taken to ensure that the other duties are subordinate. In recent years, more and more payers have implemented knowledge management tools and search engines to make access to policies and procedures easier.

Discreet policies and procedures are required for all claims capability tasks. They should have the following seven attributes:

1. They must be *written* following a well-defined format that identifies who does what, when, and how it is measured or verified. The documents should also show a history of change over time so that an adjudicator or auditor can easily determine the policy or procedure in effect at a specific time.
2. They should be *thorough* in that they account for every single step in a process. Thoroughly reviewing and documenting processes helps to reveal inconsistencies or gaps in claims processes that compromise quality and/or efficiency.
3. They should be *cross-functional* in that procedures that cross departmental lines should be developed with other departments. For example, if certain suspended claims must be reviewed by medical management personnel, procedures must be developed with the medical management staff so that each department's procedures are clearly defined.
4. They must be *current*. Production of policies and procedures is not a one-time event. It is on ongoing process that must reflect changes in the claims capability, regulatory environment, and so on. Claims personnel must feel confident that the policies and procedures are up-to-date. If found to be unreliable or outdated, personnel will not refer to them.
5. They must be *accessible*. Most payers have developed intranets or knowledge management tools to house policies and procedures that makes searching for applicable information more efficient. Search capabilities should be monitored and adjusted as needed based on user feedback.
6. They must be *consistent with external information*, that is, internal policies and procedures should correspond to the material that is printed in employer or member marketing vehicles, member handbooks, and provider guides as well as items on the payer's website.
7. They must be *shared* appropriately with trading and outsourcing partners to ensure consistent and accurate claims processing outcomes.

Staff Training and Development

Staff training and development is another discreet function that demands adequate time and resources. Like the development of policies and procedures, training is not a one-time event, but rather a process. It begins with on-boarding new employees with both knowledge and skills related to the position. It can continue to include specialty training for staff assigned to specific units that focus on behavioral health, dental, other party liability, fraud and abuse investigations, and so on.

A major pitfall of many training approaches is focusing only on the transactional processing system. Payers often fail to teach new employees the "big-picture" concepts of claims processing before teaching processing tactics. When this occurs, employees often do not understand why they should perform steps in a certain order and for specific

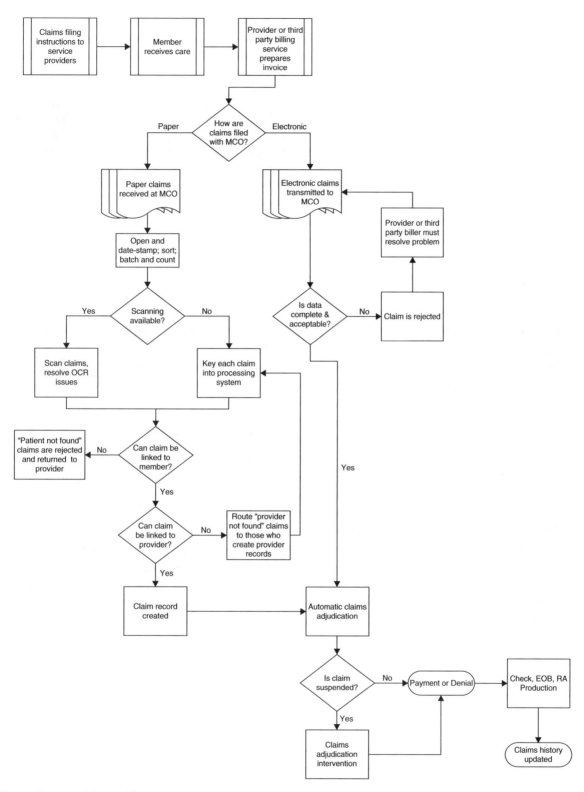

FIGURE 18-6 Claims Capability Workflow Chart

reasons. They just know how to do the steps. This ultimately limits their abilities to quickly conduct research and analysis on suspensions, errors, adjustments, and so on. "Systems" training, while vital, must be grounded in knowledge about managed health care in general and the payer in particular. New employees should understand the payer's philosophies, organization, lines of business, products, provider networks, and other basic information in order to provide context and meaning to the system processing instructions.

Training methods can include classroom training, Web-based and CD ROM courseware, conference calls, webinars, online simulations, lab-based simulations, job aids, Web pages, and/or sites, mentors, internal chats/blogs, and videos. Many organizations are also incorporating newer technologies such as podcasting, video casting, and blogging.[4] Blending a number of training delivery methods is also a current trend that allows payers to use the most appropriate delivery for the audience and topic. However, various methods must be integrated into an overall training plan aimed at addressing specific performance issues. "A blended solution doesn't occur when you just bolt on some e-learning modules to an instructor-led session. It's only when the pieces fit together logically like finely matched parts of an engine that you create a real blended solution."[5]

To be effective, training must conform to adult learning principles:

- Adults have a need to know why they must learn what is being presented to them;
- Adults approach learning in terms of problem solving; and
- Adults must see the relevance of the instruction to their immediate experience.[6]

To provide relevancy, training can be staged over a period of time, so that new hires are instructed on one aspect of claims adjudication (e.g., laboratory claims), are given time to apply the training with live claims, and are evaluated and advanced to the next level of claims adjudication. In other words, there is not a great deal of value in training all new hires on all aspects of claims adjudication when they are unlikely to be assigned to work in all aspects of claims immediately after formal training. Once new claims adjudicators become proficient with certain types of claims, they can be cross-trained on other types more easily.

Cross-training is actually one type of ongoing staff development that should be part of the claims capability total training strategy. Cross-training is vital in smaller organizations simply because there are fewer individuals to rely on when absenteeism or seasonal increased volume impact productivity. In larger organizations, cross-training is a good motivational tool and keeps staff fresh and more eager to learn and do something new. Regardless of the size of the payer, cross-training also enables career path development.

Other ongoing staff development that should be part of the total training strategy focuses on updates to policies and procedures or system processing rules. Many payers use e-mail to convey new information, but this is not a reliable method to ensure all appropriate parties, including outsourcing partners, are informed. It also does not guarantee compliance. Delivering new information requires carefully planned roll-outs that could begin with e-mails, but are followed up with workshops and updated policies and procedures. Knowledge management tools must also be kept current.

Another area of ongoing staff development has to do with softer skills training that may be offered through the payer's human resource department. Claims capability managers should take responsibility for the development of their personnel to ensure a career path and a more satisfied workforce. Time should be allotted for personnel to pursue internal as well as external training programs relevant to their responsibilities. The management team should be encouraged to attend some industry conferences to learn from other organizations and experts in the field. Such external outings should be put to good use, however, with a goal of implementing at least one new idea or process to improve productivity or quality.

■ INVENTORY CONTROL

Inventory control refers to the management of claims from receipt to final disposition. Ultimately, claims inventory is controlled by the claims capability management team; the claims capability management team should not be controlled by the inventory! Control must be based on accurate claim counts at all stages of the claims adjudication process, as well as on efficient work distribution strategies. Bottlenecks must be quickly recognized, root causes discovered, and action plans formulated and executed to eliminate the problem. The claims capability management team will always be challenged with managing inventory (production) and quality. A claims capability that does not meet this challenge will suffer from growing inventories or excessive and costly rework.

Inventory control begins with the front-end processes related to receipt and preparation of claims, electronic or paper. Management of the front-end operations should be under the direction of a single director or manager who reports to the most senior claims capability manager, as shown in the sample organization chart in Figure 18-5. The front-end process for paper claims is far more clerical in nature than that for electronically submitted claims. In either case, front-end claims handling procedures are vital to ensure that claims are promptly logged and accurately prepped for claims adjudication.

Both claim streams, electronic and paper, are dependent on other payer departments for success. Therefore, it is incumbent upon the claims capability management team to establish and nurture relationships with other payer functions to ensure coordinated processing. Consider the fact that the front-end process actually begins with instructions to providers as to how to prepare and file claims on behalf of the payer's members. Claims filing instructions, policies and procedures, and/or guidelines are usually prepared, updated, and distributed by the provider relations or provider contracting personnel. These instructions, which sometimes include certain state and federal government regulations, define what constitutes a valid or "clean" claim. The definition of a "clean" claim must address the following:

- Required claim forms and data formats,
- Minimally required data elements,
- Additional documentation requirements (e.g., emergency room or operative reports, details of anesthesia units administered), and
- Timely filing rules indicating the number of days from the date of service in which a provider must file a claim.

The claims capability management team should review claims filing instructions periodically to ensure that all pertinent information is adequately and accurately included. It is important to remember that claim turnaround rules (defined as the time allowed by government regulation and/or provider contract terms specifying the number of days the claims capability has to process submitted claims for payment or denial) depend on the definition of "clean" claims.

Claims Intake for Electronic Claims

Most claims are submitted electronically by the providers themselves or through third-party vendors known as clearinghouses. A clearinghouse establishes relationships and electronic connections with both service providers and payers to facilitate the immediate delivery of "clean" claims (those that include all of the required data elements that allow for electronic submission by the provider and receipt by the payer). There should be virtually no issues identifying the provider of service on electronically submitted claims, since each provider must have an identification number already established in order to submit electronically. Similarly, there should be no issues identifying the correct patient on the claim because the claim will not be accepted (and will automatically be returned to the provider by the clearinghouse) if the patient identification number is not recognized. It is important to recognize that any critical delays in creating or maintaining member eligibility or provider records in other payer departments will have a negative impact on the claims capability and will more than likely lead to rework or adjustments to claims later in the process.

Claims with other missing data elements are also returned to the provider, thereby ensuring that only "clean" claims are accepted electronically. Claims that do not meet criteria established by the payer are considered rejected claims. Data from these claims are never entered into claims history and never becomes part of payer reports.

An advantage of working with a clearinghouse (for both providers and payers) is that problems are identified and resolved before claims are received by the payer. Alternatively, those payers that have established direct electronic links with providers must establish strict policies and procedures to resolve electronic claims issues with the service providers directly.

Claims Intake for Paper Claims

While the volume of paper claims has decreased significantly over the two decades, there is still enough volume to require well-managed procedures to handle the paper, digitize it, and move it through the process. The inventory control process for paper claims begins with the initial handling procedures shown in **Table 18-2**.

Once paper claims are sorted, counted, and batched, they are ready to be recorded in the transactional processing system: (1) through scanning technologies or (2) through manual keying of data into the system. Operations that receive a small volume of paper claims may opt for manual keying rather than investing in scanning technology. Entry-level personnel can perform this task since they will not be making claims adjudication decisions. However, their work should be closely monitored and assessed for quality to ensure that the claims data submitted on the paper form is the data that is entered into the processing system. It should be noted that many payers have chosen to partner with other companies to perform either scanning or manual keying. These functions are often the first to be outsourced.

The payer cannot always count on paper claims being "clean" claims. Critical elements may be missing or unclearly stated. And it may be difficult to link the claim to the correct patient and/or provider of service. Specific policies and procedures must be developed to account for missing or questionable data elements and such policies and procedures must be coordinated with other payer departments.

One specific problem that has implications beyond the claims capability involves paper claims for patients who cannot be identified in the processing system. These are often referred to as "member not found" claims. If such claims cannot be linked to processing system member records (even if the member is no longer eligible for benefits), the claims can proceed no further in the process. They are typically returned to the provider of the service, indicating that the claim was sent to the wrong payer. This return process, however, may not work for claims operations administering Medicaid, Medicare, or TRICARE programs. Compliance regulations may require that the "member not found" claims be further researched

TABLE 18-2	**Initial Handling Procedures for Paper Claims within the Payer or Outsourced**
Open and date-stamp	• Allocate secure physical space • Establish detailed procedures to open, date-stamp, and count paper claims and other correspondence • Organized and equipped mailroom to move the paper through an assemblyline process ensuring no claims are lost or destroyed • Date-stamp each piece of paper • Avoid marking claims in any way (except for a date stamp and/or document control number) since they are legally binding documents • Ensure that any additional documents submitted with the paper claim (operative or emergency room reports, explanations of benefits from other insurance carriers, letters, etc.) remain with the claim • Discard envelopes except for those showing certified mail information

Sort	• Establish postal mail box numbers for each product or line of business
	  —Initial sort accomplished by the postal service
	  —Applicable claims filing address can be printed on the member's ID card to ensure compliance
	  —Coordinate with other payer departments that control the design and production of member ID cards
	
	• Sort by claim form since most transactional processing systems are designed with two separate processing tracks
	  —Claims for professional services
	  —Claims for hospital services
	
	• Sort by specialization
	  —Physician charges
	  —Durable medical expense (DME)
	  —Chiropractic and/or physical therapy
	  —Other party liability (OPL)
	
	• Sort by specific providers such as large hospitals or providers with unique contract terms
	
	Caution:
	• Too few categories may adversely impact efficiency of work distribution
	
	• Too many categories may be unnecessary and counterproductive
	
	• Sorting is never carved in stone

Batch and count	• Create batches of claims as they are sorted
	  —25–50 claims per batch
	  —Rubber-banded
	  —Labeled with a batch control sheet indicating the date of receipt, the number of claims, the type of claims, and any other important data useful to the functional area receiving the work.
	
	• Create batches of equal size to expedite overall claim count and specific claim count per sort category
	
	• Manual count in smaller operations
	
	• Automated counting methods in larger operations
	  —Use date-stamping equipment that includes automatic counters.
	  —Use a document control number that is sequentially incremented by one. The document control number not only aids the counting process, it also serves as a link between the source document and the claim recorded in the transactional processing system.
	
	• Execute a thorough physical "hard" count of paper claim forms periodically to ensure accountability and guard against intentional or unintentional misplacement.

on other databases to determine if the patient is, in fact, eligible but not yet recorded in the payer's transactional processing system. Similar issues revolve around paper claims where the "provider is not on file." If claims cannot be linked to a processing system provider record, they cannot proceed through claims adjudication. But this time, this problem must be resolved within the payer. For payers that have converted to a National Provider Identifier (NPI),

this problem may no longer be a major issue. Such claims must be worked internally by some combination of claims capability personnel and personnel responsible for creating provider records.

Beyond member and provider issues, there are other data elements that may be missing or illegible on paper claims. How these instances are handled depends on decisions made by the payer in defining a "clean" claim. The claims capability may take a hard line and return all claims with missing or questionable data elements to the submitting provider. However, it is worth considering if making telephone inquiries to clarify questionable data would better serve members, providers, and the payer. In very large operations, this may not be feasible. But in smaller operations, a few well-placed phone calls may actually be more efficient. After all, service delivery is a core component of the claims capability.

Remember, while trying to resolve paper claims with member, provider, or other data issues, the clock continues to tick in terms of claims turnaround commitments. Policies and procedures must be thoroughly thought and worked through with cross-functional teams to ensure that inventory control of paper claims is maintained and member and provider obligations are met.

Claims Intake Metrics

Whether claims are submitted electronically or on paper, inventory receipts must be measured in order to allocate adequate resources and verify financial assumptions about an insured population. Other critical measures that are also important to track include:

- Timely filing limits,
- Turnaround time based on the date the payer received the claim,
- "Claims lag," the time elapsed by comparing the date of service to the date of receipt, and
- "Incurred but not reported" (IBNR), claims measured by comparing outstanding authorization records ordering care and other unreported encounters to actual claims received. IBNR claims represent rendered but unreported services due to delays in service providers' submissions.

Turnaround time is probably the most important of these measures since claims operations must be structured to ensure that turnaround requirements, governed by provider contracts or government regulations, are met. Shorter turnaround goals are often established for electronically submitted claims (either from providers directly or through clearinghouses). Exceeding the turnaround time limits leads to customer service problems and may also result in interest and/or penalty payments to providers.

In order to produce accurate and timely reports as well as meet turnaround goals, claims should be recorded in the transactional processing system immediately upon receipt by the payer. For electronic claims, this process is automatic and, therefore, transparent to the claims capability. For paper claims, however, the front-end operations should be staffed adequately to ensure that all "clean" claims are initially processed within a day or day and a half of receipt. Volumes will vary each business day, with Mondays traditionally being the highest volume day except for weeks that include a Monday holiday. Historical reviews of daily claim receipts should help the management team adjust the staff accordingly and anticipate the need for overtime hours (e.g., for weeks following a holiday).

■ CORE CLAIMS CAPABILITY BUSINESS STEPS

Regardless of the type of claim or how it is submitted, the same core claims capability business steps apply, including determination of eligibility and liability, identification of other party liability, benefits administration, application of provider fee schedules and other contract or network terms, resubmissions, appeals and adjustments, and fraud and abuse. Each of these is discussed on the following pages.

Determination of eligibility and liability refers to decisions that establish if and to what extent the member is eligible for benefits. In determining eligibility, the payer organization must verify both the patient's record of coverage as well as the specific dates of coverage in force. Liability is directly related to underwriting considerations and premium collection. Other principles related to determining liability pertain to employer-sponsored group health benefits that direct cost-sharing as well as some waiting periods. Additionally, coverage can often be broader including benefits such as alternative medical treatments.

There are several decisions involved with determining eligibility and liability. The first decision involves the member's eligibility on the date(s) of service. The transactional processing system compares the date of service listed on the claim to the span of effective and termination (if any) dates on the member record. Members may have multiple layers of eligibility records if they have been enrolled in various benefit plans over time. The benefit plan in force on the date of service will determine the exact coverage including any cost-sharing features such as copayments, coinsurance, or deductibles as well as any limitations or maximums. Types and definitions of cost-sharing are listed in **Table 18-3.**

The member eligibility record will also indicate the member's provider network affiliation and appropriate contract terms. Whether or not the service provider on a claim is participating in the member's provider network will also have an impact on liability. If the member seeks care for certain services outside of the network, the payer may not be liable for payment or may reduce its payment according to predefined benefit rules. Benefits administration refers to applying the appropriate schedule of benefits during the claims adjudication process. The schedule of benefits consists of covered and noncovered services as well as one or more of the cost-sharing features described in Table 18-3.

For payers administering a single line of business such as a Medicaid program, the same schedule of benefits usually applies to all members. However, most payers now administer

TABLE 18-3 Benefit Plan Cost-Sharing Features, Limitations, and Maximums

Feature	Definition	Auto adjudication	EOB/RA	Balance billing
Copayment	• Usually a fixed dollar amount • Member must pay out-of-pocket directly to the service provider • Usually applies to office visits, emergency room charges, prescription drugs	• Automatically calculated and applied • Payment to the provider reduced by copayment amount	• Expressed on the member's EOB and on the provider's remittance advice with an explanatory reason code	• Provider collects copayment at the time services are rendered or by billing the patient directly
Coinsurance	• Usually a percentage such as 20% of the provider payable amount (not the billed charge) • Member must pay out-of-pocket directly to the service provider • Not as common in traditional HMO benefit plans • Usually applies to specified services	• Automatically calculated and applied • Payment to the provider reduced by coinsurance amount	• Expressed on the member's EOB and on the provider's remittance advice with an explanatory reason code	• Provider collects coinsurance, billing the patient directly
Deductible	• A dollar amount that must be paid out-of-pocket directly to the service provider before any benefits are paid by the payer • Not as common in traditional HMO benefit plans • A major feature of newer consumer-driven health plan designs with deductibles as high as $5,000 • Usually expressed as an annual amount • Can apply to specific services or globally to all services • Can be designed to apply to an individual or to a family or both	• Automatically calculated and applied • Payment to the provider reduced by deductible amount *Note:* If adjustments are made to claims where a deductible has been applied, deductible history must be reset (manually if necessary)	• Expressed on the member's EOB and on the provider's remittance advice with an explanatory reason code	• Provider collects deductible by billing the patient directly
Limitation*	• Usually expressed as the number of services that are allowed for payment during a specified period • Examples include 60 days of physical therapy per course of treatment, or 20 outpatient mental health visits per calendar year • Usually applied to specific services	• Automatically calculated and applied • Services exceeding the limitation are denied *Note:* If adjustments are made to claims where a limitation has been applied, limitation counters must be reset (manually if necessary)	• Expressed on the member's EOB and on the provider's remittance advice with an explanatory reason code	• Provider collects payment for denied services by billing the patient directly
Maximum*	• Usually expressed as a dollar amount limit for specified services or for a lifetime benefit • Examples include $5,000 limit on hospice care or $5M lifetime benefit	• Automatically calculated and applied • Payable amounts exceeding maximums are denied *Note:* If adjustments are made to claims where maximums have been applied, maximum counters must be reset (manually if necessary)	• Expressed on the member's EOB and on the provider's remittance advice with an explanatory reason code	• Provider collects payment for denied services by billing the patient directly

*The ACA eliminates lifetime limitations now and will eliminate annual limitations by 2014.

(or intend to administer) multiple programs, thus increasing the number of benefit variations. Under traditional indemnity programs, there are separate benefit structures focused on hospitalization or on physician services (sometimes referred to as "Cross" or "Shield" for the Blue Cross Blue Shield Association affiliates) or a comprehensive benefits structure referred to as Major Medical. Within traditional HMOs, there are point of service (POS) and preferred provider (PPO) benefit programs. To accurately administer benefits, each benefit plan must be assigned a unique code in the transactional processing system, and that benefit code must be attached to the member's eligibility record for a defined period of time. As a result, the transactional processing system is able to auto-adjudicate claims according to the applicable schedule of benefits.

Every enrolled member receives a document that describes the services that are covered and subject to copayments, coinsurance, deductibles, limitations, and/or maximums; this includes differences in coverage based on whether or not the provider is in the plan's network. Also included is a list of exclusions or noncovered services, as well as any requirements around utilization management and preauthorization (see Chapter 7). The detailed version of this is called the evidence of coverage (EOC), and is often also referred to as the subscription agreement. Under the ACA, payers will be required to provide this information in a new standardized document called the summary of coverage (SOC). (These documents and benefits coverage issues are discussed in detail in Chapter 20. Standardized benefits plans that go into effect in 2014 under the ACA are described in Chapter 16.)

Payer personnel must configure or "code" all covered and noncovered benefits described in the EOC into transactional processing system records used to execute auto adjudication. This is an enormous and complex undertaking and can result in thousands of business rule configuration files linked together to enable auto adjudication, which is discussed shortly in the section on auto adjudication. The heart of benefit coding are the standardized procedure (CPT, HCPCS, revenue, etc.) and diagnosis codes that include tens of thousands of items describing virtually every service a provider can bill and the medical justification underlying the claim.

Making it even more challenging is that procedure and diagnosis codes are continually updated. The American Medical Association updates CPT codes annually. New codes are added as new medical procedures are clinically approved; some procedures are marked as deleted if they are no longer accurate descriptions of current medical practice. Similarly, HCPCS codes are modified, added, or deleted as changes are made to such items as durable medical equipment or injectable drugs. Such changes to HCPCS codes are reported quarterly. Procedure code modifiers can also change over time and are important, especially as they further define surgical procedures or differentiate between professional and technical charges. For those claims capability operations that adjudicate prescription drug claims,

the U.S. Food and Drug Administration updates its directory of National Drug Codes (NDC) on a quarterly basis. As previously discussed, diagnosis codes are transitioning from ICD-9 to ICD-10, but both code sets will likely coexist for some period of time as providers and payers grapple with the complexity of parallel processing. Application of provider fee schedules and other contract or network terms refers to automatically determining the payable amount for covered services based on the service provider's fee schedule, contracts, or other payment methodology. Fee schedules, contracts, and other payment methods are recorded in the transactional processing system and linked to provider records so that the applicable payment is executed during auto adjudication. Because the same provider may be paid differently depending on the type of benefits plan (e.g., HMO vs. PPO), the system must be able to use the correct one. This may be done through the use of tables that can be updated easily.

Table 18-4 provides examples of the most commonly used payment methodologies and how they are administered. The reader is encouraged to review the relevant portions of Chapter 5 for detailed descriptions of various payment methodologies and the many ways each can be modified, particularly Tables 5-7 and 5-8, since those all come into play sooner or later.

When a claim is subjected to one or more of these payment methodologies, each line item on the claim (representing each procedure or revenue code billed) is labeled with one or more reason codes that tell a contracted provider how payment was determined. For example, an office visit procedure code of 99201 paid according to a fee schedule and subject to a copayment would most likely have two reason codes attached:

1. A code indicating that the payment was reduced by any applicable cost-sharing amount, which can be collected from the member; and
2. A code indicating that the payment was based on the contracted fee schedule and that the unpaid amount cannot be "balance billed" to the member.

Balance billing rules, applicable only to contracted providers, provide significant protection for consumers related to paying excessive charges for medical services. As discussed in Chapter 4, provider contracts prohibit them from billing the member for any amount other than copayments, coinsurance, deductibles, and amounts not paid due to limitations, maximums, or exclusions. Some states such as California also regulate the practice of balance billing to protect consumers. However, nonparticipating or out-of-network providers are not subject to balance billing policies. As such, payers must determine if covered charges are to be paid in full (subject to copayments, coinsurance, etc.) when no contract is in force with a provider. The thorny topic of what basis should be used to determine how much to pay noncontracted providers is also discussed in Chapter 5.

TABLE 18-4	**Examples of Common Provider Payment Methodologies**		
Feature	**Definition**	**Auto adjudication**	**EOB/RA**
Fee schedule	• A fixed dollar amount for each procedure code • Most common payment method for physician and most ancillary services • Some procedure codes may be labeled as special consideration and will automatically suspend for manual pricing determination	Automatically applied based on fee schedule linked to the provider record associated with the member's benefit plan	Expressed on the member's EOB and on the provider's RA with an explanatory reason code
Discount	• A percentage discount off of the billed amount • Biggest disadvantage is that providers can bill any amount • Reasonable and customary language can reduce provider abuse • A discount off the chargemaster is regularly used to pay hospitals for outlier cases when non-charge payment is used (e.g., per diems) • Discounted chargemaster fees also often used to pay hospitals even when inpatient is paid through another approach.	Automatically applied based on percentage discount linked to the provider record associated with the member's benefit plan	Expressed on the member's EOB and on the provider's remittance advice with an explanatory reason code
Per diem	• Usually applies to hospital charges for inpatient stays • A fixed dollar amount paid per each day of admission regardless of the billed amount • Multiple per diem rates can be established for various types of inpatient stays: medical, surgical, coronary care, maternity, behavioral health, etc. • Multiple per diem rates could apply to the same claim in terms of level of care: semi-private, intensive care, step-down care, skilled nursing care, etc. • Either the date of admission or the date of discharge should be paid, but not both. • If a member changes health plan coverage while admitted, the benefit plan and associated provider agreement effective on the date of admission is applicable (*Note:* This may be a plan administered by another payer.)	Automatically applied based on per diem rates linked to the provider record associated with the member's benefit plan	Expressed on the member's EOB and on the provider's remittance advice with an explanatory reason code
Case rate	• Usually applies to hospital charges for inpatient stays • A fixed dollar amount paid per a specific type of admission such as maternity or cardiac bypass surgery regardless of the number of admitted days or the billed amount • If a member changes health plan coverage while admitted, the benefit plan and associated provider agreement effective on the date of admission is applicable (*Note:* This may be a plan administered by another payer.)	Automatically applied based on case rates linked to the provider record associated with the member's benefit plan	Expressed on the member's EOB and on the provider's remittance advice with an explanatory reason code
DRGs or MS-DRGs	• Usually applies to hospital charges for inpatient stays • A fixed dollar amount paid per type of admission based on diagnosis-related group • If a member changes health plan coverage while admitted, the benefit plan and associated provider agreement effective on the date of admission is applicable (*Note:* This may be a plan administered by another payer.) • DRGs and MS-DRGS are more common in certain markets	Automatically applied based on DRG rates linked to the provider record associated with the member's benefit plan	Expressed on the member's EOB and on the provider's remittance advice with an explanatory reason code
Capitation	• A per member/per month payment for rendering specified services to members • A common payment method for primary care providers • Procedure codes associated with capitated services are programmed to result in a zero-dollar payment amount (not to be confused with denied services that also result in a zero-dollar payment amount)	Automatically applied based on capitated services linked to the provider record associated with the member's benefit plan	• Expressed on the provider's remittance advice with an explanatory reason code • May or may not be included on the member's EOB
Ambulatory surgical center (ASC) rates and ambulatory payment classifications (APCs)	• Usually applies to hospital charges for outpatient surgery • A fixed dollar amount paid per each occurrence of outpatient surgery • Total depends on multiple factors, all of which must be coded	Automatically applied based on ASC rates linked to the provider record associated with the member's benefit plan	Expressed on the member's EOB and on the provider's remittance advice with an explanatory reason code

An important policy and procedure that must be addressed by the payer is how to handle claims in the rare occurrence where the billed amount of the service is less than the contracted fee schedule or payment rate. Some payers still pay the fee schedule amount; others pay the billed amount. While this policy may be applied differently to various providers, a consistent policy across the board is preferable for the sake of both auto adjudication and customer service. It must also be determined if paying the billed amount lower than the contracted rate can be accommodated by the transactional processing system without custom programming (and if maintenance of custom programming is worth the medical cost savings in the long run).

HMOs and payers that offer HMO coverage as one of their product lines must be able to manage capitation as well as more traditional claims. Capitation is described in detail in Chapter 5. While capitation has waned over the past 15 years in favor of other payment methods, it is still important to understand how vital data capture is to the payer and member. Some capitated providers fail to report the complete record of services performed and the complete diagnosis including all comorbidities. When the member record is incomplete, it is difficult for the member to fully benefit from the payer's disease management programs. It also becomes difficult for the payer to report accurately to group, state, and federal administrators just how unhealthy its member population is.

Accurate and timely maintenance of provider payment terms in the transactional processing system are vital to the claims capability's ability to fulfill its obligations to the payer, the members, and the providers. Payer senior management must recognize that poor quality or untimely maintenance of provider payment records has an enormous negative impact on the claims capability and subsequently on members and providers. Resources must be allocated to payer personnel assigned to maintaining provider payment records so that fee schedules and other payment methods are error free and recorded before the effective dates of the payment terms. All too often, new or updated provider contracts are applied retroactively resulting in a large volume of claims adjustments. If this situation arises, the payer may find that a lump sum financial settlement outside of the transactional processing system may be more advantageous than expending the resources to adjust hundreds or thousands of claims. Of course, a lump sum financial settlement often leaves the member's claim history incomplete.

Auto Adjudication and the Use of Automated Business Rules

Auto adjudication is the process of automatically determining eligibility and correctly applying benefits and payment terms for each claim using predetermined rules without any human intervention. Virtually all transactional processing systems are capable of high auto adjudication rates, but auto adjudication is based on what seems like a million small decisions

and contingencies built into the hundreds or thousands of business rules and configuration decisions. The rules for conditional processing are called business rules, and refer to conditions that affect how a claim is adjudicated. Business rules that are not based on administrative conditions such as whether or not somebody was covered on the date the service was provided are sometimes called medical policy[*] rules. For example, a second surgeon may bill the full fee but is only paid half, or the procedure and the diagnosis must match. Those two examples are real, but business rules involving medical policy are highly complex.

As noted already, there is a hierarchy of decisions that the transactional processing system works through in order to determine if a claim is payable or if it should be denied or suspended for further attention and human decision making. Each payer determines its own "edit" hierarchy based on its specific regulations, business needs, and its customer base. Indeed, there are three outcomes of auto adjudication once a claim is accepted into the processing system: auto pay, auto deny, and suspend.

Claims that do not meet the complex (but relatively clear) criteria for payment or denial are automatically suspended for manual review by a claims adjudicator. Some claims suspend because they "get hung up" in the transactional processing system, possibly revealing some problem with the business rule configuration structure. These claims must be attended to immediately so that the problem can be rectified and inventory control, including turnaround time, is not compromised. Other claims suspend precisely because of intentional business configuration rules, such as:

- Inappropriate combinations of service type, procedure, or diagnosis codes for the patient's age,
- Illogical combinations of service type, procedure, or diagnosis codes and the patient's gender,
- Services that require specific medical management review,
- Procedure codes that must be manually priced,
- Missing or inappropriate modifier codes affecting the pricing of surgical claims,
- Suspected other party liability,
- Suspicious diagnosis codes related to accidents, and
- Suspected fraud and/or billing abuse

The business rule configuration and auto adjudication process are much more complicated than this brief description implies. Nevertheless, auto adjudication can occur almost instantaneously. The goal of auto adjudication is maximum throughput (the number of claims automatically adjudicated for payment or denial) and is achieved through

---

[*] Not to be confused with the broad activity called medical policy that is the domain of politicians, academics, think tanks, etc. Medical policy in the context of claims processing refers only to the conditional rules used for processing.

the knowledge, experience, and tenacity of the personnel assigned to create the rules, tables, and other auto adjudication files. The more complete and precise the business rule configuration files, the higher the throughput.

Those who configure the business rule configuration files must remain vigilant to changes in procedure and diagnosis and update the transactional processing system accordingly. If the processing system uses automated medical policy business rules, which virtually all of them do, those must be updated and maintained as well. If system configuration is poorly or inaccurately executed, thousands of customer service issues will erupt, requiring a massive number of claim adjustments.

Payer employees who build such files, usually a combination of information technology (IT) and claims personnel, must be knowledgeable about:

- System architecture,
- Both professional and institutional claim types,
- How claims are filed,
- How charges are reported,
- How benefits are expressed in terms of procedure and/or diagnosis codes,
- How providers are paid,
- How member liability is applied,
- How referral and/or authorization rules are applied,
- How medical policies are applied based on conditional rules,
- How ongoing medical management programs affect claims payment decisions, and
- Federal and state regulations.

Some payers place the responsibility of maintaining the business rule configuration files within the claims capability; some place it within the IT operation. Other payers place it within an integrated and centralized applications team, which includes specialists who maintain business rule files that govern eligibility, provider contracts and credentialing, medical management, and other fundamental processing functions. If the business rule configuration function is outside of the claims capability, the claims management team must maintain at least a dotted-line connection to the function to ensure accuracy and accountability.

As part of the payer's proactive management approach, the claims capability management team must insist on extensive testing of business rule configuration for auto adjudication as well as on prompt fixes to problems discovered through provider and/or member complaints and appeals. Proactive management is challenging because the skill sets and knowledge required to maintain the complex criteria for auto adjudication are often in short supply.

Payment and Issuance of an EOB and RA

Claims that are determined to by payable are then paid, but the mechanism differs for insured and self-funded accounts.

For insured accounts, the money to pay claims is held by the payer, so any checks or electronic funds transfers (EFTs) come from the payer's bank accounts. Payers do not hold the money to pay claims for self-funded accounts. Self-funded accounts set up an electronic "lock box" with a bank, and when the payer is ready to release a batch of claims payments, the account is notified of the amount and the timing, and it is the account's obligation to ensure that there are adequate funds in the lock box to pay those claims. How often such notifications take place depends on how often a payer releases payment batches. As real-time adjudication comes closer to the norm, these lock boxes will need to fund in real time as well. As a practical matter, the entire process is typically automated.

Payments themselves are made either with a check that is then mailed via the U.S. Postal Service, or funds are transferred through EFT. Facilities typically use EFT while physicians and other professionals still receive checks. Payers are pushing for all contracted providers to be paid through EFTs, however. Member-submitted claims are typically paid through a check mailed to the member.

The payment process also produces an EOB and an RA. Payments made through EFT use the HIPAA-mandated RA electronic transaction standard, the X12 835. Paper RAs provide much the same information as is found on EOBs.

The EOB is a document sent to the subscriber or the insured that provides information about how a claim was adjudicated and other relevant information. State and federal regulations usually require certain information to be provided on the EOB, as well as when an EOB must be issued and when it is not necessary to issue one. **Table 18-5** lists examples of the information usually provided in an EOB, and **Table 18-6** lists examples of when an EOB is typically issued and when it is not.

Duplicate Claims or Resubmissions

Resubmissions refer to those claims submitted for payment by providers (or sometimes members) two or more times.

TABLE 18-5	Examples of Information in an EOB
<ul><li>The provider's name</li><li>The date(s) of service</li><li>The type(s) of service</li><li>Fees charged</li><li>The amount paid</li><li>Any remaining liability payable by the member, such as cost-sharing applied against the negotiated fees for in-network providers</li></ul>	<ul><li>Reasons a claim was adjudicated the way it was, such as subject to deductible, not covered due to noncompliance, etc.</li><li>Appeal rights and procedures for requesting an appeal</li><li>Health plan contact information</li></ul>

Source: Copyright P.R. Kongstvedt Company, LLC. Used with permission.

TABLE 18-6	EOB Issuance	

Examples of when an EOB is typically issued	Examples of when an EOB is not typically issued
• Whenever the member has a cost-sharing obligation. • Whenever a claim involves a service rendered by a nonparticipating provider. • If for any reason the member submits a claim for a service rendered by any provider. • Whenever a claim submitted by a participating provider involves a denial based on the participating provider's failure to follow the plan's protocol for coverage, even where the contract between the provider and the plan contains a "hold harmless" provision. • When the plan denies a claim on the basis that the member's coverage was no longer in effect on the date of the service. • When a participating provider bills for covered services for which the provider has not contracted with the insurer. • If a member requests one. • If medical risk has been transferred to a third party such as an independent practice association (IPA), an HMO must still issue an EOB if required by law.	• When there is a prepaid capitation arrangement between an HMO and a participating provider and the provider submits a claim for a service that falls within the capitation payment. • If a claim has been suspended for further investigation prior to final adjudication. • When a global fee arrangement has been negotiated with a participating provider, but the provider itemizes or "unbundles" a claim for the services paid the global fee. • If the plan makes a level of service adjustment to the claim (down-coding or up-coding) and the participating provider contract has a provision that allows the insurer to make such adjustments (if the contract does *not* contain this provision, an EOB typically is issued). • When a participating provider bills a larger amount than the amount specified or referenced in the provider contract or when the provider was paid the contracted amount as payment in full and there is no cost-sharing. • When an exact duplicate of a claim is resubmitted to the insurer for payment provided that an initial EOB has been issued to the insured.

Source: Copyright P.R. Kongstvedt Company, LLC. Used with permission.

In some cases, providers resubmit claims automatically every 30 days or so until payment or denial is posted to their accounts receivable system. If submitted on paper, resubmitted claims may be stamped as "second" or "third" submissions. If submitted electronically, resubmitted claims will most likely be automatically denied as duplicates even if the original claim is suspended in the transactional processing system for manual intervention and resolution.

The claims capability management team must be alert to a high number of resubmitted claims from one or more providers because they signal a problem. The problem could be on the provider side in that payments and/or denials are not being properly or promptly posted. Providers have also been known to resubmit claims toward the end of their fiscal years in hopes that previously denied claims would be paid a second time around. If such trends are noticed, the claims capability managers should enlist the help of provider relations personnel to address these issues. Conversely, the problem could be on the claims capability side, indicating a backlog. This problem is self-perpetuating in that providers will continue to resubmit delayed claims, making the backlog grow even larger. The claims capability management team must keep claims inventory well within contracted turnaround times to help reduce the instances of resubmitted claims.

Task Allocation and Work Distribution

As described earlier, claims adjudicators must review suspended claims for final disposition. How suspended claims are assigned to claims adjudicators, however, varies among payers. Most large payers have either linked a workflow software application to their transactional processing system or worked to embed and integrate workflow into the transactional processing system itself. Workflow software automatically directs suspended claims to claim adjudicator work queues based on any number of factors such as claim type, suspension reason, provider specialty, dollar threshold, and so on. Managers, supervisors, or even team leaders monitor such work distribution to ensure that employees have the training and experience to manage the work assigned to them.

In previous years, many payers designed and implemented workflow applications immediately around claims processing systems to facilitate throughput. Over time, most payers have steadily expanded workflow up and down the operations continuum. This expansion began as payers reached upstream to claims intake and downstream to claims editing. Today, many payers have expanded workflow to include customer service and other key functions that are frequently outside of claims.

For those operations that do not have workflow software, the work distribution is more labor-intensive. For example, managers, supervisors, or team leaders must rely on daily reports generated from the transactional processing system that list suspended claims. The reports are either distributed via e-mail or marked up with specific names of assigned adjudicators and distributed among the staff.

In either case, claims management personnel must constantly monitor claims aging reports to ensure that suspended claims are not left untouched for unnecessary or unacceptable periods of time. Workflow not only helps with inventory control and auditing, but it also identifies many bottlenecks in the process. Detailed workflow processes as well as policies and procedures with other departments must be established and monitored to ensure that no claim is left behind.

■ COORDINATION OF BENEFITS AND OTHER PARTY LIABILITY

Identification of COB and OPL refers to the determination of whether other insurance plans (group health, government health/entitlement programs, automobile, workers' compensation, etc.) are liable or other individuals are responsible for illness or injury related to specified health care expenses. The claims capability must determine if a member is covered by any other insurance that may be considered liable in whole or in part for specific medical care, and then determine if the payer is financially responsible for any part of the care. There are generally four categories to consider: other group health insurance, automobile, workers' compensation insurance, and subrogation.

Benefits are coordinated with other group health insurance typically based on industry standard COB rules published by the National Association of Insurance Commissioners (NAIC) and defined within the member's subscription agreement. With automobile and workers' compensation, liability is shifted from the payer to another insurance carrier based on state laws or other government regulations. With subrogation, specified benefit payments are recovered from members who have been compensated for incurred health costs via legal action. See **Table 18-7** for details.

Ideally, COB and OPL claims are handled by claims specialists who have knowledge of various COB and OPL opportunities and are trained to execute decisions in the transactional processing system. The key to successful COB and OPL efforts is converting raw data into information through the use of analysis. The payer must engage employees in a variety of departments and roles to collect and record other insurance data. Most transactional processing systems provide space on the member record for other group health insurance. Business rule configuration records can be programmed to suspend claims for members who have other coverage so that benefits can be coordinated with the other program. Other group health insurance information must be updated at least once each year, although continuous updating is becoming more common. Today, as many cases of COB and OPL are identified through internal analysis as are self-reported using claims forms and provider and member identification. In addition to analysis within the claims area, information about accident-related claims is often captured by personnel in other areas of the payer. For example, utilization nurses arranging for inpatient stays or durable medical equipment are often able to determine that care is related to an automobile accident or a work-related injury. Such information can be communicated to COB and OPL specialists through an authorization record or a flag attached to the member record to suspend all claims for COB or OPL determination.

Service providers can report certain COB and OPL information when submitting either electronic or paper claims. ANSII standard transaction record layouts for electronically submitted claims include fields for communication of other party liability data. Paper claim forms also have fields specifically designed to document other coverage. Such claims can be identified in the front-end process and routed immediately to specialists for special handling. Business rule configuration records can be programmed to suspend claims submitted with such data so that benefits can be coordinated with the other program. Increasingly, COB and OPL is identified by the payer or one of its business partners using data analysis and data mining. Some identification can even occur prepayment, allowing the payer to avoid difficult "pay and chase" scenarios.

Foundational to the COB and OPL program is the decision regarding its fundamental approach: "pay and chase" or "chase and pay." In the "pay and chase" model, the payer processes claims for payment without coordinating benefits either with other group health plans or with auto carriers or workers' compensation programs. Instead, the OPL program is executed retrospectively (the "chase"). Some payers take this approach to limit prompt payment complaints from their provider community, especially when interest is calculated on late payments. Recovery, however, is both costly and challenging and may take months to realize savings. Other payers follow the "chase and pay" model in that they may suspend or even deny claims until the information is "chased" and a benefit determination is made. This approach conserves claims dollars, but it may generate more customer service issues while claims remain unresolved or denied. Over time, more and more payers have moved toward the "chase and pay" model.

Every effort should be made throughout the payer to identify COB and OPL potential, capture the information, and execute OPL policies and procedures since millions of dollars and consistency of payment are at stake. A dedicated COB and OPL unit can pay for itself with upward of a 10:1 return on investment. Financial incentives for the collection of COB and OPL overpayments should also be considered within the context of the payer's human resources and salary policies. Many payers set specific savings targets for COB and OPL personnel, a practice gaining popularity within the industry.

TABLE 18-7	Coordination of Benefits and Other Party Liability			
Feature	**Definition**	**Claims adjudication**	**EOB/RA**	**Balance billing**
Coordination of benefits in group health insurance plans	• Process by which payer determines the order of payment when a member is covered under two or more group health insurance programs • Ensures that providers and/or members are not paid twice for the same care • Industry standard rules developed and updated since 1970 by the NAIC • COB rules govern which plan is primary (pays first) and which plan is secondary (pays second) and how order is determined • Many rules apply to dependent children when covered under both parents' health plans • Birthday rule most common, indicating that parent with the birth date (month, day, not year) earlier in the calendar year is primary for children • Payer must determine calculation method (benefit less benefit or "true" COB)	• Claims for members whose payer coverage is considered secondary are suspended for COB specialist review and determination • Claims may be denied pending receipt of other health plan's EOB • Payment to the provider reduced by other health plan's payment, if any	Expressed on the member's EOB and on the provider's remittance advice with an explanatory reason code	Typically no payment balance exists for the provider since both health plans combined pay 100% of the charges
Automobile insurance	• Benefits available under an automobile insurance policy applicable to medical expenses incurred due to an automobile accident • Governed by state laws, which vary; some states do not allow coordination • Must determine if auto accident is work-related, creating different liability • Utilization management nurses or customer service reps may be alerted to auto benefits potential	• Claims incurred due to an automobile-related injury may be auto-suspended if associated with accident-related diagnosis or procedure codes • Payment to the provider may be denied until auto insurance liability is established • Once auto insurance liability is confirmed, coverage for the portion of medical care not covered by auto insurance (perhaps to policy dollar limit) is considered for payment	Expressed on the member's EOB and on the provider's remittance advice with an explanatory reason code	Payer often made aware of auto insurance settlement retrospectively if the provider refunds claims payments
Workers' compensation	• Benefits available under a workers' compensation insurance policy applicable to medical expenses incurred due to an on-the-job accident or work-related health problems occurring over time • Governed by state laws, which vary • Utilization management nurses or customer service reps may be alerted to workers' comp potential	• Claims incurred due to a work-related illness/injury may be auto-suspended if associated with work-related diagnosis or procedure codes • Payment to the provider may be denied until workers' comp liability is established • Once workers' compliability confirmed, coverage for the portion of medical care not related to work-related illness or injury is considered for payment	Expressed on the member's EOB and on the provider's remittance advice with an explanatory reason code	Payer often made aware of auto insurance settlement retrospectively if the provider refunds claims payments

continues

	TABLE 18-7	*(Continued)*			

Feature	Definition	Claims adjudication	EOB/RA	Balance billing
Subrogation	• The right of the payer to recover any damages the member may receive from a third party who assumes responsibility for an accidental injury, including those known as "slips and falls" • Usually surfaces after legal action results in a financial settlement to the member • Allows the payer to seek payment from the member for health care payments made on the member's behalf related to the injury • Must be a subrogation clause in the member's subscription agreement • Subrogation prohibited by some states, while other states require it • Self-funded plans may pursue subrogation when state prohibits it for insured plans	• Payments of claims related to subrogation settlement may be recovered from member not provider, unless there is evidence that the provider was paid twice • Payer may agree to engage third-party attorney or specialty vendor to recover funds	Expressed on the member's EOB and on the provider's remittance advice with an explanatory reason code	Payer often made aware of settlement retrospectively if the provider refunds claims payments

■ REPORTS

Well-designed, useful, and timely reports are vital to the claims capability management team. However, obtaining such reports continues to be a challenge in some payers. As previously noted, early transactional processing systems provided so-called "canned" reports that were hard-coded into the software. These were often of little use, being poorly conceived and having not only too much information, but too much useless information.

Current transactional processing systems are able to produce more customized reports and have evolved to offer a "dashboard" approach so that specific management personnel are able to focus on information of greatest interest to them. While that opportunity exists, there is still a need to design reports that provide the precise detail required for different levels of managers and for different purposes. Over time, payers have also implemented specialized reporting databases. Such operational data warehouses enable the flexibility and reporting referenced above; these warehouses allow the claims capability to perform analysis, develop statistics and trends, identify incorrectly processed claims, and identify performance improvement opportunities more quickly.

Most recently, payers have used the richness of data housed in their data warehouses to engage in advanced claims analytics and predictive modeling for both claims receipts and claims throughput. In short, reporting is evolving from a retrospective data capture activity to a prospective operational input tool, which helps payers better meet both internal and external customer needs.

Table 18-8 displays a matrix showing various types of internal and external reports and their recommended utilization. Some reports are financial in nature and are useful to senior management. Other reports facilitate operational decisions. Summary versions of such reports are usually requested by senior claims managers. The detailed versions are used by the claims capability managers, supervisors, and team leaders to monitor and distribute work. They are vital to moving claims through the process and uncovering any bottlenecks. Reports for adjudicators and adjustors are usually limited to those used for work assignments. A special report is produced for the quality assessors listing randomly selected claims for review. Additionally, ad hoc reports can be created for continuous process improvement projects as needed. External reports for employer groups and government regulators must also be produced, including those that address claims capability quality and production, group and product experience, OPL savings, and provider-specific reports related to performance and risk-sharing. The data elements included in external reports is often dictated by employer groups and government regulators.

Report design and production is as much art as science. In order to obtain the needed information in the most useful form, the claims capability management team should develop a good working relationship with report-writing personnel who are sometimes part of the IT or finance operations. If possible, report-writing positions should be staffed within the claims capability to reduce the dependency on nondepartmental resources and produce reports in a more timely fashion. Claims report writers should have the requisite technical skills, but also have claims adjudication knowledge in order to execute specifications articulated by claims management.

TABLE 18-8	**Operational Reports Matrix**

Internal reports

		Sr VP	VP	Dir	Mgr	Sup	Team lead	Adjudicator	Adjustor	Clerical staff	Other
Executive-level dashboards		X	X								
Financial											
Claims payout											
By LOB, plan, employer group, member		X	X	X							
By day, week, month, quarter, year											
IBNR											
By LOB, plan, employer group, member		X	X	X							
By day, week, month, quarter, year											
Utilization reports											Sales and marketing, medical mgmt
By LOB, plan, employer group, member		X	X	X							
By day, week, month, quarter, year											
Overpayment reports	Summary	X	X	X	X						
By LOB, plan, employer group, member	Detailed				X	X	X		X		Cost containment
By day, week, month, quarter, year											
Voluntary refund reports	Summary	X	X	X	X						
By LOB, plan, employer group, member	Detailed				X	X	X		X		Cost containment
By day, week, month, quarter, year											
Productivity/quality											
Mailroom and EDI receipts	Summary	X	X	X	X						
By LOB, plan, provider, etc.											
By day, week, month, quarter, year	Detailed				X	X				X	Network mgmt, provider relations
Claims on hand	Summary	X	X	X	X						
By LOB, plan, provider, etc.	Detailed				X	X					
By status (ready to finalize, suspended)											

continues

TABLE 18-8 (Continued)

Internal reports

		Sr VP	VP	Dir	Mgr	Sup	Team lead	Adjudicator	Adjustor	Clerical staff	Other
Claims processed through auto adjudication	Summary	X	X	X	X						
By LOB, plan, provider, etc.											
By status (ready to finalize, suspended)	Detailed				X	X					
Suspended claims	Summary	X	X	X	X						
By LOB, plan, employer group, etc.	Detail				X	X	X	X			
By assigned claims adjudicator											
Claims selected for random quality assessment or focused audit											Quality assessors
Ad hoc reports for continuous process improvements		X	X	X	X						Training, cross-functional team

External reports

		Sr VP	VP	Dir	Mgr	Sup	Team lead	Adjudicator	Adjustor	Clerical staff	Other
Quality and timeliness reports											Group/govt agency, sales and marketing
By customer		X	X	X							
Group experience report		X	X								Group/govt agency, sales and marketing
Product experience report		X	X								Group/govt agency, sales and marketing
MTM scores for BCBS plans		X	X								BCBS Association
COB and OPL reports by customer		X	X								Group/govt agency
Provider-specific reports related to performance and risk-sharing		X	X								Group/govt agency, network mgmt, provider relations
Workforce modeling and planning		X	X	X	X						Training

COST CONTAINMENT

More sophisticated quality review efforts, better analysis, strategic third-party partnerships, and more flexible reporting have enabled many payers to pursue focused but effective cost-containment programs designed to curb financial leakage such as overpayment of medical claims. Some payers have created specialized units within the claims capability to prospectively and retrospectively identify overpayments due to complex duplicates, retroactivity, inappropriate dosages, less obvious COB and OPL, inappropriate billing practices, and so on. These examples are but a few of the hundreds of causes of claims overpayments that directly impact the payer's bottom line.

To elaborate on one of the examples listed above, the term "complex duplicate" (not to be confused with a simple duplicate or resubmission) primarily refers to services that overlap. One example of the many forms of overlapping services is an emergency room visit that overlaps with a subsequent admission for an inpatient stay. Typically, a separate payment for hospital emergency room charges is not payable if the patient is admitted. The transactional processing system's duplicate logic does not always catch overlapping services, especially if the patient arrives in the emergency room during the afternoon or evening but is not admitted until after midnight. The date of service for the emergency room claim will be a day earlier than the date of admission and may avoid detection by typical business configuration rules.

Another example, retroactivity, refers to members whose termination date is reported by their employers (or government agency) well after the fact. In the interim, hundreds of claims may have been paid on behalf of such terminated members. Payment reversals (sometimes known as offsets or clipped payments) can usually be executed within transactional processing systems. However, retroactively terminated members must first be identified through analysis and their termination dates verified. Caution must also be exercised to determine how such overpayments can be collected from affected providers. Simply "offsetting" or "clipping" future payments could damage provider relationships.

A third example of financial leakage pertains to application of the correct provider fee schedule to specific health plan products. At times, a health plan may have several outstanding fee schedules that are tied to different products or networks. If the incorrect fee schedule is chosen, either automatically or manually, payments are likely to be incorrectly calculated. Often this type of incorrect payment is difficult to find and causes provider and member confusion.

The three examples provided above are intended to be illustrative. Well-managed cost containment functions are constantly looking for new examples of financial leakage. Types of financial leakage typically change with new product launches, system conversions, changes to business configuration rules, changes to state or federal legislation, and so forth. Payers participating in state health insurance exchanges created under the ACA, for example, will need to develop policies and procedures around retroactivity for members who go back and forth from Medicaid to subsidized premiums (see Chapter 25). Experience also shows that well-managed cost containment functions continue to find greater quantities of financial leakage year after year providing a long-term return on investment.

FRAUD AND ABUSE

Fraud and abuse refers to actions taken by internal or external parties that violate security and/or cause a financial loss to the payer and its customers. Payers can expect even greater government attention to fraud and abuse as expansion of health insurance coverage to new classes of insured is expected to be financed through greater control of fraudulent and abusive practices.

Instances of fraud within payers are actually rare, but the claims capability management team must be ever vigilant over security issues. Employees must be reminded not to share passwords or reveal claims-related information with anyone outside the context of their job responsibilities. Payers must also be vigilant regarding external instances of fraud and communicate their intention to investigate and prosecute fraudulent practices. A vulnerable spot within the claims operation occurs when claims are received from providers that are not yet established in the transactional processing system. Before a provider record is created, steps should be taken to verify that the provider is legitimate, especially if it is a high-dollar claim. Abuse is actually the more common and costly problem and is associated with inflated or inappropriate charges. Whether intentional or not, abuse is best tackled through analysis of claims data, provider payment practices, and anomalies in provider practice patterns within the scope of the claims capability. Fraud and abuse are discussed in detail in Chapter 19.

QUALITY ASSESSMENTS

Earlier in the chapter the core competency of quality control was described in terms of upstream and downstream controls. Quality assessment occurs within the claims capability in the form of ongoing statistical audits and temporal-focused audits; it is executed by quality assessors who should report to a nonproduction manager or director (see Figure 18-5). Quality assessors must have strong analytic and investigative skills as well as a thorough knowledge of the lines of business, products, benefit plan features, provider contracts, and policies and procedures associated with the claims they review. They must also operate with a high level of integrity so that the quality review process is not only fair, but is perceived to be fair by the claims adjudicators.

Statistical audits are typically conducted on a random sampling of claims selected by the transactional processing system. An equal number or percentage of claims are assessed for each adjudicator, and quality scores are calculated based on the number and type of errors uncovered. Some errors are regarded as financial, meaning they directly impact the payment or denial of the claim. Some errors are regarded as statistical in that the payment or denial is not affected, but some data element or aspect of processing is not correct. In the past, statistical errors were considered more of an annoyance or an indication of carelessness. However, statistical errors have taken on more significance now that claims analytics and data reporting are factors in product development, wellness and disease management programs, and government reporting (as discussed earlier in this chapter).

Focused audits are typically done when new products are introduced to ensure that all claims are being processed according to the new benefit plan(s). Similarly, if new groups are added or new provider contract terms are programmed, a focused audit will uncover quality issues early and avoid costly corrections and adjustments. Focused audits are also conducted on new hires once their training is completed and they are working on live claims. Such audits often call for 100% review of new adjudicators' work for a limited time period. Another type of focused audit occurs in preparation for a full-scale operations audit conducted by a third party such as a government agency.

Claims errors discovered via quality assessments should be traced back to determine their origins, system or human, so that steps can be taken to prevent similar errors in the future. "Systems" solutions may include correcting a provider or member record, updating a fee schedule, or adjusting a business rule configuration file. "Human" solutions may include delivering additional training, updating policies and procedures, and/or revising business processes. If the issue is specific to a small group of individuals, the claims capability management team may opt to institute performance-monitoring plans for those persons. Additional errors are also uncovered by reviewing member and provider complaints and/or appeals to discover the root causes of errors. Returned checks and other voluntary refunds are also good resources for such information. This type of research is more likely to be the responsibility of the claims capability management team. But these efforts should be coordinated with the quality assessors so that a broad picture of performance improvement issues can be constructed and attended to.

APPEALS

Appeals of a denial of benefits coverage or denial of payment are directly affected by the ACA. The process for internal review and external review of appeals are described in detail in Chapter 20, and will not be repeated here. If the appeals process reveals a problem in the claims operation, management must attend to making sure it is not repeated. In the event the appeal review processes results in a decision to pay the benefit, the typical process is to then request an adjustment in the adjudication.

Requests for adjustments should be expedited by the claims capability, especially if the claim was initially adjudicated erroneously. The claims capability management team must monitor aging and turnaround time for adjustments, just as they do for new claims. The management team should also analyze the new knowledge gained through the grievance and appeals process and use it as a basis for continuing process improvements.

INFORMATION TECHNOLOGY

Much has already been said about transactional processing systems and other technology tools used by the claims capability. This section examines the evolving nature of claims-related information technology over the last 50 years and how this evolution has impacted the management of the modern claims capability.

In the early years of claims processing, claims inventory was paper-based and manual adjudication was the vital component. Paper invoices from doctors, hospitals, and other medical providers or receipts from patients who were seeking payment were received, date-stamped, and sorted in the mailroom. This paper-based inventory was subsequently placed in staging areas. In the traditional indemnity insurance operations of the 1950s–1980s, newly received claims were inserted into file folders created for each insured individual, family, or sometimes group. Claims adjudicators compared the new claims to the collection of already processed claims in the folder to prevent duplicate payments. They verified eligibility, coverage, and coordination of benefits status based on information contained in the folder, and then they scanned the new claims for completeness. If data were missing or questionable, a form letter was generated or a phone call was made. If the new claims were cleared for payment, claims adjudicators manually calculated applicable deductibles (individual or family), out-of-pocket expenses, stop-loss amounts, annual and lifetime maximums, and other insurance benefits. Accumulators of various types were maintained on worksheets inside the claims file folder. The process concluded with the completion of a check voucher and the refiling of the patient's folder. The claims capability was an entirely manual process. Even in early managed care claims operations (usually staff model provider networks) that did not utilize the family file folder system, the process was entirely manual, including the production of an itemized list of claim payments attached to the provider's payment check.

In these early years, technology (in the form of mainframe computers housed in large temperature-controlled rooms) was in its infancy and was initially used only for check writing and financial reporting. Management of the claims capability focused on personnel. Armies of entry-level clerks were needed to sort, file, and retrieve the paper. Claims adjudicators were the keys to both production and quality. Greater emphasis on production, however, often meant that error rates were high. Greater error rates led to higher volumes of costly rework, ultimately producing a negative impact on the productivity and financial results of the payer.

Business processes revolved around an assembly line approach to the movement of claims from mailroom to check production, but were often bogged down by sheer volume. In many operations, claims adjudicators not only processed claims, but they also responded to telephone and written inquiries and complaints. Any sudden increase in claims volume easily created claim backlogs, which in turn created larger call volumes—a vicious circle that was difficult to break (without the use of overtime or temporary help).

In the early 1980s, automation led to corresponding improvements in productivity and quality. Claims continued to be submitted on paper and had to be keyed into the transactional processing system. However, the systems could now perform arithmetical calculations for copayments, coinsurance, deductibles, benefit limitations, and even coordination of benefits. Such functionality varied as large insurance carriers and payers developed proprietary systems, and software vendors developed and marketed their own applications to meet the needs of specific markets. By the mid-1990s, though, most transactional processing systems could check for duplicates, evaluate eligibility, check for required referral or prior authorization records, and calculate payments based on financial benefit rules (copayments, coinsurance, limitations, etc.) and provider contract terms.

Such automation had an enormous impact on personnel and business processes. There was no longer a need to maintain file folders of claims history once claims data were recorded in the processing systems. In many claims processing operations, tasks performed by entry-level personnel changed from chasing and organizing paper to keying claims into the processing system as they were received and identifying early in the process those claims that could not be processed due to incomplete information. Claims adjudicators were aided in determining payments with the system's financial calculators, thereby reducing errors. Productivity increased in terms of claims processed per hour. However, several challenges continued to bog down productivity, including making benefits determination at the procedure code level, linking referrals/authorizations to claims, and dealing with nonstandard provider contract payment arrangements. Such matters still had to be resolved in a manual process, requiring the expertise of experienced claims adjudicators.

Specialization of claims processing became the norm in this generation of claims capability due to the design features of the transactional processing systems. Separate system and business architectures existed for professional claims and hospital claims to comply with different billing methods for each type of claim. With increasingly diverse provider payment schemes, most claims operations divided claims processing duties by claim type. This often resulted in more senior claims adjudicators being assigned to hospital claims processing, since many aspects of hospital charges or payment methods were not initially automated. Managing two claim types required two similar but still different sets of business processes, policies and procedures, training curricula, production standards, and quality measures. Over time, various types of ancillary claims would further complicate the management and organization of the claims capability.

Another significant development during this period involved the changing relationship between the claims operation and the other departments within the payer. For example, most payers reassigned the customer service function to call centers, which were themselves evolving into higher-performing and specialized operations. The call centers responded to all types of telephone, written inquires, and complaints, including those dealing with claims. Claims production personnel, while freed from these external customer responsibilities, still retained a customer service competency for internal customers.

Additionally, the claims operations became increasingly dependent on other departments to create precise enrollment, provider contracting, and other records to ensure accurate claims processing. Those with claims processing experience were called on to educate those programming the new systems so that all aspects of claims processing would be taken into consideration as processing dictionaries were created. Contrary to some who believed that medical management would become the primary function within the evolving payer, it soon became apparent that the claims operations would remain the primary functional area within the evolving enterprise.

Over the past 10 years, we have witnessed an ongoing evolution from parameter-driven auto-adjudication technology to the use of more and more sophisticated rules and table-based adjudication. As such, a wide variety of benefit designs now can be programmed into the processing software. Rules defined by multiple combinations of various code sets (procedure, diagnosis, place of service, etc.) along with member demographics, benefit and cost-sharing calculators, and provider contract terms allow for higher and higher automatic claims adjudication. With advances in the filing of electronic claims as well as scanning technologies for the dwindling number of paper claims, most transactions are poised to sail through claims processing without human intervention. Those claims that cannot be finalized automatically are still suspended for a claim adjudicator's resolution, but the rates of auto-adjudication now exceed 90% in many payers.

This change has had a profound impact on claims capability personnel. Claims organizations have generally become smaller (fewer headcount) as auto adjudication and electronic receipt of claims continues to increase. Although total full-time equivalents (FTE) counts are lower, the skill mix is more diverse and robust. Claims adjudicators have become key problem solvers within the payer and deliver value by resolving the suspension edits that continue to occur as the simpler and even medium complexity claims have been automated. Business processes have also changed dramatically in that workflow, policies and procedures, and training need only focus on the types of claims problems the adjudicators will encounter today. Business analysts have taken an increasingly important role in improving production and quality through various quality improvement initiatives and ongoing transactional processing system enhancements.

Technological advances and their corresponding personnel and business policies have evolved to improve accuracy, avoid customer dissatisfaction, and improve the payer's financial results. Tools that enable early overpayment identification have become increasingly important as health care costs continue to escalate. Many claims capabilities have created cost containment detection filters and (where possible) prepayment adjustments. Also referred to as focused audits, such final quality checks for a known area of weakness can detect incorrect payments on processed claims that have not yet entered the final check-writing process. Consulting firms and other specialized third-party vendors have helped payers save billions of dollars through development of specialized programs to detect overpayments both prospectively and retrospectively.

There is no question that technology will continue to evolve and influence the core competencies of the claims capability, particularly in the area of self-service. Many employer groups already update employee and member eligibility information directly in the payer's eligibility system. Through the widespread usage of secure, Web-based portals, payer information is much more readily available to many customers. Virtually all claim inquiries are now made via the Internet. Many payers process authorization and administer disease management programs via their portals. For many years, billing functions also have been accomplished through electronic means.

Provider self-service has been a particular area of automation focus for payers. Because provider inquiries follow a routine pattern, payers have been able to write or purchase software that enables easy access to information related to eligibility, claims payment, provider contract and network information, and so on. Most providers enjoy the efficiency and 24-hour access to payer and patient information.

Auto-adjudication technology and processes also continue to advance, including real-time adjudication. In fact, the Blue Cross Blue Shield Association has mandated that its member plans enable real-time claims adjudication in 2014. As auto-adjudication rates and workflow management tools have improved, the standard work mix directed to claims adjudicators is more complex today than in years past (there simply are not as many "easy" claims that cannot be auto-adjudicated). Transactional processing systems continue to become more and more flexible than the legacy transaction systems used earlier, thus enabling a broader array of benefit plans, payment schemes, and products.

Many payers are beginning to explore movement of the core administrative systems to the "cloud." Hosting of core administrative systems is becoming increasingly popular. These trends enable the payer to reduce its reliance on large IT staffs and reallocate resources to other core functions. Some smaller payers could share technology with business partners to realize huge economic savings.

Finally, the analytical and reporting tools that support cost containment and payment integrity have advanced significantly. The most sophisticated payers now rely on advanced analytics and even artificial intelligence to identify specific claims and billing patterns that the business configuration rules of the past could not detect. Advances in analytics also enable far better predictive modeling for labor or staffing needs and claiming patterns. The modern payer manager has better insight than ever before into expected work volumes and work mix.

■ OUTSOURCING

The last issue to discuss in terms of managing the claims capability is outsourcing, an option exercised by many large commercial payers and more recently by smaller organizations and nonprofits. Health payers consider outsourcing as a management option not only to reduce costs, but also to improve service levels. Outsourcing is occurring across the health care marketplace, with both providers and payers participating. Many provider organizations are beginning to have X-rays and pathology reports read off-shore by U.S.-trained Indian physicians as well as paperwork completed (including operative report transcriptions and dictation) by well-educated staff in developing nations around the world.

The functions that have been traditionally outsourced by payers have been "non-customer-facing" functions, including actual claims adjudication or suspense resolution. While there are many developments that have led to an increased interest and implementation of outsourcing arrangements, the two most significant are the monumental advances in information and communications technologies, and the availability of more sophisticated workforces around the globe who are available to support American business. Just as the modern claims capability has evolved, so have outsourcing options that include the following four models: shared service, onshore, near-shore, and off-shore.

The shared service model has been operated for decades by many large regional or national payers that have consolidated "back-office" functions into a centralized office while many of the customer service, medical management, and provider relations and contracting functions remain local. Examples of shared services functions include mail intake, scanning, data entry, ID card and booklet production, and certain types of claims processing. Greater specialization, efficiencies, and economies of scale can be achieved through a shared services model. In cases in which some claims processing has been centralized, the knowledge and skills of trained, experienced claims adjudicators can be leveraged via cross-training to accommodate spikes in claims volume and serve as a critical component in contingency planning.

As the shared services model matured, many vendors emerged, enabling the payer to migrate shared functions from their own centralized offices to lower-cost third-party business partners. Over time, these lower-cost third parties began to move their own facilities to near-shore and off-shore locations to remain competitive by offering lower costs per transaction. Most of these third-party vendors were able to invest in building their own capabilities outside of the United States by entering into multiyear contracts with payers. The rise in third-party administrators (TPAs) during the 1980s and 1990s also bolstered the use of specialized third-party vendors. For example, a relatively young TPA would often outsource its clerical functions (and sometimes certain types of claims processing) to other third-party vendors in order to keep their own administrative costs low. For a new TPA, it is often more efficient to use the services of an established third-party vendor instead of building and supporting the infrastructure and staff needed for specific functions. This type of outsourcing allows the TPA to focus on product design and services that act as differentiators in the marketplace. For both TPAs and larger outsourcing organizations, services today include not only simple claims resolution, but also highly specialized claims processing for services such as home infusion therapy.

The near-shore model was the first option developed in the 1980s, with operations often located in the Caribbean, Canada, or Ireland. This model leveraged English-speaking staff trained to assume well-defined functions at a lower cost. While initially a viable option (from about 1980 to 1995), small labor pools and increasing local labor costs contributed to the migration of outsourcing from these near-shore locations to other parts of the world.

To date, Eastern Europe, India, and the Philippines have been the largest beneficiaries of the labor migration just described. Each of these labor markets includes English-speaking, educated, and highly motivated individuals eager for employment with U.S.-based firms. Even though they are physically located on the other side of the world, many of these operations work during traditional U.S. business hours. Willingness to work these hours facilitates communication and problem solving and allows outsourced production units to integrate with the payer's internal staff.

In addition to occasional information and communications technology issues, there are many other matters that must be addressed to enable off-shore outsourcing. There must be a clear delineation of responsibilities and communication protocols (electronic or telephonic) established between the payer and the outsourcing operation. This particularly applies to timely and accurate problem resolution. Corresponding policies and procedures and training materials must be designed with both parties in mind, and particular attention must be paid to materials for off-shore staff to accommodate language usage and cultural differences.

There are also legal, public relations, financial, and human resource issues to consider when outsourcing. For example, if a payer is administering government contracts, there may be contractual restrictions on both near-shore and off-shore outsourcing. Even when administering commercial business, terms may restrict out-of-state or off-shore outsourcing. Federal and state government entities, as well as politicians, may also create environments in which the payer suffers from a public relations perspective if it chooses to outsource even clerical functions. Although many payers opt for off-shore outsourcing to supplement their current workforce (not replace it), employee relations and human resource issues (often emotionally charged) arise and must be addressed with existing employees, employer groups, providers, and the business community at large.

As early as 2005, off-shore outsourcing had become a competitive requirement for many large payers and it has continued to gain traction as a means to curb accelerating health care costs. In addition to the 30–50% labor cost savings that can exist by function, there are many other benefits to outsourcing. Creation of an outsourced claims capability serves as a critical back-up for U.S. operations; this backup is particularly useful to mitigating work stoppages due to facility problems such as electrical outages, natural disasters, and local labor unrest.

Those payers that exercise due diligence, carefully plan outsourcing ventures, and more fully integrate the outsourced operations into the parent company ensure a successful outcome. In fact, most payers that outsource an initial function continue to take advantage of the better-quality results and lower costs associated with outsourcing additional functions. Regardless of political grandstanding and media hype, outsourcing will continue to have a role for payers as it will for other industries. This ongoing role presents claims management with the increasing need to work with a multicultural and broadly distributed workforce.

■ 15 RISK AREAS AND 50 TIPS

Throughout this chapter, a variety of production and quality issues were described or referenced. To provide a more pointed discussion of claims capability risks, the following list of 15 common pitfalls is shown below, along with suggested resolutions.

1. **Growing Backlog.** Claims backlogs do not develop overnight and, therefore, cannot be resolved overnight. Tight control over daily receipts and quick action when production falls behind (with the application of overtime or use of third-party support) will help prevent a backlog from growing into an enormous problem. Major undertakings such as systems conversions or adding new lines of business require advanced planning to prevent backlogs from taking root.
   - TIP 1: When planning a large new undertaking, make every effort to bring the current claims inventory down to zero, meaning that claims are resolved almost as they are received.
   - TIP 2: Be on guard for providers who resubmit claims that were previously denied. Enforce the timely filing limits to prevent old dates of service claims from entering the system again, only to be denied as duplicates.
   - TIP 3: Always attempt to reject inappropriate claims from entering the transactional processing system inventory.
   - TIP 4: When faced with a large backlog, create a "swat team," including personnel from other departments experienced in claims adjudication, to focus on the backlog while regular claims personnel focus on current claims.
   - TIP 5: If a backlog does take hold, convene a seasoned group of "configuration experts" to consider changes in the core system configuration to help the payer overcome the temporary challenge. However, always remember to reset the configuration rules once the backlog is reduced.

2. **Inadequate Front-End Control, or "Garbage In, Garbage Out" (GIGO).** EDI procedures must be strictly established to ensure only claims that are complete and with valid data elements are accepted into the system.
   - TIP 6: Enforce claim filing rules with all providers and third-party billers. Work with provider relations personnel to better educate providers on this issue.
   - TIP 7: Make sure that payer-dictated changes in billing requirements can be accommodated by front-end EDI configuration. For example, if a specific field is required for processing that is not captured by the EDI logic, claims will not be auto-adjudicated. EDI configuration may need to be modified to support the modified billing requirements.

3. **Inadequate Management of Suspended Claims.** Claims suspended through the auto adjudication process must be strictly monitored and quickly resolved.
   - TIP 8: If additional information is required from the provider, deny the claim with the applicable reason code and request the additional information. The burden is placed back on the provider, and the claim is removed from the suspended status. Be sure that providers are informed of all required data, however, so as not to cause a provider relations problem.
   - TIP 9: Use data analysis and reporting to identify aging claims and closely manage those that sit in a suspended status for an extended period of time. These claims are sometimes forgotten or ignored because claims adjudicators do not know how to resolve the problems, or their requests for assistance have not become the priority of others.
   - TIP 10: Establish and enforce pended claims procedures and turnaround times with other departments. The claims capability is ultimately responsible for all suspended claims even if awaiting action from other payer personnel. If turnaround times are not being met, alert senior management.

4. **Inadequate Focus on a Continuous Quality Improvement Process (CQIP) Effort.** Claims capability processes must be considered a work in progress. There is almost always some aspect to improve.
   - TIP 11: Designate specific claims personnel to be responsible for continuous quality improvement. As the name implies, this is not a one-time activity or task.
   - TIP 12: Involve claims adjudicators and other nonmanagement personnel in continuous quality improvement efforts. Those closest to the processes usually have the best ideas.
   - TIP 13: Create rewards or incentives for continuous quality improvement efforts including gift certificates or time off. Make sure rewards fit within the payer's human resource guidelines.
   - TIP 14: Consider using specialized outside help to establish and improve CQIP efforts.
   - TIP 15: Continue to invest in workflow and analytics tools to manage the business in a more scientific manner.

5. **Inadequate or Ineffective Workflow.** Do not allow inadequate or ineffective workflow to create bottlenecks. Claims must be pushed along the process and daily, even hourly, supervisory management is required.
   - TIP 16: Document workflow processes in minute detail using a flowchart software application. Identify every single decision point made by either the transactional processing system or by claims adjudicators.

Such detailed examination will reveal opportunities for fine-tuning the workflow.

- TIP 17: Make sure that management and supervisory staff understand how to utilize the workflow software application. The functionality of this application is not always fully leveraged.
- TIP 18: In the absence of a workflow software application, aggressively manage workflow through daily/weekly reporting.

6. **Poorly Maintained Claims Engine or Other Operational Applications.** The claims capability relies on the transactional processing system and other software applications as its tools. Poor maintenance will compromise both productivity and quality.

- TIP 19: Do not allow poor system maintenance to go unchallenged. Many claims adjudicators often find ways around system problems in order to meet productivity standards. As a result, system problems are suppressed and worked around rather than identified and resolved.
- TIP 20: Develop a working relationship with personnel who maintain the transactional processing system and other pertinent software applications. Make detailed reasonable requests for changes. If improvements are not made, enlist the support of senior payer management to determine priorities.
- TIP 21: Consider centralizing claims system configuration activities for better and more timely configuration management.

7. **Inadequate or Ineffective Data Management.** The claims capability relies on other departments' records (member, provider, pricing, authorization, etc.) to adjudicate claims. If other department files are not timely and accurately updated, claims errors will occur.

- TIP 22: Develop working relationships with other department heads to catch problems early. Cross-functional payer teams should meet regularly to identify and document expected and unexpected operational challenges.
- TIP 23: Analyze quality assessment reports and review the causes of claims adjustments to determine if poorly maintained records in other departments are the problem. Gather facts and figures to review with other department heads as needed. Avoid confrontation and use a collaborative approach to resolve problems.
- TIP 24: Participate in cross-functional teams (including third-party business partners) to address both upstream and downstream quality and performance issues.
- TIP 25: Design and implement an early warning mechanism to catch data management issues early. Most often, the type of mechanism can fit nicely

within the scope of a "claims or operations command center."

8. **Incorrect Benefit Setup and Group Installation.** The claims capability relies on business rule configuration records to process claims. If basic files associated with groups or benefits are incorrectly established, thousands of claims could be at risk. Adjusting large volumes of claims, especially if historical deductible or limitation calculations are affected, can be a nightmare.

- TIP 26: Preventative measures are the key to avoiding this risk. Whenever a new benefit plan is established or a large new group of members is ready to "go live," ask to be part of the final testing phase to ensure that the claim outcomes match the benefit specifications. Test benefit coding through a standard durable and repeatable process.
- TIP 27: Sign-off on unique benefit configuration rules to ensure accurate benefit administration within the transactional processing system should be required before such unique benefits are agreed upon by the payer.

9. **Incorrect Provider Contract Set-up and Maintenance.** The claims capability relies on all records associated with providers, including contract setup and payment methodologies to process claims. If provider files, payment methodologies, fee schedules, and so on are incorrectly established, thousands of claims could be at risk. Just as in item 8 above, adjusting large volumes of claims, especially if historical deductible or limitation calculations are affected, can be a nightmare.

- TIP 28: It is critical that claims capability personnel be proactive in participating in the initial and ongoing validation and maintenance of provider contract setups. Staff who process adjustments, in particular, have insight to cases where provider contracts are set up with the wrong payment methodology for a particular service (e.g., case rate instead of per diem for maternity delivery inpatient stay) or with the wrong variable value attached to a payment methodology (e.g., 75% of charges instead of 80% of charges).
- TIP 29: Sign-off on unique provider contracts (prior to contract execution if possible) to ensure payment will be processed correctly in the transactional processing system.
- TIP 30: For both benefit and provider contract "setups," the payer management team should employ data modeling and predictive analysis to understand future operational impacts.

10. **Inadequate Quality and Financial Controls.** The claims capability must establish and execute a quality control function. It is the flip side of its dual responsibilities of production and quality.

- TIP 31: Be sure claims adjudicators and other staff understand and agree to the quality assessment process to ensure that quality review results are accepted.
- TIP 32: Ensure that the quality assessment process is "blind" to individual adjudicators so that the process is fair and is *perceived* as fair.
- TIP 33: Quality and financial controls should be structured to simulate external audits by government regulators and third-party auditors. These simulated audits should be performed regularly to predict and ultimately prevent negative external audit findings.

11. **Poor Employee Recruiting.** Despite the advances in claims adjudication technology, claims adjudicators and other personnel are still vital to the claims capability.
    - TIP 34: Organize the claims capability with positions of increasing responsibility and salary grades to create a career path. Talented staff will seek positions outside the claims capability if that is their only path to promotion.
    - TIP 35: Be sure to reward good performance, especially exemplary performance. If budgets are tight, consider extra time off, more flexible hours, gift certificates, special award ceremonies, advanced training, and so on.
    - TIP 36: Don't forget to include third party business partners in recognition programs. Often third-party employees may provide greater value than internal staff.

12. **Inadequate Policy and Procedure Documentation.** Unwritten and/or unclear policies and procedures lead to inconsistent claims adjudication and low employee morale/motivation.
    - TIP 37: Create a space on the payer's intranet to house policies and procedures. Be sure they are searchable and are kept updated.
    - TIP 38: Assign policy and procedure responsibility to a single accountable resource, preferably someone in claims or operations.
    - TIP 39: Break the habit of communicating new information via e-mail. Rather, use e-mail to alert staff of updated information posted on the intranet.
    - TIP 40: Don't forget to update external portals for member and provider use. Consistency of policy and procedure interpretation is critical to smooth operations.

13. **Inadequate Training.** Training should not be limited to systems processing only. A comprehensive training approach that provides context and background will result in greater retention and transfer to the job.
    - TIP 41: Begin training at an industry level and proceed to payer-specific training topics. Within this context, proceed with unit and task-level training.

Keep abreast of ongoing updates associated with health reform, the transition to ICD-10, and other important developments that impact claims administration and update training materials accordingly.
- TIP 42: Employ a variety of means to train and develop staff, including any combination of classroom training, Web-based and CD-ROM courseware, conference calls, webinars, online simulations, lab-based simulations, job aids, Web pages and/or sites, mentors, chats, videos, podcasting, video casting, and blogging. Be sure to blend various methods into a cohesive and comprehensive training program.

14. **Inadequate Data Analysis and Claims Management Reports.** Data analysis and reporting should aid the management team, not impede them. In today's payer, operational insights are created through data analysis as never before.
    - TIP 43: Employ analysts within the claims capability to develop meaningful and insightful reports on demand.
    - TIP 44: Rationalize reports as much as possible to avoid report overload. In other words, more reports may not necessarily provide more insight.
    - TIP 45: Be sure to create reports and complete analysis from the same underlying data warehouse or repository. Again, be sure dashboards are built from the same underlying data structure.
    - TIP 46: Design "dashboard"-type reports to enable various levels of managers to zero in on desired information.

15. **Failure to Use the Claims Capability to Identify Customer and Operational Problems Early.** The claims capability is the repository of facts, figures, and perceptions that impact performance as well as internal and external customers. Listen to what they have to say!
    - TIP 47: Engage claims adjudicators in discussions and/or performance improvement projects. They are the closest to the work at hand and can provide great insight into the inner workings of the payer when asked.
    - TIP 48: Analyze corrections, resubmissions, voluntary refunds, and appeals to reveal root causes of problems and targets for process improvements. This rich source of information can be overlooked if it is not deliberately pulled into the continuous quality improvement process (CQIP).
    - TIP 49: Share information openly with members and providers using self-service portals and other online tools.
    - TIP 50: Treat trusted third-party business partners as if they were employees. These parties are key to the payer's success.

A final risk area that can pervade all the others is cynicism. The claims capability management team must feel that they can rely on senior payer managers for resources and cooperation, especially when thorny problems present themselves. Claims managers must remain positive and lead by example with hard work, a sense of urgency, and a commitment to high quality, integrity, and customer service.

■ CONCLUSION

The modern claims capability has multiple objectives and multiple constituencies. Its operations directly impact the corporate reputation and bottom line of the payer. This chapter has attempted to define the modern claims capability, its core competencies and business steps, and how they are managed. It has concluded with an examination of the risks that must be confronted as well as tips developed from over 50 years combined experience of the authors. Ultimately, the claims capability is a service organization. If management and business practices are executed with service to internal and external customers in mind, the

claims capability will ensure its own health and vitality as well the financial health of its payer.

Endnotes

1 Figures provided by Kaiser Family Foundation. Available at: www.kff.org.
2 *Update: A Survey of Health Care Claims Receipt and Processing Times, 2009.* Center for Policy and Research, America's Health Insurance Plans. Available at: www.ahipresearch.org/pdfs/SurveyHealthCareJan252010.pdf.
3 *Merriam Webster Online Dictionary,* www.m-w.com/dictionary/information + science.
4 The American Society for Training and Development (ASTD) is the world's largest professional association dedicated to training and development issues and provides up-to-date research and information on learning technologies at www.astd.org.
5 Zenger J, Uehlein, C. Why blended will win. *T + D.* 2001;55:54–60.
6 Knolwes M. *Self-Directed Learning: A Guide for Learners and Teachers.* Cambridge Book Company; 1988.

CHAPTER 19

Health Care Fraud and Abuse

CHRISTIE A. MOON

STUDY OBJECTIVES

- Understand the history of health care fraud and abuse, including the forces that have driven it
- Understand the challenge of defining and measuring the problem
- Understand the definitions and regulatory environment associated with fraud control
- Understand emerging and ongoing initiatives in fraud, waste, and abuse control

DISCUSSION TOPICS

1. Describe and discuss the key definitions of fraud and abuse in health care fraud.
2. Describe the challenges and forces that complicate effective health care fraud and abuse control.
3. Describe key attributes of technological systems that help detect potential health care fraud waste and abuse.
4. Discuss significant legal and regulatory issues associated with fraud prevention and control.
5. Describe the key players (persons, entities, associations) and roles that are associated with health care fraud and abuse control.
6. Understand the existence of relevant and emerging statutes, including Fraud Enforcement Recovery Act and the Patient Protection and Affordable Care Act, on health care fraud control.

■ INTRODUCTION: THE HISTORY OF HEALTH CARE FRAUD

Health care fraud is crime that over time has had a significant impact on public and private health care payment systems. However the nature and extent of the impact is difficult to discern. As the United States is working to make health care more available and affordable, more attention is being focused on activities that can prevent, detect, and mitigate health care fraud. Health care fraud as a specific type of crime initially presents most significantly in the context of the amendments to the Federal False Claims Act in 1986.[1]

Until 1986 the False Claims Act was primarily used by the government in the military and defense industry. Originally known as the "Lincoln Law," the False Claims Act presented a means by which private citizens could report fraud against the government in military contracts and then receive an award of a percentage of the ill-gotten gains recovered by the government. Its initial use was related to fraud against the Union Army during the Civil War.[2] When Congress amended the False Claims Act (FCA) in 1986, it expressed the intent that the FCA be applied to false claims against Medicare and Medicaid.[3]

The government's war on health care fraud next took center stage in 1993, when Attorney General Janet Reno declared that prosecuting health care fraud was a top priority at the United States Department of Justice, second only to violent crime.[4] This declaration was driven by the fact that health care fraud had reached epidemic proportions, with little attention being paid to its pathology or attempting to detect it or prevent it.

Then, in 1993 Janet Reno brought the matter to the attention of Malcolm K. Sparrow, a lecturer in public policy at Harvard University's John F. Kennedy School of Government. At the time, Sparrow had been working with the Internal Revenue Service on how to sort through problems in its refund system. "We need all the help we can get to understand the problem," Reno told Sparrow. "We'd be delighted if you'd take a look at it from an outsider's perspective."

Professor Sparrow's research on this topic led to his book, *License to Steal: Why Fraud Plagues America's Health Care System* (Westview Press, 1996). This book remains viable and is the best assessment of the health care fraud control situation available. Professor Sparrow also points out the increasing complexity of measuring and detecting fraud in the massive electronically automated environment as well as the surprising lack of interest in effectively addressing the problem.[5]

Sparrow's observations, in particular those associated with the lack of attention to the problem and the lack of ability to measure its cost, correctly present the complexity of the situation, which to this day contributes to the creation of the perfect storm for committing health care fraud in this country. This is true for government health care programs, but is an equal risk for private health plans.

Typical large fraud schemes include big billing scams by entities that were created only to bill Medicare. These schemes include false billing and fraudulent behavior such as upcoding, unbundling, false billing, and billing for care not performed or not medically necessary. Those seeking to commit health care fraud have cited it as an easy way to get huge amounts of money with little risk of detection, prosecution, or punishment.[6]

As fraud detection analytics have progressed and legislation around definitions and program compliance have made it easier to fight fraud, progress has been made to more effectively address the problem. For example, the Centers for Medicare and Medicaid Services (CMS) recently implemented much more rigorous standards for entry into these government health care programs.[7]

Professor Sparrow's theories regarding effectively addressing health care fraud are as viable today as when he wrote them more than a decade ago. The business of health care fraud control, also known as program integrity, has now reached a critical point in health care operations. Given its escalating cost and risk, understanding it, along with the relevant regulations and control efforts, is a critical priority for the health care system in general. As such, this topic is for the first time included in this book. Just as it is emerging in significance and finally gaining more of the attention it deserves, the health care program integrity environment is also in the process of being transformed. It is no longer acceptable to leave the fraud control problem essentially unsolved.

It is not until just the past few years, however, that significant progress has been made by the government in more effectively addressing the health care fraud problem. Since January 2009, amounts recovered under the False Claims Act "have eclipsed any previous 2-year period, with $7 billion returned to the Medicare Trust Fund, the Treasury and others. Since 1986 when Congress substantially strengthened the civil False Claims Act, recoveries now total nearly $29 billion."[8] Even so, this is still just the tip of the iceberg as far as many experts are concerned.

■ DEFINITIONS OF FRAUD AND ABUSE

The definitions of fraud and abuse vary in the detail and complexity included in the language. Health care fraud is also the subject of numerous statutory and common-law definitions. And there is not always agreement on what behaviors apply to those definitions. The main difference between health care fraud and fraud in general is that it involves conduct related to health care. This includes but is not limited to fraudulent billing of all types, suspect provider functions, medical identity theft to obtain care, plan eligibility fraud, internal fraud by health care workers, and the like.

Fraud control work on the part of payers in this area exists in various departments, depending on the nature and complexity of the organization. Departments typically involved in fraud control work include compliance, internal audit, claims, and law departments. Provider contracting is also relevant to the process because contractual arrangements with providers (where they exist) often contain provisions that change the landscape of certain billing behavior that may initially appear to be fraudulent. Therefore, it is a good idea to always check the provider contracting arrangement prior to confirming that a provider billing pattern is health care fraud.

Simple fraud and abuse definitions are as follows:

- Health care **fraud** occurs when someone misrepresents a fact related to health care services to receive— or increase—payment from a health plan or the government. Fraud also occurs when someone misrepresents details in delivery of health care services or supplies.
- Health care **abuse**, though not as well defined as fraud, typically occurs if an activity abuses the health care system but does not meet the legal definition of fraud or is not medically necessary.

It is difficult to draw a clear line between fraud and abuse in some cases. The real difference between most fraud and abuse is often the ability to prove intent. State and federal laws vary in their definitions. The National Health Care Anti-Fraud Association (NHCAA) defines health care fraud as follows:

"Health care fraud is an intentional deception or misrepresentation that the individual or entity makes knowing that the misrepresentation could result in some unauthorized benefit to the individual, or the entity or to some other party."[9]

Examples of Provider or Member Fraud

The following are examples of provider fraud, patient fraud, and provider billing abuse.

Provider:

- Billing for services not performed
- Billing to a post office box, commercial mailbox, or other suspicious address
- Billing using the provider identification of an unknowing, innocent provider
- Billing for cosmetic surgery as if it were a covered procedure
- Falsifying a patient's diagnosis to justify tests, surgeries, or other procedures that are not medically necessary
- Misrepresenting procedures performed to obtain payment for noncovered services, such as cosmetic surgery
- Unbundling, which is the practice of submitting bills for various tests or procedures individually when they are required to be billed together
- Splitting claims to avoid detection of unbundling
- Billing for more drugs than dispensed
- Billing for brand name drugs when generic are dispensed
- Upcoding, which is billing for a more costly service than the one actually performed
- Duplicate billing
- Durable medical equipment (DME) claims for equipment not provided
- DME claims for rentals that grossly exceed the value of the equipment
- Excessive lab tests and radiological examinations
- Waiving patient copays or deductibles
- Falsification of medical records to justify payment
- Billing for care provided to dead people

Patient:

- Misrepresentation on health insurance coverage applications
- Falsification of eligibility as an employee

- Filing false claims with payers
- Identity theft to obtain care
- Forging prescriptions
- Obtaining prescriptions for illegal resale
- Doctor-shopping for narcotics

Examples of Billing Abuse

- Overutilization of services, such as refilling a prescription when not needed
- Ordering more tests than medically necessary for the medical condition
- Treating patients differently, based on nature of insurance coverage
- Changing certain procedure codes and "unbundling" of services usually delivered together to increase payment
- Charging outrageous fees to third-party payers where there's no contract in place

Abuse typically leads to unnecessary cost but may not reach the level of intent necessary to prove fraud. However, in certain circumstances abusive practices can constitute fraud, particularly under the False Claims Act, as amended by the Fraud Enforcement Recovery Act (FERA) enacted in 2009. On May 20, 2009, President Barack Obama signed Public Law No. 111-21. FERA provides the federal government with more tools to investigate and prosecute health care and other financial fraud. Under the FERA amendments, False Claims Act liability can occur even without intent. For example, if a plan or provider has knowledge of an overpayment from the government and fails to notify and return the overpayment within 60 days, then there is now False Claims Act liability. The Patient Protection and Affordable Care Act (ACA), signed into law on March 23, 2010, clarified ambiguity around this issue and directly linked the retention of overpayments to false claim liability.

Abusive practices may also develop into fraud if evidence reflects that the suspect parties were engaging in this practice knowingly and willfully. This is an area where legal counsel is typically involved due to the risk and complexity.

Examples of Medicare Advantage or Managed Care Plan Fraud

Medicare Advantage (MA) plans, also called "Part C plans," are offered by private health insurers as approved by Medicare and provide beneficiaries with a full array of health care service for one capitated, risk-based rate. Medicare and MA plans, including prescription drug plans (PDPs) are discussed in detail in Chapter 24.

Although MA and other types of managed care plans are less at risk for traditional fee-for-service billing and coding health care fraud, they remain vulnerable to other types of health care fraud risks. Fraud risks for MA plans include the following:

- Beneficiary fraud, including:
  - Financial identity theft
  - Medical identity theft to obtain care or drugs
  - Prescription drug fraud including abusing drugs and reselling them
  - "Doctor-shopping" for a physician who will provide desired drugs or services, whether medically necessary or not
  - Falsely reporting loss of drugs or medical equipment such as diabetes test strips to receive replacements for resale
- Provider fraud, including:
  - Altering care schedules and medical records to make it appear as if patients are being seen who are not being seen
  - Accepting unlawful kickbacks to prescribe certain drugs or durable medical equipment
- Vendor fraud, including:
  - False billing for services not rendered
  - Sending items of lesser quality than what was contractually purchased
  - Paying plan kickbacks to receive preferential contract consideration and contracts
- Pharmacy fraud and abuse including:
  - Drug diversion by beneficiaries, family members, caregivers, providers, pharmacy staff, and others with access to covered drugs
  - Drug switching, where the plan receives an illegal payment to switch a patient or induce a provider to switch a patient from one drug to another
  - Drug shorting or splitting, where a pharmacy or pharmacy benefits manager's mail service pharmacy intentionally provides less than the prescribed quantity and does not tell the patient but bills for the fully prescribed amount
  - Drug billing fraud such as billing for brand name drugs when generics are dispensed, billing for noncovered prescriptions as covered items, and billing for prescriptions that are never picked up, often using an auto-refill process
- Medicare Advantage plans can also commit fraud against the government by:
  - Undertaking improper beneficiary marketing campaigns
  - Requiring improper premiums
  - Otherwise intentionally violating federal laws or regulations

CMS requires Medicare Advantage organizations and Part D plan sponsors to provide annual fraud, waste, and abuse training to their employees and subcontractors. In 2007, CMS published a final rule that requires these organizations provide mandatory training to all entities they associate with that provide benefits or services in Medicare Part C or Part D programs.

In 2010, CMS revised regulations to clarify that first-tier, downstream, and other related entities that have already met the fraud, waste, and abuse certification requirements through enrollment in a fee-for-service Medicare program or accreditation as a durable medical equipment provider have also met the training and education requirements for fraud, waste, and abuse.

Potential Indicators of Health Care Fraud in a Managed Care Setting

Fraud in a managed care setting used to be considered a nonissue or a minimal risk. As time has progressed it has become evident that all types of payers, even health maintenance organizations (HMOs), are not immune to fraud. Fraud in the setting of MA plans was just discussed. Some indicators of fraud in a managed care setting, regardless of plan type, include:

- Insufficient time spent by providers with patients (lack of appropriate care);
- High levels of referrals of patients to specialists (may be a sign of a kickback arrangement);
- Consistently poor care outcomes (may be a sign of lack of treatment);
- Unusual patient encounter ratios (may be a sign that patients are being scheduled fictitiously but not seen); and
- High numbers of patient claims for treatment outside the HMO service area (may be a sign that patients are not in compliance with geographic requirements or are filing claims for false or not covered care).

■ THE FRAUD TRIANGLE

People commit health care fraud for various reasons. Health care fraud falls into typical categories as noted by Joseph T. Wells, founder of the Association of Certified Fraud Examiners. Wells references has published the rationale for fraud as a Fraud Triangle. For fraud to occur, he argues, all three of the following elements must typically be present (**Figure 19-1**).

Pressure is typically one of the three reasons a person commits fraud. Just as human nature varies considerably, this can vary from more to less sympathetic. On the one hand, "pressure" can come from a need to pay medical bills and, on the other hand, it can be caused by a drug or gambling addiction or the desire for expensive designer clothing. Most often pressure comes from a significant financial issue. The recent economic downturn has also been cited as a common pressure leading to fraud. When the economy takes a downturn, fraud increases, according to an online poll conducted in 2009 by Deloitte Financial Advisory Services.

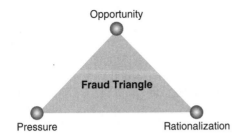

FIGURE 19-1   The Fraud Triangle

Source: Reprinted from "Occupational Fraud and Abuse," by Joseph T. Wells, Obsidian Publishing Co., 1997. Used with permission.

Opportunity is the ability to commit fraud and the second point of the fraud triangle. Unfortunately in health care, committing fraud has historically been fairly easy. Given that perpetrators don't want to be caught, they typically seek the security of system weaknesses and lack of controls. This is one area where government and payers can most effectively prevent fraud. Control and the seven elements of compliance (see later) provide significant preventive opportunities and protections in this area.

Rationalization is the third and essential element of most frauds. This typically means that a perpetrator can excuse their behavior, given commonly accepted ethical standards. To some, cheating the government or a health insurance company is acceptable. To others, conditions of employment, the economy, or unemployment provide rationalization.

CHALLENGES IN FRAUD DETECTION AND PREVENTION

Effective fraud control must include ongoing and agile enhancements for fraud detection and prevention. As technology advances, so does fraud. Once the payer gets a handle on one type of fraud scheme, fraudsters devise a new one. As soon as the payer thinks they have solved a certain type of fraud and relaxes controls around it, the same old scheme will pop back up again. This relates back to Professor Malcolm Sparrow's original analogy that fighting health care fraud is a lot like playing the "whack-a-mole" game at an arcade. As soon as you find a fraud and pound it back down, another one pops up in another area. The invisible nature of the problem must also be addressed.

The tricky thing about understanding and quantifying health care fraud is that you can only see what you detect. In Professor Sparrow's "whack-a-mole" analogy, he points out that effective fraud control demands the same three skills as the arcade game: (1) the client must have effective instruments that enable it to spot fraud early and clearly see emerging fraud patterns; (2) the client must be able to react quickly to mitigate vulnerabilities before too much loss occurs; and (3) the client must have the tools to be ready to

spot new fraud wherever and whenever it occurs.[10] These "key ingredients of fraud control" remain just as important as they were first covered in the original edition of *License to Steal*.[11]

Thus, helping government and commercial payer clients is quite dynamic and complicated. Sparrow's use of the term "fraud control" is meaningful. Because one can never really eliminate or stop fraud. The best that can be hoped for is to control fraud, optimally by deploying Professor Sparrow's three essential steps noted previously. Doing so effectively on an ongoing basis is a difficult chore. Even so, there are additional concepts and strategies that are helpful to understand.

THE FEDERAL GOVERNMENT'S EFFORTS TO CRACK DOWN ON HEALTH CARE FRAUD

It is not possible to precisely measure or assign a firm annual dollar loss amount to the fraud control problem. This is partly because, given the nature of fraud, you don't know what you don't know. All estimates place the cost of health care fraud into the billions. In his May 20, 2009, testimony before the United States Senate Committee on the Judiciary: Subcommittee on Crime and Drugs hearing on criminal prosecution as a deterrent to health care fraud, Professor Sparrow said:

> The units of measure for losses due to health care fraud and abuse in this country are hundreds of billions of dollars per year. We just don't know the first digit. It might be as low as one hundred billion. More likely two or three. Possibly four or five. But whatever that first digit is, it has eleven zeroes after it. These are staggering sums of money to waste, and the task of controlling and reducing these losses warrants a great deal of serious attention. *One of my deep regrets is to discover that academia has paid almost no serious attention to this critical problem.* I suspect this neglect is because the art of health care fraud control falls awkwardly between the traditional disciplines of health economics, health policy, crime control policy, anomaly detection, and pattern recognition. [emphasis added][12]

Professor Sparrow goes on to testify about how in 1996, he wrote his first book on the subject of health care fraud, called *License to Steal*, which analyzed the industry's approach to addressing health care fraud. His first book, Sparrow notes, can briefly be summarized by the fact that his analysis showed that the industry failed to adequately distinguish between payment accuracy and crime control. In 2000, Sparrow updated and reissued *License to Steal* to outline the progress in this area made by the Clinton administration, but also to make it clear that much more needed to be done to "properly excise the cancer of fraud from important public programs."[13] In concluding his testimony, Sparrow recommended the following:

1. As a matter of urgency, reinstate the requirement that the Office of the Inspector General (OIG) provide an independent audit of the Medicare overpayment rate on an annual basis. CMS should not be left to diagnose and report on its own failings.

2. Require the OIG, as it designs the necessary audit protocols for such overpayment measurement, to use a rigorous fraud-audit methodology, not the process-oriented desk-audit approach they used from 1996 to 2002. A fraud audit must include steps to verify with the patient or with others that the diagnosis was genuine and that the treatments actually took place. It should also include contextual data analysis sufficient to identify any suspicious patterns of incestuous or self-dealing patient referrals, diagnostic biases, or systematic padding of claims or treatments consistent with patterns of fraud.

3. Require a review of the adequacy of the Medicare and Medicaid programs' operational responses to claims submitted that are clearly implausible. Auto-rejection of claims involving dead patients, dead doctors, or previously deported persons is a terribly weak response, and actually helps perpetrators perfect their billing scams. The detection of such claims ought to trigger a presumption of the presence of serious criminal enterprise, and that presumption should then be tested through appropriate criminal investigation and law-enforcement response.

To date, these recommendations have not been fully implemented, although some progress is being made.

On March 17, 2011, the Inspector General of the United States Department of Health and Human Services (HHS), Office of the Inspector General, Daniel R. Levinson, testified before the House Subcommittee on Appropriations, Subcommittee on Labor, Health and Human Services, Education and Related Agencies. The topic of this hearing was improper payments. Levinson testified that for fiscal year 2010, HHS reported improper payments totaling $56.8 billion in just Medicare fee-for-service and Medicaid. Levinson went on to testify that his agency was now in a position to assess program risks and begin to employ data analysis to target the OIG's audits, evaluation, and investigations.

The HHS OIG reviews the work of CMS and other agencies within HHS. According to Dr. Peter Budetti, CMS Director of the Center for Program Integrity, "improper payments" are the result of a variety of circumstances, including (1) services with no documentation, (2) services with insufficient documentation, (3) incorrectly coded claims, or (4) services provided determined not "reasonable and necessary."[14] Thus, although the term "improper payments"

certainly does not always equate to health care fraud, these findings still point to these areas as high risk for fraud. And, as noted previously, there is really no common or precise measurement of what exact portion of this amount is health care fraud.

In fiscal year 2009 the OIG found that in CMS Comprehensive Error Rate Testing (CERT), six areas of health care accounted for 94% of improper Medicare payments. These six areas are therefore deserving of more intense fraud control focus.

■ PAYER AND MANAGED CARE FRAUD CONTROL EFFORTS

Health plans and related managed care organizations typically detect or learn about potential fraud through systems that hopefully enable them to quickly spot potential fraud. These are some examples of where this can take place:

- Claims analysis (prepayment, postadjudication, and postpayment);
- Calls, e-mails, or letters to leaders from patients, vendors, and even other providers;
- Coordination with other plans, task forces, or law enforcement agencies investigating the same suspect or scheme on behalf of the government or other plans;
- Data analysis tools and reports, including but not limited to scheme algorithms and predictive analytics;
- Ethics or compliance hotline calls from employees and patients.

At times, plans or plan leaders have the perception that detecting fraud is more trouble than it is worth and that a costly civil attorney is always needed to help address the issues. This is not always the case. If a plan is not open to these or other means of detecting fraud, then such an "ostrich" approach may land them in trouble with regulators and could keep them from effectively detecting health care fraud. In addition, plan leaders are often more concerned about recovering the lost revenue than they are about effective prosecution or stopping the fraud through criminal action. Another issue that contributes to failure to adequately detect health care fraud is that many people working in plans have the perception that if major fraud is detected on their watch, then this will make them look bad. "Fraud control is a miserable business. Failure to detect fraud is bad news and finding fraud is bad news too. Senior managers seldom want to hear any news about fraud because news about fraud is never good."[15]

Leaders of health plans and other payers should be counseled to adopt a culture of compliance and helped to understand that detecting health care fraud early and effectively places them in a better position with the government than if they had ignored it. Not only can detecting fraud early save them money, it can help demonstrate that they are applying the government's seven elements of compliance effectively.

To manage fraud and abuse successfully, payers, providers, facilities, and vendors must also work with their peers and regulators to prevent and identify inappropriate and potentially fraudulent practices. This can be accomplished by:

- Monitoring claims submitted for compliance with agreed-upon or established billing and coding guidelines;
- Adhering to appropriate clinical documentation standards;
- Adherence by providers and facilities to the standard of care for treatment as well as honoring medical necessity (not performing any care that is not medically necessary);
- Educating all staff members responsible for medical records (billing, coding, maintenance);
- Referring cases of suspected fraud and abuse to law enforcement and appropriate regulators.

Coding Fraud

While coding fraud (or claims fraud) can occur in any type of payer, including capitated HMOs, the risk is highest when payments are made through fee-for-service. It is the most prominent means by which providers and facilities commit health care fraud against the government and commercial payers of all types. Inappropriate or false coding is a major risk that is difficult to control. This includes upcoding and unbundling and other improper or fraudulent use of procedure codes and evaluation and management (E&M) codes, as well as applying inappropriate modifier codes. Each year in the HHS OIG Work Plan, areas of focus include aspects of coding compliance and fraud control. For example, in the HHS OIG Fiscal Year 2011 Work Plan, the Office of the Inspector General listed in its plan to review "the extent to which clinical laboratories have inappropriately unbundled laboratory profile or panel tests to maximize Medicare payments."[16]

Coding fraud can be very complicated and requires special expertise to analyze and detect. Examples including upcoding, unbundling, and modifier abuse have already been noted previously. Organizations are wise to have certified professional coders (CPC) on both sides of this issue. Hospitals and providers should use CPC to ensure that they are billing correctly and that well-intended billing is not taken out of context and presumed to be fraud. On the other hand, government and commercial payers should utilize the services of CPC to help analyze and detect anomalous coding patterns that could upon further investigation turn out to be erroneous or intentional fraud.

In addition, after more than 30 years, the *International Classification of Diseases* (ICD-9) coding system is being expanded from 17,000 code sets to new and more comprehensive (ICD-10) codes, as discussed in Chapters 18 and 23. There will be approximately 141,000 ICD-10 code sets after this update. ICD-10 is currently scheduled for implementation on October 1, 2013. The updates and additional codes will present more opportunity to detect as well as commit fraud.

Geographic Fraud Risk

There are certain geographical areas in the country that are more susceptible to health care fraud than others. For example, Florida, especially in the Miami area, is considered the "ground zero" for health care fraud. In recognition of the geographic tendencies associated with health care fraud, a few strategic thinkers in the federal government created the Health Care Fraud Prevention and Enforcement Action Teams (HEAT). HEAT was created following the successful impact of the Medicare Fraud Strike Force at ferreting out fraud in 2007, primarily in Florida. As part of the FERA and the ACA, the HEAT teams were given significant additional funding to focus on more effective fraud control efforts in cities determined to be high-risk targets for health care fraud.

The success of HEAT's focused fraud control investigative and enforcement efforts ultimately resulted in the expansion of Medicare Fraud Strike Force operations from South Florida and Los Angeles, so at the time of publication it encompasses at least nine geographic hot spots for health care fraud: South Florida; Los Angeles; Houston; Detroit; Brooklyn; Baton Rouge; Tampa; Chicago; and Dallas.

As the HEAT teams became more effective in South Florida and other cities, some fraudsters migrated from South Florida to where they could perpetrate fraud schemes without being detected. As HEAT moved into additional cities, Cuban–Americans and Cuban nationals thought to have originally worked or learned these fraud schemes in Miami were caught in the Detroit area and charged with millions of dollars in health care fraud.

The HEAT Strike Force is a partnership between the Criminal Fraud Section of the U.S. Attorneys' Offices, HHS OIG, the Federal Bureau of Investigation (FBI), and other federal, state, and local law enforcement partners. Since their inception in 2007, Strike Force operations have charged more than 1,000 defendants for Medicare fraud involving more than $2.3 billion in claims.[17]

From 2010 to the present, the HEAT teams aligned with the HHS and DOJ fraud control communications and outreach goals and coordinated across the country to arrest major health care fraud perpetrators in busts (considered by some to be "perp walks") that would typically occur across the country in one day. For example, on February 17, 2011, health care fraud task forces arrested 114 people in nine metropolitan areas across the country (all HEAT cities). This bust was called the "largest Medicare fraud crackdown in

U.S. history" by United States Attorney General Eric Holder and HHS Secretary Kathleen Sebelius. More than 700 federal, state, and local agents were involved in the bust. While the schemes varied widely, they all involved huge amounts of false claim billing. Many also involved paying kickbacks to Medicare beneficiaries who allowed their numbers to be used in the schemes. One case involved a podiatrist who billed for toenail removals but allegedly only gave footbaths or clipped toenails. This podiatrist allegedly billed Medicare approximately $700,000 and was submitting fraudulent claims for podiatry services. Essentially, the provider was charged with billing Medicare for services not performed, although he may have been giving some patients pedicures and related services.

These actions have increased in frequency over the past few years as the government strives to make sure funds spent on health care are legitimate in the face of health care reform. It can be said with 100% assurance that fraud is not confined to Medicare and Medicaid. Health plans, hospitals, and providers are strongly advised to ensure compliance with appropriate billing practices.

Types of Health Care Goods and Services at Increased Risk for Fraud

In addition to high-profile geographic areas of risk, there are also substantive high-profile areas in health care that are, based on noted detection and large cases, at higher risk for fraud. Some of these areas were recently recognized by CMS in regulations enhancing screening for acceptance into the Medicare program.

One area of health care that is at significant risk for fraud is pharmacy and drug distribution. In fact, the first formal government mandate for health plans to have a compliance program that included elements of fraud control, such as data mining, was the mandate for plan sponsors of the Medicare Part D prescription drug benefit program. The Medicare *Prescription Drug Manual* was initially released in 2006. Chapter 9 contains the provision associated with fraud control.[18]

Chapter 9 provides both interpretative rules and guidelines for Part D plan sponsors on how to implement the requirements under 42 C.F.R. §423.504(b)(4)(vi)(H) to have in place a comprehensive fraud and abuse plan to detect, correct, and prevent fraud, waste, and abuse as an element of their compliance plan. While CMS regulations require plan sponsors to implement a comprehensive fraud and abuse program, the adoption of the methods suggested within this chapter on how to implement a comprehensive fraud and abuse program are left to the discretion of each plan sponsor. Additionally, Chapter 9 outlines CMS's guidelines for operational issues such as handling complaints and coordinating with CMS and law enforcement.

Other types of health care services at risk for improper payments and potential fraud include (1) inpatient hospitals,

(2) durable medical equipment (DME) suppliers, (3) hospital outpatient departments, (4) physicians, (5) skilled nursing facilities, and (6) home health agencies. As noted by HHS OIG Inspector General Levinson, these six areas accounted for 94% of improper Medicare payments.

One of the challenges of effective fraud control within large payer programs is that, although most providers are honest, some insurance companies may unjustly deny claims or can be slow to pay them. As such there is a legitimate need for prompt payment of true and correct claims and bills. However, this must be balanced with the need to stop or at least try to control fraudulent claims. In government funded payment systems, with an improper payment rate at current levels; money is paid out before anyone even knows there is a problem. Then regulators are left with the difficult task of trying to prove the improper payment and chasing after these Medicare dollars after they have been paid out. Postpayment, retrospective fraud control is known as "pay and chase." While sometimes unavoidable, "pay and chase" is inefficient and wasteful.

In March 2011, after examining the six areas noted by the OIG most at risk for improper payments and some additional risk categories, CMS finalized regulations designed to help Medicare minimize "pay and chase" by enhancing the screening process that allows providers (including vendors and other entities that bill Medicare) into the system in the first place. CMS placed the various types of services into three risk categories with increasing levels of screening for each level, designated as limited, moderate, and high (see **Table 19-1**). The high-risk category includes home health agencies and DME suppliers, including prosthetics, orthotics, and supplies.

■ EMERGING TECHNOLOGY SOLUTIONS

Heightened interest in detecting and combating health care fraud has been accompanied by emerging technology solutions, briefly described below.

Data Analytics and Predictive Modeling

Predictive analytics or predictive modeling involves use of numerous statistical techniques that analyze current and past facts, typically in the form of data, to measure risks. Predictive analytics typically looks at patterns in historical data to identify risks and opportunities. Predictive modeling seeks to accurately capture relationships between numerous factors to allow assessment of risk or potential of risk associated with a particular set of conditions guiding assorted types of transactions.

Financial institutions, credit card companies, insurance companies, and other consumer companies are using predictive modeling tools to identify potential financial risks or fraud before it occurs. Credit scoring is an excellent example of predictive analytics. Banks and lenders use this score to

TABLE 19-1	**CMS Screening Levels by Rick Category**		
Type of screening required	**Limited risk**	**Moderate risk**	**High risk**
Verification of any provider-/supplier-specific requirements established by Medicare	◻	◻	◻
Conduct license verifications	◻	◻	◻
Database checks to verify Social Security number, National Provider Identifier, National Practitioner Databank licensure, any OIG exclusion taxpayer identification number, tax delinquency, death of individual practitioner, owner, authorized official, delegated official, or supervising physician	◻	◻	◻
Unscheduled or unannounced site visits		◻	◻
Criminal background check			◻
Fingerprinting			◻

Source: Created by author based on information in the February 2, 2011, *Federal Register* 76(22), 42 CFR Parts 405, 424, 447, 455, 457, 498 and 1007.

determine how risky it would be to extend credit to a consumer. Many health care payers in the private sector, as well as CMS, have been testing and using predictive modeling programs to facilitate early detection of possible fraudulent providers and scams based on historical information about the individual or the company with which the individual is affiliated.

Predictive analytics can also help prevent potential health care fraudsters from ever being placed in positions where they can defraud public and private sector health care payers in the first place. Effective analytics tools typically track billing patterns and other, often proprietary factors as well as other information to identify real-time aberrant trends that are indicative of fraud. "Using the most up-to-date technologies and adopting best practices across the nation's healthcare system, we have a better chance of avoiding fraudulent and abusive claims and identifying the

providers who submit these claims before they even start billing Medicare or other publicly-funded health insurance," said Peter Budetti, MD, Director of CMS's Center for Program Integrity.[19]

Stopping Pay and Chase

As analytics have progressed to where they can take place in huge volumes with millions of lines of data more quickly, it is now possible to conduct effective fraud control analysis within the parameters of prompt pay laws. This is true even when a clinical validation by a clinician, nurse, or certified coder takes place postadjudication or prepayment. It simply makes a lot more sense and is a much more efficient use of scarce fraud control resources to detect and prevent fraud payments on the front end than it does to pay the suspect claims and then chase after the money paid out to fraudsters after the fact. Thus, in the past few years most

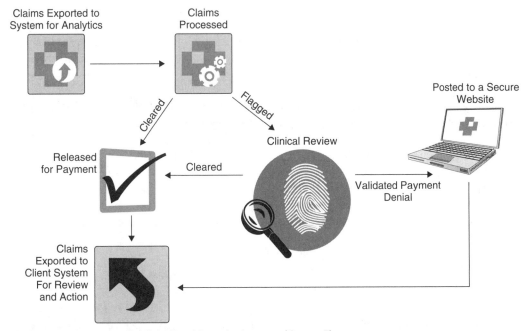

FIGURE 19-2 Recommended Claim Fraud Detection Integrated Process Flow

progressive payers in the health care industry have started to move, and some have completely moved, to prepayment fraud detection and away from pay and chase.

This does not mean that there is no post-pay fraud investigative work that will need to be done. There will still need to be some Special Investigations Unit (SIU) work in some cases; because even with more effective prepayment fraud detection systems, some types of fraud could still occur. Even so, the efficiencies of prepayment detection far outweigh the costs of waiting until after payment to work on this issue.

Software Can't Do It All

Even as technology has enhanced fraud control efforts it has also challenged them. When claims payment processes are electronic, if criminals learn the specifications of the system and learn how to bill their fraud correctly, they stand a better chance of going undetected than when a human is involved in the process and able to look at the data for signs of anomalies that might be indicative of fraud. "Virtually the only times when typical claims processing systems raise suspicions of fraud are when human beings have the opportunity to contemplate the claim in its entirety and to ask the kind of questions that only human beings can ask."[20] Despite its age, this quote is still quite true today. As such, a system that combines data-mining with human review and analysis provides better detection and prevention security than one where managers feel implementing a software-only solution has protected them.

The most effective fraud control solutions use data-mining algorithms based on emerging schemes and abnormal patterns. Then these need to be looked at by people to figure out in on what is really fraudulent and to eliminate the false-positives.

The ability to obtain, process, and look at data has come a long way in the past few years. Where this was once thought to be a rather daunting process, even the government is beginning to look at its data in ways that enable detection of fraud before the money goes out the door. **Figure 19-2** shows a recommended claim flow process that integrates data analysis and pattern detection with human review.

■ INVESTIGATION OR ACCUSATION OF HEALTH PLAN FRAUD

The focus of this chapter has been on the detection, prevention, and pursuit of health care fraud. However, any organization in health care can be accused of fraud. Although it remains as hard to measure as ever, health care fraud is a key area of attention for government enforcement officials. Every type of health care entity now faces a significant threat of being a victim of health care fraud and of being investigated for health care fraud. Health care fraud is now receiving attention at the highest levels of government; particularly in the wake of health care reform, where dollars lost to fraud are seen as inexcusable, low-hanging fruit. In particular, the stepped-up efforts by CMS to attack fraud could potentially extend to a Medicare Advantage or managed Medicaid plan.

Health care reform and related laws include provided significant fraud control focus and resources. These include:

- Significant additional financial resources for fighting fraud;

- High-level cabinet member support for the fight against health care fraud;
- Higher screening standards for billing Medicare and Medicaid;
- More coordinated exclusion between Medicare and Medicaid once a provider is kicked out of a program;
- Requirements that, in addition to hospitals and other health entities, providers also implement compliance programs;
- Allowing the government to suspend payments to certain providers suspected of fraud based on "credible allegations" of fraud (prior standard was "credible evidence");
- Numerous statutory amendments that make it easier to prosecute nefarious activities as health care fraud, including updating the False Claims Act to enable the government to charge fraud where kickbacks or overpayments are detected and not returned to the government within 60 days.

An interesting conundrum associated with fraud control is that the same entities that can be significant victims of fraud can also be accused of fraud. This is most typically by the government or by large payers. This places such entities in the unique position of being required to detect and prevent fraud but also at risk for being accused of fraud by the government. As such, an overview of some of the key players and statutes is relevant. **Table 19-2** provides a list of statutes, regulatory agencies, and professional organizations that are most significant to core knowledge of these issues.

United States Sentencing Guidelines and OIG Compliance Programs

Since about 2000, payers began addressing fraud risks through developing compliance programs. These health care compliance programs are increasingly common, largely due to the efforts of HHS OIG. However, the model compliance program concept and the rationale for implementing compliance programs originates from the Federal Sentencing Guidelines for Organizational Defendants, developed in 1991 by the United States Sentencing Commission (USSC). These guidelines were developed to promote consistent treatment of those convicted of federal crimes, including fines and restitution, imprisonment and probation, or exclusion from participation in various federally funded programs. Basically, payers or other health care entities in compliance with the Sentencing Guidelines are placed in a more desirable position should they be accused of fraud.

The Sentencing Guidelines may enable organizations to mitigate their sentences if they have adopted, implemented, and maintained an effective compliance program that includes what has become well known in health care as the "seven elements of compliance." A health care entity can reduce criminal penalties in the event that government

| TABLE 19-2 | Statutes, Regulatory Agencies, and Organizations Relevant to Health Care Fraud |

Relevant Health Care Fraud-Related Statutes

- False Claims Act (FCA), 31 U.S.C. §3729
- State false claims acts
- Anti-Kickback Statute, 42 U.S.C. §1320a-7b(b)
- Physician Self-Referral ("Stark") Statute, 42 U.S.C. §1395nn
- Deficit Reduction Act of 2005
- HIPAA of 1996, Title 18, Section 1347
- Fraud Enforcement and Recovery Act of 2009 (FERA)
- Patient Protection and Affordable Care Act (ACA)
- Health Care and Education Reconciliation Act of 2010 (HCERA)

Regulatory and Enforcement Agencies

- U.S. Department of Health and Human Services Office of the Inspector General (HHS OIG)
- Centers for Medicare and Medicaid Services (CMS)
- U.S. Department of Justice (DOJ)
- Federal Bureau of Investigation (FBI)
- State DOI/AG
- National Association of Medicaid Fraud Control Units (MFCU)

Other Resource Entities

- National Health Care Anti-Fraud Association (NHCAA)
- Accredited Health Care Fraud Investigator (AHFI)
- Association of Certified Fraud Examiners (ACFE)
- Certified Fraud Examiner (CFE)
- National Association of Insurance Commissioners (NAIC)
- National Association of Drug Diversion Investigators (NADDI)

pursues an enforcement action if they can demonstrate the proactive establishment of an effective corporate compliance program that includes all of these elements.

In fact, the Federal Sentencing Guidelines actually take into account the existence of a corporate compliance program in establishing criminal sentencing ranges and provide that an entity's culpability score will be lessened "if the offense occurred despite an effective program to prevent and detect violations of law." The seven elements were adopted specifically by the OIG for its Model Compliance Program Guidance, initially published for the health care industry in 1997.

Since March 1997, when the first OIG compliance guidance was issued specific to laboratories,[21] the OIG has issued guidance covering nearly every area of health care, including hospitals, physician practices, pharmaceutical manufacturers, clinical laboratories, home health agencies, and third-party medical billing companies.

These model plans all include seven common elements that the OIG believes provide a solid basis for health care entities to develop effective compliance programs. These elements closely follow those defined by the USSC in the Federal Sentencing Guidelines, and can be summarized as follows:

- Develop written policies and procedures;
- Designate a Compliance Officer and other appropriate bodies;
- Conduct effective training and education programs;
- Develop effective lines of communication;
- Enforce standards through well-publicized disciplinary guidelines;
- Conduct internal monitoring and auditing;
- Respond promptly to offenses and develop corrective action.

Consequently, the effective implementation of these elements can not only help prevent fraud, they can help a health care organization achieve more optimal positions with the government in the event they are ever accused of fraud, including False Claims Act violations.

What To Do When the Government Shows Up

While there is no way to capture and advise on every specific governmental audit or investigative scenario, if employed by or representing a private health care entity that is the subject of government scrutiny, there are some steps that can be taken to mitigate exposure and liability.

First, it is important to follow as closely as possible all government regulations and laws. Where an issue is unclear it is best to seek interpretive guidance from the regulating agency or counsel. Given the rapidly expanding number of regulations in this area, this is no small task. Then, in the event that you do have a situation that might be relevant to a government inquiry or the subject of mandatory reporting, it is always advisable to self-report or self-disclose the concern rather than wait until a whistleblower, perhaps with a different interpretation on the matter, does it for you.

Second, with the plethora of new laws expanding the government's power to determine that an activity (such as knowingly retaining a government overpayment) is fraud, work to be able to demonstrate that you have dedicated appropriate resources to ensure that payment processing and billing systems are accurate and not overbilling.

Third, it is important to have an implemented and effective compliance program. Better yet is to have self-assessed and audited your own program against the compliance effectiveness standards set by the government. And, if during your own assessments, you discover any impropriety associated with government billing and payments, again, coordinate with counsel to properly self-disclose them immediately and take steps toward effective systemic corrective action.

Fourth, regarding audits and investigations, it is important to be aware of the plethora of entities working on behalf of government health care payers, primarily CMS to audit programs billing the government, and what the authority or jurisdiction is for each. While these are in development and some may be in the process of being consolidated, they include:

- Medicare Administrative Contractors (MACs),
- Medicare Drug Integrity Contractors (MEDICs),
- Medicaid Integrity Contractors (MICs),
- Program Safeguard Contractors (PSCs),
- Recovery Audit Contractors (RACs),
- Quality Improvement Organizations (QIOs),
- Zone Program Integrity Contractors (ZPICs).

Fifth, when a fraud-related audit is taking place, some best processes for surviving it include:

- Centralize a location and designate an accountable person to receive all requests and related communication;
- Track all requests and be aware of due dates, deadlines, and appeal periods;
- Carefully analyze and trend results being produced to the government internally;
- Communicate regularly with key leaders, including physicians, about the audit.

Sixth, *substantive* elements necessary to survive a government fraud control compliance audit include the following:

1. Make sure your client/fraud team has clearly documented policies and procedures for detecting/preventing fraud and abuse.
2. Make sure your client/fraud team and SIU are adequately staffed and given appropriate resources to address the level of fraud detected in the program.
3. Be able to demonstrate that effective internal and external fraud control training is completed in a timely and regular manner.
4. Be sure you are conducting your own additional monitoring and oversight activities, especially in high-risk fraud areas.
5. Ensure that you are screening your client/staff against OIG Exclusion List and applicable state equivalents.

These five items were cited by the CMS Center for Program Integrity as associated with deficiencies they found during audits they conducted of fraud control programs in 2010.[22]

■ CONCLUSION

Effective fraud control or program integrity operations and appropriate strategic management of them is a core element of health plan organization and regulatory compliance. To respond to the emerging trends, fraud schemes, and regulatory scrutiny, health plans must bring this issue to where it is transparently managed and appropriately addressed.

The importance of this work cannot be overestimated, and health care executives must create a culture in which they are seen as the fraud finders and fraud fighters. Not only is this issue important to financial goals, it is also now a key to regulatory compliance. While the issues and challenges are complex, it is now more possible than ever to effectively manage fraud control from all of the conflicting directions.

Recommended Reading

1. Sparrow MK. *License to steal: Why fraud bleeds America's health care system*. Boulder, CO: Westview Press; 2000.
2. Bigelman M, Bartow J. *Executive roadmap to fraud prevention and internal control: Creating a culture of compliance*. Hoboken, NJ: John Wiley & Sons; 2006.

Endnotes

1 False Claims Act Amendments (Pub. L. 99-562, 100 Stat. 3153, enacted October 27, 1986) 31 U.S.C. §§ 3729–3733.

2 Phillips & Cohen, LLP. The False Claims Act: History of the law. 2007. Available at: www.all-about-qui-tam.org/fca_history.shtml. Accessed August 16, 2011.

3 S. Rep. No. 345, 99th Cong. 2d Sess. 21-22 (1986); H. Rep. No. 660, 99th Cong. 2d Sess.

4 Podgor ES. Criminal Fraud. *Am Univ Law Rev*. April 1999;48(4):729–768.

5 Kirsner S. Community theater. *CIO Mag*. 1997;11(5): 38–40.

6 CBS News. Medicare fraud: A $60 billion crime: "60 Minutes." October 25, 2009. Available at: www.cbsnews.com/stories/2009/10/23/60minutes/main5414390.shtml. Accessed August 16, 2011.

7 42 CFR Part 1007, pages 5862–5971, February 2, 2011 (effective March 25, 2011).

8 United States Senate Testimony of Tony West, Assistant Attorney General, Civil Division. February 15, 2011. Department of Justice before the United States Senate Committee on Appropriations, Subcommittee on Labor, Health and Human Services, Education and Related Agencies, United States Senate, entitled "Fighting Fraud and Waste in Medicare and Medicaid."

9 National Health Care Anti-Fraud Association. *The Problem of Health Care Fraud*. Available at: www.nhcaa.org/eweb/DynamicPage.aspx?webcode = anti_fraud_resource_centr&wpscode = ConsumerAndAction Info. Accessed July 19, 2011.

10 Sparrow MK. *License to steal: Why fraud bleeds America's health care system*. Boulder, CO: Westview Press; 2000, pp. 43–44.

11 Sparrow MK. License to steal: *Why fraud plagues America's health care system*. Boulder, CO: Westview Press; 1996, p. 34.

12 Testimony of Malcolm K. Sparrow to the Senate Subcommittee on Criminal Prosecution on May 20, 2009. Available at: www.hks.harvard.edu/news-events/news/testimonies/sparrow-senate-testimony. Accessed August 16, 2011.

13 Ibid., p. 2.

14 Testimony of Peter Budetti, MD, JD, to the United States House Committee on Oversight and Government Reform on April 5, 2011. Available at: www.hhs.gov/asl/testify/2011/04/t20110405b.html. Accessed August 16, 2011.

15 Sparrow MK. *License to steal: Why fraud plagues America's health care system*. Boulder, CO: Westview Press; 1996, p. 18.

16 HHS OIG Fiscal Year 2011 I-17, Work Plan Part I, Medicare Part A and Part B.

17 Department of Health and Human Services. Departments of Justice and Health and Human Services team up in Detroit to crack down on health care fraud [Press Release]. March 15, 2011. Available at: www.hhs.gov/news/press/2011pres/03/20110315a.html. Accessed August 16, 2011.

18 Centers for Medicare and Medicaid Services. Prescription drug benefit manual, Chapter 9—Part D program to control fraud, waste and abuse. Available at: www.cms.gov/PrescriptionDrugCovContra/Downloads/PDBManual_Chapter9_FWA.pdf. Accessed August 16, 2011.

19 Quotation for Peter Budetti, MD, JD, Deputy Administrator for Program Integrity, Centers for Medicare and Medicaid Services. Quoted with permission.

20 Sparrow MK. *License to steal, why fraud plagues America's health care system*. Boulder, CO: Westview Press; 1996.

21 *Federal Register*. March 3, 1997;62(41):9435–9441.

22 Moreno C. CMS Center for Program Integrity, Health Care Compliance Association (HCCA) PowerPoint slides distributed to attendees on April 11, 2011.

Member Services

KEVIN KNARR AND PETER R. KONGSTVEDT

STUDY OBJECTIVES

- Understand the basic processes and supporting technology of contact center operations
- Understand basic staffing and management issues in member services
- Understand the goals of member services in a payer organization
- Understand the basics of how a plan addresses member concerns and problems
- Understand the legal and regulatory aspects of member services
- Understand the role of the summary of coverage and the evidence of coverage
- Understand the formal internal and external review processes for an appeal of a denial of benefits coverage
- Understand the means by which member services assesses member satisfaction
- Understand proactive approaches a plan may take to measuring and maintaining member satisfaction

DISCUSSION TOPICS

1. Discuss the basic goals of a member services department.
2. Describe the typical types of steps that member services would take to address a member inquiry, a problem, a complaint, and a formal appeal.
3. Discuss how the Patient Protection and Affordable Care Act (ACA) has affected the formal appeal review processes.
4. Discuss how contact center management and technology has evolved and how it may evolve in the future.
5. Describe the legal and regulatory milieu affecting member services, and provide hypothetical descriptions of different scenarios to illustrate those effects.
6. Describe actions a plan may take to enhance member satisfaction.

INTRODUCTION

Navigating the increasingly complicated world of health care is a daunting task for the average health plan member. Ever-changing benefit structures, confusion surrounding provider networks, the nature of claims payment, explanation of benefit (EOB) and billing processes all point to an administrative complexity that can easily stump the most astute consumer. The development of consumer-directed health products (CDHPs) and high-deductible health plans further contribute to the issue. Finally, the advent of the Patient Protection and Affordable Care Act (ACA) and its associated regulations and mandates, including state-based health insurance exchanges ("exchanges"), all contribute to the increasing need for guidance from the plan itself. That guidance comes most frequently in the form of member services or, more broadly, the customer services function. The fundamental delivery approach for member services is through a customer interaction center, often referred to interchangeably as a "call center" or "customer contact center." This environment supports inbound inquiries across a broad array of media (most frequently, inbound telephone calls), blended with outbound contact and outreach transactions.

The customer interaction center enables the member to communicate directly with his or her insurer, enrolling in the plan; accessing administrative or clinical information; resolving issues; initiating complaints, grievances, or appeals; and receiving general assistance in effectively procuring coverage and care. In turn, the health plan is able to track and report problems encountered, determine the root cause of upstream issues, and help manage the member decision-making process as it relates to accessing care, obtaining the best level of coverage or defining payment responsibility.

Increasingly, plan executives understand the rich insight that the center can offer the health plan. Whereas the member services function was once considered a cost center, a "necessary evil," more forward-thinking plans realize the immense potential in developing long-term relationships with their membership through a well-designed member services function. This trend is particularly important as one considers the retail nature of the consumer-directed health plan movement that gained steam in the early 2000s, and the substantial increase in business-to-consumer (B2C) relationships being introduced through the ACA (exchanges, Medicaid expansion, Medicare/Medicare Supplemental, etc.). In mimicking a consumer products company's approach to managing the customer relationship, plans are more aware than ever of the function's ability to drive member satisfaction and, ultimately, retention, market share, and "wallet share" of the customer as they expand product and service offerings.

THE MEMBER SERVICE ENVIRONMENT

As noted previously, the bulk of member services activity takes place in the health plan's customer interaction center(s). These centers generally vary in size between 30 and 400 customer service representatives (CSRs), with the majority of centers falling in the 100-200 full-time equivalent (FTE) range. The centers are commonly located with other health plan "back-office" functions, including claims payment, provider services, enrollment and billing, and materials fulfillment. In determining an effective location for their customer interaction center(s), plans will evaluate several criteria, including:

- Commercial real estate costs (leasing/purchasing);
- Labor wage rates;
- Telecommunications and technology infrastructure;
- Availability of high school, community college, and (in some cases) college-educated CSR candidates; and
- Availability of qualified customer interaction center management candidates.

Typically, plans locate contact centers in suburban/ ex-urban locations such as in smaller towns with one or more of the following attributes:

- Plentiful availability of "flex-space" or office park real estate;
- Less expensive locations with educated and available labor pools with minimal competition for employees;
- Durable infrastructure; and
- Communities that offer the payer incentives since these centers afford stable, long-term job opportunities for their citizens.

It is important to note here that outsourcing and off-shoring of member services calls, in general, has to date received a mixed reception from the purchasing community, particularly employer groups and government entities. This can be traced to the highly sensitive nature of the calls, typically related to a member's health and finances. That stated, the tide is beginning to change, as all involved in the health care equation see the need to manage costs, assuming the quality of the interaction is not impacted, or improved.

While there is a great degree of variance in the size of health plan customer interaction centers, it is generally understood that plans derive economies of scale from pooling their labor resources in larger centers. However, client demands (such as an employer wishing to have their plan's customer interaction center near their employee base), lack of available labor pools, or structural considerations (e.g., a state-based Blues plan's requirements to keep customer interaction centers in-state) can all affect a plan's ability to scale its centers.

The customer interaction centers themselves present a unique office environment. CSRs are typically housed in cubes with low wall heights to foster teamwork and assistance, sitting with teams varying from 12 to 20, all reporting to a supervisor or team lead, who is normally located with or near the team. The ratio of CSRs to supervisors is typically determined by balancing cost with contact complexity. While more complex calls may require a smaller ratio (12:1), that ratio comes with a cost when extrapolated across a large center of 300 CSRs. These teams may be dedicated to a product line such as Medicare Advantage (MA; see Chapter 24), an account (as prescribed during the contracting phase between the plan and an employer group), or may be part of a larger pool of CSRs servicing hundreds of accounts and millions of members.

Aside from the site director and the senior management of the customer interaction center, most employees do not have enclosed offices. This usually results in a very open environment, seen as critical to collaborating to resolve their customers' issues quickly and effectively. This open environment also enables the supervisor to see when a CSR is having difficulty with a member's phone call, and also ensures that CSRs are at their station and available to take incoming calls/correspondence as scheduled. To a person more familiar with a traditional high-rise office environment, a customer interaction center has an unusual appearance.

Special Considerations Regarding the Member Services Environment

There are some special considerations that must be addressed in the provision of member services to individual members. The two that are the most important for this discussion are the hours that member services are available to members and the ability to communicate in languages other than English.

Hours of Availability

Availability is the most obvious issue to consider. While 24 hour per day, 7 days per week (referred to as 24/7) is ideal, it will not be cost-justified for any but the largest plans, and not necessarily even then. In fact, one need look no further than the arrival patterns of member calls to see that most members attempt to contact their plan's customer interaction centers between the hours of 7:00 A.M. and 6:00 P.M. (in the caller's time zone) on weekdays, with highest call volumes seen on Mondays and lower volumes as the week progresses. The size and geographic distribution of the payer organization will play a role in determining the maximum hours that member services will be available. As an example, a state-based Blues plan on the East Coast may choose to stay open from 7:00 A.M. to 7:00 P.M. in the Eastern Time Zone on weekdays, with no weekend coverage. However, a large national health insurer may choose to stay open from 7:00 A.M. Eastern Time Zone to 7:00 P.M. Pacific Time Zone, 7 days a week, in order to ensure their entire membership has coverage for their inquiries. In order to ensure the appropriate level of consumer satisfaction, plans employ several techniques to service their members during off-hours. Examples include the following.

To address the clinical (nonadministrative) call types that come in during off-hours, plans may send calls to a 24/7 nurse advice line, where a licensed nurse can help respond to a member's clinical issue or advise them to call during regular business hours to address administrative issues. It is better for some inappropriate (administrative) calls to go to the nurse advice line than for a medical problem to go unaddressed. In payers that use this approach, it is preferable for the nurse advice line organization (often an outside company that the payer has contracted with) to have direct access to the payer's systems and information, and to be able to input information for action and follow-up by the plan's member services department when it reopens. Nurse advice lines are discussed further in Chapter 7.

Plans may employ 24/7 electronic media such as web portals or an interactive voice response (IVR) system (discussed in later sections) that enable members to guide themselves through simple and moderately complex administrative questions.

Plans may choose to outsource their off-hours call volume to a customer service business process outsourcing (BPO) company, usually domestic, that hire and train representatives to handle the less-predictable off-hours volume more efficiently than the plan itself can.

Use of voice mail, once thought to be a good way to handle off-hours calls, has proven to be less effective than hoped, as iterative games of "phone tag" are carried out between the plan and the member, thus having a negative impact on customer perception. Use of voice mail is typically seen as a last-resort measure for off-hours calls.

For calls received during periods when the member services department is not open, it is critical that the automated menu heard upon connecting to the closed center makes clear that if the call is in reference to a clinical problem or medical emergency, the member should contact their physician, or in the case of a medical emergency, seek medical help directly.

Hours of operation are yet another area where the employer group purchasing the plan may have a direct impact. Some groups demand extended hours of customer interaction center operation, sometimes related to the type of business they operate. For instance, an employer group who is a manufacturing concern with round-the-clock hours may demand the same of their health plan.

Non-English Communications

The ability to communicate with members in languages other than English is becoming increasingly important, particularly in large urban areas with large populations that are not conversant in English; for example, a Spanish-speaking community. For service members who reside in such areas, payers typically employ member services representatives who speak that language. For languages that are not necessarily in high concentration, or in smaller plans, it is common for the multilingual services to be provided through externally contracted interpreter services. Via the ACA, there is an overall increase in focus on being able to service members in their preferred language, enabling improved understanding of administrative or clinical issues, and in particular consumer rights such as appeal rights, to be discussed later.

■ CUSTOMER INTERACTION SUPPORT ACTIVITIES

Payers pay a lot of attention to recruiting personnel who will ultimately work as CSRs. The team who recruits and hires the CSR and management professionals seeks to ensure the function is staffed with qualified resources. Given the potentially stressful environment, the member service function is usually one with high attrition, and requires that a steady flow of candidates be evaluated and hired when appropriate.

Beyond the ongoing recruiting needs, health plan customer interaction centers require several key support functions in order to meet the quality and service levels required by the membership base. Without these functions, questions would be answered insufficiently, CSRs would not feel empowered to do their job, contacts would not be responded to on a timely basis, and there would be no means for recognizing high performance. These activities include training, workforce management, and quality management/performance management. Each of these activities plays a key role in keeping the member service function functioning effectively and efficiently and in keeping member, groups, and plan employees satisfied.

Training

The amount of training required of member services representatives before they are allowed to interact with members varies from plan to plan. It is common for large payers to require new representatives to spend at least 40-60 working days in training before they begin actually interfacing with members, and even then the first few weeks are monitored by a supervisor. Ongoing training also occurs on a regular basis, particularly if support systems change, as well as training for increasing responsibilities for CSRs and as a means of increasing employee satisfaction. Timing of training may also be affected by workforce management issues, as discussed in the next section.

One of the difficulties in training is the ever-changing landscape of the benefits and services offered by the health plans, and the frequency of policy changes that affect the member. This places a large burden on the member services department, who find themselves having to train "on-the-fly," or by sending e-mail "blasts" to their CSRs and supervisors. Keeping training material relevant and current is an enormous challenge for member services departments.

Workforce Management

The cyclical and variable nature of the inbound customer contact environment make predicting and managing the volume demands a critical part of member services management. If there are too few CSRs on hand for the attendant call volume, contacts will go unanswered, or there will be severe delays in getting to a CSR. If there are too many CSRs, the cost structure of the member services function will be too high. The process of balancing the service level and cost structure is called workforce management (WFM).

Using an automated set of algorithms in a WFM forecasting and scheduling tool, the WFM team uses historical and projected volume data to forecast the future volume of contacts. Then, based on that projected volume, and taking into account all of the ancillary activities that occur in the center (meetings, training, etc.), the tool creates a schedule to ensure that the right number of people are ready for inbound contacts for every half-hour increment that the member services function is open.

In addition to the static planning function of forecasting and scheduling, which typically occurs every 60–90 days, the WFM team manages intraday operations to ensure that call spikes, system outages, and so on, have little to no impact on the service levels, average speed to answer (described later), for example, within the center. The WFM team is also on point to help plan for such activities as mass mailings and open-enrollment periods, ensuring that these cyclical activities are accounted for when planning the staffing need.

Performance Management and Quality Management

Member services are measured on both operational performance, generally focused on hard numbers around answering responsiveness and contact resolution times, as well as more qualitative, soft-skill metrics, such as customer satisfaction and call quality. Each of these measure sets has a direct impact on the member's view of their health plan. Holding member services personnel directly accountable for such metrics will help ensure the member has the best possible perception of the plan's service processes.

Member services departments have responsiveness requirements as part of their performance standards. Such standards generally revolve around a few simple measures, including:

- Average speed to answer (ASA)—length of time elapsed between the call leaving the IVR and the call being answered by a live CSR (common goal—an average of 30 seconds)
- Service level percentage—a specific percentage of calls to be answered within a given timeliness goal (common goal: 75–80% of all calls handled within 30 seconds)
- Abandon rates—number of calls where the caller hangs up before reaching a live CSR due to lengthy ASA times (common goal - less than 3% of all calls abandon before a live answer)

Performance standards must be tailored to meet the standards that the *members* would expect, not simply what the plan chooses to measure. For example, a plan may measure ASA by measuring how long it takes a call to be answered by a CSR once the call leaves the IVR, described later; such a measurement would fail to capture the fact that the member had to wade through several menus of an IVR in order to get there, resulting in 3 minutes of frustration by the member.

Timeliness of response and first contact resolution is also measured against goals. Examples include the percentage of calls that are resolved on the spot (i.e., no follow-up is required); for example, 90% of calls should require no follow-up. For problems or questions that require follow-up, there are goals for how long that takes; for example, 90% of outstanding inquiries or problems should be resolved within 14 days and 98% within 28 days. Similar standards apply to written correspondence. Large self-funded employer groups contracting with a payer for administrative services only also typically put similar requirements into the contract, referred to as a service level agreement (SLA).

CSRs are also measured individually for goals such as:

- Schedule adherence: Ensuring CSRs are staffed and ready for inbound contacts as scheduled by the WFM team
- Average handle time: The length of time each contact takes to complete
- First call resolution: Percentage of contacts resolved on the first call

CSRs are usually monitored not just for productivity, but for quality as well. Quality is usually monitored through silent monitoring of the calls themselves. This is usually done through relatively sophisticated systems that enable the quality reviewer to both listen to recorded calls and at the same time view what transpired on the CSR's desktop.

The answering system informs the member calling in that the call may be monitored for quality purposes. These recorded calls can be segmented by call type, CSR name, employer group name, and so on, to generate rich data for the quality personnel's focused review. The quality reviewer (which may be the CSR's supervisor, but should typically be the responsibility of an objective Quality Management team) will issue a qualitative judgment about how well the service representative handled the call, from both a call process and customer service skills point of view.

It is not enough to take and give information when a member has a problem or complaint; the representative must apply communication techniques developed for customer service in order to be optimally effective. Some plans routinely send follow-up questionnaires to members after the member services inquiry or complaint is resolved to solicit feedback on the process, as well as reinforce the notion that the member is important.

Methods of Accessing Member Services: Interaction Media

A major part of creating an enduring and positive customer experience is giving the member a variety of options in terms of how they interact with the health plan and, equally importantly, ensuring that the plan handles all interaction media effectively and efficiently. The way a member chooses to communicate varies due to several factors, most prominently:

- Reason that he or she is calling,
- Media available to the member at the time of contact, and
- Level of comfort with electronic media.

Generally speaking, members contact the interaction center through one or more of the following:

- Interactive voice response,
- Inbound telephone calls,
- Mail and paper-based communications,
- E-mail,
- Web-chat/text messaging,
- Internet/Web self-service, and/or
- Mobile devices, such as smartphones or "tablets," although the use of mobile interactive media is still in its early stages.

With each interaction medium, plans delivering a good customer experience will employ several integrated and interrelated technologies in routing and supporting the transaction, to ensure that the CSR is in the best position to handle the inquiry efficiently and with the greatest chance to drive "first contact resolution"; in other words, completing the transaction such that the member has no need to contact the plan again regarding the issue.

The first of these capabilities is known as computer telephony integration, or CTI. CTI enables the plan to take information the caller provides while in an automated menu (e.g., member ID or type of request) or other information (caller's phone number), and access the plan's underlying customer databases to identify the member who is trying to contact the customer interaction center. This is particularly helpful in both routing the contact to the appropriate location and preparing the CSR to process the contact by "popping" the contact information to the CSR's desktop screen.

Second, building on CTI, "intelligent call routing" or "skill-based routing" enables the plan to send the contact to the CSR group best prepared to handle the contact. Criteria for routing may include the issue type, severity of the issue, past history of interaction with a specific CSR or set of CSRs, employer group, or other insight/business rules that the plan deems necessary to encourage effective service. These routing mechanisms enable the plan to tailor the customer experience and increase member satisfaction with the outcomes of the contact.

Finally, effective balancing of contact volume is accomplished via the use of an automated call distributor (ACD). This is a device or switch that automatically routes contacts based on programmed distribution instructions. There may be two levels of ACDs used in a plan. The first is to serve as the initial automated answering system for inbound calls ("Hello. You have reached the member services department of XYZ Health Care"), which will then send the call on (directly or to an IVR, as discussed next), as well as serve to provide wait instructions and background content for those members put on hold. The second function is to distribute all contacts based on CSR availability; in other words, spread the workload and maximize the level of service provided. Modern ACD systems have the capability of handling all forms of interaction media, but plans typically use the ACD to balance their inbound call volume.

Note that in general, most plans are moving to the use of virtualized contact center capabilities, meaning that the majority of these functions are handled in the "cloud," as opposed to physical hardware existing on location in the contact center.

Inbound Telephone Communications Including IVR

The highest volume of interactions between a plan and its members will occur via the telephone, excluding routine mailings such as the issuance of identification cards, member newsletters, and other nonindividualized forms of communication. There are several aspects to telephone communications that must be looked at by any plan, and these are discussed next.

Placing the Call and Initial Navigation

Virtually all plans employ a toll-free line for use by members. In some cases, plans with a high incidence of local membership may opt to also publish local numbers to reduce toll charges. However, with 8nn-number (8nn refers to all toll-free numbers, including 800, 866, 877, etc.) toll charges edging as low as $0.03 per minute, it makes up a very small part of the customer interaction center cost as compared to years past. In some cases, a member's identification card or member handbook lists different numbers for different needs. For example, a plan may have an 8nn for members to select a new primary care physician (PCP), or to access a nurse line, for precertification, or to resolve a problem. In most instances, plans take the route of having one single member services telephone number, and the member then will be directed via telephone network menus or an IVR.

It is critical that these menus (either in the network or in the IVR) be clear, stripped of medical jargon, and simple to navigate. It is also important that the voice the caller hears have continuity throughout the experience. Otherwise, the plan runs the risk of consumer backlash as the service experience fails to satisfy their needs. In a very few cases, the member may be connected immediately to a service representative who will then deal with whatever issue the member has. This is particularly common in situations where the caller might be easily frustrated with the IVR menu (e.g., the senior marketplace) or in the instance of potential high-stress calls (e.g., behavioral health intake calls). Generally, though, for routing and self-service purposes, the toll-free line will first lead to automated responses.

Ensuring Capacity

It is important for the telephone "trunks" and lines to be adequate in number, and properly automated in function, depending on plan size (automatic call distribution, sequencing, etc.). These are the functions of the payer's telephone system, generally referred to as a PBX. For historical reasons, even though this system is actually a specialized computer, it is referred to as a "switch."* It is common for large payers to have more than one switch, and for some of the switches to be specialized for use by plan functional areas.

---

*A charming holdover of a 19th century term into the 21st, the computer that manages the telephone system is called a switch because in the old days of telephones, telephone operators routed calls by switching connections using a switchboard. When direct dial telephone exchanges appeared in the early 1900s, a caller spun a spring-loaded rotary dial a certain amount for each number, and the rotor would turn itself back at a set speed. As it spun back, the phone sent pairs of pulses or clicks that signaled a set of circular electromechanical switches. The first switch in the set would move one space for each pair of clicks, corresponded to the dialed number, and then move to the next switch, which would move when the dial was spun again. It's also why we still say we "dial" a phone, even though most readers of this book may never have seen an actual dial telephone except perhaps on Wikipedia®.

Because the switch is really a computer that is open to the telephone systems of the entire world, intense and specialized security precautions are required, but are beyond the scope of this chapter. Suffice it to say that the payer's telecommunications staff spends a great deal of their time ensuring that capacity exists to handle the volume of inbound calls (with contingency for spikes), that call routing programming is accurate and avoids "misdirected" calls, that security is maintained, and that failover plans are in place to ensure uninterrupted member contact response.

Routing the Call to the Right CSR

Call routing requires collaboration of the aforementioned CTI and skill-based routing capabilities, as well as use of the IVR system. The IVR is a system that provides the caller with a menu, or several menus to choose from in order to direct the call to the most appropriate department. These menus may be "touch-tone," where the caller uses the phone's key pad to interact. Payers may also take advantage of the significantly more intuitive and easy to use speech recognition programs, which employ natural language capabilities that resemble an actual voice, picking up on specific phrases spoken by the consumer to identify and help resolve the need. Due to the complexity of health insurance calls, payers have been "slow followers" in the natural language space, taking a disciplined approach so as not to upset their membership.

To illustrate a typical IVR system, the member's call is answered by the automated system. In a touch-tone or limited speech recognition environment, the member is instructed to make some basic choices; for example, "Press or say 1 if your call is about a claim, press or say 2 if your call is about an identification card, press or say 3 if your call is about selecting or changing your primary care physician . . ." and so forth. Some plans nest the menus as well; for example, after the member presses 1 because their call is about a claim, the menu may then instruct them to "Press or say 1 if your call is about an unpaid claim, press or say 2 if your call is about an incorrectly paid claim, press or say 3 if your call is to inquire about the status of a submitted claim . . ." and so forth. The general rule of thumb for best-practice touch-tone environments is to limit the menu structure to a "3 × 3" matrix; in other words, plans should offer no more than three choices at each level, and go no more than three levels deep. Also, plans must enable menu repeats and an ability to opt out to a live CSR when the member has exhausted the possibilities within the menu.

The more advanced speech recognition programs have created a paradigm shift for plans in how they employ the IVR. Rather than being beholden to a rigid touch-tone menu structure, the speech recognition IVR might prompt the caller with "Welcome to XYZ Health Care . . . what is it you are calling about today?" The IVR is programmed for hundreds of permutations of caller responses, so that

"I lost my ID card," "I need a new member ID," or "I can't understand why you don't mail my ID to me on time" are all recognized as a member who is having a problem with an ID card. The IVR might follow up with, "It sounds like you've lost or not received your ID card—is that correct?" When the member answers, "Yes," the call is either forwarded to a CSR who is now prepared to help the member with his or her lost card or else to an automated resolution of the call in a human-like manner.

IVR Self-Service

IVR systems may also provide for member self-service. This refers to providing the member with a form of self-service that does not require the intervention of a member services representative. Examples of these would include requesting a new identification card to be mailed, providing fax-back or e-mail-back information (e.g., a listing of all participating PCPs in the member's zip code or within 5 miles of their zip code or other provider listings), providing a copy of certain plan policies and procedures (e.g., how the member may receive benefits for alternative medicine), allowing the member to find out the status of a claim in process, determine the status of an authorization for services, or other information.

Self-service IVR may also be used for enrollment purposes.* In this use, the member responds to the IVR questions by entering information via the telephone, not just responding to simple Boolean-type questions. This type of self-service generally requires that the payer organization receive a base level of information from the enrolled group (i.e., the employer) ahead of time, so that the subscriber calling in (i.e., the member who is the individual actually receiving the benefit from the employer) is able to identify him- or herself by way of an identification number. The enrollment system then collects responses regarding the type of benefit plan the subscriber wants, the PCP each family member wants if enrolling in a health maintenance organization (HMO) by using a directory of PCPs in which numbers are associated with each PCP, and so forth. Additional nonhealth benefits may also be enrolled this way, but often this occurs through a party other than the payer, such as a benefits consulting firm or outsourced human resources administrator. The advantages of using this type of IVR are obvious: faster data entry, increased accuracy (the IVR simply requires reentry of incorrect data and also reads back the choices in plain language before asking the subscriber to confirm those choices), and lower costs.

There are two benefits and two limitations to effective IVR self-service usage. From a benefits perspective, the IVR

---

* While enrollment services are not part of the scope of discussion, it is appropriate to discuss this capability here since it is in the context of the overall self-service provision of member services. See Chapter 17 for a detailed discussion of enrollment and billing.

enables the member to get immediate access to answers to their inquiries without having to wait on hold for a CSR to answer their call. Additionally, the plan is able to push more call volume to the IVR for self-service, thereby reducing the number of CSRs required to handle calls, optimizing operating costs. Limiting the effectiveness is the fact that when a member calls, he or she is usually calling about issues of health or money, and the sensitive nature of those topics causes them to want to speak to a live CSR, rather than assume that the automated system is really "understanding" their needs. This is the reason for IVR completion rates (member calls satisfied through use of the IVR) have hovered in the high single-digit and low-teen percentages, although speech recognition is raising it a bit. Second, the Internet is offering a much more intuitive and easy to certify approach to completing transactions. Thus, transactions that were once problematic to complete via the IVR, even with speech recognition, are much better suited to the more visual touch-and-feel nature of the Web.

Delivering the Call to the CSR for Handling

At the point where the plan has exhausted its IVR capabilities for self-service and picked up enough information from the caller to know who he or she is and have a sense for why they are reaching out to the plan, the call is routed to a qualified CSR. Also, if the caller opts out of the IVR, the ACD makes a determination as to whom the call should be delivered. CSRs are signed into phone "splits," usually associated with a set of employer groups, a product type, call types, and so on. The ACD will deliver the call to the split, and then assign the call based on predefined parameters, often the CSR who has been available the longest.

In payers with CTI, the CSR receives the member's (non-medical) records and other data on their terminal screen at the same time the call is coming through. This is done via the switch's ability to recognize the calling number, either via caller ID or the payer's own database of numbers, as well as accepting and evaluating information the caller enters into the IVR. Although this provides the CSR with the ability to greet the caller by name, there is no way to ensure that the caller is actually who the system identifies them as, and so, to adhere to authentication regulations under the privacy and security requirements under the Health Insurance Portability and Accountability Act (HIPAA; see Chapter 29), the representative must still ask the name of the caller and generally some form of confirmation (typically a set of three to five questions). Once such identification is clear, the representative has the ability to address the caller's needs or questions rapidly since the information is already available, including, of course, notes from prior calls.

The last major type of telephone communications is the outbound, predictive dialer. This is a system in which the call center's switch is programmed to make calls to members on a proactive basis. The most common use for this in a payer's member services department is outreach to new members, as is discussed later. Another common use is for follow-up on a member's call; in other words, the payer representative calls the member to make sure that their issues or needs have been met. The effect on member satisfaction is quite positive. Other uses of outbound predictive dialing exist, particularly in the clinical arena. Examples would include regular follow-up calls to patients with serious chronic diseases (see Chapters 7 and 8) or reminders to members to use preventive services (e.g., calling women who have no record of a mammogram when they are of an age where screening mammograms are recommended; see Chapter 13).

Mail and Paper-Based Communication

Even though most of the individual-member activity in member services takes place via the telephone, mail and paper communication remains highly important, and must be managed properly. It is common that inbound mail correspondence will take place in the context of formal complaints or grievances (discussed later in this chapter) as part of a documentation effort by the individual initiating the correspondence, although it can occur in the normal course of communications from those members who simply prefer to use the mail rather than another means of communication.

All inbound correspondence must be logged and tracked, usually after being scanned and indexed in electronic format. Policies and procedures must be in place regarding the routing of correspondence, and master files need to be kept of both incoming and outgoing correspondence. Plans also frequently use imaging technology to store the massive amounts of paper documents, the originals of which may be then stored offsite for a number of years. It is important to ensure that paper correspondence receives the same attention that telephone calls do, with time standards for response. In fact, in some of the more sophisticated plans, the scanned and indexed document is then routed like a phone call through the ACD to the CSR's desktop for processing.

All payer organizations use mail and paper-based correspondence for outbound communications. This is required for any form of communication that takes place on a plan-wide or other large scale (e.g., to all members of an enrolled group). It is also used by the plan for documentation purposes when communicating important changes or notices to the members, such as a change in the pharmacy network, a change in policy coverage determinations, and so forth.

On an individual member level, outbound mail correspondence will always be used for formal communications and documentation of the complaint or grievance process discussed later in this chapter. Outbound mail is also used to reply to inbound mail from members, although that may serve as a supplement to telephone communications.

E-Mail Communication

E-mail has become ubiquitous in the office environment. Virtually every office worker in America relies on e-mail to help drive communication and resolve issues. Familiarity with this interaction media has crept into a plan's communication with their membership. On nearly every website, and at times on a member's ID card, a plan's customer service e-mail address is available as a means for interaction. Additionally, during the course of a CSR's phone interaction with a member, the CSR may ask the member to e-mail information to him or her to facilitate the closure of the issue.

Plans need to be mindful of the e-mail medium because it can actually be less efficient than live phone interaction. E-mail intent and content can be open to broad interpretation, such that a CSRs response may not exactly meet the member's needs. This can lead to unnecessary iterations of work. Generally, e-mail interaction should be focused on basic administrative issues with little need for comprehensive evaluation.

Automated e-mail response technologies have been introduced over the last decade, and are generally effective when the member request is of a basic administrative nature. Typically, the system will react to key words in the member's e-mail and attempt to answer the question using standardized responses.

Again, modern-day ACDs enable the processing of e-mails in the same way as they process and deliver inbound phone calls. The e-mail is routed to the CSR (instead of a phone call), and the CSR processes to completion. Once complete, the CSR is then ready to handle another e-mail, inbound call, or other contact medium.

Interactions between members and plans are subject to the privacy and security provisions of HIPAA, including e-mail (see Chapters 23 and 29). Therefore, the ability to encrypt data and provide for the assurance that only the member is able to electronically access confidential data about themselves is required. This is particularly relevant for both the e-mail medium as well as the next two interaction media, web-chat and Internet self-service.

Web-Chat/Text Messaging

Another increasingly common form of communication is a text messaging session, in which the member, usually on the plan's website, chooses a "Click-to-Chat" function. This enables the member to initiate a text session with the CSR, basically a written version of an inbound phone call. More effective than e-mail due to the live nature of the interaction, text chats can be used for a variety of contact reasons. It is not uncommon to see text chats used for more sensitive clinical advice discussions, as it gives the member just a little more distance between the CSR and him, enabling a more comfortable "conversation." As with e-mail and imaged paper inquiries, the ACD can be used to deliver text messaging sessions to the appropriate CSR's desktop. Like all CSR communications with members, logs and recordings are kept and securely stored.

Internet/Web Self-Service

One of the most important developments in the customer interaction center over the past decade has been the meteoric rise of the Web as a means to drive what was once inbound phone volume, to the plan's member web "portal" to enable self service. This parallels the increasing use of web portal self-service for almost all the types of transactions we make on a day-to-day basis (e.g., purchasing goods or music, booking a flight, or paying a utility bill).

While the nature of a member's inquiry is often very sensitive in nature, related to health or money, members have shown an increased propensity to use the Internet to retrieve answers to their administrative and clinical questions. Member portals have proven very effective at performing many of the basic administrative activities, including:

- Enrollment, including
  - New member enrollment commercial or MA plans and
  - Adding or removing dependent coverage due to a life event such as marriage or childbirth;
- ID Card Issuance, including
  - Obtaining a new card and
  - Entering changes to an existing card;
- Claims status/tracking;
- Provider lookup, including
  - Information about specific physicians, hospitals, labs, and so forth
  - Printing out directions;
- Benefits and eligibility lookup.

The Web has represented a significant step up from the IVR self-service option of years past, including the breadth and depth of clinical interaction available on the member portal. Treatment decision support, health risk assessments, symptom information, wellness programs, and the like are all found on a variety of plan websites. As with the IVR, the plan benefits substantially from members completing transactions online, as the cost of a Web transaction might be $0.05–0.10 versus $7–10 for a live interaction.

At the time of this publication, there is a substantial movement underfoot to offering the same administrative and clinical transactions, along with a host of other services, via applications, or "apps," that transact on mobile devices. Mobile devices, such as cell phones or tablet computers, have also become increasingly popular for health and wellness services. This enables a plan to increase the "mind share" of their consumers and more deeply weave their brand into the fabric of their customers' lives.

Accessing Member Services: Summary Points

As you have seen over the last few pages, members have many options available to them when they decide to interact with their health plan. Given the proliferation of these interaction media, there are several points to keep in mind when a plan establishes its interaction strategy:

- Not every CSR will be proficient with every transaction medium. While a CSR may be very skilled in the soft-skill techniques required to be successful on the phone, he or she may not have the requisite skills to respond to e-mail. Thus, the human capital aspect of staffing the center needs to be taken into account to ensure that members are reaching qualified CSRs irrespective of the medium they choose
- Branding of the various interaction media should be consistent. Members must feel as if they have reached the same member services department, with the same marketing and service "messaging," no matter which medium they have chosen. As a simple example, if the IVR refers to XYZ Health Care as "The Consumer's Choice in Health Plans," that same messaging should be found on the website, e-mail footer, and even in the call scripting. The plan should make every effort to appropriately promote their branding and market positioning during the member interaction.
- Issue escalation policies and procedures should be in place for every interaction type because a CSR may not be capable of handling every inbound contact to completion. The member may have a complex question that the CSR cannot answer, or may be irate from the outset of the contact. In such instances, more senior personnel must be at the ready to handle escalated issues across all interaction media.
- Plans must be able to manage the workflow of each contact type. Workflow describes the process by which contacts are forwarded throughout the organization to resolve the issue. For instance, a CSR might be required to forward a note to the claims department to review a claim (see Chapter 18). Workflow must be in place to ensure that the contact is received in claims and that the issue is resolved in a timely manner. Automated workflow technologies are typically used to support the workflow process.
- All contacts must be tracked and documented through completion, typically using a contact management system found on the CSR's desktop. Many robust technologies exist for such tracking.[*] Data and information derived from such transactions is also very valuable to drive critical insights about their members, groups, and internal business processes. This insight can be used to drive improved member administrative and clinical outcomes, improved group sales processes, and to conduct root-cause analysis to resolve upstream process issues that cause inbound contacts. By its very nature, the customer interaction center is rich with data to enable higher performance on the part of the health plan.

■ CONTACT TYPES: WHY MEMBERS CONTACT THEIR PLAN

Having looked at how members may access member services and the methods and technologies payers typically use for member interactions, the next broad topic is the reasons member contact takes place. Member services is responsible for helping members use the plan, and for disseminating information broadly to the membership. For example, new members commonly have less than complete (or even no) understanding of how the plan operates, how to access care, how to obtain authorization for specialty services (in a PCP case manager type HMO), and so forth. These are services to members as opposed to complaint and concern resolution, which is discussed later. While the broad *types* of services are generally the same across product lines, plans often find differing levels of need for each of these types of services in the commercial, Medicare, and Medicaid markets; there will also be some differences in *specific* issues depending on whether the plan or product is an HMO, a preferred provider organization (PPO), and point-of-service (POS) plan, or a CDHP (see Chapter 2 for a discussion of different plan types).

Types of Member-Specific Services

There are a variety of reasons a member contacts their health plan. It may be around any of the topics described in the new summary of coverage (SOC) document that insurers are required by the ACA to use beginning in 2012. More specifically, the following four leading types of issues that are typically addressed by payers are:

- Claims processing and payment issues;
- Enrollment issues, including ID card issues;
- Provider access issues, primarily in HMOs; and
- Benefits issues, including appeals and denials of coverage.

The first three of these are discussed in this section following a description of the SOC. Appeals of denial of coverage are discussed in a separate section later in the chapter.

The Summary of Coverage

The SOC is a document that must provide an accurate summary of benefits and coverage explanation. An SOC

---

[*]Oracle/PeopleSoft®, Pega Systems®, and SAP® are examples of vendors in this space at the time of publication.

must be provided prior to enrollment, as well as each time a policy is renewed or any substantial changes are made, and make it available both electronically and in hard copy. It does not replace the full evidence of coverage (EOC) that is described in the section on appeals, but it will likely be incorporated into the appeals process in some cases. CSRs will need to be thoroughly familiar with the language and content of any SOCs the plan issues, since it is what most members will base their understanding on.

At the time of publication, HHS had not issued final or even preliminary rules, so only a general description can be provided here, based on revised recommendations of the National Association of Insurance Commissioners (NAIC). According to those recommendations, the SOC must conform to the requirements listed in **Table 20-1**.

Because the recommendations use a highly precise language, much of it may be automated for production purposes.

TABLE 20-1	**NAIC Recommended Form and Informational Requirements for the Summary of Coverage Document**

- Form language and formatting must be precisely reproduced based on a provided model, must use 12-point (as required by federal law) Times New Roman font, and replicate all symbols, formatting, bolding, colors, and shading exactly;
- Information provided on the form must follow the exact order as the model;
- The form must be between four and six pages long, no more;
- It must use easily understood language provided in the instructions for creating the form;
- The form must provide all relevant company contact information;
- All cost-sharing, out-of-pocket costs and limits;
- Differences in cost-sharing between in-network and out-of-network services;
- Precertification for facility-care requirements;
- PCP referral authorization for specialty care requirements (HMO);
- Definitions of common coverage and cost-sharing terms;
- Examples of in-network and out-of-network coverage for common medical events;
- What is not covered;
- Any additional covered benefits;
- Continuance of coverage rights;
- Appeal rights;
- Examples using common conditions; and
- Questions and answers about the coverage examples.

Source: Adapted from "What Your Plan Covers and What it Costs, Draft Instruction Guide for Group Policies," created by the NAIC. Available at: http://naic.org/documents/committees_b_consumer_information_ACA_instructions_group_insurers.pdf. Accessed July 30, 2011.

Claims Processing and Payment Issues

Issues involving the processing and payment of claims are usually the leading reason members contact the plan. There are several aspects to claims that may prompt the call, such as denial of payment, incorrect payment, delay of payment, or other errors such as payment to the wrong provider or overpayment. Problems with claims payments will also be a major source of contacts into the provider relations or network management area, and the cost of reworking a claim is grossly higher than the cost of processing the claim correctly in the first place (see Chapters 7 and 18 for discussions of authorization systems and claims payment systems, respectively). It is no exaggeration to say the incorrectly processed claims account for a disproportionately high amount of administrative cost and dissatisfaction by members and providers.

There are myriad causes for claims to be processed incorrectly. Some of these causes are internal, some external. Examples of internal causes include:

- Key entry transpositions (for manually entered claims),
- Not correcting missing or incorrect data for claims scanned in through optical character recognition programs,
- Incorrect identification of provider,
- Incorrect medical policy application,
- Incorrect entry of member enrollment and eligibility information;
- Double payments, and so forth.

Examples of external causes include:

- Incorrect coding by the provider,
- Illegible paper claims,
- Incorrect identification of the member/patient,
- Employer or employee tardiness in sending eligibility information,
- Failure to actually file the claim,
- Duplicate claims filings that categorize the duplicate as a new claim (i.e., even paying the first claim leaves the duplicate claim marked as unpaid), and so forth.

Examples of causes that include both internal and external include:

- Claims being submitted electronically but authorizations being submitted on paper (allowing the claim to be processed immediately as though it were non-authorized),
- Lack of communication about changes in policy,
- Disputes about the application of medical necessity,
- Inconsistent interpretations of medical policy and benefits policy, and
- Issues surrounding coordination of benefits and other party liability.

As discussed in Chapter 18, payers continue to focus on those processes that will reduce error rates, including increasing the use of electronic claims, in order to address as many causes for errors as possible. Beyond any required reengineering to eliminate regular causes of claims errors, the member services department is that part of the payer that must resolve the problem on the member's behalf, while provider or network management may do so on behalf of the provider. Which department is primarily responsible for resolution will depend on who initiated the inquiry and where the cause of the problem lies.

In order for member services to resolve claims problems efficiently, several factors are important to consider. First is the ability of the CSR to access information easily and rapidly. Payers now typically provide CSRs with quick access to claims status screens, demographic information, provider information, medical policy information, and utilization management information (Chapter 7). In some older legacy systems, this is done through multiple screens that are reached through menu selection by pressing certain keys. The fewer screens and menus the representative must go through to find necessary information, the better. Those payers that are still struggling with multiple systems supporting multiple products will have the most difficult time with this, and in that case, short of replacing the old systems with a single new one, the payer may need to consider "frontware" that will perform the interface with the old systems, allowing the member services representative to access information more easily. Newer systems generally use a graphical user interface (GUI) that allows the representative to use combinations of the keyboard and mouse to rapidly access information.

It is not enough to access information, though. The CSR must also be able to do something about it. This means that the management of the payer must set policies about levels of intervention that various types of CSRs may have. For example, all CSRs may be allowed to process enrollment and ID care changes, and to correct information that was entered or submitted incorrectly in the first place, allowing the regular processing to then occur. To make a substantial change in a claim payment may require a higher level of CSR—one with more experience and training. For example, the ability of a CSR to override a claim denial based on information the member provides during the course of a telephone call must be available within the member services department, but not necessarily to all CSRs, and clearly not to an unlimited degree. For example, any claims override greater than $500 not caused by a purely clerical error may need to be approved by the medical management department. In all cases, such overrides must be tracked and patterns analyzed in order to reduce their occurrence.

In the case of self-insured benefits plans, it is not unusual for the client (i.e., the company that is self-funded and has contracted with the payer for benefits administration) to set a general tone of the latitude provided to the member services department. For example, a company may want the CSR to be able to override any claim dispute under $1,000. If this is the case, then as noted earlier, it is reasonable for those CSRs responsible for that company to be organized into a separate unit.

If the issue is a denial of payment or a denial of benefits coverage through the precertification process, CSRs must be able to provide the member with the reason for the denial and information about the appeals process, described in detail later in the chapter. Payers typically require CSRs to use precise language to avoid confusion. Members contacting the plan about a benefits denial who become emotional or upset are often transferred to a more senior CSR with the experience to maintain a cool head. If the member threatens legal action, CSRs are trained to keep careful records and if it appears that the member will indeed initiate legal action, the CSR usually notifies the supervisor who, in turn, notifies the plan's legal department. If the contact comes from an attorney, they are typically referred directly to the legal department.

Enrollment Issues and Identification Cards

This is generally a straightforward type of service in which the member needs to correct an enrollment error or make a change to his or her coverage status. The basic processes of enrollment and issuing identification cards are addressed in Chapter 17. For purposes of this chapter, it is inevitable that some members will have problems with their cards, and then member services will need to resolve those problems.

Common reasons for calls or messages include lost cards, cards that were sent to the wrong address, incorrect information on the card, the member's (or a dependent's) name being misspelled, or change of address. Changes in enrollment status may be required because of change of status; for example, adding a new dependent such as a newborn or a newly adopted child or a change in marital status. In all of these cases, the enrollment information must be updated and a new ID card(s) issued. In many cases, a payer cannot update membership information directly, but can only do so when the changes are provided from the employer; the member still contacts the payer first, but must then be redirected back to the employer's human resources function. ID card services are increasingly an automated self-service function, as described earlier in this chapter.

Primary Care Physician Selection and Network Access

In HMOs that use PCPs to access care (see Chapters 2 and 4), member services will frequently be called on to help members select a PCP. This may occur because the member failed to select a PCP in the first place, particularly in a POS plan in which the member has no intention of using the HMO part of the plan. Even in POS, it is best to require the member to select a PCP because it is not known whether the member will change his or her mind later and because the plan really does want to encourage the member to use the managed care system.

Another reason that an HMO member would need to select a new PCP is if a participating PCP leaves the network for any reason, if the PCP's practice closes because it is full but doesn't inform the plan, that information did not get into the most recent provider directory, or the member did not realize that a tiny, superscript asterisk meant that the practice was closed. Keeping the provider directory up to date is a difficult proposition, as discussed in Chapter 4. The Internet, via the Web, provides the most practical solution to this, but not all members (and potential enrollees) have Internet access or prefer to use it.

■ MEMBER COMPLAINTS AND GRIEVANCES

"Complaints" and "grievances" are the terms used when members contact the plan to express dissatisfaction for reasons other than an appeal of a denial of coverage. Because of the legal and regulatory aspects of formal appeals of a denial of coverage, that process is described in its own section. Complaints differ from grievances in that grievances are formal complaints about services provided by the plan, demanding resolution or a response. The difference between grievances and appeals is also defined for consumers in the SOC, described earlier.

Complaints

Complaints differ from routine problems that members encounter (even though those problems certainly may cause dissatisfaction) in that the routine problems are resolved by the member services department as a function of day-to-day operations. But a routine problem can evolve into a complaint if the member continues to follow up with the plan with the intent of pursuing either a different outcome, or some other action on the part of the plan. Complaints that are not resolved to the satisfaction of the member may evolve into formal grievances.

If the reason for the member expressing dissatisfaction is around benefits coverage it may still be categorized as a complaint if it does not lead to a formal appeal. For example, the benefits plan requires a higher copayment for one prescribed drug versus another, in which case there is no ground for an appeal since the benefits are what they are, even if one does not like them. Complaints about benefits that are not subject to appeal are usually not resolved to the member's satisfaction, but sometimes CSRs can assist by connecting the member with one of the plan's medical managers to address any underlying concerns.

Resolution of complaints is usually informal, although the plan should have a clear policy for investigating complaints and responding to members. Despite the informal nature of complaint resolution, it is very important for the CSR, or in fact any staff member, to document carefully every contact with a member when the member expresses any dissatisfaction. For complaints, the CSR should keep a log of even casual telephone calls from members as well as notes of any conversations with members while he or she is trying to resolve complaints. Concise and thorough records may prove quite valuable if the complaint turns into a formal grievance. Such documentation also helps in data analysis, as discussed elsewhere in this chapter.

Complaints about services are either about medical services or administrative services. Medical service complaints could include a member's inability to get an appointment, rude treatment, lack of physicians located near where the member lives, difficulty getting a needed referral in an HMO (difficult at least in the opinion of the member), and, most serious, problems with quality of care. Administrative complaints could include continually getting incorrect identification cards, not getting a card at all, poor responsiveness to previous inquiries, not answering the telephone, lack of documentation or education materials, and so forth.

Member services personnel need to investigate an administrative service complaint and to get a response to the member. Even if most of these are routine problems that are easily resolved, as discussed earlier in the chapter, in all cases of service complaints, the key to success is communication. If CSRs communicate clearly and promptly to all parties, many problems can be cleared up. Such communication must not be confrontational or accusatory.

Medical service complaints not related to quality of care are typically referred to the plan's network management department (Chapter 4), which is then responsible for determining the validity and extent of the complaint. Formal action may follow if there is evidence of a pattern or an ongoing problem. For example, complaints about medical office cleanliness or staff rudeness may result in a provider being placed under a performance improvement plan and reassessment after 3 months.

When the complaint alleges quality of care problems, the medical director needs to be notified. If investigation reveals a genuine quality of care problem, the matter requires referral to the quality management committee or peer review committee (see Chapter 14). Some states require certain types of quality complaints to be reported to a state agency, and MA requires member complaints about quality to be reviewed by a designated quality improvement organization (QIO; formerly called a peer review organization).

Finally, Medicare Advantage plans must comply with complaint tracking and reporting requirements of the Centers for Medicare and Medicaid Services (CMS), addressed in Chapter 24.

Grievances

A grievance is a formal complaint, demanding resolution or a formal response. It may come directly to the payer, but more often it comes through a regulatory agency such as a state insurance department or from the Centers for Medicare and Medicaid Services (CMS). If the member is in a self-funded benefits plan, the grievance will usually come from the employer. Examples of grievances include a formal letter to the insurance commissioner charging an insurer with deceptive sales and marketing practices, or a Medicare beneficiary writing to CMS to complain about poor service. In each case, the agency requires a response from the plan, and if it determines it necessary, may investigate further. A pattern of grievances or particularly egregious acts may lead to fines, restrictions on operations or sales, revocation of licensure, or disbarment from the program.

■ APPEALS OF DENIAL OF BENEFITS COVERAGE OR COVERAGE RESCISSION

In Chapter 7, the point was made that except for closed-panel HMOs, managed health care plans approve or deny coverage, they do not provide medical care themselves. There can be many reasons a claim does not get paid, as noted earlier and discussed in Chapter 18. But denial of coverage of a claim or a precertification request may be appealed.

On a related topic, a payer may on occasion withdraw coverage entirely from an individual or group, which is called a rescission. Prior to passage of the ACA, recessions would occur most commonly due to a payer claiming an individual or group misrepresented itself during the application process, by not disclosing a preexisting condition, for example. The ACA placed very tight limits on recession, however, limiting it to outright fraud or deliberately false statements. The ACA also created requirements on health plans to allow appeals of rescissions in much the same manner as appeals for benefits coverage denials.

Evidence of Coverage Documentation

In addition to the SOC described earlier, plans are required to provide members with access* to a much larger document called the evidence of coverage (EOC), which contains detailed information about the benefits plan, policies, procedures, rights, and more. It essentially serves as a contract. EOCs differ from payer to payer and from benefits plan to benefits plan. Fully insured plans typically use EOCs with similar language, approved by the state, for all the administrative and compliance information, and only vary coverage around differences in cost-sharing and the like. Self-funded plans typically use their own EOC language that complies

with Department of Labor (DOL) requirements and do not vary it when more than one payer is administering the plan (e.g., when employees of a national employer may choose between Blue Cross and Blue Shield, a nation payer such as Aetna, or an HMO). EOCs must also be written in a clear and understandable manner, not legalese.

Examples of information provided in detail in the EOC relevant to appeals and grievance rights are seen in **Table 20-2**.

TABLE 20-2	**Examples of the Types of Information Relevant to Benefits and Appeals that is Detailed in a Typical EOC**

- Definitions of what specific types of medical service are covered as benefits, such as
  - Physician services,
  - Hospital services,
  - Ambulatory facility services,
  - Various ancillary services, and so forth;
- Cost-sharing provisions such as
  - Copayments, coinsurance, and deductibles
    - For in-network and (if subject to it) authorized or precertified services
    - For out-of-network and/or (if subject to it) nonauthorized services
  - The maximum amount of annual per person and per family out-of-pocket spending;
- Compliance requirements such as precertification or use of network providers;
- Benefits limitations, such as
  - Actual limits (e.g., only one orthotic will be covered per year),
  - Relative limits (e.g., coverage of rehabilitation stops when the patient no longer shows improvement),
  - Based on medical necessity (see below);
- Definitions of what is excluded from coverage, such as
  - No coverage of custodial care or care that is essentially assistance with acts of daily living,
  - No coverage for experimental or investigational care, except in defined circumstances, or
  - No coverage for care not considered medically appropriate by generally accepted standards of medical practice;
- Rights to appeal a denial of benefits coverage, including the
  - Internal appeal process,
  - External review process to appeal an upheld internal denial,
  - Contact information and instructions on how to file an appeal, and
  - Compliance requirements for appeals such as how long a member has to file it;
- Any other information, definitions, limitations, or requirements applicable to benefits determinations.

---

*Because most people have Internet access and the EOC is a large document, it is usually available as a PDF file on the payer's website. Since in a self-funded benefits plan the employer is actually the health plan, the EOC may be either on the payer's site, the employer's internal employee benefits portal, or both. Members have a right to have the EOC sent to them, however.

Medical necessity is typically defined in an EOC using terms that go beyond activities that may be justified as reasonable, necessary, and/or appropriate, based on evidence-based clinical standards of care. The definition usually also includes language about services not being primarily for the convenience of the patient or physician, and not more costly than an alternative service or sequence of services at least as likely to produce equivalent results. The use of published evidence-based clinical criteria and guidelines in utilization management is described in Chapter 7.

Informal Review

While a member has the right to initiate a formal appeal process as the first step, there is often an informal review first, initiated when a member or provider requests it. It would not be considered a formal appeal. The typical processes followed for this informal re-review include:

- Appropriate documentation is reviewed by the case manager, usually a nurse.
- The information in this documentation is discussed with the medical director, who may or may not ask for additional information, depending on whether or not they require clarification or additional input.
- If coverage is approved, payment is authorized and the member so informed. The case manager may also inform the provider and member.
- If the denial of coverage is upheld, this decision is communicated to the member. Even though it is an informal process, this is often done using a form letter. The case manager may also inform the provider and member.
- The form letter contains information about formal appeal rights and how the member may exercise those rights.

The Formal Appeal Process

The Employee Retirement Income Security Act (ERISA) and laws in most states create specific consumer rights to appeal a denial of benefits coverage. The ACA further codified those rights directly and by amending ERISA, the Public Health Act, numerous provisions in the federal tax code, and several other laws. State laws and regulation is discussed in Chapter 28, federal regulation in Chapter 29, and the ACA in Chapter 30. Except for timing, appeal rights and the appeals processes are the same for precertification, concurrent review of ongoing care, denial of an incurred claim, and now, rescission. Appeals for Medicare Advantage and managed Medicaid plans are similar but not identical, and are described in Chapters 24 and 25, respectively.

Internal Review of an Appeal

The first type of formal appeal is through an internal process. States typically have specific regulatory requirements, but they generally also conform to ERISA requirements. The ERISA internal appeal requirements are listed in **Table 20-3**.

The typical operational process for an internal appeal is illustrated in **Table 20-4**.

TABLE 20-3 | **ERISA Benefits Denial Appeals Requirements Initial Filing of an Appeal**

- An individual must have at least 180 days to file an appeal.
- The plan must provide claimants, on request and free of charge, copies of documents, records, and other information relevant to the claim for benefits.
- The plan also must identify, on request, any medical or vocational expert whose advice was obtained by the plan.

Reviewer Requirements

- The appeal must be reviewed by someone new who looks at all of the information submitted and consults with qualified medical professionals if a medical judgment is involved.
- This reviewer cannot be a subordinate of the person who made the initial decision.
- The reviewer must give no consideration to the initial decision.

Timeliness Requirements

- Urgent appeals must be reviewed as soon as possible, taking into account the medical needs of the patient, but not later than 72 hours after the plan receives a request to review a coverage denial.
- Preauthorization appeals must be reviewed within a reasonable period of time appropriate to the medical circumstances, but not later than 30 days after the plan receives a request to review a coverage denial.
- Postservice appeals must be reviewed within a reasonable period of time, but not later than 60 days after the plan receives a request to review a coverage denial.
- If a group health plan needs more time, the plan must get the individual's consent. If the individual does not agree to more time, the plan must complete the review within the permitted time limit.
- An individual may obtain an independent external review of a denied appeal, and must be allowed to file for it no less than 4 months following notification of the upheld denial. External appeals review requirements are described separately.

Source: Adapted from U.S. Department of Labor Employee Benefits Security Administration. Available at: www.dol.gov/ebsa/publications/filingbenefitsclaim.html. Accessed July 27, 2011.

TABLE 20-4	Typical Health Plan Operational Processes for a Formal Internal Appeal

- Appropriate information from nursing notes, physician notes and records, and any other supporting documentation that is pertinent to the issue at hand is presented to the medical director or a physician reviewer.

- The medical director would not have been involved, or only peripherally involved, with the case under consideration for appeal.

- The medical director and case manager then discuss the case in a process similar to that described above.

- The medical director may discuss the case with the attending physician or the member when clarification is required. Such direct communication is not always necessary.

- Direct examination of the member is considered inappropriate. The medical director's interactions with an individual receiving care (or with the subscriber) are as a member of the group benefits plan, not as a patient.

- The medical director may review specific aspects of the appeal with other internal resources as appropriate. For example, the medical director may discuss the case with his or her supervisor.

- The case may be reviewed by other medical directors in the organization that were not involved with the initial determination, although that is not required.

- The case may be reviewed by a formal committee charged with the responsibility of reviewing formal appeals. This committee, when used, is usually made up of internal personnel who focus not only on clinical aspects, but on coverage issues.

- Internal legal counsel may be consulted in situations where clarification around contract language is needed, or to determine whether or not state or federal laws and regulations apply.

- A medical director makes the final decision at this level of appeal.

- If the denial is overturned, then the administrator is instructed to authorize payment and process the claims, and the member is so informed. A form letter is commonly used for this. The case manager may also informally communicate the result to the provider and member.

- If the denial is upheld, that determination is communicated to the member using a form letter. The case manager may also informally communicate the result to the provider and member.

- The denial of benefits form letter contains information about external appeal rights and how the member may exercise those rights.

External Review of an Appeal

Most states have laws and regulations that provide consumers with the right to have an external review of an upheld denial, as does ERISA. The ACA broadened that to apply to all individuals with health benefits. It does so through one of two approaches. The first is a requirement that health insurers and HMOs comply with state external review requirements, but only if the state process includes the 16 minimum consumer protection standards based on the NAIC Uniform Health Carrier External Review Model Act* (NAIC Uniform Model Act) that are listed in **Table 20-5**.

All self-insured nonfederal governmental health plans, as well as health insurance issuers in the group and individual market in states whose external review processes are found not to meet the 16 requirements listed above, must either comply with those requirements or participate in a federal external review process administered through the HHS Office of Personnel Management. Self-insured plans not participating in the federally administered program will be required to contract with at least two IROs by January 1, 2012, and with at least three IROs by July 1, 2012, and to rotate assignments among them. The federally administered external review process is shown in **Table 20-6**.

As noted in Chapter 30, an important difference between the state and federal process is the scope of adverse benefit determinations that may be submitted for external review. The state process applies to any adverse benefit determination "based on the issuer's [or plan's] requirements for medical necessity, appropriateness, health care setting, level of care, or effectiveness of a covered benefit."[1] The federal external review process applies to all benefit denials including both medically necessary decisions and a denial based on a decision that a service is not covered by the insurer or plan.[2] As a result, the federal external review process applies to a significantly larger number of issues.

Appeal Outcomes

About half of all internal and external appeal reviews result in a reversal of the coverage denial. In a March 2011 federal report to the Secretary of HHS and the Secretary of Labor, the General Accounting Office, using data from four states, reported rates of claims or precertification denials and the percentage of appeals that were overturned through the internal and external review processes. Because of differences in how the states track and report denials and appeals, the

---

* The 42-page NAIC Model Act is available through the U.S. Department of Labor Employee Benefits Security Administration web portal at www.dol.gov/ebsa/, or directly at www.dol.gov/ebsa/pdf/externalreviewmodelact.pdf (current as of July 27, 2011).

TABLE 20-5	Minimum State Regulatory Requirements for External Review of Appeals under the ACA

1. The process must provide for external review of adverse benefit determinations (and final internal adverse benefit determinations) based on medical necessity, appropriateness, health care setting, level of care, or effectiveness of a covered benefit. [Applies as well to an appeal of a rescission of coverage.[†]]

2. Issuers (or plans) must be required to provide effective written notice to claimants of their rights to external review.

3. If exhaustion of internal appeals is required prior to external review, exhaustion must be unnecessary if
   a. The issuer (or plan) waives the exhaustion requirement;
   b. The issuer (or plan) is considered to have exhausted the internal appeals process by failing to comply with the requirements of the internal appeals process except those failures that are based on de minimis violations that do not cause, and are not likely to cause, prejudice or harm to the claimant; or
   c. The claimant simultaneously requests an expedited internal appeal and an expedited external review.

4. The cost of an independent review organization (IRO) to conduct an external review must be borne by the issuer (or plan), although the process may require a nominal filing fee [not to exceed $25.00] from the claimant requesting external review.

5. There cannot be any restriction on the minimum dollar amount of a claim in order to be eligible for external review.

6. The process must allow at least 4 months to file a request for external review after the receipt of the notice of adverse benefit determination or final internal adverse benefit determination.

7. The IRO must be assigned by the state or an independent entity, on a random basis or another method of assignment that ensures the independence and impartiality of the assignment process (such as rotational assignment), and in no event assigned by the issuer, the plan, or the individual.

8. The process must provide for the maintenance of a list of approved IROs (only those that are accredited by a nationally recognized private accrediting organization) qualified to conduct the external review based on the nature of the health care service that is the subject of the review.

9. Approved IROs must have no conflicts of interest that will influence their independence.

10. Claimants must be allowed to submit to the IRO additional information in writing that the IRO must consider when conducting the external review, and the claimant must be notified of the right to submit additional information to the IRO; the IRO must allow the claimant at least 5 business days to submit any additional information and any additional information submitted by the claimant must be forwarded to the issuer (or plan) within one business day of receipt by the IRO.

11. The IRO decision must be binding on the claimant, as well as the plan or issuer (except to the extent that other remedies are available under state or federal law).

12. For standard external review, the IRO must provide written notice to the issuer (or plan) and the claimant of its decision to uphold or reverse the adverse benefit determination within no more than 45 days after the receipt of the request for external review.

13. The process must provide for an expedited external review in certain circumstances and, in such cases, provide notice of the decision as expeditiously as possible, but not later than 72 hours after receipt of the request for external review (and if notice of the IRO's decision is not in writing, the IRO must provide written confirmation of its decision within 48 hours after the date of the notice of the decision).

14. Issuers (or plans) must provide a description of the external review process in or attached to the summary plan descriptions, policy, certificate, membership booklet, outline of coverage, or other evidence of coverage provided to participants, beneficiaries, or enrollees, substantially similar to section 17 of the NAIC Uniform Model Act.

15. The IRO must maintain written records and make them available upon request to the state, substantially similar to section 15 of the NAIC Uniform Model Act.

16. The process must follow procedures for external reviews involving experimental or investigational treatment, substantially similar to section 10 of the NAIC Uniform Model Act.

[†]Different section of the same Guidance document noted as the Source.
Source: U.S. Department of Labor, Employee Benefits Security Administration, Technical Release 2010-01, Interim Guidance for Federal Review Relating to Internal Claims and Appeals and External Review under the Patient Protection and Affordable Care Act. Available at: www.dol.gov/ebsa/pdf/ACATechnicalRelease2010-01.pdf. Accessed July 27, 2011.

TABLE 20-6	**Federally Administered Process for External Review of Appeals**

Procedure for Preliminary Review

a. When the examiner receives an external review request, the examiner will contact the health insurance issuer.

b. Within 5 business days of receipt of request by the examiner, the health insurance issuer must provide to the examiner all of the documents and any information considered in making the adverse benefit determination or final internal adverse benefit determination, including:

   i. Claimant's certificate of coverage or benefit;

   ii. A copy of the adverse benefit determination;

   iii. A copy of the final internal adverse benefit determination;

   iv. A summary of the claim;

   v. An explanation of the health insurance issuer's adverse benefit determination and final internal adverse benefit determination; and

   vi. All documents and information considered in making the adverse benefit determination or final internal adverse benefit determination including any additional information that may have been provided to the health insurance issuer or relied upon by the health insurance issuer during the internal appeals process.

c. The examiner will review the information from the health insurance issuer and may request additional information that it deems necessary to the external review. If the examiner requests additional information, the health insurance issuer shall supply the information as expeditiously as possible and within five business days.

d. If the examiner determines that the claimant is not eligible for external appeal, the examiner will notify the claimant and the health insurance issuer in writing.

Procedure for External Review

a. The examiner will review all of the information and documents timely received. In reaching a decision, the examiner will review the claim de novo and not be bound by any decisions or conclusions reached during the health insurance issuer's internal claims and appeals process applicable under paragraph (b) of the interim final regulations under section 2719 of the PHS Act.

b. The examiner will forward all documents submitted directly to the examiner by the claimant. Upon receipt of any information submitted by the claimant, the examiner must within one business day forward the information to the health insurance issuer. Upon receipt of any such information, the health insurance issuer may reconsider its adverse benefit determination or final internal adverse benefit determination that is the subject of the external review. Reconsideration by the health insurance issuer must not delay the external review. The external review may be terminated as a result of the reconsideration only if the health insurance issuer decides, upon completion of its reconsideration, to reverse its adverse benefit determination or final internal adverse benefit determination and provide coverage or payment. Within one business day after making a decision to reverse, the health insurance issuer must provide written notice of its decision to the claimant and the examiner. The examiner must terminate the external review upon receipt of the notice from the health insurance issuer.

c. The examiner must provide written notice of the final external review decision as expeditiously as possible and within 45 days after the examiner receives the request for the external review. The examiner must deliver the notice of the final external review decision to the claimant and the health insurance issuer.

d. The examiner's final external review decision notice will contain:

   i. A general description of the reason for the request for external review, including information sufficient to identify the claim (including the date or dates of service, the health care provider, the claim amount [if applicable], the diagnosis code and its corresponding meaning, the treatment code and its corresponding meaning, and the reason for the previous denial, including denial codes);

   ii. The date the examiner received the assignment to conduct the external review and the date of the examiner's decision;

   iii. References to the evidence or documentation, including the specific coverage provisions and evidence-based standards, considered in reaching its decision;

   iv. A discussion of the principal reason or reasons for its decision, including the rationale for its decision and any evidence-based standards that were relied on in making its decision;

   v. A statement that the determination is binding except to the extent that other remedies may be available under state or federal law to either the health insurance issuer or to the claimant;

   vi. A statement that judicial review may be available to the claimant; and

   vii. Current contact information, including phone number, for any applicable office of health insurance consumer assistance or ombudsman established under PHS Act section 2793.

e. After a final external review decision, the examiner must maintain records of all claims and notices associated with the external review process for 6 years. The examiner must make such records available for examination by the claimant or health insurance issuer upon request.

Reversal of Health Insurance Issuer's Decision

Upon receipt of a notice of a final external review decision reversing the adverse benefit determination or final internal adverse benefit determination, the health insurance issuer immediately must provide coverage or payment (including immediately authorizing or immediately paying benefits) for the claim.

Source: Adapted from the U.S. Department of Health and Human Services, Centers for Medicare and Medicaid, Administration Interim Appeals Guidance, as amended by the Technical Release 2011-02, June 22, 2011. Available at: www.hhs.gov/ociio/regulations/interim_appeals_guidance_.pdf. Accessed July 27, 2011.

TABLE 20-7	Rates of Initial Denial of Claim or Precertification, and Percentage Reversed		
State	**Percentage of claims or precertifications denied**	**Percentage of denials reversed on internal review**	**Percentage of second denials reversed on external review**
California	24%		54%
Connecticut	14%	53%	40%
Maryland	16%	50%	54%
New York*		39%–48%	38%–42%
Ohio	11%	48%	23%
Florida			49%

* New York separated HMOs from commercial and nonprofit insurers. The lower percentages of denial reversals are in HMOs.
Source: Created by author from data in *Private Health Insurance: Data on Application and Coverage Denials*, GAO-11-268 March 16, 2011, www.gao .gov/products/GAO-11-268. Accessed July 28, 2011.

report did not provide data in all three categories except in two states, as shown in **Table 20-7**.

Further Recourse

If after exhausting the grievance and appeals process, a member wants to pursue further recourse, there are a variety of means, not all of which may be available. These are briefly described next.

Appeal to Government Agencies

In commercial insurers or HMOs, there is typically no further governmental agency recourse following the decision after external review. In self-funded employer groups, the U.S. Department of Labor does not routinely become involved with individual appeals, although may get involved after the fact if legal action finds that ERISA requirements were not met. Federal employees, or those who are covered under the Office of Personnel Management (OPM), have the right of appeal to OPM. OPM specifically reserves the right in its contract with health plans to resolve and rule on appeals and grievances by members who are federal employees. In MA and Medicaid plans, if the member is not satisfied with the results of the formal hearing, he or she has the right to appeal to CMS or the state's Department of Welfare, respectively. In fact, many beneficiaries of both programs do not use the formal appeals process at all, but go directly to the agency.

Arbitration

In some states, arbitration is allowed for cases involving insured plans. In those states where arbitration is allowed, and if the plan wishes to pursue it (or if it is required), the plan would comply with the regulations regarding arbitration in terms of selection of the arbitrator(s) and form of the hearing. With the advent of uniform appeal rights under the ACA, arbitration is likely to become even less common than it is now, or simply disappear.

Lawsuits

Although not a part of a plan's grievance procedure, the last legal remedy for a disgruntled member is legal action. If the plan carefully follows its grievance procedure, the chances of a successful lawsuit against it are small, but not zero since juries can be swayed. If the plan fails to follow proper policy and procedure, the chances of losing a lawsuit are high. The right to sue is clear and relatively unfettered for all but self-insured plans, in which ERISA limits an award to the cost of the benefit, not any additional damages.

■ RESOLVING THE CONSUMER'S ISSUE

An area getting increasing focus in payer organizations is the actual ability for a plan's member services department to actually resolve the member's inquiry. It is no longer simply good enough to have a CSR take the inbound call about the above issues within an acceptable timeframe, and to respectfully listen to the caller's concern. More important than ever, a fully satisfactory resolution to the inbound contact is a requirement, often mandated and measured by key customers. These might include employer-mandated service levels, or CMS's implementation of "STAR" ratings that in part tie payments to MA plans to the success the plans have in correctly handling their member's calls (see Chapter 24).

Thus, a great deal of emphasis is now placed on ensuring that the right infrastructure is in place to efficiently and effectively resolve the member's concern. This includes training, desktop tools, knowledge bases and workflow management systems that enable a "soup-to-nuts" review of each issue, and insight into the resolution timeframe and efficacy. On top of that, increasingly advanced systems to report individual and aggregate performance metrics related to these required service levels.

■ "CONCIERGE" APPROACH TO MEMBER SERVICES

This increased emphasis is leading payers to rethink their approach to contact center operations. At one time, the focus was on processing the call as quickly as possible, getting to the root cause of the concern quickly, attempting to resolve the issue, and moving on to the next caller. In some ways, expectations around the time required to handle calls was unfairly biased by handle times from other industries with less complex customer service needs.

At present, we are seeing a popular movement toward a "concierge" model of consumer care, increasing the level of responsibility of the CSR to resolve issues on first contact, guide the workflow for more complex issues, and to anticipate future needs that the consumer might have. While a substantially more expensive model on a "per contact" basis, the business case is being made for obviating future contacts and driving higher levels of consumer satisfaction/retention via the concierge approach.

Simply stated, a consumer's perception of a payer is not formed by comparison to other payers, but in fact to all of the other B2C relationships that the consumer experiences throughout his or her life. With companies like Amazon, USAA, Nordstrom, and others setting the bar, expectations are high, and payers, like any other business, are being put under more pressure to deliver.

■ MEMBER SATISFACTION SURVEYS AND DATA

The customer interaction center is rich with customer experience information, and the member services department should be responsible for collecting, collating, and analyzing that data. Data may be considered in two broad categories: data regarding general levels of satisfaction and dissatisfaction, and data regarding medical and administrative problems. Satisfaction data may include surveys of current members, disenrollment surveys, telephone response time and waiting time studies (these may be done in conjunction with the quality management department, but they are essentially patient satisfaction studies), and surveys of clients and accounts (although marketing rather than member services may perform many of these studies).

Member surveys are particularly useful when done properly. Even when a payer is the sole carrier in an account, surveys help the plan evaluate service levels and ascertain what issues are important to members. Surveys may be focused on a few issues that the plan wants to study, or they may be broad and comprehensive; they may be produced by the payer, or (more commonly) obtained from an outside source or commercial vendor. The survey activity itself may be conducted by plan personnel, or may be contracted out to an objective third party that specializes in consumer surveys. Of course, any protected health information as defined under HIPAA (Chapter 29) is subject to HIPAA's privacy requirements.

In an environment where members have multiple choices for their health care coverage, member surveys will be geared toward issues that influence enrollment choices. It is easier and less expensive to retain a member than it is to acquire a new one. Of special importance are those members who do not heavily utilize medical services, because their premiums pay for the expenses of those members with high medical costs, and because such members with low medical costs tend to disenroll more often than members who utilize services heavily. It must be reinforced here, though, that under HIPAA it is not permissible to specifically identify those members by name for purposes of sales, nor may utilization or cost data be made available on a member-identifiable basis to the sales and marketing department.

The Consumer Assessment of Healthcare Providers and Systems (CAHPS®), available from the federal Agency for Healthcare Research and Quality (AHRQ[*]) is a standardized survey about a member's actual experiences. There are versions that focus on health plans, Medicare, hospitals, and ambulatory care. MA and managed Medicaid plans are required to administer and report results of CAHPs surveys, and the National Committee for Quality Assurance[†] (NCQA; see Chapter 15) requires use of the CAHPS survey, and it is part of their Health Plan Employer Data Information Set (HEDIS) required for continued accreditation. Some states require its use as well. In addition to the survey itself, there are standards regarding how often it must be conducted, over what number of members, and under what conditions.

Satisfaction data and information is also frequently made available to consumers from external sources. Medicare and many states provide consumers Web-based comparative data around member satisfaction, as do a number of commercial third parties. In addition, data on participating health plans is available for purchase from NCQA under the publication title *Quality Compass*. In addition, several companies, such as J.D. Powers or Harris Interactive, perform objective third-party reviews of the customer experience.

When state health insurance exchanges become operational in 2014, qualified health plans participating or offering through the exchange will be required to submit to certain data to the exchange, HHS, and the state's insurance department. The exchange may then make that data available to the public, using "plain language" understandable to people with limited proficiency in English. Although member services may not be responsible for measuring these data, it is related to member satisfaction and CAHPS data that will also become available through the exchange. The specific data are:

- Claims payment policies and practices;
- Periodic financial disclosures;
- Data on enrollment;
- Data on disenrollment;
- Data on the number of claims that are denied;
- Data on rating practices;
- Information on cost-sharing and payments with respect to any out-of-network coverage;
- Information on enrollee and participant rights under this title; and
- Other information as determined appropriate by the Secretary.

---

[*] www.cahps.ahrq.gov.
[†] www.ncqa.org.

■ PROACTIVE MEMBER SERVICES

As is certainly apparent by this point, most member services departments are seen as complaint departments. But it is emotionally draining to listen to complaints all day. Even the satisfaction of successfully resolving the majority of complaints can be inadequate if there is nothing else the plan is doing to address satisfaction. This leads to higher personnel turnover rates in this department than in most other areas. Fortunately, member services is not only reactive, it is proactive as well. Examples include assisting a member in navigating the complexity of the new health care environment or providing consumers the information and decision support tools to enhance their participation in health care decision making.

A number of forces have either required that a CSR take a more proactive approach to member services, or have actually enabled that advanced interaction:

- Consumer-directed health plans, with their corresponding savings/investment accounts and debit/credit card solutions (see Chapter 2);
- The advent of personal health records (PHRs), enabling a longitudinal view of the member's health (see Chapter 23);
- Deeper integration of disease management and other health and wellness functions into the health plan, either through internal care management or through relationships with external vendors (see Chapters 7 and 8);
- Publicly available provider and facility quality data, evidence-based medicine and outcomes data, and provider/facility unit cost data for procedures;
- Easy-to-use decision support tools, enabling the front line to assist members in their treatment choices; and
- Robust customer insight and analytics tools, enabling the identification and segmentation of member populations for targeted interventions.

The member services function is perhaps the most logical arena to execute on a plan's consumerism strategy, given the volume of interaction that takes place between the plan's membership and their CSRs. Given the tools available to them, CSRs will be able to guide a member's decision making throughout the member's health care life cycle. The most proactive activity is new member outreach, which is discussed next, followed by other examples of proactive member services.

Outreach

An outreach program can be of great benefit in preventing member complaints and problems, especially in HMOs and MA plans (see Chapter 24). An outreach program is one that proactively contacts new members and discusses the way the plan works. By reaching out and letting members know how the authorization system works, how to obtain services, what the benefits are, and so forth, the plan can reduce confusion.

Virtually all payers mail some form of an information pack to new members, although as a practical matter it may instead be sent from the employer. This pack typically includes not only the new identification card, but descriptive language about how to use the plan, accessing care, how the authorization or precertification system works, information about coordination of benefits (see Chapter 18), how to access urgent or emergency care, in some cases a provider director, and a description of how the pharmacy benefit works (see Chapter 11). Some plans may also include a copy of the benefits description and even possibly the evidence of coverage, described later. Closed panels, medical groups in open-panel plans, and integrated delivery systems (IDSs; see Chapter 2) may also include hours of operation and telephone numbers for their health centers. The various telephone numbers, mailing addresses, and website addresses are also provided. Increasingly, employers post the information pack virtually, meaning most of the information is electronically accessible and not sent as printed documents, although even then the ID card is sent by mail.

Many plans (particularly HMOs, Medicaid, and MA plans, as noted earlier) accomplish a more aggressive and effective outreach program by conducting a telephone-based outreach program. Telephonic outreach requires a carefully scripted approach during the contact. Development of scripts allows the plan to use lesser-trained personnel to carry out the program; when questions arise that are not easily answered from the script or when problems are identified, the member may be transferred to an experienced member services representative.

Outreach also gives members a chance to ask questions about the plan, especially when those questions do not come up until the member has heard about the plan from the outreach personnel. It is worthwhile to bear in mind that for many members who do not access medical services frequently, this contact may be the most important one; clearly it is in the plan's interest to retain such members. Outreach is most effective when carried out during both daytime and early evening hours to ensure that contact is made.

Member Education Programs

Member education may be clinically oriented or administratively oriented. For the latter topic, that occurs most commonly during new member orientation meetings or seminars where a group of new members are educated on how best to use the health plan, questions are answered, and so forth.

Health education is usually the responsibility of the medical management function of the plan, but it is common for member services to be involved, and in some cases, even be primarily responsible. The two broad categories of health education are general preventive educational services, and disease- or condition-specific education, as described in

Chapter 7. These programs are often accompanied by medical self-help literature, interactive videos, and other consumer-oriented information. The actual content of these programs may be provided by medical management or an outside vendor, but it is member services that organizes the programs and manages communications with the members.

Member Decision Support Tools

Payers are providing more information than ever to members to help them make informed decisions regarding their health care. While health plans have long made access to self-care information, as well as health risk appraisals, available (see Chapter 7), the provision of information and decision support tools has taken new directions. Data about actual costs is being made available, as well as automated tools accessed via the Web that help members with factoring in the financial impact of medical care. Alternatives to various types of clinical services are described, although final decision making ultimately falls to the member and her or his physician.

Member Suggestions and Recommendations

Soliciting member suggestions and recommendations can be valuable. This may be done along with member surveys, or the plan may solicit suggestions through response cards in physicians' offices, in the member newsletter, or via the Internet. There are times when the members will have ways of viewing the plan that provide valuable insight to managers. Although not all the suggestions may be practical, they may at least illuminate trouble spots that need attention of some sort.

Special Services, Affiliations, and Health Promotion Activities

Managed care plans frequently develop affiliations with health clubs and other types of health-related organizations. This usually takes the form of discounts on membership to health clubs, discounts on purchases of health-related products such as safety equipment or home medical equipment, and discounts on medical self-help products such as books or computer programs. This serves to underscore the emphasis on prevention and health maintenance, allows for differentiation with competitors, and provides value-added services to the member. Payers often affiliate with other organizations to sponsor or provide special services or health promotion; for example, working with a grocery store chain to provide consumers with easy-to-use means to make healthy food purchasing choices.

■ CONCLUSION

Member services are a requirement of any managed care plan. The primary responsibilities of member services include providing information to the membership in general, helping guide members through the system, and helping members resolve any problems or questions they may have. Member services also manages the formal appeals and grievances processes. Member services must also track and analyze member problems and complaints so that management can act to correct problems at the source. Management of the full range of contacts between members and the health plan requires sophisticated systems support and management processes. Finally, proactive member services provide significant value to health plans, so member services should not be confined to reacting to member contacts.

Endnotes

1   29 C.F.R. §2590.715-2719(c)(2), 45 C.F.R. §147.136 (c)(2).
2   29 C.F.R. §2590.715-2719(d)(1), 45 C.F.R. §147.136(d)(1).

Operational Finance and Budgeting

DALE F. COOK AND CHRISTOPHER R. CAMPBELL

CHAPTER 21

STUDY OBJECTIVES

- Understand the basic flow of funds in a typical managed care organization
- Understand the basic types of revenues and expenses
- Understand the impact of the Patient Protection and Affordable Care Act on financial statements
- Understand some of the key issues involved in statutory accounting
- Understand basic regulatory requirements as they pertain to financial activities
- Understand the budgeting processes

DISCUSSION TOPICS

1. Discuss what regulatory agencies/organizations govern financial reporting and solvency of different types of managed care organizations, and describe the different aspects of their governance.

2. Discuss how profit and loss and forecast information might be segregated and why. Why is it important to analyze the results using per member per month data?

3. Describe and discuss the key elements a health maintenance organization finance officer needs to properly set the claims accruals.

4. Discuss what is on a lag report and what completion factors are. What are the strengths and problems associated with completion factors?

5. Discuss how premiums are billed and received.

6. Discuss what a premium deficiency is, why its identification is important, and how this should be reflected in the accounting records.

7. Discuss the more significant issues related to risk pool liabilities.

8. Discuss the minimum capital requirements and risk-based capital requirements under the National Association of Insurance Commissioners Model Act.

9. Discuss the key differences between statutory accounting principles and generally accepted accounting principles. Why is this important to a managed care plan?

◼ INTRODUCTION

To manage successfully a managed care organization or payer organization, the value financial managers provide their organizations starts with their ability to interact with operational and medical managers, to manage changes in the regulatory environment, and gather timely information to facilitate communication of financial results to the organization and its constituencies to react appropriately to sustain or exceed financial goals. Present-day payers employ a comprehensive financial management process, combining short-term and long-term planning techniques in a manner that allows for measured progress against goals. The organization's actual results will be compared on a timely basis, typically monthly, quarterly, and annually comparing key performance metrics of reported actual results to their forecasted values. This variance analysis serves as the basis for informing leaders of the need for corrective action, or to highlight emerging opportunities.

Accuracy of the reported financial results is affected by significant accounting estimates that are based on historical trends and results and appropriately adjusted for recent changes affecting such estimates. The interaction between operational managers and financial managers is key to developing timely, accurate financial results and projections. Overall financial management of a payer organization begins with the payer's organizational design, and product pricing strategy employed for each line of business, and government regulation. Commercial, Medicare, or Medicaid populations are the most common organizational separation, depending on the size, scope, and complexity of the organization, then geography and/or groupings of customer segment, based on employer size, may also be pivotal.

State and federal regulation has significant influence of organizational and financial reporting design; for example, the Patient Protection and Affordable Care Act (ACA)[1] along with the assistance of the National Association of Insurance Commissioners (NAIC) provided specific guidelines for regulating organizations in segments defined as large group, small group, and individual as described in Chapter 16. Given various state and federal reform, the fundamentals of each business unit's strategy will result in different strategic pricing decisions for each unit. Product pricing will be based on an assessment of the competition, targeted profitability, the payer's estimate of volume and cost incurred for the provision of health care, and the costs to support the operation of each line of business, all elements requiring financial management skills and focused reporting.

Changes in the provider sector also affect payers, both directly and indirectly. Many varieties of integrated delivery systems (IDSs) have appeared and are described in Chapter 2. With some exceptions such as California, there may be little or no legislation governing these non-health-plan organizations. Prior to passage of the ACA, the Centers for Medicare and Medicaid Services (CMS) launched a pilot program for patient-centered medical homes (PCMHs), and contained within the ACA are passages directing CMS to promote yet another type of IDS, the accountable care organization (ACO), which will be paid through a "value-based payment" model that had not been finalized at the time of publication, but that would contain elements of risk.

Managing and controlling costs and reacting to the medical cost trends as well as the construct of administrative costs are vital to achieving desired results and preserving profitability. Detailed operating budgets, forecasts, and strategic plans are then developed under the same assumptions used in the pricing strategy. Financial managers rely significantly upon information captured and monitored by operational departments to develop detailed budgets. Said another way, financial management is heavily dependent on both a robust information technology (IT) system and on the timely and accurate entry of data by all operational areas.

The focus of this chapter is a review of the components of the financial statements of a payer, key information and the operational procedures that the financial manager will need and rely upon, addresses typical problems that occur in gathering information, and provides insight into the challenge of the integrity of information.

◼ REGULATORY BACKGROUND

State regulation of managed health care plans is discussed in more detail in Chapter 28, federal regulation is discussed in Chapter 29, and the ACA is the sole topic of Chapter 30. Nevertheless, it is worthwhile here to briefly summarize some examples of key regulatory elements that bear directly on the financial management and reporting for all payer organizations.

Accounting policy for payers is set by many regulatory entities. Payers are primarily regulated by the states through the Department of Insurance. Health maintenance organizations (HMOs) may also be regulated by the state's Department of Health Department of Managed Health Care. Historically, the state's Department of Insurance was generally concerned with the fiscal solvency of the payer to ensure that the health benefits of enrollees will be provided. The state's Department of Health (to the extent that it is involved at all) is generally concerned with quality of care issues as well as access to care issues, including the location of providers within specific geographic boundaries and the mix of primary care physicians and specialists to serve the population within these boundaries.

In the past, federal oversight generally focused on the regulation of Medicare risk contracts by the Centers for Medicare and Medicaid Services (CMS). The ACA, however, contains a great deal of language that will result in substantial new regulations for payers, either directly through federal regulation or indirectly through new state regulations. Examples include limits on the medical loss ratio (MLR) and oversight of premium rate changes; the MLR limitation is discussed later in the chapter. Publicly held payers are also subject to the rules and regulations of the Securities and Exchange Commission (SEC). This more recently includes the Public Company Accounting Oversight Board, which was created, as discussed later in this chapter, when the Sarbanes-Oxley Act of 2002 was introduced into law.

Financial management of payers must consider the interests of each of the users of financial information, whether they be senior management, the board of directors, regulators, the SEC, tax authorities, or investors. Balancing the concerns of each interested party represents a challenge for the financial manager. Senior management is concerned with the profitability and viability of products and market segment performance. Management will require internal reporting that focuses on line of business management and also meets regulatory reporting requirements. Regulators are concerned with protecting the insured members and focus on both the liquidity of the payer and the rate at which the payer desires to increase premium on the products it sells. The SEC is concerned with the protection of investor interests. Balancing conservatism and positive performance with the best return on investment is a difficult task.

The NAIC is an organization comprising the state commissioners of insurance who set guidelines at a national level. The NAIC has no governing authority over the individual states, however. Generally, states will introduce legislation modeling NAIC guidelines. The NAIC has adopted an annual statement report format that has been adopted by most states. The financial information is prepared in accordance with statutory accounting practices (SAP). Other financial statement users (lenders, the SEC, and investors) require that financial statements be prepared in accordance with generally accepted accounting principles (GAAP). The American Institute of Certified Public Accountants (AICPA) issued an audit and accounting guide for health care providers that provides additional guidance on audit, accounting, and reporting matters for prepaid health plans.

Other developments include the NAIC's development of risk-based capital requirements for health insurers, including HMOs, which imposes strict minimum capital requirements on their insured or at-risk business. Also in the past few years, expanded financial disclosure requirements regarding changes in claims reserves have been imposed on health insurers and HMOs.

A successful financial manager needs to be aware of the continuous changes taking place in the regulatory arena. More common than ever before are legislative acts that are passed with uncertainty surrounding the regulatory details for which the payer often depends on in order to understand the true implications and costs associated with the regulations. For many states, managed care market penetration has historically been minimal, and legislation has not kept pace with recent growth in managed care.

▓ COMPONENTS OF THE FINANCIAL OPERATING STATEMENT

The financial operating statement refers to financial reports that provide information on profit and loss, or in the case of nonprofit payers, surplus and loss.[*] Summary information is backed up by progressively more detailed operating statements, allowing plan managers to focus their efforts properly. A typical high-level profit and loss statement for an HMO is depicted in **Table 21-1**.

The Impact of the ACA on Financial Statements

One of the provisions of the ACA that went into effect early was limitations on the MLR.[2] It affects only insured business, not self-funded. Enforcement is left to the states, but the federal Department of Health and Human Services (HHS or DHHS) has asserted the authority to step in if necessary.

The MLR is simply the percentage of the premium dollar that is spent on health care services, not administrative services. Under the ACA, the MLR can be no lower than 80% for small employer groups and individuals and no lower than 85% for large insured groups. If the MLR is below those thresholds, the payer must rebate the difference to the customers. A state may apply to HHS for a waiver on the MLR requirement if their insurance department believes the MLR limit will destabilize the individual market that year.

For purposes of calculating the rebate, individuals' policies are pooled, small groups are pooled, but large groups are not pooled, meaning an expensive large group cannot be subsidized by less expensive large groups. Also, all

TABLE 21-1	Example of a High-Level Profit and Loss Statement for an HMO	
Percentage revenue		
Premiums earned		95%
Other income		5
Total revenue		**100**
Percentage expenses		
Health care expenses		84
General and administrative expenses		11
Total expenses		**95**
Percentage income or loss before income taxes		**5%**

---

[*]The term "profit" is used from here on to refer to either profit or surplus.

MLR calculations and rebates are confined to a single state, meaning an insurer or HMO cannot pool or average the MLR for companies with employees in more than one state; said another way, if a multistate company has a low MLR in one state but a high MLR in another state, the insurer would have to rebate the company in the low MLR state but absorb the loss in the high MLR state.

Based on recommendations by the NAIC, HHS has defined what can and cannot be counted as a medical expense, and any cost not considered a medical expense is considered administrative and subject to the 20% or 15% limitations. Not all medical costs are directly paid to providers. Some costs associated with quality may be added to the benefits costs for purposes of calculating the MLR. Non-benefits-related costs that may be included or are excluded from the medical cost calculation are shown in **Table 21-2**. Finally, insurers and HMOs may deduct federal and state taxes (except taxes on investment income and capital gains), and licensing or regulatory fees from premiums received when calculating the MLR.

Financial Statements by Line of Business or Market Segment

For internal management reporting purposes, the ability to develop profit and loss reports by product line/market segment is critical to the financial management process. Assumptions and financial benchmarks may vary widely by product or market segment.

For example, medical cost estimates are based on utilization patterns and provider payment strategies that will differ by product and market segment. Likewise,

administration of lines of business may be different; for example, the costs associated with supporting a Medicare or Medicaid product will differ from those associated with the commercial population because the customers have unique service needs and because dedicated staff with specific skill sets will be needed to service Medicare and Medicaid enrollees. Similarly, the ACA recognizes that the large group market has some economies of scale, which is why the MLR limit is higher in the large group insured market.

Costs and therefore premium pricing will also vary significantly by commercial line of business, based on many factors. Examples include:

- Whether or not the product is guaranteed issue;
- Whether medical underwriting guidelines are in force, subject to exclusions for preexisting conditions;
- What kind of payment methodologies such as fee-for-service (FFS) or capitation are being used; and
- How costly it is to administer.

Financial management by line of business may seem like a simple concept, but it is one of the most important success factors of any business, let alone the managed care industry where the products, benefit plan designs, segments, and lines of businesses within an organization can represent thousands of dimensions that may each be operating under differing levels of revenue, expense, margin, capital, and regulatory scrutiny.

Warren Buffet has long endorsed the writings of investment author Philip A. Fisher, who in 1958 authored the following excerpt from *Common Stocks and Uncommon Profits* that consummately describes the importance of this type of financial management practice:

No company is going to continue to have outstanding success for a long period of time if it cannot breakdown its overall costs with sufficient accuracy and detail to show the cost of each small step in its operation. Only in this way will a management know what most needs its attention. Only in this way can management judge whether it is properly solving each problem that does need its attention. Furthermore, most successful companies make not one but a vast series of products. If the management does not have a precise knowledge of the true costs of each product in relation to the others, it is under an extreme handicap. It becomes almost impossible to establish pricing policies that will insure the maximum obtainable over-all profit consistent with discouraging undue competition. There is no way of knowing which products are worthy of special sales effort and promotion. Worst of all, some apparently successful activities may actually be operating at a loss and, unknown to management, may be decreasing rather than swelling the total over-all profits. Intelligent planning becomes almost impossible.[3]

TABLE 21-2	Additional Activities Considered Medical Costs When Calculating the MLR	
Quality-improving expenses specifically added to benefits expenses for MLR calculation	**Expenses specifically excluded as benefits costs**	
• Expenses designed to measurably improve health outcomes	• Retrospective and concurrent utilization review	
• Prevent hospital readmissions	• Fraud prevention activities	
• Improve patient safety	• Developing and maintaining provider networks and contracting	
• Increase wellness		
• Enhance the use of health care data to improve quality, transparency, and outcomes	• Provider credentialing	
	• Sales costs and commissions	
	• Profit or retained earnings	
• Health information technology costs that are clearly attributable to the above		

Source: Created using information in the *Federal Register*, December 1, 2010;75(230):45, CFR Part 158, "Health Insurance Issuers Implementing Medical Loss Ratio (MLR) Requirements under the Patient Protection and Affordable Care Act."

Within each line of business (LOB) the payer will also be differentiating its product offerings by the size and type of purchaser. And it will reach each member it serves through a diverse set of distribution channels, each with its own unique cost structures and complexities. Most commercial products are sold to employer organizations, municipal and state governments, large business enterprises, mid-size commercial ventures (all defined as having over 100 employees), or to small businesses (defined by ACA as less than 100 covered lives, but by many states under 50 lives), and/or to individuals and sole proprietors. Within each customer segment, the payer will typically offer a tailored set of these commercial products, and on each product set there typically will be varying benefit plan designs that allow for the same product to be tailored for economic preferences. On top of this, a payer may also have Medicare and Medicaid products that are even more different. With ACA a reality, the advent of minimum loss ratios, resulting rebate liabilities, age band, and other rating restrictions that will inevitably force the subsidization of certain cohorts from others, there are certain to be many micro aspects of a payer's total book of business that will become unprofitable and unsustainable if not properly managed to keep balance with viable cohorts. It will be up to the finance manager to develop the correct level of management reporting necessary to manage a successful outcome.

In the following discussion of the components of the financial statement, keep in mind the importance of segregating the reporting by product line or market segment, and even by distribution channel within a given segment. Analyzing financial results by line of business not only enhances management's ability to understand the fluctuations from budgeted results, but provides the information needed to redirect strategies or to preserve the overall success of the operation.

Premium Revenue

Premium revenue is the primary revenue source for payers. This is the case even though as pointed out in Chapter 2, the majority of commercial coverage is self-funded, meaning the payer receives only an administrative fee, not premiums. However, premiums are so much higher than administrative fees that even if less than half of a payer business is insured or at risk, the total amount of premiums can still dwarf the total amount of fees. Premiums are generally received in advance of the coverage period, which is usually monthly, while premium rates are generally effective for a 12-month period. Rates or rating methodologies are usually filed with and must be approved by the state's Department of Insurance. Insurers may file revisions to the rates or methodology, which will also be subject to approval by the Department of Insurance. New rates will not be effective for existing groups until the renewal of the annual contract.

Premiums are intended to cover all medical and administrative expenses as well as to provide a profit margin, but also be competitive in the marketplace. Premium rates are therefore directly related to medical expense and administrative expense projections, or if a Medicare Advantage product, then the relationship is to the risk scores of the covered life. If the premium rates are not adequate to cover the actual medical expenses and administrative costs, expected profit margins will diminish. If losses for a line of business are anticipated, a premium deficiency exists. Under GAAP accounting, because premium rates are fixed until the end of the coverage period, the aggregate anticipated net loss for the line of business may need to be recorded immediately, not ratably over the remaining coverage period.

Determination of Premiums Rates

Actuarial and underwriting functions, including the determination of premium rates, are discussed in detail in Chapter 22. The varied approaches to premium rate determination are summarized as follows. If the summaries are not sufficiently explanatory, it is enough for now to understand how many different factors may apply and how many different approaches to rate development may be used.

For most commercial lines of business, premiums are derived from a complex set of rating methodologies that set rates based on an evaluation of demographic data (e.g., the age and gender mix or geographic location) of the population to insure. Rates may be determined using a community rating methodology or an experience rating methodology. Community rating is often used for small groups (less than 50 subscribers) or individuals, and experience rating is used for large groups. In several states, pure community rating is mandatory for small groups and individuals. However, in the majority of states modified community rating allows for medical underwriting and enables premiums to be "rated up" for taking additional risk. This will change in 2014 when the ACA's requirements for community rating in the small group and individual markets will go into effect.

Basic community rating entails the application of a standard rate to all groups within the community being underwritten. The standard rate is applied to groups on the basis of the number of rate tiers quoted, the average family size, and the contract mix assumed for the group. Rate tiers are developed based on the age and sex of members as well as the classification of single versus family. Community rating by class considers an adjustment to the basic rate for specific demographics and/or industry classification of the group. Adjusted community rating allows for adjustments to the base rate for group-specific information other than demographics and industry classification.

The experience rating methodology develops a group rate based on a group's actual experience. After determining actual past experience, expenses are trended forward. Experience-rated contracts can be retrospectively rated or prospectively rated. Retrospective rate adjustments allow for an adjustment to the current period premium based on actual experience. The premium adjustment should be accrued in the current financial statement period and may need to be estimated if the settlement date is subsequent to the end of the accounting period. Prospectively rated premiums provide for increases in rates in the next contract period based on the actual experience of the previous period. When premium adjustments are prospectively rated, there are no accounting entries required in the current reporting period. Since the ACA does not address rating other than as it applies to the small group and individual markets, it has no impact on rate adjustments for larger groups.

Certain premium rates may not be in part or in total controlled by the payer, such as those for Medicare risk or Medicaid contracts. These rates are subject to review and final determination by the government, as discussed in Chapters 24 and 25, respectively. For example, premium rates for Medicare Advantage (MA) programs are especially complex because a significant proportion of the total premium for the products comes not from the statutorily defined components (relating to the county rates of each member and the bid savings as submitted by the plan to CMS) but by the progression of each covered life's risk score. These risk scores are the key variable in forecasting and understanding Medicare revenue and how it will behave over time. In addition to the CMS portion of premium that an MA plan receives, there can be supplemental premium that the member pays, as well as an amount that the MA plan may need to recognize (and perhaps accrue for) in order to account for changes in the risk score that may be driven by CMS's midyear payment practice (whereby it will true up for changes in each covered member's risk score). Medicare Part D Prescription Drug Programs (PDPs) come with a couple more complexities because of the added components of risk corridor and reinsurance that essentially links the amount of premium that a plan will receive from CMS to the claims experience of the covered lives.

Billing and Payment of Premiums

Revenues are recorded in the financial statements as a function of the underlying billing process; enrollment and billing are also addressed in Chapter 17. The effectiveness of the billing process is further dependent upon the membership or enrollment process. Membership data must be gathered in sufficient detail from the enrollment forms to allow for the proper classification of the enrollee to ensure that the appropriate rates are charged. Timely updating of enrollment records for changes in membership status not only ensures the accuracy of rates charged but also ensures that medical services are only provided to active enrollees. Furthermore, compliance with billing and enrollment procedures may affect whether the payer will incur costs for health care services provided to inactive enrollees.

Subscribers, providers, and the payer each have contractual obligations related to updating and verification of the enrollee's status. Failure to meet contractual obligations to maintain enrollment records properly and accurately could result in additional costs to the payer. Therefore, the financial manager should have the information needed to ensure that revenue is being billed for all active enrollees and that business processes are functioning in a manner to prevent loss as a result of noncompliance with contract terms.

Premium billing may occur under two methods: self-billing or retroactive billing. The self-billing method permits the subscriber (or the group) to adjust the invoice for changes in enrollment. In this situation, the amount billed and recorded as premium revenue receivable will differ from the actual amounts paid by the group. Differences in the amount billed and received require adjustment to revenue and accounts receivable records. A secondary process should include communication of changes to ensure timely updating of enrollment records and notification of enrollment changes to providers. If processes are not in place to ensure that such differences are reconciled and resolved on a timely basis, revenue and accounts receivable may not be recorded properly in the financial statements, and health care benefits may be provided to individuals who are no longer insured.

The retroactive billing method results in adjustments to be recorded in the next month's billing cycle. Under this method, payments made by the group should equal amounts billed. Any changes in enrollment will be adjusted on the next billing. Any changes in enrollment noted should also be forwarded to the appropriate department to ensure updating of enrollment records.

For either billing method, the financial manager must develop a methodology of estimating adjustments affecting the current accounting period. Because the actual adjustments are not known until payment is received or reported in the next billing cycle, an estimate of expected adjustments should be accrued in the current reporting cycle.

Certain large commercial or government clients remit payment without detailed hard copy explanation of the adjustment. These customers often request electronic data transfer for billing purposes. Financial managers should be aware that significant resources may be needed to service these customers. Information systems personnel will be needed to deal with technical aspects of the electronic data transfer process. Support personnel with specific training will be needed to handle the unique challenges associated with large accounts. The Health Insurance Portability and Accountability Act (HIPAA) mandated certain electronic transaction standards for use by covered entities, including Benefit Enrollment and Maintenance–834 and Payroll Deduction and Group Premium Payment for Insurance Products–820. However, employers are not covered entities and are not required to use these standards even though payers are.

The process of reconciling the payer's records with the customer's records can be time-consuming but is absolutely necessary. The financial manager should monitor the status (timeliness and completeness) of the reconciliations of these accounts to ensure that any potential problems with the reconciliations do not also affect other financial statement components, such as medical expense accruals. An additional new burden provided to financial managers is to be able to properly account for the proportion of premium that is used to cover premium taxes, as well as other state and federal taxes, as specified in ACA; items relating to state and federal tax activities can be deducted from the denominator used in the minimum loss ratio calculation.

Other Revenue Sources

There are several additional sources of revenue other than premiums. The most common ones are administrative fees, coordination of benefits (COB), and other party liability (OPL), reinsurance recoveries, and interest and investment income.

Administrative Fees

Fee revenue is typically the largest component of other revenue. Fee revenue is charged to self-funded accounts under administrative services contracts (ASC, also sometimes referred to as administrative services only, or ASO contracts). The account managers typically select a managed care product and pay a variety of specified per member per month (PMPM) fees depending on the type and number of administrative services being provided.

To begin with, there is a base fee for accessing the provider network in whatever product the account chooses; for example, a preferred provider organization (PPO) product or an HMO. Pricing of access fees should consider costs of performing administrative functions related to maintaining the provider network, such as credentialing, contract negotiations, and monitoring physician practice patterns. Examples of additional PMPM fees typically added to the access fee for an ASO account include:

- Claims processing
- Member services
- Utilization management
- Case management
- Disease management
- Providing a primary care physician "gatekeeping" function for an HMO product
- Various reports and analytics

Coordination of Benefits and Other Party Liability

COB recoverable is another source of revenue for the payer, as is OPL. Payers must have sufficient procedures in place to identify recoveries or of costs under COB and OPL. COB usually exists when there is a two-wage-earner family and individuals will have insurance coverage under two policies with a different insurer or health plan. Policies and procedures are established by insurance organizations to determine which insurer or health plan will serve as the primary or secondary payer for COB. Procedures need to be in place to ensure that costs that are the responsibility of the other carrier are recovered. The data necessary to perform this procedure are usually gathered during the enrollment and billing process. Again, accuracy and completeness during the enrollment process are key to securing the data necessary to determine the amounts recoverable.

OPL refers to a nonhealth insurer responsible for medical costs. The two most common sources of OPL are workers' compensation and automobile liability policies. These cases may be identified first through the utilization management function of the plan, or the information may come from the provider, or through billing codes. Like COB, policies and procedures must be in place to detect potential OPL.

There are two primary methods of recovering COB and OPL: pay and pursue and pursue and pay. Under the pay-and-pursue method, claims are paid, and recovery is sought later from the other carrier. Under pursue and pay, the claim net of any COB is paid. To ensure that medical expenses are not recorded net, it is important that gross claim costs and COB recoverable are identifiable by the financial manager. (See Chapter 18 for a detailed discussion of COB and OPL.)

Reinsurance Recoveries

Reinsurance recoverable is another source of income to the payer. Reinsurance against catastrophic claims or claims in excess of specified dollar limits is often obtained to reduce the risk of individual large losses for the payer. Payers may forgo obtaining reinsurance based on the cost versus benefit of the coverage. The financial manager, often in conjunction with the payer's actuaries, needs to perform a risk assessment to determine whether stop-loss insurance is appropriate. Of note, self-funded groups typically also purchase reinsurance, but the recovery goes to the group, not the payer.

Procedures need to exist to ensure that costs recoverable under reinsurance are identifiable, so that the payer receives the full benefit to which it is entitled under the reinsurance arrangement. Reinsurance premiums should be recorded as health care costs, and reinsurance recoverable should be shown net of health care costs.

Interest and Investment Income

Another source of income for payers is interest and investment income. Excess cash is generally invested in short-term instruments to ensure cash availability for the payment of claims. If an insurer has more than adequate statutory reserves, which are described later, it may invest some of that excess in more traditional ways. In the past, income from interest and investments actually accounted for the difference between profit and loss for some smaller payers, but economic conditions since 2007 have almost eliminated it as a significant revenue source.

Medical Expenses

Medical expenses are made up primarily of payments to providers. In a closed-panel HMO, that would include the costs of operating the medical group, including physician compensation. The other category of medical costs are those allowed under the ACA to be added to provider payments for purposes of calculating the MLR.

Provider Payments

Table 21-3, from Chapter 22 (Table 22-3, Sample Actuarial Cost Model), provides an example of a summary breakdown of medical costs among hospital, physician, and ancillary services.

Medical expenses may be incurred by payment through capitation, fee schedules, per diems, case rates, or any of the other arrangements described in Chapter 5. Another form of payment that is similar to capitation is percentage of premium, but that is far less common than it once was. Capitation and percentage of premium represent risk transfer arrangements and are typically only used by HMOs. Risk transfer arrangements place the providers at risk if utilization exceeds expected results, reducing the risk exposure of the HMO, although there are usually limits to the degree of risk that is transferred.

Medical expenses reported in the financial statements should represent paid claims plus accruals for claims reported but unpaid and claims incurred but not reported (IBNR). The development of the accruals for both reported and unreported claims is an accounting estimate whereby the accuracy of the estimate is dependent upon the data captured by operations personnel and communicated to financial managers.

For reported claims, the incidence of claims is known (e.g., estimated length of stay for inpatient service, number of referred visits for outpatient services) and the type of claim is known (e.g., inpatient procedure codes, type of outpatient service). The costs related to the claim incident must be estimated. For reported claims there is less unknown, and there can be more accuracy when ultimate costs are projected, although the ultimate disposition of the claims must still be estimated.

For IBNR claims, both the incidence of claims and the type of claims are unknown and must be estimated. IBNR estimates are often developed with the assistance of actuaries. A preferred methodology for estimating IBNR is the development of loss triangles, an example of which is seen in **Table 21-4**. The triangles graphically depict the lag between either the date of service and the payment date or the date of service and the date the claim is reported. From the lag analysis, completion factors are developed to estimate the remaining claims to be reported or paid at each duration. Claim severity, or the estimated average claim costs, is then used to calculate the total projected costs yet to be incurred. The total projected costs are the basis for accruals to be recorded in the financial statements for the IBNR claims.

Loss triangles are often developed separately for hospital, ambulatory facility, and physician claims. Physician claims can also be further analyzed by type of specialty claim where appropriate. Also IBNR claims analysis should be segregated by line of business. Although greater levels of detail can assist in a more refined estimate, caution should be used when one is developing estimates from small population sizes. The smaller the base population, the less precise the estimates. It is prudent to limit the level of detail used in the analysis.

As discussed earlier, the adequacy of the estimates for reported claims developed by financial managers is dependent upon the availability of data from the operating areas within the payer. These data are usually developed from the utilization management program. Inpatient and ambulatory facility care, excluding emergency care, typically requires preauthorization; therefore, if the utilization managers are keeping accurate records of ambulatory procedures, and admissions and length of stay statistics, the data needed by the financial managers to estimate the cost of those services should be readily available. In HMOs, referrals are usually required for most specialist services, but not in other types of plans. For HMOs at least, if the utilization management program is properly monitoring outpatient and specialist utilization and is maintaining accurate records of referrals, the data needed to estimate outpatient and specialist visits should be readily available to financial managers. To be usable, the authorization information must be carefully controlled so that authorizations unlikely to be used are eliminated before ultimate utilization is estimated. It is important that the utilization managers understand the significance of their responsibilities in that utilization managers not only are vital to controlling overall utilization but also provide necessary information to predict medical costs accurately, prepare reports on financial results, and develop budgets and financial forecasts.

Because the tools used by financial managers to estimate medical costs also rely heavily on claims data, the claims processing department plays a critically important role in financial management because the accuracy of claims data and the timely processing of claims will affect the reliability of the data used to develop the loss triangles. The extent of any backlogs in claim processing must be communicated in a timely fashion to the financial manager. (See Chapter 18 for a detailed discussion of claims.)

Loss triangles represent the most frequently used method to estimate claims costs. Other analyses can also be performed to substantiate further the reasonableness of the estimates for IBNR claims. Analyzing the monthly trends in

| TABLE 21-3 | Sample Actuarial Cost Model | | | | | | | |

Medical service category	Medical service	(1) Annual utilization per 1,000 members	(2) Allowed average charge per service	(3) PMPM medical cost	(4) Copay frequency	(5) Copay amount	(6) Cost-sharing PMPM	(7) Net claim costs PMPM
Hospital inpatient	Medical/ surgical	170 days	$7,000.00	$99.17				$99.17
	Psychiatric/ substance abuse	50days	2,000.00	8.33				8.33
	Skilled nursing care	20 days	1,000.00	1.67				1.67
	Subtotal	240 days	$5,458.33	$109.17				$109.17
Hospital outpatient	Emergency room	150 cases	$2,500.00	$31.25	145	$100.00	$1.21	$30.04
	Surgery	60 cases	6,000.00	30.00	55	50.00	0.23	29.77
	Radiology/ pathology	350 cases	750.00	21.88				21.88
	Other	300 cases	455.00	11.38				11.38
	Subtotal	860 cases	$1,318.60	$94.50			$1.44	$93.06
Physician	Office and inpatient visits	4,500 visits	$100.00	$37.50	4,000	$25.00	$8.33	$29.17
	Preventive care	2,000 visits	80.00	13.33				13.33
	Surgery	500 procedures	1,000.00	41.67				41.67
	Radiology/ pathology	3,500 procedures	100.00	29.17				29.17
	Other	3,000 services	130.00	32.50				32.50
	Subtotal			$154.17			$8.33	$145.83
Other	Prescription drugs	10,500 scripts	$65.00	$56.88	10,100	$25.00	$21.04	$35.83
	Home health care	50 visits	500.00	2.08				2.08
	Ambulance	30 cases	800.00	2.00	27	100.00	0.23	1.78
	Durable medical equipment	150 procedures	300.00	3.75				3.75
	Subtotal			$64.71			$21.27	$43.44
Total medical costs PMPM				$422.54			$31.04	$391.50
Retention load PMPM (10% of the required rate)								$43.50
Required rate PMPM								$435.00

Source: Milliman as Table 22-2 in Chapter 22. Used with permission.

TABLE 21-4	**Example of Loss Triangles**

Inpatient services

Claims paid by month of receipt service

Month	Jan	Feb	Mar	Apr	May	June	July	Aug	Sep	Oct	Nov	Dec
Jan	10	100	150	50	35	2	1		1		4	1
Feb		7	126	164	44	22	1	1		6		
Mar			24	89	201	33	46	53			5	1
Apr				12	109	177	3	25	2	2	1	
May					1	188	156	45	59	3	4	2
June						3	255	189	67	55	4	1
July							9	163	198	84	54	8
Aug								33	127	199	87	62
Sep									27	244	149	88
Oct										17	155	205
Nov											5	104
Dec												12
Total	10	107	300	315	390	425	471	509	481	610	468	484

Completion factors by month of receipt

Month	Cur	+1	+2	+3	+4	+5	+6	+7	+8	+9	+10	+11	Total
Jan	0.03	0.31	0.73	0.88	0.97	0.98	0.98	0.98	0.99	0.99	1.00	1.00	
Feb	0.02	0.36	0.80	0.92	0.98	0.98	0.98	0.98	1.00	1.00	1.00		
Mar	0.05	0.25	0.69	0.77	0.87	0.99	0.99	0.99	1.00	1.00			
Apr	0.04	0.37	0.90	0.91	0.98	0.99	1.00	1.00	1.00				
May	0.00	0.41	0.75	0.85	0.98	0.99	1.00	1.00					
June	0.01	0.45	0.78	0.90	0.99	1.00	1.00						
July	0.02	0.33	0.72	0.88	0.98	1.00							
Aug	0.06	0.31	0.71	0.88	1.00								
Sep	0.05	0.53	0.83	1.00									
Oct	0.05	0.46	1.00										
Nov	0.05	1.00											
Dec	1.00												
Jan–June	0.02	0.36	0.78	0.87	0.96	0.99	0.99	0.99	1.00	1.00	1.00	1.00	

claims costs or loss ratios by service type (inpatient, outpatient, physician services by specialty, etc.) within product lines and on a per member per month basis provides a foundation for determining whether the overall trends in claims costs are consistent with expected results and, where appropriate, industry benchmarks. Factors that may affect the trends include the following:

- Significant changes in enrollment;
- Unusual or large claims (isolated occurrences vs. changes in utilization/cost patterns);
- Changes in pricing or product design;
- Seasonal utilization or reporting patterns;
- Claim processing backlogs; and
- Major changes to the provider network or payment methods.

Each of these factors provides a basis for explaining fluctuations when one is preparing trend analyses. It is important to note, however, that significant changes in enrollment also affect the financial manager's ability to determine reasonable estimates used in financial statements. For example, during periods of enrollment growth, it is difficult to estimate medical cost trends because there is little history associated with the current enrollment base and revenue begins on the first day of enrollment but medical costs generally do not; this may lull an inexperienced financial manager into believing that the medical costs ratio is low. In times of significant disenrollment, there is a risk of adverse selection. Adverse selection exists when the characteristics of the remaining population of insureds is weighted toward a high-risk group. Significant disenrollment often occurs when it is generally not an optimal condition for the enrollee to maintain the current coverage. Usually, those insureds with less choice (e.g., those who are unable to opt for other coverage because of current health status) remain enrolled. Medical cost estimates must be adjusted under these circumstances.

Additionally, as the competitive landscape changes and pressures increase to contain premium costs to employers and members, payers need to continuously look to be innovative in product design, for example, consumer-directed health plans as discussed in Chapter 2. The rising cost of health care continues to challenge the ability to market profitable and reasonably priced products. New product initiatives often affect the claims activity and can increase the difficulty in measuring and estimating medical cost trends.

Medical Costs Other Than Payments to Providers

As noted earlier and seen in Table 21-2, HHS has defined which quality improvement activities may be considered as medical costs and added to provider payments for purposes of calculating the MLR. Those costs do not appear on any lag table or actuarial break out of provider costs. But they are added to the schedule or report that insurers must submit to their state departments of insurance when reporting MLR ratios. These costs are not discussed further here.

Administrative Expenses

Administrative expenses include salaries as well as sales, marketing, and other operating expenses; sometimes they are collectively referred to as sales, governance and administration (SG&A). Administrative expenses also vary by product and market segment. Administrative expenses can be measured using percentage of premium and per member per month benchmarks. Administrative expenses are also tracked by functional area (finance, sales, underwriting, member services, etc.). Administrative expenses will vary with volume as a result of economies of scale. In growth periods, administrative expenses tend to be high as a percentage of premium.

Tracking of administrative expenses by product and market segment enables management to identify whether the appropriate resources are being allocated to product lines. Additionally, if the payer experience rates certain groups, management needs to track adequately costs associated with a particular group's business to ensure that costs are appropriately allocated to the group and are recovered.

In addition to the MLR limits on insured business discussed earlier, federal accounts, Medicare, and Medicaid also typically place limits on the administrative expense allocations to these product lines. Given these limits, one of the only levers available for payers to expand margin in a postreform marketplace is for the lowering of administrative expense ratios through increased SG&A efficiency.

■ BALANCE SHEET

Cash and Investments

Cash and investments represent a significant balance sheet account for a payer. As already noted, the major source of cash is premium revenue. A payer's investment portfolio usually consists of short-term investments because cash outlays for claims are frequent. Because cash does churn quickly through the payer, management may benefit from implementing strong cash management practices, such as using lock-box arrangements for premiums. Maximizing the investment in short-term instruments is the main focus of the investment risk.

Premium Receivable

Another significant balance sheet account is premium receivable. Premiums are generally collected monthly; therefore, problems with the aging of accounts will probably arise from old items that are not reconciled. Unreconciled differences may occur when billing problems exist or as a result of discrepancies in the enrollment records of the payer in comparison with customer records.

Timely update of membership records ensures the accuracy of premium billings and further ensures that claims are paid appropriately. Policies and procedures to ensure timely updating of membership records protect the payer from paying claims for terminated members or ensures the recoverability of amounts paid incorrectly. In general, if membership records are not up-to-date and the payer bills incorrectly for terminated or inactive members, upon remittance a group will adjust the payment accordingly. If the payer does not have procedures in place to reconcile remittances to billed amounts, premium receivable records will show amounts outstanding and past due. Because of the large number of individual members within a group and the potentially large number of billings, management must monitor closely the status of premium reconciliation procedures. The reconciliation process related to premium receivable for government accounts is usually a more complex problem. For example, federal and state employers often remit premium on a cycle that differs from the normal billing cycle of the payer. The remittances by these institutions are consistent with the institution's payroll cycles. Premium is remitted only for those employees noted as active on the payroll.

There are many events that affect the active status of federal and state employees (e.g., leave of absence, summer recess for educators), but these employees may still be eligible for health benefits. For this reason, the payer will bill and accrue for premiums that will not be paid until the employee's status on the institution's records is reinstated to active status. Often, payers that provide coverage to federal and state groups will have dedicated resources to support the reconciliation process. The reconciliation process for certain large groups may also be complex. The high enrollment volume or the need to accept enrollment data in compatible electronic format may present a challenge for the payer.

Other Assets

The significance of other assets of a payer will vary. A typical large asset may be fixed assets, for example, an HMO is organized as a staff model HMO that owns and operates physician offices. Because of standards under SAP regarding what may or may not be counted as an asset for purposes of calculating the statutory net worth of the payer as discussed later in this chapter, it is relatively uncommon for payers to own property, however, since it is not considered liquid. Statutory net worth is an extremely important concept for insurers and HMOs, and is discussed in a later section.

Unearned Premiums

Unearned premiums are premiums received by the insurer that at the close of the financial reporting period have not been earned, principally because the premiums are for an ensuing time period, and are in actuality premiums received in advance. Because most payers bill on a monthly basis, unearned premium is generally not a major accounting issue. If premiums are billed and collected other than monthly (e.g., quarterly), an unearned premium reserve would be required.

Claims Payable and IBNR

As discussed earlier, the basis for the recording of claim reserves, including IBNR, is dependent upon information provided by other operating areas of the payer. Claim liabilities are separated between hospital claims and physician claims. In addition to the matters discussed for medical expenses, the financial manager should prepare further analyses of claim reserves and IBNR estimates.

The financial manager should compare the actual claim payments since the close of the accounting period with the original estimates. Significant differences in the actual results compared with estimated results should be investigated. Information obtained from the investigation should be considered when the sufficiency of current estimates is evaluated.

Risk Pool Liabilities

As discussed in Chapter 5, payment strategies may provide for risk pools, which will require the payer to maintain accurate records of payment withholds from hospitals and physicians. Amounts payable to the providers from the withhold should be maintained in separate accounts. In addition, shortfalls in the risk pool that must be recovered from the providers need to be evaluated to ensure that the amounts are recoverable, and where necessary the financial manager should consider the need for a provision for unrecoverable amounts. Additionally, any contributions to be made by the payer for its participation in a risk pool should be appropriately accrued in the financial statements.

Equity

The payer will need to track its SAP and GAAP basis equity. SAP equity generally differs from GAAP equity as a result of certain assets being nonadmitted, and also where permitted, certain liabilities being recognized as equity. For example, the statutory balance sheet may permit certain surplus notes to be classified as equity for purposes of determining statutory net worth (issues regarding statutory net worth are discussed later). Surplus notes are obligations to investors that meet certain requirements of the state insurance laws, which are generally subordinated to all obligations of the payers. Repayment of surplus notes is subject to the approval of the state's commissioners of insurance. Other transactions affecting equity that are generally subject to the approval of the state's commissioners of insurance include restrictions on the payout of dividends.

■ REGULATORY REQUIREMENTS AND REPORTING

Generally, HMOs and health insurance companies are required to file quarterly financial statements with the state Department of Insurance, which are due 45 days after the close of the quarter. An annual statement filing is also required. The annual filing is due March 1. Effective with the reporting for calendar year 1998, changes were made to the NAIC annual statement format. The changes to investment reporting (Schedule D to the NAIC annual statement) resulted in HMOs reporting of investment activity, which is identical to that reported by other types of insurance organizations (e.g., life and health insurers and property/casualty insurers). Previously, HMOs were not required to submit such detailed information of their investment activity and holdings at the end of the reporting period.

Another important change included the addition of Schedule L to the NAIC annual statement, which reports information and activities with intermediaries, including the concentration of business with intermediaries and whether or not the intermediaries are subject to regulatory oversight, including risk-based capital requirements, and provides an indication as to whether the requirements have been met. Schedule L provides the regulators with more up-to-date information on the extent of risk transfer arrangements between the payer and an intermediary organization that may not in turn be subject to regulatory oversight. This is particularly important to the regulators because when risk is transferred to unregulated entities, there is an increased risk that the assuming entity may not have adequate capital to sustain adverse underwriting risk. In these situations, the funds for the provision of care have already been disbursed by the payer. If the intermediary is in financial distress, the funds may no longer be available, further increasing the financial risk to the payer. The information provided on both Schedules D and L also facilitated the development of the data to be reported in the payer's risk-based capital (RBC) filing, which is discussed shortly.

Many states also require the filing of a certification on claims reserves prepared by a licensed actuary. Audited financial statements are also required; the filing deadline may vary by state but is generally June 1. Any differences in the amounts reported in the audited financial statements and the annual filing due on March 1 must be disclosed in the footnotes to the audited financial statements. Depending on the applicable state's requirements, the audited financial statements may be prepared on either an SAP basis or a GAAP basis.

SAP versus GAAP

GAAP focuses more on the matching of revenue and expenses in a given reporting period to measure the earnings of an entity. SAP, on the other hand, represents a specific set of rules applicable only to insurance companies, health service plans, HMOs, or other entities that take risk; it is how state insurance departments assess an insurer's or HMO's ability to pay claims in the future. For example, certain expenditures (e.g., capital assets) may benefit future earnings ability and therefore are likely to be capitalized and expensed ratably over future periods for GAAP. However, such costs are expensed immediately in accordance with SAP because moneys expended are no longer available to pay future liabilities.

Many differences between SAP and GAAP accounting are generally based on the premise of the state insurance department's ability to determine liquidity of the payer.[*] Some of the major differences include the following:

- Treatment of certain assets and investments as non-admitted under SAP (e.g., fixed assets other than electronic data processing equipment, past due premium receivables, certain loans and other receivables, and

---

[*] Another way to think of this is as a type of "fire sale" accounting in which the only thing that counts as an asset is cash and whatever can be converted to cash at a moment's notice.

investments not authorized by statute or in excess of statutory limitations);
- Deferred tax accounts; and
- Carrying value of investments in subsidiaries (which are primarily affected by limitations in the carrying amount and the amortization period of goodwill).

The entire purpose of SAP rules is to determine the statutory net worth of an insurer or HMO, which is different to how a company's net worth would be calculated under GAAP rules. This leads to the next topic: statutory reserve requirements and risk-based capital.

Statutory Reserve Requirements and Risk-Based Capital

Each state's Department of Insurance imposes minimum statutory capital requirements for HMOs and insurance companies. While each state is free to set its own requirements, as a practical matter they are mostly similar from state to state. For example, the NAIC adopted a model act for HMOs that specified that minimum capital for HMOs should be determined as follows:

- The greater of $1 million, or
- Two percent of annual premium as reported on the most recent annual financial statement filed with the commissioners of insurance on the first $150 million of premium and 1% of annual premium on premium greater than $150 million, or
- An amount equal to the sum of 3 months' uncovered health care expenditures as reported on the most recent financial statement filed with the commissioners, or
- An amount equal to the sum of:
  1. Eight percent of annual health care expenditures except those paid on a capitated basis or a managed hospital payment basis as reported on the most recent financial statement filed with the commissioner, and
  2. Four percent of annual health care expenditures paid on a managed hospital payment basis as reported on the most recent financial statement filed with the commissioner.

(Managed hospital basis means agreements wherein the financial risk is primarily related to the degree of utilization rather than to the cost of services. Uncovered expenditures means the costs to the HMO for health care services that are the obligation of the HMO, for which an enrollee may also be liable in the event of HMO insolvency and for which no alternative arrangements have been made that are acceptable to the commissioner.)

Although the states' minimum requirements have provided a means to measure the financial viability of an insurance entity, the states' requirements were often a flat minimum and disregarded the size of an entity or the differing degrees of risk to which different entities are exposed. Insurance entities' exposure to risk has become more diverse, and although some are conservative in investment and underwriting practices, others have been more aggressive.

Risk-Based Capital

The NAIC began examining existing capital requirements and concluded that consumers should be further protected by having companies that assume a more aggressive, risk-taking approach be subject to higher capital requirements. RBC requirements were first required for life and health insurers and property/casualty insurers. A working group was formed in 1993 to develop a separate risk-based capital formula for health organizations, including traditional health insurers, HMOs, Blue Cross and Blue Shield plans, and health service plans. The working group completed its assignment and now, the Risk-Based Capital (RBC) for Insurers Model Law published by the NAIC[4] (the Law) covers the RBC requirements for such health organizations.

In the final stages of development of the Law, payers were required to complete model filings using financial information reported in prior reporting periods. For the calendar year ending 1998, payers were required to file electronic and paper filings with the NAIC and to respective state regulators, and beginning with the calendar year 1999, payers needed to complete the "RBC Plan" to be submitted as required by the Law in the event the reporting payer's RBC requirements are not met. Consistent with the deadline for filing the payer's NAIC annual statement, the RBC filing is due on March 1.

RBC is a method of measuring the minimum amount of capital appropriate for an insurer or HMO to support its overall business operations based on its size and degree of risk taken in each of the five major categories of risk: (1) asset risk—affiliates, (2) asset risk—other, (3) underwriting risk, (4) credit risk, and (5) business risk.

An insurer's RBC is calculated by applying factors to various asset, premium, and reserve items that result in a charge to the payer's actual capital and arrives at adjusted capital. The payer's actual capital is compared to varying levels of the adjusted capital to determine levels of actions, if any, to be taken to improve actual capital, as discussed later.

Of the five categories of risk, underwriting risk results in the largest charge to adjusted capital. The development of this charge was to protect against the risk of fluctuation in underwriting experience. The net charge for underwriting risk is offset by credits that are based to a great extent upon the positive effect that management care arrangements may have on underwriting risk.

There is a presumed benefit from certain managed care arrangements that may reduce the uncertainty about future claims payments. For example, HMO capitation with no risk-sharing by the HMO is generally fixed costs PMPM that therefore reduce the HMO's risk associated with adverse fluctuations in utilization or intensity, thus providing for a more defined estimate of the cost of the capitated fee arrangement. Case rates and fixed global fees, while not the same as capitation, may also ameliorate the level of risk. Conversely, if there are excessive percentages of outlier cases as described in Chapter 5, that would imply that some level of risk is also borne by the plan.

The impact on a payer's RBC for the other categories of risk include protection against investments in assets of affiliates, including subsidiary entities with their own RBC requirements, investments in other assets whose value may be subject to fluctuation in market value, credit risk associated with the recoverability of amounts owed to the payer (i.e., premium receivables and recoverables from providers), and business risk including the effect of excessive business growth on the payer's capital.

The regulatory environment under which payers operate is continuously changing to meet market changes, and entities need to prepare themselves in particular to meet the challenges imposed by new or expected legislation and regulation.

Impairment or Failure

The requirements of each of the states generally call for plans of action when an entity's capital falls within a close range of the minimum requirement. If the payer's actual capital is greater than 200% of the adjusted capital, typically no action is required, although if it has been steadily trending downward, the department may initiate meetings with management.

At or around 200% of adjusted capital, an insurer or HMO typically is required to develop and submit a plan of action about how it will improve reserves to specified levels within a specified time period; for example, it will boost reserves above 200% within 90 days. Insurance departments are typically reluctant to make public this or prior steps so as to avoid a sudden loss of customers or revenue to the insurer.

Should the insurer's or HMO's reserves fall below 150%, the insurance commissioner will usually place it under tight control of the department. The commissioner may declare the plan to be impaired, but not always. In some cases, declaring an insurer to be impaired is reserved for the next and final stage.

If the reserves are below the required minimum or fall to 70%, mandatory control of the plan by the insurance department is usually required. At that point, the department will usually either request a larger and healthier insurer or HMO to absorb the failed plan, or else liquidate it and distribute its members to other insurers. The department will also enforce the network's provider hold harmless clauses (see Chapter 4).

Recall from Chapter 1 that there were a considerable number of failures of early HMOs and other health plans in the 1980s and 1990s. Since then it has settled down considerably, most likely as a result of market consolidation and the absorption of smaller plans into larger and better managed companies. Failures still do occur, however, although typically confined to small local insurers. **Table 21-5** lists the number of Health, Property and Casualty, and Life and Annuity insurance failures from 2008 up to August 2011.

Sarbanes-Oxley Act of 2002

In July 2002, the Sarbanes-Oxley Act of 2002[5] was signed into law. The act came in response to a string of corporate scandals, including the collapse of a number of businesses that negatively affected the confidence of investors in the capital markets of the United States.

Focusing primarily on investor-owned companies (not specifically on health insurance), the Act contains 11 titles (sections) that range from board responsibilities, to "whistleblower" protections, to penalties. Most important, it created the Public Company Accounting Oversight Board, a quasi-government agency that oversees the audits of public companies, intending to protect the interest of investors and other users of an "issuer's" financial statements. The board, which is subject to SEC oversight, is empowered to establish auditing standards for public company audits, inspect accounting firms that audit public companies, investigate possible rule violations, and sanction violators.

In passing the Act, Congress reasoned that the restoration of investors' trust in public companies would depend on demanding that public companies possess strong internal control over financial reporting (ICOFR) and then report on that assessment at the close of its fiscal year. The Act also requires a company's external auditor to attest to and report on the assessment made by management.

Specifically pertaining to financial management, Section 404 of the Act has two parts:

- Section 404(a) describes management's responsibility for establishing and maintaining an adequate internal control structure and procedures for financial reporting. It also outlines management's responsibility for assessing the effectiveness of internal control over financial reporting.
- Section 404(b) describes the independent auditor's responsibility for attesting to and reporting on management's internal control assessment.

■ BUDGETING AND FINANCIAL FORECASTING

The importance of maintaining detailed budgets has been discussed throughout this chapter. Financial forecasts, which project activity and results beyond the current period, are also important management tools. Financial forecasts, budgets, and plans are often developed several months in advance of the actual reporting period. In developing the forecasts, a balance between complexity and simplicity is sought by the financial manager. Although it is essential to capture much detail to develop the overall forecast, the detail information must roll up to a summary level that will facilitate presentation to senior decision makers within the organization and to provide ease for monitoring variances in actual results. At the early stages of development, if the financial forecast evolves from the appropriate level of detail, the overall summaries discussed by senior management teams will be more meaningful.

At the highest level, membership data priced at blended premium rates (for at-risk business) must be presented. The development of both the aggregate membership growth and the blended premium rates is based on input from personnel within sales and marketing, underwriting, and actuarial functions and should have considered specific assumptions for the different array of products offered by the payer. It is important to verify assumptions with the sales function's expectations and the organization's underwriting policies and pricing strategies.

Because both new and renewal membership and premium rate changes are affected by seasonal patterns, the assumptions should trend from quarterly, if not monthly, baseline data. Developing the overall financial forecasts from this level of detail will assist the financial manager in providing the most accurate report of actual versus budgeted results. Understanding variances in planned to actual premium revenue will support whether expected rate changes or net membership growth assumptions were achieved. Sometimes the rate increase by product and the net membership growth may meet expected targets; however, changes in the membership by product type could still result in the aggregate premium levels not being achieved.

TABLE 21-5	Insurer Failures, 2008–Mid-2011		
Year	**Health insurer/ HMO**	**Property and casualty**	**Life and annuity**
2011*	0	6	0
2010	1	15	4
2009	6	14	11
2008	7	3	7

*As of August 2011.
Source: Created by author from data at Weiss Ratings. Available at www.weissratings.com/ratings/track-record/insurer-failures.aspx. Accessed August 18, 2011.

The ability of the financial manager to identify the root cause of variances between forecast and actual results is essential to achieving an organization's overall financial goals.

The baseline for the medical expense component of the financial forecast is generally developed from a historical "look back" of the results. At the time that financial forecasts are being developed, there is still some level of estimation in the historical results, which further complicates the development of the baseline estimate of medical expenses. This baseline must then be adjusted for expected changes including but not limited to medical inflation trends, expected changes in regulations (e.g., new benefit mandates), changes in provider contracting arrangements, enhancements to patient management programs, and introduction of new plan designs. The effects of changes in provider contracts may be dependent upon whether the changes affect a significant portion of the overall membership. Additionally, the effects of patient management programs often require a period of time before the financial impact of the benefit is achieved and/or measurable. It may also be beneficial, to the extent it is practicable, to segregate average medical costs by types of provider contract arrangements. For example, identifying expected PMPM costs for global contract arrangements, fee-for-service arrangements, specialty capitation, and other ancillary arrangements could provide critical information for monitoring the success of the various types of provider arrangements. If it is difficult to identify expected or actual costs for these arrangements, one may question the appropriateness of the arrangement and the viability of the rate that was negotiated with the provider.

Other key components of forecasting medical expenses include the impact of risk-sharing arrangements with providers and the cost and/or benefit of the historical settlement in additions to regulatory imposed costs, such as interest assessed on late payment of claims or surcharges assessed as subsidies to finance the cost of individual and small employer insurance and care for the uninsured. When forecasting medical costs, it is important to consider the complexity that seasonality of medical expenses can exhibit, especially as it relates to benefit plan design features, such as calendar year deductibles.

Administrative costs need to be forecasted. Consideration of the cost to invest in planned growth as well as sustain existing membership volumes is necessary. The most significant component of the administrative costs is typically salary and selling expenses relating to commissions paid to producers. A less visible, but material determinate of SG&A-related expenses is to understand any shifts in the composition of the business relating to its distribution channel. Though it is too soon to tell at the time of publication, the ACA will likely reduce broker commissions due to the MLR limits discussed earlier.

Whether the financial manager is developing premium revenue, medical expense, or administrative costs, the development of the financial forecast is an iterative process and the financial model must be flexible to facilitate this process while at the same time be responsive and not unreasonably complex.

The financial forecasting process must also include the development of a projected balance sheet. This is particularly important to evaluate the impact of the projected growth in operations on minimum capital requirements. Additionally, the forecasting process should require variations from the baseline projections to determine the risks and exposures if the actual results fall short of the baseline and also to project the impact if actual results are better than expected. Cash flow analyses are also important to ensure that cash will be generated from operations or to determine the extent to which cash reserves will be needed, particularly as new lines of business are pursued.

■ CONCLUSION

Whether the financial manager is developing budgets or financial forecasts or preparing financial statements, he or she must depend on the information prepared and maintained by the operating departments. This information is an integral part of the financial manager's decision-making process. Communication among the various functional areas in the payer will be key to the successful operation of the entity. Timely financial reporting enhances management's ability to determine performance against anticipated results and redirect its strategies to minimize exposure to loss and preserve favorable financial performance.

Endnotes

1 The Patient Protection and Affordable Care Act (P.L. 111-148) as amended by the Health Care and Education Reconciliation Act of 2010 (P.L. 111-152), which was signed into law on March 30, 2010. For purposes of this chapter, the ACA includes both laws.

2 ACA Section 2718, 42 U.S.C. §300gg-18, Bringing Down the Cost of Health Care Coverage.

3 Fisher P. *Common Stocks and Uncommon Profits*. Hoboken, NJ: John Wiley & Sons; 1996. First published by Harper & Brothers; 1958.

4 See www.naic.org/committees_e_capad.htm. Accessed August 18, 2011.

5 Pub. L. No. 107-204, 116 Stat. 745, also known as the Public Company Accounting Reform and Investor Protection Act of 2002 and commonly called SOX or SarbOx.

Underwriting and Rating

MICHAEL G. STURM AND TROY M. FILIPEK

STUDY OBJECTIVES

- Understand the basic forms of premium rate development in managed care plans
- Understand the basic issues involved in underwriting
- Understand the basic elements that go into rate development
- Understand how per member per month medical costs are calculated
- Understand the impact of the Patient Protection and Affordable Care Act on underwriting and rating

DISCUSSION TOPICS

1. Describe and discuss the differences between rating and underwriting.
2. Describe and discuss the basic forms of premium rates used by payers.
3. Describe and discuss the basic elements that go into typical rate development formulas.
4. Describe at what points that underwriting may occur, and discuss the importance of each point.
5. Discuss the positive and negative effects of the ACA's requirements on underwriting and rating, both intended and unintended.

■ INTRODUCTION

Underwriting and rating are two very important related, but distinct, functions for any health plan. Successful underwriting and rating strike a balance among adequacy, competitiveness, and equity of rates. It can be a difficult and delicate balance to achieve. Moving too far in any direction can lead to financial disaster for a health plan. The focus of the chapter is on insured or at-risk business for health maintenance organizations (HMOs) and health insurers, regardless of the actual type of plan [e.g., preferred provider organizations (PPOs), point of service (POS), consumer-directed health plans (CDHPs)].

Similar issues arise for self-funded employer groups and many techniques described in this chapter may be applicable to them as well, although not all. Certainly underwriters and actuaries assist self-funded plans in calculating an imputed premium, meaning a figure that corresponds to what the actual premium would be if it were insured, but this is done for purposes of determining employee payroll deductions and the employer's budget for health care benefits. It also helps in looking at plan design alternatives. With that said, the remainder of the chapter focuses primarily on underwriting and premium rating for insured plans.

Adequate rates are high enough to generate sufficient revenue to cover all claims and other plan expenses and to yield an acceptable return on equity. Competitive rates are low enough to sell enough policies and enroll enough members to meet health plan volume and growth targets. Equitable rates will approximate any given group's costs without an unreasonable amount of cross-subsidization among groups. Equitable rates are achieved through applying various rating factors appropriately and result in higher persistency, meaning groups may not change health plans if they realize they are being charged a fair amount for their insurance.

A health plan should continually assess its success in each of these areas. Although always important, this is particularly true for a newly established plan or product offering. For example, a plan cannot be sure whether a high volume of sales is good or bad until adequacy and equitability are assessed because competitive rates are not necessarily adequate or equitable.

This chapter discusses underwriting and rating functions common to most major health insurance markets, as well as discussing implications of the Patient Protection and Affordable Care Act (ACA). Major markets include private individual, commercial group (both small and large), and government business (Medicare and Medicaid). Several core underwriting and rating functions are common to these markets, which are addressed in this chapter. However, each major market segment also has several components with unique risk characteristics that require different approaches to underwriting and rating. These unique to market topics are outside the scope of this chapter and are not addressed here; Medicare and Medicaid are addressed in Chapters 24 and 25, respectively; the ACA is further addressed in Chapter 30; and certain concepts such as incurred but not reported (IBNR) claims reserves are addressed as well in Chapter 21.

■ UNDERWRITING

Underwriting involves gathering information about applicants or groups of applicants to determine an adequate, competitive, and equitable rate at which to insure them. The type of underwriting and level of scrutiny depend on many factors, including the time at which the underwriting is done (at issue, during the plan year, or renewal), the group size (individual, small, or large), and the risk arrangement (fully insured or self-insured).

Underwriting is a function that often is specific to the market being served. For example, individual and small group underwriting generally requires review of individual medical records, whereas large group underwriting does not require this level of depth. As a result, this section provides only a high-level discussion of underwriting techniques and philosophies, without delving deep into the technical details specific to a particular market. Carrier actions based on underwriting information include issuing coverage at the base

rate, issuing coverage at a higher rate, excluding certain services, or declining coverage (where allowed by law); most of these options will become unavailable beginning in 2014 under the ACA sure it prohibits health status underwriting.

At Issue

Effective underwriting at issue determines the following information for the individual or group: health status, ability to pay the premium, availability of other coverage (if any), and historical persistency (applies mainly to groups with high start-up costs).

Health Status

Until ACA provisions take effect in 2014, health status information is still used for underwriting. Information gathered to determine health status varies. The following examples are the types of information that might be requested:

- Physical exams and/or attending physician statements (individual),
- Prescription drug histories (individual and small group),
- Individual medical questionnaires (individual and small group),
- An employer disclosure listing major health conditions (large group),
- Medical cost experience (large group), and/or
- No health status information (Medicare and Medicaid risk contracts).

Under the ACA, health status is no longer allowed as a rating variable in the individual and small group markets beginning in 2014, which would change these markets to using only two health status proxies age and smoking status.

Some carriers historically have used health status information in certain markets (where allowed by law) to apply a preexisting condition limitation or exclusion, meaning a temporary or permanent limit on medical payments for existing health conditions. Preexisting condition limitations have historically been used in conjunction with underwriting to limit antiselection and therefore provide incentives to prospective enrollees to apply for coverage prior to becoming sick. This ensures appropriate risk pooling occurs, which is essential for a successful insurance arrangement. With that said, preexisting condition limitations and exclusions are not allowed under ACA beginning in 2014 for everyone and shortly after the passage of ACA for children only.

Other underwriting policies are used to screen for health status at both issue and renewal, such as ensuring a valid employer–employee relationship exists and a minimum percentage of employees participate in the medical plan. These policies, along with others, prevent groups with higher than average morbidity, meaning level of illness, from being issued coverage at average rates (i.e., adverse selection).

The propensity to purchase coverage is dictated by several factors, including cost concerns, the need to attract and retain employees with health benefits, and whether health insurance premiums are tax-deductible. The chance of adverse selection increases as group size decreases because individual and small group applicants are likely to buy insurance only if they need it. In addition, large groups typically submit claims experience, which enables the underwriter to better estimate a specific group's rates. Therefore, underwriting with medical questionnaires to determine health status is common for individuals and small groups and uncommon for large groups.

Other markets, such as Medicaid and Medicare risk, and individual and small group beginning in 2014, do not allow medical underwriting for rate-setting. Risk-adjusted revenue payments from the federal and state governments help address adverse selection issues.

Ability to Pay

Information gathered to determine an applicant's premium-paying ability might include income and credit history. Income can be verified through tax returns or audited financial statements. Credit history can be verified through independent credit agencies. Credit history is particularly important for employers in industries facing financial hardship, new employers, or employers first offering medical coverage to employees.

Insurers do not necessarily decline coverage to applicants with poor credit histories. However, some insurers require groups with a poor credit rating to produce some form of collateral or a letter of credit (for up to 2 months of premium) instead of declining coverage. Insurers nearly always require individual policyholders to pay premiums in advance of the coverage period to ensure their ability to meet premium requirements.

Other Coverage

Insureds, meaning the individuals who are covered by the health insurer or HMO,[*] are often asked on the application, or are surveyed during the plan year, if they have other health insurance coverage. The presence of other coverage should be noted, so that the claim adjudicator can determine which insurer is responsible for payment of claims based on coordination of benefits (COB) rules. Coordinating payment for benefits enables insurers to reduce their premiums, as also noted in Chapter 21.

Furthermore, it is important to ensure that workers' compensation insurance is in place for commercially insured groups. This insurance provides for coverage in the event

of a workplace injury. The coverage enables the medical insurer to avoid payment of claims for which the workers' compensation coverage is responsible, which is called other party liability (OPL), or to subrogate for claims it pays initially that occur in a workplace setting. Premium loads of 10–20% are common for employers without workers' compensation insurance. (COB, OPL, and subrogation are discussed in detail in Chapter 18.)

Persistency

Insurers should be cautious when writing groups that frequently change carriers because there can be a significant amount of fixed costs associated with writing a new group. The group should appear to be committed to a multiyear relationship, as demonstrated by a history of persistency with prior carriers. Small groups that frequently change carriers could be placed in the highest rating tier, as allowed by state rating limitations. Large groups with more than two carriers in the past 5 years might not be offered coverage at all, although because of the ACA, states will likely close that option beginning in 2014.

Underwriting During the Plan Year and at Renewal

Underwriting during the plan year and at renewal varies greatly by major market segment and, therefore, is not discussed in depth here. However, in general, underwriting during the plan year involves a stringent review to prevent adverse selection. At renewal, the underwriter usually has more information on the insureds (possibly including claims experience) and implements rate changes based on this additional information and any projected changes that could affect future experience. Although the ACA will limit what insurers can do about adverse selection beginning in 2014, it does not prohibit the use of underwriting for purposes of calculating experience rates for large employer groups, which is discussed in the next section.

■ RATING

Rating uses information gathered through underwriting to calculate the premium for a specific individual or group. The premium calculation is generally done using a rate formula, historical experience, predictive underwriting tools, or some combination of the three. The result of the rate formula is sometimes called the manual or book rate. The manual rate is developed using the experience of all individuals or groups in a specific block or pool (i.e., a base rate). The starting base rate is adjusted through the rate formula for demographics, area, group size, industry, and other characteristics (as allowed by law) to arrive at a manual rate specific to a group or individual.

The rate formula should recognize all health plan costs, be easy to apply in most situations, and result in an appropriate

---

[*]This is synonymous with the term "subscriber" as used in Chapter 18.

premium rate. Health plans' costs include medical services, prescription drugs, sales and marketing expenses, administrative expenses, and profit. The rate formula typically expresses rates on a per member per month (PMPM) basis that must be transformed into contract rates for each employee based on the average number of covered members per contract.

The rate formula is updated through various analyses that measure carrier experience. These analyses can also be helpful in establishing budgets by medical service category or department, measuring cost and utilization trends, establishing funding for provider-based risk pools, and identifying, quantifying, and prioritizing medical management opportunities within the health plan. Timely analyses will allow the health plan to establish the proper provider-based education and incentives necessary to realize opportunities within the health plan.

Community Rating versus Experience Rating

A basic split between types of premium rates is the one between community rating and experience rating. Community rating means the experience of a group or individual is not taken into account when calculating rates, only the collective experience of all who are in the same risk pool such as all small employer groups.

In experience rating, the manual rate is blended with group-specific historical experience depending on the group size and credibility of the data. Generally, group sizes of more than 50 are rated at least partially based on experience, while 50 and under are strictly community rated. State regulation and carrier practices dictate the level of this threshold. Beginning in 2014, the ACA will place the limit at 100 employees, but a state may elect to reduce it back down to 50 until 2016. Carriers offering coverage through the new state health insurance exchanges, which are discussed later, will not be allowed to separate groups into those in the exchange and those outside the exchange, but the ACA does not require carriers to offer plans through the exchange.

Experience rating can be thought of as the converse of pooling experience because recognizing a group's experience in its rate calculation reduces the extent to which groups subsidize each other. Experience rating will still be allowed under the ACA for groups with over 100 employees, although beginning in 2017 states may elect to open the exchange to groups over 100.

Adjusting an individual's rate (whether the individual has individual or group coverage) based on the individual's experience is not allowed by law. In some states, and then only until 2014, individuals may be placed into different risk pools corresponding to when and how they accessed coverage, for example, through a state's mandatory open enrollment period, or the year the individual purchased coverage. Rates are then developed for that particular risk pool, although not for each individual in it. Beginning in 2014, the ACA requires that all individuals be placed in the

same risk pool, although it does not require individuals and small groups to be placed in the same pool.

Rate Formula

The rate formula provides the mechanism to adjust the base rate to a group-specific premium to quote. The formula adjusts the base rate for demographics, area, group size, industry, and other characteristics (as allowed by law) to arrive at the manual rate specific to a group or individual. Then, upon adding the retention costs and converting to a per contract rate, the group-specific quote is determined.

Base Rate Development

Most rate formulas start with a base rate, developed from PMPM-incurred medical costs over a historical experience period. The base rate generally reflects the specific information seen in **Table 22-1**.

The projection period base rate is developed by analyzing historical incurred medical costs for a given time period, called the base period, and trending it forward to the projection period, recognizing actual and anticipated changes in the block of business. Historical medical costs are often summarized in 12-month segments of incurred medical costs to provide a credible experience base and to avoid any seasonal variations. Multiple years of experience are commonly used to develop the base rate.

Claims data are generally summarized according to when payments are made. Paid claims data should be converted to an incurred basis, including IBNR reserves, using various estimation techniques such as claim lag analyses and loss ratio techniques, as discussed in Chapter 21. Incurred claims are then matched with health plan exposure, as

TABLE 22-1	Historical Experience Information Typically Reflected in the Base Rate

- Population (e.g., commercial, Medicare, Medicaid, or other population)
- Covered services, including service-specific limits
- Cost-sharing provisions
- Provider payment arrangements
- Demographics such as age and gender
- Average members per contract
- Geographical area
- Occupation or industry
- Health status
- Degree of health care management
- Coverage effective date
- Level of out-of-network usage, if applicable
- Presence or absence of workers' compensation insurance
- Underwriting practices
- Claim administration practices
- Distribution methods such as agents or brokers
- Other variables affecting medical costs

generally measured in member months, to develop a base period PMPM medical cost.

Incurred claim estimation techniques should account for a health plan's unique payment arrangements. The actuary should know whether the paid claim triangles include capitations, withhold payments, stop-loss recoveries, and/or COB savings. If these are not included, the actuary should make the necessary adjustments to account for these plan provisions as part of the incurred claims. In addition, the actuary may need to modify incurred claims for any accrued medical incentives, such as provider bonuses.

Projection adjustments should be made to recognize and account for changes in health plan operations between the base period and projection period. **Table 22-2** presents elements to consider that may change between the base period and projection period; note that these are similar but not identical to the information reflected in the historical base rate in Table 22-1. The elements listed in Table 22-2 may be offsetting. For example, the underlying demand to use more health care services, as the U.S. population ages and technology advances, may be offset by anticipated medical management improvements.

TABLE 22-2	Adjustments to Convert a Historical Base Rate to a Projection Period Base Rate

Actual and/or anticipated changes in incurred claims as a result of changes in:

- The underlying demand for medical services
- The mix of medical services (e.g., because of new technologies or treatment procedures)
- Intensity (i.e., the amount of services per day or visit)
- Level of out-of-network usage, if applicable
- Medical management
- Provider payment methodologies
- Wellness and preventive care programs (now mandatory under the ACA)
- Covered services, including service-specific limits
- Contractual benefit levels or member cost-sharing
- The level of consumer involvement in directing and paying for care
- The average amounts contained in consumer-directed health spending accounts
- Average members per contract
- Occupation or industry
- Coverage effective date
- Presence or absence of workers' compensation insurance
- The demographics of the insured population (e.g., age, gender, Medicare/Medicaid eligibility)
- The geographical area of the insured population
- Claims administration
- Underwriting requirements
- Distribution methods such as agents, brokers, direct, or (beginning in 2014) insurance exchanges
- Other variables affecting health care costs

The projection period base rate can be summarized in an actuarial cost model. **Table 22-3** displays a sample abbreviated actuarial cost model. The model contains, by service category, the following information:

- Annual utilization per 1,000 members (column 1);
- The allowed average charge per service (column 2);
- PMPM medical costs (column 3 = (column 1) × (column 2) / 12,000), which do not reflect cost-sharing provisions;
- Cost-sharing adjustments (columns 4, 5, and 6), which should be composited across the underlying benefit plans offered; and
- PMPM medical costs net of cost-sharing (column 7).

Each service category is defined by a unique set of procedure codes. For example, hospital inpatient services can be grouped by diagnosis-related groups (DRGs) or Medicare severity-adjusted diagnosis-related group (MS-DRGs), and physician services can be grouped using current procedural terminology (CPT). Prescription drugs are generally analyzed separately, using the national drug code (NDC).

One major component of the cost model is the rate at which the population is assumed to use medical services, or utilization. Utilization can vary substantially depending on the efficiency of network providers. Two or more utilization scenarios are often developed to estimate medical costs under current levels of health care management and well-managed levels for use in benchmarking. Utilization can also vary depending on the benefit designs in place, the level of consumer involvement in directing and paying for care, demographics, and area, among other variables.

The other major cost model component, the average charge per service, is based on the provider payment negotiated and specified in the health plan/provider contracts. The average charge per service can be in the form of discounts from billed charges, per diems, case rates, negotiated fee schedules, capitation payments, or other forms of payment. Payment of providers is discussed in Chapters 4 and 5.

The impact of copays on the cost model depends on the benefit plan design and the plan's policy for copay collection. The PMPM medical cost equals the annual utilization per 1,000 members, multiplied by the average charge per service, divided by 12,000 less the value of cost sharing (i.e., the copay frequency multiplied by the copay, divided by 12,000). The values in the actuarial cost model will differ for each group depending on the group's characteristics, as discussed previously.

Rate Determination

Table 22-4 contains a sample rate formula with case-specific adjustments to the base rate. Steps 2–5 in the formula adjust the projection period base rate to reflect the specific group and plan characteristics because the projection period base

| TABLE 22-3 | **Sample Actuarial Cost Model** | | | | | | |

		(1)	(2)	(3)	(4)	(5)	(6)	(7)
Medical service category	Medical service	Annual utilization per 1,000 members	Allowed average charge per service	PMPM medical cost	Copay frequency	Copay amount	Costsharing PMPM	Net claim costs PMPM
Hospital inpatient	Medical/ surgical	170 days	$7,000.00	$99.17				$99.17
	Psychiatric/ substance abuse	50 days	2,000.00	8.33				8.33
	Skilled nursing care	20 days	1,000.00	1.67				1.67
	Subtotal	240 days	$5,458.33	$109.17				$109.17
Hospital outpatient	Emergency room	150 cases	$2,500.00	$31.25	145	$100.00	$1.21	$30.04
	Surgery	60 cases	6,000.00	30.00	55	50.00	0.23	29.77
	Radiology/ pathology	350 cases	750.00	21.88				21.88
	Other	300 cases	455.00	11.38				11.38
	Subtotal	860 cases	$1,318.60	$94.50			$1.44	$93.06
Physician	Office and inpatient visits	4,500 visits	$100.00	$37.50	4,000	$25.00	$8.33	$29.17
	Preventive care	2,000 visits	80.00	13.33				13.33
	Surgery	500 procedures	1,000.00	41.67				41.67
	Radiology/ pathology	3,500 procedures	100.00	29.17				29.17
	Other	3,000 services	130.00	32.50				32.50
	Subtotal			$154.17			$8.33	$145.83
Other	Prescription drugs	10,500 scripts	$65.00	$56.88	10,100	$25.00	$21.04	$35.83
	Home health care	50 visits	500.00	2.08				2.08
	Ambulance	30 cases	800.00	2.00	27	100.00	0.23	1.78
	Durable medical equipment	150 procedures	300.00	3.75				3.75
	Subtotal			$64.71			$21.27	$43.44
Total medical costs PMPM				$422.54			$31.04	$391.50
Retention load PMPM (10% of the required rate)								$43.50
Required rate PMPM								$435.00

rate assumes that all characteristics of a particular insured individual/group are the same characteristics as the average historical medical costs of the block of policies the base rate represents.

The rate formula adjustments should consider relevant, measurable factors that predict medical cost differences among individuals/groups, but the formula should still be easy to measure and apply as well. The adjustments might be additive or multiplicative, depending on the type of adjustment and user's preference. For example, the base rate may need to have costs added to it to reflect additional covered services for mandated benefits in certain states. Conversely, the base rate may need to be multiplied by a factor to reflect lower utilization of services as a result of an efficient health care provider network (i.e., degree of health care management).

Retention

Retention items are usually built into the rate formula once medical costs are calculated. Retention can include administrative expenses, a buildup of contingency reserves, coordination of benefit savings, and profit. Retention is combined with medical costs to arrive at the PMPM premium by dividing the medical costs by a target loss ratio (fixed or variable by group size) or adding specific PMPM retention costs.

Retention must be sufficient to cover all functions performed by the carrier, including claims administration, distribution, and underwriting, among others. Retention

TABLE 22-4	Sample Rate Formula
Step 1:	Incurred medical costs PMPM (i.e., the base rate)
Step 2:	Add or subtract: – Covered services [not] reflected in the base rate – Reinsurance costs
Step 3:	Multiply by: – Benefit plan factor – Geographical area factor – Age/gender factor – Degree of health care management factor – Provider payment factor – Health status factor – Trend factor – Other factors
Step 4:	Retention load (multiply or add) – Administrative expenses – Contingency reserves – Coordination of benefits savings – Profit
Step 5:	Convert the member rate to a contract rate

might only include a subset of a normal carrier's costs if the targets are developed for a physician–hospital organization or other provider-based group that is responsible for only a portion of the administrative duties. This may increase over time due to the ACA's limits on the MLR since delegation of certain responsibilities such as managing a portion of the network or managing utilization is transferred to providers as part of their payment for medical services.

Conversion of Rates from Member to Employee Level

Last, the PMPM manual rate must be converted from a member rate to a contract rate, meaning the rate for the employee/subscriber. Individual and some small group contracts covering multiple members are generally rated by adding together the appropriate rates for each member based on their age and gender, called list bill rating. Conversely, large groups and some small groups are often charged rates according to specific contract tiers such as employee only, employee plus spouse, and family, without varying rates by age or gender; this is also referred to as composite rates. Composite rates need to be set such that the total premium generated for the group reflects the average number of members per contract tier in the group. Medicare and Medicaid rates are nearly always stated on a per member basis, reflecting the fact that coverage is almost always based on the individual. However, Medicaid for Temporary Assistance to Needy Families may be a composite rate covering parent and children.

Data Sources

The best data source for any health plan is its own experience because it implicitly recognizes all of the plan-specific characteristics. However, some carriers have trouble collecting their experience in the necessary format. Alternatively, some carriers have recently been established or are expanding into new markets or products. As a result, many health plans look to published data sources or actuarial consulting firms to provide initial medical cost targets, calibrated to be relevant to the situation. The carrier can substitute experience for the estimates with data from their own health plan over time as it becomes available and is credible.

Consumer-driven health plans (CDHPs; Chapter 2), which are high-deductible health plans using health payment accounts (HRA) or health savings accounts (HSA) are an example of when historical experience data may not be directly usable for predicting future experience. This type of coverage pairs a high-deductible health plan with a consumer spending account that can be used to offset member cost-sharing or is allowed to accumulate over time. Given the uncertainty of consumer behavior with the high-deductible plan and the associated account, a health plan would not want to use traditional plan experience, such as their HMO and PPO products that do not use HRAs or

HSAs, to predict utilization behavior under CDHPs. Many health plans are working through this issue now as the CDHP experience, although growing, is still relatively new and oftentimes is not credible all by itself. In addition, many of the enrollees that voluntarily elect a CDHP plan when they also have a more traditional alternative such as a PPO are healthier than the average book of business across all benefit plans. Some carriers recognize this in their benefit adjustment factors. Other carriers set their benefit adjustment factors assuming the individuals electing the plan have average morbidity.

Managing the Business

The rate formula should be routinely updated. Most health plans review and update the formula at least once per year, with some carriers doing quarterly updates. Updates are done using analyses and data accumulated in various management reports. These reports can assist the health plan in analyzing experience and updating the rate formula on a consistent basis. Examples of management reports include those listed in **Table 22-5**.

Most carriers also produce traditional accounting reports such as the income statement, balance sheet, and cash flow reports. These reports help measure health plan success in reaching its financial goals. One measure might be return on equity, a popular and universal measure of the value of a business. Return on equity is universal because it enables a business to compare its value to other types of investments, such as investing the carrier's surplus in a money market account, bonds, or the stock market. It is also easily comparable across different companies and industries. Other carriers instead target a percentage of premium and, as a result, might find it difficult measuring the value of the business versus non-insurance-oriented businesses. (Accounting reports are discussed in Chapter 21.)

■ THE IMPACT OF THE ACA ON UNDERWRITING AND RATING

The ACA includes provisions that could have far-reaching implications for health plans and their approaches to underwriting and rating. Most of these provisions do not take effect until 2014. Chapter 30 includes a full discussion of the changes and the timeline for implementation. Some of the changes that will most affect underwriting and rating through 2014 and beyond are listed in **Table 22-6**.

Most of these provisions add regulatory or operational burdens that health plans will need to navigate and address successfully. Underwriting and rating processes will need to be modified accordingly for plans to compete and succeed in the post-ACA environment.

An unknown issue at the time of publication is around how states will address the open-enrollment period. The ACA only requires states to have an annual open-enrollment

TABLE 22-5	Examples of Typical Ongoing Actuarial Reports

Financial gain/loss summaries by:	**IBNR development containing:**
• Total block of business	• Paid claim triangles
• Line of business (commercial vs. Medicare)	• A lag development of incurred claims
• Product line (HMO vs. PPO, traditional vs. CDHP)	• A projection development of incurred claims
• Group size (large group vs. small group)	• Paid claim lags to monitor the speed of claim processing
• Type of business (new vs. renewal)	• Analysis of seasonality/ working days
• Type of medical service (hospital inpatient, hospital outpatient, etc.)	• Medical cost trends, along with monthly, quarterly, and annually incurred claim estimates
• Calendar year or quarter	
• Each group individually (usually large group)	

Incurred claim costs by:	**IBNR reports by:**
• Total block of business	• Line of business (commercial vs. Medicare)
• Line of business (commercial vs. Medicare)	• Product line (HMO vs. PPO, traditional vs. CDHP)
• Product line (HMO vs. PPO, traditional versus CDHP)	• Type of medical service (hospital inpatient, hospital outpatient, etc.)
• Group size (large group vs. small group)	
• Type of business (new vs. renewal)	
• Funding arrangement (fully insured vs. self-insured)	
• Geographical area	
• Policy duration of the individual/small group (not usually applicable to large groups)	

Large group–specific reports including:	**Membership by:**
• Earned premium	• Line of business (commercial vs. Medicare)
• Paid claims	• Product line (HMO vs. PPO, traditional vs. CDHP)
• Medical loss ratio	• Group size (large group vs. small group)
• Large claim information	• Type of business (new vs. renewal)
• Benefit plan changes	• Contract tier
• Subscriber and membership counts by contract type	• Geographical area
	• Age and gender

TABLE 22-6	Impact of the ACA on Underwriting and Rating through 2014 and Beyond

Year	Provision
2010	• Beginning in September 2010, extension of dependent coverage to age 26.
	• Prohibition on rescissions except in cases of outright fraud.
	• Prohibition on exclusions for preexisting conditions for children.
	• Elimination of lifetime policy coverage limits.
	• Require first-dollar coverage for preventive services rated A or B by the U.S. Preventive Services Task Force; recommended immunizations; preventive care for infants, children, and adolescents; and additional preventive care and screenings for women.
	• States must establish a process for reviewing increases in health plan premiums and require plans to justify increases.
	• Require states to report on trends in premium increases and recommend whether certain plans should be excluded from the exchange based on unjustified premium increases.
2011	• Minimum loss ratios of 85% for large group and 80% for individuals and small groups (i.e., maximum retention loads of 15% and 20%, respectively).
2014	• Insurers will be required to guarantee availability and renewability of coverage to individuals and groups.
	• Insurers will not be allowed to use health status as a rating variable for individuals and small groups.
	• Only the following will be allowed to vary premiums: • Age-related pricing variations are limited to a maximum of 3 to 1. • The number of people covered under the policy (e.g., "single" vs. "family" coverage). • Tobacco use (except rates may not vary by more than a ratio of 1.5 to 1).
	• Complete phase-out of all annual policy coverage limits.
	• Prohibition of preexisting condition exclusions and coverage rescissions.
	• Reduce the out-of-pocket limits for those with incomes up to 400% of the federal poverty limit.
	• Insurers must offer an "essential" health benefits package at one of four minimum coverage levels.
	• Limit deductibles for health plans in the small group market to $2,000 for individuals and $4,000 for families unless contributions are offered that offset deductible amounts above these limits.
	• Limit any waiting periods for coverage to 90 days.
	• States will be required to establish health care exchanges to facilitate the purchase of coverage for individuals and small groups.
	• States must establish a risk adjustment mechanism for the individual and small group markets.
Beyond 2014	• Beginning in 2018, excise tax for plans with premiums exceeding a certain level.
	• States may expand insurance exchanges to groups over 100.

period, meaning insurers and HMOs must accept all applicants. This period could be as short as one month per year, although a state could elect to have multiple open-enrollment periods in a year or even continuous open enrollment. Since the risk of adverse selection rises when individuals can opt in and out of a market at will, the most likely scenario is something other than continuous open enrollment. On the other hand, the ACA requires insurers and HMOs to issue coverage without regard to health status. Whether or not states, or the federal government, will allow underwriting based on health status during periods without open enrollment is unknown.

CONCLUSION

The underwriting and rating functions seek to achieve an optimal balance between adequate, competitive, and equitable rates. Underwriting involves gathering information to analyze applicants' risk characteristics. Rating includes using the information gathered through underwriting and management reports to develop a final rate.

Recommended Reading

Bluhm WF. *Group Insurance.* 5th ed. Winstead, CT: Actex Publications; 2007.

Bluhm WF. *Individual Health Insurance.* Winstead, CT: Actex Publications; 2007.

Rosenbloom JS. *The Handbook of Employee Benefits.* 6th ed. New York: McGraw-Hill; 2005.

Information Systems and Electronic Data Interchange in Managed Health Care

James S. Slubowski

STUDY OBJECTIVES

- Understand the role of information services in a payer organization
- Understand the basic information systems functionalities
- Understand different approaches to delivering services, and the advantages and disadvantages of those approaches
- Understand privacy and security requirements for protected health information

DISCUSSION TOPICS

1. Describe and discuss the key attributes for the information systems area in a payer organization.
2. Discuss the different aspects of technology required by a health plan.
3. Discuss the merits of in-house or owned versus outsourcing.
4. Describe and discuss the data warehouse and its key attributes.
5. Describe and discuss how systems have evolved and how they might evolve in the future.
6. Discuss the role of systems in providing information to health plan executives, to regulators, to providers, and to consumers.

■ INTRODUCTION

Managed care organizations (MCOs) recognize the paramount importance of information technology to power their business. Focusing on administrative cost reductions, health improvement, and customer service are a few of the key elements that enable MCOs to be successful and thrive. To that end, MCOs are best positioned because of their holistic insight into the entire health care process. All patient activity, both administrative and clinical, flows through the MCO for financial and medical management activity. The potential of this information has not yet been fully tapped to improve care delivery, outcomes and financial results, but must be fully leveraged to abate the annual growth rate of the national health expenditure, which is projected to be 6.3% through 2019.[1]

MCOs have leveraged technology for automation of key business processes, sales and distribution of products, informatics, and enabling consumerism in health care. To offset increasing medical costs, automation is critical to promote MCO growth, while also decreasing administrative costs. MCOs do not produce a physical good, but provide a service, whether it be insurance, wellness, or consumer-driven information. Without information technology, delivery of these services would be impossible.

Information technology adoption trends over the last decade have been favorable. The participation in electronic connectivity and data transmissions, with the rooting of the Health Insurance Portability and Accountability Act (HIPAA), has increased greatly. MCO software vendors have improved and increased their functionality to provide holistic automation and integration for the MCO, therefore decreasing the need to purchase independent software to integrate. Most notably is the increase of member demand and usage of consumerism and self-service tools on the Web and mobile devices. The movement toward a paperless environment is becoming a reality for MCOs, which drives efficiencies in services and cost structures.

Another evolving trend is the sales model of the MCO has evolved with legislative changes and economic conditions. An increasing portion of MCO products and services are being sold directly to individuals versus employer groups. In 2014, this will be further expanded when the Patient Protection and Affordable Care Act (ACA) enables health care exchanges, including:

- Federal tax credits to low- to moderate-income people (133–400% of the federal poverty level) for those who do not receive employer-provided health benefits.
- Authorization for states to establish a health benefit exchange so that individuals buying insurance using the federal tax credits have access to high-value health plans.[2]

In preparation for this burgeoning business opportunity, MCOs' systems and processes must be elastic and scalable to handle the increasing individual market. This market expansion will tax core processes such as sales, member enrollment, premium billing, and customer servicing. Readiness is paramount for this true consumer-driven market requirement.

This chapter provides an overview of the foundational information systems and their key functionality required within MCOs to grow the business and reduce costs. The systems reviewed include:

- Core administration (managed care) system;
- Electronic data interchange (EDI) capabilities;
- Customer service system;
- Medical management system; and
- Data warehousing.

The MCO must remain nimble to react quickly to a constantly shifting market and legislative landscape, while delivering an exceptional experience to all customers. The chapter will continue with a review of systems, which provides value-added services into the future to support the trend in consumerism. These services offer distinction in the marketplace and engage the member, while strengthening the partnership with the provider and employer. Most importantly, success in this arena will transform the value of the MCO to the health care equation. As MCOs automate core business functions, dollars can be freed to invest in these new initiatives:

- Participating in health information exchanges and meaningful use with providers;

- Leading in provider and employer informatics with predictive modeling;
- Becoming consumer-focused in services; and
- Selling to the individual market.

Lastly, the chapter reviews privacy and security requirements for MCO information systems. As for all organizations that handle protected health information (PHI), the MCO must be steadfast and vigilant in this regard.

Information technology remains a key driver for success within MCOs and investments will continue to grow. The U.S. market for health care information technology is expected to increase to $9 billion in 2014, an annual growth rate of 17.5%.[3] MCOs are keenly aware of their dependency on information technology to not only reduce administrative costs, but most importantly, transform the value they can deliver to the health care equation. The winners will have recognized this from the onset.

■ FOUNDATIONAL INFORMATION SYSTEMS

An MCO's core managed care system is synonymous with a manufacturing company's enterprise resource planning (ERP) system, defined as an integrated information system that serves all departments within an enterprise. There are a small number of top managed care administration vendors in the marketplace today, which have significant market penetration. Only one known vendor has a complete and integrated health care product suite from core provider systems (e.g., electronic medical record) to core MCO administration systems, thus fully supporting an integrated delivery system.

Over the last decade, managed care system vendors have made great strides to expand the functionality of their software platforms. The marketplace for whole new system sales has dried so vendors have expanded functionality and worked to integrated third-party applications into their managed care system offering. Moreover, software vendors have adopted new development tools and system architectures such as service-oriented architecture (SOA) to "open" their software to improve and ease integration. Providing these new modules and integration points has provided new revenue streams for vendors to replace whole system sales. MCOs may decide to pursue a best of breed strategy for certain functionality niches; if so, the open architecture of the managed care software system will allow for easier integration. For example, a third-party financial or enterprise resource planning system (e.g., Lawson or PeopleSoft) will be interfaced with the managed care system to support the general ledger, accounts payable, accounts receivable, and purchasing requirements of the MCO.

The foundational or administrative systems are reviewed in this section. Managed care systems have a series of integrated functions or modules that work together to support the operations of the MCO. The modules may be included in the core software or may be integrated with third-party solutions. The modules that are reviewed include:

- Benefit configuration;
- Employer group and member enrollment;
- Premium management;
- Provider enrollment, contracting, and credentialing;
- Claims payment;
- Electronic data interchange (EDI);
- Document imaging and workflow;
- Customer servicing;
- Medical management; and
- Data warehousing.

Benefit Configuration

The benefit configuration module is one of the most important and critical setup functions to ensure claims payment accuracy and meeting customer expectations and provide the foundation for effective medical cost management. With this module, benefits are set up so they can be used by the member enrollment, claims payment, and customer servicing modules. During the configuration process, the following attributes will need to be affixed to the benefit package to control future processing:

- Product selection, such as
  - Health maintenance organization (HMO),
  - Preferred provider organization (PPO), or
  - Point of service (POS);
- Services covered, such as inpatient, outpatient, pharmacy, home care, wellness, and the like;
- Member liabilities, meaning copays, co-insurance, and deductibles;
- Member liability limits such as maximum out-of-pocket spend;
- Benefit maximums such as limits on the number of visits;
- Provider network accessibility and levels of coverage for each; and
- Primary care physician requirements for HMOs.

Benefit packages can be reused multiple times. Benefit standardization is encouraged as much as possible as this is one of most complex configuration activities within the managed care administrative system. System capabilities and limitations should be known to the Product Development team to ensure accuracy and automation can occur for new products that are designed and sold.

Employer Group and Member Enrollment

As described in Chapter 17, employer group enrollment establishes the employer group and its employees within the system. Basic demographic information is captured along with the appropriate product(s) and benefit package(s) that the group has agreed to offer their employees through the MCO. At this point in the process, the employer will be configured as self-funded or fully funded. Employer group information is important so the health plan can bill for coverage premiums, referred to as premium billing, or obtain funding for claims payment if it is a self-funded client. This process is typically a manual entry process.

Understandably, member enrollment is the largest volume portion. Basic demographic information is captured into the system for the contract holder, spouse, and dependents, if applicable. Demographic information captured includes name, address, date of birth, gender, and Social Security number; however, systems must be flexible to capture new demographic information such as e-mail address and mobile phone numbers to support text messaging. The benefit package is linked on the member's selection and, if applicable, an employer group linkage is also established. If required, a primary care provider selection will be entered. To minimize financial loss to the plan, it is critical to capture coordination of benefits (COB) information if another MCO is liable either primarily or secondarily. For annually renewing employer groups, an enrollment roster can be sent to the MCO with as-is, updated, and/or new information for the upcoming benefit year.

As mentioned earlier in the chapter, the use of electronic transactions has increased, especially with large employers (over 500 contracts). Data entry is typically automatic with only exceptions being processed manually. Once all of the member information is entered, fulfillment can take place, which is the creation and distribution of member materials such as member handbooks, certificates of coverage, and identification cards. The request for materials is automatically generated by the managed care system and typically sent to a third-party fulfillment company, if paper distribution is requested by the employer group and/or member. Electronic distribution is increasing in customer popularity.

The membership module will allow for retroactivity, adding the member with an earlier enrollment date. This is a frequent occurrence. When retroactivity occurs, claims payment, provider payment, and premium billings need to be adjusted accordingly in the next billing and accounts payable cycle. Retroactivity is generally limited to 90 days prior. Absent this limitation, reconciliation with claims payment, provider payment, and premium billing would be extremely difficult due to a large encompassing time span.

Managed care systems may allow for the automatic processing of flexible spending accounts (FSA) and health payment arrangements (HRA). When medical or dental claims are received by the MCO, payment can automatically occur to the provider (for the HRA) or member (for the FSA) if funds are available in the account. For example, if a member has a deductible and a claim for a qualified medical expense is received by the MCO, a check can be automatically generated to the member deducting funds from the FSA. A submitted form with receipts is not necessary. The member's preference on using this feature will need to be captured in the enrollment process.

Moving toward consumerism opens the door for the MCO to reinvent the enrollment process to better understand their customers. The MCO can use this information to create appropriately targeted and tailored messaging. Moreover, MCOs can use this information immediately to identify high-risk members, which may benefit from the assignment of a health navigator. Managed care systems should allow for the addition of customized fields so enrollment information captured can be expanded to include:

- Education level
- Ethnicity
- Areas of health interest
- Identification of current health issues (e.g., asthma, diabetes, obesity)
- Preferred mode of communication (e.g., e-mail, text, phone)
- Preferred date/time of communication

Premium Management

The primary source of income for a health plan is premium billing of individuals, employer groups, and the government, as described in Chapter 21. Premium rate development is determined by the Underwriting and Actuarial departments based on a number of factors that are discussed in great detail in Chapter 22.

The system will determine who is eligible for the coming month, the benefit package selected, and spouse/dependent count. The information is summarized, listing number of contracts at each benefit and premium amount quoted. A detailed list of policyholder names is also available to assist the employer in reconciling the bill. Premium billing is performed for the following month and an accounts receivable record is generated. Premium bills can be distributed electronically with electronic funds transfer (EFT) to accept payment in a paperless fashion. Payment can be automatically posted to the managed care system for tracking.

Within this module, broker or agent commissions are calculated based on the commission rate and active membership. Rates are determined though a number of ways that are agreed upon at the onset of the broker relationship with the MCO. Typical commission calculation examples include percent of premium, per member fee, or flat fees. An accounts payable record is generated for the broker/agent on a predetermined basis and an EFT can be initiated. Operational reports created by the premium billing module include billing status, accounts receivable aging, and billing summaries.

Provider Enrollment, Contracting and Credentialing

The provider enrollment modules of managed care systems will capture the necessary information about the provider and contracting terms to ensure accurate claim payment. Information captured about the provider includes name, address, clinic, phone numbers, fax number, website address, and so on, and also contracted payment terms as described in detail in Chapter 5. Based on contracting methods, providers may be aligned to only certain product offerings (e.g., HMO and/or PPO) so that information will need to be captured. The provider enrollment function also captures the provider's tax identification number for the generation of 1099s for tax purposes and group affiliation. Hospitals, professional providers, and equipment suppliers are enrolled within this module to allow appropriate adjudication of claims received from these entities. This module will also allow for the identification of providers that want electronic or paper remittance advice (or explanation of payment) and electronic funds transfer or paper checks.

Some managed care system vendors are expanding the provider enrollment modules to support credentialing; however, this is an area where a third-party solution may better suit the health plan. The credentialing process has very specific data needs and is very different than the provider payment process. Based on the approach adopted within the health plan, a provider database "source of truth" will need to be identified. That system will then be used for provider information data feeds to other systems. Maintaining provider information is a laborious task within all health plans as many provider databases generally exist. Without identifying and maintaining a provider database source-of-truth, a relatively simple task such as producing a provider directory can become very difficult. Since managed care systems are ultimately designed to pay claims, provider enrollment modules mainly focus on data collection to support the claims payment process and not necessarily the credentialing process; however, new managed care system releases are offering more features to support credentialing. Specific credential data elements include medical license information, malpractice data, and schooling credentials in addition to pertinent member-requested information such as gender, age, languages spoken, and so on. (This is further discussed in elements in Chapters 4 and 5.)

Claims Payment

Claims processing is the core feature of all managed care systems. It is addressed in detail in Chapter 18, so it is only summarized here.

Because of HIPAA, the majority of claims submitted are through an electronic data feed (EDI is discussed later in this chapter) and automatically loaded into the managed care system. The EDI process provides a precheck to ensure that the submitted claim is complete; if not, it is rejected at the point of submission to the health plan and returned to the provider. Systems will accept a variety of claims forms such as the CMS-1450 for hospital charges or CMS-1500 for professional services and dental. Paper claims received are scanned and converted to an electronic data feed for automatic loading. Manual data entry has been virtually eliminated in the Claims Departments of MCOs.

Key data elements captured during the claims entry process include:

- Member identification;
- Provider identification;
- Date of service(s);
- Procedure code(s);
- Diagnosis code(s);
- Place of service code(s);
- Type of service code(s); and
- Quantity.

After the claim is entered, it will go through a process of adjudication, which validates the claims information and approves or denies payment for the service or product. This adjudication process relies on configuration of approval rules established by the MCO. The outcome of the adjudication process is validation of the claim and the calculation of the provider payment and member liability, which is directly aligned with the member's benefit package and the provider payment contracts. Claims systems allow for both real time and batch adjudication processing. On schedule, the system will automatically process each batch through the adjudication review process and send the information directly to the accounts payable system if approved or will hold (usually referred to as pend) the claim for review by an examiner. If the claim is pended, a claims examiner must manually open each claim to review the status and determine if the system properly adjudicated it. If so, the examiner will deny the claim or override the pend code by repairing the claim to pay it. Automatic adjudication rate is calculated as those claims that are automatically approved or denied.

Adjudication rules within the claims system can be extensive or minimal. Checks for age, gender, eligibility, authorizations, accumulators, benefit maximums, special holds, and so on, can be taken into account as the system determines if and how the claims should be paid. These rules and checks are determined by the MCO in the initial system configuration process.

Claim modules will allow for integrated medical editing, either real-time or through batch processing, which checks all physician-generated claims for coding errors. This claim review process focuses on the appropriateness of billing versus the payment policies or cost of claims. Medical cost savings, realized through claim denials, are experienced from daily claim reviews, historical claims analysis, multiple procedure hierarchy, and correct use of claim modifiers. The claim review process evaluates the common practice of bundling or unbundling of submitted charges in a clinically and professionally responsible manner. For example, it verifies if the services were already paid as part of an earlier billing (e.g., postoperative office visit). Third-party software can

be licensed to interface with the claims system to validate provider billing appropriateness. If the claim meets any of the criteria, it is held for manual review or denied outright.

For utilization and health management reporting, the claims modules will accept encounter information, which is claims experience data for capitated members (a set monthly fee paid to a provider to care for a member). The claims system will recognize the data as an encounter and will not generate a payment transaction (check request) to the accounts payable system. The encounter information is written to the system database tables as if it were a regular claim, although the system treats it as prepaid.

Operational reports that the core module will generate include:

- Pended claims (e.g., authorization mismatch, procedure/gender mismatch);
- Daily claim volumes and automatic adjudication rates;
- Claim examiner productivity; and
- Inventory and aging analysis.

The ideal situation is for claims to be received electronically, automatically adjudicated by the system, and culminating with a record being sent to the accounts payable system for a check to be mailed or an electronic payment transfer to occur. In this situation, there is little or no manual intervention required, thus reducing labor expense for an ongoing process while improving volume scalability. MCOs have experienced an increase in automatic adjudication from 37% in 2002 to 75% in 2009. Also, 44% of claims were electronically submitted in 2002 versus 82% in 2009. To further highlight the efficiency gains of electronic commerce, 80% of claims submitted electronically could be adjudicated automatically compared to just 37% of claims submitted on paper.[4]

The key output for claims processing is provider payment and support of managed care reporting. Managed care information systems support a myriad of provider payment methodologies, as described in Chapter 5, although not equally well for all types. It should be noted here that those responsible for provider contracting will agree to a form of payment that, while possibly logical or rational, is not supported by the existing information systems without considerable programming or "work-around" solutions. In such cases, the administrative cost of administering payment becomes high as the value of automation is decreased. For this reason, it is incumbent on those in network contracting to understand the capabilities and limitations of the managed care software to ensure automation can be obtained for new payment methodologies.

For services that are not capitated, payments will be calculated based on the provider's contract. The appropriate fee schedule or payment method is chosen within the system and the payment is calculated. An explanation of payment (EOP) or remittance advice (RA) is included, which shows the specific claims that were processed with the payment. The provider can then use the EOP to close the open accounts receivable records within their billing system.

Electronic Data Interchange

To assist with automation and to lower the administrative ratio, EDI has been a low-hanging fruit opportunity. EDI allows the MCO to streamline its internal processes and improve its service levels for claims payment and enrollment. In the case of claims, manual data entry is eliminated and the claims information is entered sooner; as a result, the claims payment cycle is shortened and providers are paid quickly. The Administrative Simplification provisions of HIPAA require the Department of Health and Human Services to adopt national standards for electronic health care transactions and national identifiers for providers, health plans, and employers.

The passage of HIPAA's Administrative Simplification Rule has been instrumental with advancing electronic data interchange and a paperless work process since their required adoption in 2003. As stated earlier, 83% of claims were submitted electronically in 2009. Transactions are electronic exchanges involving the transfer of information between two parties for specific purposes. For example, a health care provider will send a claim to a health plan to request payment for medical services. HIPAA named certain types of organizations as covered entities, including health plans, health care clearinghouses, and certain health care providers. HIPAA also adopted certain standard transactions for EDI of health care data. These transactions standards follow the American National Standards Institute (ANSI) X12 version 4010 (at the time they were adopted) standards and are as follows:

- 834 for enrollment, which includes adds, updates, and terminations;
- 837 for claims;
- 270, 271, and 271R for eligibility inquiry request, eligibility reply, and eligibility roster, respectively;
- 835 for remittance advice or explanation of payment;
- 278 for referral and authorization;
- 276 and 277 for claims inquiry request and claims status reply, respectively; and
- 820 for premium payments.

Under HIPAA, if a covered entity conducts one of the adopted transactions electronically, they must use the adopted standard. This means that they must adhere to the content and format requirements of each standard. HIPAA also adopted specific code sets for diagnosis and procedures to be used in all transactions. They are:

- *International Classification of Diseases*, 9th Revision, Clinical Modification (ICD-9 CM) for hospitals and facilities;

- Healthcare Common Procedure Coding System (HCPCS) for ancillary services and procedures;
- Common Procedural Terminology, Version 4 (CPT-4) for physician's procedures;
- Common Dental Terminology (CDT); and
- National Drug Codes (NDC) for drugs.

Finally, HIPAA adopted standards for unique identifiers for employers and providers, which must also be used in all transactions.[5]

Effective January 2012, the new ANSI X12 version 5010 transaction set replaces the 4010 version. This new version of the HIPAA transaction set will have three major changes, including many transaction improvements, support for ICD-10, and clarification of the national practitioner instructions. Covered entities can begin testing of the transaction in mid-2011 and must be ready to receive transactions under the new version by January 2012. Provisions under the ACA will further increase the adoption of electronic data transmissions. The ACA includes requirements to adopt:

- Operating rules for each of the HIPAA transactions;
- A unique, standard Health Plan Identifier (HPID); and
- A standard for electronic funds transfer (EFT) and electronic health care claims attachments.

In addition, health plans will be required to certify their compliance with the adopted standards and operating rules. The Act provides for substantial penalties for failure to certify and comply with the new standards and operating rules.

With the acknowledgment of the EDI standards as outlined by HIPAA, the health care community can rally around a common set of data transmissions. Moreover, managed care system vendors can develop interfaces to these standards, thus minimizing the plans needed to develop the interfaces internally to a proprietary standard.

MCOs benefit greatly from EDI transactions for obvious reasons. The need for hired staff is lessened when the information does not need to be manually entered. Second, accuracy increases because data entry allows for the potential for human error. Third, internal processes can be shortened, thereby releasing payment sooner, generating ID cards faster, ensuring accurate cash collections at the provider office, and so on. In addition, most employers are now expecting the MCO's ability to fully process electronic files. Employers expect to see higher quality, faster turnaround, and greater efficiencies within the MCO, so premiums do not increase. The benefits of EDI are substantial and now embedded in many MCO processes.

Without industry-wide standards for consistency, EDI could be a costly and laborious task for the health plans. This is becoming true for enrollment and eligibility with employer groups. Note that employers are not "covered entities" by the HIPAA Administrative Simplification requirements. As a result, the health plan has very little influence with the employer to send the file in the X12 format. Most employers will send the enrollment file in a format that is convenient for them, expecting the MCO to conform. This causes the health plan to develop and maintain custom interfaces for each employer, requiring high-cost technical staff. Consequently, cost efficiencies could be reduced to the health plan. For example, most employers will use their human resources information systems to generate enrollment files to the health plan. Human resource systems manage many portions of benefits for their employees—health care coverage being one of them. Any change to the employee's record on the employer's human resources system could generate a record to be sent to the health plan. This requires sophistication in the health plan's enrollment system to detect if a pertinent change has occurred. These "edits" must be uniquely programmed for each employer that exchanges files with the health plan.

Many companies called clearinghouses have been established over the years to support health plans, provider, and employers with their EDI transmissions. The clearinghouse has relationships with many practice management system vendors and providers. The providers submit their claims electronically to the clearinghouse for distribution to the appropriate payer. Clearinghouses provide value-added services such as claims editing and reformatting. The provider who submits claims and the MCO that receives claims pay a per claim fee to the clearinghouse, which ranges from $0.25 to $0.75.

Document Imaging and Workflow

To further support the operations and efficiencies of the MCO, technology such as scanning, imaging, and workflow technology can be leveraged for all processes. When paper is received by the MCO, it can be scanned and converted to an electronic image and attached to a case within the managed care system. Not only does this eliminate the need for paper files, but retrieval is instantaneous, thus providing comprehensive insight on the case for the MCO employee.

In the case for data entry, a scanner supported by an Optical Character Recognition (OCR) application can interpret alpha-numeric characters on paper documents and write this information to an electronic file. The accuracy of OCR has become reliable. Paper claims received at the health plan can be scanned, with the data transferred to an electronic file. The file is read into the system automatically as is any EDI file that the plan would receive directly from a provider or clearinghouse. The document image is also stored so it can be easily retrieved and referenced when needed, thus eliminating the need for paper files. The process requires a scanner, OCR application, network servers, stations, and an electronic image storage device.

Workflow is yet another application that can electronically route work within an MCO. This work can contain electronic data, document images, or both. Workflow applications have rule tables that instruct the system as to where to route the work, either to an individual or to a work team queue. The workflow system controls inventory by monitoring queues and refilling them continually. Management monitors within the workflow application provide constant measures for productivity and inventory levels. The following are scenarios of applied workflow applications:

- Enrollment and claims for a specific self-funded customer are routed to one specific queue. Team members are assigned to the queue to process work. If one team member is absent, the system automatically distributes the work to the other members in the queue.
- Specific pended claim codes can be routed to specific individuals that have greater experience.
- Medical review cases can be sent to designated clinical staff based on the submitting physician or diagnosis.

Customer Services

Customer service is especially important to MCOs as it is an opportunity to distinguish itself from the competition. MCOs offer services, not physical products, so exceptional customer service is critical to its success. Accreditation by the National Committee on Quality Assurance (NCQA) and by URAC requires that health plans track contacts (calls, letters, or in-person visits), issues/grievances, resolution, and turnaround times. The MCO must demonstrate continuous improvements to member and provider issues by utilizing this contact and resolution data. To do so, an MCO must engage a customer servicing system to track this information for all customer contacts via phone calls, written correspondence (both U.S. Mail and e-mail) or face-to-face encounters. Data to be captured should include reason for the contact, date, resolution, and close date. Also, the customer service system should allow a case to be forwarded to another person or team for resolution if the customer services representative is unable to resolve the issue due to lack of knowledge (e.g., clinical issue). Needless to say, the customer service system is extensively used by the customer service department for its day-to-day operations; however, all MCO departments will interact with the system.

Many managed care software systems contain a customer servicing module; however, the MCO must determine if it will meet its current and future needs to exceed customer expectations. Customer servicing solutions are generally not the core competency of a managed care system vendor, so a third party or internally developed solution is often sought. These applications are referred to as customer relationship management (CRM) systems, which focus exclusively on integrating customer servicing, marketing, and sales.

Timely informatics from the customer service system is vital. Customer service departments must religiously review data of open cases to ensure that they are being completed in a timely manner. Recurring issues must be investigated to determine if they can be prevented or if additional education, either for the MCO or its customers, is needed on a specific topic. Resolution time reports should be analyzed to determine if the cycle time can be shortened, if not eliminated. Satisfaction surveys indicate that customers want issues resolved within the first call or they experience dissatisfaction with the MCO.

To properly service the Customer Services team, the customer service system must be easy to use, quick to capture information, and self-contained. If the customer service representative must jump to many other systems for information and reenter member, provider, or employer data, the process will become laborious and time-consuming, thus disappointing customers by adding time to the call and increasing costs. Inquiries for eligibility, claim, and authorization/referral must be integrated within the customer service module for quick reference and seamless transition.

To compliment customer services systems and many other MCO processes, intranet systems (Web-based systems that are only accessible by employees) are useful to provide electronic policy or reference information that is up-to-date and easily obtained. Intranets allow the easy distribution of reference material to the MCO staff. Resources available on the MCO intranet can include:

- Summary plan descriptions for each enrolled group;
- Certificates of coverage;
- Member handbooks;
- Medical policies;
- Clinical guidelines;
- Key performance indicators; and
- Departmental policies (e.g., claims, enrollment, premium billing).

Telephone technologies obviously play a major role within customer service departments. Full telephony integration with the customer service system is paramount for a good experience. For example, when prompted to enter your ID card number by phone, the information should transfer with the caller to the agent, so it does not need to be repeated, with the customer information automatically displayed for the agent. Also, interactive voice response (IVR) tools are valuable to provide self-service opportunities for members and providers to obtain information or service (e.g., eligibility inquiry, ID card request) without requiring an agent.

Providing options for customers to interact with the MCO is vital to assist customers at various points of the technology adoption spectrum. Customer service systems, intranet Web-based solutions, and telephony/IVR systems, when combined, can assist the health plan in providing excellent customer service that is quick and efficient.

(The customer service, or member services, process is discussed further in Chapter 20.)

Medical Management

The largest opportunity to improve health care utilization, quality, and cost is through proactive and intensive medical or care management. The medical expense is the single largest expense managed by the MCO, averaging about 80–92% of premiums received. The medical management system can assist with containing costs for the MCO, but it can also be a key enabler to assist the health plan with proactive health management.

The Medical Department of an MCO requires the use of an information system to help with utilization, case, and disease management. Contained within the medical management system will be all membership and utilization based on claims and clinical information. The medical management system goes beyond the claims payment system (or administrative data as it is sometimes referred) for member utilization and case profiling since it allows the Medical Department staff to enter clinical information obtained through their participation in the member's case or via electronic interfaces with providers' clinical systems. This critical information cannot be obtained from a claim.

The medical management system allows the Medical team to build a case either through an event such as an admission or through proactive management such as disease management or a member registry. The system allows the user to capture a predefined set of clinical information (e.g., blood pressure, peak flow meter readings) and ensures a certain protocol of intervention or activity is followed by the MCO's case manager or disease management nurses. Intervention dates can be set to notify the user of a key intervention point for themselves or anyone on the team. Clinical cases can be forwarded to the Medical Director for review and approval.

Authorization management is another key component of a care management system. If this module is not provided by the managed care software vendor, interfaces between the managed care system and the care management system will be needed to ensure authorization data is available for appropriate claims payment. Membership, provider, and claims interfaces will also need to be built into the care management system from the managed care system, if not a single integrated system.

Ideally, care management systems allow for true integration with a delivery system since a common system is used for medical management of a population. The medical management system allows the MCO to leverage clinical information, along with claims information for analysis and reporting. For example, clinical information is critical to enhance the plan's ability to stratify patients based on disease severity, as discussed in detail in Chapter 10.

Data Warehouse

MCOs are uniquely positioned as they are able to supply holistic information about the continuum of care based on administrative and clinical information. No other entity in the health care process can do this. The importance and dependency on this information is paramount since it can influence behavior, especially for efficient care delivery and improved outcomes. This wealth of information has not yet been fully tapped by the provider community. However, with the piloting of accountable care organizations (ACOs) and new payment methodologies such as bundled payments, this will certainly change.

Data warehouses can be created through purchased solutions or internal development efforts. By utilizing the information captured by all of the aforementioned systems within this chapter, MCOs can leverage a series of data sets for analytical purposes. These data sets create the continuum of care that was previously mentioned. The data sets that the MCO can leverage for analysis include:

- Medical claims, within network and out of network;
- Authorizations and specialty referrals;
- Prescription drug claims;
- Home care, durable medical equipment, skilled nursing, and behavioral health claims;
- Case and disease management data, including nonclaims-based clinical information such as vital signs, body mass index, and blood pressure results;
- Pathology and radiology results;
- Immunization data;
- Health risk appraisals;
- Personal interests, captured from evolving consumer-based systems; and
- Personal health information such as self-reported medical history information provided by the member, for example.

This information is captured by the foundational MCO information system and Internet-based systems utilized by the MCO and its members. The data is extracted to a warehouse system that is solely dedicated to financial, utilization, customer servicing, and outcomes analysis and reporting. This allows the MCO to easily analyze and report on this information while ensuring that production functions such as claims and enrollment are not impacted due to demanding computer resource queries. The data warehouse can support both production report queries and ad hoc queries; for MCOs, the data warehouse must support both.

In addition to storing the information in a separate environment, the MCO can develop or purchase data "enhancers" that add new characteristics to the claims records to aid with the analytical process. These third-party solutions can enhance the data in a way that it can predict certain utilization trends or health risks of the defined population. Discussed in detail in Chapter 10, examples of some "enhancers" might include:

- Episode of care creation (e.g., treatment of asthma, hip replacement);
- Event creation (inpatient, obstetrical event, emergency event, outpatient, etc.);
- Diagnostic categories;

- Case severity adjusting; and
- Therapeutic drug class categories.

In determining how the data warehouse and reporting environment should be designed, it is critical to engage a multidisciplinary team with the MCO. Users of the data warehouse must trust the data and understand how the data pieces fit together. The creation of a Data Governance Committee should be created to oversee the design, normalization, validity, and attributes of the data warehouse. This committee will approve source systems to be used, calculations, and the appropriate audience of the data.

The data warehouse can be leveraged to produce various reports that can be used by the MCO, providers, and/ or employers. Examples include:

- Medical utilization reports such as inpatient, outpatient, and specialty referrals;
- Provider profiling, which utilizes a common denominator such as episode of care;
- Specialty profiling;
- Hospital profiling;
- Physician Key Indicator Reports;
- Registries–member listings based on predefined present or nonpresent medical indicators, predictive and stratified;
- Drug utilization profiling including alternate prescribing opportunities;
- Employer group utilization reports such as employer demographics, medical and pharmacy utilization, inpatient analysis, and expenses by relationship to policyholder with comparisons to the health plan and the employer group's industry; and
- Required data extracts for the creation of Healthcare Effectiveness Data and Information Set (HEDIS®) reporting for NCQA accreditation. These reports could be created by the MCO or a third-party service or software solution.

ICD-10 Readiness

The importance and magnitude of the ICD-10 conversion warrants a brief mention. The implementation data of ICD-10 nationwide is October 1, 2013. An overview of the change is provided in Chapter 10. Diagnosis coding is pervasive in all MCO processes and systems, especially in pricing, medical management, and claims payment. The effort to prepare for this conversion is daunting and should not be underestimated. A full impact analysis of all processes and systems should be undertaken. Remediation efforts can be minimized by leveraging a conversion utility; however, the valuable potential of the expanded coding scheme would be lost and MCO performance improvement opportunities missed. The new ICD-10 version provides expanded specificity of diagnostic conclusions. This additional specificity can segment resource-intensive populations. ICD-10 information can be leveraged to improve MCO performance with:

- Medical management by improved population stratification and predictive modeling,
- Pricing through increased knowledge of diagnosis severity, and
- Provider contracting and payment terms since payment can be adjusted based on resource-intensive diagnosis.

■ TRANSFORMING THE VALUE OF THE MCO

As mentioned at the start of this chapter, MCOs are indeed uniquely positioned to help transform the health care delivery system for a host of reasons. First, and most importantly, the MCO is positioned to provide holistic insight into the health care process with its myriad data, as outlined earlier in the chapter. Second, MCOs have been proactive with consumer-driven transparency by providing information to members regarding cost, quality, and utilization of health care. Third, MCOs have provided consumer-based services such as direct-to-consumer sales, Web-based "member centers," and telephonic consumer service departments. Lastly, MCOs have been continually focused on prevention and wellness, not just episodic care. By leveraging the inherent skills of the MCO, care delivery and the health experience can be greatly enhanced. This section of the chapter provides an overview of those services that can separate the MCO from its competitors as well as establish itself as a leader in the transformation of health care delivery.

Health Information Exchanges and Meaningful Use with Providers

The United States government thrust health care into the national spotlight with the Health Information Technology for Economic and Clinical Health (HITECH) Act in its landmark legislation, the American Recovery and Reinvestment Act (ARRA) of 2009. The HITECH Act creates sweeping programs that aim to improve the health of Americans along five health care priorities:

- Improve the quality, safety, and efficiency of care while reducing disparity.
- Engage patients and families in their care.
- Promote public and population health.
- Improve care coordination.
- Promote the privacy and security of electronic health records.

The act uses the existing payment structures of Medicare and Medicaid to incent and penalize participating providers based on their attainment of key objectives for the meaningful use of a certified electronic health record (EHR). The three main components of meaningful use are:

1. The use of a certified EHR in a meaningful manner, such as e-prescribing.
2. The use of certified EHR technology for electronic exchange of health information to improve quality of health care.
3. The use of certified EHR technology to submit clinical quality and other measures.

Simply put, "meaningful use" means providers need to show they're using certified EHR technology in ways that can be measured significantly in quality and in quantity.[6] Moreover, to support interoperability, the State Health Information Exchange (HIE) Cooperative Agreement Program funds states' efforts to rapidly build capacity for exchanging health information across the health care system both within and across states. Awardees are responsible for increasing connectivity and enabling patient-centric information flow to improve the quality and efficiency of care. Key to this is the continual evolution and advancement of necessary governance, policies, technical services, business operations, and financing mechanisms. This program is building on existing efforts to advance regional and state-level health information exchange while moving toward nationwide interoperability.[7]

Electronic interfaces can be customized by the MCO to support meaningful use and the HIE. The MCO is well positioned to share information about a population since it receives information about utilization that occurs anywhere in the world. Utilization includes medical services and pharmaceuticals or products such as durable medical equipment. This information can be analyzed for potential high utilization or simply as a notice to the primary care provider regarding the holistic needs and activities of the patient. For providers leveraging an EHR, electronic information or "notices" can be transmitted to the provider by the MCO. Information could include:

- Instantaneous reminders for preventive care action;
- Notifications of admissions outside of the health system;
- Emergency room encounters;
- Disease management member registries;
- Predictive modeling of high-, medium-, and low-risk patients based on past medical consumption;
- Complete pharmaceutical profile of the member;
- Immunization information; and
- Insight into health risk appraisal results that could be a flag for high risk (e.g., inactivity, depression, family medical history).

Upon signing onto the EHR, the provider could have a managed care population profile available to engage its assigned membership when appropriate.

Leveraging the HIPAA EDI transactions reviewed earlier, real-time connectivity can occur for administrative functions. Electronic connectivity with the provider's practice management system (registration, billing, and appointment scheduling) can include member eligibility and claims submission. This allows health insurance status and copayment information to be verified by one system while the member is present for service at a provider's office. This supports the provider by streamlining their clinical processes and improving cash collections.

Examples of actions taken to date to improve information interoperability are as follows.

> The members of **Michigan Association of Health Plans (MAHP)** have decided to not compete on data needed to enhance the care delivery process. To that end, the Association and its membership collaborated to create a centralized Web solution, called "MAHP Connect." This solution enables the sharing of information from MAHP member health plans to their respective communities. Service offerings include a centralized portal with security and messaging, multipayer and Medicaid eligibility validation, multipayer claim status check, federated single sign-on capability from the MAHP portal to participating health plan portals, and secure file exchange services.[8]
>
> **United Health Group** is leveraging swipe-card technology with ID cards. This magnetic strip added to ID cards can be read through a standard card-reader machine. This feature will provide patient eligibility information and access to a personal health record, as well as process health care transactions. The capabilities are:
>
> - Confirmation of the plan participant's benefit eligibility and coverage information;
> - Access to the patient's personal health record, providing critical up-to-date information about medical history, current and past prescriptions, and diagnoses from other care providers; and
> - Real-time claim adjudication, allowing physicians to submit UnitedHealthcare claims online and receive a fully adjudicated response in seconds.[9]
>
> **Humana** has partnered with practice management systems and clearinghouses to develop an integrated real-time adjudication solution allowing physicians to collect the patient's share at the time of service. This real-time access means that a provider can give patients a statement listing the total cost of their service, including their copay, deductible, and out-of-pocket expense at

the time of their appointment, resulting in fewer delays, fewer overdue balances, and less time spent with collections.[10]

Some efforts began well and appeared to be gaining traction, but experienced setbacks. One example is Minnesota's HIE, which was a statewide secure electronic network designed to share clinical and administrative data among providers in Minnesota and bordering states. At one point, they reported over 4.2 million Minnesota residents being included in their secure patient directory. However, the Minnesota HIE terminated its business on June 30, 2011, consolidating its business operations with the Community Health Information Collaborative (CHIC) under the HIE-Bridge™ trademark.[11] HIE-Bridge is now seeking to provide electronic information exchange in Minnesota and Wisconsin.[12]

Even though the current interoperability efforts and vision are promising, the industry is years from full implementation. Technology adoption will truly transform medicine from a reactive to a proactive state of delivery, improving quality and eliminating redundancy. The patient-centered medical home initiatives are depending on this technological infrastructure to be in place. According to a 2009 study, physician practices spend $23–31 billion each year interacting with MCOs, approximately $68,274 per physician.[13] This is an amount better directed to improved care delivery due to information technology.

Provider and Employer Informatics and Predictive Modeling

The MCO will need to take its investment to the next level, which is informatics. The data warehouse is a consolidation of disparate data into common identifiers and agreed calculations. However, the data needs to be presented as key indicators and/or mined into actionable information, which is informatics. Software can be purchased and configured to allow for up-to-date common indicators or dashboards with the ability to drill into the indicators for additional information. For example, a dashboard indicator could be membership. Further drill-down could reveal membership breakdowns by gender, age, geography, industry, and so on. Informatics software has greatly improved to provide customized graphical dashboards with very responsive drill-down capabilities.

One critical tool in the informatics arsenal is the use of predictive modeling. This is a tool that combs through many sources of information including membership, demographics, claims, health risk appraisals, drug information, lab result data, and so on, to predict future health care costs and disease states for a defined population. For individuals, it can recommend intervention opportunities using clinical guidelines and a comprehensive overview of a member's health, including retrospective and predictable future issues that present a risk to a member's future care. Thus, members can be flagged for intervention before their health becomes catastrophic by using transparent predictive modeling, evidence-based medicine, and tailored clinical and business rules to identify, stratify, and assess members. This information can enable the MCO to design new disease/case management programs, initiate new interventions, or make better care decisions.

With the advent of accountable care organizations (ACOs) as part of the ACA, the importance and dependency on information has grown significantly since it can influence behavior, especially with care delivery. The vast amounts of information within an MCO are valuable, as it can supply 360-degree information about the continuum of care for the member. This information can be used by providers to proactively engage in the care for their members. For example, a physician can be notified by the MCO that their member was admitted or had an emergency encounter out of the service area because the MCO is notified on a timely basis. This offers many advantages to the provider such as very early awareness of the event and the opportunity to contact the member and coordinate any additional care if needed. Another example is a patient listing (or registry) of members that are health-risk-stratified by disease state so the provider can devote time to the appropriate population for disease state management initiatives. MCO information systems can truly aid the delivery of managed care by providing timely, complete information to the provider with the goal of improving the quality of life for their population.

The MCO's greatest strength is the ability to influence provider behavior based on well-rounded experience and cost data formed from claims (both medical and drug), membership, and clinical information. With the data manipulated through third-party algorithms, utilization or health predictions can be determined. The MCO's enrollment and utilization information allows the member's needs/risks to be identified by the provider—and possibly prior to becoming a patient. By proactively analyzing the member's utilization, MCOs can provide their greatest assistance to a provider by ensuring a population remains healthy and is appropriately utilizing their health benefits.

Concurrently, the interest by employers to assist in health management is increasing. Employers are interested in promoting wellness initiatives within their organization to reduce health care consumption and costs. As a result, they are requesting assistance from MCOs either through population profiles (e.g., high rate of obesity or smoking) or with member assessments/health risk appraisals. Survey data obtained through health risk appraisals coupled with claims experience data can successfully identify a high-risk population needing provider intervention. Please note there are confidentiality limitations with the amount of detailed data that can be shared with an employer. In a world with advanced technology and longer life spans,

employers, providers, and the MCO must partner to ensure appropriate, high-quality, and cost-effective health care is delivered.

Self-funded employers are very engaged in the health management of their employees to effectively manage their medical cost exposure and to increase employee attendance and productivity. Employers are requiring informatics tools from MCOs. Key indicators that self-funded employers should have about their employees include:

- Multiyear medical cost trends;
- Comparison trends to similar industries;
- Population trending by age and gender;
- Prevalent disease risks such as cardiovascular disease;
- Provider rates and utilization, both in-network and out-of-network;
- Future cost trends, including leveraging predictive modeling;
- Wellness/healthy living trends; and
- Health risk trends such as smoking, obesity, and inactivity.

Leading MCOs will provide this information to employers through informatics solutions that provide indicators with drill-downs, but are easily understood and actionable by the employers. This is a true value-added service that only MCOs can provide.

Consumerism and the Individual Market

Because of the ACA, the individual market will be ripe for significant expansion for MCOs. The accessible market will increase substantially with the creation of tax credits for certain incomes and the introduction of regulated statewide exchanges. To that end, the MCO business will become normalized and geographical market differences will be blurred. There will be little room for distinction among competitors. MCOs will truly need to transform to the consumer-based model for service and transparency to win business in the new world of legislative mandates. The type and use of information technology will be a key advantage to be seen as a distinctive leader.

The first significant change that all MCOs will need to make is learning to sell and service individual purchasers versus an employer group. MCOs will need to leverage phone and Web-based sales systems to:

- Display product information in consumer-oriented terms based on life stages such as single and healthy, married with children, retired, and so forth;
- Allow for the customized building of insurance and wellness products with instantaneous pricing quotes;
- Provide side-by-side product and service comparisons, again in consumer-oriented terminology;
- Allow quotes to be saved and reopened later when calling the MCO or through the Web;

- Enable the entire enrollment experience to be facilitated electronically or by phone once the consumer decides to buy; and
- Provide member materials such as ID cards, the evidence of coverage and summary of coverage schedule of benefits, and so forth electronically with the member's option to print, if desired.

These sale systems will need to leverage "open" technology architectures so interoperability can be reached once state health exchanges are operational. To secure future business, the experience between the state exchange and the health plan should be seamless. If the MCO's technology causes impediments with that experience, members will choose the route of least resistance, which could mean choosing a competitor's product. Guidelines on state exchanges are not yet published so MCOs will need to be mindful of the future as systems and technologies are selected to support the individual/consumer market.

To support consumerism with existing members, MCOs will need to provide access to services and support electronically either through Web-based or IVR-based services in addition to call centers. The experience must be exceptional or it will offer no differentiation to competitors. Members want to obtain help 24/7/365. The following are self-service tools that MCOs provide for members to:

- Review their benefits in greater detail;
- Determine how much of their deductibles and out-of-pocket expenses have been met;
- Review provider directory with greater search capabilities including geography, gender, areas of interest, specialties and quality score;
- Review pharmacy formularies;
- Review health care consumption for themselves and their families;
- Review and/or request member materials as described earlier; and
- Schedule wellness classes and services.

To improve the health care equation, members must be supported and engaged since MCOs and providers cannot change it alone. Members must be mindful and active to maintain healthy lifestyles and become actual consumers of health care. Providing customized education, direction, transparency, and self-servicing tools will be foundational expectations. To that end, the MCO can provide the following tools to differentiate themselves from the competition:

- Full transparency to cost and quality information for physicians, hospitals, and pharmaceuticals in easy-to-understand terms and life event scenarios;
- Cost information that is specifically aligned to the member's benefit at the time it is being requested; in other words, true out-of-pocket costs based on current coverage and deductibles;

- Treatment options such as alternatives to surgery;
- Medical encyclopedias for disease and treatment research;
- Automatic reminders for preventive health such as immunizations, physicals, cervical smears, and so forth;
- Awareness of disease management services within the MCO; and
- Recommendations as to how to save money through alternatives for health care services and products such as using in-network providers, using over-the-counter medicine alternatives, and the like.

MCOs can further leverage technologies to improve service and the overall experience for the member by doing the unexpected, for example, by using informatics, proactively outreaching to educate members when a change in benefits has occurred in the new plan year. Other examples would be calling the member when they convert to a high-deductible product to remind them that the provider may want to collect for the entire visit so they are prepared to pay or outreaching to the member on their birthday to offer a greeting, and to also proactively ask if they have any questions about their benefit or have feedback on their experience with the MCO.

Some plans are trying to provide a seamless transition between the Web, phone, and in-person experiences. For example, while using online chat, you request that a customer service agent calls you. When the phone rings, it is the same individual that you were chatting with online. They know exactly what you are inquiring about with no need to repeat anything. Related to that would be to provide a "call back when convenient" feature by providing the date, time, and phone number that is best for you.

With further sensitivity to being green, members are becoming less tolerant to unnecessary documents being printed and mailed. Many times, a member only has a single question and wants it answered immediately during their life event. The proliferation of mobile devices such as tablet computers and smartphones are the ideal tool for the MCO to be "green" while also providing timely and personalized service. Examples of MCOs that have embraced mobile technology include:

- UPMC Health Plan provides MyHealth Connect, a search for health care providers. From primary care physicians and specialists to hospitals and urgent care centers, the site will let you search based on location or name and then connect you to a phone number and even a map to give you directions.[14]
- eHealthInsurance has released its eHealth mobile platform to provide health insurance quotes for those on the go. Consumers interested in purchasing health insurance can now use their hand-held mobile devices. Mobile users can get quotes from a selection of eHealthInsurance's best-selling individual and family

health insurance plans, look up coverage details, create an account, and start an application. Shoppers can then call the eHealthInsurance call center or log in to the website from their home computer, complete the insurance application, and submit it for approval.[15]

- Priority Health offers account information on the go. The smartphone apps for iPhone, BlackBerry, and Android allow the member to view their ID card, find contact information for their doctor's office, view copays, and fax the ID card and copay information to their doctor, hospital, or pharmacy.[16]
- HealthPartners offers short-term paperless policies. The product is aimed at younger members in transition or just out of school. Enrollment and transactions are completed exclusively online. Members can print out an ID card, but the card can also be accessed on a smartphone and faxed to a provider.[17]

A few MCOs will set the bar for leading products and services aimed at the individual market. By doing so, they will effectively engage their membership and partner to improve the health care equation.

■ INFORMATION SECURITY

Systems and information is of paramount importance to MCOs and other companies that work with or maintain PHI. The MCO will assign a security officer to work with the information technology department to provide reasonable, yet extensive, safeguards against data loss and system breaches.

HIPAA required the Secretary of the U.S. Department of Health and Human Services (HHS) to develop regulations protecting the privacy and security of PHI. To fulfill this requirement, HHS published the HIPAA Privacy Rule and Security Rule. The Privacy Rule (or Standards for Privacy of Individually Identifiable Health Information) establishes national standards for the protection of PHI. The Security Rule (or Security Standards for the Protection of Electronic Protected Health Information) establishes a national set of security standards for protecting PHI that is held or transferred in electronic form. The Security Rule implements the protections contained in the Privacy Rule by addressing the technical and nontechnical safeguards that organizations must put in place to secure individuals' "electronic protected health information" (e-PHI). Within HHS, the Office for Civil Rights (OCR) has responsibility for enforcing the Privacy and Security Rules with voluntary compliance activities and monetary civil penalties.[18]

The Security Rule requires covered entities to maintain reasonable and appropriate administrative, technical, and physical safeguards for protecting PHI. Specifically, covered entities must:

- Ensure the confidentiality, integrity, and availability of all PHI they create, receive, maintain or transmit;

- Identify and protect against reasonably anticipated threats to the security or integrity of the information;
- Protect against reasonably anticipated, impermissible uses or disclosures; and
- Ensure compliance by their workforce.

The Security Rule defines "confidentiality" to mean that PHI is not available or disclosed to unauthorized persons. The Security Rule also promotes the two additional goals of maintaining the integrity and availability of PHI. Integrity means that PHI is not altered or destroyed in an unauthorized manner while availability means that PHI is accessible and usable on demand by an authorized person.[19]

Three categories of controls can be followed for the effective implementation of security controls for information systems and environments. The categories of prevention, auditing, and monitoring are outlined below with examples of actions that can be taken to ensure information system security.

Prevention

The following three elements are typically used for prevention:

- A firewall, which is a network filtering and monitoring device that is used to protect trusted systems from untrusted systems;
- Antivirus software that runs on a computer and scans files as they are saved or opened for patterns ("signatures") and deleting known "bad" files; and
- Intrusion prevention systems, which are network "sniffing" devices that sit on the network and works like antivirus software, but for network information ("packets") instead of files, ensuring that "bad" traffic is dropped before it reaches sensitive systems.

Auditing

Auditing is the next major element typically used to address security. Two examples are:

- Vulnerability scanning, which is software that scans addresses and ports on a network looking for known vulnerabilities and reports on them in order to find weak spots before attackers do; and
- Penetration testing, which is done by hiring specially skilled consultants to try and hack and "social-engineer" their way into systems to replicate a hacker attack.

Monitoring

Monitoring systems encompasses a broad array of reports and logs. Examples specific to systems security include:

- Security information and event management using software that collects log data from multiple sources (firewall, intrusion prevention, servers, etc.) and correlates the data looking for suspicious behavior or policy violations; and

- Investigate security incidents.

Access Control

The information technology department of an MCO is responsible for ensuring that there is only authorized access to e-PHI, either directly by people or by automatic interfaces. The following are examples of additional efforts that can be taken to ensure the security of the MCO's systems:

- Creating a secure e-mail system for PHI, which will automatically detect and encrypt all e-mails containing PHI;
- For each and every job change within the MCO, the human resources department and security officer obtains authorization from leadership that the employee's new job function requires access to PHI and, if not, appropriate system access is revoked; and
- All laptop and mobile device information is constantly encrypted in case of loss or theft. Once encrypted, PHI cannot be accessed without an ID and password should the device fall into the wrong hands.

■ CONCLUSION

The information systems in a payer organization of any type supports nearly every function and transaction the company performs. As the health sector becomes increasingly complex, systems must keep up and even exceed the market. More and more sophistication is being incorporated into MCO systems, and there is no end in sight.

Endnotes

1   Centers for Medicare and Medicaid Services. National Health Expenditure Projections 2009–2019. September, 2010. Available at: www.cms.gov/NationalHealthExpendData/downloads/NHEProjections2009to2019.pdf. Accessed August 18, 2011.

2   California Health Care Reform. Developing a health benefit exchange to make it easier to shop for and buy insurance. 2010. Available at: www.healthcare.ca.gov/Priorities/HealthBenefitExchange.aspx. Accessed August 18, 2011.

3   BCC Research. Healthcare Information Technology. 2009. Available at: www.bccresearch.com/report/healthcare-information-technology-hlc048b.html. Accessed August 18, 2011.

4   Webb J. New payment methods drive advanced claims processing. *Managed Healthcare Executive* (April 26, 2011).

5   Centers for Medicaid and Medicare Services. Transaction and code sets standards overview. Available at: www.cms.gov/TransactionCodeSetsStands/. Accessed August 18, 2011.

6   Centers for Medicaid and Medicare Services. EHR meaningful use overview. Available at: www.cms.gov/EHRIncentivePrograms/30_Meaningful_Use.asp#TopOfPage. Accessed August 18, 2011.

7   Office of the National Coordinator for Health Information Technology. State Health Information Exchange Cooperative Agreement Program. 2011. Available at: http://healthit.hhs.gov/portal/server.pt?open = 512&objID = 1488&parentname = CommunityPage&parentid = 58&mode = 2&in_hi_userid = 11113&cached = true. Accessed August 18, 2011.

8   Michigan Association of Health Plans. Health Information Exchange Leveraging a Single Platform: Connecting a Statewide Healthcare Ecosystem. June 29, 2010. Available at: www.mahp.org/media/HIEWebinarSlides062910.pdf. Accessed August 18, 2011.

9   UnitedHealthcare Group. UnitedHealthcare Groups makes it easier for physicians to administer health care with updated customer ID cards. 2009. Available at: www.unitedhealthgroup.com/newsroom/news.aspx?id = 788061b5-d650-441b-9046-1e10e2b9b49f. Accessed August 18, 2011.

10 Webb J. New payment methods drive advanced claims processing. *Managed Healthcare Executive* (April 26, 2011).

11 Minnesota Health Information Exchange. Available at: www.mnhie.org/index.html. Accessed August 18, 2011.

12 www.hiebridge.org/about.html. Accessed August 18, 2011.

13 Webb J. New payment methods drive advanced claims processing. *Managed Healthcare Executive* (April 26, 2011).

14 UPMC Health Plan. UPMC MyHealth Connect. 2011. Available at: www.upmchealthplan.com/about/mobile.html. Accessed August 18, 2011.

15 eHealthInsurance. eHealth mobile platform providers health insurance options for customers on the go. 2009. Available at: http://news.ehealthinsurance.com/pr/ehi/PRN-get-health-insurance-on-your-mobile-102611.aspx. Accessed August 18, 2011.

16 Priority Health. Your mobile ID card. Available at: www.priorityhealth.com/memberservices/your-account-online/mobile?WT.ac = aheadcurve&WT.ac = droid. Accessed March 14, 2011.

17 Hoisington A. Paperless policy show glimpse of health plans' digital future. *Managed Healthcare Executive* (April 10, 2011).

18 Health and Human Services. Summary of the HIPAA Security Rule. Available at: www.hhs.gov/ocr/privacy/hipaa/understanding/srsummary.html. Accessed August 18, 2011.

19 Ibid.

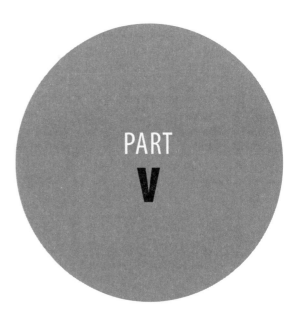

PART

V

Special Markets

"We're One
But we're not the same."

Bono [1991]

CHAPTER 24

Health Plans and Medicare

John K. Gorman, Jean D. LeMasurier, William A. MacBain, Stephen J. Balcerzak, Wendy K. Burger, and Amy Huang

STUDY OBJECTIVES

- Understand the impact of both the Medicare Modernization Act and the Patient Protection and Affordable Care Act on Medicare managed care plans
- Understand the different types of Medicare D and Medicare Advantage programs
- Understand what the ongoing contract requirements are for organizations that have entered into contracts
- Understand the factors the government uses in determining payments to Medicare Advantage organizations, including the STARS program
- Understand the rights and responsibilities of Medicare enrollees of health plans
- Understand some of the issues related to how an organization administers a Medicare contract
- Understand how the government monitors and tracks Medicare Advantage and Part D plans

DISCUSSION TOPICS

1. Discuss state licensure requirements that an organization must comply with to become a Medicare Advantage plan, any exceptions to the state licensure requirement, and any cases in which special consideration is given to particular types of entities.

2. Discuss the different types of Medicare Advantage plans, the key differences between them, and why such differences exist.

3. Discuss the impact of the Medicare D drug benefit and how that benefit affects the market.

4. Discuss the kinds of consumer rights and protections available to enrollees, or prospective enrollees, of Medicare Advantage plans.

5. Discuss how Medicare Advantage plans have been paid in the past, are paid now, and how they may be paid in the future.

■ INTRODUCTION

On March 23, 2010, President Barack Obama signed sweeping health care reform legislation into law. The bill represented the biggest expansion of federal health care guarantees in more than four decades, and its enactment was a giant victory for the President and Democrats after a brutal legislative battle dating back to the start of his presidency. Not a single Republican supported the measure, and when Republicans gained a majority in the House in the 2010 mid-term elections, they vowed to "repeal and replace" the Patient Protection and Affordable Care Act (ACA). At the time of publication, no significant element of the ACA has been repealed or blocked, but readers should note that every single major federal law has been amended, over and over again. Whether or not the ACA will be overturned is unknown, but the odds are very high that it will be amended in ways that cannot comfortably be predicted as of August 2011.

The ACA, with a near $1 trillion price tag and fundamental changes to health care financing and delivery, also made dramatic changes to Medicare Advantage (MA), the program in which Medicare contracts with private insurance companies, health service plans, and health maintenance organizations (HMOs) to provide benefits to seniors and the disabled. MA plans suffered significant cuts ($136 billion over 10 years), saw the introduction of a new payment methodology, witnessed the advent of performance-based bonuses, and had their enrollment season cut in half. In the wake of the largesse of the Bush administration and the Medicare Modernization Act (MMA) of 2003, with its payment increases and the introduction of the Medicare Part D drug benefit, the ACA felt like a cold shower for many MA stakeholders. Yet the program continues to grow.

This chapter provides a summary of MA and Part D contracting provisions for all types of health plans, as modified by the ACA and subsequent regulations and guidance. It starts with an explanation of the various types of health plans that can contract with Medicare, then to a discussion of how payment works in MA and Part D plans (PDPs). Following that is a discussion about how the Centers for Medicare and Medicaid Services (CMS) contracts with these companies, how the agency regulates virtually every aspect of plan operations, and how beneficiaries' and providers' rights are protected.

One way of thinking about this chapter is that it describes the "farm team" of health reform. In MA and Part D, the government created subsidized individual and group markets for insurance, and through a tight framework of regulation and guidance, it delivered a public good with great value to one in four Medicare beneficiaries. Health reformers have much to learn from this experience.

■ BACKGROUND

For the last 30 years, a political "pendulum effect" has characterized the relationship between the Medicare program and the health plans contracting with it to provide benefits to older adults and individuals with disabilities. The core of enrollment in Medicare plans is disproportionately lower-income and minority beneficiaries—a typically Democratic constituency that trades some reduced choice of providers in exchange for less costly benefits. But free-market Republicans remain the program's staunchest supporters, while most Democrats rail against profiteering insurance companies and seek greater accountability for their performance. The increase in publicly traded health plans participating in the program in the 1990s and rising to prominence in the 2000s fanned partisan passions. For the past two decades, usually in conjunction with a change of leadership in either the White House or the Congress, legislation has been enacted that reflects Washington's mixed feelings about private companies organizing all health care services for those in Medicare. As a result, every several years the pendulum swings from free markets and competition to regulation and accountability.

Chapter 1 provided background on the early days of Medicare and managed health care. Recall that the origins of the HMO Act of 1973 were initially aimed at controlling the rising cost of traditional fee-for-service (FFS) Medicare, but when it came time to act, Congress passed the law but focused it on the employer-based sector, and provisions applicable to Medicare failed to accomplish much. It took until 1982, when Congress passed the Tax Equity and Fiscal Responsibility Act (TEFRA), to authorize the Medicare program to pay HMOs on a capitated basis, provided that they met Medicare's participation requirements; regulations were not finalized until 1985, however. The hope was that Medicare HMOs would lower costs and use the savings to offer more comprehensive benefits than FFS Medicare, for example, less cost-sharing and coverage of prescription drugs, something that FFS Medicare didn't cover at all. For the most part, that is exactly what happened.

Plan participation and enrollment in Medicare Risk and Cost (Section 1876) programs grew steadily until the late 1990s, propelled by investments made in the program by publicly traded companies such as Humana and United Healthcare. The trend was halted when President Bill Clinton signed the Balanced Budget Act (BBA) of 1997, which made significant changes to Medicare health plan payments and instituted a number of aggressive operating requirements. Dozens of plans and approximately half of the beneficiaries in the program (then called Medicare + Choice) exited over the ensuing 4 years.

The signing of the MMA of 2003 by President George W. Bush reignited enrollment with:

- The new Medicare Part D drug benefit, administered entirely by the private sector through either free-standing PDPs or Medicare Advantage Part D Plans (MA-PDPs);
- Renaming Medicare's managed health care program Medicare Advantage;
- Creating new regional MA preferred provider organization (PPO) plans;
- Creating new special needs plans (SNPs);
- Dramatically increasing payment for MA plans; and
- Introducing competitive bidding and risk-adjusted payments.

The MMA was successful in that it made Medicare plans available to almost all beneficiaries and significantly increased enrollment. As of August 2011, out of 47.7 million Medicare beneficiaries, enrollment in some type of private health plan, not counting Medicare supplemental insurance or MediGap, is as follows:

- Part D plans: 27.9 million enrollees
  - Stand-alone PDPs: 18.3 million enrollees
  - MA-PDPs: 9.7 million enrollees
- Other MA plans: 11.5 million enrollees
- SNPs: 1.2 million enrollees[1]

Medicare Part D has proven to be an unqualified success, with over 85% of enrolled beneficiaries stating they are satisfied or very satisfied with their plan, and with the overall program costs coming in at $100 billion less than projected.

The pendulum swung back again when Congressional Democrats balanced much of the cost of health care reform in the ACA on to MA. Much of the cost of the ACA was paid for by Medicare payment reductions, with health plans taking $136 billion in payment cuts over 10 years. The ACA also ushered in a new era of value-based purchasing of health care by government: a data-driven rush to the highest-rated MA and PDP products at the lowest price. By 2017, the average MA plan will see payments cut by 17% relative to projections under the MMA, and will face unprecedented scrutiny of most aspects of their Medicare operations in near real-time. Furthermore, plans will see growing proportions of their revenues contingent on performance against dozens of quality and satisfaction measures.

Still, plan participation remains steady because MA and Part D have become staple products for many regional and local insurers like Blue Cross and Blue Shield plans, and the publicly traded companies now dominating the program. These large private payers derive an average of 26% of their revenues from Medicare—double the share of revenue in 1997. Medicare and private insurers are now codependent—the plans are in too deep to withdraw, and politicians are reliant on the private sector to "bend the cost curve" of Medicare's unsustainable expenditures, especially on chronic diseases. Private health plans are entrenched in Medicare, and policymakers may always be ambivalent about that reality.

■ TYPES OF MEDICARE ADVANTAGE PLANS

The Medicare law defines three categories of MA plans that private health companies can offer to Medicare beneficiaries: Coordinated care plans that have contracted provider networks; medical savings account (MSA) plans that are Medicare's version of consumer-directed plans; and private FFS (PFFS) plans that are a model unique to Medicare. Since the inception of Medicare managed care in 1972, Congress has amended the program by adding plan types to increase the choices available to Medicare beneficiaries. Organizations that have an MA contract may offer different types of plans in a given service area; for example, a payer may offer an HMO-based plan and a PPO-based plan. As noted already, Part D plans are offered by private plans including stand-alone PDPs and MA-PDs. Approximately two-thirds of Medicare beneficiaries enrolled in Part D plans are enrolled in PDPs and one-third in MA-PDs.

Coordinated Care Plans

Coordinated care plans use a network of providers to deliver the benefit package approved by Medicare. CMS must approve the provider network to ensure that enrolled Medicare beneficiaries will have sufficient access to covered services. Coordinated care plans may use financial incentives or utilization review to control the use of services and must meet quality requirements. Other than in an emergency or urgently needed situation, a coordinated care plan has no obligation to cover the cost of care if a non-network provider is used, even if the care would have been covered under FFS Medicare. Coordinated care plans include HMOs, regional and local PPOs, and SNPs, all of which are discussed briefly below. Other types of coordinated care plans such as Religious and Fraternal Benefit Society plans and senior housing facility plans are not discussed due to their limited availability.

Health Maintenance Organizations

Medicare HMOs are similar to HMOs in the commercial market; for example, they offer more controlled and limited networks. Medicare HMOs are the oldest coordinated care plan type and have the highest enrollment (65% of all MA enrollments in 2010). Medicare offers a point-of-service (POS) option where HMOs can cover services out-of-network.

Preferred Provider Organizations

Medicare PPOs are similar to PPOs in the private sector, in that they do not use primary care physician "gatekeepers," typically have larger networks and provide some coverage for noncontracting providers. Unlike many purely commercial PPOs, MA-PPOs must meet MA quality requirements but only for services provided in-network. PPOs must have a maximum out-of-pocket limit for in-network services and a catastrophic limit on in and out-of-network services.

Medicare offers two types of PPOs: local PPOs and regional PPOs (RPPOs). *Local PPOs* have the flexibility to choose the service area where they will operate (e.g., one or multiple counties). *Regional PPOs* were added to Medicare by the MMA to provide increased access to private plans, particularly in rural counties. RPPOs must serve all counties in one or more of 26 statewide or multiple state regions designated by CMS. Because of the difficulty in setting up networks in broader geographic areas, RPPOs have more flexibility; for example, they can meet access standards by paying FFS rates and Medicare will pay for "essential" hospitals in rural areas if providers refuse to contract with the RPPO. RPPOs also have other requirements that are different than local PPOs; for example, if they chose to impose a deductible, it must be a single deductible for Part A and Part B services (unlike Medicare FFS). The single deductible may be different for in-network and non-network services.

Under the MMA, a moratorium was placed on new MA plans other than RPPOs during 2006 and 2007, in order to support their creation and growth. Since then, local MA PPOs also appeared, and by 2010 PPOs had increased their market share, with local PPOs enrolling 12% of the market and RPPOs enrolling 7%.

Special Needs Plans

SNPs are coordinated care plans (usually offered by HMOs) that limit enrollment to individuals with special needs. There are three types of SNPs:

- D-SNPs—Dual-eligible SNPs enroll beneficiaries that are eligible for both Medicare and Medicaid ("dual eligibles"). There are different types of D-SNPs based on Medicaid eligibility criteria. New and expanding D-SNPs must have a contract with the state Medicaid agency that meets a number of requirements intended to ensure that Medicare and Medicaid benefits and requirements are coordinated.
- I-SNPs—Institutional SNPs enroll beneficiaries who are institutionalized in a SNF, NF, ICF/MR, or psychiatric facility for 90 days as assessed through CMS-approved assessment tools. I-SNPs may also enroll a person with similar needs living in the community as assessed by a state assessment tool administered by an independent party. I-SNPs may also restrict enrollment to individuals that reside in a contracted assisted-living facility.
- C-SNPs—Chronic care SNPs enroll beneficiaries with one or more severe or disabling chronic conditions.

The benefit plans offered by C-SNPs must include benefits beyond Part A and B services and the minimum care coordination requirements for other types of MA plans, including supplemental health benefits related to the chronic condition, specialized provider networks, and appropriate cost-sharing.

The SNP authority was enacted in the MMA for a limited period of time to allow SNPs to improve care for vulnerable groups through improved coordination and continuity of care. The SNP program has been extended through December 2013 with new requirements. For example, the Medicare Improvements for Patients and Providers Act of 2008 (MIPPA) required a specific definition of "severe or disabling" chronic conditions for C-SNPs. Based on the recommendations of a panel of clinical providers, CMS specified 15 chronic conditions:

1. Chronic alcohol and other drug dependence;
2. Certain auto-immune disorders;
3. Cancer, but excluding precancer conditions;
4. Certain cardiovascular disorders;
5. Chronic heart failure;
6. Dementia;
7. Diabetes mellitus;
8. End-stage liver disease;
9. End-stage renal disease requiring dialysis;
10. Certain hematological disorders;
11. Human immunodeficiency virus/acquired immunodeficiency syndrome (HIV/AIDS);
12. Certain chronic lung disorders;
13. Certain mental health disorders;
14. Certain neurological disorders; and
15. Stroke.

A C-SNP can target multiple chronic conditions that are clinically linked and comorbid in one of five specified CMS groupings (e.g., diabetes and chronic heart failure) or customized into groupings of the 15 conditions. Beneficiaries only need to have one qualifying condition to enroll.

CMS has contracted with the National Committee for Quality Assurance (NCQA; see Chapter 15) to develop specific quality measures for the Healthcare Effectiveness Data Information Set (HEDIS®; see Chapter 15) and structure and process measures that evaluate the quality of care provided by SNPs. SNPs began reporting on the first phase of these measures in 2009. The measures will be refined over time and will eventually include outcomes measures. Beginning in 2012, SNPs are required to be certified by NCQA.

By 2010, 1.3 million beneficiaries were enrolled in SNPs, with most enrolled in dual-eligible SNPs.

Private Fee-for-Service Plans

PFFS plans were authorized in 1997 and are a model unique to Medicare. Enrollees are permitted to self-refer to any

Medicare provider willing to accept the individual as a patient (known as "deemed providers") consistent with the rules of the plan regarding coverage. The PFFS plans pay providers on a FFS basis at Medicare fee schedule rates, do not place the provider at financial risk, and do not vary rates by utilization. A PFFS plan is permitted to vary the payment rates based on the provider specialty, location, or other factors not related to utilization. PFFS plans may increase payment rates to a provider based on increased utilization of specified preventive or screening services.

PFFS plans and enrollment grew very rapidly beginning in 2006 when MMA payment rates went into effect. Because there was no cost in establishing provider networks, there was little barrier to entry and by 2008 PFFS plans were available to almost all Medicare beneficiaries. Beneficiaries were attracted to PFFS plans because they were cheaper than MediGap policies, which most beneficiaries buy to supplement FFS Medicare. Often PFFS plans were the only choice in rural counties and this rapid expansion accomplished the goal of the MMA to expand choices, especially in rural areas.

However, Congress became concerned about the performance of many of the PFFS plans; for example, the failure to pay providers correctly or in a timely manner, marketing abuses, and beneficiary confusion. PFFS plans also received a high payment rate, despite not having a requirement to add value; for example, there were no quality improvement or care coordination requirements for PFFS plans. Congress amended the authority beginning in 2011 to require PFFS plans to operate as full network plans in areas with at least two coordinated care plans. This amendment preserved the open access model in rural counties where it was difficult for plans to contract with sufficient providers to meet Medicare access requirements. In response to this new network requirement, many PFFS plans chose to exit the market. As a result, PFFS enrollment, which had peaked at 2.3 million in 2009, declined to 1.5 million enrollees in 2010.

Special Rules for Group Retiree Plans

CMS has historically offered MA plans wide latitude to negotiate with employers and unions for retiree coverage under MA. The MMA went farther by including a very broad waiver provision to encourage employer- or union-sponsored plans to offer retiree coverage through MA plans and PDPs, and added a new option where employers or unions could directly contract with CMS as MA plans or Part D plans. By 2010, one-sixth of MA enrollees were in employer group plans and 8% of PDP enrollees were in employer group plans.

CMS waivers allow group retiree MA plans to:

- Enroll only retirees in MA plans following the employer or union's eligibility rules;
- Group enroll and disenroll retirees;

- Disregard the minimum enrollment requirement;
- Extend service areas to where retirees reside;
- Enroll beneficiaries with end-stage renal disease (ESRD) and Part B-only retirees;
- Modify websites, call centers, and marketing;
- Vary cost-sharing levels and premiums (e.g., by markets and different employer subsidy levels);
- Offer noncalendar year plans;
- No requirement to submit a Part D bid; and
- Provide flexibility on state licensure and administrative and management requirements for employer-direct contracting plans.*

Medical Savings Account Plans

Medicare MSA plans combine a high-deductible MA plan and a medical savings account, which is an account established in conjunction with an MSA plan for the purpose of paying the qualified medical expenses of the account holder on a pretax basis. These plans offer a high-deductible insurance plan similar to commercial health payment accounts (HRAs) and health savings accounts (HSAs) described in Chapter 2. The primary difference is that only Medicare, and not the beneficiary or another party on their behalf, may make a deposit into the account.

MSAs have not had much success in the Medicare market. As of January 2011, CMS had approved only two contracts and there were only around 1,000 beneficiaries enrolled in MSA plans. The plans are confusing to beneficiaries and the insurers and the plan design do not allow beneficiaries to contribute to their tax-free accounts.

Medicare Cost Plans

A Medicare Cost Plan is not an MA plan, and its roots go back decades. It is a type of Medicare HMO that works in much the same way, and has some of the same rules, as an MA-HMO, with two key differences. First, it is paid based on the actual costs incurred by the plan, not through the payment methodology described later in the chapter. Second, Medicare beneficiaries enrolled in a Medicare Cost Plan may go to a non-network provider, and the services are covered under traditional FFS Medicare. They are only included here for the sake of completeness since there are still enrollees, but are not discussed any further except in the section to follow that provides background to how MA plans are paid.

Trends in Medicare Advantage Enrollment and Plan Availability

The year 2010 saw an all-time high for the number of Medicare beneficiaries enrolled in an MA plan when 24% of all Medicare beneficiaries chose these private plans. This steady

---

*As noted in Chapter 30, the Employee Retirement Income Security Act (ERISA) allows single-employer benefits plans to operate without state licensure.

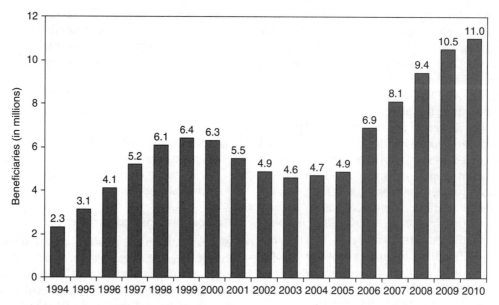

Note: MA (Medicare Advantage).

FIGURE 24-1 Enrollment in MA plans, 1994–2010

Source: Data from Medicare Payment Advisory Commission, "A Data Book: Healthcare spending and the Medicare program, June 2010," p. 159.

rise in MA enrollment from 2005, when 4.6% of Medicare beneficiaries were enrolled in MA plans, can be attributed to the MMA. The MMA increased payments to private plans, leading to a dramatic increase in enrollment. **Figure 24-1** displays the enrollment in MA plans from 1994 to 2010.[2]

The number of MA plans has also increased since the enactment of the MMA. From 2006 on, all Medicare beneficiaries had access to an MA plan. A drop in PFFS plans and CMS rules encouraging consolidation of low enrollment and duplicative plans decreased the number of total MA plans available nationwide in 2011 by 13%. However despite the decline in total number of plans nationwide, Medicare beneficiaries in 2011 have on average 24 plans to choose from. The distribution of MA enrollees by plan type as of February 2011 can be seen in Figure 1-2 in Chapter 1.

■ MEDICARE ADVANTAGE BENEFITS

MA plans can offer multiple "benefit plans" such as a high option and low option. Each benefit plan must have a uniform premium and benefit structure and with the exception of SNPs, must be available to all residents of the service area of the plan. MA plans must offer at a minimum the FFS level of Medicare services and cost-sharing, and with the exceptions noted below, they must also offer at least one benefit plan with Medicare Part D drug coverage throughout their service area.

PFFS plans have the option of including Part D drug coverage, but MSA plans are not permitted to include Part D coverage as part of the plan. All benefit plans offered by SNPs, a type of coordinated care plan that serves the most vulnerable beneficiaries, must include Part D drug coverage. Most MA coordinated care plans also offer benefit plans that do not include drug coverage to serve beneficiaries that decline Part D coverage or obtain it elsewhere; for example, beneficiaries who receive drug coverage from their employer can elect an MA-only plan.

Beneficiaries who are enrolled in a coordinated care MA plan can only get Part D drug coverage from the MA plan. If they enroll in an MA plan without Part D, they cannot enroll in a stand-alone PDP. Beneficiaries who enroll in a PFFS plan without Part D or an MSA plan may enroll in a stand-alone PDP for drug coverage.

The Medicare Part D Benefit Design

The statute specifies the basic Medicare Part D drug benefit design that plans use to submit competitive bids. Most MA-PDs do not use the standardized basic benefit design (other than as the basis for submitting Part D bids, as discussed below). MA-PDs typically offer an actuarially equivalent benefit design (e.g., copayments in lieu of cost-sharing). Many MA-PDs offer an enhanced benefit design that fills in the deductible and/or the "donut hole" (described below), or use rebate dollars (described earlier in this chapter) to buy down the Part D premium.

Under the basic Part D plan, drugs are covered after the enrollee pays an annual deductible (see **Figure 24-2**). In the first phase of coverage the enrollee pays 25% coinsurance and the government pays 75% up to an initial coverage limit. In the second phase between the initial coverage limit and a catastrophic limit, there is a coverage gap referred to as

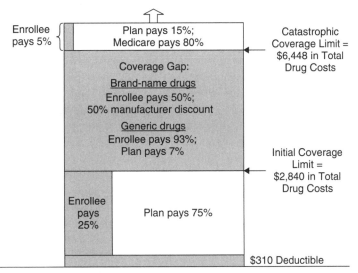

FIGURE 24-2 Standard Benefit Design, 2011

Source: Modified from "Standard Medicare Prescription Drug Benefit, 2011." Kaiser Slides, The Henry J. Kaiser Family, January 2011. http://facts.kff.org/chart.aspx?ch=1929.

"the gap" or the "donut hole," where the enrollee had been responsible for 100% of the costs of the drugs. In the third or catastrophic phase after the out-of-pocket threshold is met, the beneficiary pays 5%, the government pays 80%, and the Part D plan pays 15%. The reason for this unusual benefit design is that at the time the MMA was enacted, there was insufficient funding to offer a comprehensive drug benefit design that was typical in the commercial market. Plus, it mimicked the consumer-directed health plan (CDHP; see Chapters 1 and 2) design that was becoming popular.

The primary difference between an MA-PD and a PDP drug benefit is that the MA-PD plan can use savings from their Part C bid to make the Part D drug more attractive to beneficiaries, for example, by offering better drug coverage or lower cost-sharing. MA-PDs can meet Part D access standards through pharmacies that they own and operate.

As part of health reform, the ACA begins to close the coverage gap between 2011 and 2020. If a beneficiary without a low-income subsidy (LIS) reaches the coverage gap beginning January 1, 2011, he or she will have a 50% discount on brand name drugs at the point of sale. Cost-sharing will be phased down for generic drugs beginning in 2011 and for brand name drugs in 2014. Cost-sharing will be reduced each year until beneficiaries pay only 25% of the cost of covered Part D drugs by 2020. Figure 24-2 shows the standard benefit design for 2011. **Table 24-1** shows enrollee cost sharing as phased down under the ACA.

Formularies

Part D plans are allowed to develop formularies that limit the number of drugs that are covered under the plan. The formularies are developed by a Pharmacy and Therapeutics

(P&T) Committee that includes pharmacists and practicing physicians. Part D formularies must include drug categories and classes that cover all disease states. Each category or class must include at least two drugs (unless only one drug is available for a particular category or class, or only two drugs are available but one drug is clinically superior to the other for a particular category or class). Part D formularies must include all or substantially all drugs in the following classes: immunosuppressant (for prophylaxis of organ transplant rejection), antidepressant, antipsychotic, anticonvulsant, antiretroviral, and antineoplastic. The formularies are

TABLE 24-1	Enrollee Cost-Sharing in the Coverage Gap under the ACA	
Year	Generic drugs	Brand name drugs
2010	100%	100%
2011	93%	50%
2012	86%	50%
2013	79%	47.5%
2014	72%	47.5%
2015	65%	45%
2016	58%	45%
2017	51%	40%
2018	44%	35%
2019	37%	30%
2020	25%	25%

Source: HHS FY 2012 budget. Available at www.hhs.gov/about/hhsbudget.html#HHSBudgetinBriefandPerformanceHighlights.

submitted to CMS in April and are reviewed to ensure that they are "adequate" and include a range of drugs in a broad distribution of therapeutic categories and classes. CMS also reviews the formulary to ensure that it does not substantially discourage enrollment by any group of beneficiaries. Part D plans typically have four or five tier formularies, where the fifth tier is a specialty tier.

The P&T Committee also recommends formulary management activities that limit beneficiary access to drugs including prior authorizations, step therapies, quantity limitations, generic substitutions, and other drug utilization review.

Medication Therapy Management Programs

Part D plan sponsors also are required to offer a medication therapy management (MTM) program that targets beneficiaries with multiple chronic diseases and high drug costs. Currently, MTM programs must target four of seven specified chronic conditions such as hypertension, heart failure, or diabetes. In addition, MTM programs must target beneficiaries who incur annual drug costs of $3,000 or more. MTM programs include a comprehensive medication review, ongoing monitoring, and beneficiary or prescriber interventions, if necessary.

■ MEDICARE ADVANTAGE PAYMENT

The MMA laid the groundwork for significant changes in how private Medicare managed health care plans are paid. It is useful to know the background about payment of Medicare plans, which was only briefly touched upon in Chapter 1.

Background

Recapping from Chapter 1, the original Medicare program as enacted in 1965 was based on the Blue Cross and Blue Shield plans as they operated in the mid-1960s. Medicare benefits provided under Part A of the Medicare act cover hospital claims and claims for services from a number of other institutional providers of care, like the original Blue Cross plans; while Part B of the act covers claims from physicians and other individual health care providers, like the original Blue Shield plans. Part A paid providers on the basis of "reasonable cost," while Part B paid on the basis of historical charges.

From the beginning, Medicare paid the few HMO-like organizations then in existence for the reasonable cost of caring for Medicare beneficiaries. Since these organizations provided care either through a salaried physician staff or a capitated medical group, there was no claim history on which to base payment, and Medicare followed the established path of part cost-based payment. This is the origin of the Medicare Cost Plans briefly noted earlier.

In 1972 and actually preceding the HMO Act of 1973, amendments to the Social Security Act authorized per capita payments to HMOs either on a risk basis or a cost basis.

The amendments allowed for continuation of the cost-based payment model. Two cost-based models emerged. Prepaid group practice plans (PPGP) were paid for the professional services provided by the medical group's physicians, while Medicare paid all other services under the standard FFS payment methodology. As of 2011, both models still exist, with a combined enrollment of about 400,000, less than 3.4% of total Medicare enrollment in private health plans. However, beginning in 2010 cost plans located in areas where there is adequate competition from other organization types, as defined in 42 CFR 417.402, will not be renewed by CMS.

Risk plans envisioned in the 1972 amendments were to be fully at risk for any amount by which their costs exceeded their payments. However, they were required to share any profits with the Medicare program. Plans could retain 50% of the profit up to 20% of the estimated amount that Medicare would have paid for beneficiaries in the same counties on an FFS basis. Savings in excess of 20% were retained by Medicare. The local county-based estimate of FFS costs was dubbed the adjusted average per capita cost (AAPCC) and, as will be seen later in this chapter, that estimate still plays a major role in determining how Medicare health plans are compensated today.[3]

This asymmetrical risk, with unlimited potential for loss and limited potential for gain,* was not successful in attracting health plans, and cost-based contracts continued to be the norm until the enactment of TEFRA in 1982.

■ TEFRA AND MMA

When regulations under TEFRA were published in 1985, health plans had the opportunity to contract with Medicare for risk-based monthly payments under new rules. Payment would be set equal to 95% of the AAPCC, and plans were fully at risk. Medicare assumed a guaranteed savings by retaining 5% of the AAPCC. In addition, plans were allowed to earn the same profit margin they earned on their commercial business. If a plan's projected per capita costs, including the allowed profit margin, were less than 95% of the AAPCC, the excess had to be used to subsidize other benefits, or to be returned to the Medicare program.

The AAPCC was calculated as a 5-year average, trended to the contract year using estimates developed by Medicare. The rate paid to health plans was further adjusted by the age and sex of enrolled beneficiaries, with an additional adjustment for SNF residents and dual eligibles; there were 142 rate cells in all, although not every category of Medicare beneficiary was eligible to enroll in a Medicare HMO.

Two problems with the AAPCC became apparent in the years following the enactment of TEFRA. First, the risk adjustments for age, sex, institutional status, and Medicaid

---

*This concept is echoed in the limits the ACA now places on the medical loss ratio for commercially insured business, as described in Chapter 21.

proved to be poor predictors of cost variation among beneficiaries, although an additional adjuster for beneficiaries who originally qualified for Medicare due to disability was added later. But these risk adjusters only accounted for about 1% of the variation in beneficiary costs.[4] Additionally, large variations were observed in the AAPCC values from year to year within certain counties, and between neighboring counties, making long-term commitments to the program unpredictable.[5] Still, during the TEFRA years Medicare experienced a measure of success in contracting with private plans, and private plan enrollment grew to 1.4 million by 1991, and 6.8 million by 2000.

The BBA introduced several reforms in the program, including reforms in the payment methodology. It would be an understatement to say that the BBA reforms failed to promote further growth of the new Medicare + Choice program and, as noted earlier, enrollment dropped from the 2000 high of 6.8 million to 5.3 million by 2003.

The MMA once again made substantial changes to the Medicare program. The most dramatic change was the establishment of Part D of Medicare, the prescription drug benefit, which was discussed earlier in the chapter. To the point of this section, the MMA also introduced a better risk adjustment methodology for the new "Medicare Advantage" program. The new risk adjustments began in 2004, and were fully phased in by 2007. The new methodology added hierarchical condition categories (HCCs) to the other risk adjustments used since the passage of TEFRA. The MMA also established a new approach to determining the payment to MA plans, based on bids submitted by each plan and the relationship of that bid to a county benchmark. The benchmark was based on the old AAPCC, although a number of legislative changes resulted in benchmarks in many counties that exceeded the county AAPCC.

Payment Calculation and Bidding Process

The calculation of payments and the bidding process for MA and PDP plans is complex compared to the commercial market. A summary of the key elements follows.

The Bid

In June of each year, MA plans are required to submit bids to CMS. These bids represent the average per capita projected cost for Part A and B services net of cost-sharing, plus the plan's administrative costs to provide those benefits, plus a profit. Generally health plans will cover additional benefits, such as some or all of the beneficiaries' cost-sharing amounts, but the cost of these added benefits is not included in calculating the bid.

For plans with a prior claim history, bids are based on prior experience, adjusted for anticipated changes in utilization and unit costs of services. Since plan bids are due at the beginning of June, plans will be calculating their bids in April and May. This means that a plan is required to forecast claims expense for next year based primarily on last year's data, with relatively complete current-year data only for January and perhaps February. This requires estimating trends in utilization and unit costs for 2 years into the future.

Plans without sufficient claims history—such as new plans, plans that have been in operation only a short time, and plans entering new service areas—will need to substitute a manual rate, based on average Medicare cost data, for actual claim experience. Common sources of these average cost data are 5% claim samples available from Medicare and proprietary data bases maintained by actuarial firms.

The bid is normalized to a risk score of 1.0. This means that the claim history upon which the bid is based needs to be adjusted by the risk score of the population that generated the data, so that the bid represents the anticipated cost for a beneficiary of average risk, where a score of 1.0 is average. For instance, assume that a plan projects next year's revenue requirement, including projected claim costs, administrative cost, and profit, to be $1,000 per member per month, and the average risk score of the population that generated the claim data upon which that projection is based is 1.1. Then a normalized bid, normalized to a risk score of 1.0, would equal $1,000 ÷ 1.1 = $909.09. The normalized bid would be $909.09. Risk scores are discussed in more detail below. Benchmarks as published by CMS are already normalized to a 1.0 risk score.

The bid is then compared to the benchmark. If the bid exceeds the benchmark, the plan must charge beneficiaries the difference in the form of a monthly premium. Since the bid represents the cost of providing only Part A and Part B benefits, this situation would require beneficiaries to pay to the plan an extra amount that they would not pay under traditional Medicare FFS, in order to receive the same benefits. Not surprisingly, MA plans seek to achieve bids that are less than the benchmark to avoid this financial disincentive for beneficiaries.

If the bid is less than the benchmark, the difference is referred to as "savings." Plans receive a percentage of the savings as a rebate, and CMS retains the rest. Through 2011, the percent of savings paid to plans was 75%. The ACA reduces this rebate percentage in future years, as described below. Plans must use rebates to provide additional benefits, such as covering part of the beneficiary cost share or providing dental or vision benefits. Plans may also use rebate dollars to pay beneficiaries' Part B premiums or to subsidize their Part D drug benefit premiums if the plan offers the Medicare prescription drug benefit as part of the benefit package. See **Figure 24-3**.

When a plan bid covers more than one county, the bid and the benchmark are both calculated as the weighted average of the county-specific amounts, weighted by projected enrollment in each county.

RPPOs calculate their benchmark somewhat differently. After bids are submitted, CMS determines the average

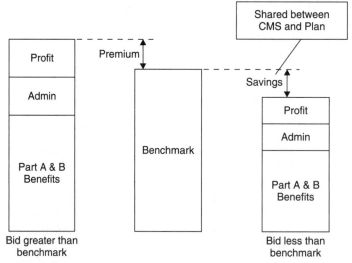

FIGURE 24-3 Bids and Benchmarks

RPPO bid and calculates a blended benchmark. The blend is weighted by the relative percentages of Medicare beneficiaries in the FFS program and in MA, as follows:

(Weighted average RPPO bid ×
    percentage of beneficiaries in MA plans) +
(Weighted average county benchmarks ×
    percentage of beneficiaries in FFS Medicare) =
RPPO Benchmark

Bids are not automatically accepted by CMS. Plans may be required to submit revised bids if CMS determines that their year-to-year total beneficiary cost (premium plus cost-sharing) would increase by an unacceptable amount, or if the proposed profit margin exceeds what CMS considers reasonable. Also, plans must avoid benefit designs that are discriminatory, for instance by imposing unusually high copayments on certain service categories with the effect of discouraging enrollment of sicker beneficiaries. Plans must also present cost-sharing designs that are no less generous than FFS Medicare, from an actuarial standpoint. Plans may have cost sharing that differs in the specifics, compared with FFS Medicare, but the aggregate value must be actuarially equivalent or better. To use a simplified example, consider Medicare's 20% coinsurance on physician fees. A health plan may have a $15 copayment on physician fees. If the projected weighted average of all physicians' fees is $75, then the $15 copayment is actuarially equivalent to the FFS Medicare benefit, since $15 is 20% of $75. Failure to meet these standards may result in rejection of a bid by CMS.

Risk Adjustment

As noted earlier, the original attempt to risk-adjust payments from Medicare to private plans based on the AAPCC was little better than no adjustment at all, and at best had a predictive value of about 1%.[6] Under the MMA, CMS began in 2004 to phase in a more sophisticated risk adjustment system, adding diagnosis information to the other adjusters.

CMS now uses what is known as the CMS Hierarchical Condition Category model, or CMS-HCC. The CMS-HCC model maps ICD-9 diagnosis codes to groups of diagnoses called condition categories. The condition categories are ranked in a hierarchy, in which a higher category trumps a lower category for a patient whose diagnoses map to both categories. Each category is assigned a value (risk adjustment factor, or RAF) based on the statistical relationship between that category and the following year's claim costs. The risk factors are based on the coefficients in a multiple regression calculation that expresses the statistical relationship between the presence and absence of a given condition category for a patient, and that patient's claim cost the following year. Over 13,000 ICD-9 codes are mapped to 189 condition categories.

For instance, a diagnosis of a sprained ankle in Year 1 would have no association with claim costs in Year 2. A diagnosis of diabetes would have some association with the following year's claims, and diabetes with complications would be associated with higher costs than uncomplicated diabetes. So the sprained ankle would have no risk score attached to it. Uncomplicated diabetes has a risk score of 0.162. There are several categories for diabetes with various complications, ranging as high as 0.508.[7] For a patient with diabetes diagnoses that mapped to both uncomplicated and complicated condition categories, the complicated category would trump the uncomplicated category on the hierarchy.

Figure 24-4 shows in more detail how the CMS-HCC model assigns risk scores.

The CMS-HCC model explains about 10% of the variation in medical costs among Medicare beneficiaries.[8] While this is a ten-fold improvement over the prior methodology, 10%

**Clinical vignette for CMS-HCC (version 12) classification
community-residing, 76-year-old woman with AMI, angina pectoris,
COPD, renal failure, chest pain, and ankle sprain**

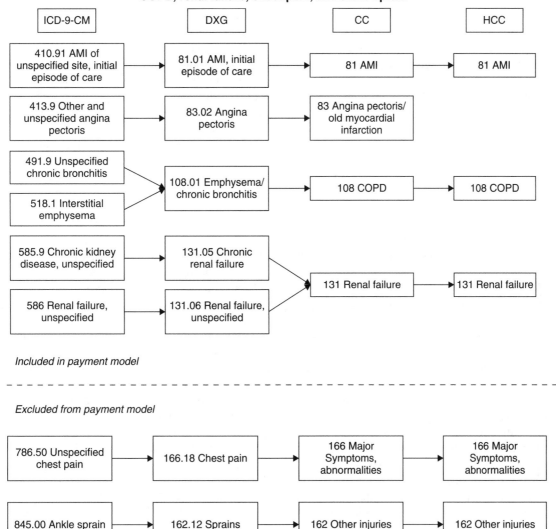

Note: AMI, acute myocardial infarction; CC, condition category; COPD, chronic obstructive pulmonary disease; DXG, diagnostic group; HCC, hierarchical condition category; ICD-9-CM, *International Classification of Diseases*, Ninth Revision, Clinical Modification.

FIGURE 24-4 Clinical Vignette of CMS-HCC Model Assigning Risk Scores

Source: Evaluation of the CMS-HCC Risk Adjustment Model, Final Report. March 2011. Prepared for Melissa A. Evans, PhD, Centers for Medicare & Medicaid Services, Medicare Plan Payment Group, Division of Risk Adjustment and Payment Policy, Prepared by Gregory C. Pope, MS, John Kautter, PhD, Melvin J. Ingber, PhD, Sara Freeman, MS, Rishi Sekar, BA, Cordon Newhart, MA, RTI International; CMS Contract No. HHSM-500-2005-00029I; www.cms.gov/MedicareAdvtgSpecRateStats/06_Risk_adjustment.asp#TopOfPage. Accessed August 19, 2011.

is still a low correlation. There are several problems with the CMS-HCC model that result in the improved but low correlation.

The first is the nature of the diagnosis data in the sample of Medicare claims that are used to determine the risk co-efficients. With the exception of inpatient claims that are paid on the basis of diagnosis-related groups (DRGs), the diagnosis codes on Medicare claims have little effect on payment. Hence, there is no incentive to be complete and accurate for most of the claims submitted to Medicare. For instance, in the year that a patient has a heart attack, that diagnosis will be present on a hospital DRG claim. But in the following year, the diagnosis may or may not appear on physician claims. Since the risk scores are based only on prior year data, each member, in effect, begins each year in perfect health, as far as the risk adjustment model is concerned. The lack of persistence in the data from year to year hinders the predictive power of the model.

Additionally, the standard professional claim form, the CMS-1500, collects a maximum of four diagnosis codes. A patient may have more coexisting conditions and, even if a physician uses all four positions to report diagnoses, those that are more germane to risk adjustment may be omitted from the claim form. So a diabetic with complications may appear to be an uncomplicated diabetic based on the claim data. Unlike the paper-based CMS-1500, the 837 Professional standardized electronic claim (see Chapters 18 and 23) can accept up to eight diagnoses, but until physician payment is affected by the accuracy of diagnostic coding, there is no incentive to use all the fields.

Similar data problems exist for health plans when they collect diagnostic data for the purpose of risk-adjusting their payments from CMS. Claim forms may or may not have complete and accurate information. Furthermore, even though the risk coefficients in the CMS-HCC model are determined from error-prone claim data, health plans are expected to be able to substantiate the risk adjustment data they submit with information from patients' medical records. Arguably, the most accurate system would use plan data that contains the same degree of error as the data used to calibrate the model. However, there is no way to determine this, since the FFS claim data used to set the risk coefficients are not audited.

It is not clear whether this requirement to substantiate diagnostic data from medical records increases or decreases risk scores and payments. Many health plans screen their claim data for indications of missing or inaccurate diagnosis codes, using software and logic rules to correlate claims by member. For instance, a member who has claims for a beta blocker may have had a heart attack in the past. If the current year's record doesn't include a code for the heart attack, the plan may review that member's medical record to determine whether the member is being reported correctly for risk adjustment purposes. Plans that do this report significant increases in revenue per member as a result of correcting coding errors. However, this is a search for missing and underreported diagnoses, and does not include the impact of unsubstantiated codes that would increase payment. On the other hand, CMS has conducted risk adjustment data validation (RADV) audits, looking at a sample of members in the audited plan for unsubstantiated claims, specifically looking for overpayments. Although CMS has not published the results of these audits as of this writing, anecdotal reports indicate that the error rate is significant. CMS has also proposed to extrapolate the audit findings to the entire plan. If the sample shows an overpayment rate of 10%, extrapolation of that finding to the whole plan would mean that the plan would have to refund to CMS 10% of the payments it received from CMS in the audited year. Since MA plans generally have a financial margin in the range of 3.6 to 4.5%,[9] a refund of that magnitude could wipe out several years' margins and could erode financial reserves below the levels required by state regulators (see Chapters 21 and 28).

These two audit activities, one undertaken by health plans looking for missing or incorrect codes that result in underpayments and the other undertaken by CMS to find unsubstantiated overpayments, may cancel each other out, but there are not sufficient data at present to know what the net impact will be on health plans. However, the high error rates that appear to be identified in both types of audits point out a weakness in the current CMS-HCC calibration methodology, and its reliance on unaudited FFS claim data.

Another challenge for health plans that are subject to a RADV audit is the need to produce the one best medical record to substantiate their risk score reports. For many patients, the information needed to substantiate all of their diagnoses may be scattered across several records maintained by several different providers of care. Nor is it clear how health plans can respond when a record is not available because a physician had died, or closed his or her practice, or when a record has been destroyed.

Some health plans are responding to this audit requirement by conducting annual risk assessments for those members who appear to be most likely to have diagnoses that map to HCCs, using physicians and mid-level practitioners who have been trained to record medical conditions to CMS standards. In this way, the health plan is assured of possessing the one best record, since it directs its creation each year. More significantly, the annual risk assessments ensure that the plan has an up-to-date register of high-risk members, so it can provide appropriate care management and support services to reduce the incidence of high-cost complications of chronic illness. This one approach can improve the accuracy and audit readiness of the risk adjustment data, contribute to a reduction in claim costs, and improve the quality of life of high-risk members.

A related approach is to flag claims that contain diagnostic codes that map to HCCs, for members who have not had a risk assessment, so that the plan can obtain the necessary medical record information to substantiate the diagnostic code.

As noted above, health plans are becoming adept at reducing errors in diagnostic coding, to avoid being underpaid through the CMS-HCC model. CMS studies indicate that, by reducing the error rate relative to the error rate implicit in the FFS data that are used to calibrate the HCC model, health plans have increased their average risk scores above what they would have been using uncorrected data. CMS contends that this results in increased payments that are not related to increased risk, but to increased coding accuracy. To offset this, CMS introduced a coding intensity adjustment in 2010. This adjustment reduced payments to all health plans by 3.41%. The ACA mandates CMS to increase this adjustment to at least 5.71% in gradual annual steps through 2018. This mandatory payment reduction makes it even more important for health plans to ensure that the data they submit to CMS for risk adjustment are complete and accurate since they are being paid less on the assumption that they are making these corrections, and that the corrections have the effect of increasing risk scores.

Impact of the ACA on Payment

The ACA makes substantial changes to MA payments, as has already been shown in earlier sections. In this section, the most significant changes are summarized in one place. The need for change arose as a result of Congressional actions between 1997 and 2003 that increased the county payment rates. Through the mid-1990s, health plans were paid 95% of the county average FFS cost (95% of the AAPCC). The Congressional increases in county payment rates following 1996 resulted in a patchwork of rates. By 2010, rates ranged from just slightly better than the AAPCC, to more than 150% of local FFS in a few counties (and over 200% of local FFS in some Puerto Rican *municipios*). The Medicare Payment Advisory Commission (MedPAC) calculated that, nationwide, the average payment to MA plans exceeded the average FFS cost by about 12%.[10]

Congress sought to correct this through provisions in the ACA, and return the average payment to health plans to something close to the average FFS cost. However, the approach adopted by Congress in the ACA recognized that some counties appear to have more efficient patterns of medical care than others, and the benchmark payments set by the ACA vary by county based on a measure of efficiency. Counties are ranked by quartile, based on their average FFS cost. The cost estimate is adjusted for risk, so that all counties' costs are projected at a theoretical risk score of 1.0. Benchmarks in counties in the lowest cost quartile will be set at 115% of local FFS, while payments in the highest cost quartile will be reduced to 95% of local FFS. The quartiles for 2011, based on 2009 FFS costs, are presented **Table 24-2**.[11]

Only $103 separates counties at the top of the first quartile, with the best payment rates, from the bottom of the

fourth quartile, with the worst rates, relative to local FFS costs. Relatively small variations in local cost will have substantial impacts on benchmark payments. The new payment rates will be phased in over a number of years, and will be completely phased in by 2017. The phase-in schedule will vary from one county to another. Counties that will incur the greatest payment reductions, relative to what they would have expected under the pre-ACA payment formula, will see the new rates phased in over 6 years. Counties with smaller reductions will be phased in over 2 or 4 years, depending on the size of the reduction. The weighted average payment, weighted by MA enrollment in each county, will be approximately 100% of FFS. While this represents a 12% reduction from the rates analyzed by MedPAC in 2010, it is still an improvement over the pre-1997 rates, which were set at 95% of the local FFS cost.

The ACA also introduces a bonus payment for MA plans that meet certain quality standards. Starting in 2014, under the ACA, high-quality health plans will receive a bonus of 5% of the benchmark payment specified under the ACA. This bonus is calculated only for the ACA rate, so counties where the new ACA rate is still being phased in will receive a lower bonus, until the phase-in is complete. For instance, in a county with a 6-year phase-in schedule, the ACA "specified amount" will account for only one-half of the payment rate in 2012. The other half will be based on the "applicable amount" that would have been paid under the pre-ACA rules. The bonus in such a county would be 5% of the ACA rate, not 5% of the total rate. **Table 24-3** illustrates the 2014 calculation for a county on a 6-year phase-in schedule.

The ACA also provides for double bonuses for counties that meet the following criteria:

- Paid at the urban floor rate in 2004 (the urban floor is one of the steps that Congress took to improve payment rates for certain counties, by setting a minimum payment in excess of 95% of the AAPCC)
- MA penetration of a least 25% of all Medicare beneficiaries in the county
- Average FFS costs below the national average

The bonuses will be paid to health plans that achieve a quality score of at least four stars on a scale of one to five (the Star Rating system is discussed later in this chapter). CMS has proposed to use its demonstration authority to start the bonus program in 2012, instead of waiting until 2014. The CMS demonstration would also expand the bonuses to plans with three stars or higher as an incentive to improve quality.

Bonus payments must be used to provide additional benefits, reduce cost-sharing, or reduce beneficiary premiums. They will not contribute directly to profit, although improvements in benefits and reductions in cost are expected to give bonus-eligible plans a market advantage.

It is not yet clear at the time of publication how loss of a bonus will affect the CMS review of bids that show

TABLE 24-2	Quartiles for 2011			
Quartile	Min	Max	Range	% of FFS
1	$ 419.27	$ 634.49	$ 215.22	115%
2	$ 634.50	$ 685.09	$ 50.59	107.5%
3	$ 685.10	$ 737.77	$ 52.67	100%
4	$ 737.78	$ 1,295.83	$ 558.06	95%

Source: Author's calculation, based on the methodology described in the CMS publication "Advance Notice of Methodological Changes for Calendar Year (CY) 2012 for Medicare Advantage (MA) Capitation Rates, Part C and Part D Payment Policies for 2012 Call Letter," February 18, 2011.

TABLE 24-3	2014 Calculation on a Six-Year Phase-in Schedule					
	Rate	Blend Factor	Blended rate	5% Bonus		Total
ACA rate ("specified amount")	$ 800	50%	$ 400	5%	$ 20	
Pre-ACA rate ("applicable amount")	$ 900	50%	$ 450	0%	–	
Blended rate paid in 2004			$ 850		$ 20	$ 870

significant increases in total beneficiary cost (TBC). For instance, if a plan has received a 5% bonus worth $40 for the current year, and uses this bonus to reduce total beneficiary cost, how will CMS view a bid for the following year, if the plan has lost its bonus? Loss of the $40 will mean an increase in TBC. It is not yet clear whether that will trigger CMS criteria that seek to limit large increases in TBC.

The ACA rewards health plans in another way for high-quality ratings. Under prior law, a health plan was allowed to retain 75% of the savings that were attributable to a bid that was less than the plan's benchmark payment. These "rebates" are used to provide additional benefits, or to reduce beneficiary costs. Under the ACA, the rebate will be reduced to 50% by 2014, with the reductions being phased in at one-third each year starting in 2012. However, plans with high-quality ratings will receive a greater rebate. Plans with a rating of 4.5 or 5 stars will receive a 70% rebate. Plans with ratings between 3.5 and 4 will receive 65%. Plans below 3.5 stars will receive the 50% rebate.

The ACA also imposes a minimum medical loss ratio (MLR) standard on MA plans. While the Medicare Advantage MLR provision does not specifically reference the requirements for commercial plans (see Chapters 21 and 30), at present it appears likely that CMS will apply the same MLR regulations and definition to MA as applied to commercial insurance. This will mean that MA plans will probably be allowed to count activities that improve the quality of care as medical costs rather than administrative costs and be able to deduct certain tax payments from revenues; all of these are described in Chapter 21, including Table 21-2. On average, MA plans operated in the range of the new 85% floor prior to passage of the ACA.[12] However, approximately one-third of

beneficiaries in 2010 were in plans with loss ratios less than 85%.[13] In addition to the adjustments to the MLR calculation allowed for commercial insurance, the payment reductions mandated by the ACA should drive loss ratios up, as revenues increase more slowly than health care costs while the new rates are phased in.

Medicare Prescription Drug Payment

Payment under Medicare Part D has some superficial similarities to the MA payment, but there are critical differences in how the payments are calculated. Part D plans may be free-standing PDPs, or may be offered by MA plans as MA-PDs. Both types of sponsors are paid under the same rules.

PDPs submit bids to CMS to provide the standard Part D package of benefits for the coming year. The bids are due at the same time as MA bids. Bids are based on historical data, or manual rates for new plans, and include administrative costs and a reasonable profit. CMS calculates the weighted national average monthly bid. This is the average of all PDP bids received, weighted by the current enrollment of each bidder. Consequently, the large PDPs with the greatest number of members have the greatest influence on the national average bid. CMS then calculates the base beneficiary premium. This is the national average monthly bid multiplied by 25.5%, and divided by 1 minus the ratio of projected average reinsurance payments to Part D plans to the total payments received by PDPs. Reinsurance is a payment from CMS for beneficiaries whose total out-of-pocket cost in a given calendar year exceeds a maximum out-of-pocket threshold calculated by CMS each year. **Figure 24-5** illustrates the calculation of the base premium.

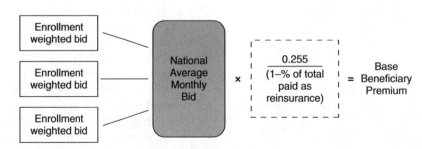

FIGURE 24-5 Calculation of the Base Premium

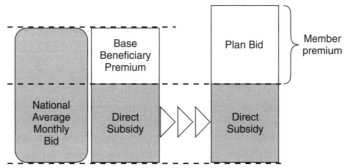

FIGURE 24-6 Calculation of Member Premium

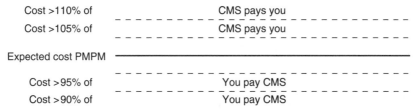

FIGURE 24-7 Risk Corridors

Each PDP receives a direct subsidy toward the cost of benefits that is equal to the national average monthly bid minus the base beneficiary premium. The plan then must charge beneficiaries a premium that equals the difference between the plan's bid and the base beneficiary premium. **Figure 24-6** illustrates the calculation of the member premium for a PDP whose bid is greater than the national average monthly bid.

Payments to PDPs are risk-adjusted, using a variant of the CMS-HCC model known as the RxHCC model. Like the HCC model used for MA plans, the RxHCCs are calibrated by a multiple regression analysis of the relationship between diagnoses on medical and hospital claims and prescription drug costs in the following year. Since prescriptions don't include diagnosis codes, medical claims are used as a proxy source of the diagnosis information. Since there is less inherent variability in drug costs than in medical costs, the RxHCC model is a better predictor of the following year's costs than the CMS-HCC model, with a predictive power (R^2) of 25%.

The Part D program includes a risk-sharing provision that is not part of the MA program. An allowable cost per capita is calculated from the plan's bid and represents the expected cost for covered prescription drugs, less reinsurance payments and other nonpremium subsidies. If a plan's actual adjusted costs for a given year exceed the projected cost by more than 5%, CMS will pay the plan 50% of the amount in excess of 5%. If the plan's costs exceed 10% of the expected amount, CMS will pay 80% of the amount in excess of 10%. Conversely, the plan must pay CMS 50% or 80% of any amount by which costs are less than 5% or 10% of the expected cost. These corridors reduce both a plan's

potential profit and potential loss on prescription drugs. **Figure 24-7** illustrates the risk corridors.

In calculating gains or losses for purposes of the risk corridor payments, CMS will disallow any prescription claims (known as prescription drug events, or PDEs) for members whose enrollment is not recorded correctly on the PDP's records. This places a premium on regular reconciliation of enrollment records with CMS, to ensure that the plan is being paid properly for its members, that it is not paying claims for people who are not its members, and that all valid claims will be counted when it reconciles the risk corridors with CMS.

CMS also pays PDPs for beneficiaries who qualify for "extra help," whose income is below stated levels. The extra help consists of low-income premium subsidies (LIPS) and low-income cost-sharing subsidies (LICS). LIPS pay most or all of the low-income beneficiary's premium, up to a maximum amount that equals the weighted average premium in each Part D region. Regions may be a single state or multiple contiguous states, depending on population. LICS pay all but a few dollars of the 25% coinsurance for covered prescriptions that is part of the standard benefit package, and pay for prescriptions in the coverage gap (the "donut hole").

CMS also pays PDPs a reinsurance amount, to cover 80% of the cost of benefits for members whose total out-of-pocket costs exceed the current year's threshold.

■ APPLICATION AND CONTRACTING PROCESS

The process for an MA or PDP plan to apply for a contract with CMS follows defined rules. The most important elements are described next.

Eligibility Requirements for a Medicare Contract

An organization must meet certain basic requirements to be eligible for a Medicare contract. These requirements are related to the organization's licensure and financial solvency, premiums, provider network, and administration and operations. In particular:

- All organizations must be licensed as risk-bearing entities to offer health insurance or health benefits in the state(s) in which they will operate, or hold a certificate of authority or operation in states that do not license such entities. RPPOs can obtain a temporary waiver of the requirement.
- All organizations must demonstrate financial solvency and a positive net worth.
- Plan premiums may not exceed the actuarial value of Medicare cost-sharing, although the organization can offer supplemental benefits at an additional cost to the member. Plan benefits and premiums must be uniform throughout the contracted service area to prevent discrimination.
- Organizations must use Medicare-certified providers to provide health care services to members. These organizations must demonstrate network adequacy within the contracted service area. This means that within the MA plan network, services must be made available to members through staff providers or providers under contract with the organization, the organization must be capable of providing 24-hour emergency care and paying for out-of-area emergency and urgently needed services, and the plan must meet CMS access standards for medical and pharmacy services.
- MA organizations must meet specific minimum enrollment requirements. The organization must have at least 5,000 members or, in rural areas, at least 1,500 members.
- All organizations must demonstrate an ability to administer the contract. This includes adequate staffing and management, meeting Medicare quality and care coordination requirements, and having a compliance plan that ensures the organization can meet Medicare requirements and avoid and/or correct fraud and abuse.

The Application

The process for obtaining any type of MA or Part D contract begins almost 13 months before the effective date of the contract. It begins when applicants file a required Notice of Intent to Apply. While CMS does not require the organization filing the notice to complete an application, it allows CMS to begin preparation for processing the steps necessary for managing the application throughout each step of the application process.

For the most part applicants must make substantial preparations for filing the contract in late February. This means that both strategy and operational details along with contracting for provider and administrative services has been completed by the applicant well before an application is submitted to CMS.

Applications are completed through the Health Plan Management System (HPMS). This is a fully electronic submission process that every initial applicant and current contractor seeking to expand their service area or add an SNP must use. Applications that are not filed by the deadline date are not reviewed.

The application is a series of attestations or questions that reflect requirements that the applicant must meet. These are supported by required uploads of documentation that provide evidence of compliance. These cover state licensure, organization structure and management, financial solvency, service area, provider and administration contracting, and a quality improvement plan. A second set of attestations cover requirements for compliant Medicare operations. These include marketing, eligibility and enrollment, working aged, claims, grievances and appeals, and communication with CMS.

An applicant that wishes to provide a prescription drug benefit must submit additional materials that are unique to the requirements for the Part D program. This addendum requires attestations and uploaded material that address the requirements for operation of a Part D benefit program. These include 25 additional areas unique to prescription drug regulations that focus on benefit design, pharmacy access, and beneficiary protections.

For both Part C and Part D, CMS has also developed sophisticated methods for evaluating access to contracted provider services that are proposed in each application. For Part C, applicants are required to upload provider contracts and CMS compares this information to information collected in the FFS system. Networks must meet two critical adequacy criteria: minimum number of providers/beds and time/distance requirements. Criteria vary by specialty type. With a geo-mapping tool, CMS identifies any areas where access standards are not met. For Part D, CMS will use information gathered from the pharmacy list uploaded by the applicant to identify pharmacy addresses. With this information, CMS can geo-code the street-level locations of the pharmacies to determine retail pharmacy access.

CMS reviews the information that is submitted and identifies any deficiencies. When CMS identifies deficiencies, applicants receive a Notice of Intent to Deny. Applicants have 10 days to provide information necessary to address the deficiency. If it is not corrected, CMS will issue a denial notice to the applicant. Applicants who receive a denial can appeal this determination by filing a request for a hearing within 15 days. The hearing will be held within 30 days and allows the applicant to present evidence that CMS made an incorrect determination. If the hearing officer upholds the CMS decision, the applicant can appeal to the CMS Administrator. The timing of these processes is critical to ensure that all approved contracts meet each step needed to publish information for the Annual Election Period beginning on October 15.

After CMS releases a formulary submission tool in late March for Part D, applicants must submit a formulary by mid-April. CMS releases information necessary for completion of bid pricing in April with the annual payment notice. By late May, CMS notifies all applicants who have submitted acceptable applications. Following the approval, applicants and all contracted health plans complete their bids and benefit packages and submit them on the first Monday of June. Bids are reviewed and approved, and CMS executes contracts by mid-September.

CMS may verify an applicant's readiness and compliance with Medicare requirements through onsite visits at the applicant's facilities as well as through other program monitoring techniques throughout the application process. During this period, applicants prepare operations and marketing information and submit it as necessary to CMS for review and approval.

The Contracting Cycle

The majority of health plans choose to renew their contracts. Renewing contractors must still submit acceptable bids and meet all required timelines for updates to benefit packages and marketing materials. However, CMS reviews performance measures and makes a determination that allows the renewal to occur.

Health plans that choose to not renew their contract must send notice in June, approximately 6 months before the termination date, to allow for appropriate steps to remove the health plan as an option in the CMS systems and to notify beneficiaries about their options for coverage in other plans. Health plans that do not renew are prohibited from applying for a contract or expansion in the service area for a 2-year period unless CMS determines that there are extenuating circumstances.

CMS may also choose to not renew a health plan consequent to performance or failure to reach minimal enrollment. CMS has also announced its intention to evaluate plans for nonrenewal if they maintain a 2.5 star rating for 3 consecutive years (star rating is described later in the chapter). CMS notifies plans of its intention to not renew their contract by August 1 of each year.

Contracts can be terminated by mutual consent or involuntarily by CMS. Generally, mutual consent occurs when an organization ceases to exist, a contract is modified, or a new organization has been approved to provide services to the enrolled beneficiaries. There are required notice procedures that the health plan must follow to inform beneficiaries of any changes or modifications. As in nonrenewals, health plans are prohibited from applying for a service area expansion in the area for 2 years.

Involuntary terminations occur when CMS determines that a health plan failed to meet one or more of 13 regulatory requirements that are cause for termination. Termination can be expedited if there is a determination that there is an imminent and serious risk to the health of the enrolled beneficiaries, or if there are financial difficulties so severe that services to beneficiaries could be curtailed. In any CMS termination action, the health plan has the ability to appeal the determination. As in any adversarial action taken by CMS, the health plan must prove that the determination made by CMS was in error.

ENROLLMENT OF MEDICARE BENEFICIARIES INTO MA PLANS

There are specific rules that MA plans must follow with respect to enrollment and disenrollment of Medicare beneficiaries.

Who May Enroll

The BBA established some very specific rules regarding who may enroll in an MA plan. With some exceptions, any Medicare beneficiary permanently residing in the MA plan's service area may enroll in the plan as long as the person has both Medicare Part A and Part B, and as long as the request to enroll is received by the plan during an election period. Medicare beneficiaries who are also Medicaid recipients may also enroll in an MA plan. Medicare beneficiaries who do not have Medicare Part D cannot enroll in MA-PD plans, but they can enroll in MA-only plans (i.e., plans that do not cover Part D).

There are some exceptions to the eligibility rules that prevent individuals from enrolling in MA plans. If the plan is not open for enrollment, because it has a capacity waiver or has been closed by CMS, for example, then the Medicare beneficiary may not enroll in the plan. In addition, if enrollment in the plan is limited to special needs individuals or to employer group members, then the Medicare beneficiary may only enroll in the plan if the individual meets the special needs or employer group requirements for the plan.

The only Medicare beneficiaries not entitled to enroll in MA plans are beneficiaries who have ESRD, but there are exceptions to this rule. If the plan is a special needs plan offered to individuals with ESRD, then enrollment is allowed as long as the individual meets all other eligibility requirements. Enrollees who acquire ESRD after enrollment in a plan may not be disenrolled from the plan because they have ESRD. In addition, individuals who have ESRD and who were enrolled as non-Medicare members of a plan may be retained as Medicare enrollees on becoming eligible for Medicare.

Enrollment and Election Periods

Prior to the BBA, Medicare beneficiaries could enroll in Medicare managed care plans at any time during the year. The BBA began a trend toward structuring enrollment and disenrollment periods to more closely (but not completely) resemble the more limited enrollment periods that employers tend to offer to their employees and retirees. The ACA further limited enrollment periods, cutting the enrollment season in half.

There are several election periods during which a Medicare beneficiary may enroll in or disenroll from a plan. These include the Annual Election Period, the Medicare Advantage Disenrollment Period, Special Election Periods, Initial Coverage Election Periods, and an Open-Enrollment Period for Institutionalized Individuals.

Annual Election Period

The Annual Election Period runs from October 15 through December 7, for enrollments effective on January 1 of the following year. This is the election period most widely advertised by CMS and the MA plans as it is open to all eligible Medicare beneficiaries, involves allowing individuals to choose to join or switch plans based on how benefits and cost-sharing will change in the coming year, and most closely mimics an "open season" offered by employers and unions.

Medicare Advantage Disenrollment Period

During the Medicare Advantage Disenrollment Period, MA plan members can disenroll from an MA plan and return to Medicare FFS between January 1 and February 15 of each year. Note that this election period does not allow for enrollment in a new MA plan. Individuals who switch to Medicare FFS during this time period have the option to join a PDP to add drug coverage.

Special Election Periods

MA plans are required to be open during Special Election Periods. As with most private health insurance election periods, Special Election Periods tend to center around certain events, such as when an individual changes residence, loses employer/union health coverage, loses MA coverage because another organization in the service area terminates a Medicare contract, or gets Medicaid. CMS has the authority to define additional Special Election Periods for "exceptional conditions" on an as-needed basis. These Special Election Periods tend to be unique to Medicare, such as periods when individuals want to leave MA plans as a result of sanctions imposed by CMS on the plan or when individuals lose their eligibility for Medicaid or other low-income subsidy programs.

Initial Coverage Election Periods

The Initial Coverage Election Period is intended to allow individuals newly eligible for MA to join an MA plan. The period begins 3 months before an individual's first entitlement to Medicare Part A and B and ends the later of the last day of the month before entitlement to Parts A and B, or the last day of the individual's Part B initial enrollment period. There is an additional Initial Coverage Election Period for Part D that allows individuals newly eligible for Part D to join a Part D plan.

Open-Enrollment Period for Institutionalized Individuals

The Open-Enrollment Period for Institutionalized Individuals is continuous. It only applies to individuals who move into, reside in, or move out of certain institutions such as skilled nursing facilities, nursing facilities, long-term care hospitals, and so forth. It ends 2 months after the individual moves out of the institution. MA plans are not required to be open for this enrollment period.

Involuntary Disenrollment

An MA organization must involuntarily disenroll a Medicare beneficiary if the person leaves the service area permanently (defined by regulations as an absence lasting more than 12 months), is incarcerated, or loses entitlement to either Medicare Part A or B. An MA organization has the option to involuntarily disenroll a Medicare beneficiary if the person has committed fraud in enrolling in a plan or permits others to use his or her enrollment card to obtain care; for failure to pay premiums in a timely manner including optional supplemental premiums unless there is a demonstration of good cause; or because of disruptive or abusive behavior, subject to CMS approval.

Capacity Limits and Age-Ins

While a plan is ordinarily required to be open for enrollment during the election periods described above, a plan may limit or close its enrollment if it does not have the capacity to accept new members. In such a case, a plan may discontinue or limit enrollment with CMS approval, but may still set aside a specified number of vacancies to enroll members who "age-in" from the plan's commercial product into its Medicare product. Capacity limits may be based on several different reasons and the limit may apply to specific plan benefit packages or counties in different configurations, for example by plan or by county.

■ MARKETING AND SALES RULES

The scope of marketing in the MA program goes well beyond the public's general understanding of advertising, and reflects the government's desire to maintain a level of control over MA plan marketing practices. In addition to advertising, MA marketing requirements cover all informational materials and activities targeted to Medicare beneficiaries, including sales activities, member communications, and any other activities or materials that are intended to attract Medicare beneficiaries to enroll in private plans. Serious marketing abuses by plans that used agents or brokers without sufficient oversight resulted in even more enhancement of marketing requirements; for example, for the first time Medicare introduced regulation of commission structures and required training for brokers and agents.

Prohibited Marketing

Prohibited marketing activities include door-to-door solicitation, discriminatory marketing (avoiding low-income areas, for example), and misleading marketing or misrepresentation. These activities are subject to sanctions, including suspension of enrollment, suspension of payment for new enrollees, or civil monetary penalties. MA plans are prohibited from giving monetary incentives as an inducement to enroll and from completing any portion of the enrollment application for a prospective enrollee.

Prior Approval

All marketing and enrollment material, including enrollment forms, must have CMS approval prior to public use. CMS has 45 days to review materials. If 45 days pass without CMS comments on the material, it is deemed approved. If an MA plan's marketing materials were approved for one service area, they are deemed approved in all of the plan's service areas, except with regard to area-specific information. For certain marketing and enrollment documents, CMS has developed optional model language. Use of the model language reduces the approval time period to 10 days. Under certain circumstances, CMS also allows a "file and use" approach, whereby no prior approval is required.

Required Notifications to Prospective Enrollees

Prospective enrollees must be given descriptive material sufficient for them to make an informed choice. One of the required pre-enrollment marketing documents is a Summary of Benefits form that uses standard benefit definitions and a standardized format to allow beneficiaries to make "apples to apples" comparisons among MA offerings and between MA and FFS; it is similar in concept to the Summary of Coverage document now required under the ACA for commercial coverage. Plans must also provide information about their plan star ratings to current and prospective enrollees by referring them to www.medicare.gov in all enrollment kits. They must also provide enrollment instructions and forms, customer service contact information, and an explanation of the plan's appeals and grievances process.

Required Notifications to Enrollees

MA plan enrollees must be notified at least 30 days in advance of changes in plan membership rules, which must be approved by CMS. However, for the change in benefits and cost-sharing occurring from one year to the next, an Annual Notice of Change must be sent to enrollees by September 30.

The statute specifies the kind of information an MA member must receive on enrollment and annually thereafter. The document containing this descriptive information, like its counterpart for commercial coverage, is called the Evidence of Coverage (EOC). The EOC includes information on benefits and exclusions; the number, mix, and distribution of plan providers; out-of-network and out-of-area coverage; emergency coverage—how it is defined and how to gain access to emergency care, including use of 911 services; prior authorization or other review requirements; grievances and appeals; and a description of the plan's quality assurance program. On request, the organization must provide information on utilization control practices, the number and disposition of appeals and grievances, and a summary description of physician compensation. The organization must also provide all members annually with provider directories and member identification cards, and MA plans offering Part D coverage must provide pharmacy directories and drug formulary information.

Sales

Plans or their subcontractors are allowed to conduct "marketing or sales events" to promote the benefits and services of the plan. At these events, sponsors distribute brochures and pre-enrollment materials such as a Summary of Benefits and approved sales materials. Sponsors may also accept enrollment application forms. Plan sponsors are responsible for overseeing all marketing activities used by their subcontractors including agents and brokers and must approve materials they use, including sales scripts.

Plans and other entities may also conduct "educational events" provided there are no sales activities such as distribution of marketing materials or distribution or collection of enrollment applications.

Agents and Brokers and Commissions

An organization may employ or contract with agents or brokers to market and sell its plans. Agents and brokers must be appointed according to the laws of the state(s) in which the agent or broker operates. The organization must train and test all of its agents and brokers annually on Medicare rules and regulations and on details specific to the plans they are selling. CMS has established rules on agent or broker compensation to prevent agents and brokers from steering Medicare beneficiaries into plans providing higher payment.

Website and Call Center Requirements

All organizations must have a website or web page dedicated to each product they offer. The website or web page must include certain information, such as a plan description, contact information, and links to member materials.

CMS specifies a variety of call center operations that the organization must operate. All organizations must also operate a toll-free call center for current and prospective enrollees. If the organization offers plans that cover Medicare Part D, it must also operate a pharmacy technical help call center to respond to inquiries from pharmacies and providers. The organization must also provide a call center available to providers inquiring about coverage determinations and Part D appeals.

■ CONSUMER PROTECTIONS

MA plans are subject to certain requirements relating to access to services for beneficiaries and appeal rights that must be provided to Medicare members.

Access Standards

With regard to access to care standards, the regulations have a number of requirements, including:

- Maintaining an adequate provider network, including minimum provider-to-enrollee ratios and maximum travel times and distances as specified by CMS;
- Using the "prudent layperson" definition of what constitutes an emergency, the liability of the MA organization for the cost of such care, and a requirement to cover appropriate maintenance and poststabilization care after an emergency;
- Limiting copayments for emergency services to amounts specified by CMS, for example $65 in 2011;
- Covering out-of-area dialysis during an enrollee's temporary absence from the service area;
- Specifying that the decision of the examining physician treating the individual enrollee prevails regarding when the enrollee may be considered stabilized for discharge or transfer; and
- Requiring plans to permit female enrollees to choose direct access to an in-network women's health specialist for women's routine and preventive health services.

Member Appeals and Grievances

MA enrollees have the right to an administrative and judicial appeals process and a grievance process. These rights are similar to the appeal rights under ERISA and the ACA for commercial coverage (Chapter 20), but have shorter timeframes and more avenues for pursuit. Medicare appeals (referred to in regulations as "organization determinations")

pertain to adverse decisions regarding coverage or cost of an item or service included in the Medicare contract (Medicare-covered items and services and additional and supplemental benefits). Grievances are complaints or disputes falling outside the definition of "appeal" related to a member's dissatisfaction with provision of health care services, including the way the service was provided, or the appropriateness, timeliness, or setting of the health service.

Appeals

The steps of the appeals process include:

- The determination by the organization (or a subcontracted entity);
- Reconsideration by the organization, or, if the organization proposes a reconsideration decision adverse to the enrollee, review of that decision by an independent review entity under contract to CMS;
- Review by an administrative law judge (ALJ) for claims valued at $130 or more (for 2011) if the independent review entity's decision is adverse to the enrollee (the MA organization is not entitled to appeal a decision by the independent review entity when the decision is in favor of the enrollee);
- Review of the ALJ's decision by the HHS's Medicare appeals council, a right available both to members and to the MA organization; and
- Judicial review in federal court for claims valued at $1,300 or more (for 2011).

The first-level determination is to be made by the MA organization within 14 days (or "as expeditiously as the enrollee's health condition requires" but no later than 14 days), and a reconsideration decision (by the organization or the review entity) is to be made within 30 days (with the same requirement for expeditious processing). For expedited appeals, the standard is that a decision must be rendered within 72 hours.

Quality improvement organizations (QIOs) under contract with CMS also review enrollee complaints, including appeals, about the appropriateness of a hospital discharge. Expedited timeframes similar to those of Medicare FFS apply in such a case. QIOs are described later in the chapter.

Grievances

Grievances against a plan, as opposed to Medicare appeals, are subject to different standards. Enrollees must currently be afforded a "meaningful" grievance right, which includes requiring the MA plan to respond to grievances on a timely basis and provide appropriate notification of investigation results to all concerned parties. The statute requires organizations to provide data on the number of grievances and their disposition in the aggregate on an enrollee's request.

Prescription Drug Coverage Determinations and Exceptions

Enrollees with prescription drug coverage have the right to take certain steps to ensure coverage of a particular drug even before they fill their prescription. In particular, they can get a "coverage determination" by their plan to determine whether a particular drug will be covered. The enrollee or the prescriber may request an exception to have the drug covered if the plan states that it will not cover the drug or if the drug is not on the plan's formulary. The enrollee or prescriber may also ask for an exception to have the enrollee pay less for the drug if the drug is in a higher (i.e., more expensive tier) but the enrollee or prescriber believes the enrollee cannot take the lower tier drugs for the same condition. If the enrollee disagrees with the plan's coverage determination or exception decision, then the enrollee can follow the appeals process described above.

Cultural Competence

MA plans are required to ensure that services are provided in a "culturally competent" manner (i.e., with sensitivity toward cultural, ethnic, and language differences) to all members. This includes members with limited English proficiency or reading skills, hearing incapacity, or those with diverse cultural and ethnic backgrounds. Translator services, interpreter services, or TTY connections are all examples of services that would help MA plans meet this requirement.

■ PROVIDER PROTECTIONS AND RIGHTS

MA organizations are required to afford certain rights to contracting providers, and plans are required to make timely payment on claims from noncontracting providers.

Basic Provider Rights

The MA statute contains provider protections, including:

- Prohibition of discrimination against particular providers, in selection of providers or payment or indemnification provisions, solely on the basis of the provider's licensure status;
- Appeal rights afforded to providers in the event of suspension, termination, or nonrenewal of a contract; and
- A requirement that MA organizations consult with plan physicians regarding medical policy, quality assurance programs, medical management procedures, and credentialing policies.

Provider Payment

Providers are afforded a number of rights and protections related to payment. All contracting providers must receive reasonable payment for covered services. Also, MA plans are required to meet the same prompt payment standards that apply to FFS Medicare carriers and fiscal intermediaries with respect to the timeliness of payments made to noncontracted providers. The standards apply to "clean" claims; that is, claims having no "defect or impropriety" as the law says and not lacking "substantiating documentation" or "requiring special treatment." The standard is that 95% of clean claims must be paid within 30 days, and that interest must be paid on clean claims not paid within 30 days.

By regulation a physician incentive plan is "any compensation arrangement to pay a physician or physician group that may directly or indirectly have the effect of reducing or limiting the services provided to any plan enrollee." If a plan has a physician incentive plan that places physicians at substantial financial risk (SFR; defined in Medicare regulations) for the care of Medicare or Medicaid enrollees, then it must provide for continuous monitoring of the potential effects of the incentive plan on access or quality of care. According to CMS, monitoring should include the review of utilization data to identify patterns of possible underutilization of services that may be related to the incentive plan. Organizations should consider concerns identified as a result of this monitoring when developing focus areas for quality improvement projects. SFR and its associated requirements are described in detail in Chapter 5.

■ QUALITY AND PLAN PERFORMANCE

MA plans have specific quality and performance requirements that have evolved over time. As discussed below, CMS uses quality and performance data to monitor plans, to administratively reward plans, and to provide information to beneficiaries to facilitate plan choice. As provided by the ACA, beginning in 2012 high-performing plans will receive a quality bonus and enrollees in high-performing plans will receive extra benefits. CMS uses quality and performance data as part of its performance assessment system and CMS denies new applications or service area expansions for poor-performing plans. CMS will soon use quality metrics to terminate poor-performing plans from the program, but has not begun to do so at the time of publication.

Quality Requirements

MA coordinated care plans must have a quality improvement program that measures performance under the program and that includes the following:

- Chronic Care Improvement Program (CCIP)—CCIP programs focus on beneficiaries with multiple or severe chronic conditions and include measures to assess performance such as clinical, cost, and beneficiary satisfaction. An example of a CCIP is a disease management program. Plans must monitor enrollee participation in the program.

- Quality Improvement Projects (QIPs)—QIPs are focused on improving health outcomes and enrollee satisfaction and include both clinical and nonclinical projects. Projects include an intervention with quality indicators and performance measurement, and periodic follow-up on the effect of the interventions. MA plans are responsible for selecting QIPs that are relevant to their populations. An example of a clinical QIP is a project that focuses on improving the rate of eye exams and blood sugar control in enrollees with diabetes. An example of a nonclinical project is a project that focuses on reducing health disparities.
- Plans must have a health information system that collects, analyzes, and reports data.
- Plans must have and follow written policies and procedures that reflect current standards of medical practice and mechanisms to detect both underutilization and overutilization of services.

The plan must perform a formal evaluation at least annually of the impact and effectiveness of its program and all problems that are revealed through internal surveillance, complaints, or other mechanisms must be corrected.

CMS requires the annual submission of the QIP and the CCIP from all except new plans in July. Since regulations vary according to contract type, each program is reviewed according to the requirements that apply. Projects are reviewed at the contract level to identify those that show some level of improvement. Health plans receive feedback and technical assistance based on the outcomes of the review. CMS receives reports about the information received and makes any determination about compliance with the requirements. Failure to make these submissions may result in compliance or enforcement action.

Plan Reporting

MA plans report the following specific data sets to CMS:

- HEDIS: Measures reported by MA plans are built off of the measures reported by commercial plans and have been adapted for the characteristics of the Medicare population. Most of the measures are process measures or intermediate outcomes measures. MA plans report HEDIS measures at the contract level. PPOs report on a subset of HEDIS measures that rely on a review of claims; however, they have the option to report on certain measures using medical records to be consistent with HMOs.
- The Consumer Assessment of Healthcare Providers and Systems (CAHPS®): Measures enrollee and disenrollee satisfaction with MA plans and provides the beneficiary perception of the quality of care. The MA plan selects a vendor to conduct the survey. Samples are selected to

reach 300 completed surveys. CAHPS originally stood for Consumer Assessment of Health Plan Survey, and this initial version was related to Medicare + Choice (today's MA plans) with physician payment models that met the definition of SFR. It has since branched out into versions applicable to MA plans, managed Medicaid plans, commercial plans, hospitals, and physicians. CAHPS is maintained by the federal Agency for Healthcare Research and Quality (AHRQ). It comes in several versions besides the version applicable to MA plans (e.g., CAHPS Hospital).

- Health Outcomes Survey (HOS)[*]: Measures a random sample of 1,200 MA enrollees enrolled for at least 6 months and resurveys the same sample 2 years later. The survey focuses on health status and use of services and is intended to measure improvement or declining physical and mental health from the enrollee's perspective.
- Plan Information: Plans report on contract performance measures (e.g., call center performance, appeals, and grievances rates).

As discussed in the next section, CMS summarizes the data from these data sets and ranks plans according to a five-star rating system. There are fairly wide variations in plan performance based on quality reporting. For example, high-performing plans may have HEDIS scores that are five times higher for outcomes measures than low-performing plans. However, there may be underlying reasons beyond quality differences that explain this variation (e.g., different geographic areas served by the plans or a higher rate of disabled beneficiaries enrolled in RPPOs).

CMS also expects plans to use the data, including HOS data, for internal quality improvement. The data should help plans identify some of the areas where their quality improvement efforts need to be targeted and may be used as the baseline data for quality improvement projects.

Health plans are required to submit additional reports about benefit utilization and plan operations. There is some overlap between these reports and data collected for star ratings (discussed in the next section), but these reports are somewhat less detailed and are generally aimed at providing overall rates by membership. Reported data are used for comparative purposes both between health plans as well as with the greater FFS system. Part D reports are required by statute while Part C reports are governed by regulation. Although some reports are made on a quarterly basis, most reports are due on an annual basis. In 2011 there are 13 reports for Part C (such as Benefit Utilization, Provider Network Adequacy, and Grievances) and 16 reports for Part D (such as Enrollment, Medication Therapy Management Programs, and Long-Term Care [LTC] Utilization).

---

[*] It was initially named the Health of Seniors survey, but was renamed in 1999, one year after its launch.

For 2011, CMS has initiated data validation audits. This new regulatory requirement ensures that health plans provide Part C and Part D data to CMS according to a standardized methodology that will ensure comparability. Data validation requires health plans to obtain the services of an external data validation auditor. The validation auditors conduct the required audit yearly by evaluating data programming inputs along with the processes and programming used to query databases and develop reports provided to CMS.

Star Ratings

Plans report required quality and performance measures to CMS and CMS creates a Part C and Part D Report Card using a five-star rating (one star is a poor-performing plan while five stars is an excellent-performing plan). Medicare displays Plan Ratings in the Medicare Plan Finder used by beneficiaries to select health plans on www.medicare.gov. The data are displayed prior to the open-enrollment period every year in a star format similar to *Consumer Reports*.

For 2011, Part C Plan Ratings are reported at four levels, which allow the beneficiary to drill-down and get more detailed information:

- Overall rating for MA-PD contracts—average of Part C and D stars
- Summary level—star rating for a contract
- Domain—nine groups of similar measures assigned a star rating based on an average of each of the individual measures
- Individual measures—53 quality and performance measures (36 MA and 17 Part D of which one-third are contract performance measures)

In addition, in the Medicare Plan Finder CMS includes a warning symbol for low-performing contracts that have a 3-year average summary rating of 2.5 stars or lower. The star assignment methodology adjusts for minimum time in the MA program, missing data, and mean and variation of individual measures.

Table 24-4 displays an example of a domain and measures with data sources for 2011.

The other domains for 2011 include Managing Chronic Care Conditions; Health Plan Responsiveness and Care; Member Complaints, Appeals, and Disenrollment; and Telephone Customer Service.

CMS considers organizations that fail to achieve at least a three-star summary rating on Part C or D for 3 straight years to have ignored their obligation to meet program requirements and to be substantially out of compliance with their Medicare contracts. In 2011 CMS has announced that it expects to initiate action to terminate these contracts in 2012 once they publish the third consecutive summary rating of less than three stars and after confirming that the star data reflect the health plan's substantial noncompliance.

TABLE 24-4	Domain 1 Measures and Data Sources, 2011

Domain 1: Prevention—Staying Healthy: Screenings, Test, and Vaccines	
Measure	**Data source**
Breast cancer screening	HEDIS
Colorectal cancer screening	HEDIS
Cardiovascular care cholesterol screening	HEDIS
Diabetes care—cholesterol screening	HEDIS
Glaucoma testing	HEDIS
Appropriate monitoring for patients taking long-term medication	HEDIS
Annual flu vaccine	CAHPS
Pneumonia vaccine	CAHPS
Improving or maintaining physical health	HOS
Improving or maintaining mental health	HOS
Osteoporosis testing	HEDIS/HOS
Monitoring physical activity	HEDIS/HOS
At least one primary care doctor visit in the last year	HEDIS

Source: CMS.

With regard to future measures, more emphasis will be placed on outcomes measures and new measures will be developed for older beneficiaries.

External Quality Review

The QIOs that are under contract to CMS to review the quality of care of hospitals in Medicare FFS also review the quality of care among MA enrollees. QIOs review complaints by MA enrollees about the quality of care in an MA plan. As in Medicare FFS, QIOs process beneficiary requests for review of hospital discharge decisions. Generally, QIOs review care to ensure that it meets the general standard for professional services and that appropriate services were delivered in an appropriate setting.

Finally, QIOs play a significant role in the appeals process. QIOs review a determination by a health plan whenever a beneficiary disputes the health plan's denial for continued services in an acute care hospital, skilled nursing facility, home health agency, or comprehensive rehabilitation facility.

Performance Assessment

CMS monitors a plan's compliance with regulatory requirements through data analysis, audits, beneficiary appeals, and complaints. In recent years CMS has moved from a plan oversight process that relies on routine onsite audits of all plans to a performance assessment system that is quantitative in nature. The Performance Assessment System arrays information from HEDIS, HOS, CAHPS, beneficiary complaints, audits, sanctions, and other sources to identify outliers and organizations whose performance is very poor compared to the rest of industry. CMS may target areas that warrant further review based on the data, prohibit an organization from expanding its service area, or deny a new application for a new contract.

Annual Performance Assessment

Each year CMS performs a review of all contracts' past performance covering a 14-month period. Each plan is provided a rating based on a weighted scale related to the seriousness of the finding. For example, a notice of noncompliance is the mildest with a weight of negative 1 while a corrective action plan (CAP)–ad hoc compliance event based on continuing and severe systemic problems is weighted at a negative 6. A plan with a CMS-imposed termination is weighted at a negative 8. Overall, CMS considers a poor-performing MA plan as one with a negative score of 4 points and Part D plan with a negative score of 5 points.

In 2011, CMS reviewed the following performance categories:

- Compliance Letters;
- Performance Metrics;
- Multiple Ad Hoc CAPs;
- Ad Hoc CAPs with Beneficiary Impact;
- Financial Watch List;
- One-Third Financial Audits;
- Performance Audits;
- Exclusions;
- Enforcement Actions;
- Terminations; and
- Outstanding Compliance Concerns Not Otherwise Captured.

Contracts in good standing have certain privileges, for example, inclusion in the *Medicare & You Handbook*, participation in the online enrollment center, allowing formulary updates, and receiving LIS enrollee reassignments and auto-enrollment.

Plan Performance Data

MA plans must report operational data, and CMS monitors and tracks several types of performance data from external sources. These different data are described next.

Operational Data

CMS uses a number of performance data points for purposes of conducting an annual performance assessment to track plan operations. With this data, CMS conducts outlier analysis by reviewing performance across all contracting organizations, which results in the identification of potential noncompliance and the need for further investigation.

This tracking process is ongoing. Whenever a plan demonstrates that it is outside of expected performance, CMS institutes an inquiry and potentially initiates a compliance action such as a compliance letter, an audit that results in an ad hoc compliance action, or an outstanding compliance concern. Generally, this occurs when CMS identifies outliers in plan operations or receives information from day-to-day operational interactions with the health plans. CMS tracks data submissions from health plans on a monthly basis; for example, failure to provide proper secondary payer information and failure to match enrollment with proper LIS rates (indicating an inability to ensure that beneficiaries do not pay higher copayments than they should pay).

Active Monitoring

CMS takes a more active role in the receipt of information from beneficiaries and from contracted resources that actively monitor how health plans communicate with beneficiaries. These are complaint tracking, sales surveillance activities, and customer service monitoring.

Complaint Tracking

With the implementation of Part D, CMS noted that beneficiaries' calls to CMS about obtaining prescribed medication required immediate action from health plans. The Complaint Tracking Module (CTM) process evolved as CMS received complaints and raised them to plans for action. The process now considers all types of complaints including marketing misrepresentation, enrollment errors, copayment for prescribed medications, and so on. The CTM process classifies complaints and assigns a range of time-required responses up to immediate need, which must be resolved within 2 calendar days. With the enactment of the ACA, the CTM process was formalized to require a complaint system that allows for the collection and maintenance of complaints against PDPs and MA-PD plans. As opposed to other types of information and data that takes time to accumulate, CTM information is current and CMS takes action to ensure that health plans are taking corrective action.

Sales Surveillance

CMS conducts ongoing surveillance of health plan sales and marketing functions, including observations of sales presentations, secret shopping calls, and reviews of marketing materials. Health plans receiving information about surveillance activities are expected to review their results and implement any corrective action plans to address any issue of noncompliance before CMS issues a compliance letter to the plan about the findings.

Call Center Surveillance

CMS monitors hold times, disconnect rates, and the time it takes for an interactive voice response (IVR) or live customer service representative (CSR) to answer the phone. Monitoring mostly occurs during the Annual Election Period and the 60 days following. While this is especially important to the ability of beneficiaries to resolve issues related to receipt of prescription drugs, CMS also requires the timely response to beneficiaries with questions regarding any benefit or question they could have about their health plan membership. Call centers or contact centers are discussed in detail in Chapter 20.

Audits

CMS conducts financial, actuarial, and performance audits using both CMS personnel and contracted resources. By law, CMS must conduct financial and actuarial audits of one-third of the plans each year. This review includes financial records, including documentation used to develop plan bids, administrative costs, and provider payment. CMS uses a Financial Watch List to track organizations with actual or potential financial solvency problems.

A performance audit is an in-depth review of a health plan's documentation related to the operation of their Medicare contracts. CMS conducts performance audits during which reviewers assess whether the health plan is complying with regulatory requirements in such areas as legal, quality of care, marketing practices, enrollment/disenrollment, claims payment, and grievance and appeals procedures.

CMS uses risk analysis to select plans for audits. The risk assessment is based on the performance categories and combines a number of factors, including each organization's compliance history, enrollment levels, and the rate of growth of plan enrollment. If the audit has findings, the organization is required to submit a corrective action plan to correct any deficiencies. Close monitoring of the plan continues until CMS is satisfied that the problems have been resolved. Contracts with audit scores in the worst 25th percentile are subject to further compliance and enforcement actions.

Prevention and Detection of Fraud, Waste, and Abuse

CMS regulations specifically direct health plans to implement a program that prevents, detects, and corrects fraud, waste, and abuse. While misbehavior may be committed by providers (e.g., billing for services that were not provided), beneficiaries (e.g., misuse of a plan ID card), or employees (e.g., paying claims that are known to be false), it has not been as prevalent in health plans as in the traditional Medicare FFS system. In addition, the use of periodic financial and actuarial audits of health plans have provided a sentinel system for ensuring that health plan cost estimates and bids closely follow requirements. However, with full risk adjustment and Part D, opportunities for fraud, waste, and abuse have significantly increased. These opportunities exist at each level within the health plan organization and warrant increased vigilance within health plans so that all actions necessary can be taken by the health plan as well as

government agencies. Fraud and abuse are discussed more fully in Chapter 19.

Compliance Program

All health plans must operate a compliance program for oversight of the MA and Part D programs. By regulation, the program must consist of seven elements:

1. Written Policies and Procedures;
2. Compliance Officer and Compliance Committee;
3. Training and Education;
4. Effective Lines of Communication;
5. Enforcement of Standards through well-publicized disciplinary guidelines;
6. Monitoring and Auditing; and
7. Corrective Action Procedures.

The regulations for the compliance program are explicitly detailed, having evolved from their initial introduction as a regulatory requirement in 1998. The program must describe the health plan's commitment to compliance with regulatory standards, include a code of conduct, provide guidance to employees and others on processes to communicate compliance issues, and include procedures to investigate and resolve them. Finally, it must state a policy of nonintimidation and nonretaliation for good faith participation in any aspect of the compliance program or reporting potential issues.

The compliance officer must be an employee of the contracted organization, its parent, or a corporate affiliate and must report to the CEO or other senior management. In addition, periodic reports must be made by the compliance committee to the health plan's governing body, usually the Board of Directors, who must exercise reasonable oversight. The regulation cites the types of personnel who must receive compliance training as well as those who serve in downstream entities. Processes must ensure that communication of compliance issues is confidential and can be anonymous. Disciplinary standards must be effectively applied to all levels within the health plan. Audit and monitoring programs must be effective in identifying compliance issues.

CMS expects regular monitoring activities as well as periodic audits of all operations, including delegated first-tier operations. Audits can be conducted by outside auditors if necessary. The compliance program must also demonstrate that compliance issues are promptly investigated and corrective actions are undertaken to quickly resolve any noncompliant issue. This includes repayment of overpayments and disciplinary actions against responsible employees in response to the potential violation. While self-reporting is not a required process, the health plan must have processes to voluntarily self-report potential fraud or misconduct related to the MA program to CMS, the Office of the Inspector General, or other federal agencies.

To emphasize its interest in the proper operation of compliance programs, CMS has conducted audits of each health plan's compliance program in 2010 to evaluate their effectiveness. Audits focused on the examination of the evidence of compliance program operations. These included records of compliance committee meetings, reports to the governing body, audits, investigations, and corrective and disciplinary actions.

Enforcement

Over the last several years, CMS has implemented a graduated system of compliance notices to make organizations aware of when they are not in compliance. These notices use an outlier-based standard for the lower-level notices. These notices reflect the earlier stages of CMS compliance efforts and afford organizations reasonable opportunities to take corrective action.

Whenever noncompliance is identified, the notice generally allows for an opportunity for corrective action. The health plan is solely responsible for the identification, development, and implementation of a CAP and for demonstrating that the underlying deficiencies have been corrected. Health plans have at least 30 calendar days to develop and implement a CAP. However, in some cases where the corrective action might take more time, CMS can allow a longer period for corrective action to be completed. CMS does not approve the corrective action but will focus only on determining that the noncompliance has been corrected. The health plan must develop and implement the corrective action prior to CMS issuing a notice of intent to terminate or nonrenew.

Administrative and Intermediate Sanctions

CMS can use other enforcement options short of termination and nonrenewal to address health plans that are noncompliant. First, CMS can reject applications from health plans who have demonstrated a pattern of noncompliance. CMS believes that a pattern of noncompliance indicates operational difficulties and that the health plan should focus on improving its existing operations before expanding into new types of plan offerings or additional service areas. This action would be based on the most recent 14-month period and would apply even if the applicant currently meets all of the application requirements. For 2012 applications, CMS provided a point system based on the performance categories that would be used to determine if a health plan demonstrated noncompliance that would warrant rejection of an application. Health plans that had a score of four points for Part C or five points for Part D could see their application for expansion rejected. CMS would also apply this rule to any plans that withdrew bids after the benchmark was announced as well as ones that terminate a contract for an upcoming benefit year after the organization had executed the contract.

Second, CMS can implement three intermediate sanctions when issues of noncompliance have risen to a serious and significant level. They are: (1) suspension of acceptance of applications for enrollment, (2) suspension of marketing activities to Medicare beneficiaries, and (3) suspension of payment for new Medicare beneficiaries during the sanction period.

Most frequently, CMS imposes intermediate sanctions that suspend marketing and enrollment. CMS keeps sanctions in place until the health plan has corrected its deficiencies and they are not likely to recur. Health plans can rebut CMS findings and can also request a hearing to demonstrate that CMS made an incorrect determination, but these actions do not affect the effective date of the sanction.

Between 2008 and 2010 CMS cited numerous reasons for enforcement actions. They included denial of critical prescription drugs, marketing misrepresentation, inappropriate enrollment and/or disenrollment, and insufficient improvement despite warnings.

Termination

For the ultimate sanction, CMS can terminate or nonrenew a contract. CMS takes into account the nature and extent of the failure of the noncompliant regulatory requirements and their materiality in relation to all other requirements. As noted above, CMS allows at least 30 days following a notice of noncompliance for correction of the deficiency before the notice of termination or nonrenewal is issued to the health plan.

For termination, CMS can cite any one of 13 regulatory reasons for termination. These range from very general failure to carry out the terms of the contract to 11 other specific operational requirements, such as the failure to comply with the prompt payment rules. CMS can expedite a termination when there is an imminent and serious risk to the health of enrollees or evidence exists that fraud has been committed. As in an intermediate sanction, the health plans can request a hearing where the health plan must provide the preponderance of the evidence that CMS has made an incorrect determination. The process for the hearing does not delay the termination action.

Civil Monetary Penalties

CMS and the HHS Office of the Inspector General (OIG) can impose civil money penalties on health plans based on noncompliance with the regulations. The basis for these penalties is the same as the reasons for imposing an intermediate sanction on the health plan. CMS imposes all civil money penalties except for cases that involve creditable evidence that the health plan has committed or participated in false, fraudulent, or abusive activities.

There are four different types of civil money penalties:

- $25,000 for each CMS finding where one or more beneficiaries was adversely affected or could have been of adversely affected;

- $25,000 for each beneficiary who was adversely affected or could have been of adversely affected by a deficiency;
- Up to $10,000 for each week that a deficiency remains uncorrected after CMS notice of noncompliance; and
- $250 per Medicare enrollee or $100,000, whichever is greater, from when a health plan has failed to follow proper procedures for terminating its contract with CMS.

In its capacity to address fraud, waste, and abuse, the OIG levies all civil money penalties whenever there is credible evidence that a health plan has committed or participated in false, fraudulent, or abusive activities. In addition, to a civil money penalty, health plans can be required to agree to a corporate integrity agreement that will detail additional requirements for continued participation in federal programs.

Exclusion from all Federal Programs

Health plans and individuals can be excluded from federal programs. The HHS OIG is mandated to operate the program to exclude individuals and entities from participating in federal programs. The OIG conducts these activities under various legal authorities, contained in sections 1128 and 1156 of the Social Security Act. In addition, the OIG maintains a list of all currently excluded parties, called the List of Excluded Individuals/Entities.

Generally, exclusion from federal programs follows conviction of a felony, misdemeanor, license revocation, or similar offense. However, it could also include defaults on health education loans or scholarship obligations. Conviction of a crime can result in imprisonment. The nature of each violation drives the period of exclusion. Exclusions have minimal periods that must be applied or can be permanent.

Of particular note is that exclusions of corporate officers have been upheld since prosecutors have demonstrated that an executive has a duty to know about the actions of subordinates and that the executive must move to stop any wrongdoing upon learning of it.

■ SUBREGULATORY GUIDANCE

The operation of the Part C and Part D programs requires the development of additional requirements and guidance. This guidance is used to explain the letter and intent of a requirement and to provide information necessary for the proper management of the program. With this guidance, health plans can conduct day-to-day operations as well as communicate with CMS about required processes, formats, timeframes needed to maintain compliant operations for enrollment, payment, risk adjustment, marketing approvals, and so on.

CMS uses the HPMS as the vehicle for communicating with and sending information to contracted health plans. CMS provides additional guidance and information that clarifies regulatory requirements in the form of manuals,

notices, monitoring guides, an annual call letter, and updates to requirements. The subregulatory guidance further explains how CMS will regulate specific regulation that is the basis for the guidance.

Separate Part C and Part D manuals are used as the basis for subregulatory guidance and reflect the current CMS interpretation of the requirements and related provisions. Manuals evolve over time as regulators and health plans address questions and new circumstances. Each manual has multiple chapters that define terms discussed in the chapter and provide direction on the application of any regulation.

CMS provides periodic updates to the provisions in the manual via HPMS. These periodic notices become the operational understanding for the subject of the HPMS notice. Generally, these notices are annual updates to a process for timeframes, definitions, category, revised standards, and so on. An example of this type of notice is the annual announcement of calendar year payment rates, which announces changes to payment rates as well as annual due dates and effective dates for new requirements. Typically, CMS obtains comments from health plans before implementing a new subregulatory requirement.

CMS follows a process for updating manual chapters by soliciting comments to draft changes from health plans and other interested parties. This process allows for the development of common understanding about the application of requirements to the operation of the Part C and Part D programs.

■ CONCLUSION

This chapter is, in effect, only a fleeting snapshot of MA and Part D. These two programs—consistent with their history—are bound to change and likely dramatically so. At the time of publication:

- Baby Boomers are enrolling in Medicare at a rate of 3,600 *per day*. They will double Medicare's enrollment over the next 25 years, and double its expenditures in the next decade. The steady drumbeat of demographics will force Congress to reform the program further.
- Boomers are familiar with health plans from their employer-sponsored health care coverage—over 90% of the working insured are in HMOs, PPOs, or POS plans. Most will want to continue their coverage into their retirement, and therefore will seek to enroll in MA in growing numbers. Indeed, in both 2010 and 2011, over 40% of beneficiaries aging-in to Medicare have chosen health plans over the traditional FFS program. And let's not forget the two truisms of Medicare beneficiaries: if they're not sick today, they will be and they vote in overwhelming numbers in defense of the program.
- Some publicly traded health insurance companies have grown dependent on Medicare revenues and will continue to play a major role in administering the program. When the BBA passed, publicly traded

companies derived, on average, 13% of their revenues from Medicare. Today that number has doubled to 26%, with several companies seeing more than half of their revenues from Medicare. Said another way, health plans are here to stay in Medicare.

- There is broad consensus that Medicare is unsustainable in its current form. Medicare's Trustees point out the program will become insolvent in the next decade without structural reforms. The program is literally dying under its own weight. The aging of the population only accounts for 2% of that doubling in Medicare's expenditures this decade. The other 98% is due to the costs of chronic disease and the proliferation of medical technology and procedures, as described in Chapter 7. Today 1 in 4 Medicare dollars is spent on diabetes, 1 in 4 on cardiovascular disease, and 1 in 4 on end-of-life care. CMS will continue to "raise the bar" on plans to deliver more cost-effective chronic care.
- The federal debt is issue #1 in Washington and Medicare is at the center of that debate. How this will play out is, as is always the case with politics, nearly impossible to predict. Sooner or later it will be addressed, whether we like it or not.

For the life of this version of the book, MA and Part D will continue to be a political football tossed between the two parties as they battle for their respective visions of the future for this massive and essential entitlement program. Don't blink or you might miss the latest in the annals of Medicare reform.

Endnotes

1 Kaiser Family Foundation Medicare Plan Tracking data, available at http://healthplantracker.kff.org/georesults .jsp?r = 1. Accessed August 19, 2011.

2 Medicare Payment Advisory Commission. *A Data Book: Healthcare Spending and the Medicare Program*. June 2010, p. 159.

3 Zarabozo C. Milestones in Medicare Managed Care – Statistical Data Included. *Health Care Financ R*. Fall 2000; 61–67.

4 Pope GC, Kautter J, Ellis RP, et al. Risk Adjustment of Medicare Capitation Payments Using the CMS-HCC Model. *Health Care Financ R*. 2004;25(4):119–141.

5 McBride TD, Penrod J, Mueller K. Volatility in Medicare AAPCC rates: 1990–1997. *Health Affairs*. 1997;16(5): 172–180.

6 Pope GC, Kautter J, Ellis RP, et al. Risk Adjustment of Medicare Capitation Payments Using the CMS-HCC Model. *Health Care Financ R*. 2004;25(4):119–141.

7 Risk scores are those in effect in 2011, from the CMS file "HCC_Coefficients_2011.csv" included in the CMS 2011 Ratebook at: www.cms.gov/MedicareAdvtgSpecRateStats/ RSD/itemdetail.asp?filterType = none&filterByDID = .99&sortByDID = 1&sortOrder = descending&itemID = CMS1237871&intNumPerPage = 10.

8 Pope GC, Kautter J, Ellis RP, et al. Risk Adjustment of Medicare Capitation Payments Using the CMS-HCC Model. *Health Care Financ R*. 2004;25(4):119–141.

9 Government Accountability Office. Medicare Advantage: Comparison of Plan Bids to Fee-for-Service Spending by Plan and Market Characteristics. February 4, 2011.

10 Medicare Payment Advisory Commission. *A Data Book: Healthcare Spending and the Medicare Program*. June 2010, p. 157.

11 Author's calculation, based on the methodology described in the CMS publication: "Advance Notice of Methodological Changes for Calendar Year (CY) 2012 for Medicare Advantage (MA) Capitation Rates, Part C and Part D Payment Policies and 2012 Call Letter." February 18, 2011.

12 Government Accountability Office. Medicare Advantage: Comparison of Plan Bids to Fee-for-Service Spending by Plan and Market Characteristics. February 4, 2011.

13 Government Accountability Office. Medicare Advantage: Comparison of Plan Bids to Fee-for-Service Spending by Plan and Market Characteristics. February 4, 2011.

CHAPTER 25

Medicaid Managed Health Care

Rodney C. Armstead, Catherine K. Anderson, and Elizabeth Cabot Nash

STUDY OBJECTIVES

- Understand the legislative history of Medicaid and managed care
- Understand the challenges associated with access and the necessary solutions to meet the needs of the Medicaid consumer
- Understand Medicaid managed care's growth and the opportunity with health reform
- Understand Medicaid managed care and its application to other vulnerable populations (long-term care; behavioral/substance abuse; aged, blind, disabled, and other special populations)

DISCUSSION TOPICS

1. Should managed care organizations (MCOs), including health maintenance organizations (HMOs)* be leveraged by states as primary options for program effectiveness?
2. What are the implications for more costly populations like long-term care? Should they be transitioned into MCOs?
3. Health reform is leveraging Medicaid for a significant part of the expansion. Is this good public policy?
4. Who are the new eligibles covered under health reform?

■ INTRODUCTION

Medicaid has been the vehicle relied upon to provide coverage for the uninsured for over 45 years. This entitlement program, established in 1965 as part of President Johnson's "Great Society," was initially intended as a health coverage supplement for those receiving cash assistance (predominantly women of childbearing age and children).[1] Over time, Congress has expanded eligibility substantially to fill

coverage gaps left by private insurance. Therefore, states have expanded their programs by (1) raising the income eligibility levels for aid categories; and (2) adding and/or expanding new populations.[2] Medicaid pays for nearly 40% of all newborn deliveries and covers 1 in 4 children, and provides benefits to more people than any other public program, including Medicare, or any single private insurer.

When the Balanced Budget Act (BBA) was passed in 1997, it created Title XXI, or the State Children's Health Insurance Program (SCHIP or CHIP)—a grant in aid statute, expanding eligibility for states to cover uninsured children who did not qualify for Medicaid. States were incentivized

---

*Most Medicaid MCOs are HMOs or HMO-like organizations. Both of these terms are used except when a particular type of MCO is being discussed.

TABLE 25-1	**Medicaid and CHIP Enrollment as a Percentage of the U.S. Population, 2010**		
	Administrative Data		**Survey Data (NHIS)**
Medicaid and CHIP Enrollment	**Ever enrolled during the year**	**Point in time**	**Point in time**
Medicaid	66.7 million	52.9 million	Not available
CHIP	8.1 million	5.4 million	Not available
	74.8 million	58.3 million	45.8 million
U.S. Population	**2010 Census**		**Survey Data (NHIS)**
	308.7 million		303.4 million, excluding active-duty military and individuals in institutions
Medicaid and CHIP Enrollment as a Percentage of U.S. Population			
	24.2 percent	18.9 percent	15.1 percent
	(74.8/308.7)	(58.3/308.7)	(45.8/303.4)

Notes: Excludes U.S. territories. Enrollment from administrative data includes individuals who received limited benefits. Survey data shown here are 2010 National Health Interview Survey (NHIS), which excludes individuals in institutions such as nursing homes. NHIS point-in-time estimates were as of survey interviews taken between January and June 2010. Administrative data are for fiscal year 2010 (October 2009 through September 2010). By combining administrative totals from Medicaid and CHIP, some individuals may be double-counted, if they were enrolled in both programs during the year. Overcounting of enrollees in the administrative data may occur for other reasons—for example, because a person moves and is enrolled in two states' Medicaid programs during the year. The 2010 census number was as of April 1, 2010, but was also applied in the calculation of the percentage ever enrolled during the year.

Source: Medicaid and CHIP Payment and Access Commission (MACPAC). www.macpac.gov/.

to increase coverage for children with an enhanced federal financial participation (FFP) rate of at least 70% for those children enrolled and receiving benefits and services, which are in parallel with the Medicaid definition of "medical assistance." From December 1999 to December 2010, SCHIP enrollment has grown from 2.7 million to approximately 8 million consumers, respectively, and overall, Medicaid enrollment has increased from 31.7 million consumers in June 2000 to 58 million in 2010.[3, 4] See **Table 25-1**.

The average increase in monthly enrollment over this period of time was 2.7%. For the period June 2007–June 2010 and June 2009–June 2010 (coincident with the start of the recession in December 2007 and recovery), the average increase in monthly enrollment was higher as expected—3.1% and 3.3%, respectively.[3] Between June 2009 and June 2010, Medicaid enrollment grew 7.2%, or 3.37 million enrollees. From December 2007 to June 2010, unemployment went from 5% to 9.5%, as shown in **Table 25-2**.

Many people lost jobs and access to employer-sponsored health coverage. Finding they qualified for Medicaid thus resulted in explosive growth in the program over the past several years. This phenomenon of growth, which inversely correlates to unemployment in the state and lost revenue, places significant fiscal pressure on states. Medicaid spending on average is about 20% of states' budgets and is always a target for cuts, particularly when there is a fiscal crisis.

On March 23, 2010, President Barack Obama signed the Patient Protection and Affordable Care Act (ACA). The ACA is the single most significant piece of social legislation since 1965. It seeks to dramatically close the gap of those without health care coverage by (1) creating access to affordable care instituting a legal obligation for individuals to obtain coverage; and (2) leverage a national framework of universal coverage aimed at improving care and decreasing cost. A tenet of reform is expansion through Medicaid—essentially absorbing half of the newly covered or 16 million additional enrollees.

Within the past 15 years, state agencies have been very proactive and aggressive about building upon the successes of Medicaid MCOs and HMOs, utilizing the federal waiver process across all products (acute, behavioral, long-term care, special populations, SCHIP) as solutions to not only bend the cost trend curve to mitigate their risk and exposure, but, more important, to assist with the development and implementation of integrated comprehensive programs, sensitive to the ethnic, linguistic, cultural, and social attributes, to improve the health outcomes, functional status, and the overall member experience for their consumers. This will be important in preparation for the anticipated growth from health reform.

After reviewing the legislative history for Medicaid and the challenges presented by the Medicaid population, this chapter examines growth of Medicaid managed care and solutions afforded states by leveraging full-risk models and the implications of health reform for Medicaid managed care, including the role of exchanges for Medicaid, SCHIP, and the subsidized uninsured.

TABLE 25-2	National Economic Data, 2000–2009									
	2000	**2001**	**2002**	**2003**	**2004**	**2005**	**2006**	**2007**	**2008**	**2009**
GDP[a]										
in billions % change	9,951.50	10,286.20	10,642.30	11,142.10	11,867.80	12,638.40	13,398.90	14,061.80	14,369.10	14,119.00
Unemployment %[b]	3.97%	4.74%	5.78%	5.99%	5.54%	5.08%	4.61%	4.61%	4.82%	9.28%
Income[c]										
Real Median Household	52,388	52,301	51,161	50,563	50,519	50,343	50,899	51,965	50,112	49,777
Real Per Capita[d]	27,833	27,685	27,177	27,145	27,507	27,507	28,034	27,728	26,862	26,530

Source: Reproduced from Holahan, John. "The 2007–09 Recession and Health Insurance Coverage". Health Affairs, January 2011, Vol. 30, No. 1, available online at http://content.healthaffairs.org/content/early/2010/12/07/hlthaff.2010.1003.full.pdf+html
[a]Bureau of Economic Analysis: National Economic Accounts. U.S. Department of Commerce. www.bea.gov
[b]Bureau of Labor Statistics: Current Population Survey: Labor Force Statistics. U.S. Department of Labor. www.bls.gov/data
[c]Income measurements are from U.S. Census Bureau, Current Population Survey, Annual Social and Economic Supplements.
[d]The per capita income data presented in this report are not directly comparable with estimates of personal per capita income prepared by the Bureau of Economic Analysis, U.S. Department of Commerce. The lack of correspondence stems from the differences in income definition and coverage. For further details, see www.census.gov/hhes/www/income/compare1.html
Source: "Medicaid Spending Growth over the Last Decade and the Great Recession, 2000–2009" (#8152). www.kff.org/medicaid/upload/8152.pdf, p. 4. This information was reprinted with permission from the Henry J. Kaiser Family Foundation. The Kaiser Family Foundation is a non-profit private operating foundation, based in Menlo Park, California, dedicated to producing and communicating the best possible analysis and information on health issues.

■ LEGISLATIVE HISTORY OF MEDICAID

The Medicaid program is a federal/state shared publicly funded entitlement program signed into law in 1965 initially intended to provide coverage for women receiving cash assistance and their children. Between 1965 and 2010, there have been numerous amendments expanding Social Security Amendment Public Law 89-97 that have been both calculated and deliberate in an effort to expand coverage for women, children, and eventually childless adults.[2-5] The chronology of key legislative amendments is as follows:

1. Social Security Amendments of 1967
   a. Enacted early, periodic, screening, diagnosis, and treatment (EPSDT) benefit requiring regular periodic health screening for children with details on how physical exams were to be performed (i.e., unclothed thorough physical)
   b. Required states to allow Medicaid beneficiaries to use any provider willing to accept Medicaid payment
2. Omnibus Reconciliation Act (OBRA) of 1981
   a. Limited Aid for Dependent Children (AFDC) eligibility, thus limiting Medicaid eligibility
   b. Enacted 1915(b) freedom of choice waivers to allow mandatory managed care in Medicaid
3. Tax Equity and Fiscal Responsibility Act (TEFRA) of 1982—allowed states to impose nominal cost-sharing on certain beneficiaries and services but exempted pregnant women and children as well as other groups
4. Deficit Reduction Act (DRA) of 1984—changed coverage for children and pregnant women; allowing infants born to mothers covered by Medicaid automatically eligible for 1 year
5. Consolidated Omnibus Budget Reconciliation Act (COBRA) of 1985
   a. Dropped the AFDC unemployed parent criteria
   b. Required coverage of children up to age 5 for families meeting AFDC income and resource standards
6. Omnibus Budget Reconciliation Acts of 1986 and 1987—expanded coverage for pregnant women, allowed states to use presumptive eligibility and continuous eligibility for pregnant women, and required coverage for children up to age 8 meeting certain AFDC criteria
7. Omnibus Budget Reconciliation Act (OBRA) of 1989
   a. Expanded coverage of pregnant women and children under age 6 to 133% of the federal poverty level (FPL)
   b. Expanded EPSDT to children under age 21
   c. Required coverage of services provider by federally qualified health centers
8. Omnibus Budget Reconciliation Act (OBRA) of 1993—established the Vaccines for Children program, providing federally purchased vaccines to states
9. Personal Responsibility and Work Opportunity Reconciliation Act (PRWORA) of 1996
   a. Repealed AFDC and replaced it with a block grant to the states, Temporary Assistance for Needy Families (TANF), and severed the link between eligibility for cash assistance and Medicaid
   b. Established Section 1931 of the Social Security Act, essentially covering families meeting July 1996 AFDC income standards

c. Barred Medicaid coverage for most illegal immigrants who entered the United States on or after August 22, 1996

10. Balanced Budget Act (BBA) of 1997
    a. Established SCHIP, providing coverage for low-income children, with incomes above March 1997 level
    b. Allowed states to require most Medicaid beneficiaries to enroll in HMOs without states obtaining Section 1915(b) "freedom of choice" waivers
    c. Allowed presumptive and continuous eligibility for children
    d. Shifted prescription drug responsibility for dually eligible individuals to Medicare

11. Deficit Reduction Act (DRA) of 2005
    a. Requires that people applying for Medicaid must provide proof of citizenship (such as a birth certificate) and identity (such as a drivers' license)
    b. Created opportunities for states to expand community-based alternatives for costly populations

12. Children's Health Insurance Reauthorization Act of 2009 (CHIRA)—reauthorized SCHIP and expanded coverage for an additional 4 million children with enhanced payments to states through 2013

13. Patient Protection and Affordable Care Act (ACA) of 2010—single largest social reform legislation since 1965—expanding coverage to approximately 16 million childless adults in 2014 leveraging Medicaid infrastructure; incremental 16 million uninsured will receive federal subsidy and purchase health care through state exchanges

Medicaid enrollment grew substantially in the early years of the program but began to slow considerably in the mid-1970s. This was largely due to the fact that Medicaid eligibility was linked to AFDC and cash assistance. During that period of time, the number of women qualifying for AFDC declined, resulting in a decline in the enrollment of low-income children with a corresponding increase in infant mortality rates, which prompted Congress to improve pregnant women and children's access to health care by delinking receipt of welfare and Medicaid eligibility for these two groups. From 1984 through the early 1990s, federal legislation was very effective at expanding coverage for these two groups by aligning Medicaid eligibility to family income status and access to two-parent families as well. Changes in legislation also gave states the latitude to cover children at higher income levels and still receive federal matching funds.

Figure 25-1 demonstrates the impact of legislation on Medicaid enrollment growth for children.

Medicaid experienced the most significant growth when the Personal Responsibility and Work Act of 1994 (PROWA) delinked eligibility in 1996 from cash assistance and aligned it with family income. In repealing AFDC and replacing it with block grants to the states, now defined as TANF, it capped an individual's financial assistance at 5 years and coupled eligibility for Medicaid to family income. Prior to the passage of welfare reform, there were attempts to repeal Medicaid as an entitlement program and replace it with a federal block program (very similar to SCHIP today) that was materially different than Medicaid in design and coverage;[6] however, a threat of a residential veto resulted in its removal from the final bill as signed into law.

President George W. Bush signed the Balance Budget Act into law on August 5, 1997, which created SCHIP. Between 1997 and 2009, this grant program has accounted for approximately 8 million additional children with comprehensive health coverage, as shown in Figure 25-1. Interestingly,

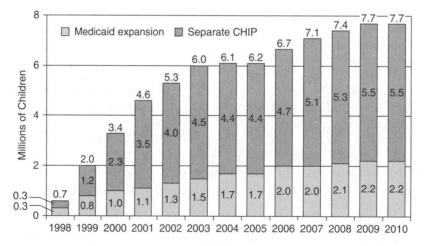

Note: Numbers are children ever enrolled during the year, even if only for a month. Components may not add to total due to rounding.

FIGURE 25-1 Child Enrollment in CHIP, FY 1998–2010

Source: Medicaid and CHIP Payment and Access Commission (MACPAC). https://7737438414307547177-a-macpac-gov-s-sites.googlegroups.com/a/macpac.gov/macpac/reports/ MACPAC_March2011_web.pdf?attachauth=ANoY7cqji2nzfoaw3_z_3nc5rT56nfcGY5gJvxH4M2N2Oxh02o7RRwVo1ZMVeL9x0jB-Zno279uU-5P3YdtuV-k_EuZ6Kh7SJRBJpX0AjX 2c3lsnuXGtg50Fqi5d36q3vaOyll9CpkLPTDrqzrKV4qXX-xGW_axe5EQMgGt30fJUaZ1dD0OET2TxliDoUrp50OM6wXPCZtF864xgE2dX8SR001gQhEybZQ%3D%3D&attredirects=0. Report to the Congress on Medicaid and CHIP, March 2011, p. 55.

<table>
<tr><td rowspan="2">**TABLE 25-3**</td><td colspan="3">**Sources of Coverage Among Children and Nonelderly Adults with Family Income from 100–199% of the Federal Poverty Level, 1997 and 2010**</td></tr>
<tr><td>**Private**</td><td>**Public**</td><td>**Uninsured**</td></tr>
</table>

	Private	Public	Uninsured
Children			
1997	55.0 percent	24.3 percent	22.8 percent
2010	30.8	57.6	13.5
Change	−24.2	+33.3	−9.3
Nonelderly Adults			
1997	52.6	14.6	34.9
2010	34.9	22.5	43.9
Change	−17.7	+7.9	+9.0

Source: National Health Interview Survey (NHIS), Martinez and Cohen 2010. Note: For this table, the federal poverty level (FPL) is based on the U.S. Census Bureau's poverty thresholds. Children are between the ages of 0 and 1 years, and non-elderly adults are between the ages of 18 and 64. "Public" coverage includes CHIP, Medicaid, and Medicare. Federal surveys such as NHIS do not publish separate results for Medicaid and CHIP enrollment; child enrollment in Medicare is relatively small.
Source: Medicaid and CHIP Payment and Access Commission (MACPAC). https://7737438414307547177-a-macpac-gov-s-sites.googlegroups.com/a/macpac.gov/macpac/reports/MACPAC_March2011_web.pdf?attachauth=ANoY7cqji2nzfoaw3_z_3nc5rT56nfcGY5gJvxH4M2N2Oxh02o7RRwVo1ZMVe\L9x0jB-Zno279uU-5P3YdtuV-k_EuZ6Kh7SJRBJpX0AjX2c3lsnuXGtg50Fqi5d36q3vaOyll9CpkLPTDrqzrKV4qXX-xGW_axe5EQMgGt30fJUaZ1dD0OET2TxliDoUrp50OM6wXPCZtF864xgE2dX8SR001gQhEybZQ%3D%3D&attredirects=0. Report to the Congress on Medicaid and CHIP, March 2011, p. 53.

between 1997 and 2010, Medicaid has surpassed private insurance as the primary payer of health services for children in the United States, as shown in **Table 25-3**.

The Children's Health Insurance Program Reauthorization Act (CHIPRA) of 2009 reauthorized SCHIP to 2013 and further expanded eligibility to cover up to 4 million additional children. Finally, as discussed later in the chapter, the ACA is extraordinary in its expansion of coverage to include up to 32 million uninsured adults.

The sustained legislative effort to improve access resulted in tremendous growth for the Medicaid program through the mid-1990s and generated fiscal concerns for states that were managing large fee-for-service (FFS) programs. In an effort to achieve predictable costs in these rapidly expanding programs, the states began to leverage prepaid health plans or HMOs, appreciating the benefit of their robust contracted networks and their ability to mainstream many of the Medicaid consumers.

This growth in HMO enrollment was certainly accelerated by legislation favorable to state flexibility as they recognized the cost-controlling attributes of HMOs. In the mid-1990s, Medicaid managed care enrollment grew five- to six-fold and BBA 1997 provided further flexibility to states to do mandatory enrollment without requiring permission from the Secretary of the Department of Health and Human Services.

Two remaining pieces of legislation generated tremendous growth in Medicaid and HMOs. PROWA, or welfare reform, completely delinked Medicaid eligibility from welfare and aligned eligibility with family income. In doing so, it increased significantly the number of Medicaid eligibles. BBA 97, authorized SCHIP and expansion of coverage to children who did not qualify for Medicaid.[2, 4, 7]

■ BARRIERS THAT CAN AFFECT ACCESS TO CARE

On the surface, one might conclude that Medicaid consumers should not have any problem with access to health care, as shown in **Figure 25-2** and **Table 25-4**, given the comprehensiveness of the Medicaid benefit package.

In 2009, consumers covered by Medicaid and private insurance appeared to have an equally low percentage of no usual source of care when compared to the uninsured. The evaluation of benefits reveals that only 60% of the covered services are federally mandated—40% are optional services (i.e., prescription drugs, dental, eyeglasses, private-duty nursing, transportation) that states decide that they want to cover; however, they do receive the federal medical assistance percentage (FMAP).[*5]

The states have decided to cover these optional services for a variety of reasons. The common thread is that these optional services mitigate benefit gaps that would, if not covered, result in suboptimal care and poorer outcomes for Medicaid consumers.

Physician Payment

Despite this comprehensive benefit package, Medicaid consumers still have significant barriers to receiving health care services. Historically low provider payment rates when compared to commercial and Medicare has limited consumer access to many of the mainstream primary care and specialty physicians as well as treatment in many of the centers of excellence around the country. For example, California, New York, and New Jersey physician Medicaid FFS payment was 56%, 43%, and 37% of Medicare, respectively, for 2006. The national average for that year was 72% of Medicare.[7] Physician participation in Medicaid is voluntary, and national surveys suggest that while Medicaid consumers have better access to care than the uninsured, they have considerably less access than those covered by private insurance. There is limited information on the number of physicians who participate in the Medicaid program nationally. This broadly held assumption is supported by a University of California, San Francisco, survey developed and conducted in 2008 to determine the level of physician participation in Medi-Cal, (California's Medicaid program), which revealed the following findings.[5]

---

*The FMAP is the percent of program expenditures paid by the federal government, commonly known as the match ratio. The formula for determining the rate is based on the states' per capita income.

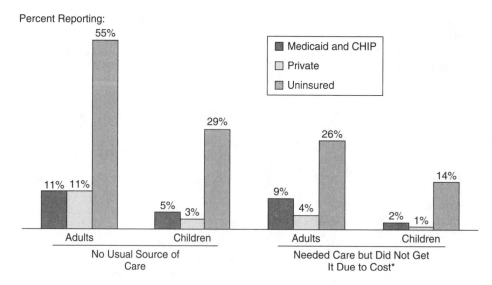

Percent Reporting:

* In the past 12 months
Note: Respondents who said their usual source of care was the emergency room were included among those not having
a usual source of care.

FIGURE 25-2 Access to Care: Medicaid and CHIP Enrollees Compared to Persons with Private Insurance, 2009

Source: Medicaid and CHIP Payment and Access Commission (MACPAC). https://7737438414307547177-a-macpac-gov-s-sites.googlegroups.com/a/macpac.gov/macpac/reports/
MACPAC_March2011_web.pdf?attachauth=ANoY7cqji2nzfoaw3_z_3nc5rT56nfcGY5gJvxH4M2N2Oxh02o7RRwVo1ZMVeL9x0jB-Zno279uU-5P3YdtuV-k_EuZ6Kh7SJRBJpX0AjX
2c3lsnuXGtg50Fqi5d36q3vaOyll9CpkLPTDrqzrKV4qXX-xGW_axe5EQMgGt30fJUaZ1dD0OET2TxliDoUrp50OM6wXPCZtF864xgE2dX8SR001gQhEybZQ%3D%3D&attredirects=0.
Report to the Congress on Medicaid and CHIP, March 2011, p. 134.

- California physicians were less likely to have Medi-Cal consumers in their practices (68%) than to have patients with private insurance (92%) or Medicare coverage (78%), with varied participation among specialties.
- While 90% of physicians in California were accepting new patients and 73% were accepting new Medicare patients, only 57% reported accepting new Medi-Cal patients.
- Medi-Cal patients are concentrated within a small share of practices, with 25% of physicians providing care to 80% of Medi-Cal patients.

The most common reason cited by physicians for limiting their practice to Medicaid consumers was low payment rates. Low payment rates from Medicaid have been attributed to both states' fiscal pressure and the changing practice environment. Changes in their income and practice arrangements make physicians less willing to accept Medicaid and uninsured patients.[8, 9] However, an interesting observation was that a physician would stop accepting new Medicaid consumers, yet continue to provide the same level of charity care.

While it is clear that low rates of payment may have contributed to lower Medicaid consumers' access, Medicaid physician fees did increase 15.1 percent, an average annual rate of increase of 2.6%, between 2003 and 2008.[9] This was below the general rate of inflation—the consumer price index (CPI) increased 20.3%, or 3.4% per year on average, and the Medical Care Services component, which includes physician services, grew 28.15, or 4.6% per year

on average. Simply stated in real terms, Medicaid physician fees, on average, declined 1 percent annually relative to general inflation and 2% annually relative to Medical Care Services inflation from 2003 to 2008.[9] However, states did invest in primary care, including obstetrical services, as fees grew at the rate of inflation—20% between 2003 and 2008. While the gap between Medicaid and Medicare fees continued, it did close slightly over the period of time due to slower growth in Medicare fees—growing from 69% to 72% of Medicare.

Experts in Medicaid policy would suggest that adequate payment is the linchpin to physician access; however, research is mixed on how fees influence physicians' participation. Anecdotal and retrospective data has shown that payment delays can offset any advantages that states try to achieve by paying higher rates.[9] Higher payment can enhance the chances of a consumer's access to a physician, but this is often setting-specific (i.e., office vs. hospital/academic clinic). Payment is extremely important to getting the door open for Medicaid consumers, but alone cannot ensure the door remains open.

Physician Supply

Provider supply and physician supply, in particular, will continue to be an ongoing concern. Physicians and other health care professionals are unevenly distributed across the country. Physicians tend to distribute where population is dense and income opportunity is high.[4] While some will migrate to areas of lower provider/population ratios, they generally have a tendency to migrate to areas where there is higher per

TABLE 25-4	**Mandatory and Optional Medicaid Benefits**

Mandatory	
• Inpatient hospital services	• Home health services
• Outpatient hospital services	• Laboratory and X-ray services
• Physician services	• Nursing facility services (for ages 21 and over)
• Early and Periodic Screening, Diagnostic, and Treatment (EPSDT) services for individuals under age 21 (screening, vision, dental, and hearing services and any medically necessary service listed in the Medicaid statute, including optional services that are not otherwise covered by a state)	• Nurse midwife services (to the extent authorized to practice under state law or regulation)
	• Rural health clinic services
	• Tobacco cessation counseling and pharmacotherapy for pregnant women
• Family planning services and supplies	• Nonemergency transportation
• Federally qualified health center services	
• Freestanding birth center services	

Optional (number of states covering benefit)	
• Medical or remedial care provided by licensed practitioners under state law. (Specific provider types, as well as all optional benefits states cover, are listed in Table 12 in MACStats.)	• Emergency hospital services (40)
	• Dentures (37)
	• Preventive services (37)
• Intermediate care facility services for individuals with mental retardation (51)	• Personal care services (35)
	• Private duty nursing services (33)
• Clinic services (50)	• Rehabilitative services (33)
• Skilled nursing facility services for individuals under age 21 (50)	• Diagnostic services (32)
• Occupational therapy services (50)	• Program for All-Inclusive Care for the Elderly (PACE) services (31)
• Optometry services (50)	• Screening services (30)
• Physical therapy services (50)	• Chiropractic services (29)
• Prescribed drugs (50)	• Critical hospital services (22)
• Targeted case management services (50)	• Respiratory care for ventilator-dependent individuals (22)
• Prosthetic devices (49)	• Primary care case management services (14)
• Hospice services (48)	• Services furnished in a religious nonmedical health care institution (13)
• Inpatient psychiatric services for individuals under age 21 (48)	
• Dental services (46)	• Tuberculosis-related services (13)
• Eyeglasses (45)	• Home and community-based services (HCBS) (4)
• Services for individuals with speech, hearing, and language disorders (45)	• Sickle cell disease-related services (2)
	• Health homes for enrollees with chronic conditions (new benefit as of January 1, 2011)
• Audiology services (43)	
• Inpatient hospital services, nursing facility services, and intermediate care services for individuals age 65 or older in institutions for mental diseases (42)	

Note: This table provides a list of mandatory and optional state plan benefits for the 50 states and the District of Columbia. It does not include services provided under a Medicaid waiver, for example, while four states provide HCBS under the state plan option; all states offer home and community-based services through waivers.

Source: Medicaid and CHIP Payment and Access Commission (MACPAC) https://7737438414307547177-a-macpac-gov-s-sites.googlegroups.com/a/macpac.gov/macpac/reports/MACPAC_March2011_web.pdf? attachauth=ANoY7cqji2nzfoaw3_z_3nc5rT56nfcGY5gJvxH4M2N2Oxh02o7RRwVo1ZMVeL9x0jB-Zno279uU-5P3 YdtuV-k_EuZ6Kh7SJRBJpX0AjX2c3lsnuXGtg50Fqi5d36q3vaOyll9CpkLPTDrqzrKV4qXX-xGW_axe5EQMgGt30fJUaZ1dD0OET2TxliDoUrp50OM6wXPCZtF864xgE2d X8SR001gQhEybZQ%3D%3D&attredirects=0. Report to the Congress on Medicaid and CHIP, March 2011, p. 33.

capita income and lower unemployment. Disincentives to choose primary care practice continue. Solutions are needed such as aggressive loan repayment programs like that proposed by New York State (Proposal to Redesign Medicaid to "Establish the Public Health Services Corps") and practice incentives so that physicians/providers will relocate to less economic communities, where many of the Medicaid consumers reside.[10]

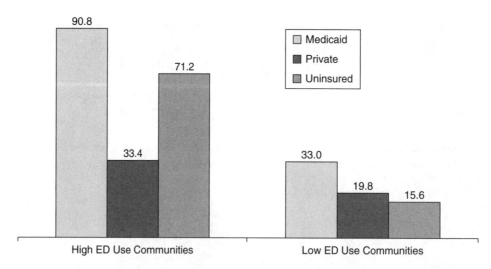

Note: High ED use communities are defined as the 25 % of Community Tracking Study (CTS) communities with the highest number of ED visits per 100 people. Low ED use communities are defined as the 25 % of CTS communities with the lowest number of ED visits per 100.

FIGURE 25-3 Emergency Department (ED) Visit Rates by Coverage Type, 2003

Source: Medicaid and CHIP Payment and Access Commission (MACPAC). https://7737438414307547177-a-macpac-gov-s-sites.googlegroups.com/a/macpac.gov/macpac/reports/MACPAC_March2011_web.pdf?attachauth=ANoY7cqji2nzfoaw3_z_3nc5rT56nfcGY5gJvxH4M2N2Oxh02o7RRwVo1ZMVeL9x0jB-Zno279uU-5P3YdtuV-k_EuZ6Kh7SJRBJpX0AjX2c3lsnuXGtg50Fqi5d36q3vaOyll9CpkLPTDrqzrKV4qXX-xGW_axe5EQMgGt30fJUaZ1dD0OET2TxliDoUrp50OM6wXPCZtF864xgE2dX8SR001gQhEybZQ%3D%3D&attredirects=0. Report to the Congress on Medicaid and CHIP, March 2011, p. 138.

Limited primary care services do influence the place of service where Medicaid consumers decide to receive services. As shown in **Figure 25-3**, Medicaid consumers receive a disproportionate amount of health care services in the Emergency Department.

Low payment, low physician/provider to population ratio, inadequate diversity of the physician/provider community, and geographic imbalance of physicians/providers in urban and rural communities are just some of the gaps that exacerbate primary care capacity. Over the past 40 years, many safety net providers such as federally qualified health centers (FQHCs), rural health centers (RHCs), community clinics, mental health clinics, and outpatient clinics associated with many community and academic teaching institutions have developed primary care practices in an attempt to bridge and close the access gap. FQHCs, FQHC look-alikes, and RHCs have received significant support from Congress. Incremental federal legislation has been passed that has both expanded the number of health centers nationally and stabilized them financially by modifying the payment structure—health center state-specific cost-based payment for both Medicaid and Medicare consumers seeking services in their facilities. The permanent authorization of FQHCs and RHCs passed as part of the ACA, and investment in excess of $11 billion for expansion and infrastructure (physical plant and technology) codified Congress' commitment to the centers and their role as core to primary care delivery in anticipation of Medicaid expansion in 2014. With health centers totaling 4,500 + nationwide, serving 18.7 million patients in 2009,[7] many providing comprehensive services (medical, dental,

behavioral, social services, and coordination with specialty care) for very diverse Medicaid consumers, there continues to be significant primary care access gaps for the reasons stated above. Medicaid consumers are important to health centers, accounting for in excess of 37% of health centers' revenue in 2009 as noted in **Table 25-5**.

The absence of these key critical safety net providers would only worsen an already very challenging problem.

TABLE 25-5	**Distribution of Revenue by Source for Federally Funded FQHC, 2009**	
United States	**Percent**	**0.0%–100.0%**
Federal Grants	21.9%	
State & Local Grants/Contracts	12.1%	
Foundation/Private Grants/Contracts	3.9%	
Medicaid	37.1%	
Medicare	5.9%	
Other Public Insurance	2.9%	
Private Insurance	7.3%	
Patient Self-Pay	6.0%	
Other Revenue	2.9%	

Source: www.statehealthfacts.org/profileind.jsp?ind=428&cat=8&rgn=1. This information was reprinted with permission from the Henry J. Kaiser Family Foundation. The Kaiser Family Foundation is a non-profit private operating foundation, based in Menlo Park, California, dedicated to producing and communicating the best possible analysis and information on health issues.

Social Determinants

There are a number of social determinants that negatively affect access to health care such as poverty, health literacy (complicated by language, cultural diversity, and ethnicity), gender bias, racial bias, complex health care needs, and unemployment, to name a few. Poverty is the single largest factor contributing to poor health outcomes, with a direct correlation between poverty level and health outcomes.[11] While many Medicaid consumers have comprehensive health benefits coverage, their ability to access needed medical services is complicated by the fact that many live in poverty, which often means poor housing and crowded living conditions, limited access to adequate and nutritious food, personal safety issues, limited access to technology such as telephone and the Internet (which is widely used for dissemination of information), and suboptimal primary and secondary education, to name a few. **Figure 25-4** demonstrates the negative impact of poverty on health status, with Medicaid beneficiaries demonstrating poorer status compared to privately insured individuals.

Health literacy is as equally important as poverty as a predictor of poor health status and outcomes. The Institute of Medicine defines health literacy as "the degree to which individuals have the capacity to obtain, process, and understand basic health information and services needed to make appropriate health decisions" or value-based health decisions.[12] Recent research and empirical evidence support this model of health literacy and its influence on health care expenditures and health outcomes. Specifically:

- Nielsen-Bohlman, Panzer, and Kindig (2004) found that individuals with limited health literacy reported poorer health status and were less likely to use preventive care.
- Baker et al. (1998, 2002) and Schillinger et al. (2002) found that individuals with low levels of health literacy were more likely to be hospitalized and to experience bad disease outcomes.
- Howard (2004) estimated that inpatient spending increased by approximately $993 for patients with limited health literacy.
- Baker et al. (2007) found that, within a Medicare managed care setting, lower health literacy scores were associated with higher mortality rates, after controlling for relevant factors.
- Friedland (2002) estimated that low functional literacy may have been responsible for an additional $32–58 billion in health care spending in 2001. A substantial part of these expenditures is financed by Medicaid and Medicare.
- Weiss (1999) found that adults with low health literacy are less likely to comply with prescribed treatment and self-care regimens, make more medication or treatment errors, and lack the skills needed to navigate the health care system.[12]

Health literary transcends insurance status. In fact, this study suggests that 75% of the low literacy population is, in fact, insured. Therefore, recommendations and interventions

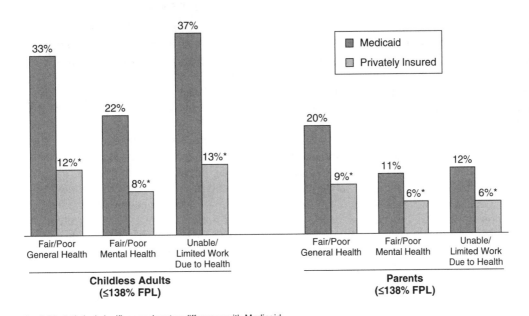

*p<0.05 statistical significance denotes difference with Medicaid.

Note: FPL is federal poverty level. In 2011, 138% of FPL is $15,028 for an individual. Adults are 19–84 years of age.

FIGURE 25-4 Health Status of Low-Income Adults: Medicaid Enrollees Compared to Persons with Private Insurance, 2005–2006

Source: Medicaid and CHIP Payment and Access Commission (MACPAC). https://7737438414307547177-a-macpac-gov-s-sites.googlegroups.com/a/macpac.gov/macpac/reports/MACPAC_March2011_web.pdf?attachauth=ANoY7cqji2nzfoaw3_z_3nc5rT56nfcGY5gJvxH4M2N2Oxh02o7RRwVo1ZMVeL9x0jB-Zno279uU-5P3YdtuV-k_EuZ6Kh7SJRBJpX0AjX2c3lsnuXGtg50Fqi5d36q3vaOyll9CpkLPTDrqzrKV4qXX-xGW_axe5EQMgGt30fJUaZ1dD0OET2TxliDoUrp50OM6wXPCZtF864xgE2dX8SR001gQhEybZQ%3D%3D&attredirects=0. Report to the Congress on Medicaid and CHIP, March 2011, p. 130.

are designed to reach all persons, regardless of health insurance status. Some of these solutions include the following:

- Ensuring that patients understand instructions and are able to navigate throughout the health care system.
- Incentivizing health care providers (medical, behavioral, dental, pharmacy, hospitals, and clinics) and systems to provide comprehensive services that assist people in adapting to the health care environment; these interventions might include language translation and interpreters and the development of materials in multiple languages.
- Leveraging existing programs and health care settings to develop best practices for improving health literacy with a parallel goal of decreasing health disparities.
- Encouraging payment from both the private and public sector (insurers, government, and foundations) to fund innovative solutions targeted at the elimination of health illiteracy.

Many Medicaid consumers find themselves having to rely on public transportation to get back and forth to the provider's office as well as to have diagnostic tests. While transportation is an optional Medicaid benefit, every state Medicaid program covers it. These services are usually provided by taxis, bus, or rail (with use of vouchers) and special vehicles for individuals with certain clinical conditions like ESRD requiring dialysis or physical limitations secondary to stroke. States may choose to contract with a single vendor or multiple vendors to provide transportation services for the entire state or by region, like urban, rural, and/or county-specific. In the managed care setting, the states will require the MCO to manage the transportation benefit or carve the benefit out and manage it directly between the state and the vendor(s). Without the transportation benefit, many Medicaid consumers would not be able to get the necessary services, thus worsening health outcomes and functional status.

While it is acknowledged that there are many social determinants that impact access to health care, poverty and health literacy are two of the most important that, if understood, identified, and adequately addressed will significantly close the health disparity gap, resulting in improved and sustained health outcomes, improved functional status for the most chronically ill, decrease in disease burden, and lower health care cost. Medicaid managed care has and continues to provide systems and solutions that are innovative and addresses many of the social determinants outlined above.

■ FEDERAL WAIVER AUTHORITY

OBRA 1981 authorizes multiple waiver and demonstration authorities to allow states flexibility in operating Medicaid programs (see **Table 25-6**). Each authority has a distinct purpose and distinct requirements. As states experience and contemplate how to address improving health outcomes and decreasing cost for some of the most diverse and vulnerable

TABLE 25-6	Medicaid Waivers and Research Demonstrations			
Authority	Waiver Period	Renewal Period	Number Active	Number of States with Waiver/ Demonstration
1915(b)	2	2	44 (as of 2009)	25
1915(c)	3	5	287 (as of 2008)	all
1115	5	3	66 (as of 2011)	41

Note: Section 1115 numbers include comprehensive statewide health care reform demonstrations, as well as those that are more limited in scope such as family planning
Source: Medicaid and CHIP Payment and Access Commission (MACPAC). https://7737438414307547177-a-macpac-gov-s-sites.googlegroups.com/a/macpac.gov/macpac/reports/MACPAC_March2011_web.pdf? attachauth=ANoY7cqji2nzfoaw3_z_3nc5rT56nfcGY5gJvxH4M 2N2Oxh02o7RRwVo1ZMVeL9x0jB-Zno279uU-5P3YdtuV-k_EuZ6Kh7SJR BJpX0AjX2c3lsnuXGtg50Fqi5d36q3vaOyll9CpkLPTDrqzrKV4qXX-xGW_ axe5EQMgGt30fJUaZ1dD0OET2TxliDoUrp50OM6wXPCZtF864xgE2dX8S R001gQhEybZQ%3D%3D&attredirects=0. Report to the Congress on Medicaid and CHIP, March 2011, p. 44.

populations, waiver authority is the vehicle utilized to provide innovative solutions. As of March 2011, there are a total of 451 unique waivers either approved or pending approval by the Secretary of HHS.

Summary and brief explanations of the waivers most often used by states follow.[13]

Section 1115 Research and Demonstration Projects

This Section provides the Secretary of Health and Human Services broad authority to approve projects that test policy innovations likely to further the objectives of the Medicaid program.

Section 1915(b) Managed Care/Freedom of Choice Waivers

This Section provides the Secretary authority to grant waivers that allow states to implement managed care delivery systems, or otherwise limit individuals' choice of provider under Medicaid with the exception of emergency services. States can waive freedom of choice by enrolling Medicaid consumers into primary care case management programs (PCCMs) or HMOs. States can also waive state wideness requirements and provide services in a limited geographic area. The waiver must be cost-effective and show federal expenditures are not greater under the waiver. The waivers are approved for 2 years with 2-year renewal periods.

Section 1915(c) Home and Community-Based Services Waivers (HCBS)

This Section provides the Secretary authority to waive Medicaid provisions in order to allow long-term care services to be delivered in community settings. This program is the Medicaid alternative to providing comprehensive long-term services in institutional settings such as institutional care in nursing homes, intermediate care facilities for people with mental retardation (ICFs-MR), and hospitals. The states use this as a rebalance for long-term care services and supports in their Medicaid programs from institutional settings to community settings. Statute identifies those services that can be home- and community-based, including case management, homemaker/home health aide services, personal care services, adult day health, habitation services, and respite care. States can provide a targeted set of services to specific populations including seniors, people with physical disabilities or HIV/AIDS, people with developmental disabilities, and people with traumatic brain injury. HCBS waiver programs must be "cost neutral" or, in other words, cannot have federal expenditures be no greater than if an individual had resided in an institution.

Section 1115 Waivers Expanded Explanation

Section 1115 of the Social Security Act provides the Secretary of Health and Human Services broad authority to authorize experimental, pilot, or demonstration projects likely to assist in promoting the objectives of the Medicaid statute. Flexibility under Section 1115 is sufficiently broad to allow states to test substantially new ideas of policy merit. These projects are intended to demonstrate and evaluate a policy or approach that has not been demonstrated on a widespread basis. Some states expand eligibility to individuals not otherwise eligible under the Medicaid program, provide services that are not typically covered, or use innovative service delivery systems.

There are two types of Medicaid authority that may be requested under Section 1115:

- Section 1115(a)(1)—allows the Secretary to waive provisions of Section 1902 to operate demonstration programs.
- Section 1115(a)(2)—allows the Secretary to provide federal financial participation for costs that otherwise cannot be matched under Section 1903.

Projects are generally approved to operate for a 5-year period, and states may submit renewal requests to continue the project for additional periods of time. Demonstrations must be "budget neutral" over the life of the project, meaning they cannot be expected to cost the federal government more than it would cost without the waiver.

Application Process

There is no standardized format to apply for a Section 1115 demonstration, but the application must be submitted by a single state Medicaid agency. States often work collaboratively with the Centers for Medicare and Medicaid Services (CMS) from the concept phase to further develop the proposal. A demonstration proposal typically discusses the environment, administration, eligibility, coverage and benefits, delivery system, access, quality, financing issues, systems support, implementation timeframes, and evaluation and reporting.

Proposals are subject to CMS, Office of Management and Budget (OMB), and Department of Health and Human Services (HHS) approval, and may be subject to additional requirements such as site visits before implementation. CMS does not have a specific timeframe to approve, deny, or request additional information on the proposal. Additionally, CMS usually develops terms and conditions that outline the operation of the demonstration project when it is approved.

Examples of Current State Initiatives

The Arizona Health Care Cost Containment System (AHCCCS), approved in July 1982, was the state's solution for Medicaid. As the last state to implement Medicaid in 1982, Arizona utilized the waiver authority to introduce a full-risk capitated model for acute, behavioral, and long-term care services. While the state agency does manage the three programs under separate contracts and request for proposal (RFP) cycles, all three full-risk capitated models utilize comprehensive provider networks to deliver services.

Rhode Island's 1115 Global Consumer Choice Compact waiver, approved in January 2009, provides the state with greater administrative flexibility than is available under existing program guidelines. Rhode Island will use the additional flexibility afforded by the demonstration program to redesign the state's Medicaid program to provide cost-effective services that will ensure beneficiaries receive the appropriate services in the least restrictive and most appropriate setting. Accordingly, Rhode Island will operate its entire Medicaid program under a single Section 1115 demonstration program. All Medicaid-funded services on the "continuum of care," from preventive care in the home and community to care in high-intensity hospital settings to long-term and end-of-life-care, will be organized, financed, and delivered through the demonstration program. Rhode Island's Section 1115 RIte Care and RIte Share programs for children and families, the 1915(b) Dental Waiver, and the Section 1915(c) HCBS waivers will be subsumed under the Global Consumer Choice Compact waiver.

HCBS Waiver 1915(c) Expanded Explanation

States may offer a variety of services to consumers under an HCBS waiver program and the number of services that can be provided is not limited. These programs may provide a combination of both traditional medical services (i.e., dental services, skilled nursing services) as well as nonmedical services (i.e., respite, case management, environmental modifications). Family members and friends may be providers of waiver services if they meet the specified provider qualifications. However, in general spouses and parents of minor children cannot be paid providers of waiver services. States have the discretion to choose the number of consumers to serve in a HCBS waiver program. Once approved by CMS, a state is held to the number of persons estimated in its application but has the flexibility to serve greater or fewer numbers of consumers by submitting an amendment to CMS for approval.

Application and Approval Process

The State Medicaid agency must submit to CMS for review and approval an application for an HCBS waiver, and the state Medicaid Agency has the ultimate responsibility for an HCBS waiver program, although it may delegate the day-to-day operation of the program to another entity. Initial HCBS waivers are approved for a 3-year period, and waivers can be renewed for 5-year intervals.

Provisions Waived

Section 1902(a)(1), regarding state waivers, allows states to target waivers to particular areas of the state where the need is greatest, or perhaps where certain types of providers are available.

Section 1902(a)(10)(B), regarding comparability of services, allows states to make waiver services available to people at risk of institutionalization, without being required to make waiver services available to the Medicaid population at large. States use this authority to target services to particular groups, such as older adults, technology-dependent children, or persons with mental retardation or developmental disabilities. States may also target services on the basis of disease or condition, such as AIDS.

Section 1902(a)(10)(C)(i)(III), regarding income and resource rules applicable in the community, allows states to provide Medicaid to persons who would otherwise be eligible only in an institutional setting, often due to the income and resources of a spouse or parent. States may also use spousal impoverishment rules to determine financial eligibility for waiver services.

Program Requirements

Within the parameters of broad federal guidelines, states have the flexibility to develop HCBS waiver programs designed to meet the specific needs of targeted populations. Federal requirements for states choosing to implement an HCBS waiver program include:

- Demonstrating that providing waiver services to a target population is no more costly than the cost of services these individuals would receive in an institution.
- Ensuring that measures will be taken to protect the health and welfare of consumers.
- Providing adequate and reasonable provider standards to meet the needs of the target population.
- Ensuring that services are provided in accordance with a plan of care.

Olmstead and HCBS Waivers

In the 1999 *Olmstead v. L.C.* decision, the Supreme Court affirmed the right of individuals with disabilities to receive public benefits and services in the most integrated setting appropriate to their needs. The *Olmstead v. L.C.* decision interpreted Title II of the Americans with Disabilities Act (ADA) and its implementing regulations. Medicaid can be an important resource to assist states in fulfilling their obligations under ADA. The HCBS waiver program in particular is a viable option for states to use to provide integrated community-based long-term care services and supports to qualified Medicaid-eligible recipients.

Current Status

Forty-seven states and the District of Columbia offer services through HCBS waivers, and Arizona, Hawaii, and Tennessee operate similar programs under Section 1115 research and demonstration authority. There is no federal requirement limiting the number of HCBS waiver programs a state may operate at any given time, and currently there are approximately 287 active HCBS waiver programs in operation throughout the country.

Combined 1915(b)/(c) Waiver Expanded Explanation

States may opt to simultaneously utilize Section 1915(b) and 1915(c) program authorities to provide a continuum of services to older adults and individuals with disabilities. In essence, states use the 1915(b) authority to limit freedom of choice, and 1915(c) authority to target eligibility for the program and provide home- and community-based services. By doing this, states can provide long-term care services in a managed care environment or use a limited pool of providers.

In addition to providing traditional long-term care state plan services (such as home health, personal care, and institutional service), states may propose to include nontraditional home- and community-based "1915(c)-like" services (such as homemaker services, adult day health services, and respite care) in their managed care programs. States can implement 1915(b) and 1915(c) concurrent waivers as long as all federal requirements for both programs are met. Therefore, when submitting applications for concurrent 1915(b)/(c) programs, states must submit a separate application for each waiver type and satisfy all of the applicable requirements. For example, states must demonstrate cost neutrality in the 1915(c) waiver and cost effectiveness in the 1915(b) waiver.

States must also comply with the separate reporting requirements for each waiver. Because the waivers are approved for different time periods, renewal requests must be prepared separately and submitted at different points in time. Meeting these separate requirements can be a potential barrier for states that are considering going forward with such a program. However, the ability to develop an innovative managed care program that integrates home- and community-based services with traditional state plan services is appealing enough to some states to outweigh the potential barriers.

Examples of Current State Initiatives

The Texas STAR+PLUS program, approved in January 1998, was the first concurrent 1915(b)/(c) program to be implemented. This mandatory program serves older adults and individuals with disabilities in Harris County (Houston) and integrates acute and long-term care services through a managed care delivery system, consisting of three managed HMOs and a PCCM. The majority of STAR+PLUS enrollees are dually eligible for Medicaid and Medicare. Although STAR+PLUS does not restrict Medicare freedom of choice, an enhanced drug benefit is provided as an incentive to dual eligibles that elect to enroll in the same HMO for their Medicaid and Medicare services. Care coordination is an essential component of the STAR+PLUS model.

Michigan's Medicaid Prepaid Specialty Mental Health and Substance Abuse Services and Combination 1915(b)/(c) Medicaid Prepaid Specialty Services and Supports for Persons with Developmental Disabilities program were approved in June 1998. Unlike the STAR+PLUS program, which integrates acute and long-term care, Michigan's program "carves out" specialty mental health, substance abuse, and developmental disabilities services and supports and provides these services under a prepaid shared risk arrangement. The purpose of this program is to provide beneficiaries an opportunity to experience "person-centered" assessment and planning approaches that provide a wider, more flexible, and mutually negotiated set of supports and services, thus enabling such individuals to exercise and experience greater choice and control.

Future Initiatives

As discussed earlier in this chapter, Medicaid HMOs gained significant popularity in the early to mid-1990s as a solution to states in their effort and desire to control burgeoning program costs. States have used waiver authority liberally and extensively in an effort to introduce innovation in their Medicaid programs to coordinate care and services for vulnerable populations, gain predictability in program costs, consolidation of financing streams in the case of dual-eligibles, and expansion, reform, and transformation of programs. Given the additional flexibility provided states under the ACA and the continued challenge of increases in health care costs (new therapies, medical technology, etc.), more populations will be transitioned into managed care as MCOs have proven program effectiveness in both cost savings and quality.

■ COST TRENDS

The CMS chief health actuary projects that national health care spending is set to increase from $2.6 trillion to $4.6 trillion—19.6% of the gross domestic product (GDP) by the end of the decade. **Table 25-7** demonstrates health insurance enrollment and enrollment growth rates under the ACA, which is projected to significantly increase overall Medicaid spending annually to $826 billion by 2019.[7]

Table 25-8 demonstrates average annual Medicaid growth from 1990 to 2009, with a high of 10.9, reflecting an explosive membership growth period. Between 2004 and 2007, there was much slower growth in Medicaid and in fact, some programs had membership contraction. However, with the onset of the great recession beginning in December 2007, Medicaid spending increased on average 7.1% between 2007 and 2009.

Figure 25-5 further demonstrates the impact of the economy on Medicaid medical services spending, with a high at 8.2%,

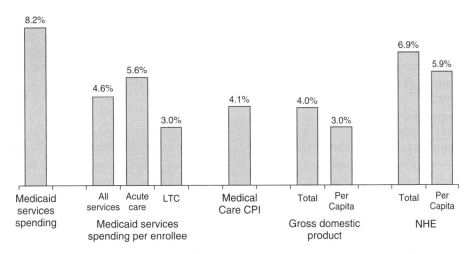

Notes: All expenditures exclude prescription drug spending for dual eligibles to remove the effect of their transition to Medicare Part D in 2006. Prescription drug spending for non-dual eligibles is included in acute care Medicaid spending per enrollee.
LTC is long-term care. CPI is Consumer Price Index. NHE is national health expenditures.

FIGURE 25-5 Average Annual Medicaid Spending Growth versus Growth in Various Benchmarks, 2000–2009

Source: Kaiser Commission on Medicaid and the Uninsured. Medicaid Spending Growth over the Last Decade and the Great Recession, 2000–2009 (#8152). Washington, DC; February 2010. Available at www.kff.org/medicaid/8152.pdf, p. 2. This information was reprinted with permission from the Henry J. Kaiser Family Foundation. The Kaiser Family Foundation is a non-profit private operating foundation, based in Menlo Park, California, dedicated to producing and communicating the best possible analysis and information on health issues.

TABLE 25-7	**Health Insurance Enrollment and Enrollment Growth Under the ACA**

Health Insurance Enrollment and Enrollment Growth Rates Under the ACA (Sept. 2010 Projections) versus Prior Law (Feb. 10 Projections), Calendar Years, 2009–2019[1]

Enrollment under ACA (in millions)	2008	2009	2010	2011	2012	2013	2014	2015	2016	2017	2018	2019
Medicare	45.2	45.9	46.8	47.9	49.3	50.9	52.4	53.9	55.4	57.1	58.8	60.5
Medicaid/CHIP	53.6	57.1	60.4	61.8	62.6	63.4	85.2	84.8	83.8	81.2	81.6	82.2
Other Public	11.6	11.8	12.5	12.8	12.8	13.1	13.4	13.7	14.1	14.4	14.8	15.1
Employer-sponsored Private Health Insurance	169.4	166.6	162.1	160.8	162.4	164.8	168.0	169.3	166.9	165.2	164.2	165.1
Other Private Health Insurance[2]	26.0	26.6	27.1	26.3	26.0	25.9	14.3	13.7	13.0	12.4	11.9	11.4
Exchanges	0.0	0.0	0.0	0.0	0.0	0.0	15.8	17.6	23.8	26.8	30.4	30.6
Uninsured	44.3	44.3	49.7	52.0	51.1	49.9	25.5	23.4	22.1	23.1	23.9	24.4
Insured Share of US Population[3]	85.5	85.6	84.0	83.4	83.8	84.3	92.1	92.8	83.2	93.0	92.8	92.7
Enrollment Under Prior Law (Feb. 10 Projections) (in millions)												
Medicare	45.2	45.9	46.8	47.9	49.3	50.9	52.4	53.9	55.4	57.1	58.8	60.5
Medicaid/CHIP	53.6	57.1	60.4	61.8	62.6	63.4	61.9	60.3	60.6	60.9	61.4	61.9
Other Public	11.6	11.8	12.1	12.4	12.8	13.1	13.4	13.7	14.1	14.4	14.8	15.1
Employer-sponsored Private Health Insurance	169.4	166.5	160.5	159.5	160.9	163.3	165.1	165.6	165.7	165.6	165.3	165.2
Other Private Health Insurance[2]	26.0	26.6	27.1	26.9	26.6	26.5	26.5	26.6	26.6	26.7	26.7	26.7
Uninsured	44.3	44.5	51.7	53.2	52.1	50.9	51.1	52.3	53.3	54.4	55.6	56.9
Insured Share of US Population[3]	85.5	85.5	83.3	83.0	83.5	84.0	84.1	83.8	83.7	83.5	83.2	83.0
Annual Growth Rate Under ACA												
Medicare		1.5%	1.9%	2.3%	3.0%	3.1%	3.0%	2.9%	2.9%	2.9%	3.0%	3.0%
Medicaid/CHIP		6.5%	5.9%	2.3%	1.4%	1.3%	34.2%	−0.4%	−1.2%	−3.1%	0.5%	0.7%
Other Public		2.3%	5.8%	2.5%	−0.5%	2.5%	2.5%	2.5%	2.4%	2.4%	2.4%	2.3%
Employer-sponsored Private Health Insurance		−1.7%	−2.7%	−0.8%	1.0%	1.5%	1.9%	0.8%	−1.4%	−1.1%	−0.6%	0.5%
Other Private Health Insurance[2]		2.2%	1.8%	−2.8%	−1.3%	−0.4%	−44.8%	−3.9%	−5.2%	−4.5%	−4.6%	−4.0%
Exchanges		–	–	–	–	–	–	11.2%	35.2%	20.8%	5.6%	0.6%
Uninsured		0.2%	12.1%	4.7%	−1.7%	−2.4%	−48.9%	−8.2%	−5.5%	4.4%	3.6%	1.9%
Insured Share of US Population[3]		0.1%	−1.9%	−0.7%	0.5%	0.6%	9.2%	0.8%	0.5%	−0.3%	−0.2%	−0.1%
Annual Growth Rate Under Prior Law (Feb. 10 Projections)												
Medicare		1.5%	1.9%	2.3%	3.0%	3.1%	3.0%	2.9%	2.9%	2.9%	3.0%	3.0%
Medicaid/CHIP		6.5%	5.9%	2.3%	1.4%	1.3%	−2.4%	−2.6%	0.4%	0.6%	0.8%	0.8%
Other Public		2.3%	2.6%	2.6%	2.5%	2.5%	2.5%	2.5%	2.4%	2.4%	2.4%	2.3%
Employer-sponsored Private Health Insurance		−1.8%	−3.5%	−0.6%	0.9%	1.4%	1.1%	0.3%	0.1%	−0.1%	−0.1%	−0.1%
Other Private Health Insurance[2]		2.2%	1.8%	−0.9%	−1.1%	−0.1%	−0.1%	0.4%	0.2%	0.1%	0.1%	0.1%
Uninsured		0.6%	16.1%	3.0%	−2.1%	−2.4%	0.4%	2.5%	1.8%	2.1%	2.3%	2.2%
Insured Share of US Population[3]		0.1%	−2.6%	−0.4%	0.6%	0.6%	0.1%	−0.3%	−0.2%	−0.2%	−0.3%	−0.3%

[1]The September 2010 health spending projections were based on the 2008 version of the National Health Expenditures released in January 2010, updated to take into account the impact of health reform and other relevant legislation and regulatory changes.

[2]In the prior-law baseline, other private health insurance includes private Medicare supplemental coverage and individual coverage. In the new-law estimates, other private health insurance includes only those with Medicare supplemental coverage.

[3]Calculated as a proportion of total U.S. population, including unauthorized immigrants.

Note: Numbers may not add to totals because of rounding.

Source: Centers for Medicare & Medicaid Services, www.cms.gov/NationalHealthExpendData/downloads/NHEProjections2009to2019.pdf. Accessed August 22, 2011.

TABLE 25-8	Medicaid Growth 1990–2009		
United States	**Percent**	**0.0%–100.0%**	
FY 1990–2001	10.9%	▬▬	
FY 2001–2004	9.4%	▬▬	
FY 2004–2007	3.6%	▬	
FY 2007–2009	7.1%	▬	

Source: www.kff.org/statefacts. This information was reprinted with permission from the Henry J. Kaiser Family Foundation. The Kaiser Family Foundation is a non-profit private operating foundation, based in Menlo Park, California, dedicated to producing and communicating the best possible analysis and information on health issues.

significantly exceeding other key economic indicators like GDP, CPI, and national health care expenditure per capita.

As depicted in **Figure 25-6**, Medicaid expenditures exceeded $400 billion, distributed across the type of services represented. In excess of 30% was spent on long-term care services including HCBS and institutional nursing homes. Today, Medicaid is the primary payer of nursing home services in the United States. Older adults and those with disabilities represent 30% of Medicaid consumers; however, states spend in excess of 60% of program funds on this population. Unfettered FFS spending in long-term care and behavioral services are the Achilles' heel of Medicaid programs and require innovative reform and transformation to arrest unsustainable health cost trends.

Cost Containment through Medicaid Managed Health Care Plans

Between 2000 and 2009, Medicaid managed care enrollment increased materially in number and type of health plans with most consumers enrolled in full-risk comprehensive health plans. The decrease in the average growth in Medicaid spending from 2000 to 2009, as depicted in **Figure 25-7** and **Figure 25-8**, is largely attributable to the transition of the majority of Medicaid consumers to HMOs and capitation and away from FFS payment.[*]

The TANF population accounts for about 70% of the Medicaid consumers and 40% of the expenditure, with the largest cost drivers being obstetrical and neonatal services. States have mitigated cost trends with these services through full-risk payment to HMOs. For most clinical conditions, the states pay

_____
[*]Payment methodologies are discussed in detail in Chapter 5.

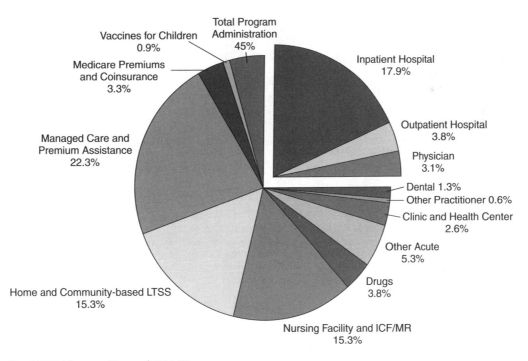

Total FY2010 expenditures: $406 billion

Note: See Tables 6 and 7 in MACStats for information on the categories of spending shown here. Collections from third-party liability, estate recovery, and other recoveries ($7 billion) are distributed proportionately among benefit categories. Percentages in MACStats Table 7 differ because that table includes benefits spending only.

FIGURE 25-6 Distribution of Medicaid Spending, FY 2010

Source: Medicaid and CHIP Payment and Access Commission (MACPAC). https://7737438414307547177-a-macpac-gov-s-sites.googlegroups.com/a/macpac.gov/macpac/reports/MACPAC_March2011_web.pdf?attachauth=ANoY7cqji2nzfoaw3_z_3nc5rT56nfcGY5gJvxH4M2N2Oxh02o7RRwVo1ZMVeL9x0jB-Zno279uU-5P3YdtuV-k_EuZ6Kh7SJRBJpX0AjX2c3lsnuXGtg50Fqi5d36q3vaOyll9CpkLPTDrqzrKV4qXX-xGW_axe5EQMgGt30fJUaZ1dD0OET2TxliDoUrp50OM6wXPCZtF864xgE2dX8SR001gQhEybZQ%3D%3D&attredirects=0. Report to the Congress on Medicaid and CHIP, March 2011, p. 150.

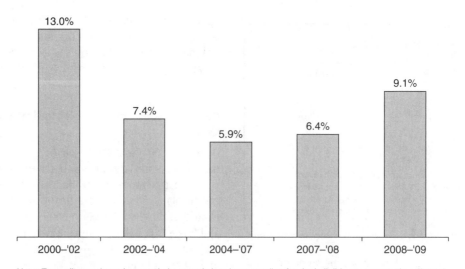

Note: Expenditures shown here exclude prescription drug spending for dual eligibles to remove the effect of their transition to Medicare Part D in 2006. See Table 3 for Medicaid medical service spending growth including dual eligibles.

FIGURE 25-7 Average Annual Growth in Spending on Medical Services, 2000–2009

Source: Kaiser Commission on Medicaid and the Uninsured. Medicaid Spending Growth over the Last Decade and the Great Recession, 2000–2009. Washington, DC; February 2010. Available at www.kff.org/medicaid/8152.cfm. This information was reprinted with permission from the Henry J. Kaiser Family Foundation. The Kaiser Family Foundation is a non-profit private operating foundation, based in Menlo Park, California, dedicated to producing and communicating the best possible analysis and information on health issues." Medicaid Spending Growth over the Last Decade and the Great Recession, 2000–2009," (#8152) p. 4. The Henry J. Kaiser Family Foundation, February 2011.

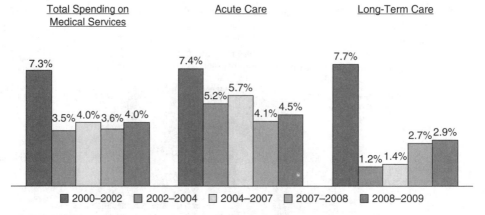

Notes: Expenditures exclude prescription drug spending for dual eligibles to remove the effect of their transition to Medicare Part D in 2006.
Prescription drug spending for non-dual eligibles is included in acute care Medicaid spending per enrollee.

FIGURE 25-8 Average Annual Growth in Medicaid Spending Per Enrollee, 2000–2009

Source: Kaiser Commission on Medicaid and the Uninsured. Medicaid Spending Growth over the Last Decade and the Great Recession, 2000–2009. Washington, DC; February 2010. Available at www.kff.org/medicaid/8152.cfm. This information was reprinted with permission from the Henry J. Kaiser Family Foundation. The Kaiser Family Foundation is a non-profit private operating foundation, based in Menlo Park, California, dedicated to producing and communicating the best possible analysis and information on health issues.

HMOs an actuarially sound per member per month capitation rate and the HMO assumes full financial risk for all medical services unless they are carved out (pharmacy and behavioral health are often carved out depending on the state).

Some states may choose to augment payment to MCOs in the form of a kick payment, which is often the case for maternity and associated deliveries. Other clinical conditions such as transplants and HIV/AIDS may be carved out and managed in the FFS program or states may choose to provide catastrophic payment in the form of reinsurance. In many circumstances MCOs will purchase stop-gap coverage from a third-party vendor to mitigate catastrophic exposure.

The number of Medicaid consumers in managed care, which rose significantly during the 1990s, nearly doubled in the most recent decade.[14, 15] As of June 2009, the total Medicaid population was 50.5 million, with 38.3 million, or 72%, enrolled in managed care.[15] Most of this membership was enrolled in comprehensive full- or partial-risk plans; 7.2 million were enrolled in PCCMs. States have achieved predictable cost trends with the TANF populations, which in most states have been mandatorily enrolled in MCOs. Increasingly, the more costly aged, blind, and disabled (ABD) populations have been enrolled in MCOs for better case/care management and coordination of services for consumers with chronic conditions yielding cost predictability for the states. Behavioral health and long-term care continue to be the areas representing the highest cost proportionately, the least integrated and coordinated. There is a huge opportunity for states to improve quality and achieve cost savings by expanding populations into mandatory managed care.

The Need to Demonstrate Improvements in Quality while Containing Costs

To succeed, Medicaid managed care must demonstrate that consumers are receiving a higher quality of care, not just containing costs. Medicaid managed care has demonstrated success as it relates to quality measurement as determined by the Healthcare Effective Data and Information Set (HEDIS®) and consumer satisfaction as determined by the Consumer Assessment of Healthcare Provider and Systems (CAHPS®) survey. Specifically, Medicaid HMOs performed on par with commercial HMOs in 2009 on:

- Avoidance of antibiotic treatment in adults with acute bronchitis, 26.5% versus 24%;
- Advising smokers to quit, 74.3% versus 79.5%;
- Chlamydia screening in women, 56.7% versus 43.1%;
- Beta-blocker treatment for first-time heart attack survivors, 76.6% versus 74.4%;

- Diabetes care including
  - Blood pressure control,
  - Eye exams,
  - Hemoglobin A1c (HbA1c) screening, and
  - Nephropathy monitoring.

There are areas where Medicaid HMOs did worse than commercial HMOs. Specifically, commercial health plans had better rates for:

- Discussion of smoking cessation strategies as well as discussion of smoking cessation medications;
- Timeliness of prenatal care, 83.4% versus 93.1%;
- Postpartum visits, 64.1% versus 83.6%; and
- LDL cholesterol screening and control.

Medicaid HMOs do an extraordinary job with childhood immunization rates (see **Table 25-9**)—success attributed to the vaccine for children program and EPSDT coupled with pay for performance to providers.

Medicaid consumers for the most part are happy with the services that they receive from their HMO and providers, as demonstrated in key CAHPS results shown in **Table 25-10**.

Having demonstrated both improved quality and a cost-savings proposition, states, and policymakers are focusing

---

TABLE 25-9   HEDIS Effectiveness of Care Measures—Historical Trends

CHILDHOOD IMMUNIZATION STATUS			
Combination 3: HMO Means			
YEAR	COMMERCIAL	MEDICARE	MEDICAID
2009	73.4	N/A	69.4
2008	76.6	N/A	67.6
2007	75.5	N/A	65.4

CHILDHOOD IMMUNIZATION STATUS			
HIB: HMO Means			
YEAR	COMMERCIAL	MEDICARE	MEDICAID
2009	94.8	N/A	93.7
2008	94.8	N/A	93.4
2007	93.1	N/A	87.7

CHILDHOOD IMMUNIZATION STATUS			
MMR: HMO Means			
YEAR	COMMERCIAL	MEDICARE	MEDICAID
2009	90.6	N/A	91.2
2008	93.5	N/A	90.9
2007	93.5	N/A	90.4

CHILDHOOD IMMUNIZATION STATUS			
DTAP/DT: HMO Means			
YEAR	COMMERCIAL	MEDICARE	MEDICAID
2009	85.4	N/A	79.6
2008	87.2	N/A	78.6
2007	86.9	N/A	77.8

CHILDHOOD IMMUNIZATION STATUS			
IPV: HMO Means			
YEAR	COMMERCIAL	MEDICARE	MEDICAID
2009	91.1	N/A	89.0
2008	92.1	N/A	87.9
2007	91.5	N/A	87.3

CHILDHOOD IMMUNIZATION STATUS			
VZV: HMO Means			
YEAR	COMMERCIAL	MEDICARE	MEDICAID
2009	90.6	N/A	90.6
2008	92.0	N/A	89.7
2007	91.9	N/A	88.7

CHILDHOOD IMMUNIZATION STATUS			
Hepatitis B: HMO Means			
YEAR	COMMERCIAL	MEDICARE	MEDICAID
2009	90.1	N/A	89.1
2008	91.8	N/A	88.3
2007	91.3	N/A	87.2

CHILDHOOD IMMUNIZATION STATUS			
Pneumococcal Conjugate (PCV): HMO Means			
YEAR	COMMERCIAL	MEDICARE	MEDICAID
2009	84.6	N/A	77.6
2008	84.8	N/A	75.6
2007	83.6	N/A	73.8

Source: NCQA State of Health Care Quality 2010. www.ncqa.org/portals/0/state%20of%20health%20care/2010/sohc%202010%20-%20full2.pdf . Used with permission.

TABLE 25-10	Select CAHPS HMO Member Satisfaction Measures, 2009		
Measure	Commercial	Medicare	Medicaid
Consumer and Patient Engagement and Experience			
Rating of Health Plan of 9 or 10	38.3%	59.0%	52.5%
Rating of Health Care: Rating of 9 or 10	48.7	56.2	47.0
Getting Needed Care: Usually or Always	85.4	89.1	75.0
Getting Care Quickly: Usually or Always	86.4	86.7	79.5
How Well Doctors Communicate: Usually or Always	93.4	93.5	87.0
Personal Doctor: Rating of 9 or 10	63.2	73.3	60.1
Specialist: Rating of 9 or 10	61.8	69.3	60.5
Customer Service: Usually or Always	84.5	86.5	79.5

The data reported to and by National Committee for Quality Assurance (NCQA) only includes data collected from managed care plans. Comparisons among the populations need to be viewed with caution because important differences between the commercial, Medicare and Medicaid populations may affect the results (i.e., health status and benefit designs of the different programs).
Source: Medicaid and CHIP Payment and Access Commission (MACPAC). https://7737438414307547177-a-macpac-gov-s-sites.googlegroups. com/a/macpac.gov/macpac/reports/MACPAC_March2011_web.pdf? attachauth=ANoY7cqji2nzfoaw3_z_3nc5rT56nfcGY5gJvxH4M2N2O xh02o7RRwVo1ZMVeL9x0jB-Zno279uU-5P3YdtuV-k_EuZ6Kh7SJRBJ pX0AjX2c3lsnuXGtg50Fqi5d36q3vaOyll9CpkLPTDrqzrKV4qXX-xGW_ axe5EQMgGt30fJUaZ1dD0OET2TxliDoUrp50OM6wXPCZtF864xgE2dX8 SR001gQhEybZQ%3D%3D&attredirects=0. Report to the Congress on Medicaid and CHIP, March 2011, p. 136.

their attention on Medicaid MCO expansion for acute, behavioral, and long-term care as the solution.

Key Characteristics of an Effective Medicaid Managed Health Care Plan

The UnitedHealth Group Center for Health Reform and Modernization has modeled potential Medicaid-only savings from providing coordinated care for all Medicaid consumers of approximately $580 billion over the next 25 years, of which $350 billion are federal savings. Additionally, the Center further calculates a savings estimate of $1.62 trillion, including $1.27 trillion for the federal government through coordinating care for the "dually eligible".[16] These savings could be attained by states and the federal government more broadly embracing existing and evolving managed care models. The following are the key characteristics of an effective Medicaid MCO:

- A comprehensive network of providers[*] that are sensitive and responsive to the demographics and vulnerability of the Medicaid consumer;
- Effective utilization programs for cost control;
- Targeted and effective disease management programs;
- Targeted and effective case management programs for
  - OB, including normal and high-risk pregnancies;
  - Neonatal services;
  - Chronic illnesses such as diabetes, HIV/AIDS, coronary artery disease, chronic obstructive pulmonary disease, and so forth;
  - Childhood illnesses such as asthma;
- Excellent and effective call center support reflective of the populations managed;
- Effective outreach that is both culturally and linguistically sensitive and addresses health literacy;
- Coordination of any service that may be carved out such as behavioral, pharmacy, long-term care, and others;
- Patient-centered medical home and health homes capability;
- Ability to work with and integrate accountable care organizations into a network framework;
- Robust quality program to meet and exceed state requirements for EPSDT, HEDIS, and other state-specific measures;
- Operational excellence for providers such as claims payment accuracy and timeliness;
- Innovation with providers as it relates to use of electronic medical records, including pay for performance; and
- Compassion as first thought, not after thought.

The ideal structure that is most effective and efficient is a full-risk integrated model that pays an MCO for all mandatory and optional benefits. While there are only a few states that have adopted this comprehensive integrated model (Tennessee), it is very important that any MCO that is at risk for acute medical services have the capacity to coordinate any carved-out service so that care to the consumer is as seamless as possible.

■ COMPLEX POPULATIONS: LONG-TERM CARE, BEHAVIORAL CARE, AND SPECIAL POPULATIONS

States have historically excluded some of the most costly and complex Medicaid consumers from managed care models. ABD beneficiaries disproportionately drive Medicaid expenditures, representing only 25.3% of the total population, but accounting for 67% of total Medicaid expenditures.[7] This population is, therefore, five and a half times the cost of nondisabled adults and more than three times the cost of children.[7] Even with the daunting costs associated

---

[*] See Chapter 4 for full descriptions of different provider types.

with caring for ABD beneficiaries, only 25% are in managed care,[17] the vast majority only in programs targeted at acute or non-long-term care Medicaid benefits. While these individuals have the benefit of managed care for services such as hospitals and physicians, some of the most costly services remain largely unmanaged.

Long-Term Care

Medicaid long-term care costs account for 33% of the total Medicaid budget.[7] These costs are driven by a broad spectrum of benefits, including those defined by the Medicaid State Plan such as nursing home care and home health care. Long-term care also represents benefits that are waiver benefits (HCBS) such as home-delivered meals, personal care, and home modifications. These benefits differ substantially state by state and are extremely complex to manage. Medicaid long-term care has become a complex policy issue due to several factors, including the cost of services; an aging population with more chronic and comorbid conditions; eligibility criteria that results in institutional bias; and lack of systemic delivery systems. As a result, states have become heavily reliant upon the most costly form of long-term care: nursing homes. Nursing homes drive 49% of total long-term expenditures and are significantly more expensive than other types of care than are often used to support individuals in need of long-term care.[7] See **Table 25-11** for a list of state long-term care programs.

Ten states have developed programs designed to provide support to individuals in need of long-term care through managed care. The programs in four of these states—Massachusetts, Minnesota, New York, and Wisconsin—are discussed later. The programs in the remaining six states (there are two programs in New York, one of which is discussed later) differ in design but are all focused on managing the costs associated with caring for individuals in need of long-term care through targeted individual care management. Reduction in the use of nursing homes, as well as hospitals and emergency rooms, is demonstrated in successfully managed long-term care programs.

TABLE 25-11	Types of State Long-Term Care Programs
State	**Program**
Arizona	Arizona Long Term Care System (ALTCS)
Florida	Long Term Care Community Diversion Program Frail Elderly HMO Program
Hawaii	QUEST Expanded Access Program
New York	Managed Long-Term Care
New Mexico	Coordination of Long Term Care Services
Tennessee	TennCHOICES
Texas	STAR+PLUS

Effective managed long-term care models include specific program design elements that ensure programmatic success. The most important elements are described next.

Population

The broadest populations should be included in a managed long-term care program, meaning states should include as many ABD consumers as possible, which results in less impactful models. In other words, programs that include only individuals deemed eligible for nursing home placement—a higher eligibility threshold than ABD—miss the opportunity to manage individuals who have yet to become eligible for nursing homes and, thereby, reduce the comprehensiveness of the program design.

Benefits

Similar to the populations included in a managed long-term care program, the broadest possible spectrum of benefits should be considered to ensure a highly flexible and effective system. Including all Medicaid benefits—acute and long-term care—as well as all waiver benefits allows for a comprehensive approach to individual care.

Program Authority

A managed long-term care program requires state authority, either through a state plan amendment or a waiver. The structure of the authority can have a dramatic impact on the effectiveness of the program; for example, in many nonmanaged long-term care programs, states have placed participation limits (or slots) on the ability to access waiver services, which limits states' liability. In a managed long-term care program, these same slots can inhibit the use of waiver services such as HCBS. If a state maintains a very low participation limit on HCBS, the ability of managed care to offer services outside of the nursing home can be dramatically limited, resulting in a need to maintain costly nursing home placement instead of providing care in a more cost-effective and restrictive setting. States must be very cognizant of the goals of the program and ensure program design that supports those goals.

Program Design

Certain program design elements can affect program success and cost-effectiveness. For example, managed long-term care programs deploy cost-effectiveness measures to ensure that the program can demonstrate success against an unmanaged FFS model. Cost-effectiveness measures on an individual result in personalized evaluation to determine appropriate placement and allocation of services, thereby reducing the risk of an individual costing more to maintain in the community than in the nursing home.

Rate Design

Rates should be structured in such a way as to incentivize appropriate utilization. For many programs, a goal of "rebalancing" long-term care away from nursing homes to a more cost-effective setting is a fundamental goal. In order to incentivize rebalancing, rates should encourage health plans to place as few people in nursing homes as possible and look for opportunities to move individuals already placed in nursing homes back to community settings.

Clinical Delivery

Given the complexities of individuals served in managed long-term care programs, clinical delivery is fundamental to successful program design. These models rely heavily on care managers—nurses and social workers—to develop comprehensive care plans and work with multiple traditional and nontraditional providers to ensure reduced utilization of costly services, such as overly prescribed care management models, and to ensure adequate staffing levels, for example.

These and other program design elements are vital to creating a strong foundation on which to build a system that rebalances long-term care and provides increasing options and infrastructure for individuals to be cared for in less restrictive environments.

Identification and Intervention

Given the complexity of individuals served by Medicaid long-term care systems, it is extremely important to identify individuals who are at risk of needing services as early as possible. In many instances, identification following an acute episode may be too late to effectively impact community placement. By using analytic tools such as claims reviews and risk stratification as well as employing comprehensive assessment—often face-to-face—of current and future needs can be identified.

Comprehensive Care Management

The presence of chronic and comorbid conditions can provide an indication of the likelihood of accessing services at some future point. In addition, assessing and fully understanding social and behavioral limitations alongside physical conditions is fundamental in rebalancing long-term care systems over time. An individual with three chronic conditions living with a spouse and having access to numerous community and family supports represents a significantly different risk to Medicaid utilization than an individual with three chronic conditions living in an apartment with no transportation and a history of substance abuse. Understanding these differences on an individual basis allows for maximum impact. At its core, managed care relies heavily on care management. Unlike other populations, however, those in need of long-term care require care management that stretches beyond coordination of traditional health care. In many instances, individuals can be maintained in the community only with the presence of nontraditional benefits and services. By developing a care plan that ties primary

care to specialty care to home supports, individuals are much more likely to be successfully treated in a less restrictive setting.

Transition Management

Many managed care models rely heavily on utilization management to control costs and reduce lengths of stay in costly settings. Managed long-term care also relies on transition management. Transition from an acute episode is often the point at which an individual becomes reliant on nursing home placement. Understanding each individual's circumstances and needs results in effective transition management that can ensure community placement. In this way, it is similar to transition management for patients with multiple chronic conditions, discussed in Chapter 7.

Network Development and Increased Access

Like all managed care models, managed long-term care relies on networks of providers; unlike other managed care models, managed long-term care must ensure support of a broad spectrum of providers that moves beyond traditional acute and physician services. In certain instances, individuals are better managed through the use of social workers than nurses. Particularly for individuals who have dynamic social needs that directly affect their health, social workers can support them in ways that would otherwise drive them to costly utilization of hospitals, emergency rooms, and nursing homes. Networks in managed long-term care programs must also include nontraditional providers such as personal care, contractors, adult day care, Section 8 housing, and home-delivered meals.

In many instances, nontraditional providers are not available in the market, not available in the quantity needed to support aggressive rebalancing, or not organized in an efficient manner. Managed long-term care health plans must dedicate significant resources to developing access to community-based services and tying resources within communities that have otherwise not been a part of comprehensive program delivery. As such, the health plan becomes responsible for developing comprehensive networks from a patchwork of local services.

The Impact of Managed Long-Term Care Programs

While managed long-term care programs have been limited to a small number of states, those that have developed such programs have benefited from program success. Many factors have been reviewed to determine program success. Both utilization and costs have been affected by managed long-term care and member satisfaction has demonstrated the benefit of comprehensive managed care as compared to a highly fragmented and ineffective FFS system.

The longest standing managed long-term care program is the Arizona Long Term Care System (ALTCS). In existence since 1989, Arizona has demonstrated reduced reliance on

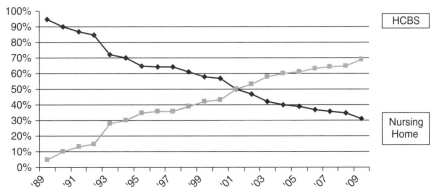

FIGURE 25-9 Arizona's Long-Term Care System (ALTCS)

nursing homes year after year. In 1989 the state placed 95% of its eligible beneficiaries in a nursing home while only 5% were cared for in the community. As of 2009, only 31% of eligible beneficiaries were treated in nursing homes, representing significant savings to the state and a systemic shift in delivery for complex consumers.[18] These data are shown in **Figure 25-9**.

Other programs have demonstrated positive results. Texas STAR+PLUS reduced avoidable inpatient care by 22%, acute outpatient care by 15%, emergency room visits by 38%, and long-term care by 10%.[19, 20] STAR+PLUS saved the state 8% relative to the FFS program.[21]

Florida's Nursing Home Diversion Program has demonstrated both cost savings as well as an ability to keep people from entering nursing homes as well as helping them transition to community settings. Program participants had a 12% probability of entering a nursing home as compared to 26% for FFS waiver participants. Additionally, participants were four times as likely to leave nursing homes for community settings as compared to FFS beneficiaries.[22] Participants in Florida's program saved the state between $10,000 and $15,000 per beneficiary per year.[23]

Dual-Eligibles*

Dual-eligibles, those who qualify for both Medicare and Medicaid, pose unique challenges for Medicaid programs as compared to non-dual-eligible ABD beneficiaries. As dual-eligibles, certain benefits are the responsibility of the Medicare program. As a federal program, Medicare is funded and regulated outside of state control. Individuals who are eligible for Medicare, either due to their age or a permanent disability, have the majority of their acute benefits provided through Medicare. Each Medicare beneficiary may choose to participate from private health plans offering MA or SNPs based on geography. Likewise, beneficiaries can opt to remain in FFS Medicare.

Of the total Medicare-eligible beneficiaries, only 21% are also eligible for Medicaid, making the intersection of the two programs less of a concern to Medicare.[7] Conversely, dually eligible individuals represent 60% of the total number of ABD beneficiaries,[7] making the intersection of the two programs a much more significant challenge to states. The complexities of the two programs, however, have led most states to avoid including dually eligible individuals in managed care models. Participation by dual-eligibles in managed Medicare plans remains very low as compared to the total number of individuals who are eligible for Medicare.

Programmatic Complexity

Benefit design between Medicare and Medicaid has historically created a reluctance to develop managed care models for these beneficiaries. Whether participating in an MA or SNP plan or in FFS Medicare, beneficiaries access services such as hospitals, physicians, and short-term skilled nursing care through Medicare. Medicaid is responsible for any Medicaid benefits outside of the Medicare benefit set. Unlike a nondual Medicaid beneficiary, the state frees itself of financial responsibility for acute benefits. While there are varying levels of eligibility, for fully eligible duals, the state is also responsible for any cost-share amounts—premiums, copayments, and deductibles—on Medicare benefits. Medicaid remains responsible for long-term care and waiver benefits.

Medicare and Medicaid effectively work as parallel systems with very little interaction (with the exception of cost-share amounts, described previously). In many instances, the state is unaware of services being rendered due to the fact that Medicare is the primary payer. Unfortunately, this separation leads to increased reliance on long-term care services due to the inability of the state to intervene early given the lack of claims information and ability to stratify individuals for future risk.

Added to this complexity, many Medicare beneficiaries do not become eligible for Medicaid until an acute episode occurs. In many instances, an individual experiences an

---

*Dual-eligibles are also discussed in Chapter 24.

acute admission followed by transition to a nursing home. Once admitted to a nursing home they have limited physical and financial resources to return to their own homes. Many people apply for Medicaid and deplete any resources they do have in order to qualify. This whole process results in permanent placement with limited ability for return to a less restrictive environment. There is nothing in the current, fragmented, and separate systems of Medicare and Medicaid to proactively intervene with, provide support for, and transition back to the community individuals who are dually eligible or likely to become dually eligible.

Both Medicare and Medicaid are are managed and regulated in a silo structure within CMS, which results in the parallel payment systems described earlier as well as systems that have their own regulatory requirements that affect all the parties involved. A dually eligible beneficiary is subject to two unique processes for enrollment: grievances and appeals, and member materials. Beneficiaries are required to manage these two systems even though their benefits are intertwined. It is quite possible that a beneficiary could be enrolled in a Medicare managed care plan and in FFS Medicaid, or vice versa. There are also instances where a beneficiary may be enrolled in separate managed care programs, one for Medicare and one for Medicaid. There is little within the current system to encourage cooperation, much less integration.

Four State Programs for Dual-Eligibles

While attempts have been made to create a more integrated approach to caring for individuals who are dually eligible, in certain states these attempts have been limited. Some states have adopted models in which a capitation payment is made to the Medicare managed care plan for all Medicare cost-sharing amounts. This limited relationship allows for single payments to providers for Medicare services without the administrative burden for providers and states to collect the minimal cost-sharing amount due.

In other states, capitation has been developed to include a small subset of Medicaid benefits. These "Medicare wrap" models allow for the Medicare managed care plan to assume financial responsibility to certain Medicaid benefits, improving coordination and, again, reducing administrative burden to certain providers as well as the state. Due to the regulatory requirements, in instances where non-cost-sharing benefits are included in capitation, participation by the beneficiary is voluntary and Medicare health plans must comply with Medicaid managed care regulations. This is often problematic for health plans with limited experience and desire to accept the regulatory burden of Medicaid managed care. As shown in **Table 25-12**, four states—Massachusetts, Minnesota, New York, and Wisconsin—have developed programs specifically designed for individuals who are eligible for both Medicare and Medicaid. (Texas STAR+PLUS expansion into Dallas and Fort

TABLE 25-12	Medicare and Medicaid State Programs
State	**Program**
Massachusetts	Massachusetts Senior Care Options (SCO)
Minnesota	Minnesota Senior Health Options (MSHO)
New York	Medicaid Advantage Plus (MAP)
Wisconsin	Family Care Partnership

Worth in 2010 required plans to participate in Medicare at a future date with a stated commitment to create an integrated program.)

These programs created integration at the plan level by requiring the health plan to coordinate benefits across the two programs and administer the regulatory requirements concurrently. While these approaches have improved coordination and demonstrated an ability to improve utilization of costly services, they remain limited in impact due to specific program constraints.

First, participation in these programs must be voluntary, which results in lower levels of participation compared to standard Medicaid programs. Second, even though managed care programs for dual-eligibles are significantly more coordinated and has an increased flexibility in benefit allocation, it does not make them immune to the problem of regulatory silos; for example, beneficiaries who choose to participate in any of these programs receive two sets of member materials, each describing the single benefit set, and in some cases contradicting one another. Similarly, beneficiaries are subject to a separate grievance and appeals process for Medicare and Medicaid.

Even with the weaknesses of these programs, they have proven effective, at least in two of the programs listed in Table 25-12. Massachusetts' SCO has demonstrated an ability to decrease reliance on nursing homes while treating a more complex population in a community setting: 8.7% of SCO members access nursing home services as compared to 12% of individuals in the control group. Of those who entered a nursing home, SCO clients had a higher frailty level.[24] In the other program, Minnesota's MSHO, participants had a lower rate of inpatient and emergency room use for community members versus the control group.[25]

Obstacles to State Program Development

Many states are interested in developing integrated approaches in caring for dual-eligibles, but have been reluctant to date. Many obstacles have stood in the way of program development from states' perspective. The first obstacle is any savings to date achieved by improving utilization of Medicare benefits have been returned to the Medicare program. This holds true even when the improvement occurs based on an integrated approach. In order to implement an integrated program, states must incur significant startup costs and in many cases Medicaid savings occur over a longer timeline than Medicare savings. For example, reducing emergency room and hospital admissions occur much faster than rebalancing long-term care. This results in program savings to Medicare much sooner than Medicaid. When you couple the delayed Medicaid savings with startup costs, many states have concluded they can ill afford to incur costs that primarily benefit Medicare only.

Second, there is no easy waiver process to develop an integrated program. Programs such as Massachusetts' SCO took numerous years to receive approval from CMS. The protracted timeline and lack of a specific waiver process for integration has resulted in additional reluctance for states given limited administrative resources within state Medicaid agencies.

The third obstacle is the administrative inefficiencies of the combined program, resulting in reluctance by Medicaid officials to create integrated models. Until the passage of ACA, there was not a single resource within CMS to assist states in developing integrated approaches to caring for dually eligible individuals. The ACA created the Federal Coordinated Health Care Office with the specific purpose to promote synergies between Medicare and Medicaid and assist states and other interested parties in developing integrated approaches, so in time perhaps this obstacle will diminish or even disappear.

Behavioral Health

Behavioral health is a significant issue for state Medicaid programs. Nearly 60% of the most complex Medicaid beneficiaries have co-occurring behavioral and physical health needs.[26] Psychiatric conditions are linked to a chronic physical condition in three of the top five most prevalent comorbid conditions for Medicaid beneficiaries, and behavioral and physical health is inextricably linked to each other for many complex beneficiaries served by Medicaid.[26] One recent study, for example, showed that of individuals with disabilities under age 65 served by Medicaid, a diagnosis of depression was present in only 2.32%, whereas depression was diagnosed with another chronic condition 37.36% of the time.[27] In the case of congestive heart failure, disabled Medicaid beneficiaries experience 0.92 hospitalizations per year, but this increased to 1.39 with the presence of a mental illness, and to 2.96 with the presence of both mental illness and substance abuse.[27] The presence of behavioral health comorbidities is also associated with increased inpatient hospitalizations, as seen in **Figure 25-10**.

While growing evidence suggests that management of behavioral health needs for Medicaid recipients would be best served in an integrated approach with physical health, there are few examples of integrated behavioral/physical managed care Medicaid programs. Behavioral health is provided in Medicaid programs through a variety of structures.

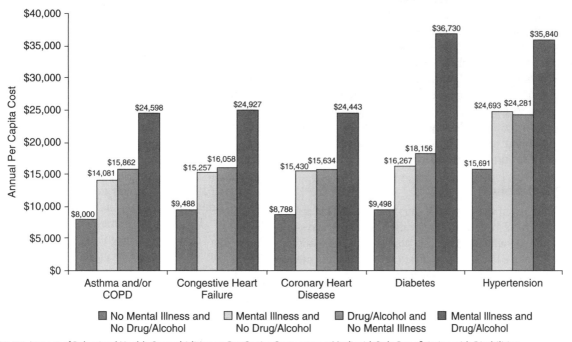

FIGURE 25-10 Impact of Behavioral Health Comorbidities on Per Capita Costs among Medicaid-Only Beneficiaries with Disabilities

Sources: Centers for Health Care Strategies, Inc. and Johns Hopkins University. Used with permission. www.chcs.org/usr_doc/clarifying_multimorbidity_patterns.pdf.
Clarifying Multimorbidity Patterns to Improve Targeting and Delivery of Clinical Services for Medicaid Populations by Cynthia Boyd, Bruce Leff, Carlos Weiss, Jennifer Wolff, Allison Hamblin, and Lorie Martin, December 2010.

In many states, it is managed through a separate behavioral health organization (BHO). BHOs operate similarly to HMOs, but responsibility and financial risk are limited to behavioral health services.

Other states have behavioral health carve-outs in which service is provided through an FFS model—even when physical health is provided through a capitated managed care model. Still other approaches include regionalized or localized behavioral health delivery through established mental health providers including both private and government support programs. Furthermore, the delivery system may vary in each state based on the population being served. For instance, specific populations such as severely and persistently mentally ill (SPMI) beneficiaries may be carved out of any Medicaid managed care program and managed through a unique waiver program.

This variability of delivery systems for behavioral health and substance abuse results in fragmentation in most states between behavioral and physical health. Given both recent economic pressures as well as growing evidence of the linkages between behavioral and physical health, attention is being given to improve the management and, thereby, the coordination of services for individuals with comorbid conditions.

There are emerging models of integration worth noting that are currently addressing the need to integrate physical and behavioral health. With the development of TennCare, Tennessee chose to create a fully integrated approach to Medicaid managed care, which included behavioral health. TennCare MCOs are responsible for providing a comprehensive benefit structure for both behavioral and physical health needs. TennCare MCOs utilize behavioral health providers as part of comprehensive care plan development to address beneficiaries holistically. Pennsylvania created a pilot program to incentivize collaboration between its HealthChoices MCOs and the BHO. Through the program, an incentive pool was funded by both the MCOs and the BHO and payment to the entities is made based on improved quality for predetermined measures.

Special Populations

There are unique subsets of populations that are eligible for Medicaid that have historically had differing delivery systems compared to traditional Medicaid populations. Generally states have developed waiver programs to deliver specific care to these populations, given the uniqueness of their needs. Examples are individuals with developmental disabilities, HIV/ AIDS, or spinal cord injuries and children with special needs. In many instances waiver services for these populations are managed either by the state Medicaid agency or by specialized providers and/or care managers. Understandably, the care for a young adult with a developmental disability would differ dramatically from an adult with HIV/AIDS.

While creation of unique waivers and services for highly specialized populations makes sense, there is potential to create fragmentation in some of these programs. For example, a developmentally disabled Medicaid beneficiary may have their acute Medicaid benefits provided in an FFS or managed Medicaid program while their developmental disability benefits would be provided through the waiver contractor. While specialized, this approach has potential for lack of coordination and nonintegrated plans of care.

Some states have tried to address the problem of fragmentation in these populations by including requirements for Medicaid managed care plans to coordinate with waiver service providers. In other instances, states have created specialized managed care programs to address special populations; for example, Arizona's Children's Rehabilitative Services (CRS) creates a unique managed care approach to specialized populations requiring comprehensive management with sensitivity to their needs.

Given the current economic conditions in many states, cost savings from waiver programs are being closely evaluated. In many instances changes in these programs do not affect any maintenance of effort (MOE) requirements and may allow states to achieve certain, but limited, cost savings. It is conceivable that states may evaluate the administrative burden of administering programs for special populations and explore opportunities to achieve managed care efficiencies even within these groups.

■ MEDICAID AND THE ACA*

The most comprehensive health reform law since 1965, the ACA put in place consumer protections for all Americans, an individual requirement to obtain health insurance, and a framework to expand coverage to nearly 32 million individuals, including 16 million Medicaid consumers. Medicaid, an established and scalable program, was leveraged as the foundation for expansion.

In its March 2011 estimates, the Congressional Budget Office (CBO) projected that the provisions of the ACA that expand health coverage would increase the deficit between 2012 and 2021 by $1.3 trillion over that period. "Those effects are only a part of the total budgetary impact of the legislation. The previous estimate by CBO and the staff of the Joint Committee on Taxation (JCT) showed that the effects of the other provisions on mandatory spending and revenues, taken together, will reduce the deficit by roughly $1.25 trillion over the 2012–2021 period—meaning that the legislation, as a whole, was projected to reduce the deficit over 10 years. The budgetary effects of all of those other provisions cannot be separately identified in the new baseline."[28] This is shown in **Table 25-13**.

---

* The ACA is discussed in succinct detail in Chapter 30.

TABLE 25-13	Effects on the Federal Deficit of Insurance Coverage Provisions in ACA and Provisions of the Reconciliation Act Related to Health Care (Billions of Dollars; Estimates from CBO and the Staff of the Joint Committee on Taxation)					
	March 2010		February 2011		March 2011	
	2010–2019	2012–2019	2012–2019	2012–2021	2012–2019	2012–2021
Insurance Coverage Provisions						
Gross Effect	938	931	934	1,390	971	1,445
Net Effect	788	778	733	1,042	794	1,131
Other Provisions Affecting Direct						
Spending and Revenues	−912	−910	−853	−1,252	n.a.	n.a.
Net Increase or Decrease (−)						
in the Budget Deficit	−124	−132	−119	−210	n.a.	n.a.

Source: Congressional Budget Office, Directors Blog, "Revisions to CBO Estimates of the Cost of Law Year's Major Health Legislation," March 23, 2011.

Medicaid Expansion in 2014*

Medicaid is leveraged as a foundation for at least half of the coverage expansion contained within the ACA. Estimated costs and savings as a result of the Medicaid expansion and other programmatic modifications in ACA are substantial. According to an analysis provided in a report by the nonprofit and nonpartisan Kaiser Family Foundation:

The Congressional Budget Office (CBO) estimates that the legislation will increase Medicaid/CHIP coverage by 16 million from a baseline of 35 million by 2019 with a federal Medicaid/CHIP federal cost of $434 billion from 2010 to 2019 due to coverage related changes. CBO estimates that the coverage related changes in the legislation will increase state spending over baseline spending by $20 billion over the 2010 to 2019 period. Other significant federal Medicaid costs over the 2010 to 2019 period are related to improving payments to primary care practitioners ($8.3 billion) and the Community First Choice Option ($6.09 billion). Significant federal Medicaid savings over the 2010 to 2019 period are related to Medicaid prescription drug coverage (−$38.14 billion) and reductions in Medicaid disproportionate share hospital (−$14.0 billion).[29]

Prior to 2014, the federal government requires states to cover minimum categories of eligibility up to various levels of poverty, as described earlier, but the eligibility requirements and application processes are complex and vary by state. Many states provide coverage beyond the minimums with federal approval of waivers, as described earlier in the chapter, but even then, eligibility is more generous to children than adults.

In 2014 and beyond, the ACA expands Medicaid eligibility in all states to at least 133% of FPL, which was approximately $14,404 for an individual or $29,327 for a family of four in 2009.[29] It eliminated categories of eligibility and state-by-state variation, with the exception of persons dually eligible for Medicaid and Medicare based on their age (65 and older) and/or health status (disability). Furthermore, the law requires a simplified application and eligibility determination criteria based on a household's modified adjusted gross income (MAGI). The new standard is consistent with criteria to determine a consumer's eligibility for subsidies on an exchange, discussed next.

Newly eligible individuals covered through the Medicaid expansion will receive "Benchmark Benefits." The specific benefits are to be defined by the Institute of Medicine (IOM), but at the time of publication, the IOM had not yet released a draft of the specific benefits. However, these are broadly defined in the ACA to include:

- Inpatient and outpatient hospital services;
- Physician services;
- Lab and X-ray services;
- Prescription drugs;
- Well-baby and well-child care;

---

*The discussion of the impact of the ACA on Medicaid, including its expansion, is based on the author's best knowledge at the time of publication. The ACA, like all major laws in the history of the United States, is continually subject to amendments and regulatory interpretations. Therefore, the reader will want to seek out current information from time to time. An excellent source for regularly updated information about Medicaid, Medicare, and the ACA overall is the nonprofit Kaiser Family Foundation, available at www.kff.org.

- Mental health and substance abuse services; and
- Mental health benefits parity (for commercial plans).

At the time of publication, it is yet to be determined how states will implement the new Medicaid eligibility standards and/or apply the benchmark benefits package since no federal guidance has been issued.

For the first 3 years of the Medicaid expansion (2014–2016), the federal government will provide states with full federal financing for its costs. In 2017, however, states will begin to take on a share of the cost, increasing to 10% by 2020. The ACA funded the SCHIP program through 2015, but authorized it through 2019. SCHIP eligibles above 133% FPL in 2014 may transition to an exchange or the Basic Health Plan, both of which are discussed later, if a state reaches its enrollment cap and/or if the program funding is not extended.

States are required to maintain eligibility levels for adults from the time the ACA was passed until 2014, or until their exchange is operational. Eligibility for children enrolled in Medicaid and SCHIP must be maintained through September 2019. Furthermore, states may not modify eligibility or enrollment standards or methodologies or procedures in an effort to decrease enrollment; for example, they cannot require more frequent recertification. This MOE requirement effectively restricts a state's ability to reduce benefits, reduce eligibility for optional populations (i.e., those covered above federal minimum requirements), increase enrollment fees or premiums, or establish more restrictive enrollment procedures.

State Medicaid programs have been struggling, as the worsening economy resulted in lower tax revenues, combined with growing enrollment and costs as the safety net for the newly jobless. Expansion of Medicaid under the ACA only serves to increase the strain. States that were already reliant on managed care plans will likely increase their reliance as they seek the capacity to meet the increased demand for medical services of all types.

Medicaid and Health Insurance Exchanges

The ACA requires the establishment of health insurance exchanges in all states by 2014.* Exchanges will serve as an organized marketplace through which consumers and small employers may shop for and purchase insurance. The requirements placed on the exchange, including the functions it must provide, eligibility for coverage, and the ACA's requirements for "essential health benefits" and "qualified health plans," are addressed in detail in Chapter 30 and are also summarized in Chapter 16.

Individuals between 133% and 400% of the FPL will receive subsidies to purchase coverage. Those below 250% will receive cost-sharing subsidies. Each will be based on a sliding scale and provided in the form of tax credits, as

---

*In states that do not establish an exchange, the federal government will do so.

TABLE 25-14	**Premium and Cost-Sharing Limits for Individuals up to 400% of FPL under Health Reform**	
Income (% FPL)	**Coverage**	**Premiums and Cost Sharing**
≤138% FPL	Medicaid	• No premiums
		• Cost sharing limited to nominal amounts for most services
139%–250% FPL	Exchange	• Sliding scale tax credits limit premium costs to 3–8.05% of income.
		• Sliding scale cost-sharing credits
251%–400% FPL	Exchange	• Sliding scale tax credits limit premium costs to 8.05–9.5% of income.
		• No cost-sharing credits

Source: "Focus on Health Reform" (#8168), p. 1 www.kff.org/healthreform/upload/8168.pdf. This information was reprinted with permission from the Henry J. Kaiser Family Foundation. The Kaiser Family Foundation is a non-profit private operating foundation, based in Menlo Park, California, dedicated to producing and communicating the best possible analysis and information on health issues.

seen in **Table 25-14**. The exchange will serve as an entry point for the determination of eligibility for exchange subsidies, Medicaid, and SCHIP.

The ACA adopted the "no wrong door" approach to ensure that any individual who entered through an exchange was directed to the program for which they are eligible. Consumers determined eligible for Medicaid, SCHIP, or another state program may not enroll in an exchange, however. The federal government has offered states increased federal matching dollars (90%) to modernize Medicaid enrollment and eligibility systems and (75%) for ongoing maintenance, recognizing that many state systems are decades old and will require modernization to work effectively with the exchange.[30]

Figure 25-11 provides a high-level flow chart of how the "no wrong door" approach to eligibility determination may function in an exchange.

It is anticipated that there will be a great deal of movement between Medicaid and the exchange as consumers experience changes in income and circumstances. One study published in *Health Affairs* estimated that 28 million people, representing 50% of adults below 200% of the FPL, will experience a shift in eligibility from Medicaid to an insurance exchange within a year.[31] This is an important factor as states address the design of systems, linkages with Medicaid, and eligibility, enrollment, and recertification rules and processes within the exchange. The goal will

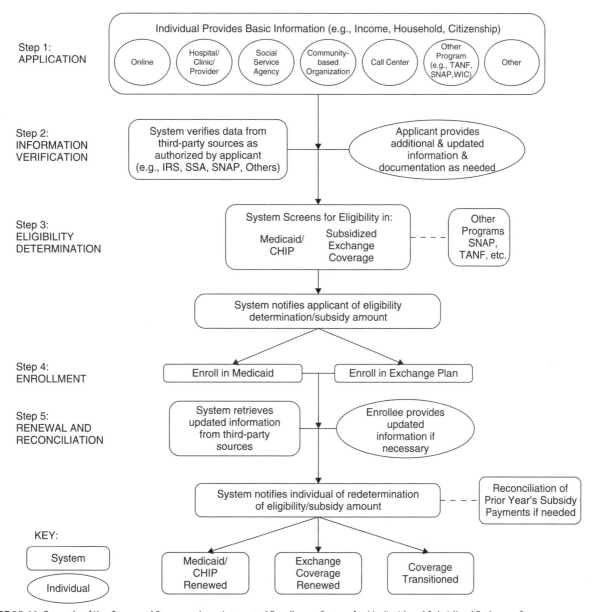

FIGURE 25-11 Example of Key Steps and Processes in an Integrated Enrollment System for Medicaid and Subsidized Exchange Coverage

Source: "Kaiser Commission on Medicaid and the Uninsured" (#8118), p. 4. www.kff.org/healthreform/upload/8118.pdf. This information was reprinted with permission from the Henry J. Kaiser Family Foundation. The Kaiser Family Foundation is a non-profit private operating foundation, based in Menlo Park, California, dedicated to producing and communicating the best possible analysis and information on health issues..

be to minimize the need to transition consumers between programs, and to do so seamlessly when they must.

There are also programmatic options to address the movement between Medicaid and the exchange, though whether or not states will pursue them is unknown at the time of publication. These options include:

- Allowing a period of continuous eligibility on the exchange and/or Medicaid, requiring recertification on an annual (or more frequent) basis;
- Requiring or allowing managed Medicaid plans to participate in the exchange;

- Requiring or allowing commercial plans in the exchange to participate as Medicaid plans; and
- Establishing a Basic Health Plan, discussed next.

Basic Health Plan Option

The ACA allows states to establish and offer a Basic Health Plan (BHP) to uninsured individuals with incomes between 133% and 200% FPL who would otherwise be eligible to receive premium subsidies in the exchange. States would receive 95% of the federal cost-sharing and premium subsidies that would have been provided to an individual on the exchange. They must offer at least the minimum essential benefits and must use program savings to reduce enrollee premiums, provide cost-sharing, or increase benefits. This may also be a natural vehicle for transitioning SCHIP eligibles once program funding expires in 2015.

The BHP option may be a mechanism for states to improve continuity of care by:

1. Offering the same or a subset of plans and/or provider networks offered to Medicaid and CHIP enrollees;
2. Reducing "churn" between Medicaid and the exchange as incomes fluctuate;
3. Allowing families to enroll in the same plan/program; and/or
4. Offering a low or no-cost option.

At the time of publication, states are awaiting federal guidance and rules about the exchange and the BHP. These rules, combined with economics, politics, and availability of resources, will influence the extent to which states choose to expand state-managed programs such as the BHP, and pursue policy options that would help to ensure continuous coverage of consumers.

The ACA and Long-Term Care

The ACA provides opportunities for states to address long-term care. In some instances, the reform law created new programs while in others it either fixed or extended programs designed to address long-term care needs. The following highlights the ACA's impact on long-term care programs.

1915(i) Community-Based Services Waiver

1915(i) waivers, originally created in the Deficit Reduction Act of 2005, were amended to increase the scope of the HCBS and included behavioral health services. The waiver now allows states to serve expanded populations and/or targeted populations, and allows for home-and community-based service availability at higher-income categories. This could allow states to intervene earlier with broader populations to avoid future nursing home placement.

The ACA also included new requirements that states cannot adopt slots as a mechanism to control participation in the waiver nor can they create a geographically limited program. HCBS services created through the 1915(i) waiver would essentially be considered "entitlement" benefits and thereby states would have limited ability to provide utilization management criteria once benefits have been authorized.

Medicaid Community First Choice Option

This provision allows states to create a home- and community-based service program through a State Plan Amendment rather than a traditional HCBS waiver (e.g., 1915(c)).

States have flexibility in service design and can make HCBS services available to beneficiaries who do not meet nursing home eligibility criteria. This would expand the ability for states to proactively provide HCBS services with the hope of avoiding future nursing home care.

The ACA set specific requirements for approval of a Community First Choice Option: services must be consumer controlled, states may not implement a waiting list of slots to control access; states must develop an Implementation Council to provide program guidance; states must maintain benefits for a 1-year period; and states must create a comprehensive quality assurance program for the option. States have the ability to receive an additional 6% FMAP to support development of a Community First Choice Option.

Long-Term Care Balancing Incentives

As mentioned above, states are striving to rebalance their long-term care systems to become more reliant on community-based care and less reliant on nursing home care. This provision of ACA allows for increased FMAP match to achieve rebalancing. Varying amounts of increased match are available depending on the reliance on nursing homes at the time of program implementation.

States must agree to certain things in order to receive additional match. They must create a single-entry point system to encourage ease of eligibility determination and application for eligible individuals. Additionally, they must demonstrate "conflict-free case management" and adopt a standardized assessment tool. States may not adopt more restrictive eligibility criteria for HCBS supports than were in place on December 31, 2010.

Health Homes for Chronic Conditions

States will have access to $25 million in planning grants for the development of State Plan Amendments that create comprehensive care management. This is essentially the same concept as the PCMH, which was first piloted by CMS in 2010, and which is addressed in the ACA as well for Medicare.

Payment Demonstrations

CMS has the authority to work with up to five states to develop large capitated systems or networks, and to create global at-risk payment structures. These global payments would include acute, post-acute, and long-term care services and could have lasting impact on payment for Medicaid services. Demonstrations can be granted to up to eight states to create bundled payments for physician and post-acute services related to an acute stay. These payment methodologies, along with other possible approaches, as well as specific payment approaches mentioned in the ACA in conjunction with the new Center for Medicare and Medicaid Innovation, are described in detail in Chapter 5.

The Federal Coordinated Health Care Office

Finally, the ACA also authorized the creation of the Federal Coordinated Health Care Office with the specific charge to address fragmentation between Medicare and Medicaid. State planning grant opportunities have already been publicized for up to 15 states and ongoing demonstration authority exists within the office to create demonstrations to improve care, quality, and cost associated with dual-eligible individuals.

■ EMERGING TRENDS IN MEDICAID MANAGED CARE

Given the proven effectiveness of Medicaid managed care, it is likely to play a significant role in Medicaid expansion. What is yet to be determined is the scope in which various managed models will be explored. For many years, certain states relied upon PCCM models to provide enhanced care as compared to FFS, since they provide a level of care management and can support improved care coordination for Medicaid beneficiaries—albeit less comprehensive than a fully managed Medicaid plan. It also may be somewhat effective at improving quality, depending on quality requirements included in the state's participation agreement with primary care providers. However, PCCMs provide limited protections to states because they are nonrisk.

Emerging trends indicate that there is a desire to move beyond a very limited management approach of PCCMs to a model that encourages increased quality, alignment, and utilization, resulting in a continuum of managed care options. Along the continuum and with increasing financial incentives are health homes. These models ensure identification and active participation of a care manager and coordination of services, resulting in improved outcomes. In some instances, health homes will be created from primary care practices or safety net providers such as FQHCs and in other instances, it is conceivable that managed care programs for specific populations will be treated as health homes. The designation is important in light of ACA due to opportunities to garner additional FMAP match.

Further along the continuum are accountable care organizations (ACOs), as described in Chapters 2 and 4. As envisioned both in the ACA and by CMS, ACOs would be paid through a form of shared savings payment model with risk corridors, as described in Chapter 5. However, at the time of publication there are no final federal rules or regulations, and the only operational prototype ACOs are large health systems with a successful history of risk through their own HMO.

Medicaid managed care is the most comprehensive in design along the continuum, with substantial financial incentives to improve quality and utilization through capitation and contractual requirements and incentive programs to systemically improve quality. The continuum offers states the ability to create program flexibility that might address challenges to traditional managed care posed by such things as rural geographies or unique populations. It is highly likely that the number of individuals served in FFS Medicaid will continue to decline as increasing numbers of individuals or subsets of the total population move into models with built-in incentives to ensure improvement in the entire Medicaid program.

■ CONCLUSION

Medicaid managed care has had extraordinary growth over the past 15 years that has been largely attributable to federal legislation targeting uninsured children. Welfare reform and BBA 97 allowed for significant growth in the program in the mid to late 1990s, with states mandating most of the TANF enrollment into HMOs. HMOs appreciated significant growth in type (commercial vs. Medicaid only), enrollment, and revenue. From 2000 to 2009, states have mandated more complicated and costly populations into HMOs with resultant predictability of cost and better outcomes as measured by HEDIS and CAHPS surveys.

CHIPRA has been reauthorized through 2013 and expanded coverage to an additional 4 million children. Under the ACA, almost 32 million uninsured childless adults will have health care coverage, of which half, or 16 million, will be covered through Medicaid expansion in 2014, and some portion of another 16 million newly covered individuals will be subsidized through premium or cost-sharing depending on family income level. Exchanges will be the vehicle used by states to inform consumers about their choices so that they can be informed prior to making an enrollment decision in a product and/or health plan.

Embedded in the legislation are several key managed care models, such as ACOs, PCMHs, and health homes that seek to get better alignment of the health care system through the redesign of clinical delivery model and payment. In addition, ACA provides opportunities to demonstrate innovative approaches to Medicaid through CMS's Center for Medicare and Medicaid Innovation.

There will be a huge demand on the existing health care system by 2014. This creates a significant opportunity for Medicaid MCOs to work closely with ACOs, PCMHs, and health homes by acting as an accelerator and/or facilitator leveraging technology and other resources to assist many of the providers that will be in existing MCO networks providing services to current and new members—new members who may have similar or different demographics. Medicaid managed care has an undeniable history of improving quality and controlling cost for some of the most vulnerable populations, and embodies the compassion necessary to recognize, address, and mitigate access issues. Medicaid MCOs are well positioned to scale and absorb the anticipated future growth while maintaining high quality and predictable cost, thereby playing a major role in sustainable health care delivery for the states.

Endnotes

1   Kaiser Commission on Medicaid and the Uninsured. *Medicaid: A Primer: Key Information on Our Nation's Health Coverage Program for Low-Income People.* Washington, DC; June 2010. Available at: www.kff.org. Accessed March 30, 2011.

2   Mann C, Rowland D, Garfield R. Historical Overview of Children's Health Care Coverage. *The Future of Children.* Spring 2003;13(1):31–53.

3   Kaiser Commission on Medicaid and the Uninsured. *Medicaid Enrollment: June 2010 Data Snapshot.* Washington, DC; February 2011. Available at www.kff.org. Accessed March 18, 2011.

4   Medicaid and CHIP Payment and Access Commission (MACPAC). *Report to the Congress on Medicaid and CHIP.* March 2011. Available at: www.macpac.gov. Accessed March 18, 2011.

5   California Healthcare Foundation. *California Health Care Almanac: Medi-Cal Facts and Figures.* September 2009. Available at: www.chcf.org/publications/2009/09/medical-facts-and-figures. Accessed March 18, 2011.

6   Rosenbaum S, Markus A, Sonosky C. Public Health Insurance Design for Children: The Evolution from Medicaid to SCHIP. *J Health Biomed Law.* 2004;1(1):1–47.

7   Kaiser Family Foundation. *States health facts.* Available at: www.statehealthfacts.org. Accessed March 2011.

8   Cunningham P, Hadley J. Effects of Changes in Incomes and Practice Circumstances on Physicians' Decisions to Treat Charity and Medicaid Patients. *Milbank Q.* March 2008;86(1). Available at: http://hschange.org. Accessed March 18, 2011.

9   Zuckerman S, Williams A, Stockley, K. Trends in Medicaid Physician Fees, 2003–2008. *Health Affairs.* 2009;28(3):w510–w519. Available at: www.content.healthaffairs.org. Accessed March 18, 2011.

10 New York State Department of Health. *Redesigning the Medicaid program.* Available at: www.health.state.ny.us/health_care/medicaid/redesign. Accessed March 2011.

11 Foege W. Social Determinants of Health and Health-Care Solutions. *Public Health Reports.* 2010;125(Suppl 4):8–10. Available from Association of Schools Public Health. Available at: www.ncbi.nlm.nih.gov/pmc/articles/PMC2882969. Accessed March 18, 2011.

12 Vernon J, Trujillo A, Rosenbaum S, DeBuono B: Low Health Literacy: Implications for National Health Policy. Available at: www.npsf.org/askme3/download/

UCONN_Health%20Literacy%20Report.pdf. Accessed March 18, 2011.

13 Kaiser Commission on Medicaid and the Uninsured. *The Role of Section 1115 Waivers in Medicaid and CHIP: Looking Back and Looking Forward.* Washington, DC; March 2009. Available at: www.kff.org. Accessed March 12, 2011.

14 Kaiser Commission on Medicaid and the Uninsured. *Medicaid and Managed Care: Key Data, Trends and Issues.* Washington, DC; February 2009. Available at www.kff.org. Accessed March 18, 2011.

15 Centers for Medicare and Medicaid Services. *National Summary of Medicaid and Managed Care Programs and Enrollment.* June 2009. Available at www.cms.gov. Accessed March 18, 2011.

16 UnitedHealth Center for Health Reform and Modernization. *US Deficit Reduction: The Medicare and Medicaid Modernization Opportunity.* Working Paper 4. October 2010.

17 Centers for Medicare and Medicaid Services. *Medicaid Statistical Information System (MSIS) State Data Mart.* 2008. Available at: www.cms.org. Accessed March 18, 2011.

18 Arizona Cost Containment System: Arizona Long Term Care System, Annual HCBS Report CY 2009, March 2010. Available at: www.azahcccs.gov.

19 Shenkman E. *STAR + PLUS Enrollees' Satisfaction with Their Health Care.* Institute for Child Health Policy. University of Florida, October 2003.

20 The Lewin Group. *Actuarial Assessment of Medicaid Managed Care Options.* Prepared for the Texas Health and Human Services Commission. December 15, 2003.

21 Houser A, Frox-Grage W, Gibson MJ. Across the States; Profiles for Long-Term Care and Independent Living. *AARP.* 2009.

22 Florida Office of Program and Policy Analysis & Government Accountability. *The Nursing Home Diversion Program Has Successfully Delayed Nursing Home Entry.* May 2006.

23 Salmon JR, Mitchell G II. *Preliminary Evaluation of Medicaid Waiver Managed Long-Term Care Diversion Program: Final Report.* Florida Policy Exchange Center on Aging, University of South Florida, November 27, 2001.

24 JEN Associates, MassHealth SCO Program Evaluation, Pre-SCO Enrollment Period CY2004 and Post-SCO Enrollment Period CY2005: Nursing Home Entry Rate and Frailty Level Comparisons. Boston, MA: Department of Health and Human Services, 2008. Available at: www.mass.gov/Eeohhs2/docs/masshealth/sco/sco_evaluation.pdf.JEN Associates, Inc. Accessed March 18, 2011.

25 Kane RL, Homyak R, Bershadsky B, et al. Patterns of Utilization for the Minnesota Senior Health Options

Program. *Journal of the American Geriatrics Society.* December 2004;52(12):2039–2044.

26 Kronick RG, Bella M, Gilmer TP. *The Faces of Medicaid III: Refining the portrait of people with multiple chronic conditions.* Center for Health Care Strategies. October 2009.

27 Boyd C, Leff B, Weiss C, Wolff J, Hamblin A, Martin L. Clarifying multimorbidity patterns to improve targeting and delivery of clinical services for Medicaid populations. Center for Health Care Strategies. December 2010.

28 Congressional Budget Office, Director's Blog. Revisions to CBO Estimates of the Cost of Law Year's Major Health Legislation. March 23, 2011.

29 Kaiser Family Foundation. Medicaid and Children's Health Insurance Provisions in the New Health Reform Law. April 7, 2010.

30 Center for Medicare and Medicaid Services, Department of Health and Human Services. Medicaid; Federal Funding for Medicaid Eligibility Determination and Enrollment Activities. Notice of Proposed Rulemaking. *Fed Regist.* November 23, 2010;75(215): 68583–68595.

31 Sommers BD, Rosenbaum S. Issues in Health Reform: How Changes in Eligibility May Move Millions Back and Forth Between Medicaid and Insurance Exchanges. *Health Affairs.* 2011;30(2):228–236.

The Military Managed Care Health System

M. Nicholas Coppola, Ronald P. Hudak, Forest S. Kim, Lawrence Fulton, Jeffrey P. Harrison, and Bernie J. Kerr, Jr.

STUDY OBJECTIVES

- Understand the difference between direct care and purchased care
- Understand the importance of readiness in the military health system
- Understand the governance process in military managed care
- Understand TRICARE performance metrics
- Understand the influence of outside stakeholders on military health care policy
- Understand the current and future challenges faced by the military health system
- Understand the relationships and competing priorities of actors within the Managed Care Quaternion

DISCUSSION TOPICS

1. Discuss the following statement made by a former Assistant Secretary of Defense for Health Affairs, "The military health system operates the only health maintenance organization that goes to war." Why is this statement important in understanding the military health system?

2. Discuss key legislative events in military health care that resulted in the implementation of the current TRICARE program.

3. Discuss key differences and advantages of TRICARE Prime, Extra, and Standard. What other TRICARE programs are available for specific beneficiaries?

4. Discuss the historical events that resulted in "TRICARE for Life" becoming a right for eligible beneficiaries.

5. Discuss opinions on how best to ensure the survival of the military health system.

6. Discuss and describe the Parity of Healthcare.

■ INTRODUCTION

This chapter discusses the Military Health System (MHS). The MHS operates a specialized form of managed care called TRICARE and responds to the challenge of maintaining medical combat readiness while providing health services for all eligible beneficiaries. TRICARE brings together the worldwide health resources of the Army, Navy, Air Force, Coast Guard, and Commissioned Corps of the Public Health Service (often referred to as direct care) and supplements this capability with network and non-network civilian health professionals, hospitals, pharmacies, and suppliers (referred to as purchased care) to provide better access and quality service while maintaining the capability to support military operations. In essence, TRICARE can be considered a group of health plans within the MHS.

On the direct care side, the MHS, worldwide, oversees over 50 military hospitals and medical centers, 364 medical clinics, and 282 dental clinics at the time of publication. The MHS also operates a fully accredited medical school, graduate programs, and 36 medical research laboratories. It also offers scholarships at a number of major universities as well as broad programs in medical research and development. Each service's medical department is headed by a Surgeon General who is the senior officer, meaning general officers in the Army and Air Force and an admiral in the Navy.* Each military Surgeon General is responsible for the care provided in his or her respective service's military treatment facilities (MTFs). MTFs are analogous to civilian medical centers, hospitals, and health clinics.

In the purchased care side, there are over 380,000 network providers and over 60,000 retail pharmacies. In a typical week, the MHS does more than 23,000 inpatient admissions; 1.8 million professional encounters (outpatient); 2,400 births; 230,000 behavioral health outpatient services; and fills 2.6 million prescriptions. In addition, over 3.5 million claims are processed and 12.6 million electronic health record messages are completed.[1]

TRICARE offers a range of primary, secondary, and tertiary care health services to almost 10 million eligible beneficiaries with an annual cost of over $49 billion. Approximately 3.7 million are enrolled in the direct care system, 1.6 million are enrolled in TRICARE's purchased care contractor networks, and the remainder are in other TRICARE programs. A unique aspect of military managed care is the MHS's readiness mission. Readiness is defined as the ability of forces, units, technical systems, and equipment to deliver the output for which they were designed.[2] Readiness is also associated with maintaining the health status of active duty personnel well above the health standing associated with nonmilitary personnel. Furthermore,

readiness is synonymous with ensuring efficient supplies are available for national disasters and war, and ensuring that appropriate processes are in place to support mobilizations. This means that readiness is associated with the ability of certain elements of brick-and-mortar health care facilities to become mobile and deploy worldwide when necessary. Finally, readiness is concerned with operations management processes and the efficient and effective use associated with the transformation of inputs into outputs. No other managed care plan in the United States—or the world—has a similar focus and responsibility. Former Assistant Secretary of Defense for Health Affairs Dr. Sue Bailey once said that the military health system operates the only health maintenance organization (HMO) that goes to war.[3]

To understand the current structure and process of military managed care, it is first necessary to review the seminal events in military managed care evolution. Factors affecting military managed care evolution stem from issues in war, directives from Congress, beneficiary demands, and adoption of civilian best practices over 200 years. In contrast, some civilian managed care practices may have antecedent roots in earlier military health programs. The end result is a civilian managed care system with undeniable ties to military initiatives and a military managed care system that is similar to civilian managed care in many ways while still maintaining distinctiveness in mission and purpose. In essence, the MHS can be considered:

- A provider of health care;
- An employer of health care professionals;
- An insurer of beneficiaries;
- An educator of clinical and nonclinical personnel, unique within the U.S. health care industry;
- A military component prepared to go anywhere, anytime in defense of our nation.

■ BRIEF HISTORY OF THE MILITARY HEALTH SYSTEM

Military health care began when the country did, and has undergone considerable and continual change. The history of the military health system is briefly described next.

The Revolutionary War through Post World War II

The history of military health care traces its origins to the establishment of the Army Medical Department on July 27, 1775. During the American Revolution, military health care was delivered in the field, often in churches and barns. After 1777, several fixed facility hospitals were established in various northern states. On March 2, 1799, Congress established *An Act to Regulate the Medical Establishment*. This legislation gave the Physician General (renamed from the Director General and Chief Physician) the authority

---

*The Navy is also responsible for providing medical care to the Marine Corps.

and responsibility of overseeing the development of (primarily) Army hospitals. That same year, General George Washington approved the construction of one of the first military hospitals in the Colonies, in Morristown, New Jersey. Although the act did not provide for dependants of one service to be treated in the hospital of another branch of service, both the Army and the Navy routinely took care of members from their sister service.[4, 5]

One of the other unique features of the 1779 Act was a directive to collect prospective payments for health care services. The 1779 Act also directed the Secretary of the Navy to deduct 20 cents a month from the pay of sailors and marines for their care in civilian treatment facilities. Proceedings suggest that the practice of collecting money for health care services not received—but promised at some future time and place—may represent the first time in U.S. managed care history that prospective health services were established in the United States health system.[6]

From the Revolutionary War through the Civil War, the military attempted to differentiate between care for dependants and active duty access. However, the westward growth of the nation required Army posts to be located in remote areas with no alternative access to health care. As military posts expanded west, families accompanied soldiers. Although departmental regulations prohibited military surgeons from treating civilians, some exceptions were granted. Finally, in 1834, the Adjutant General ruled that military surgeons had permission to treat civilians when it did not interfere with their required military duties.[7] This policy established the benefit—and later entitlement—to free health care for authorized dependants of the military that currently exists. More important, this may also be the first instance in U.S. health care that nonmonetary benefits, specifically health care benefits, were granted by an organization to family members of the employed person. The preponderance of the civilian sector did not adopt a similar provision for providing free health care to an employed person's family on a regular basis until the next century, as described in Chapter 1.

CHAMPUS and the Modern Military Health Care Era

In 1956, in an effort to keep up with a growing civilian trend to offer health care benefits and entitlements to retired persons, Congress enacted the Dependants Medical Care Act. This act provided that "medical and dental care in any medical facility of the uniformed services may, under regulations prescribed jointly by the Secretaries of Defense and Health, Education and Welfare, be furnished upon request and subject to the availability of space, facilities, and capabilities of the medical staff, to retired members of uniformed services." The act additionally applied to dependants of uniformed retirees. The significance of the Act was that it legitimized standing policies already in widespread application throughout the military health system.[8] In 1965, Congress

created Medicare and Medicaid. One of the original goals of Medicare was to provide health care for retired workers who were no longer covered by a health plan after retirement. However, a problem existed for many military personnel who often retired from a military career in their mid- to late 40s. As a result of the space availability clause of the Dependants Medical Care Act, a problem arose where some military retired members could not gain access to MTF—and were too young to participate in Medicare. As a result, some service members found themselves paying for medical care in civilian institutions out of pocket.

In an effort to address the inability to gain access to health care for some categories of beneficiaries, Congress amended the Dependants Medical Care Act and created the Civilian Health and Medical Program of the Uniformed Services (CHAMPUS). CHAMPUS was created under Public Law 89-614, the Military Medical Benefits Amendments Act of 1966. Modeled after the Blue Cross and Blue Shield options of the time, CHAMPUS was a fee-for-service benefit that provided for comprehensive medical care when there was no space available in the MTF.[9] For the first time in the history of the military, two different systems existed to provide care to beneficiaries. The resulting composite organization was composed of a direct military care system for active duty personnel that used all available military hospitals and clinics, and a second system monitored through CHAMPUS that acted as a gatekeeper to the civilian care system.[10] Although CHAMPUS did not require a monthly premium like Medicare did (for Part B only; see Chapter 24), CHAMPUS had an annual deductible and a cost share for care received outside of the MTF.

Through the late 1980s, CHAMPUS benefits remained relatively stable and unchanged. However, spiraling health care costs in the 1980s affecting civilian health care organizations also began affecting CHAMPUS. As a result, the Department of Defense (DOD) began to explore options and alternatives to control costs, monitor access, and maintain health care quality. One option centered on closing inefficient military hospitals. The second option focused on reengineering military health care.

The first option implemented by Congress to control military health care costs was the Base Realignment and Closure (BRAC) initiative. From 1987 through 1997, Congress mandated a 35% reduction of military health care assets.[11] The second option focused on quality and access and resulted in a series of five notable demonstration projects initiated from 1986 through 1993. These demonstration projects were conducted to validate the ability to use defined civilian networks effectively to treat military beneficiaries as well as to conduct a cost-benefit analysis between purchased civilian health care services and CHAMPUS expenditures. These demonstrations included the CHAMPUS Reform Initiative (CRI), the New Orleans managed care demonstration, Catchment Area Management (CAM) projects, the Southeast

Region Preferred Provider Organization (PPO) demonstration, and the Contracted Provider Arrangement (CPA) in Norfolk, Virginia.[12-14] For a more detailed review and historical presentation of these projects, readers are referred to the third edition of *The Managed Health Care Handbook*.[15]

CHAMPUS Demonstration Project Outcomes and the Creation of TRICARE

In 1993, the CHAMPUS demonstration projects suggested a reorganization of military health care by providing some evidence that civilian managed care techniques could help the military contain costs, improve quality, increase access, and advance patient satisfaction. In 1994, Congress enacted the National Defense Authorization Act (NDAA). The NDAA directed the DOD to prescribe and implement a health benefit option for beneficiaries eligible for health care under Chapter 55 of Title 10, United States Code (USC). The NDAA also directed the military health system to implement health programs modeled on managed care plans in the private sector.

In response to the DOD and Congress, the military health system developed the military managed care plan called TRICARE. TRICARE's name was coined to represent the three primary military services involved in providing health care to DOD beneficiaries (Army, Navy, and Air Force). The name also represents the three managed care options originally developed to administer care, called TRICARE Prime, TRICARE Extra, and TRICARE Standard (**Table 26-1**). Although several others have been added since TRICARE's inception, most MHS beneficiaries are enrolled in these three options. Overall, TRICARE adopted several successful managed care features, such as primary care managers, gatekeeper access, enrolled beneficiaries, and empanelled providers. The program also includes case, disease, risk, and utilization management principles.

Enhanced TRICARE Benefits

TRICARE continually seeks to enhance the benefit offered to uniformed service members, their families, and retirees and their families. As a result, in addition to the managed care options of Prime, Standard, and Extra, several niche-specific programs and adaptations have evolved to provide benefits to a larger population of beneficiaries. The preponderance of these programs resulted from initiatives in Congress to improve health care access and quality of care. One of the most significant changes to TRICARE came about with the signing of Public Law 106-398 as part of the 2001 NDAA. Dr. J. Jarrett Clinton, the acting Assistant Secretary of Defense for Health Affairs in 2001, said, "Collectively, this act represents the most significant change to military healthcare benefits since the implementation of CHAMPUS in 1966."[16] The 2001 NDAA authorized several key TRICARE improvements, including the following:

1. Established TRICARE as the secondary payer for Medicare-eligible military retirees (MEMR);
2. Established a pharmacy benefit for MEMR called TRICARE Senior Pharmacy Program (TSPP);
3. Established a MEMR Healthcare Trust Fund (HCTF);
4. Eliminated copayments for TRICARE Prime active duty family members;
5. Expanded TRICARE Prime Remote;
6. Introduced chiropractic care for active duty soldiers;
7. Established the Individual Case Management Program (ICMP) for persons with extraordinary conditions; and
8. Reduced the catastrophic cap from $7,500 to $1,000 for active duty families and $3,000 for all others.[17]

Other mentionable benefits included in this Act were permanent health benefits for Medal of Honor recipients and their families, extension of medical and dental benefits for survivors of deceased active duty soldiers, and authorization of payment for school physicals. The 2001 NDAA also authorized the DOD to expand TRICARE health benefits to niche-specific programs. The significant programs that were eventually enacted as a result of the original 2001 NDAA—and subsequent amendments—included TRICARE for Life, TRICARE Reserve Select, and the TRICARE Dental Program.

■ THE TRICARE PROGRAM

The components of the TRICARE program are discussed next.

TRICARE and the Patient Protection and Affordable Care Act

TRICARE is an entitlement program, meaning anyone who qualifies as eligible can enroll in TRICARE (eligibility is discussed next). Because it is an entitlement program, it is not affected by the Patient Protection and Affordable Care Act (ACA). The two other major entitlement programs, Medicare (Chapter 24) and Medicaid (Chapter 25), are addressed specifically in the ACA, but as separate Titles within the Act, not by inclusion with the new nonentitlement health benefits coverage requirements; TRICARE, however, is not addressed in the ACA at all.

Long before passage of the ACA, TRICARE already met all but one of the major coverage requirements, benefits, and prohibition on various limitations that the ACA now requires for commercial coverage by 2014. The only one it didn't meet, extending coverage to children of covered individuals up to age 26 if those children do not have access to coverage through their own work, was resolved when the NDAA of fiscal 2011 authorized the premium-based Young Adult Program that provides for this type of coverage extension. The ACA is not addressed further in the chapter.

		TABLE 26-1 TRICARE Beneficiary Costs, 2010	

	TRICARE Prime	TRICARE Extra	TRICARE Standard
Active Duty and Their Family Members			
Annual deductible	None	$150/individual or $300/family for E-5 and above; $50/$100 for E-4 and below	$150/individual or $300/family for E-5 and above; $50/100 E-4 and below
Annual enrollment fee	None	None	None
Civilian outpatient visit	No cost	15% of negotiated fee	20% of allowed charges for covered service
Civilian inpatient admission	No cost	Greater of $25 or $16.30/day	Greater of $25 or $16.30/day
Civilian inpatient behavioral health	No cost	Greater of $20 per day or $25 per admission	Greater of $20 per day or $25 per admission
Civilian inpatient skilled nursing facility care	$0 per diem charge per admission No separate cost share for separately billed professional charges	$16.30/day ($25 minimum) charge per admission	$16.30/day ($25 minimum) charge per admission
Retirees, Their Family Members, and Others			
Annual deductible	None	$150/individual or $300/family	$150/individual or $300/family
Annual enrollment fee	$230/individual $460/family	None	None
Civilian cost shares		20% of negotiated fee	25% of allowed charges for covered service
Outpatient emergency care mental health visit	$12 $30 $25 $17 (group visit)		
Civilian inpatient cost share	Greater of $11 per day or $25 per admission; no separate copayment for separately billed professional charges	Lesser of $250/day or 25% of negotiated charges for institutional services plus 20% cost share for separately billed services	Lesser of $535/day or 25% of billed charges for institutional services, plus 25% cost share for separately billed services
Civilian inpatient skilled nursing facility care	$11/day ($25 minimum) charge per admission	$250 per diem cost share or 20% cost share of total charges, whichever is less, for institutional services, plus 20% cost share for separately billed services	25% cost share of allowed charges for institutional services, plus 25% cost share for separately billed services
Civilian inpatient behavioral health	$40 per day; no charge for separately billed professional charges	20% of total charge, plus 20% cost share for separately billed services	High-volume hospitals—25% hospital-specific per diem Low-volume hospitals—$197 per day or 25% of the billed charges, whichever is less

Source: TRICARE: Summary of Beneficiary Costs, www.tricare.mil/mybenefit/Download/Forms/Bene_Cost_Br_L_011510.pdf. Accessed November 2, 2010.

TRICARE Eligibility

TRICARE is the health care program serving active duty uniformed service members, National Guard and Reserve members, retirees, their families, survivors, and certain former spouses worldwide of the U.S. Army, U.S. Navy, U.S. Air Force, U.S. Marine Corps, U.S. Coast Guard, as well as the Commissioned Corps of the U.S. Public Health Service and the National Oceanic and Atmospheric Administration. Family members include spouses, unmarried children under age 26, and stepchildren adopted by the sponsor. National Guard and Reservists become eligible for TRICARE when called to active duty for more than 30 days. All who are eligible for TRICARE must be listed in the Defense Department's worldwide, computerized database, the Defense Enrollment Eligibility Reporting System (DEERS). The following are not eligible for TRICARE benefits: parents and parents-in-law of active duty service members, or retirees and people who are eligible for health benefits under the

Civilian Health and Medical Program of the Department of Veterans Affairs (CHAMPVA). Out-of-pocket costs for each TRICARE option are provided in **Table 26-1**.

TRICARE Governance

To implement and administer TRICARE, in 1994, the DOD originally reorganized the military health system into 12 joint-service regions. All 12 regions were subordinate to the TRICARE Management Agency (TMA). The decision to separate contracts for different TRICARE regions was made in an effort to prevent any one contractor from having too much control over the care delivered to DOD beneficiaries.

In 2004, the Assistant Secretary of Defense (Health Affairs) and the services' Surgeons General established a governance structure consisting of three TRICARE regions. The new governance structure is designed to monitor performance and resolve problems at the lowest possible level for managing the military health benefit with force readiness as the first priority, followed closely by beneficiary satisfaction. Each of the three TRICARE regions in the United States has a regional contractor to coordinate medical services available at the MTF and the civilian network. The regional contractors work with the TRICARE regional offices (TROs) to manage TRICARE at a regional level. Both the regional contractors and the TROs receive overall guidance from the TMA. The three TRICARE regions are organized geographically into a North, South, and West region, as depicted in **Figure 26-1**.

Governance of the three TRICARE service regions remains complex. The TRICARE regional offices are responsible for planning, coordinating, and monitoring all health care delivered throughout their region. Additionally, each region establishes contracts with civilian health care organizations to provide medical care to beneficiaries. However, both military commanders and civilian contractors struggle with dual missions to maintain wartime readiness requirements and peace time beneficiary health care with limited budgets in a not-for-profit environment.

TRICARE Program Options

The TRICARE program has three main options: TRICARE Prime, TRICARE Standard, and TRICARE Extra. There are also three additional options available under certain circumstances: TRICARE for Life, TRICARE Reserve Select, and TRICARE Retired Reserve.

TRICARE Prime

TRICARE Prime is the HMO-like plan in which beneficiaries enroll in this benefit option where it is offered. Each enrollee chooses, or is assigned, a primary care manager (PCM), a health care professional who is responsible for helping the patient manage his or her health, promoting preventive health services (e.g., routine exams, immunizations), and arranging for specialty provider services as appropriate. Prime offers enrollees additional benefits such as access standards in terms of maximum allowable waiting times to obtain an appointment, emergency services (24 hours per day, 7 days per week), and waiting times in doctors' offices, as well as preventive and wellness services (routine eye exams, immunizations, hearing tests, mammograms, Pap tests, prostate examinations). A point-of-service (POS) option permits enrollees to seek care from non-network providers, but with significantly higher cost-sharing.

Active duty service members must enroll in TRICARE Prime and must receive all health care benefits at an MTF unless

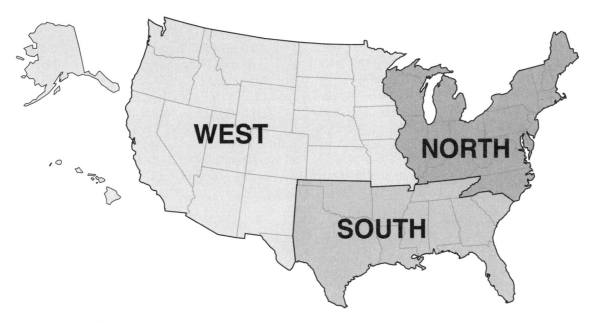

FIGURE 26-1 TRICARE Regions

Source: TRICARE Choices: Your Guide to Selecting the TRICARE Program Option That's Best for You. Available at: www.tricare.mil/mybenefit/Download/Forms/Choices_Handbook.pdf. Accessed November 2, 2010.

otherwise authorized. All health care benefits are free, and there are no out-of-pocket costs to service members. TRICARE Prime is also available to other eligible beneficiaries, such as family members of active duty service members and retirees under age 65. If enrolled in TRICARE Prime, active duty family members must also receive health care at an MTF unless otherwise directed. Retirees not eligible for Medicare can enroll in TRICARE Prime; however, they must pay an annual enrollment fee as well as copayments for care received in civilian facilities. TRICARE Prime enrollees must follow well-defined rules and procedures. Failure to follow strict TRICARE Prime guidelines may result in refusal of care, refusal of payment, and costly POS option charges.

In addition to low to no out-of-pocket costs, an advantage of being enrolled in TRICARE Prime is the policy-directed access to care standards for appointments. Access to care standards differ by the level of care sought. For emergency care, MHS beneficiaries have the right to access emergency health care services when and where the need arises. For urgent (acute) care, the standard is an appointment within 24 hours and within 30 minutes travel time; routine care within 7 calendar days and within 30 minutes drive time; for wellness and specialty care, the appointment must be within 28 days and within 1 hour drive time from the beneficiary's residence. If these access standards cannot be met, TRICARE offers the beneficiary a referral and authorization to seek care in the civilian network. Moreover, TRICARE access standards state that office waiting times in nonemergency circumstances shall not exceed 30 minutes for Prime enrollees.

For service members and their families who do not live near an MTF, TRICARE offers TRICARE Prime Remote (TPR). TPR is specific to certain geographic locations, and eligibility is based on residence and/or work address. To be eligible for TPR, active duty members and their families must live and work more than 50 miles—or approximately 1 hour drive time—from the nearest MTF. TPR offers the same access standards and low out-of-pocket costs as TRICARE Prime. Like TRICARE Prime, enrollment in TPR is required.

Another TRICARE Prime option is the Uniformed Services Family Health Plan (USFHP) and is available to active duty family members, retirees, and their eligible family members (including those age 65 and older regardless if they are enrolled in Medicare Part B). The USFHP is available through networks of community-based, not-for-profit health care systems in six areas of the United States. Enrollment in USFHP is required and enrollment fees apply for retirees and their eligible family members. If enrolled in USFHP, access to care at an MTF or use of MTF pharmacies is excluded. This managed care option has the same coverage and costs as Prime, but also offers additional services at the local level.

TRICARE Standard

TRICARE Standard is the traditional indemnity benefit, also known as fee-for-service (FFS), and formerly known as CHAMPUS. It is open to all eligible Department of Defense beneficiaries, except active duty service members and, until recently, Medicare eligibles. No enrollment is required to obtain care from civilian providers. TRICARE Standard gives beneficiaries the option to see any provider. Advantages include a wider selection of providers and health care facilities and the option to participate in TRICARE Extra. There is no required annual enrollment, and the option offers comprehensive health care coverage for beneficiaries not enrolled in TRICARE Prime.

While Standard offers the greatest flexibility in choosing a provider, the plan also has the most out-of-pocket cost-sharing by the beneficiary; for example, TRICARE Standard requires that the beneficiary satisfy a yearly deductible before TRICARE cost-sharing begins. Furthermore, the plan requires beneficiaries to pay copayments or cost shares for outpatient care, medications, and inpatient care. Another disadvantage is that the patient may also be required to file his or her own claims. Finally, the option also does not provide a PCM benefit.

TRICARE Extra

TRICARE Extra is based on a civilian PPO model in which beneficiaries eligible for TRICARE Standard may decide to use preferred civilian network providers on a case-by-case basis (they may switch between the Standard and Extra benefits). TRICARE Extra is open to any TRICARE-eligible beneficiary who is not active duty, not otherwise enrolled in Prime, and not eligible for TRICARE for Life (discussed next). TRICARE Extra requires no enrollment and there is no enrollment fee. Under this option, beneficiaries can see civilian providers and go to civilian health care organizations that are on an approved list of TRICARE providers called the TRICARE Provider Directory.

TRICARE Extra is essentially an option for TRICARE Standard beneficiaries who want to save on out-of-pocket expenses by making an appointment with a TRICARE Prime network provider. TRICARE Extra requires the same deductible as TRICARE Standard; however, by using network providers, beneficiaries reduce their cost-sharing by 5%. An advantage of TRICARE Extra is that the Extra option user can expect that the network provider will file all claims forms—similar to TRICARE Prime. An additional advantage is that the access to the authorized provider may be more geographically convenient to the Extra user. However, disadvantages include extra fees associated with deductibles and copayments, the loss of a PCM, some restrictions on specialty care access, and limited provider choice.

TRICARE for Life

Over the years, military recruiters marketed "free health care for life" to potential recruits, promising this benefit for the recruit and certain family members if they served a certain amount of time in uniform.[18] However, in 1956, Public

Law 569 changed the century-old, quasi–health care for life entitlement to a benefit. PL 569, Section 301, changed from: "Hospital space *SHALL* be made available" to "Hospital space *MAY* be made available [sic]."[19] Despite the change in law, retirees and family members continued to receive benefits well into the early 1990s. However, in the mid-1990s, under congressional and presidential guidance, these beneficiaries were required to use a civilian health care provider, use a civilian organization, and rely on Medicare or other health insurance (OHI) as payers.[20]

The Pentagon estimated that approximately 1.5 million personnel, approximately 20% of the beneficiary base, were locked out of the military health system in the late 1990s.[21] Based partially on the grassroots response to restricted access to health care options, TRICARE for Life (TFL) was signed into public law (PL 106-398) as part of the 2001 NDAA.

TFL effectively fulfills the promise of lifetime health care made to older retirees for a career in uniform. TFL restores TRICARE coverage for all Medicare-eligible retired beneficiaries regardless of age or place of residence who are enrolled in Medicare Parts A and B.[22] Congress established TFL as a "fully funded entitlement program" by means of a new Medicare-Eligible Retiree Health Care Trust Fund.[23] To qualify for TFL, a retiree must have served at least 20 years in the uniformed services (including retired members of the National Guard and the Reserves). There are no enrollment fees, premiums, or deductibles for TFL. Beneficiaries receive most of their care from civilian providers and Medicare is the first payer, whereas TRICARE (or other health insurance) serves as the secondary payer. TFL makes TRICARE a secondary payer to Medicare at no cost to a retiree.

Another option available to eligible TFL beneficiaries is TRICARE Plus. TRICARE Plus affords beneficiaries the opportunity to receive primary care and specialty care at their local MTF, provided that facility has space available. There are no charges or fees for TRICARE Plus, if offered by the MTF. Another benefit of TRICARE Plus is that beneficiaries are entitled to the same primary care access standards as beneficiaries in TRICARE Prime. For example, the beneficiary would be assured of a primary care appointment within one week. However, TRICARE Plus is not available at all MTFs due to the availability of care. Also, the MTF commander may limit the program to only certain beneficiary categories, again based on local staffing and other considerations.

Another limitation is that beneficiaries already enrolled in TRICARE Prime, a purchased care HMO, or a Medicare HMO are not eligible. Basically, TRICARE for Life (benefits received from civilian providers) and TRICARE Plus (care received at MTFs) give beneficiaries more coverage while simultaneously allowing the military health system the ability to control costs and access due to local, medically related considerations. The enactment of TFL represents one of the many military managed care outcomes that can be traced to antecedent activist actions by constituents.

TRICARE Reserve Select

The NDAA of 2005 authorized a program called TRICARE Reserve Select (TRS). TRS is a premium-based health plan for eligible Reserve component members. TRS offers comprehensive health care coverage similar to TRICARE Standard and TRICARE Extra. TRS members and covered family members can access care by making an appointment with any TRICARE authorized provider, hospital, or pharmacy or TRICARE network or non-network. TRS members may access care at an MTF on a space-available basis only; however, pharmacy services are available from an MTF pharmacy, the TRICARE Mail Order Pharmacy, or TRICARE network and non-network retail pharmacies. Medical coverage (direct care at the MTF) is available when the member is activated. When ordered to active duty for more than 30 consecutive days, Reserve component members and their families have comprehensive health care coverage under TRICARE.[24]

TRICARE Retired Reserve

TRICARE Retired Reserve (TRR) provides comprehensive coverage for a specified group of beneficiaries. Eligibility for this program is limited to retired Reserve individuals who are qualified for nonregular retirement and their families. Also, they must be under the age of 60 and not eligible for, or enrolled in, the Federal Employees Health Benefits Program (FEHBP).[25]

In addition, survivors of retired Reserve members may be qualified if they meet certain requirements: the Reserve member was covered by TRR at time of death; the survivors must be immediate family members and the spouse must not have remarried; and the coverage would begin before the Reserve member would have turned 60. However, eligibility for FEHBP is not necessary for the survivors.

TRR is a premium-based plan that offers TRICARE benefits worldwide by TRICARE-authorized providers. Similar to other TRICARE programs, there are annual deductibles and copays. However, unlike some of the other TRICARE plans, the law does not provide any government subsidy, therefore, enrollees pay the full cost of the program. Nevertheless, the cost is less if the providers are in the TRICARE network.

Other advantages of the program include beneficiaries being authorized to receive care in military hospitals on a space-available basis. Also, the beneficiary may visit any TRICARE-authorized provider whether or not that provider is in the network. However, if the provider is in the network, the beneficiary will pay less and the provider will file the claim on behalf of the beneficiary. There is no referral, although some medical services may require preauthorization by TRICARE. Finally, continuity of care may be enhanced because there is no requirement for eligible Reserve personnel to change providers if they already have one. A description of all of the TRICARE program options is provided in **Table 26-2**.

TABLE 26-2	**TRICARE Program Descriptions**

Program	Type of program	Enrollment and fees	Medical provider choice
TRICARE Prime	• Similar to a managed care or HMO option available in specific geographic areas	• Enrollment required • Retirees, their families, survivors, and qualifying former spouses pay annual enrollment fees • Offers lowest out-of-pocket costs	• Receive most care from PCM at an MTF or within the TRICARE network • PCM referrals required for most specialty care
TRICARE Prime Remote	• Benefit similar to TRICARE Prime for active duty service members living and working in remote locations and eligible family members residing with the service member	• Enrollment required • No annual enrollment fee • Offers same low out-of-pocket costs as TRICARE Prime	• Receive care from TRICARE network providers (or a TRICARE-authorized provider if a network provider is unavailable)
TRICARE Standard	• FFS option available worldwide	• No enrollment required • No annual enrollment fee or enrollment applications • Annual deductibles and cost-shares apply	• Receive care from TRICARE authorized non-network provider • No referrals required • Some services require prior authorization • May enroll in TRICARE Plus where available
TRICARE Extra	• Preferred provider option in areas with established TRICARE networks • Not available overseas	• No enrollment required • No annual enrollment fee or enrollment applications • Annual deductibles and discounted cost-shares apply	• Receive care from TRICARE network providers • No referrals required • Some services require prior authorization
TRICARE Reserve Select (TRS)	• Premium-based health care plan that qualified National Guard and Reserve members may purchase • Available worldwide • Offers member-only and member-and-family coverage	• Must qualify for and purchase TRS to participate • Monthly premiums, annual deductibles, and cost-shares apply	• Receive care from any TRICARE-authorized provider (network or non-network) • No referrals required • Some services require prior authorization
TRICARE Retired Reserve (TRR)	• Premium-based health care plan that qualified Retired Reserve members may purchase • Available worldwide • Offers member-only and member-and-family coverage	• Must qualify for and purchase TRR to participate • Monthly premiums, annual deductibles, and cost-shares apply	• Receive care from any TRICARE-authorized provider (network or non-network) • No referrals required • Some services require prior authorization
TRICARE for Life	• TRICARE's Medicare-wraparound coverage available to all Medicare-eligible TRICARE beneficiaries, regardless of age, provided they have Medicare Part A and Medicare Part B	• No enrollment fees • Must be entitled to premium-free Medicare Part A and have purchased Medicare Part B	• Receive care from Medicare providers • Can use TRICARE Pharmacy Home Delivery option to meet prescription needs • May enroll in TRICARE Plus where available
U.S. Family Health Plan (USFHP)	• TRICARE Prime managed care option available through networks of community-based, not-for-profit health care systems in six areas of the United States	• Enrollment required • Enrollment fees for retirees and their eligible family members	• Receive care from primary care providers in the health care system to which you are enrolled • Primary care providers will refer you for specialty care

Source: TRICARE Choices: At a Glance. Available at: www.tricare.mil/tricaresmartfiles/Prod_539/TRICARE_Choices_At_a_Glance_Br_10_LoRes.pdf. Accessed November 2, 2010.

TRICARE Pharmacy Program

The MHS provides comprehensive prescription drug coverage to all its beneficiaries including active duty service members and their families, retirees and their families, and beneficiaries who are over age 65. Also, this coverage is the same regardless of the TRICARE program in which the beneficiary is enrolled. Pharmaceuticals may be obtained at MTFs or through the TRICARE Pharmacy program (TPharm), which includes home delivery, retail network pharmacies, and non-network pharmacies.

TPharm is a contractor-provided benefit, which provides convenience and low cost to beneficiaries. TPharm has the combined features of a home delivery (by mail order) service and a retail pharmacy. In addition to not requiring enrollment, there are several other advantages to beneficiaries:

- A single call center and a help desk are available for convenience;
- Prescriptions are easily transferred between pharmacies regardless of whether they are retail, military, or mail order; and
- Although the prescription drug coverage is the same regardless of health plan, there are financial incentives for beneficiaries to utilize home delivery (mail order) rather than retail pharmacies.[26]

TRICARE Dental Programs

The TRICARE Dental Program (TDP) is a voluntary dental insurance program that is available to eligible active duty family members, select reserve component personnel, Individual Ready Reserve (IRR) members, select retirees, and other eligible beneficiaries. This premium-based program has annual costs and deductibles for both family members of active duty personnel as well as other classes of beneficiaries.[27] The plan covers ordinary dental procedures such as annual screenings, preventive care, and standard dental treatments.

Another dental program exists solely for active duty and activated Reserve and National Guard service members. This program, the Active Duty Dental Program (ADDP), is administered by a civilian contractor who provides care for service members who live and work more than 50 miles from a military dental clinic as well as service members in the U.S. Virgin Islands, Puerto Rico, as well as the Pacific islands of Guam, American Samoa, and the Northern Mariana Islands. Although there is no enrollment feature, treatment must be provided by the contractor's network provider.

Other TRICARE Programs

Beyond the programs that have already been discussed, other TRICARE programs include TRICARE Overseas, transitional health care benefits such as the Transitional Assistance Management Program and the Continued Healthcare Benefit Program (CHCBP), and programs for special needs beneficiaries.

TRICARE Overseas

Because there are over 500,000 TRICARE beneficiaries living overseas, TRICARE contracts exist in three geographical regions: Latin America-Canada, Eurasia-Africa, and the Pacific. In these areas, MTFs provide primary care to beneficiaries but the host nations provide specialty care. The contract vendors are responsible not only for ensuring care is provided to the beneficiaries, but also for provider relations in the host nations and some medical evacuations. TRICARE Prime Overseas allows service members and their families who live overseas to get their health care under a TRICARE Prime–like option. Active duty service members must enroll in TRICARE Prime Overseas; however, family members can select between two options: TRICARE Overseas Prime and TRICARE Standard Overseas. TRICARE Standard Overseas also extends to military retirees and their families. TRICARE Extra is not available in overseas locations.

Transitional Assistance Management Program and the Continued Healthcare Benefit Program

Individuals who lose TRICARE eligibility or other coverage under the military health system are eligible for two transitional health care options: the Transitional Assistance Management Program (TAMP) and the Continued Healthcare Benefit Program (CHCBP). TAMP provides 180 days of transitional health benefits after leaving active duty with the option to enroll in TRICARE Prime or receive coverage under TRICARE Standard and TRICARE Extra. CHCBP is a premium-based health care program administered by a private contractor that provides temporary transitional health coverage (18–36 months) after TRICARE eligibility ends. CHCBP offers similar benefits and operates under most of the rules of TRICARE Standard. To obtain this coverage, the member must enroll in CHCBP within 60 days after separation from active duty or loss of eligibility for military health care.[28, 29]

Extended Care Health Option

TRICARE offers three enhancements to the traditional TRICARE program for active duty family members with special needs: TRICARE Extended Care Health Option (ECHO), ECHO Home Health Care (EHHC), and EHHC Respite Care. ECHO delivers financial assistance and additional benefits, including supplies and services, beyond those available from the basic benefit in TRICARE Prime, Standard, or Extra. The benefit increased from $1,000 (through the Program for Persons with Disabilities) to $2,500 per eligible family member in fiscal year 2004 under ECHO. Additionally, beneficiaries who are homebound may qualify for extended in-home health care through ECHO.

ECHO Home Health Care provides medically necessary skilled services to eligible homebound beneficiaries who generally require more than 28–35 hours per week of home health services or respite care. This benefit helps eligible beneficiaries stay home rather than having to go to an institutional/acute-care facility or skilled nursing home. Similarly, the EHHC Respite Benefit provides temporary relief or a rest period for the primary caregiver to promote well-being for both the caregiver and the homebound beneficiary. This benefit offers 8 hours of respite care per day up to 5 days per calendar week.[30]

■ MONITORING MHS PERFORMANCE

Like all managed health care plans, the performance of the MHS is continually monitored, often using the same metrics and measures used by commercial payers. But the MHS is not exactly the same as all other managed health care plans, so it must monitor performance in some unique ways.

The MHS Quadruple Aim

In 2009, MHS leaders recognized that the MHS strategic plan was consistent with the concept of the Triple Aim proposed by the Institute for Healthcare Improvement (IHI). The Triple Aim describes the results that can be achieved when all the elements of a health care system work together to serve the needs of a population. Because the MHS is a system dedicated to the health of the military family, it was appropriate to adopt the Triple Aim as its strategic vision with the addition of one key element: readiness. Readiness reflects the core mission of the MHS and its reason for being. **Figure 26-2** shows the MHS Quadruple Aim.

The MHS Quadruple Aim is comprised of the following elements:

- *Readiness*—ensuring that the total military force is medically ready to deploy and that the medical force

is ready to deliver health care anytime, anywhere in support of the full range of military operations, including humanitarian missions.

- *Population Health*—improving the health of a population by encouraging healthy behaviors and reducing the likelihood of illness through focused prevention and the development of increased resilience.
- *Experience of Care*—providing a care experience that is patient and family centered, compassionate, convenient, equitable, safe, and of high quality.
- *Per Capita Cost*—creating value by focusing on quality, eliminating waste, and reducing unwarranted variation and considering the total cost of care over time, not just the cost of an individual health care activity.

The MHS monitors a number of metrics to assess its strategic performance. When appropriate, the MHS uses existing measures found in the civilian sector in order to benchmark its performance. Some examples of these measures include those taken from the Healthcare Effectiveness Data and Information Set (HEDIS®), the Consumer Assessment of Health Plans Study (CAHPS®), and the Overall Hospital Quality Index (ORYX®). Emphasis on specific metrics changes as the needs of the population change.[*]

Performance Metrics for TRICARE Contractors

TRICARE contractors are charged with providing or arranging for delivery of high-quality, timely health care services and accurate, timely processing of claims received into their custody, whether for network or non-network care. In addition, the contractor must provide courteous, accurate, and timely response to inquiries from beneficiaries, providers, the TMA, and other legitimately interested parties. TMA has established standards of performance that are monitored by TMA and other government agencies to measure contractor performance. Key performance standards include such measures as preauthorizations/authorizations, referrals, and claims processing timeliness requirements.[31]

Outcomes of the TRICARE Program

Initial results of the TRICARE reengineering initiative, combined with other improvements within the military health system, suggest that cost containment and quality improvement were achieved through (at least) 2004.[32] However, from 2001 through 2010, expenses associated with military health care rose 167%, resulting in an increase of costs from $19 billion to $51 billion in the same period of time. This increase represents over 10% of the defense budget.

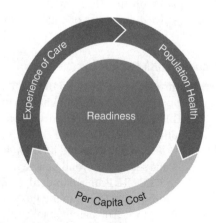

FIGURE 26-2 The MHS Quadruple Aim

Source: 2011 MHS Stakeholders' Report, www.health.mil/About_MHS/ StakeholdersReport.aspx. Accessed March 2, 2011.

___

[*] HEDIS is maintained by the National Committee on Quality Assurance (NCQA), and CAHPS is maintained by the federal Agency for Healthcare Research and Quality (AHRQ); both are addressed in Chapter 15. ORYX is maintained by The Joint Commission and is not within the scope of this book.

Projected costs are estimated to reach $65 billion by 2015. To compound issues, TRICARE fees have not increased since 1995. The result has been a less cost-efficient military health system.[33, 34]

However, quality indicators suggest that military hospitals have higher Joint Commission scores than civilian organizations. Additionally, military report cards suggest that military hospitals have a higher percentage of board-certified doctors, administrators, and allied health personnel than civilian hospitals.

Beneficiaries who are enrolled in the purchased care plan are generally more satisfied than those enrolled in the direct care plan. Issues being addressed include aligning incentives for both beneficiaries and providers, enhancing continuity of care, and maintaining access standards in both military health care facilities and the civilian network.[35, 36]

Although there is mixed research and opinion on whether military health care is more or less cost effective per quality outcomes than civilian health care, Congress, the DOD, TMA, and the beneficiary base largely consider TRICARE a success. As a result, in an effort to maintain satisfaction with key stakeholders, the military health system is continually developing process improvement initiatives and incorporating progressive management practices to maintain optimal cost, quality, and access. Such examples in recent years have included the adoption of both a balanced scorecard and lean six sigma initiatives.

■ CURRENT AND FUTURE CHALLENGES

Many of the current and future challenges for the MHS parallel those in the commercial sector, but some are unique.

Continually Rising Costs

Like health care benefits in the commercial sector, and in Medicare and Medicaid, the biggest threat to the military health plan is its cost. Between fiscal year 2007 and 2010 alone, costs increased almost 10%. About half of this increase was in the purchased care part of TRICARE, meaning private sector providers. Major causes of this increase were the retail pharmacy network, the TFL benefit, and an increased number of beneficiaries. In response, the pharmacy benefit has been restructured to encourage home delivery. However, there are limited options to reduce the cost of TFL. Similarly, it can be expected that there will be more beneficiaries as the population's life span increases and more National Guard and Reserve beneficiaries enroll.

In 1995, beneficiaries paid approximately 27% of their health care costs; however, in 2010, beneficiaries paid only 12% of their own health care costs. The result is a more generous military medical benefit to beneficiaries. Unfortunately, in an effort to control health care costs in the civilian market, many employers of military beneficiaries (including state agencies) have encouraged them to forgo participating in the employee health plan in lieu of extra wages and income. The new employer avoids an increase in the company's benefits costs, but only because the burden of providing medical care to the military beneficiary base remains with TRICARE.

In addition to benefit enhancements, increased use by an increased number of beneficiaries and no increases in cost-sharing have resulted in the MHS experiencing the same health care inflation as all health plans in the nation. The MHS implemented a number of management initiatives designed to reduce the costs of delivery and to enhance performance within its health system. For example, an Outpatient Prospective Payment System has been implemented. This seeks to leverage the Medicare program by aligning hospitals' outpatient payment rates with the rates approved by Medicare. Similarly, tighter management controls have been implemented to constrain per member per month costs as well as emergency department utilization.

Having the enormous responsibility and accountability to be a good steward of taxpayers' dollars often makes the MHS a keen concern of Congress. Because the health care industry is the largest service industry in the United States, and health care costs have historically shown a trend of rapid increase, it is little wonder that health care expenditures are a significant issue in terms of the annual military budget and a potential threat to the TRICARE program.

The Next Generation of Tricare Contracts

The military health system is continually adapting the structure of its health care delivery system to meet DOD requirements. The current contracts were awarded in 2010 for a maximum of 5 years. Soon after these contracts were awarded, the DOD began an initiative to assess the requirements for the next generation of TRICARE contracts. To determine the scope of the contracts, this initiative assessed national security, health care, and the economic climate as well as such factors as various health care delivery and finance models, scope of coverage, leveraging best practices and knowledge management, and individual choice and financial implications. Throughout the assessment, key considerations were maintaining the military's readiness, strengthening continuity of care, and focusing on health vis-à-vis health care.[37]

Caring for Wounded Warriors

In addition to providing health care through the direct care and purchased care TRICARE program, the MHS remains focused on optimizing the health and quality of life of wounded service members and their families. To accomplish this, MHS centers of excellence (CoE) have been established for research and treatment. These CoEs are addressing how to treat the most serious injuries including psychological health and traumatic brain injury, amputations, neuroscience and regenerative medicine, and vision.[38]

Representative of the comprehensive approach to research and treatment is the Defense Centers of Excellence for Psychological Health and Traumatic Brain Injury (DCOE). This center is the focal point for a number of interdisciplinary resources to assist the families in understanding and coping with the injuries of their service members. In addition to providing information on the nature of psychological and traumatic brain injuries, this assistance includes providing state-of-the-art advice regarding issues including preventing suicide, helping children whose mother/father has deployed or just returned, adjusting to changes, taking care of family members, and understanding the stress of service members who are transitioning in their careers (e.g., relocating or returning to civilian life). DCOE also provides a free, 24/7 outreach center, which consists of experts who provide information by telephone, e-mail, or online chat.

Since the beginning of hostilities in Iraq, the MHS has treated substantial numbers of severely wounded, ill, and injured (WII) service members. However, subsequent to the 2007 media coverage regarding the quality and effectiveness of care, management, and support systems for the WII, a number of additional initiatives were implemented. Also, the National Defense Authorization Act of 2008 required the Secretaries of Defense and Veterans Affairs to develop policies regarding the WII's care, management, and transition into the civilian community.

Within the Department of Defense, there are several organizational elements to accomplish these goals. The Office of Wounded Warrior Care and Transition Policy (WWCTP) was established in November 2008 and was charged with providing oversight, establishing policy, and collaborating with other agencies to ensure that WII service members receive quality health care while in a patient status and, when appropriate, the necessary support during their transition to either civilian life or return to active duty.

The office has a number of responsibilities, including providing recovery care coordinators, administering the Disability Evaluation System (DES), and maintaining the National Resource Directory as well as the Transition Assistance Program. The DES initiative is administered in coordination with the Department of Veterans Affairs. The intent is to ensure that the WII service member is provided only one medical examination that will ensure a faster, more equitable, and more transparent disability determination.

The Recovery Coordination Program consists of recovery care coordinators who work with the military departments' recovery care teams to ensure that all nonmedical needs of WII service members are met in a timely and comprehensive manner. The Transition Assistance Program is responsible to ensure that WII service members are connected with a comprehensive range of services and resources. These include counseling and briefings in such areas as benefits, transition to civilian life, post-military employment and career changes, and resources for WII service members with disabilities. The National Resource Directory is a robust website that offers information pertaining to important topics such as benefits and compensation, employment, family and caregiver support, health care, housing and transportation, and education and training.[39]

In support of the WWCTP and the military services, the MHS provides health care as well as coordination and transition services for its WII service members through the services' wounded warrior programs. The core attribute of these programs is the comprehensive and personalized health care and nonmedical case management of each WII service member and his or her family.

The largest program is the Army's Wounded Warrior Program (AW2), with the mission to assist and advocate for its severely wounded, ill, and injured soldiers, veterans, and their families for as long as it takes. It provides individualized services to this population by means of a designated advocate whose responsibility is to provide personal assistance. Although this advocate is a nonmedical manager, he or she is also responsible to ensure that appropriate health care is received as indicated. The second largest program is the Marine Corps Wounded Warrior Regiment. Similar in mission to the AW2, the Wounded Warrior Regiment "provides and facilitates assistance to wounded, ill, and injured Marines, Sailors attached to or in support of Marine units, and their family members in order to assist them as they return to duty or transition to civilian life."[40]

Although supporting a substantially smaller WII population, the Navy's Safe Harbor and the Air Force Wounded Warrior programs also provide individualized and enhanced assistance to their service members and families during and after active duty.

The features of AW2 are representative of the other services' programs, although there may be differences in some operational aspects due to service philosophy, numbers of WII service members, or other service-specific considerations. As noted above, AW2's key feature is individualized support provided to WII service members, who are defined as those Army soldiers who are expected to require at least 6 months of rehabilitation as well as complex medical management. Each soldier is assigned a nonmedical case manager who is called an AW2 Advocate. This Advocate is located in an area as close as possible to the soldier. Typically, the Advocate is located where there are large concentrations of WII service members, including military installations, VA facilities and polytrauma centers, and urban areas. The Advocate is required to personally maintain contact with the soldier and assist him or her for the long term, hence the AW2's philosophy of "for as long as it takes." The Advocate's assignment is not limited by the soldier's recovery or rehabilitation time and, if the soldier moves, another local Advocate will be assigned.[41]

Balancing Stakeholder Priorities

The most significant struggle the military managed care system has grappled with from the inception of TRICARE to the present is the careful balance between elements of the Coppola's Managed Care Quaternion (MCQ)[42–44] and Kissick's Iron Triangle.[45]

When juxtaposed together, the two models create a new decision-making paradigm Coppola coined, "The Parity of Health Care,"[46] as shown in Figure 26-2. Coppola developed the Parity of Health Care concept and model to assist in explaining to military health care leaders why consensus on any single aspect of health care is difficult. The model has gained popular support within governmental organizations, as well as some state Medicaid agencies, as an aid to health planning and policymaking. It has also been used to forecast future health care needs in many civilian organizations and entities as well.[47]

Managed Care Quaternion

The term *Managed Care Quaternion* was coined in the Army-Baylor Graduate Program in Health and Business Administration in 2003. The Army-Baylor Program has been responsible for training and educating the next generation of military health care executives since 1953. The Quaternion has been used for several years to help explain the complex interactions among employers, patients, providers, and payers in regard to partisan and competing views about health care.

Understanding the careful balance between stakeholders in military health care policy and strategy formulation is critically important. This reality becomes more important as leaders rise in positions of increased responsibility, from running health care organizations to directing policy for entire health systems. Key stakeholders in the military are similar to any civilian health care entity, and are comprised of military and civilian individuals, groups, and associations. While the numbers of stakeholders in health organizations can be numerous, there are four main types of stakeholders to consider in any health care decision making: patients, payers, providers, and employers.

The Iron Triangle

The concept of the Iron Triangle was developed by Kissick in the early 1990s during the managed care revolution in America. Kissick coined the term Iron Triangle to demonstrate the difficulty in selecting priorities for health as they relate to health care costs, quality, and access.[*] Kissick suggested that an understanding of these resource elements would assist managed care organizations in setting

logistical priorities. Kissick's model is a vital tool to health leaders; however, the model itself fails to take into account outside actors and agents. In this regard it is incomplete by itself for dynamic organizational analysis.

Parity of Health Care

The Parity of Health Care model juxtaposes the Managed Care Quaternion and the Iron Triangle models together in a manner that allows military and civilian leaders to strategically plan and forecast the impact of new policy decisions that may affect the organization, such as patient care, payment arrangements, external costs, outside stakeholder satisfaction, program efficiency and effectiveness, quality, and other policies affecting organization survivability. Patients, payers, employers, and providers all play a vital role in the operations of any health organization. With any one of the four major stakeholders of the Managed Care Quaternion omitted in the decision-making process for a health care entity, failure at some level is sure to occur. For example, a military primary care clinic without extended and weekend office hours may be regarded as low quality to the patient because of the inconvenience factor; however, the same clinic may be regarded as high quality to the DOD (i.e., the payers) because of the cost efficiency of the clinic. However, if patients continue to perceive lack of extended and weekend office hours as low quality, dissatisfaction with the overall clinic may result regardless of the quality of provided care. As a result, health professionals must be cognizant of the constant struggle between stakeholders to maintain high satisfaction with all elements of the Managed Care Quaternion.

As seen from in **Figure 26-3** and **Figure 26-4**, even a slight variation in the prioritization of Iron Triangle options results in myriad interrelated and intrarelated competing priorities that can be hard for even the stakeholders to resolve themselves, let alone in tandem with other stakeholders along the continuum of care.

Sword of Damocles

In continuing to understand the difficult nature of the relationships between the Iron Triangle and the Managed Care Quaternion, we offer a metaphor from classical literature called the *Sword of Damocles*. In Greek mythology, the Sword of Damocles represents "ever-present peril." It is also used as a metaphor to suggest a "frailty in existing relationships." For example, in the Parity of Health Care, the Sword of Damocles represents an inability of any one stakeholder to reach sustained consensus for priorities of cost, quality, and access.

With health priorities constantly changing due to environmental demands, it is no wonder why agreements on health policy are difficult to reach. However, an understanding of the Parity of Health Care can be helpful to health leaders for strategically forecasting threats to relationships

---

[*] A variation of this was used by the consulting firm Ernst & Young, LLP around the same time: cost, access to all providers, and high level of benefits coverage.

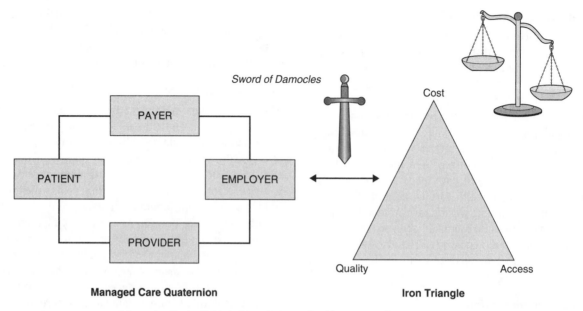

Managed Care Quaternion   Iron Triangle

Measuring the ineffable balance between healthcare paradigms

FIGURE 26-3 Parity of Health Care

Payer	Patient
Cost-Quality-Access	Access-Cost-Quality
Access-Cost-Quality	Quality-Access-Cost
Quality-Access-Cost	Quality-Cost-Access
Quality-Cost-Access	Access-Quality-Cost
Access-Quality-Cost	Cost-Access-Quality
Cost-Access-Quality	Cost-Quality-Access
Employer	**Provider**
Access-Quality-Cost	Quality-Cost-Access
Cost-Access-Quality	Access-Quality-Cost
Cost-Quality-Access	Cost-Access-Quality
Access-Cost-Quality	Cost-Quality-Access
Quality-Access-Cost	Access-Cost-Quality
Quality-Cost-Access	Quality-Access-Cost

FIGURE 26-4 Parity of Health Care Competing Priorities and Possible Combinations

amid stakeholders, while also balancing priorities among those stakeholders. If anything is apparent, continuous external and internal assessment and evaluation and relationship building among stakeholders are critical to leadership success.

As a result, both military and civilian health planners must be cognizant that solutions developed to solve health problems in the current environment may not be valid solutions to tomorrow's new issues. As environmental demands continue to place pressures on the relationships within the Parity of Health Care, health leaders must renegotiate priorities. Health planners and leaders should be aware of this fact and view change as a new opportunity for success and not simply problems of the dynamic environment. Always consider the *Sword of Damocles* represents the frailty of established relationships among stakeholders, and that constant maintenance and attention is required. An understanding of the Parity of Health Care can be helpful in the military health system for strategically forecasting threats to relationships amid actors—and also balancing priorities among actors.

A Different Health Care Environment

The military health system operates in a unique cost environment. MTFs operate in a typical government fiscal bureaucracy. Under this paradigm, health care dollars are allocated to the MTF at the beginning of the fiscal year on October 1. The hospital commander (similar to a civilian hospital CEO) is then encouraged to spend all the allocated monies prior to September 30 of the following year. Typically, hospital commanders attempt to exhaust all allocated dollars by the end of August—and then request more year-end funds. Under this federal bureaucracy and paradigm, military health leaders have little incentive to conserve resources, seek synergies, or save money. All money not used by September 30 of the fiscal year is lost. Ironically, then, commanders and health leaders failing to spend all their allocated dollars may be considered poor financial managers under this paradigm. However, a significant advantage of this philosophy is that MTFs are able to consider aspects of quality and access over costs in some cases.

Until September 11, 2001 (9/11), this placed the military health system in a unique situation where it was able to focus attention and resources on matters of self-interest first rather than key stakeholder and actor priorities. Since 9/11 and the Global War on Terror, priorities have changed.

Congress closely monitors military health care budgets and major health care expenditures. Although MTFs still operate on a 12-month exhaustible account, MTFs' budgets are closely reviewed for superfluous spending. Additionally, under revised financing initiatives, MTFs are moving toward a value-based financing system whereby facilities are paid based on the quantity and quality of services delivered rather than traditional budget allocations.[48] Additionally, as the retiree and beneficiary population continues to increase, non–active duty beneficiaries have found they have a voice in Congress and the power to influence military health policy. The passing of the TRICARE for Life and the TRICARE Reserve Select options are only two of the examples of stakeholder influence on the modern military health system.

Finally, the local MTF commander now finds him- or herself in competition with the local TRICARE network. Because certain classifications of beneficiaries have a choice of enrolling in TRICARE Prime (care at the local military treatment facility) or choosing TRICARE Extra or Standard (care rendered through the civilian network), for every one patient that elects not to enroll (or disenroll) in TRICARE Prime, the local MTF commander loses money. As a result, contrary to the friendly relationship that existed between the TRICARE contractor and the local MTF in the 1990s, both the TRICARE contractor and the military hospital are competing more and more for the same health care dollars that are associated with every one DOD beneficiary.

As a result, if the military health system is to continue to survive, military health leaders must understand the parity of health care. Furthermore, the military health system must, in essence, discontinue thinking "military" and adopt best practices and processes used by civilian peers. Military health leaders must consider aspects of the Managed Care Quaternion when formulating policy. Additionally, federal health care leaders must consider the consequences of cost, quality, and access to care actors. Failing to consider the complex relationships associated with the parity of health care will affect the efficiency, effectiveness, and survival of military health care in the future.

CONCLUSION

The MHS operates the oldest form of organized health care delivery in the United States. Originally founded in 1775, the military health system has more than 235 years of experience in the effective operation and delivery of military medicine and management. The success of the military health system is caused in part by its ability to adapt to changes in the internal and external environments to maintain effectiveness.

Developing initially as colloquial health programs designed to treat specific categories of beneficiaries and active duty service personnel, the military medical system eventually developed comprehensive direct care and purchased care systems. The purchased care system, called CHAMPUS, provided health care to a large standing military throughout the Cold War era. However, in response to changes in the health care environment, the military developed and implemented TRICARE. TRICARE is the DOD's managed care model that delivers health care to approximately 10 million beneficiaries worldwide.

Although it struggled through its initial growing pains during the late 1990s, the TRICARE program has become a viable model of success. Significant advantages of TRICARE include high-quality care and the lowest out-of-pocket costs as compared to civilian managed care models. Threats include costs associated with implementing TRICARE, providing care to an aging retiree population, and the additional mission of providing care to select Reserve members. Additional threats include a loss of stakeholder satisfaction and the stretching of scarce military health assets and dollars. Finally, the military health system is grappling to achieve equifinality with Coppola's *Parity of Health Care*. However, if past success predicts future behavior, the military health system will continue to be a relevant and ready health care entity for the rest of the century.

ACKNOWLEDGMENTS

The authors wish to thank Army-Baylor University Graduate Program in Health and Business Administration (Joint MBA/MHA program) classes of 2005 and 2006 and Army-Baylor students Eric McClung, Joseph Edger, and Joe Phillips for contributions to the chapter version used in the fifth edition of this book, which is still valuable. Our thanks are also extended to Lieutenant Colonel (Ret) Dawn Erckenbrack, PhD, as an author and contributor to the fifth edition's chapter. We kindly appreciate the contributions of Captain Cheryl Anne Borden from the United States Public Health Service, and Michael Dinneen, MD, PhD, from the Office of the Assistant Secretary of Defense (Health Affairs) for their assistance as subject-matter experts in verifying the content of this chapter. Finally, a small portion of this chapter detailing issues with the CHAMPUS Reform Initiative was adapted from Boyer and Sobel's chapter, "CHAMPUS and the Department of Defense Managed Care Programs." In: Kongstvedt PR, ed. *The Managed Health Care Handbook*. 3rd ed. (Gaithersburg, MD: Aspen Publishers; 1996), which is now out of print.

DISCLOSURE

The opinions or assertions contained herein are those of the authors and do not necessarily reflect the view of the Department of Defense.

Endnotes

1 2011 MHS Stakeholder's Report. Presented at: The 2011 MHS Conference; January 24, 2011; National Harbor, MD.

2 Joint Chiefs of Staff. Policy Memorandum of Policy No. 172. Pentagon, Washington, DC; 1983.

3 Bailey S. Keynote address. Presented at: TRICARE Conference; 1999; Washington, DC.

4 Holcolm RC. A Century With the Naval Hospital in Portsmouth. Portsmouth, VA: Printcraft Publishing Company; 1930, p. 543. Cited by: Garrigues RM. *The Serendipitous History of Discovery and Development Surrounding the Hospital Point Area and Its Naval Hospital in Portsmouth*. Available at: www-nmcp. mar.med.navy.mil/aboutus/nmcphist/nmcphist.asp. Accessed December 10, 2010.

5 Coppola MN. Correlates of military medical treatment facility (MTF) performance: Measuring technical efficiency with the structural adaptation to regain fit (SARFIT) model and data envelopment analysis (DEA). Doctoral dissertation; Medical College of Virginia Campus, Virginia Commonwealth University, Richmond, VA; August 2003.

6 Gillett MC. *The Army Medical Department 1775–1818*. Washington, DC: Government Printing Office; 1981.

7 Ibid.

8 Military Healthcare Reclamation Group. Detailed history of healthcare issues. White Paper. Military Grass Roots Group Priorities 2003/4 (Tab E); 2002. Available at: http://rebel.212.net/mhcrg/tabe.htm. Accessed February 15, 2004.

9 Burrelli DF. Report for Congress on military healthcare: The issue of "promised" benefits. 2002. Congressional Research Service Publication No. 98–1006F; Washington, DC: Library of Congress.

10 Government Accountability Office. DOD's managed care program continues to face challenges. Washington, DC: GAO; 1995.

11 Zwanziger J, Hart KD, Kravitz RL, Sloss EM. Evaluating large and complex demonstrations: The CHAMPUS reform initiative experience. *Health Serv Res*. 2001;35(6):1229–1244.

12 Boyer JF, Sobel LS. CHAMPUS and the Department of Defense managed care programs. In: Kongstvedt PR, ed. *The Managed Health Care Handbook*. 3rd ed. Gaithersburg, MD: Aspen; 1996. [Editor's note: This book is out of print.]

13 Sloss EM, Hosek SD. *Beneficiary access and satisfaction*. Santa Monica, Calif: RAND National Defense Research Institute; 1993. Evaluation of the CHAMPUS Reform Initiative; vol. 2, R-4244/2-HA.

14 RAND National Defense Research Institute. Evaluation of the CHAMPUS Reform Initiative. Vols. 3 and 6. Santa Monica, CA: RAND National Defense Research Institute; 1993 and 1994. R-4244/3-HA and R-4244/6-HA.

15 Op cit: Boyer JF and Sobel LS.

16 Mientka M. TRICARE for Life in need of supplemental. US Medicine. 2021 L Street, #400, Washington, DC. April 2001. Available at: www.google.de/search?hl = de&q = %22TRICARE + for + Life + in + need + of + supplemental%22&btnG = Google-Suche&meta. Accessed February 22, 2004.

17 TRICARE Management Activity Policy Memo, TRICARE Management Activity. Sky 5, Suite 810, 5111 Leesburg Pike, Falls Church, VA 22041-3206; Washington, DC, 2006.

18 Coppola MN, Hudak R, Gidwani P. A theoretical perspective utilizing resource dependency to predict issues with the repatriation of Medicare eligible military beneficiaries back into TRICARE. *Mil Med*. 2002;167(9):726–731.

19 Public Law 569, The Dependants Medical Care Act (37 USC, Chapter 7); 1956.

20 The Retired Enlisted Association (TREA). July, 2001. History of lost benefits: The creation of the military health care system. Unpublished white paper. Legislative Affairs Office, 909 North Washington Avenue, Suite 301A.

21 Op cit.: Coppola MN, Hudak R, Gidwani P.

22 National Defense Authorization Act of 2001.

23 US Medicine Institute. TRICARE for Life—Roundtable forum addressing the impact of provisions of the National Defense Authorization Act for 2001. Washington, DC: Charles Sumner Museum and Archives; January 16, 2001.

24 Op Cit: TRICARE Management Activity Policy Memo.

25 Army Reserve Non-regular Retirement Information Guide. Compiled by United States Army Reserve Command and Retirement Services, USAR LNO, February 12, 2009. Available at: www.armyg1.army.mil/rso/docs/ARReserveRetirementGuide.doc. Accessed January 5, 2011.

26 TRICARE Operations Manual 6010.56-M, February 1, 2008; Chapter 23, Section 1, TRICARE Pharmacy (TPharm), TRICARE Management Activity; Washington, DC.

27 Op cit.: TRICARE Management Activity Policy Memo.

28 Op cit.: TRICARE Management Activity Policy Memo, and TRICARE Operations Manual.

29 TRICARE Operations Manual 6010.56-M, February 1, 2008; Chapter 23, Section 1, TRICARE Pharmacy (TPharm), TRICARE Management Activity; Washington, DC.

30 TRICARE Management Activity, Extended Care Health Option. Available at: www.tricare.mil/mybenefit/ProfileFilter.do;jsessionid = Nn6QLhR1qS8yL4kXM1XBGL1YdZGRXTXNWT9fj3dn4V3nppBhFLhK!1467275286?puri = %2Fhome%2Foverview%2FSpecialPrograms%2FECHO. Accessed January 2, 2011.

31 TRICARE Operations Manual 6010.51-M, August 1, 2002, Chapter 1, Section 3, TRICARE Processing Standards. TRICARE Management Activity; Washington, DC.

32 Op Cit: TRICARE Management Agency Policy Memo.

33 Ackerman S. Daily Pentagon jackpot: Health care edition. *WIRED*. July 14, 2010. Available at: www.wired.com/dangerroom/tag/daily-pentagon-jackpot/. Accessed January 2, 2011.

34 Bumiller E, Shanker T. Gates seeking to contain military health costs. *New York Times*. November 29, 2010. Available at: www.nytimes.com/2010/11/29/us/29tricare.html. Accessed January 2, 2011.

35 Evaluation of the TRICARE Program, Fiscal Year 2010 Report to Congress.

36 Gillette B. Vulnerable system no longer taking chances on claims. *Managed Healthcare Executive*. February 2003:38–39.

37 The Future of TRICARE Regional Contracts: T-4 Kickoff Meeting. September 20, 2010. Available at: www.health.mil/libraries. Accessed January 2, 2010.

38 Gagliano DA. 2010 military health system conference, lessons learned: CoE support to families and wounded through a patient center approach. Sharing knowledge: Achieving breakthrough performance. A Joint DoD/VA vision center of excellence. January 25, 2010. Available at: www.health.mil/Libraries/2010_MHS_Conference_Presentations/Lessons_Learned_CoE_Support_to_Families_and_Wounded_Through_a_Patient-Centered_Approach.pdf. Accessed January 2, 2010.

39 Warrior Care: We stand together. Available at: www.warriorcare.mil. Accessed January 2, 2010.

40 Wounded Warrior Regiment. Available at: www.woundedwarriorregiment.org. Accessed January 2, 2010.

41 Hudak RP, Morrison C, Carstensen M, Rice JS, Jurgersen BR. U.S. Army wounded warrior program (AW2): A case study in designing a nonmedical case management program for severely wounded, injured, and ill service members and their families. *Mil Med*. 2009;174(6): 566–571.

42 Coppola MN, Harrison J, Kerr B, Erckenbrack D. The Military Managed Care Health System. In: Kongstvedt PR, ed. *Essentials of Managed Care*. 5th ed. Sudbury, MA: Jones and Bartlett; 2007: 633–653.

43 Ledlow J, Coppola MN. *Leadership in The Health Professions: Classics of Leadership Theory, Practical Applications and Essential Skills*. Boston: Jones and Bartlett; 2011.

44 Coppola MN, Erckenbrack D, Ledlow GR. Stakeholder Dynamics. In: Johnson JA. *Health Organizations: Theory, Behavior, and Development*. Boston: Jones and Bartlett; 2009: 255–278.

45 Kissick WL. *The Past Is Prologue in Medicine's Dilemmas: Infinite Needs versus Finite Resources*. New Haven, CT: Yale University Press; 1994.

46 Op cit.: Coppola MN, Harrison J, Kerr B, Erckenbrack D.

47 Op cit.: Ledlow J, Coppola MN; and Coppola MN, Erckenbrack D, Ledlow GR.

48 West TD, Cronk MW, Goodman RL, Waymire TR. Increasing accountability through performance-based budgeting. *J Gov Financ Manag*. 2010;59(1): 51–55.

Managed Care in a Global Context

JONATHAN P. WEINER, EMILY ADRION, JOANNA CASE FAMADAS,
DJORDJE GIKIC, AND HUGH R. WATERS

STUDY OBJECTIVES

- Understand, compare, and contrast the financing and organization of the United States health care system with the health care infrastructures in other selected nations
- Understand paradigms and typologies useful in framing a global comparative analysis in the managed care arena
- Understand some of the international experience to-date of U.S. managed care companies and U.S.-inspired, but locally grown, managed care models
- Identify and understand some of the promises and pitfalls of U.S.-style managed care for other nations in the arenas of financing, organization, and care management

DISCUSSION TOPICS

1. Discuss what types of system measures/indicators are used to describe the financing and organization of health care systems. What do these measures tell us about different systems? What other information would you like to have?
2. Discuss some of the aspects of one or more international health care systems of interest to you and discuss how they provide an opportunity or challenge for systems organized using managed care principles.
3. Discuss what some of the biggest challenges are that U.S. managed care organizations (MCOs) have faced in operating abroad. What are some of the ways that these MCOs have dealt with these challenges?
4. Discuss some of the current opportunities for U.S. MCOs abroad. If you were the CEO of a U.S. MCO that had decided to operate abroad, what type of services would you try to offer? Why?
5. Discuss what you think U.S. MCOs and policymakers can learn from other health care systems.

■ INTRODUCTION

This is the global century. Although more "local" than other sectors, health care must increasingly be viewed from a global perspective. International boundaries are becoming porous; on a daily basis health-related goods, information, staff, financial capital, services, patients, pathogens and, of course, ideas and innovations are exchanged. The global dimension of health care has implications for health systems around the world, particularly as policymakers increasingly look to the experiences of other nations when considering how best to formulate health policies in their own countries.

This chapter provides an international context for managed health care. It is relevant to those in the United States who are interested in sharing their knowledge or services with others abroad, and to persons in other nations wishing to learn from the U.S. managed care experience. Moreover, those leading the U.S. managed health care industry have something to gain by stepping back and comparing and contrasting our system to those in other lands. Cross-national comparative analysis of multiple health care systems is not an easy undertaking. Therefore, the goals of this chapter must be broad out of necessity. The specific objectives for this chapter include discussion of the various types of health systems around the globe; the role, or potential role, of managed care in other nations; the experience of U.S. managed care companies abroad; and future opportunities for the cross-national export of managed care methods. While this chapter focuses on issues and frameworks that may primarily be useful to those in the United States and other higher income nations, aspects of this analysis are for a wide variety of countries.

As described in detail in Chapter 1, managed care organizations (MCOs) were developed in the United States largely as a response to escalating health care costs. Like "traditional" health insurers (such as Blue Cross and Blue Shield plans), most MCOs function as third-party payers; but unlike traditional insurers, some MCOs, specifically closed-panel health maintenance organizations (HMOs), have legal responsibility for both the financing and delivery of care.[1] Other types of MCOs and HMOs contract with independent physicians, hospitals, and other providers, but more closely manage cost and pricing than do traditional third-party payers. Finally, MCOs have spread from the commercial sector where their primary focus was on the employer market (see Chapter 16), to the public sector where they are rapidly growing in both the Medicare (see Chapter 24) and Medicaid (see Chapter 25) markets.

The structure of MCOs is constantly evolving, as seen in Chapter 2, but the core functions of managed care organizations include maintaining provider networks, negotiating contracts and pricing, monitoring and influencing service utilization and care management, managing information flow, and measuring quality and outcomes. Another core function is bearing and managing financial risk, but recall from Chapter 2 that a little over half of all employer-sponsored group health coverage is now self-funded, meaning the employer is at risk for medical costs, not the MCO, although bearing and managing financial risk are still core MCO functions. For that reason, self-funding has little real impact on the content of the chapter except to underscore the ability of U.S. MCOs to succeed whether they bear financial risk or not.

All of these operational issues are described and discussed in detail in other chapters in this book. Although managed care is sometimes considered a uniquely American invention, all public and private health systems around the globe face similar trade-offs between cost, quality, access, and ever increasing consumer needs and demands.

In the United States, MCOs are typically thought of as a private, often investor-owned organization with which employers or governments contract to provide health care to an enrolled population. Among health economists in the United States and internationally, much has been written about the potential competition that can ensue when MCOs vie for consumers in a given market.[2, 3] In fact, the United States' Patient Protection and Affordable Care Act (ACA) includes provisions establishing health insurance exchanges that are designed to facilitate such competition among plans. These exchanges are described in detail in Chapters 16 and 30. Outside the United States, there has been substantial international interest, at least among market-oriented parties, in the importation of MCO-based American-style competition as well.[3, 4] In early 2011, England's health secretary, Andrew Lansley, with support from Prime Minister David Cameron, introduced legislation aimed at reforming the National Health Service by expanding the role of private care management companies and promoting competition among providers.[5] Under the legislation, providers would form organizations that are similar in many ways to a type of provider-sponsored HMO.

However, witnessing the runaway costs in the United States, accompanied by mediocre health outcomes and strong public sentiments associated with the "managed care backlash" of the 1990s as described in Chapter 1, policymakers and managers in other developed nations are not so keen on adopting U.S. models on a wholesale basis. Rather, they tend to be interested in the possibility of carefully grafting selected managed care tools onto their existing universal government or social insurance models.

Although not without controversy, some policymakers in high-income nations have been calling for the expansion of private health insurance as a way to supplement or complement the services provided through public health care systems. This "topping-up" of publicly provided or coordinated health care programs is especially appealing to higher-income members of society who may wish to purchase coverage for services beyond the basic levels of care. And as will be seen shortly, private health insurance is already present in a great many countries in some degree or another.

In emerging markets and middle-income countries with rapidly growing economies, the possibility of using private sector health plans as a vehicle for increasing the middle class's investment in the health sector, while allowing government to focus on care for those with lower incomes, is also gaining some degree of attention.[6] These types of potential cross-national exchange issues are explored further in this chapter.

A QUICK AROUND-THE-WORLD REVIEW OF HEALTH CARE

This section begins with a high-level overview of how major nations structure and finance their health care delivery systems. Following that is an overview of the role of private health insurance in other nations.

For selected nations from several continents, **Table 27-1** presents some key demographic, economic, and health care cost descriptors, illustrating the diversity of economies and of the sources and levels of health care system financing around the world. These particular countries were chosen both because they represent a variety of health care financing and organizational models, but also because they integrate private health insurance into their systems in different ways and to varying degrees. This table not only summarizes the size of the overall health care economies, it also offers some basic markers of the health of these nations.

TABLE 27-1	Economic and Health Indicators for Selected Countries									
	(1)	(2)	(3)	(4)	(5)	(6)	(7)	(8)	(9)	(10)	(11)
Country	GDP per capita, PPP (current U.S. $)	Total population (millions)	Life expectancy at birth (years)	Under-5 mortality rate (per 1,000)	Health expenditure per capita (current int'l $)	Total expenditure on health as % of GDP	Private expenditure on health as % of total expenditure on health	Out-of-pocket expenditure as % of total expenditure on health	Private prepaid plans as % of total expenditure on health	General government expenditure on health as % of total expenditure on health	% of population covered by government/ social insurance (OECD countries)
Argentina	$14,700	39.9	75.2	16.3	$1,665	0.101	0.545	0.239	0.297	0.455	–
Australia	$41,300	21.4	81.3	5.7	$3,122	0.087	0.323	0.182	0.106	0.677	100.0
Austria	$40,300	8.3	80.0	4.4	$3,545	0.102	0.241	0.158	0.055	0.759	98.8
Canada	$39,600	33.3	80.6	5.7	$3,672	0.100	0.296	0.145	0.088	0.704	100.0
Chile	$15,500	16.8	78.4	9.0	$697	0.053	0.473	0.259	0.224	0.527	73.5
China	$7,400	1,326	73.0	21.9	$342	0.046	0.593	0.493	0.343	0.407	–
Czech Republic	$26,600	10.4	76.7	3.9	$1,696	0.069	0.120	0.115	0.066	0.880	100.0
France	$33,300	62	81.0	4.3	$3,554	0.110	0.203	0.067	0.041	0.797	99.9
Germany	$35,900	82.1	79.7	4.4	$3,328	0.106	0.231	0.132	0.054	0.769	89.4
Hungary	$19,000	10	73.1	6.8	$3,319	0.083	0.291	0.226	0.049	0.709	100.0
India	$3,400	1,140	64.7	71.8	$87	0.036	0.750	0.686	0.372	0.250	–
Israel	$29,500	7.3	80.6	5.0	$2,263	0.080	0.400	0.331	0.153	0.600	–
Japan	$34,200	127.7	82.5	3.5	$2,514	0.081	0.187	0.151	0.033	0.813	100.0
Mexico	$13,800	106.3	74.9	34.7	$756	0.066	0.558	0.524	0.316	0.442	70.8
Netherlands	$40,500	16.4	80.2	5.2	$3,383	0.094	0.200	0.059	0.0364	0.800	98.8
New Zealand	$28,000	4.3	80.1	5.8	$2,447	0.093	0.222	0.166	0.049	0.778	100.0
Singapore	$57,200	4.8	80.5	2.7	$1,228	0.033	0.669	0.628	0.444	0.331	–
South Africa	$10,700	48.7	50.5	59.0	$869	0.080	0.623	0.109	0.362	0.377	–
Sweden	$39,000	9.2	80.9	3.2	$3,119	0.092	0.183	0.161	0.034	0.817	100.0
Switzerland	$42,900	7.6	81.7	4.9	$4,312	0.108	0.409	0.308	0.162	0.591	100.0
United Kingdom	$35,100	61.4	79.3	5.8	$2,784	0.082	0.127	0.116	0.016	0.873	100.0
United States	$47,400	304	78.0	7.6	$6,714	0.153	0.542	0.127	0.294	0.458	28.5
Uruguay	$14,300	3.3	75.9	14.0	$989	0.082	0.565	0.176	0.319	0.435	–

Sources: Column 1: United States Central Intelligence Agency (CIA) World Factbook, 2010; Columns 2–10: World Bank. *World Development Indicators 2010.* Washington, DC: World Bank; 2010; Column 11: Organisation for Economic Co-operation and Development (OECD) Health Data, 2010.

Basic System Structure and Health Levels

The first column of Table 27-1 presents the income of each country in gross domestic product (GDP) per capita in U.S. dollars, measured in purchasing parity units, and the second shows the size of the country's population. Columns 3 and 4 show health outcomes in terms of life expectancy at birth and the rate of child (under age 5) mortality. Column 5 presents total estimated health care expenditure per capita from all sources capita (in U.S. $), and column 6 presents this figure as a percentage of the nation's GDP.

Although low-income countries with low health care outlays tend to have poor health measures, as has often been observed, among higher-income countries there is not always a strong correlation between spending on health and health outcomes. For example, the life expectancy and child mortality outcomes of Singapore, Australia, and the United Kingdom are all significantly better than the U.S. outcomes, although the resources spent on health care per capita in those countries are less than half of what the United States spends (and these countries currently insure all residents, unlike the United States).

The remaining columns of Table 27-1 focus on the role of government and nongovernmental sources in financing health care. Column 7 shows the percentage from all nongovernmental sources. Column 7 (used as the base) is broken down further in the next two columns into the two major "private" components: column 8 presents the percentage of total outlays that is paid out-of-pocket from consumers, and column 9 shows the same for prepaid plans.

Prepaid private plans include social insurance funds (generally sponsored by unions and other social collectives) as well as private sector health insurance companies and managed care plans, which are usually considered distinct from private social insurance funds. For example, take the first row for Argentina: slightly less than half of all nongovernmental outlays, representing 54.5% of all health care costs in that nation, are made up of direct payments. So, for Argentina, approximately 24% of all health care outlays are paid for out-of-pocket.

Column 10 presents the approximate percentage that the government-sponsored health care or health insurance program represents of the total outlay for health care expenditures. Column 11 shows the percentage of the population covered by government-sponsored health care or health insurance programs, but only for nations that are members of the Organisation for Economic Co-operation and Development (OECD), for which data are available.

Tables like this one can be used to make broad comparisons among countries. For example, Singapore and New Zealand have similar population sizes and GDP per capita, but New Zealand spends about twice as much as Singapore on health, in absolute terms. In addition, New Zealand health expenditures are financed primarily by the government, whereas private expenditures constitute the bulk of Singapore's health spending. Moreover, Singapore compares quite favorably with New Zealand in terms of life expectancy and under-5 child mortality, two common health indicators. This comparison shows that there is no one "right" way to design a health system.

For U.S. readers not familiar with such broad comparisons as those outlined in Table 27-1, the difference between the U.S. system and those of other high-income countries on this list is stark. The U.S. spends more on health than any other nation, both per capita and in terms of percentage of GDP, yet our health outcome measures are middling. Furthermore, until key provisions of the ACA go into effect in 2014, the United States remains the only high-income nation on the list without universal or near-universal coverage.

The Role of Private Insurance

In this single chapter, it is not feasible to discuss even this limited subset of 22 health care systems along all dimensions. However, it is possible to add to the reader's understanding of these selected systems by categorizing them along several organizational and functional dimensions relevant to this chapter's discussion on health care delivery, financing, and care management.

Table 27-2 expands upon the information presented in Table 27-1 by offering a categorization of the type of health care system financing and organization found in each nation, as well as the role and estimated market share of private health insurance. Although there are many variations within each category, the first dimension on Table 27-2 (column 1) classifies the system by whether it is primarily government-sponsored, run by independent or quasi-independent social insurance funds, or the private health insurance sector.

The *government-sponsored systems* include both systems where many or most providers are employees or contractors of a government or quasi-governmental entity, for example, the United Kingdom and Sweden, as well as "single-payer" models such as Canada where the national or regional government pays independent providers. Most systems of this type have compulsory universal coverage, financed from general tax revenues. Health care delivery in these countries is often organized around distinct geographic administrative units, which have the added value of providing the potential, which is not always realized, of a population-based orientation based on place of residence.

In a *social insurance model*, health care is predominantly financed through payroll taxes rather than general taxation. Social insurance is not a right of every citizen, although in many countries social insurance is combined with other mechanisms to ensure that universal coverage is achieved. Purchasing social insurance may be mandatory for a designated population, but eligibility is based on payment of a

TABLE 27-2	Summary of System Structure and Role of Private Insurance in Selected Countries			
	(1)	(2)	(3)	(4)
Country	Primary type of health coverage	Main administrator(s)	Role of private insurance	Est. % with private primary/ secondary health insurance
Argentina	Private sector/government sponsored	Private plans and social insurance funds	Primary/ supplementary	NA
Australia	Government sponsored	Regional and national government	Complementary and supplementary	0%/51%
Austria	Social insurance	Regional government	Complementary and supplementary	NA
Canada	Government sponsored	Regional government	Supplementary	0%/68%
Chile	Social insurance	Private plans and social insurance funds	Primary/ supplementary	NA
China	Private sector/government sponsored/social insurance	None/national government	None	NA
Czech Republic	Social insurance	National government	None	0%/0%
France	Social insurance	Social insurance funds	Complementary and supplementary	0%/94%
Germany	Social insurance	Social insurance funds	Primary/ complementary and supplementary	11%/19%
Hungary	Social insurance	National government	None	0%/0%
India	Private sector	None/national government	Primary	NA
Israel	Social insurance	Social insurance funds	Complementary and supplementary	0%/80%[*]
Japan	Social insurance	Social insurance funds	None	NA
Mexico	Social insurance/private sector	National government/private plans	Supplementary	0%/NA
Netherlands	Social insurance	Private plans and social insurance funds	Complementary/ supplementary	0%/92%
New Zealand	Government sponsored	National government/ QUANGOs	Complementary and supplementary	0%/32%
Singapore	Government sponsored/mixed	National government	Primary/ supplementary	NA
South Africa	Government sponsored/mixed	Government/private plans	Primary/ supplementary	NA
Sweden	Government sponsored	Regional and national government	Complementary and supplementary	0%/NA
Switzerland	Social insurance	Private plans and social insurance funds	Supplementary	0%/30%
UK	Government sponsored	QUANGOs/national government	Supplementary	0%/10%[†]
U.S.	Private sector/ government Sponsored	Private plans/national and regional government	Primary/supplementary	57%/8%[‡]
Uruguay	Private sector/ government sponsored	Private plans and social insurance funds	Primary/ supplementary	NA

Definitions:
Government-sponsored, government provides care and/or is the principal payer for care; social insurance, compulsory participation, or contribution in health insurance scheme for designated population; private sector, reliance on individuals and private corporations for the purchase and provision of health insurance; QUANGOs, quasi-autonomous nongovernmental organizations; NA, data not available.

[*]*Source:* Rosen B, Samuel H. Israel: Health system review. *Health Systems in Transition.* European Observatory. 2009;11(2):1–226.
[†]*Source:* Organisation for Economic Co-operation and Development (OECD). Health Data, 2006.
[‡]In the United States, supplementary private insurance includes private plans contracting with the government Medicare program for older adults.
Source: Columns 1–3: Organisation for Economic Co-operation and Development. *Private Health Insurance in OECD Countries.* OECD; 2004. Column 4: Organisation for Economic Co-operation and Development (OECD). Health Data, 2010.

contribution, much like an insurance premium. Social insurance funds are financially autonomous and must maintain solvency. These funds are generally not-for-profit collectives, sometimes known as "sickness funds," often linked to individuals' places of employment. Under a social insurance model, the government directly provides care or subsidizes the premiums for those who cannot afford the payments on their own, such as persons who are unemployed, poor, or disabled. Examples of countries with social insurance systems include Germany and Japan. Several other countries, including France, have "hybrid" health insurance systems that are primarily based on social insurance, but also incorporate substantive elements paid through general taxation and private insurance.

Only a few countries in the world have national systems based primarily or heavily on multiple private insurers mixed with government insurance providers. Among high-income countries, a national system based on multiple private insurers exists only in the Netherlands and in the United States; even in the United States, public sources account for 45% of health expenditures nationwide.[7] Other nations with a substantial private insurance market include Switzerland, Chile, South Africa, and the Philippines.

Although the sources of health care financing are important, so too are the structure and locus of the management of care and resources. Column 2 of Table 27-2 provides a summary of the type of administrative entity that dominates key policy and management decisions. The way that a particular health care system is organized and administered will impact whether and how the various managed care tools described in this book might be applicable. The most common administrators of health benefits include national government, regional government, social insurance funds, private insurers/MCOs, and quasi-autonomous nongovernmental management units, such as locally controlled primary care trusts put in place under Prime Minister Tony Blair, and the current proposals for general practice commissioning consortia in the United Kingdom.[8]

Categorizing health systems in this way can be challenging, particularly for countries with no nationalized system. In Mexico, for example, although the majority of the population has access to basic health services, many Mexicans choose to pay out-of-pocket for health services because of dissatisfaction with public programs.[9] The system is divided among the social security system, the ministry of health, a government program for poor rural populations (*Seguro Popular*), and the private sector.

Even in countries with universal national systems, private insurance may play a significant role; columns 3 and 4 of Table 27-2 provide a summary of the role and scope of private insurance in this subset of countries. The role of private insurance is classified in one of three ways: (1) as a "primary" plan or *substitute* for the public program, meaning enrollees can opt out of an available public plan in favor of a private one; (2) as a *complement* to public programs, meaning coverage for out-of-pocket outlays for the government program; or (3) as a *supplement* to public programs, meaning coverage for services not provided under the public system are offered by private health insurance and private health care providers. The latter two types of secondary coverage are sometimes referred to as "topping-up" one's coverage above and beyond what is offered through the public system.

Column 4 provides an estimate of the percentage of the resident population of each country that relies on private insurance on a primary or secondary basis. Note that non-nationals in a country, U.S. expatriates for example, that may have private insurance as a primary type of coverage are not included in these figures. It is estimated that there are hundreds of thousands of U.S. citizens living abroad with such coverage. Although difficult to count, individuals working for American companies are increasingly insured by a number of U.S. and global insurance companies in a similar fashion.

The wide variety of approaches to paying and organizing health care provide many opportunities for managed care approaches and organizations. But this also adds significantly to the complexity involved in assessing the scope, appropriateness, and viability of those opportunities around the globe. The diversity also complicates, but does not eliminate, some lessons that can be learned from some of these settings.

■ MANAGED CARE AS A TOOL FOR DEVELOPMENT

The predominant source of health financing in lower-income countries is direct out-of-pocket consumer payments to doctors, hospitals, and other providers. Although some level of out-of-pocket payment is appropriate in any health system to deter overutilization, out-of-pocket payments are generally a regressive type of financing that leaves the most vulnerable groups particularly susceptible to financial shocks.

As a nation's economy progresses (as can be seen in China) public sector insurance schemes are introduced, though these systems often face challenges because of a lack of sufficient resources to provide basic coverage to all of the population. Many believe that the introduction of private insurance in this context allows the public sector to focus on delivering services that benefit the people most in need, while those that can do so, meaning the middle class, purchase coverage on their own.[10-13] Thus, in countries with growing middle classes, MCOs can complement the public system by providing coverage to those who can afford to purchase it, leaving public programs for those most in need. Such plans may be purchased either by employers or by the individuals themselves.

This is illustrated in the Philippines where unsuccessful attempts were made in 1978 to establish the first HMO.

However, a few years later, five HMOs were created, a number that grew to 35 companies by the year 2000.[14] This growth occurred without government regulation or promotion, but rather through private sector initiatives. The primary driving force was the need for financial access to quality health services in the private sector. A mechanism for risk pooling was strongly needed in the private sector, as opposed to the public sector, where free medical care was being dispensed generally to the poor. As in many lower-income countries, the Philippines has limited resources for health care and spends just 3.8% of its GDP on health.[15] With the introduction of managed care, HMO enrollees could access private providers without risking bankruptcy. In addition, the government has been able to reallocate its limited resources and strengthen its programs for the poor.

Although there is great opportunity for private plans to play a role in the expansion of access to affordable care in middle-income developing nations, among some camps there is concern that the problem of limited management capacities in these developing countries will only be exacerbated by the expansion of the private sector and the need to regulate it. For example, managers may leave the public sector to work for these private plans, and some of the remaining ones will need to divert some of their time toward regulating the private plans rather than managing care for the poor.

On the other hand, while one managed care company may become an alternative insurer in a developing nation, another may choose to offer its expertise to government to help regulate the growing private sector. Private companies usually have good institutional capacity, well-developed information systems, and skills that can be transferred to the public sector to help in this regulation process to enable them to more effectively manage expanding publicly funded schemes.

Case Study: Managed Care in Chile

The Chilean health system[16] is financed through the public National Health Fund (FONASA) and a group of regulated private insurers (ISAPREs). Since reforms put into place in 1982, employed individuals not otherwise covered are required to contribute 7% of their income to FONASA or to purchase health insurance from an ISAPRE. The ISAPREs currently cover approximately 17% of the population (increased from 2% in 1983); 69% of the population is covered by FONASA.[17] The remainder either lacks health insurance or obtains it through particular public agencies, for example, the Military Health Services.

The ISAPREs offer subscribers and their dependants a package of health services, subject to copayments, in their own health care facilities or through contracts with other providers; in this regard, they have some similarities with closed-panel HMOs in the United States. Affiliates pay the obligatory 7% salary deduction and may also make additional payments to improve the coverage of their plan. The ISAPREs also benefit from a series of public subsidies. One of these is a tax rebate to employers, who contribute an additional 2% of payroll to complement the compulsory 7% salary deduction used to pay ISAPRE premiums for low-income employees. Other subsidies correspond to public health programs—maternity leave payments, free distribution of vaccines, and food supplementation products to ISAPREs' members.

Several ISAPREs have implemented another type of managed care using networks of preferred private health providers paid on a fee-for-service basis, which are both attributes of preferred provider organizations (PPOs) in the United States. In some cases, ISAPRE affiliates are also referred to public health facilities, in which case the ISAPRE must pay the public sector for the care.

In 1990, the *Superintendencia de ISAPREs* was created as a regulatory body. In order to reduce wide variations in pricing among private plans, and to reduce cream skimming, the ISAPREs were required to set premiums at community rates—by age, sex, and family size. Other private insurance companies offer differentiated plans that vary according to the premium paid and the health risk of the insured family. For those covered by FONASA, contributions are calculated as a percentage of salary. Individuals may move between FONASA and the ISAPREs. The Ministry of Health, which supervises the private insurance system through the *Superintendencia de ISAPREs*, regulates both subsectors. The ISAPREs offer a wide range of premiums, copayments, and coverage plans; there are many thousands of different coverage plans. In October 2004, there were 16 active ISAPREs.

The dual Chilean health care system is subject to adverse selection, as seen from the income distribution between FONASA and the ISAPREs. In 2003, FONASA covered 90.9% of individuals in the first (poorest) income quintile, compared to 33.2% in the fifth (wealthiest) quintile, according to analyses of the Chilean Socioeconomic Household Survey (CASEN). This trend is reversed for the ISAPREs, which covered just 1.6% of the population in the poorest quintile compared to 51.2% in the wealthiest.

Beyond issues of adverse selection, differences in the quality and availability of care between the ISAPREs and FONASA have been an issue. Up until the early 2000s, persons covered by FONASA had limited access to many services outside of primary care, and when access was obtained it was often of variable quality and potentially high cost.[17] In recent years, the Chilean Ministry of Health has implemented a number of reforms in an attempt to address inequities between the populations covered by ISAPREs and FONASA; for example, the Explicit Guarantees and Universal Access (AUGE) law established a set of 56 priority health conditions that must be covered under law by both the ISAPREs and FONASA.[17]

■ MANAGED CARE WITHIN DEVELOPED HEALTH CARE SYSTEMS

Over the last several decades, market-oriented policymakers within many developed nations have argued that competing health insurance plans, patterned after U.S. MCOs, could offer certain benefits to socialized models of care. The belief that efficiency in health care can be improved through competition has led several nations to introduce elements of competition via what is sometimes termed "internal markets." According to this school of thought, properly regulated competition leads to more efficient use of resources, controls health care expenditures, and improves quality.[2, 3] For example, in a national health system, independent or semi-independent plans or sickness funds could offer additional services, price reductions, and/or higher quality services on top of mandated benefits.

Beyond the introduction of competition into national health insurance systems, many developed countries have thriving private health insurance markets for complementary, supplementary, and/or substitutive insurance plans. Some of those private insurance plans already utilize managed care techniques and tools, while others could potentially learn from the methods applied by U.S. private health insurers, HMOs, and other types of MCOs.

Introducing Managed Care in Existing Government-Sponsored Systems

For several reasons, the results of introducing competition into government-sponsored health coverage programs have not been as dramatic as proponents might have hoped.[3] First, because the allocation of monies by government is based on average cost, one difficulty with the introduction of competition into health care systems is the temptation for "cream-skimming" or "gaming" to attract enrollees that are younger and healthier than average. This is a particularly pronounced problem when payments to plans are not properly adjusted for risk.

In Germany, for example, when the sickness fund playing field was made more competitive, the health plans competed on price, not on the comprehensiveness of services. Unsurprisingly, the plans with the lowest premiums, and not the most comprehensive services, had the largest increase in members.[18] This inequity led to the introduction of a risk-adjusted transfer of revenue between sickness funds to discourage risk selection; said another way, unless adequate risk adjustment systems are put in place, as Israel, Germany, and the Netherlands have done, sickness funds try to select members with the lowest risk, threatening the integrity of the system. The health insurance exchanges that will function as part of the U.S. ACA reform are expected to use similar risk adjustment methods.

Second, there is limited opportunity to influence quality and efficiency of health care because provider payments and practices are heavily regulated and thus plans may not be able to offer appropriate incentives to clinicians. In other words, to achieve efficiency and effectiveness gains, these competing health insurance plans ideally need the flexibility to influence providers in a number of ways. This flexibility may be limited by system structure, such as the availability of providers, the mix of doctor specialties, and lack of non-inpatient alternatives (e.g., ambulatory surgery).[3]

Finally, the higher administrative cost of a system with multiple competing plans—arising from fewer economies of scale—is often troublesome to policymakers. These extra transaction costs need to ultimately be shown to translate to added value, if the devolved competing plans are to be accepted within socialized settings.

To experienced U.S. MCO managers or observers, none of these issues is new; they are are on the list of real or perceived challenges faced over the last few decades in the United States. Furthermore, none of these issues means that managed care cannot succeed. This is illustrated by its use in Israel, which is described next.

Case Study: Managed Care and Private Health Insurance in Israel

The Israeli health care system is a prime example of a system where competition and managed care mechanisms are being applied in a national health insurance scheme, as well as a prime example of a system with a flourishing private health insurance market.

Israel introduced a national health insurance (NHI) system in 1995. Today, all Israeli citizens and permanent residents have a choice of four tax-financed, nonprofit NHI plans. Each NHI plan is required by law to provide a standardized benefit package covering hospital care, ambulatory care, and certain prescription drugs. To avoid cream-skimming, plans receive prospective, age-adjusted capitation payments from the government, which they use to provide care to their enrollees.[19]

All four NHI plans have incorporated some managed care mechanisms into the organization and delivery of care, such as the use of restricted provider networks. Clalit, the largest Israeli NHI plan, has developed a model similar to a prepaid, closed-panel, staff-model HMO in the United States, owning and operating a large network of hospitals and clinics across Israel. Clalit also directly employs their physicians, nurses, researchers, and administrators and has recently begun developing telemedicine and electronic medical records programs.[20] Like a mixed-model HMO in the United States, however, Clalit members may select a privately practicing primary care physician other than a physician at a Clalit-owned clinic, although approximately 80% select a Clalit physician.[19]

Beyond NHI plans, Israel also has a flourishing private health insurance market. Because the benefit package offered through the public system is somewhat limited, over

80 percent of Israelis also have some form of voluntary supplementary and/or complementary health insurance coverage. Voluntary health insurance can be obtained through one of the four NHI plans (essentially quasi-public insurance) or through private, commercial health insurance companies. The NHI plans offering complementary and supplementary health insurance coverage are legally prohibited from risk-rating or denying coverage because of preexisting conditions.[19] All of these elements have played a role in the expansion of voluntary health insurance in Israel.

International Potential for Managed Care

Managed care and private health insurance plans also have considerable international potential, even for those nations with little interest in having competing plans. As described in this chapter, private plans can act as a complement, supplement, or even partial substitute for existing government-sponsored systems; they may also provide important care management expertise to existing insurance schemes.

In the European Union, private health insurance accounts for less than 5% of total health expenditures, but plays a more significant role in specific member states, as illustrated previously in Table 27-2. In France, for example, more than 90% of the population has complementary private insurance, primarily to help cover high cost-sharing under the public system. In addition, European consumers wanting faster access to elective services and freedom from restrictions can often purchase supplementary private insurance, as more than 10% of the British population do.[21]

■ THE EXPERIENCE OF U.S. MANAGED CARE ABROAD

Despite the many potential roles for private plans and MCOs outside the United States, in most nations there is more than a bit of political anxiety associated with the question of balancing private sector involvement with a national commitment to equity and access for all. In part because of this challenge and also because of the limited market potential and other political barriers, few U.S. MCOs have elected to operate independent supplementary or complementary plans as an overlay to the national health program. Rather, U.S. insurers' forays abroad have tended to focus on substitute plans, targeting relatively wealthy population segments.

Another option for managed care companies is not to offer risk-bearing insurance services at all. For example, they can enter into collaborative arrangements where they contract with government agencies (or their agents) to provide management or even clinical services. Given that all nations have a long way to go before they reach optimal care efficiency and effectiveness, appropriate use of managed care may offer some solutions to these issues. In terms of actual experience, over the past few decades most U.S.

MCOs and health insurance companies have found that exporting their product overseas has proved to be challenging. In the late 1990s, faced with a saturated domestic market, many companies looked for markets abroad as a source of growth. During that period, as many as 13 U.S. MCOs had significant business abroad;[4] today, only a few still operate those businesses and are now often targeted at U.S. expatriates or for employees working for U.S. companies.

The Challenges Faced Abroad by U.S. Managed Health Care Companies

The good news is that the U.S. managed care community can offer other nations—such as Germany or the United Kingdom—some solutions to these issues as these countries move forward with delivery and financing models that involve alternative risk-bearing health plans or MCO-like entities. The bad news is that some challenges are such that despite a company's best efforts, they cannot be successfully overcome. Furthermore, because the financing and provision of health care the world over is so closely tied to the political and cultural environment of each nation, challenges can shift in ways that reduce or eliminate the likelihood of success for a U.S. company.

Companies found that the challenges confronting them abroad are complex and require careful analyses and preparation. They have generally learned to be wary of such an uncertain enterprise and the resource commitment that may be required for success. This section summarizes some of the experiences and lessons learned from the executives and individuals involved in managed care enterprises abroad.

It has been suggested that at the most basic level, prerequisites for success abroad by U.S. companies in the managed care and health insurance domains include the need for these domains to be dedicated lines of business (and not a sideline to a broader insurance or financial services offering); strong incentives for local providers to participate; adequate middle-income population of target market consumers; and the ability to collect adequate premiums to build a reasonable infrastructure.[22]

Other experts have suggested a number of other factors that should be considered when developing products for a specific nation. These include the state of the existing provider and health information infrastructures, consumer expectations and preferences, regulatory barriers, and local culture and perceptions associated with private insurance and managed care.[23] Some of the strengths of U.S. MCOs lie in claims processing, utilization management, care management, quality improvement, and the design and implementation of provider payment schemes. But implementing these programs is a significant challenge when overlaid onto existing complex systems found in other nations. For example, in most other countries (at least those not yet using electronic medical records), there are few standardized codes that describe services provided. In Argentina, for example, a U.S./local managed care joint venture decided it would be easier to incorporate the Argentine service/procedure coding system into the MCO's claims processing system rather than try to change systems or "translate" between the local and international system.[24] However, the lack of a usable coding infrastructure created great difficulty in getting clinical information from providers and limited the ability of the MCO to implement even the most basic functions of managed care.

The tactical decision of the Argentine joint venture to use the local coding system rather than trying to be an "agent of change" illustrates the importance of recognizing existing institutional power and resistance to change. In Latin America, MCOs often experienced resistance from providers, unions, and political organizations.[25, 26] One of the most important sources of potential resistance is the provider community. In the first place, there must be enough providers to support the managed care plans. In addition, plans must be able to build relationships and offer meaningful financial incentives. For example, in many low- and middle-income countries an informal economy (i.e., off the books) provides sources of income for many providers and other stakeholders; thus, a more formal payment system introduced by an MCO might represent a serious threat to their livelihood. MCOs that fail to take these societal factors into account may face strong resistance from providers.

Like other cross-national business or social policy exchange, cultural sensitivity is essential to export managed care concepts or products successfully. Historically, failures have often been caused by lack of understanding of all facets of the market, often because the local context was viewed through a North American frame of reference.[27]

For example, one of the features of managed care is that it frequently requires restrictions on services or consumer choices in exchange for lower costs. If consumers are not ready for this or do not see the benefit of this trade-off, MCO models are not likely to succeed. Although social trade-offs are the norm for many international social welfare programs, some consumers in those settings are wary of such trade-offs in the corporate context. It is not uncommon for international consumers to be uncomfortable with a shift from a view that health care or health insurance is a public good to that of a market commodity.[25] U.S. MCOs doing business abroad must be cognizant that there is a delicate balance between corporate and social contexts when it comes to health care in most nations outside the United States.

To the extent that the introduction of managed care results in inequities in access, it will be perceived negatively in countries that value solidarity. In Argentina, for example, a public hospital had to provide 1.25 million outpatient visits for elderly patients covered by a privately administered social insurance fund. These patients were denied access to private providers because of nonpayment by the private insurer and some bureaucratic confusion.[28]

Case Study: UnitedHealth Group in South Africa

Perhaps the greatest challenge MCOs have faced abroad is the negative public perception of managed care. Both internationally and domestically, this has been referred to as "managed care backlash." Even when great efforts are made to be a "good corporate citizen," things do not always go according to plans. For example, UnitedHealth Care engaged in careful analysis before entering the South African market. The company formed a joint venture and built up the necessary infrastructure. However, this initiative was not successful in large part due to negative media reports promoted—some say for political reasons—by the local South African press. In the early 1990s, UnitedHealth Care Corporation (now UnitedHealth Group) was enjoying domestic success and believed that "its expertise in successfully managing diverse health care systems was an exportable asset." UnitedHealth believed that it understood the importance of adapting to local conditions through its experience with acquiring regional health plans. United's success in this area was a result of its focus on three core competencies: (1) strong centralized financial management, (2) efficient and automated claims-driven data systems, and (3) a doctor-friendly but expert medical-managed capability. Internationally, UnitedHealth believed that managed care could reduce costs by reducing the inefficiencies inherent in Western-style scientific and technical medicine and changing the mechanism of coverage decisions to one of medical appropriateness. After much analysis, UnitedHealth selected South Africa for its foray into international managed care because it believed the health system was most similar to the United States.[26] UnitedHealth formed a joint venture with Southern Life, a South African insurance company, and Anglo American Corporation, a huge mining and financial services conglomerate in South Africa. The plan for the joint venture was that the South African companies would provide local market expertise, actuarial experience, and local relationships, and UnitedHealth would contribute managed care systems and programs and expertise. At first, responsibilities would be shared, but eventually management would be transferred entirely to the South Africans.

Despite the careful planning and successful implementation of the information system for the new company, Southern HealthCare Limited, the joint venture faced several insurmountable challenges, including negative physician response and bad press. When Anglo American made an independent business decision to divest of its nonmining businesses, the joint venture was effectively abandoned. In the final analysis, several factors have been identified as contributing to the failure: (1) overcommitment of resources, (2) failure to recognize the importance of direct-patient-pay pharmaceuticals as a source of revenue for South African physicians (eliminated in the new plan), (3) failure to gain the support of employers, and (4) lack of cultural sensitivity to the complex racial divide in South Africa, which ultimately led to the failure to gain black physicians' support for the plan.

Recent analyses of the health system in South Africa describe ongoing structural issues in the South African system that could continue to impede such efforts. These include many of the difficulties that plagued United's venture, such as social inequality, particularly with respect to public/private health care access; workforce shortages; and great variation in local and regional standards and resources.[29] More broadly, the South African health care system remains highly fragmented, with a large number of insurance companies covering only small numbers of individuals. Such small risk pools have prevented insurance companies from successfully negotiating substantial discounts in rates from physicians and hospitals and, as a result, the costs of health insurance have been rising rapidly while covered benefits have been shrinking. The rising costs of health insurance coverage in South Africa—known locally as "medical schemes"—have led to a decline in private health insurance coverage from about 17% of the population in 1997 to 14% in 2008.[30] Equity, access, and affordability issues continue to plague the health care system in South Africa and could impede future market entry by U.S. MCOs.

Case Study: Shifting Challenges in the United Kingdom

Rather than the full-scale exportation of their risk-bearing health insurance product lines, recently MCOs have found more receptive markets for their expertise and specific managed care tools, such as information technology applications and care management quality-enhancing techniques.

Despite the rocky start that U.S. health insurers and MCOs have experienced with their international exportation attempts, these companies have developed expertise and on-the-ground experience that is of considerable relevance abroad. In particular, many U.S. MCOs have found success by offering global consulting in areas ranging from information technology applications to utilization and care management techniques, as well as by supporting local provider and administrative organizations as they work to adopt other managed care tools and methodologies. This has very much been the case in the United Kingdom over the past decade. U.S. managed care techniques received considerable attention during Tony Blair's time as prime minister[31]—in fact, Blair's key health adviser left to head United's European, and then international, divisions.[32] As a result, during the Blair years and beyond, several U.S. companies, including Aetna, UnitedHealth, and Humana, offered a wide range of consulting and care management services in the United Kingdom, primarily consulting with local primary care trusts (PCTs) and regional strategic health authorities working with the National Health Service.[33] The role of such U.S. (and other U.K.-based) commercial corporations

within the United Kingdom's PCTs was quite controversial and viewed by many as a back-door mechanism for privatizing the public system.[34] Despite the controversy, some analysts have also cited the benefits of transplanted managed care approaches, including efforts to improve financial responsibility at the primary care level.[35]

The return of a Conservative-controlled government with the election of David Cameron as prime minister in 2010 has led to a number of changes to the National Health Service that will give more power to general practitioners and less power to government-employed managers. Given the dramatic changes that may soon be taking place within the National Health Service, future demand for commercial consulting and care management services remains unclear. Most likely as a result of this uncertainty, in early 2011 Humana announced that it will be closing its operations in the United Kingdom.[36] However, given the general direction of the reforms, the need for American-style managed care tools will likely continue.

◼ MANAGED CARE READINESS AND ORIENTATION

The United Kingdom's NHS is not the only system that has a potential need for the types of administrative and care management services that U.S. MCOs have to offer. As discussed earlier, a nation's (or a region's) health financing and organization infrastructure will have considerable implications for how, or even if, U.S.-style managed care tools might be applied. The focus of this section, therefore, is on a framework for assessing managed care "readiness" in a given jurisdiction, based on the authors' collective knowledge of managed care in the United States and other health care systems.

The framework focuses on selected characteristics of the systems in the United States, both fee-for-service and current MCOs, and six other selected nations, as shown in **Table 27-3**. In addition to a 2011-based assessment of the characteristics of these nations from within a managed care–centric framework, Table 27-3 suggests a model for how this typology might be applied beyond these countries to characterize a health care system along a continuum of managed care readiness.

Managed Care Readiness Characteristics

The framework of Table 27-3 is an assessment of eight distinct relevant managed care dimensions, grouped into four broad categories: overall system structure, consumers, providers, and clinical management.

Each of the eight measures for the health care system of each nation is rated along a continuum of four levels of attainment, from uncommon/very weak to widespread/very strong. What follows next is a description of each dimension, including the rationale for some of the ratings in Table 27-3.

TABLE 27-3	**Characteristics Associated with Managed Care Readiness and Orientation in Selected Nations**						
	Overall system structure		**Consumers**		**Providers**		**Managed care**	
	Degree of central/regional government control	Autonomy of health plan/management organization	Choice of health plan	Choice of provider	Degree of provider/integration/organization	Degree of financial controls/incentives	Population orientation	Use of UR/EBM and care management*
U.S.†	–/–	+/++	++/++	++/+	+/++	+/++	–/++	+/++
UK	++	+	—	–	+	+	++	+
Chile	+	+	+	+	–	+	–	—
Canada	++	—	—	+	—	–	–	—
Sweden	++	–	—	–	+	+	+	—
Germany	+	–	+	++	–	+	–	—
France	+	–	+	+	–	–	–	—

Rating Key, relative to other nations:
++ Widespread/very strong;
+ Not uncommon/strong;
– Not widespread/weak;
— Uncommon/very weak.
*Care management includes DM and CM programs.
†In the case of the United States, both nonmanaged FFS and MCO-based systems are summarized.

Degree of Central/Regional Government Control

The first structural dimension is the extent of control that the central or regional government exerts over the health care system's day-to-day management and care processes. Characteristics considered include the degree of government control of the overall budget, level of centralized or regional planning, and the management of care delivery processes. For example, in the United Kingdom, Canada, and Sweden—the nations rated as having very strong central or regional government control—most resources are budgeted by governmental units, and there is a high degree of central goal setting and operational guidance. Both the U.S. fee-for-service and MCO systems are rated in the weak (though not very weak) category, given that the majority of health care is not controlled or guided by government. Moreover, the U.S. government payers are fairly laissez-faire by international standards, and neither the federal Medicare nor the state/federal Medicaid programs have fixed budgets or mandate that providers and health plans practice collective planning or standardized care delivery.

The roles of the German and French governments fall midway. In these nations there is a fairly high degree of global budgeting and central planning, but nongovernmental sickness funds and health plans and providers do most of the day-to-day management, within broad boundaries.

Autonomy of Private Health Plans/Organizations

There are a variety of potential roles for nongovernmental insurance plans or care management organizations. The second structural dimension is an assessment of the extent to which private plans or organizations play a significant and largely independent role within each country as the main source of coverage. The term private includes non-governmental (or quasi-nongovernmental) organizations, social insurance funds, and private insurance or managed care companies (either investor-owned or not-for-profit). The degree to which these private entities are allowed to set their own operational objectives, select or hire providers, interface with consumers directly without a high level of regulation, and set their own standard operating procedures are the factors considered when rating within this dimension.

The U.S. MCOs are the model at the high end of the continuum, and are rated as "++." These private (usually investor-owned) companies function on a very independent basis relative to government. The UK—with its increasingly independent PCTs—and Chile, with a large number of ISA-PREs, or private health plans, are rated as having a strong role for private organizations that intermediate between the other parties (government, consumers, and providers). The single-payer system of the Canadian provinces is rated the lowest on this health plan autonomy dimension. Other than a few small pilots (and supplementary private insurers, which are not considered here), currently there is no major role for MCO-like organizations as the main manager of care in Canada. Other nations in Table 27-3 (e.g., Germany and France) do have independent sickness funds that play key roles, but they have not, until very recently, been involved in setting their own independent goals, care delivery mechanisms, or provider networks; therefore these organizations are rated as not having widespread autonomy, although this may change moving forward.

Choice of Health Plan

The first consumer-oriented dimension assessed is the degree to which consumers have significant alternative options with respect to their primary health insurance plan and system of care. The type of health care plan or program can potentially play an important role in the quality and amenities of care that consumers receive. Consumer choice is often cited as the central tenet of a market economy in health care.

In the United States consumer choice is high, but it varies by market segment. For employer-sponsored group coverage, which represents the largest market, large groups typically offer multiple options to employees, including more than one carrier and more than one plan design; small employers typically offer only one option to employees, but the employer has multiple options from which to choose. Medicare Advantage members typically have many options available, and can change each year. Beginning in 2014, individuals and small groups will also be able to select coverage through new health insurance exchanges, but will not be confined to purchasing through the exchange, further broadening their options.

In the United Kingdom and Sweden, there are no real choices in this regard, as the organization of care (even within the autonomous PCTs) is almost always delivered on a geographic basis, and virtually all persons in the same area are "enrolled" in the same program. In Chile, Germany, and France, many or most consumers do have a real choice of alternative health plans. However, given that these plans generally offer options that are similar to one another, these systems are rated as having as much true choice as employers and consumers served by the U.S. MCOs.

Choice of Provider

The second consumer-oriented characteristic assessed is the ability of patients to choose their provider (e.g., generalist or specialist physician and hospital) at the time they seek care. The number of alternative provider options available to the consumer will affect satisfaction and potentially the quality of care. The dynamics of choice can also have an impact on the degree to which providers feel the effects of market pressures. For this dimension U.S. MCOs are rated lower than traditional fee-for-service indemnity plans, as provider network limitations are a hallmark of U.S. managed care, albeit with far fewer restrictions now than in the past, as described in Chapter 1.

In the United Kingdom and Sweden, consumers usually choose from among a limited number of capitated/ salaried primary care doctors within their neighborhoods.

Their choice of specialists and hospital is often even more limited, as they usually reach these secondary-care providers based on referral by their general practitioners and then most usually based on geographic availability. The rating for Germany—where all consumers have direct access to mainly community-based specialists paid on a fee-for-service basis—is higher than other nations. For the most part, German consumers have direct access to almost any generalist, specialist, or hospital in the nation. In Canada and France, and in Chile (at least for those enrolled in the private plans), consumers may choose from a wide number of providers, assuming they are taking new patients.

Degree of Provider Integration and Organization

The first provider-oriented dimension considered is the degree of organizational interconnectedness or "integration," defined as cohesiveness of function, particularly between primary and specialty care, and between ambulatory and hospital care. The level of integration can directly affect efficiency and effectiveness of health care. The degree to which clinicians and their support structures view themselves as an interconnected unit with singular goals has great implications for how influential providers can be relative to government and health plan administrators.

U.S. MCOs are rated highly on this dimension, as integration is often considered a hallmark of "good" managed care. This is demonstrably the case for many of the long-established organizations such as Kaiser Permanente, the Geisinger Clinic and Health Plan, the Johns Hopkins Health System (JHHS),[*] and others. The rating is not unreservedly high, however, for reasons discussed in detail in Chapter 7, including evidence of a growing disconnection between facility-based care and community-based care that is having a negative impact on the chronically ill in the nonmanaged fee-for-service (FFS) system. Exceptions exist in which specialists and primary care physicians work together, such as large multispecialty medical groups or health systems with large numbers of employed physicians (see Chapter 4), but so far those do not make up the majority of the FFS system.

The British NHS with its PCTs, as well as the care networks developed by the Swedish country councils, are "purpose built" as rational integrated systems. The other nations' FFS systems are rated somewhat lower on this dimension, as generalists, community-based specialists, hospital-based specialists, and hospitals are often fairly autonomous, and it is not always common for clinical pathways and patient support systems to cross these providers' organizational boundaries. In Germany and France interoperable electronic health records (EHRs) and other care integration initiatives are attempting to address this issue.

---

[*] All of the authors of this chapter are part of or associated with the JHHS.

Degree of Provider-Directed Financial Controls and Incentives

The second provider-oriented dimension focuses on the extent to which financial incentives and controls are targeted at clinicians in support of efficient and effective practice. Examples include special payments to foster preventive care to minimize the use of inappropriate medical technology or to maximize adherence to evidence-based medical guidelines. This dimension attempts to gauge the presence of payer incentives beyond the simple ratcheting-down of fees, intended to constrain overall costs. U.S. MCOs are rated most highly, as many of them apply numerous mechanisms that link cost-effective practices and guideline adherence to payments, including pay for performance (P4P; see Chapter 5). Also, many HMOs share some degree of gains and losses with at least some of their physicians through capitation or other forms of limited risk-sharing. Practice-based incentives do exist in the U.S. non-MCO FFS environment, but they are not widespread at the time of publication; however, as discussed in Chapters 5 and 30, the ACA calls for Medicare to institute performance-based payments for FFS Medicare, so this could change.

All general practitioners in England are now eligible for significant bonuses that are awarded based on their attainment of the Quality and Outcomes Framework (QOF) indicators. This may be the largest P4P program in the world, in terms of budget and scope. In Germany physicians are paid extra for achieving certain "disease management program" (DMP) criteria for their patients with selected chronic disease. For these reasons these nations are rated at the " + " level. The other nations in Table 27-3 have pilot projects in this domain and make use of various salary, bonus, and FFS incentives to induce productivity and to mitigate above-average FFS billings; at the time of publication, however, there is no evidence of any widespread payment incentives linked to the provider's attainment of cost effectiveness or quality-linked targets.

Population Orientation

Economists often note the difficulty associated with distributing finite health resources among members of a population, so this characteristic is an assessment of the degree to which each nation has adopted a "denominator" approach in structuring its delivery system. Specifically, are public health and epidemiologic principles applied in conjunction with economic incentives to maximize benefits across the society, or at least the enrolled group? Population-based systems tend to emphasize primary, preventive, and community-based services and minimize high-technology services without clear-cut benefit. Many leading U.S. MCOs and HMOs in particular have developed sophisticated population-oriented programs with targeted outreach both for screening and for chronic-disease care management. They use tools such as health risk appraisals and "data-mining" methods of case finding (often termed predictive modeling). (Population-oriented programs, targeted outreach, data use, and related subjects are all addressed in Part III of this book.)

U.S. MCOs are rated highly along with the British NHS, which is applying many of these same techniques within their PCT catchment areas. The United Kingdom also has "public health doctors" assigned to each region. The British, like the Swedes, pay their providers capitation and salaries, which fosters the idea that the population is being served, in addition to single patients. In Sweden, care systems are all designed with a clear geographic dominator in mind, and effective outreach for screening is quite common. In the U.S. FFS system and other nations, programs like this may be present for some subgroups and for some conditions. However, the other systems are given a "−" rating where FFS payment dominates, since single patients with a presenting symptom or problem are the focus rather than the broader population.

Use of Utilization Review and Care Management

The last dimension in Table 27-3—and the second clinical management dimension—focuses on what is generally considered the essence of managed care: the widespread use of various methods to actively manage utilization in differing populations, using computerized decision support systems populated with evidence-based clinical guidelines and criteria. The basic form of this is utilization management (UM), including utilization review (UR), and most U.S. MCOs also use disease management (DM) and complex case management (CM) programs that focus on the small percentage of individuals with chronic conditions that incur the vast majority of costs, a phenomenon that is not confined to the United States and thus applicable to the other columns of Table 27-3. (All of these approaches and activities in the United States are discussed in detail in Part III of this book.)

Many nations are increasingly sharing evidence-based guidelines with clinicians, and nurse-led care coordination for selected patients is seen in most developed nations. However, the wide-scale use of sophisticated evidence-based care management is not widespread outside U.S. MCOs, and is used unevenly, at best, in U.S. FFS settings. As nations increasingly apply computerized clinical decision support systems linked to EHRs, it is likely that these types of UR/UM tools will be applied more widely around the globe.

Managed Care Readiness Characteristics of Seven Nations

It is difficult to fully and accurately characterize all aspects of care in these seven large nations, and a full review of the research evidence summarizing what is known about each of these managed care dimensions goes beyond the scope of this chapter. However, these caveats aside, the framework just described and the assessment shown in Table 27-3 provides at least one approach for identifying priority areas and challenges that might be addressed in these nations and others, using key managed care principles and tools.

Table 27-3 illustrates that not counting the United States, among the six nations assessed there has been only limited uptake of the methods and approaches found within leading U.S. managed care plans. For example, across the Canadian provinces, the managed care readiness matrix suggests strong centralized control, limited population orientation, limited provider integration, and few provider incentives linked to care improvement. For this reason there is considerable potential for the introduction of managed care tools within the Canadian system.

Furthermore, in many nations there is considerable opportunity for U.S. managed care plans to collaborate for the benefit of both parties. Alternatively, as has been done in places like the UK and Germany, local organizations can learn from the experiences of the U.S. health plans. The Recommended Reading section at the end of this chapter offers many such "lessons in reverse" discussions.

■ CONCLUSION

The chapter's conclusion provides the opportunity to summarize a few likely global trends and their key implications for both the United States and international health care communities.

Given that all high-income OECD countries other than the United States (as of 2011) already provide health insurance for virtually all of their populace, most of the international growth in health insurance enrollment will take place within low- and middle-income nations, particularly where there is a growing middle class. This presents considerable opportunity for the expansion of private health plans in these settings. But this approach is not without controversy; some social policy analysts are troubled by the prospect of parallel delivery systems for those with and without means, and by the potential waste associated with the overhead of multiple competing private plans. On the other hand, self-pay or employer-sponsored private health insurance plans may be more efficient and responsive than government programs are, and they can free limited public resources that can best be used to target the programs to those with the greatest need.

Even wealthy countries will never be able to collect enough taxes or insurance premiums to provide all of the health care services that their citizens may need or want. Thus, policymakers (or consumers) in at least some countries with universal government-sponsored or mandated health plans are likely to come to conclude that supplementary or complementary private health insurance

should be fostered, or at least tolerated, as a way to expand health coverage and bring additional, nongovernmental financial resources into the health sector. Such private sector expansions might represent a possible role for U.S. managed care companies or the transnational partnerships they form.

Even if a nation's health care leaders do not embrace secondary private health plans, with certainty they will still find many useful lessons and practical techniques from within the vast managed care tool kit described throughout this book. As described in this chapter, possible innovations can focus on care management, provider payment models, or the organizational structure of health care providers. Each of these is a complex and challenging domain. Although U.S. managed care firms have not had runaway success abroad because of the overwhelming dual challenges of cost containment and optimal quality attainment, the global need for managed care tools and principles remains considerable. Anecdotal evidence suggests that many other nations remain interested in managed care techniques and that U.S. managed care companies are always looking to expand into new markets.[37, 38] The question is not whether managed care approaches will be implemented internationally, but rather which are the most relevant, what processes are required for their local adaptation and implementation, and what the role might be for U.S. managed care organizations.

Whatever the case, the goal of this chapter was to facilitate the sharing of the tremendous trove of information contained in this book by providing a quick comparison of the health care systems of many nations, reviewing recent history, and offering future-oriented paradigms and frameworks. The intent behind that goal is to help guide the way for those working toward the technically and culturally appropriate transfer of managed care innovations around the globe.

Recommended Reading

European Observatory on Health Systems and Policies. Available at: www.euro.who.int/en/home/projects/observatory.

Kane NM, Turnbull NC. *Managing Health: An International Perspective*. San Francisco: Jossey-Bass; 2003.

Organisation for Economic Co-operation and Development. Available at: www.oecd.org.

Powell FD, Wessen AF, eds. *Health Care Systems in Transition: An International Perspective*. Thousand Oaks, CA: Sage Publications; 1999.

Saltman RB, Busse R, Figueras J, eds. *Social Health Insurance Systems in Western Europe*. Open University Press; 2004.

Timmons N. Letter From Britain: Across the Pond, Giant New Waves of Health Reform. *Health Affairs*. December 2010;29(12):2138–2141.

Wieners W, ed. Global Health Care Markets. *A Comprehensive Guide to Regions, Trends, and Opportunities Shaping the International Health Arena*. San Francisco: Jossey-Bass; 2000.

World Health Organization. Available at: www.who.int.

Endnotes

1 Weiner JP, deLissovoy G. Razing a tower of Babel: A taxonomy for managed care and health insurance plans. *J Health Polit Policy Law.* Spring 1993;18(1): 75–103.

2 Enthoven AC, Singer SJ. The managed care backlash and the task force in California. *Health Affairs.* July–August 1998;17(4):95–110.

3 Saltman B, ed. *Social Health Insurance Systems in Western Europe.* Berkshire, UK, and New York: Open University Press; 2004.

4 Katzman CN. Managed care poised to take Europe. *Mod Healthc.* 1998;28(44):38–40.

5 Coombes R. Briefing: Health and Social Care Bill. *Brit Med J.* January 26, 2011;342:d507.

6 Pauly MV, Zweifel P, Scheffler RM, Preker AS, Bassett M. Private health insurance in developing countries. *Health Affairs.* March–April 2006;25(2):369–379.

7 World Bank. *World Development Indicators 2006.* Washington, DC: World Bank; 2006.

8 Weiner JP, Gillam S, Lewis R. Organization and financing of British primary care groups and trusts: Observations through the prism of U.S. managed care. *J Health Serv Res Policy.* January 2002;7(1):43–50.

9 Sekhri N. Mexico. In: Wieners WW, ed. *Global Health Care markets: A comprehensive guide to regions, Trends, and Opportunities Shaping the International Health Arena.* San Francisco: Jossey-Bass; 2001:247–262.

10 Bassett M. *Background paper for conference on private health insurance in developing countries.* World Bank; Wharton Business School; 2005.

11 Colombo F, Tapay N. *Private Health Insurance in OECD Countries: The Benefits and Costs for Individuals and Health Systems.* Paris: OECD Publishing; 2004. OECD Health Working Papers, No. 15.

12 Organisation for Economic Co-Operation and Development. The Reform of Health Care: A Comparative Analysis of Seven OECD Countries. Paris: Organisation for Economic Co-operation and Development, Health Policy Studies; 2002.

13 Gwatkin DR. *Are Free Government Health Services the Best Way to Reach the Poor?* Washington, DC: World Bank; 2004. Health, Nutrition, and Population Discussion Paper.

14 Reverente B. Philippines. In: Wieners WW, ed. *Global Health Care Markets: A Comprehensive Guide to Regions, Trends, and Opportunities Shaping the International Health Arena.* San Francisco: Jossey-Bass; 2001:247–262.

15 World Health Organization. WHO estimates for country national health accounts data. Geneva, Switzerland. March 2010. Available at: www.who.int/nha/country/phl/en/. Accessed May 3, 2011.

16 Baeza CC, Packard TC. *Beyond Survival: Protecting Households from the Impoverishing Effects of Health Shocks in Latin America.* Washington, DC: World Bank; 2005.

17 Vargas V, Poblete S. Health prioritization: The case of Chile. *Health Affairs.* 2008;27(3):782–792.

18 Gress S, Groenewegen P, Kerssens J, Braun B, Wasem J. Free choice of sickness funds in regulated competition: evidence from Germany and the Netherlands. *Health Policy.* 2002;60(3):235–254.

19 Rosen B, Samuel H. Israel: Health system review. Health Systems in Transition. *European Observatory.* 2009;11(2):1–226.

20 Website for Clalit health plan. Available at: www.clalit-global.co.il/en/. Accessed May 9, 2011.

21 Thomson S, Mossialos E. Private health insurance and access to health care in the European Union. *Euro Observer.* 2004;6(1):1–8.

22 Beichl L, Gunnery L, Navarro JA. A formula for successfully competing in non-U.S. health insurance markets. *Manag Care Q.* 2003;11(2):22–28.

23 Kahn H, Ware M. Critical issues in evaluating global markets. In: Wieners WW, ed. *Global Health Care Markets: A Comprehensive Guide to Regions, Trends, and Opportunities Shaping the International Health Arena.* San Francisco: Jossey-Bass; 2001:43–51.

24 Wieners WW. Setting up camp . . . overseas. If you're thinking about a foray abroad, IT implementations in Latin America and elsewhere offer constructive lessons. *Healthc Inform.* 1999;16(2):52–54, 56, 58.

25 Stocker K, Waitzkin H, Iriart C. The exportation of managed care to Latin America. *N Engl J Med.* 1999;340(14): 1131–1136.

26 Gould BS. When managed care doesn't travel well: A case study of South Africa. In: Wieners WW, ed. *Global Health Care Markets: A Comprehensive Guide to Regions, Trends, and Opportunities Shaping the International Health Arena.* San Francisco: Jossey-Bass; 2001:52–65.

27 Kahn H, Li L. Crossing borders: Considerations in delivering health insurance products and services. *Manag Care Q.* 1999;7(2):57–64.

28 Iriart C, Frarone S, Quiroga M, Leone F. *Atencion Gerenciada en Argentina: Informe Final.* Buenos Aires, Argentina: Universidad de Buenos Aires; 1998.

29 Coovadia H, Jewkes R, Barron P, Sanders D, McIntyre D. The health and health system of South Africa: Historical roots of current public health challenges. *Lancet.* 2009;374:817–834.

30 McIntyre D, Garshong B, Mtei G, Meheus F, Thiede M, Akazili J, Ally M, Aikins M, Mulligan J, Goudge J. Beyond fragmentation and towards universal coverage: insights from Ghana, South Africa and the United Republic of Tanzania. *Bulletin of the World Health Organization.* 2008;86:871–876.

31 Feachem R, Sekhri, White K. Getting more for their dollar: A comparison of the NHS and California's Kaiser Permanente. *Brit Med J.* 2002;324(7330):135–143.

32 Day M. UK Government Accused of Privatizing NHS. *Brit Med J.* 2006;333(7558):61.

33 Department of Health (England). New Framework for PCTs to Deliver Services Locally [Press Release]. Government News Network Ref. No. 152385P. October 5, 2007.

34 Pollock A, Price D. Privatising primary care. *Brit J Gen Pract.* 2006;56(532):555–566.

35 Donaldson C, Ruta D. Should the NHS follow the American way? *Brit Med J.* 2006;331(7528):1328–1330.

36 Timmins N. Humana pulls out of UK as another private provider admits reforms are no "gold rush." *Brit Med J.* 2011;342:d490.

37 Meads G. The organisation of primary care in Europe: Part 1 Trends—position paper of the European Forum for Primary Care. *Qual Primary Care.* 2009;17(2):133–43.

38 Johnson A. Cigna travels abroad for its financial health. *Wall Street Journal.* September 14, 2010.

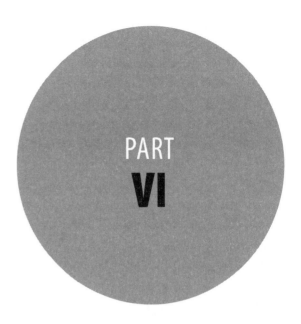

PART
VI

Laws and Regulations

"A wise government knows how to enforce
with temper or to conciliate with dignity."

George Grenville (1712-1770)
Speech against expulsion of John Wilkes,
in Parliament [1769]

State Regulation of Managed Health Care

TOM WILDER

STUDY OBJECTIVES

- Understand how states came to be the primary regulators of insurance
- Understand which types of state laws and regulations apply only to insured or at-risk business, and which apply equally to insured and self-funded business
- Understand how various types of payers are regulated by state agencies
- Understand how health maintenance organizations are licensed compared to health insurers
- Understand the steps state regulators take to safeguard the interest of consumers
- Understand how state laws affect provider contracting
- Understand how regulators oversee the market

DISCUSSION TOPICS

1. Discuss the most critical components of state oversight of HMO operations. How might this differ for different types of health plans?
2. Discuss when state regulation does and does not apply to health coverage sold by different types of managed care plans and arrangements.
3. Discuss how state regulation is driven by what is best for consumers and when it is driven by what is best for special interest groups.
4. Discuss possible ways to create a seamless regulatory system for all managed care organizations.

■ INTRODUCTION

Traditionally, most regulation of health insurers, health benefits service plans, preferred provider organizations (PPOs), point of service (POS) plans, health maintenance organizations (HMOs) and other managed care organizations (MCOs) described in Chapter 2 has occurred at the state level.

In most cases, state regulation is triggered if a payer is at risk for the cost of medical services, either as a health insurer or an HMO or POS plan. The authority of states to regulate health benefits plans for self-funded business, meaning benefits plans that do not involve insured or at-risk products, is circumscribed by the preemption provisions of the federal Employee Retirement Income Security Act of 1974 (ERISA), as addressed in Chapters 2 and 29. For the sake of simplicity, this chapter addresses state oversight as though all of a payer's business is fully insured or at risk, and only differentiate self-funded business in the event a state requirement applies to self-funded benefits plans as well.

Notwithstanding increasing federal oversight of managed care, as discussed in Chapters 29 and 30, states retain significant authority over the operation and activities of payers. States have enacted a broad range of laws affecting managed health care, including requirements for the cooperate structures of payers, types of products sold in the individual and group insurance markets, information disclosures and other consumer protections, coverage mandates, contracting with health care providers, and solvency standards.

This chapter discusses the state oversight of payers and managed care in the commercial market. In addition, the chapter reviews the powers and duties of agencies with regulatory responsibility for payer operations, including state insurance agencies and departments of managed care. Additional detail on some topics discussed is also found in other chapters, which are identified. Not discussed in this chapter are state managed laws pertaining to government programs such as Medicaid, a topic addressed in Chapter 25.

■ LEGISLATIVE HISTORY

Although there is a long history of insurance regulation at the state level (generally with respect to life insurers and property and casualty products such as automobile or homeowner's coverage), the primary emphasis on state oversight of insurance traces its origins to a 1944 decision by the United States Supreme Court and Congressional reaction to that court ruling. In the Supreme Court case *U.S. v. South-Eastern Underwriters Association*,[1] the court determined that state insurance contracts were subject to the Commerce Clause of the U.S. Constitution and, as a result, Congress had the authority to regulate insurance. The court found that the Sherman Antitrust Act was applicable to the operations of an underwriters' association that accounted for 90% of the fire insurance policies sold in a six-state area.[2]

In response to the Supreme Court decision, Congress enacted the McCarran-Ferguson Act in 1945.[3] In general, McCarran-Ferguson states that "(n)o Act of Congress shall be construed to invalidate, impair, or supersede any law enacted by any State for the purpose of regulating the business of insurance . . . ."[4] The federal statute specifically provided that federal antitrust laws do not apply to insurance carriers, unless state law does not address antitrust issues or in situations involving boycott, coercion, and intimidation, in which case federal law may be applicable.[5]

As health insurance became more prevalent, states began passing laws to govern the operations of health insurers and the products sold to individuals and businesses. State oversight of managed care gained ground with the passage in 1973 of the federal HMO Act, which was discussed in Chapter 1 and again in the next chapter on federal regulation. The Act established conditions for the operation of federally qualified HMOs and provided loans and loan guarantees for HMO startup costs.[6] States began regulating payers not only with respect to the traditional aspects of health insurance operations (e.g., laws applicable to licensing, insurance agents, and solvency) but also in terms of the provision of managed care (e.g., regulation of health care provider network contracts, utilization review, and medical necessity requirements). Today, managed care techniques are used by all health insurers and the lines of distinction between "traditional" indemnity-type insurance, PPOs, and HMOs is increasingly blurred. As discussed later in this chapter, however, some states (e.g., California) maintain separate statutory and regulatory provisions applicable to HMOs.[7]

To some degree state regulation of payers is influenced by legislation enacted at the federal level and, in turn, federal managed care law draws on state requirements. For example, the Health Insurance Portability and Accountability Act of 1996 (HIPAA)[8] established new rules for the guaranteed availability of coverage in the individual and small group insurance markets and limited the use of preexisting condition exclusions. States reacted to HIPAA by enacting their own versions of these requirements. In the same manner, federal laws such as the Genetic Information and Nondiscrimination Act (GINA)[9] and Michelle's Law[10] are based on laws previously approved in many states. As discussed more fully in Chapter 30, many states are starting to incorporate provisions of the Patient Protection and Affordable Care Act (ACA)[11] into state laws regulating managed care and payers.

■ REGULATORY STRUCTURE

State oversight of managed care generally focuses on two aspects: the techniques and processes used by a payer, and in particular an HMO, to deliver or arrange for the delivery of health care services to enrollees, and the organizational structure of the payer. As discussed in prior chapters, managed care techniques include the selection of a panel or network of health care providers such as physicians and hospitals that deliver services to payer enrollees, use of preventive care services, and requirements for utilization review and medical necessity determinations with respect to medical services and treatments. Enrollees are provided incentives to steer them toward the health care provider network and to utilize certain types of services, settings of care, and prescription drugs.

Recapping from Part I of this book, MCOs are typically divided into three broad types of structures:

- HMOs, which provide coverage of physician services either directly as a closed-panel plan (group or staff model) or through a network of contracted physicians as an open-panel plan (independent practice association [IPA] or direct contract model). Enrollees must receive care from one of the physicians or hospitals participating in the HMO network. Nonemergency care received outside the network is typically not paid. In the HMO structure, members usually must select a primary care physician (PCP) who is then responsible for the individual's care, and must approve any referral of a patient for services provided by a specialist provider.

- PPOs, which provide coverage through a contracted network but also covers services obtained out-of-network. Medical services outside of the PPO network will be paid at a lower rate by the payer, with the enrollee responsible for any cost difference.
- POS plans, which have the structure of an HMO but will also cover some level of out-of-network care, with the enrollee responsible for the cost that is not paid by the POS plan.

In addition, although not generally considered a type of payer, IPA model HMOs make up the majority of open-panel HMOs, and are subject to some level of regulation in some states. Other forms of integrated delivery systems (IDSs), which assume some degree of insurance risk, may also fall under state licensing and other requirements.[12] Detailed descriptions of types of MCOs and IDSs are found in Chapter 2.

Almost all health insurers utilize managed care techniques today and payers offer insurance products and are subject to licensing and other requirements imposed on insurance carriers by states. Many states have incorporated managed care provisions directly into the general insurance code. If a state has enacted a separate set of laws applicable only to one type of MCO such as an HMO Act, it will include many of the same requirements as applied to health insurers generally. As a result, this chapter uses the terms "payer" and "health insurer" interchangeably, unless a specific law or regulation is applicable only to a specific type of MCO such as an HMO.

Much of the state regulation of managed care is based on the Health Maintenance Organization Model Act released by the National Association of Insurance Commissioners (NAIC) in 1972. The NAIC is the national association representing state insurance regulatory agencies. To date, 50 states, the District of Columbia, and Puerto Rico have adopted the NAIC Model Act in whole or in part.[13] States have also enacted other NAIC model laws and regulations affecting managed care and payers including requirements for the individual and small group insurance markets, utilization review provisions, standards for health care provider networks, and consumer protections such as procedures for resolving claims appeals and grievances.

State regulation of PPOs is more varied, and states have applied provisions from several NAIC models to PPOs. In general, states permit insurers to enter into preferred provider arrangements that ensure reasonable access to covered services under the network and include mechanisms to control the cost of the health benefit plan. Risk-bearing PPOs are generally regulated by departments of insurance, either under the laws applicable to all insurance carriers or a special section of state insurance law.

■ LICENSING AND CORPORATE STRUCTURE

In general, states require insurers and HMOs to submit to licensing requirements to ensure there is a valid corporate structure and that the payer has sufficient management, health care provider network, and financial capacities to conduct operations. Health insurers are typically required to obtain an insurance license, while HMOs are required to obtain a certificate of authority (COA) from the state, a similar but distinct type of license granting them approval to engage in operations. Health insurers with HMO subsidiaries will have to obtain both. State licensure is one of the few (but not the sole) areas that apply equally to insured and self-funded business.

The application generally includes the names, titles, and biographical information on corporate officers, financial statements and projected balance sheets, enrollment and cash flow projections, information on health care provider networks, description of utilization review and quality assurance programs, and copies of marketing materials, provider contracts, and operational policies and procedures.[14] State laws also spell out the powers of payers such as the ability to purchase and operate hospitals and other medical facilities, enter into contracts with individuals and employers for health coverage, provide health care services, and market health insurance products.

Many states require PPOs to be licensed, registered, or certified. In the states with such a requirement, the standards imposed on PPOs tend to vary depending on whether the PPO is risk-bearing or not. Risk-bearing PPOs are likely to be subject to solvency and other requirements similar to those for HMOs and insurers. PPOs that do not bear risk may only have to register. Some states require the insurer with which a PPO contracts (most often an indemnity plan) to document that the PPO complies with certain state laws. Generally, the discussion of PPO regulation in this chapter focuses on risk-bearing PPOs.

In addition, states generally impose licensing and other requirements on agents that sell or market payer and other health insurance products to individuals and employers. The term "insurance agent" has been replaced with "insurance producer" in most state laws. These laws are intended to ensure that insurance producers are knowledgeable about the products they are selling (including continuing education requirements in some states), meet financial solvency standards, and disclose the commissions or other compensation they receive from the payer.[15] In 1999 a federal law, the Gramm-Leach-Bliley Act,[16] made a number of changes to the financial services industry, including banks, insurance companies, and securities dealers. One provision of that law required states to modify their requirements with respect to insurance producers to make it easier for out-of-state residents to obtain a license, and these changes have been enacted by most states.

States also regulate holding companies that own or have a controlling interest in an insurer or payer. Holding company laws govern financial reporting, transactions between the holding company and subsidiary or affiliated companies, responsibilities of officers and directors, and oversight of holding company operations.[17] A primary purpose of holding company laws is to ensure that a group of insurers owned or controlled by a holding company does not dominate a particular insurance market in a state. In addition, the laws are designed to make sure the holding company has sufficient financial capacity to handle the risk assumed by the insurer subsidiaries.

■ CONSUMER PROTECTIONS

States have enacted a wide range of provisions affecting how managed care is provided to consumers. These laws typically govern the types of information given to individuals about their health coverage, procedures for resolving grievances and appeals of coverage denials, protections for access by enrollees to health care providers, and mandates for the coverage of certain types of medical conditions and health services.

Consumer Disclosures

State laws govern the disclosures to enrollees, including information provided when individuals or businesses are purchasing coverage and on enrollment. Typically, these provisions require enrollees to be informed about the extent of coverage that will be provided, a directory of health care providers that are included in the network (including information about professional designations, languages spoken, and whether they are accepting new patients), cost-sharing requirements (deductibles, copayments, and co-insurance), a description of any limits on coverage (e.g., where services must be prior approved or subject to medically necessary requirements), and procedures for submitting grievances and appeals of claim denials.[18] Payers are also required to disclose the drug formulary indicating which prescription drugs are covered, cost-sharing requirements, and the process for appealing if a prescribed drug is not included on the formulary. The ACA requires the development of a standard evidence of coverage (EOC) document to be given to all purchasers of insurance coverage describing the coverage and any limitations or cost-sharing requirements, as well as a shorter standardized summary of coverage (SOC) document that must be provided to anyone considering purchasing coverage, and to existing members annually.[19] Descriptions of both documents are provided in Chapter 20. States have

also established laws governing disclosures included in explanation of benefit (EOB) statements provided to enrollees. EOBs indicate the date and type of medical treatments that were provided, the name of the health care provider, the cost of the service, the amount paid by the payer, and the responsibility, if any, of the individual. If a claim for benefits is denied, the EOB typically indicates the reason for denial, a reference to any plan provisions related to the denial (e.g., any policies or procedures tied to a medical necessity determination), and a description of how the decision by the payer may be appealed. To date, 23 states have enacted laws regarding EOB statements.[20] Further detail about EOBs is found in Chapter 18.

Many states require health insurers to submit policy forms, EOBs, and other types of disclosure documents for approval by the insurance regulatory agency before use. In addition, a number of states have enacted requirements dictating the wording that must be used in certain disclosures, type size for printed materials, and "readability" standards to ensure consumers understand the terms and conditions of coverage.[21] A number of states have also imposed provisions requiring disclosures of information to be provided in other languages to non-English-speaking enrollees. For example, California requires all HMOs to offer language assistance services, including interpreters, to individuals with limited English proficiency and to translate vital documents into other languages for certain populations of non-English-speaking enrollees.[22]

Insurance Applications

States may require health insurers and HMOs to use a uniform application form for coverage sold to individuals or businesses. The requirements specify what types of information may be requested from applicants and how the application form is worded.[23] In some cases, the state law defines when a health insurer may void the insurance coverage based on misstatements made by the enrollee on the application.[24] Generally, these provisions require the insurer to prove that they relied on the information in the application in their decision to offer coverage and that the misstatement was intentional (e.g., an applicant for health insurance coverage in the individual market is asked if they have had any surgery in the past 5 years and they respond negatively even though they recently had a heart bypass operation).[25] The use of this form is called medical underwriting and is described in Chapter 22. The guaranteed issue requirement in the ACA will diminish its use beginning in 2014.

The laws addressing insurance applications and reliance on statements made by an applicant are intended to restrict the ability of a health insurer to rescind coverage once it is provided (i.e., the insurer argues there was not a valid contract because of the misstatements or failure to include information on the application and, as a result, they are not responsible for paying for any health care services).

The ACA further limits the ability of health insurers to rescind coverage based on the information provided during the application process.[26]

Health Information Privacy

States have extensive requirements governing the collection, use, and sharing of information by payers. These laws generally provide protections for an individual's health information and restrict when the information may be disclosed without their consent. In some cases, the laws place additional protections on so-called "medically sensitive" information such as evidence that they were treated for a mental health condition, substance use disorder, or sexually transmitted disease.[27] Many of these laws are intended to provide additional consumer protections to supplement the federal privacy standards included in the Health Insurance Portability and Accountability Act (HIPAA)[28] discussed in Chapter 29.

In addition, a growing number of states have enacted data security laws that require notification of consumers if their personal information maintained by a business has been lost or stolen. To date, 37 states have such requirements that address the types of information subject to protection (e.g., identifiable financial or health data), determine when a breach has occurred, and provide the timing and content of notices that must be made to the public. Some states also require entities such as payers that have a data breach to pay for credit monitoring services for the individuals whose information was lost or stolen.[29] Federal data breach notification requirements included in the Health Information (HITECH) Act are reviewed in Chapter 30.[30]

A majority of states have also enacted a law governing when Social Security numbers may be collected or displayed by businesses including health insurers. These provisions directly affect payers, who routinely use Social Security numbers as the primary identifier for enrollees in processing claims, health insurance plan identification cards, and other situations. In general, these laws prohibit the public display of an individual's entire Social Security number (e.g., an ID card can only use the last four digits of the number).[31] As a practical matter, payers have moved away from using the Social Security number as an identifier for ID cards and the like, but will still use it to verify identity in some situations, such as a telephone call.

Coverage Mandates

Almost all states require payers to provide coverage for specific medical services or health conditions. Mandated coverage may include certain types of health care providers (e.g., chiropractors, midwives, physician assistants), benefits (e.g., bone marrow transplants, home health care, maternity), and medical devices or drugs (e.g., hearing aids, diabetic supplies, hair prostheses).[32] For example, 37 states require coverage for autism spectrum disorders or provide that such coverage, if offered, must be at "parity" with coverage for other medical and surgical services. ("parity" means that any financial requirements or treatment limitations for autism spectrum disorders are the same as or less restrictive than similar requirements or limits for medical and surgical coverage.)[33]

States typically mandate coverage of nonauthorized urgent or emergency care, even from an out-of-network provider, using a "prudent layperson" standard under which an individual believes their health or life is in danger, mirrored in the ACA. Some states also require HMOs to cover some portion of the cost of out-of-network care, essentially making HMOs into POS plans. State mandate laws also address situations when certain individuals must be provided coverage. For example, a number of states require that children up to a specified age or up to the time they graduate from college must be covered under a parent's health insurance policy.[34] As discussed in Chapter 30, the ACA requires coverage for children up to age 26 in most cases.[35]

Many states, however, recognize that mandated coverage requirements have cost implications for individuals and employers and have responded in two ways. First, a number of states require that any legislation that would impose a coverage mandate include cost projections.[36] This information is intended to inform the legislative process about the additional premium that will be required if the coverage or service is mandated. In addition, at least 19 states allow health insurers, including payers, to sell "mandate-lite" policies to individuals or small employers (typically businesses with up to 50 employees).[37] These laws exempt such policies from some or all of the state coverage mandates.

Network Access Requirements

Network adequacy standards apply to HMOs (and in some states, to PPOs as well), and typically impose requirements intended to promote access to PCPs and specialist providers (e.g., oncologists), and to hospitals or other care settings. In general, these provisions require that the health care provider's office or facility is located within reasonable proximity to enrollees who need medical services and access to emergency services is provided 24/7. For example, Colorado requires payers to maintain adequate provider networks that are sufficient to ensure that benefits are available to all enrollees "without unreasonable delay."[38] Access is measured based on the ratio of health care providers to enrollees, the location of a physician's office or in-patient facility, and waiting times for appointments. (Access is discussed in detail in Chapter 4.)

Most, though not all, HMOs require enrollees to select a PCP, who provides services to the individual and their family members. In such HMOs, enrollees are required to get authorization from their PCP or from the HMO before seeing a specialist. Some states have reacted to these managed care requirements by enacting laws that allow enrollees to designate certain types of health care providers as their PCP, for example, permitting a woman to name a pediatrician as the PCP for a child. Other state laws may allow patients to access specialists without having to first obtain approval from the HMO. As discussed in Chapter 30, the ACA also contains provisions allowing the designation of a health care provider such as a pediatrician as the enrollee's PCP.[39]

Consumer Protection from Balance Billing

All states plus the District of Columbia* have laws applicable to a payer's provider contract terms around balance billing practices and, as described in detail in Chapters 3 and 4, there are two forms this takes, although they are really manifestations of a single concept. The first form prohibits a contracted provider from billing an enrollee for any difference between the provider's charges and the fees or payment terms used by the payer. The second form prohibits the provider from billing an enrollee for anything that is the responsibility of the payer, even if the payer doesn't pay anything or goes out of business. Forty-one states and the District of Columbia have balanced billing requirements for HMO provider contracts.[40] Some states have also imposed balanced billing requirements with respect to all health insurers, Medicaid programs, or provider-sponsored health care organizations, such as IPAs.

In addition to balance billing laws, a number of states regulate the usual, customary, and reasonable (UCR) rate for payments by a payer to a health care provider. As described in detail in Chapter 5, the UCR rate is what the payer typically uses to calculate the payment amount to an out-of-network provider for medical services for an enrollee. The UCR rate may be based on a percentage or the average charges for a specific medical service in a geographic region, and UCR schedules are often licensed from third-party vendors. Because the patient is typically billed for any out-of-network charges not paid by the managed care organization, the UCR rate is important for both the health care provider and the enrollee. A majority of states require health coverage documents to define the term and a few states require the disclosure of UCR data.[41]

Grievances, Appeals, and External Review

State laws governing grievances and the internal appeal and external review of benefit denials provide consumers with a process to resolve disputes with a payer. In general, a grievance is any matter not involving a claim for benefits, for example, a disagreement over the adequacy of a health care provider network. The laws typically require payers to handle grievances within a specific timeframe and to inform consumers of their rights to have a grievance addressed by the payer. In addition, state insurance and managed care regulatory agencies generally have consumer assistance offices or staff to work with individuals and their payers to resolve grievances.

The appeal of a denial of coverage for a medical service is generally subject to separate regulatory requirements. Such coverage denials are typically defined by state law as prior authorization requests (i.e., the payer denies a health care provider's request for a service), postservice claims, concurrent review (i.e., where there is an ongoing course of treatment), and urgent care claims involving serious medical conditions that must be handled on an expedited basis. The state laws will define how quickly the health insurer must respond to a request to reconsider a denial, establish the process used to review the appeal (e.g., provisions giving individuals the right to present additional evidence or testify at a hearing), and provide the individual with access to the information regarding the claim. In addition, most states require the payer to provide the enrollee with a copy of any medical criteria or other policies and procedures that serve as the basis of the denial.

In addition, almost all states provide an external review process for claim denials if the internal appeal is not resolved in the enrollee's favor. According to the U.S. Department of Labor, as of March 2011, only three states (Alabama, Mississippi, and Nebraska) do not provide for external review of adverse benefit decisions.[42] External review is generally available under state law when the denial is for reasons of medical necessity or because it is a noncovered investigational or experimental treatment.[43] In a few states, all coverage decisions may be submitted to external review.

The review is usually handled by an independent review organization (IRO) that is not affiliated with the payer (in a few states, the state insurance regulatory agency may conduct the review). States' external review laws also address the independence and qualifications of IROs, require medical staff responsible for reviews to have educational training and experience in the medical issue that is the subject of the appeal, give the individual the right to submit information for consideration during the review, and provide that the decision will be binding on the payer and the enrollee.[44] The ACA has established national, uniform standards for internal appeals and external review, which are reviewed in Chapters 20 and 30.[45]

Utilization Review

In general, utilization review (UR) is the process used by a health insurer or HMO to determine if coverage of a particular medical service is appropriate given the needs of the individual enrollee, based on a determination of the medical necessity of the treatment and availability of effective alternatives. In some situations, the payer may require a precertification review before authorizing the service and in other cases a retrospective review may be applied. In all cases, the UR is based on a consideration of the medical

---

*The exception is Alaska.

records and other history of the individual, treatment guidelines, and other information about the individual's condition. The UR process, including medical necessity determinations and the use of evidence-based clinical criteria, is extensively described in Chapter 7.

Managed care organizations conduct UR using medical experts who are employed by the payer or may contract with a third-party entity (such as a physician practice) to handled the review. Almost all states require the individuals conducting UR to have training and experience in the field of medicine that is the subject of the review, establish time frames for how quickly a review must be completed, and provide that a decision may be appealed by the enrollee or his or her treating health care provider. In addition, states typically apply accreditation standards to the payer or third-party organization that conducts the review.[46] Almost all UR accreditation is done through either URAC or the National Commission on Quality Assurance (NCQA), which are independent organizations that have developed UR standards and conduct reviews at payers or UR entities, as described in Chapter 15. For example, URAC has established CORE Standards for UR functions that focus on the criteria for UR contracts, confidentiality of information used in the review, quality management standards, and the credentialing of medical review staff.[47] In addition, many states have enacted requirements regarding the medical licensing of health care providers that conduct UR. For example, 33 states require that the reviewer be licensed to practice medicine in the state in order to conduct such reviews.[48]

Market Conduct

Market conduct involves the regulation by a state of the practices of a payer that directly affects consumers, such as marketing, advertising, and language used in documents provided to prospective purchasers and enrollees. Many states have enacted laws prohibiting unfair or deceptive trade practices such as not promptly handling a claim for benefits or engaging in misleading advertising.[49] State insurance regulatory or managed care agencies will periodically carry out market conduct examinations at payers to review how complaints are handled, products are marketed, and other processes affecting consumers. The NAIC has developed a *Market Conduct Examiners Handbook* to guide these reviews and provide a uniform approach among the states to examinations.

States have the authority to conduct market conduct examinations. The focus of these examinations is intended to be on general business patterns or practices and not on random or isolated errors. If a payer is found to have engaged in unlawful market practices, regulators usually provide an opportunity for the payer to take corrective and/or remedial action. Serious misconduct and consumer harm can result in the suspension or revocation of a payer's license or COA if necessary to protect the public from

further harm. The seven main areas that may be reviewed as part of a market conduct examination are:

1. Company operations and management;
2. Complaint handling;
3. Marketing and sales;
4. Producer licensing;
5. Policyholder service;
6. Underwriting; and
7. Claims.

A number of states, such as California, make the results of the market conduct exams public,[50] while others may provide information on the number of appeals or grievances handled by the health insurer and the percentage resolved in favor of the enrollee. The examination results or other data is intended to inform consumers about the business practices of the insurer.

■ PROVIDER CONTRACTING

Provider contracting laws establish requirements for payer agreements with physicians and hospitals that are part of the provider network. These laws range from requirements for specific contract provisions to establishment of restrictions on consumer cost-sharing, as described earlier. Some states have enacted laws prohibiting a payer from offering incentives to a health care provider to limit or not provide medically necessary care, and restricting "gag clauses" in health care provider contracts that ban physicians and other providers from discussing certain treatments or care options with their patients.[51]

Another issue that has arisen in states concerns "most favored nation" clauses that may be used in some payer agreements. These clauses generally limit the contracting physician or hospital from charging the payer more than is charged by the provider to any other payer. The use of a most favored nation clause has been found to not violate the federal antitrust laws.[52] However, a number of states ban the use of such contract provisions or classify them as an unfair or deceptive trade practice.

States also typically establish requirements around provider rights. For example, in many states a payer must give at least 60 days notice before terminating a provider contract "without cause," and some states give a terminated provider the right to appeal the termination. Most states impose requirements on how quickly claims must be paid by a payer. For example, 41 states apply deadlines for payment of "clean claims" (i.e., claims that include all necessary information needed to process a claim for payment). These deadlines typically range from 15 to 60 days.[53] In most cases, health insurers are required to pay claims filed electronically within a shorter time period (generally 30 days). Penalties and interest may be imposed if the payment deadlines are missed.

In addition, a number of states have enacted "any willing provider" (AWP) laws, which require the payer to accept into a network any health care provider that is willing to accept the contract terms and meet quality standards established by the MCO. States may also extend the AWP requirements to pharmacies or to certain categories of health care providers such as dentists or providers specializing in treatment of behavioral or substance use disorders. Based on a 2003 ruling by the U.S. Supreme Court, AWP laws are one of the few types of state laws that are not preempted under ERISA because they apply to laws regulating insurance.[54]

■ INSURANCE MARKET RULES

All states have laws governing health insurance markets, including restrictions on premium rating factors, requirements that coverage must be guaranteed available and renewable, and limits on the use of preexisting condition limitations. As discussed in Chapter 29, many of these laws are based on the federal HIPAA provisions that were enacted in 1996.[55] Many state insurance market rules will be superseded in 2014 by rules embodied in the ACA, which are discussed in Chapter 30.

In general, the state requirements divide the health insurance market into individual coverage, small employer groups (typically businesses with 2–50 employees), and large employer groups.[56] Two additional variations must be noted. First, a number of states also extend the small group market to include self-employed individuals or "groups of one."[57] In addition, as discussed further in Chapter 30, the ACA defines the small group market as employers with up to 100 employees (although states are permitted to continue defining small groups as businesses with up to 50 employees until January 1, 2016).[58]

States take the following approaches to allowing variation of rates within a particular market:

- Pure community rating—in pure community rating each enrollee or policyholder (i.e., a business purchaser) is charged the same rate. Variations are only permitted for certain factors such as family size or geographic location of the purchaser. Two states, New York and Vermont, require pure community rating in the individual and small group markets.[59]
- Adjusted community rating—under this structure states permit variations in rates for demographic and other factors (other than health status factors). Eight states permit adjusted community rating in the individual market and nine states allow this approach in the small group market.[60]
- Rating bands—these allow the use of health status and claim experience in the rating process but limit the rates that may be charged to a specified percentage above or below an index rate (e.g., the percentage rate is the average rate charged to all small employers

in a particular market by the health insurer). Eight states allow rating bands in the individual insurance market and 38 states permit rating bands in the small group market.[61]

States impose the fewest premium rating restrictions in the individual insurance market. For example, most states do not impose any rating requirements for coverage sold in the individual market. In other words, health insurers are permitted to charge any premium amount based on their estimate of the health risks of the purchaser. In addition, at the time of publication, most states permit insurers in the individual market to medically underwrite the coverage, which means the health insurer may deny coverage or may restrict coverage for certain medical conditions (e.g., the individual market policy may exclude coverage for diabetes). Only a few states require insurance sold in the individual market to be guaranteed issued (i.e., any individual that applies for coverage must be sold a policy).[62] (Underwriting and rating are discussed in detail in Chapter 22.)

As noted above, coverage sold in the small group market is generally subject to state regulation. The state small group insurance market requirements typically mirror the federal provisions in HIPAA applicable to the small group market:[63]

- Coverage must be "guaranteed available." This means that any employer or employee that applies for health insurance coverage must be insured.[64]
- Coverage must be guaranteed renewable. This means the coverage must be extended for an additional term unless the employer fails to pay premiums or commits an act of fraud.[65]
- The health insurer may not impose any preexisting condition exclusions (i.e., limits on coverage for medical conditions that were diagnosed or treated prior to the date of enrollment) unless the condition occurred 6 months prior to enrollment. Coverage for such preexisting medical conditions may only be excluded for 12 months after enrollment. In addition, the enrollee must be given "credit" against any limits for prior insurance coverage (i.e., an individual who previously had insurance or other health coverage for 12 months may not have any preexisting condition exclusions under the new policy).[66] Some states further restrict or prohibit the use of preexisting condition limitations in the small group market.
- Health insurers may not deny coverage to an individual and may not charge them premiums based on health status such as a medical condition or claims history. In other words, an individual with diabetes may not be charged more than the other individuals who receive health insurance coverage from a small group. The business, however, may be charged a rate based on the claims history of all enrollees in the group.[67]

- Most states define the rating factors that may be used in the small group market. Typical factors include age, gender, family composition, geographic area, and the type of business.[68]

States also exercise authority over the premiums that may be charged to individuals or employers through laws requiring rates to be submitted for approval. These requirements generally fall into three categories. States with "file and use" provisions require the payer to submit its premiums to the state regulatory authority and then permit use of those rates without further action by the state. "Prior approval" laws provide that the payer send their rates to the regulatory agency and may not charge the new premium rates until approved. "Deemer" requirements mean that the payer files their rates and then may start charging the new premiums if they are not disapproved by the state after a period of time (i.e., they are deemed approved). Premium rate filings generally must include information about the market that will be affected (e.g., protected claims and other financial data) and an actuarial justification for the increase. States that require payers to submit premiums for approval generally require that rates be reasonable in relation to the benefits provided under the coverage and that the premiums are not excessive or inadequate.[69]

As discussed more fully in Chapter 30, the rating requirements in the individual and group markets will change over the next few years as the federal government implements the ACA. For example, the ACA requires that beginning in 2014, all coverage in the individual and small group markets must be guaranteed available. In addition, the ACA limits the types of rating restrictions that may be applied (e.g., health insurers may vary premiums based on family size, the individual's age, or tobacco use).[70]

Almost all states provide coverage to individuals with chronic health conditions through a "high-risk" pool. These pools typically accept applicants if they have been turned down for coverage on the private market. The pool will limit the premiums charged for coverage through the pool and may impose other restrictions on coverage such as annual or lifetime benefit limits. In most states, coverage in the pool is funded by an assessment on health insurers to the extent that the premiums collected do not pay for claims incurred by the participants in the program.[71]

■ SOLVENCY

States require health insurers and payers to meet solvency standards using accounting based on statutory accounting principles (SAP). SAP differs from generally accepted accounting principles (GAAP) in regard to what may be considered as capital to meet those standards. The typical method is based on "risk-based capital" (RBC) standards developed by the NAIC. These standards are intended to measure the potential exposure to an insolvent condition that an insurance company or managed care organization may have based on the types of coverage offered and the general financial condition of the insurer.[72] Companies that fail to meet certain RBC target levels may be subject to various regulatory actions including increased monitoring or a takeover of the business operations by the state regulator. Solvency and RBC as well as monitoring and possible sanctions are discussed in detail in Chapter 21.

States also require payers to undergo periodic financial examinations by and reporting to the state regulatory agency. These exams and reports focus on the RBC levels at the managed care organization, the amount of surplus available to pay claims, and other factors affecting the financial condition of the payer.

Most states require insurers and HMOs to maintain insurance or other coverage that will pay claims in the event of the insolvency of the payer.[73] In addition, 13 states have established specific guaranty funds that will apply in the case of a payer insolvency. These funds are intended to cover claims if the MCO is unable to continue business. In some cases, the laws provide that other health insurers or MCOs must take enrollees of the failed payer.[74]

■ OVERSIGHT AND REGULATION

Regulation of payers and managed care is generally handled through a state Department of Insurance that has responsibility for oversight with respect to insurance companies, insurance products, and agents. The type of state regulatory structures include an independent agency with an elected insurance commissioner, a cabinet-level department reporting to the state governor, or an agency within a larger department responsible for banking, securities, or other financial services.

In some states, the oversight of managed care is provided by the Department of Health or Department of Managed Health Care. For example, the California Department of Managed Health Care is responsible for regulating MCOs licensed under the state's Knox–Keene Act.[75] In Pennsylvania, the Department of Health provides oversight to HMOs with respect to licensing and the provision of health services.[76]

Multistate Operations

Payers operating in more than one state must comply with the regulations of each jurisdiction. Other multistate payers can face the same regulatory challenge when complying with the rules in more than one state as well. Most states mandate that "foreign" payers, meaning payers that are domiciled in another state (not another country), meet the same requirements applicable to domestic MCOs. States also may require that out-of-state MCOs register to do business under the appropriate foreign corporation law and appoint an agent in the state for receipt of legal notifications.

Secondary Types of State Oversight

States usually also exercise a second form of oversight by contracting with one or more HMOs to manage health care services to low-income individuals. This adds new requirements, which are described in Chapter 25. State and local governments also provide health benefits to their employees, which means contracting with one or more payers as an employer to purchase health insurance or arrange for the payer to provide administrative services for their self-funded health benefits plan; like all large group employers, any contract will contain additional oversight requirements.

Other state agencies may also have some involvement in payer oversight. For example, California has created a regional health information organization (CalRHIO) that oversees the exchange of health information between health care providers and payers and other health insurance entities. In addition, a number of state attorneys general have engaged in litigation or other actions challenging managed care practices such as the development of UCR rates,[77] health insurance rate increases,[78] and rescissions in health insurance contracts.

■ CONCLUSION

States continue to exercise significant control over the operations of MCOs and the provision of managed care to consumers. These requirements concern almost every aspect of managed care, from the types of organizations that may be licensed as payers to the products offered to enrollees and the premium rates that may be charged for insured coverage. While the federal government has an important role with respect to health insurance and managed health care, as discussed in Chapters 29 and 30, it is clear the states will remain as the primary regulatory authority over health insurers and HMOs in regard to their at-risk business.

Endnotes

1   322 U.S. 533 (1944).
2   322 U.S. 535.
3   15 U.S.C. §1011 et seq.
4   15 U.S.C. §1012(b).
5   15 U.S.C. §§1012 and 1013.
6   42 U.S.C. §§300e et seq.
7   See, e.g., California's Knox–Keene Act, Cal. Health and Safety Code §1340 et seq. (2008).
8   P.L. 104-191.
9   P.L. 110-233.
10 P.L. 110-381.
11 P.L. 111-148.
12 See, e.g., N.Y. Comp. Codes R. & Regs., Title 10, §98-1.5 (2005).
13 National Association of Insurance Commissioners (NAIC), "Health Maintenance Organization Model Act" (2010).
14 NAIC, "Health Maintenance Organization Model Act," Section 5 (2003).
15 See, e.g., Col. Rev. Stat. §10-2-401 et seq.
16 P.L. 106–102.
17 See, e.g., Del. Code. Ann. Title 18, §5001 et seq.
18 See, e.g., Kan. Stat. Ann. §40-2202.
19 ACA Section 1001, 42 U.S.C. §300gg-15.
20 America's Health Insurance Plans (AHIP), "Explanation of Benefits (EOB) Statements: Summary of State Requirements" (August 9, 2010).
21 See, e.g., Mass. Gen. L. Ch. 175, §2B.
22 Cal. Admin. Code Title 28, §1300-67.04 (2011).
23 See, e.g., Ariz. Rev. Stat. Ann. §20-2206.
24 See, e.g., Cal. Admin. Code Title 10, §10.2274.70 et seq.
25 See, e.g., Or. Rev. Stat. §742.013.
26 ACA Section 1001, 42 U.S.C. §300gg-12.
27 Agency for Healthcare Research and Quality, "Privacy and Security Solutions for Interoperable Health Information Exchanges: Report on State Medical Record Access Laws" (August 2009).
28 See 45 C.F.R. Part 164.
29 AHIP, "Data Security Breaches: Summary of State Requirements" (September 13, 2010).
30 P.L. 111-5, Title XIII.
31 See, e.g., Me. Rev. Stat. Ann. Title 10, §1272.
32 Victoria Craig Bunce, J. P. Wieske, "Health Insurance Mandates in the States 2008," Council for Affordable Health Insurance (2008).
33 AHIP, "Autism Spectrum Disorders: Summary of State Requirements" (December 27, 2010).
34 See, e.g., Mich. Stat. Ann. §550.1807.
35 ACA Section 1001, 42 U.S.C. §300gg-14.
36 See e.g., Kan. Stat. Ann. §40-2248.
37 AHIP, "Mandate-Lite Health Insurance Plans: Summary of State Requirements" (January 19, 2009).
38 Col. Rev. Stat. §10-16-704.
39 ACA Section 1001, 42 U.S.C. §300gg-19a.
40 AHIP, "Restrictions on Provider Balance Billing: Summary of State Requirements" (August 1, 2010).
41 AHIP, "Disclosure of Usual, Reasonable and Customary Information: Summary of State Requirements" (September 14, 2009).
42 U.S. Department of Labor, "Technical Release 2011-01" (March 18, 2011).
43 See, e.g., Ill. Rev. Stat. Ch. 215, Para. 180, §1 et seq.
44 NAIC, "Uniform Health Carrier External Review Model Act" (2010).
45 ACA Section 1001, 42 U.S.C. §300gg-19.
46 See, e.g., N.H. Rev. Stat. Ann. §420-J:6.
47 See URAC CORE Standards, Version 3.0 accessed at: www.URAC.org.

48 AHIP, "Same-State Licensure and Utilization Review as the Practice of Medicine: Summary of State Requirements" (July 17, 2008).

49 See, e.g., Del. Code Ann. Title 38a, §38a–816 et seq.

50 See Market Conduct Exam Reports at: www.insurance.ca.gov/0100-consumers/0275-market-conduct/.

51 See, e.g., Del. Code Ann. Title 38a, §38a–478k.

52 Ocean State Physicians Health Plan v. Blue Cross Blue Shield of Rhode Island, 883 F. 2d 1101 (1st Cir. 1989).

53 AHIP, "Prompt Payment of Claims: Summary of State Requirements" (January 23, 2009).

54 538 U.S. 329 (2003).

55 P.L. 104-191.

56 See, e.g., N.Y. Ins. Law §3231.

57 See, e.g., Colo. Rev. Stat. §10-16-102.

58 ACA Section 1304, 42 U.S.C. §18024.

59 AHIP, "Individual Comprehensive, Major Medical Health Insurance: Summary of State Guarantee Issue and Rating Requirements" (November 9, 2009) and "Small Group Premium Rating Rules: Summary of State Requirements" (November 5, 2009).

60 Ibid.

61 Ibid.

62 AHIP, "Individual Comprehensive, Major Medical Health Insurance: Summary of State Guarantee Issue and Rating Requirements" (November 9, 2009).

63 42 U.S.C. §300gg et seq.

64 42 U.S.C. §300gg-11.

65 42 U.S.C. §300gg-12.

66 42 U.S.C. §300gg.

67 42 U.S.C. §300gg-1.

68 See, e.g., Idaho Code §41-4706.

69 See, e.g., Ala. Code §27-52-20.

70 ACA Section 1201.

71 Schwartz, T. "State High Risk Pools: An Overview," Kaiser Family Foundation (January 2010).

72 See, e.g., N. J. Stat. Ann. §26:2J-18.2 et seq.

73 See, e.g., Colo. Rev. Stat. §100-16-411.

74 AHIP, "Guaranty Fund Coverage and Insolvency Assessments: Summary of State Requirements" (January 5, 2009).

75 Cal. Health and Safety Code §1340 et seq. (2008).

76 See Pa. Stat. Ann. Title 40, §1551 et seq.

77 See New York Attorney General, "The Consumer Payment System is Code Blue" (January 13, 2009).

78 See Connecticut Attorney General, "Attorney General Says Anthem Rate Hearing Must Be Delayed Or Denied Until Critical Data Provided" (November 15, 2010). Accessed at: www.ct.gov/ag/cwp/view.asp?A = 2341&Q = 468474.

CHAPTER

29

Federal Regulation of Health Insurance and Managed Health Care

Tom Wilder

STUDY OBJECTIVES

- Understand how the Employee Retirement Income Security Act (ERISA) regulates employee-benefit plans
- Understand the differences between insured benefits and self-insured benefits
- Understand the documentation, reporting, and disclosure requirements under ERISA
- Understand the fiduciary duties required under ERISA
- Understand the effect of the Consolidated Omnibus Budget Reconciliation Act (COBRA) as it relates to "qualified life events"
- Understand the concept of health insurance "portability" as established by the Health Insurance Portability and Accountability Act (HIPAA)
- Understand the meaning of administrative simplification and be able to explain why it is an important term in the health care industry
- Understand the privacy and security requirements included in HIPAA's administrative simplification provisions
- Understand two important amendments to HIPAA: the Genetic Information Nondisclosure Act (GINA) and Mental Health Parity
- Understand the role of Tax Code on health benefits plans
- Understand federal oversight of payers and health plans, and the interaction between state and federal laws, including preemption

DISCUSSION TOPICS

1. Describe what is included under the administrative simplification portion of HIPAA. Why is it important to the health care industry?
2. Describe the electronic transactions performed in the health care industry and how they are affected by HIPAA. Discuss the positive and negative consequences and implications of this.
3. Discuss how HIPAA privacy requirements might differ from state laws about confidentiality of health information. Discuss when either HIPAA requirements or state requirements might prevail.
4. Explain why confidentiality of health information has been a controversial public policy issue.
5. Describe ERISA preemption of state insurance laws and mandates. Discuss the implications of this preemption.

6. Discuss when an employer would or would not choose to self-fund a health benefits plan for employees.

7. Describe the fiduciary responsibility aspect of ERISA. Discuss the implications of those responsibilities.

8. Describe how a benefits claims denial may be challenged under ERISA. Discuss how a benefits plan might avoid successful challenges, and the implications of such actions.

9. Discuss how conflicts between state and federal laws might be addressed.

■ INTRODUCTION

Managed care has traditionally been regulated at the state level. As discussed in Chapter 28, states impose significant oversight of the operations of health insurers and managed care organizations (MCOs). However, starting in 1973 with the passage of the Health Maintenance Organization (HMO) Act,[1] followed by the enactment of the Employee Retirement Income Security Act (ERISA) in 1974[2] and the Health Insurance Portability and Affordability Act (HIPAA) in 1996,[3] Congress and federal regulatory agencies have increasingly assumed responsibility for laws affecting managed care and MCOs. This trend toward federal regulation of managed care has continued through the present with the Patient Protection and Affordable Care Act (ACA), which President Barack Obama signed into law on March 23, 2010.[4]

This chapter discusses the primary federal laws governing managed care and the oversight of MCO operations provided through federal agencies such as the Departments of Health and Human Services (HHS), Labor (DOL), and the Treasury. This chapter is intended to outline the federal regulation of managed care in the commercial market. Not discussed are the operations and oversight of MCOs in federal government health care programs such as Medicare or Medicaid, which are covered in Chapters 24 and 25.

In some cases, the laws directly govern MCO products and services, for example, requirements under HIPAA prohibiting health insurance issuers (including MCOs) from setting premium rates based on a health status factor.[5] Other laws, such as ERISA, governing group health benefit plans sponsored by employers and employee organizations, and the Emergency Medical Treatment and Active Labor Act (EMTALA),[6] establishing guidelines for the provision of emergency care by hospitals, affect the employers that purchase MCO products and services and the physicians and hospitals that provide medical care to MCO enrollees.

Regardless of the type of legislation and whether the law directly or indirectly affects MCOs, it is clear the federal government plays an important role in determining how managed care is provided to Americans. Additionally, the interaction with, and potential conflicts between, federal and state oversight of managed care poses continuing challenges for MCOs.

■ HISTORY OF FEDERAL REGULATION

Starting in 1973, Congress has approved a series of legislative initiatives governing all aspects of managed care, and they are listed here in chronological order (excluding laws focused on Medicare, Medicaid, and the military health system). The laws that significantly affect MCOs are discussed in more detail later in this chapter

1973 – The HMO Act

The HMO Act established conditions for the operation of federally qualified HMOs and provided loans and loan guarantees for HMO startup costs.[7] This Act was described in more detail in Chapter 1, and is summarized here.

Federally qualified HMOs were required to provide "basic" and "supplemental" health services to their enrollees, including inpatient, outpatient, home health, laboratory, preventive, and emergency care.[8] The Act required federally qualified HMOs to meet solvency standards, provide procedures for handling member grievances, and establish programs for quality assurance.[9] In addition, the HMO Act required employers that offered health benefits to their employees through a federally qualified HMO to not financially discriminate against employees that choose the HMO option (i.e., the employer's contribution toward the cost of coverage had to be reasonable and designed to ensure the employee had a fair choice among benefit plan options).[10]

1974 – The Employee Retirement Income Security Act

ERISA provides comprehensive standards for group health plans offered to workers and their family members. Group health plans may provide managed care through either an insurance policy purchased by the plan or a self-funded arrangement administered by a payer ("self-funding" means that the plan sponsor assumes the risks of paying claims). As discussed in more detail later, ERISA exempts self-funded plans from many, but not all, state laws. It also sets out requirements for group health plans with respect to solvency, procedures to resolve appeals of benefit denials, disclosures of information to plan participants and beneficiaries, reporting to federal regulatory agencies, and the responsibilities of plan fiduciaries and administrators.[11]

1985 – The Consolidated Omnibus Budget Reconciliation Act (COBRA)

COBRA included provisions on a variety of subjects including Title X, which established rules for the continuation of health coverage to employees and qualified family members because of certain qualifying life events such as termination of employment or where an individual loses coverage because of the death of, or divorce from, a covered spouse.[12] The COBRA continuation coverage requirements apply to employers with 20 or more employees.[13]

Another section of COBRA enacted the EMTALA, which requires hospitals to provide services to patients with emergency medical conditions.[14] EMTALA affects decisions by MCOs to pay medical services at hospital facilities.

1990 – The Americans with Disabilities Act (ADA)

The ADA prohibits discrimination against individuals on the basis of a disability in employment and public services and accommodations.[15] In the context of employment decisions, the ADA restricts discrimination in hiring, promotion, compensation, training, and "other terms, conditions, and privileges of employment."[16] Although the Act recognizes an exception for "risk classification programs" such as health insurance coverage,[17] the ADA has implications for how MCOs provide wellness programs and other services to employers. For example, the Equal Employment Opportunity Commission (EEOC), which is responsible for ADA enforcement, has determined that a wellness program such as a smoking cessation initiative that requires employee participation or penalizes employees who do not participate violates the ADA.[18]

1993 – The Family and Medical Leave Act (FMLA)

The FMLA requires certain employers with 50 or more employees to allow workers to take unpaid leave of up to 12 weeks a year for recovery from a serious health condition, for the birth or adoption of a child, or for care of a sick family member.[19] Upon returning to work, the individual must be restored to their old job or an equivalent position, including all benefits such as health coverage.[20] The Act affects how MCOs provide coverage to individuals both during their leave and after return to work.

1994 – The Uniform Services Employment and Reemployment Rights Act (USERRA)

USERRA protects the employment and benefit rights of service personnel such as members of the National Guard who are working in the public or private sectors and are called to active duty.[21] The law requires, among other protections, that individuals have the right to return to their jobs and to reenroll in the employer's health coverage without penalty.[22] As with the FMLA, USERRA affects how managed care coverage is provided to service personnel and their family members during deployment and after return from active duty.

1996 – The Health Insurance Portability and Accountability Act

As discussed in greater detail later in this chapter, HIPAA establishes requirements for the guarantee availability and renewability of health coverage, prohibits the use of health status factors in setting premium rates, sets out safeguards for health information privacy and the security of electronic data, and provides standards for the exchange of electronic health information.[23] The Act has a significant impact on how MCOs operate in the individual and group insurance markets and with respect to the administration of self-funded group health plans.

Congress approved two additional provisions to HIPAA that same year:

- The Newborns' and Mothers' Health Protection Act, establishing requirements for the coverage of minimum hospital stays after the birth of a child;[24] and
- The Mental Health Parity Act, requiring parity between coverage for medical and surgical benefits and mental health benefits with respect to annual and lifetime dollar limits.[25]

1998 – The Women's Health and Cancer Rights Act (WHCRA)

The WHCRA requires health insurers and group health plans to provide coverage for reconstructive breast surgery after a mastectomy.[26]

2008

In 2008, three laws were passed that have a direct bearing on how MCOs and health benefits plans operate. The first two were passed as amendments to HIPAA, while the third was passed as an amendment to HIPAA and ERISA. They are:

- **The Genetic Information Nondiscrimination Act (GINA)**—As discussed further below, GINA prohibits health insurers and group health plans from denying health coverage or setting premium rates based on genetic information.[27] Additionally, the law places restrictions on the use and sharing of genetic information.[28]
- **The Mental Health Parity and Addiction Equity Act (MHPAEA)**—The law amended the 1996 Mental Health Parity Act by extending the parity requirements

to include substance use disorder benefits. In addition, the MHPAEA requires parity with respect to all financial requirements (cost-sharing such as deductibles, copayments, and co-insurance) and treatment limitations (day or visit limits) between medical and surgical benefits and benefits for mental health and substance use disorder services.[29]

- **Michelle's Law**—The law requires health insurers and group health plans that provide family coverage to continue covering dependent children for up to 12 months after the child leaves school for a medically necessary leave of absence.[30]

2009 – The Health Information Technology for Economic and Clinical Health Act (HITECH)

The HITECH Act amended the privacy protections and data security standards contained in HIPAA.[31] It established new requirements for notifying individuals if their health information has been wrongfully disclosed due to a data breach and increases the penalties for violations of the HIPAA privacy rule.[32] In addition, the HITECH Act provided funding to states and public entities for health information technology (IT) initiatives, created a new federal office to coordinate health IT programs, and established a process to develop standards for electronic health records (EHRs) and interoperability standards to facilitate data-sharing between health information systems.[33]

2010 – The Patient Protection and Affordable Care Act (ACA)

As is explained further in Chapter 30, the ACA is the most comprehensive federal law affecting MCOs and other entities providing health coverage since the passage of HIPAA in 1996.[34] The law includes immediate insurance market reforms (including requirements to cover preventive and emergency services, the extension of health coverage for dependents up to age 26, and restrictions on annual and lifetime benefit limits) and imposes additional requirements with respect to health insurers and group health plans beginning in 2014, including guaranteed issue of coverage and restrictions on the use of age and other rating factors. The ACA also establishes new mechanisms to expand access to health coverage, including the creation of state health insurance exchanges and mandates for employers to offer and individuals to maintain health coverage.

■ ERISA

ERISA was enacted to provide uniform national protections for participants and beneficiaries of group health and pension plans. The purpose of the law is to protect "the interests of participants in employee benefit plans and their beneficiaries, by requiring the disclosure and reporting to participants and beneficiaries of financial and other information with respect thereto, by establishing standards of conduct, responsibility, and obligation for fiduciaries of employee benefit plans, and by providing for appropriate remedies, sanctions, and ready access to the Federal courts."[35]

ERISA applies to group health plans sponsored by employers and employee organizations.[36] A group health plan may be "fully insured" by providing benefits through an insurance policy purchased from a health insurance issuer. Alternatively, the group health plan may choose to "self-fund" by assuming the risk of losses through funds set aside by the plan sponsor.

Payers interact with group health plans through insurance coverage purchased by the group health plan or where the payer provides administrative services to employers or employee organizations that sponsor self-funded group health plans. These administrative functions may include the processing and paying of claims, providing access to networks of physicians and hospitals, and conducting utilization review and other medical management functions.

This also points out an issue in semantics that has a great deal of substance when used in the legal, regulatory, and legislative sense, but is generally ignored in common usage: technically speaking, a health plan is the benefits plan itself, including the sponsor. For fully insured or at-risk business underwritten and sold by a health insurer or HMO, the insurer or HMO is indeed the health plan. But when a payer of any type is administering a self-funded benefits plan, the payer is not the health plan, the self-funded plan sponsored by the employer is. In common usage, however, including in this book, the term "health plan" or "plan" is used interchangeably with "payer," "HMO," or any other type of payer.

Applicability of ERISA

While ERISA applies to group health plans sponsored by employers and employee organizations, in some situations, more than one employer or employee organization may be involved with the group health plan. A "multi-employer plan" is a group health plan established pursuant to a collectively bargained agreement between one or more employers and employee organizations. Although involving more than one employer, coverage applies through a single-plan document. These are sometimes referred to as "Taft-Hartley plans" after a 1947 federal law that, among other provisions, established requirements for the use of employer funds for employee health and pension benefits.[37] Coverage through a labor union is an example of a common type of Taft-Hartley plan.

Another form of multi-employer plan is group coverage offered through an association such as a business chamber, which is not the same as individual coverage sold through an association. Another form is multiple employers grouping together in order to be collectively large enough to sustain a self-funded benefits plan and thus avoid state benefit mandates and premium taxes (discussed in the section on preemption); these are referred to as multi-employer welfare associations (MEWAs) or multi-employer trusts (METs).

ERISA specifically exempts some types of group plan arrangements. The statute does not apply to nonfederal governmental group health plans such as health coverage provided to state employees or coverage offered to employees of religious organizations (known as church plans).[38] In addition, ERISA does not govern arrangements established for the purposes of complying with certain state laws requiring compensation for employees in the case of an accident, disability, or unemployment.[39]

Plan Funding

As noted, plan sponsors may choose to provide benefits to participants and beneficiaries through health insurance coverage purchased from an HMO or other insurer. Alternatively, the sponsor will assume the risk for the cost of medical claims and administrative costs by self-funding the group health plan. In this situation the sponsor contracts with a payer or a third-party administrator (TPA) to handle certain administrative functions.

Most sponsors of self-funded group health plans purchase stop-loss insurance coverage or reinsurance. The policy will pay a portion of costs incurred by the plan during the year above a certain "attachment point" that is determined on either an individual or aggregate basis. In the former situation, the policy will pay the sponsor if the claims of any one individual exceed a certain dollar amount. In the case of an aggregate attachment point, the policy pays if the claim losses of the entire group exceed a specific dollar threshold.

There are several different types of stop-loss or reinsurance, including differing rules around how and when the reinsurer is liable or not. The policy also typically only covers a percentage of covered costs, such as 80%, and typically has a maximum payout ceiling as well. Finally, the policy is not health insurance, meaning the insurer can change what and how they cover excess liabilities each year, including declining to cover them at all, since they operate under different insurance rules. All of these issues are addressed in more detail in Chapter 2.

Fiduciary Standards

ERISA requires the group health plan to appoint a fiduciary with responsibility for the operation of the plan.[40] Fiduciaries are required to discharge their duties in the interests of plan participants and beneficiaries and in accordance with the documents establishing plan governance.[41] In addition, a fiduciary is prohibited from engaging in certain types of prohibited transactions that are considered contrary to the interests of the plan; for example, an agreement between the fiduciary and the plan involving the sale, lease, or exchange of any plan assets.[42] If the fiduciary breaches their duty, they are subject to civil liability or enforcement actions by the DOL.[43]

Disclosure of Plan Information

ERISA requires that plan sponsors inform participants and beneficiaries of information about the plan in a document called the Summary Plan Description (SPD). Information provided in the SPD includes the following:[44]

- The name of the ERISA plan and the type of plan administration (e.g., insurer or TPA).
- Whether a health insurance issuer is responsible for funding, financing, or administration of the plan and the contact information for the insurer.
- Contact information for the plan sponsor (including address, phone number, and Employer Identification Number).
- Names, titles, and addresses of any plan trustee.
- A summary description of the benefits.
- A description of any cost-sharing provisions, including premiums, deductibles, coinsurance, and copayment amounts.
- Any annual or lifetime benefit limits.
- Coverage of preventive services, medical tests, devices, procedures, and emergency care.
- The composition of any health care provider networks and terms governing the use of in-network and out-of-network providers.
- Information on any provisions requiring preauthorization or utilization review as a condition for receiving services.
- Procedures for making claims for benefits.
- Information about the Department of Labor office from which participants and beneficiaries may seek assistance or information regarding their rights.

In cases where the coverage is provided through a health insurance or HMO policy, the insurer typically provides the document that describes many of these items such as the types of benefits, any limits on coverage, and the cost-sharing responsibilities of plan enrollees.[45]

The document must be written in a manner calculated to be understood by the average plan participant and in certain situations, the SPD must include a statement advising individuals with limited English proficiency how to obtain language assistance and become informed about their rights.[46] The SPD must be issued to participants within the first 90 days of becoming covered under a plan.[47]

Group health plan beneficiaries and participants also must be notified of modifications to the plan. This information must generally be provided within 210 days after the end of the plan year in which the change was made or adopted.[48] If there is a "material reduction" to covered services or benefits (e.g., eliminating benefits or increasing copayments or premiums), a Statement of Material Modification (SMM) must be provided within 60 days after the adoption of the change.[49] As discussed in the next chapter, however, the ACA requires additional disclosures to group health plan enrollees and shortened timeframes for providing information.

In addition to SPD and SMM statements, a number of federal laws, including ERISA and HIPAA (discussed below), require that plan enrollees receive specific notices in response to certain events, including the following:

- Adverse Benefit Determinations—as discussed below, group health plan participants and beneficiaries have the right to appeal certain adverse benefit determinations. They must be notified of their right to appeal a claim denial, the time limits for filing an appeal, how to request an appeal, and other rights such as the ability to review the claim file and present information to be considered by the group health plan.[50]
- Consolidated Omnibus Budget Reconciliation Act—COBRA provides individuals with the right to continue coverage under a group health plan under certain circumstances. A group health plan enrollee must be given notice of their right to continuation coverage after a "qualifying event" (the exercise of COBRA rights is discussed in more detail later as well as in Chapter 17).[51]
- HIPAA Notice of "Creditable Coverage"—HIPAA includes provisions allowing individuals to "credit" prior health insurance or group health plan coverage when obtaining new coverage under a group health plan or health insurance policy for purposes of waiving limits on preexisting medical conditions. Group health plan enrollees must be provided a creditable coverage certificate when they terminate coverage or upon request.[52]
- Medical Child Support Order—The MCSO is any judgment, decree, or order that provides for the support of a participant's child under a group health plan or provides for a child's health benefit coverage as required by state domestic relations laws or federal medical assistance laws.[53]
- Mental Health Parity—As discussed below, the Mental Health Parity Act and the Mental Health Parity and Addiction Equity Act establish rules with respect to financial requirements and treatment limitations on coverage for mental health and substance use disorder benefits. These provisions allow employers to obtain an exemption from the application of the parity requirements under certain conditions. In such cases, the group health plan enrollee must be provided a notice that the employer is choosing to exercise the exemption.[54]
- Newborns' and Mothers' Health Protection Act—Group health plan participants must be given an annual statement advising them about their rights under the Act. This statement may be included as part of the SPD, if distributed annually.[55]
- Privacy Practices—Individuals who are enrolled in health insurance coverage or with a group health plan must be provided a Notice of Privacy Practices detailing how their health information is collected, used, or shared by the insurer or plan.[56]
- Women's Health and Cancer Rights Act—group plan enrollees must be given a statement each year of their rights under the Act. This statement may be included in an annual SPD that is given to participants and beneficiaries.[57]

Reporting Requirements

In general group health plans with 100 or more participants must file an annual report (called the Form 5500 report) with the DOL and the Internal Revenue Service (IRS). The report includes information on plan administration and operations, funding, agreements with and compensation paid to third parties such as TPAs, and insurance contracts or agreements. In most cases, the report must be filed electronically.[58] Two attachments to the Form 5500 report directly involve MCOs: Schedule A, listing insurance contracts providing coverage to participants and beneficiaries, and Schedule C, detailing agreements with third parties to provide services to the group health plan.

Appeals of Denial of Coverage

Group health plans are required to establish "reasonable" procedures for resolving the appeal by a plan enrollee of a decision to deny a claim for benefits. An "adverse benefit determination" that may be appealed is any denial, reduction, or termination of a benefit or a failure to make payment for a benefit.[59] The plan must respond to appeals of adverse benefit decisions within specified timeframes, depending on the type of claim for benefits; for example, a request for approval of urgent care services must be decided within an expedited timeframe.

Claimants must be given a notice of their rights to appeal and informed of the process for submitting a request to the plan to review an adverse benefit determination. In addition, individuals submitting an appeal have the right to review the claim file and present evidence. If the decision to deny a claim for benefits is based on an internal plan rule, guideline, protocol, or other criterion, the claimant must be provided a copy. In addition, if the denial is based on an exclusion for medically necessary or experimental treatments, the claimant has the right to obtain the medical criteria upon request.[60] As discussed in Chapters 20 and 30, the ACA expanded the right of group health plan enrollees to appeal adverse benefit determinations, including a new provision allowing submission of certain disputes to an independent external review process.

■ COBRA

As already noted and as described in Chapter 17, COBRA provides group health plan enrollees with the right to continue coverage after employment ends or where an individual loses coverage because of the death of or divorce from a spouse who was covered by the group health plan.[61] COBRA requirements apply to employers with 20 or more employees (many states have so-called "mini COBRA" laws applicable to businesses with fewer than 20 workers, although the individual's right to continue coverage may not be as extensive and the continuation period may be shorter).[62]

In general, COBRA provides the ability for an individual to have continuing coverage under a group health plan in the event of certain "qualifying events" or "life events" as follows:

- The involuntary termination of employment, provided it is not for "gross misconduct";
- A reduction in the number of hours worked such that the enrollee no longer qualifies for coverage;
- In the case of a covered spouse or dependent children, the death of or a divorce or legal separation from a covered employee;
- Loss of coverage due to a layoff, strike, lockout, or medical leave; or
- In the case of a dependent child, he or she is no longer eligible to continue under a parent's coverage.[63]

Continuation coverage is generally permitted for up to 18 months. If the individual is determined by the Social Security Administration to be disabled, COBRA coverage may be continued for up to 29 months. If there is a legal separation, divorce, or death of a covered spouse, coverage may continue for up to 36 months.[64]

The cost of COBRA continuation coverage is borne entirely by the individual—unlike most group health plans, where a portion of the cost is paid by the employer. The law permits the group health plan or health insurer providing coverage to the plan to add a 2% administrative fee to the cost of the premium.[65]

■ HIPAA

HIPAA affects payers by establishing requirements for health insurance and group health plan coverage; setting limits on the collection, use, and disclosure of health information; creating safeguards for the security of electronic data; and establishing standards for the exchange of electronic health information between MCOs and physicians and hospitals.

The law was intended to expand access to health coverage and streamline the administration of health insurance and medical services.

HIPAA is divided into five titles:

- Title I—"Health Care Access, Portability, and Renewability";
- Title II—"Preventing Health Care Fraud and Abuse, Administrative Simplification, Medical Liability Reform";
- Title III—"Tax-Related Health Provisions";
- Title IV—"Application and Enforcement of Group Health Plan Requirements"; and
- Title V—"Revenue Offsets."

As described below, the first two titles have the most direct impact on payers. HIPAA applies to payers through amendments to three federal laws:

- The Public Health Service Act, which applies to health insurance issuers such as MCOs;
- ERISA, which applies to group health plans; and
- The Internal Revenue Code, which imposes excise tax penalties on health insurers and group health plans that violate certain HIPAA provisions.

Health Coverage Provisions (HIPAA Title I)

Title I of HIPAA establishes conditions for the provision of health coverage by health insurance issuers (including MCOs) in the individual and group insurance markets and by group health plans sponsored by employers and employee organizations.

Preexisting Condition Limitations

Health insurers in the group market and group health plans are prohibited from denying coverage for a preexisting medical condition that was manifested more than 6 months prior to the start of the plan or insurance policy. A condition is "manifested if it was present before the date of enrollment whether or not any medical advice, diagnosis, care, or treatment was recommend or received."[66] If a preexisting condition limit is imposed for conditions that arise within 6 months of enrollment, the plan may only prohibit coverage for that condition for up to 1 year.[67]

In addition, enrollees must be given credit against any preexisting condition limits for each month of any prior "creditable coverage" such as health insurance, an employer health plan, Medicaid, or other specified health coverage.[68] The creditable coverage waiver of preexisting condition limits applies only if there is a 63-day or shorter period between the prior and new coverages. For example, a payer or health plan cannot apply any preexisting condition limitations to an individual who enrolls within 45 days of dropping a prior health insurance policy that had covered the individual for 12 months.

Prohibiting Health Status Discrimination

Health insurance issuers in the group market and group health plans are not permitted to use the following factors as a basis to deny coverage or for purposes of setting the premium rates paid by an individual:[69]

- Health status;
- Medical condition, meaning physical and mental illnesses;
- Claims experience;
- Receipt of health care;
- Medical history;
- Genetic information;
- Evidence of insurability, including conditions arising out of acts of domestic violence; or
- Disability.

For example, an MCO that provides group health insurance may not use the fact that an enrollee was treated for cancer to deny coverage or in determining how much the individual pays for health coverage. Health insurers and group health plans may, however, use claim history and other medical information in determining how much the entire group is charged for coverage.[70]

Guaranteed Availability of Coverage

Health insurance issuers in the small group market must provide coverage to an employer group or individual that wishes to obtain coverage as long as they meet the insurer's eligibility requirements.[71] HIPAA defined "small group" as any employer with up to 50 employees, although, as discussed in Chapter 30, the ACA is expanding the definition to include employers with 100 employees.[72]

Guaranteed Renewability of Coverage

Health insurance issuers are required to renew coverage for any group health plan as long the plan sponsor continues to pay premiums, has not committed any fraud or intentional misrepresentation of fact under the terms of coverage, and meets any participation or contribution requirements. An example of a participation requirement would be a minimum number of employees that must sign up for health insurance coverage.[73]

Special Enrollment Periods

The HIPAA provisions with respect to the restrictions on preexisting condition limits are intended to apply to enrollees who obtain coverage during the annual open-enrollment periods that are offered by health insurers in the group market and group health plans (see Chapters 16 and 17). In addition, HIPAA extends these protections to individuals who enroll during certain special periods. For example, an MCO must provide a special enrollment period so that a covered employee can add a new spouse or a newborn or adopted child. Special enrollment periods are also provided to allow an individual to obtain coverage through their employer if they lose other coverage they previously had through a spouse in the event of a legal separation or divorce or the death of the spouse.[74] These are further examples of the qualified live events discussed earlier.

Individual Market Requirements

HIPAA requires health insurers selling policies in the individual market to guarantee the availability of coverage to any individual that wishes to enroll.[75] States were given flexibility, however, to develop "alternative mechanisms" to provide individuals with access to health insurance in the individual market. For example, states that did not adopt the HIPAA provisions could either require health insurers to make certain types of coverage available or establish a "high-risk pool" to provide insurance for individuals that were unable to obtain coverage because of illness or their medical histories.[76] In addition, health insurance issuers are required to renew coverage sold in the individual market unless the individual fails to pay premiums, the individual commits an act that is fraudulent or an intentional misrepresentation of material fact under the terms of coverage, or the insurer decides to stop offering the particular policy or withdraws from the insurance market in the state.[77]

Administrative Simplification (HIPAA Title II)

Title II of HIPAA establishes "administrative simplification" requirements that govern the collection, use, and disclosure of health information; provide protections for the security of electronic health data; and establish standards for electronic health care transactions. The administrative simplification provisions apply to health care providers, health insurers, group health plans, and health care "clearinghouses" (entities that facilitate the exchange of health information). These providers, plans, insurers, and clearinghouses are defined as "covered entities" in HIPAA. In addition, the HIPAA requirements with respect to health information privacy and data security apply to "business associates" that are third parties that collect, share, or use protected health information on behalf of a covered entity.[78]

Health Information Privacy

"Protected health information" that is subject to the HIPAA provisions is information in any form (electronic, written, or oral), that is created or received by a covered entity, employer, life insurer, or educational institution and that relates to (1) the past, present, or future health of the individual; (2) health care provided to the individual; or (3) payment for health care. The privacy provisions establish protections for health information that is "individually identifiable," which means it directly identifies the person or where there is a reasonable basis to believe you can use the information to identify the individual. For example, disclosure by an MCO of a medical claim that identifies a medical diagnosis or treatment and the address of the patient would be individually identifiable because it is possible to determine the patient's name from the address.[79] In general, individuals must first give consent before their health information may be used or disclosed unless the use or disclosure is for purposes of treatment, payment, or certain designated health care operations.[80] For example, a doctor may share information with a nurse (treatment), a hospital may submit a claim to an insurer (payment), and an MCO may share information with an outside vendor for data-processing purposes (health care operations) without having to obtain permission.

The HIPAA privacy law and regulations set limits on the use of health information for other purposes such as marketing, establishes requirements for the disclosure of health information for specific purposes such as law enforcement or public health activities, defines how information may be collected or used for medical research, and establishes standards for the encryption of data in certain circumstances.[81] In addition, individuals have the right to review their health information maintained by a covered entity and request amendments to correct any inaccuracies.[82] Individuals may also request that their health information not be disclosed under certain circumstances.[83]

Covered entities are required to establish policies and procedures to govern the collection, use, and disclosure of protected health information and training programs for workforce members must be provided. HIPAA-covered entities and business associates may be subject to civil or criminal penalties for violating these requirements.[84]

As noted earlier in this chapter, health insurers and group health plans must provide enrollees with a notice of privacy practices in certain circumstances. The notice must include a description (including an example) of the types of uses and disclosures permitted by the HIPAA provisions for payment, treatment, and health care operations. In addition, individuals must be informed of any restrictions on the use or disclosure of their information under applicable law, the right to inspect and amend their protected health information, and the contact information for the person or office at the covered entity to address any complaints or inquiries. The notice must also inform the individual that they will not be penalized for exercising their rights under the HIPAA privacy provisions.[85]

Electronic Transaction and Code Set Standards

As described more fully in Chapter 23, and noted in Chapters 17 and 18, the HIPAA Title II administrative simplification provisions require covered entities to use standardized electronic transactions and billing code sets for defined types of electronic exchanges. These standards apply primarily to business-related transactions, not electronic medical records. The intent of mandatory standardization was to encourage

and streamline the use of electronic transactions such as health care claims, verification of an individual's enrollment in health coverage, and the coordination of benefits (situations where more than one insurer or group health plan may be responsible for a covered medical service).[86] In addition, the standards establish systems for identifying covered entities using electronic health transactions through uniform employer, health care provider, and health plan identifiers. As is discussed in Chapter 30, the ACA made a number of modifications and improvements to the electronic transaction standards.

The HIPAA standards are developed by private sector "standards organizations" and approved by HHS. Once approved, the standards must be used by covered entities after a specified timeframe for implementation (in general, 24 months).[87] The standards apply to the following health care transactions:

- Health claims or equivalent encounter information;
- Health claims attachments;
- Enrollment and disenrollment in a health plan;
- Eligibility for a health plan;
- Health care payment and remittance advice;
- Health plan premium payments;
- First report of injury;
- Health claim status; and
- Referral status.

For claims submissions or other billing-related transactions, standard existing code sets are required, as delineated in Chapter 23. In addition, standards have been developed for the National Provider Identifier (NPI) and the National Employer Identifier (NEI) that engage in health care transactions, and a National Health Plan Identifier is under consideration for health insurers and group health plans at the time of publication.[88]

In addition to transaction standards, Title II of HIPAA requires protections for the security of electronic health care data, which was also described more fully in Chapter 23. In general, covered entities must ensure the confidentiality and integrity of electronic protected health information, protect against any anticipated threats, and ensure compliance by its workforce.[89] Covered entities and business associates must put in place policies and procedures to safeguard the storage and transmission of electronic health information.[90] Covered entities must also establish administrative and technical safeguards for data and provide training for workforce members that are responsible for handling electronic information.[91]

Significant Amendments to HIPAA

Like all major laws, Congress has amended HIPAA from time to time. HIPAA amendments within the ACA are discussed in Chapter 30, while three particularly significant amendments are described next.

GINA

GINA was enacted in 2008 as an amendment to HIPAA. GINA limits the collection and use of genetic information and the use of genetic tests by health insurers in the individual and group markets and group health plans.[92] Genetic information is defined to include information about the individual's genetic tests, tests of family members, and the manifestation of a disease or disorder in a family member (e.g., family history). Health insurers and group health plans are prohibited from establishing rules for eligibility of coverage or to vary premium rates based on genetic information. In addition, health insurers and group health plans are restricted from requesting genetic information or requiring enrollees or applicants to take a genetic test.[93]

■ MENTAL HEALTH PARITY

As noted earlier, as part of the original HIPAA statute in 1996, Congress passed the Mental Health Parity Act. This law required health insurers in the group market and group health plans that imposed annual or lifetime limits on the dollar value of benefits to have annual and lifetime limits for mental health coverage that were the same as or not less than the limits imposed for medical and surgical benefits. Group health plans were not mandated to provide mental health coverage, but were expected to treat any annual or lifetime dollar limits at "parity." For example, a health plan cannot limit coverage for mental health benefits on an annual basis to $1 million while imposing no annual limits for medical and surgical coverage.[94]

Significant amendments to the parity requirements were enacted in 2008 through the MHPAEA,[95] which added substance abuse disorders to the parity requirements. In addition, the law requires health insurers in the group market and group health plans to provide the following with respect to medical and surgical coverage and coverage for mental health or substance use disorder benefits:

- Any financial requirements applicable to mental health or substance use disorder benefits such as co-payments, coinsurance, or deductibles must be the same as or less than financial requirements imposed for medical and surgical coverage; and[96]
- Any treatment limitations such as day or visit limits imposed for mental health or substance use disorder benefits must be the same as or less than the limits applied for medical and surgical benefits.[97]

The parity requirements do not apply to "small employers" with 50 or fewer employees. In addition, if the group health plan can demonstrate that the application of the parity provisions has increased the cost of coverage under the plan by more than 2%, the provisions will be waived for the following plan year.[98]

HITECH

The HITECH Act was enacted in 2009 and placed further restrictions on the use of health information for marketing purposes, increased the civil penalties for HIPAA violations, and extended certain privacy requirements to business associates.[99] Additionally, HIPAA-covered entities must notify individuals if they are responsible for an unauthorized disclosure of their health information, for example, if the data is lost or stolen.[100] If the breach involves more than 500 residents of a state or jurisdiction, the covered entity must notify the news media serving the area.[101]

■ FEDERAL TAX CODE

The federal Internal Revenue Code (IRC) affects decisions by individuals and employers to purchase and maintain health coverage. For example, the costs paid by employers and their employees for health coverage, whether through health insurance or self-funded group health plans, are fully deductible for income tax purposes.[102] The cost of health insurance purchased on the individual market is also deductible to the extent it exceeds 7.5% of the individual's adjusted gross income.[103] The deductibility of health coverage provides a major incentive for individuals and employers to purchase coverage.

In addition, the IRC and regulations and guidance promulgated by the Treasury Department have encouraged the development of products such as health flexible spending accounts (FSAs)* and consumer-directed health plans (CDHPs) with savings options such as health reimbursement accounts (HRAs) and health savings accounts (HSAs).[104] The intent of CDHPs is to increase consumer awareness of costs and to facilitate their making cost-conscious decisions, as discussed in more detail in Chapter 2.

The HRAs or HSAs associated with CDHPs are tax-favored accounts funded by individuals or employers that may be used to pay certain types of medical expenses. The accounts are considered tax-favored because contributions to, and qualified expenditures from, a health care spending account are deductible for federal tax purposes. In the case of HRAs and HSAs, the account is coupled with a qualified high-deductible health plan (HDHP)[105] offered through a health insurer or by a self-funded group health benefits plan. The minimum deduction to qualify as an HDHP for tax code purposes is annually determined by the U.S. Department of the Treasury based on a number of indexes. For calendar year 2012, an HSA qualified HDHP is defined under § 223(c)(2)(A) as a health plan with an annual deductible that is not less than $1,200 for self-only coverage or $2,400 for family coverage.[106]

---

*FSAs are straightforward pretax accounts for use in paying out-of-pocket costs, are not linked to a specific health benefits plan, and are not addressed any further in this chapter.

The ACA will make significant changes in the dynamics of the federal tax code impact on health coverage by providing tax credits to assist with the purchase of health coverage, penalizing certain employers that do not provide and individuals that do not maintain coverage, and imposing additional taxes on health insurers and providers of medical services. These changes are discussed further in Chapter 30.

■ FEDERAL REGULATORY OVERSIGHT

Oversight of HMOs, health insurers, and group health plans is carried out by a number of different federal agencies. These agencies are responsible for developing regulations to implement the federal laws discussed in this chapter, providing civil and criminal enforcement of regulatory requirements, and working with stakeholders such as consumers, employers, payers, and health care providers to carry out the legislative directives of Congress. Below are the key federal regulatory agencies with oversight of managed care activities.

The **Department of Health and Human Services** has primary responsibility for federal laws affecting managed care, including HIPAA, GINA, and the ACA. Within HHS, three agencies provide oversight:

- The Centers for Medicare and Medicaid Services' (CMS) Center for Consumer Information and Insurance Oversight (CCIIO), which enforces the HIPAA, GINA, MHPAEA, and ACA insurance market requirements;
- The CMS Office of E-Health Standards and Security (OESS), which is responsible for HIPAA electronic transaction standards; and
- The Office for Civil Rights (OCR), which has responsibility for HIPAA health information privacy and data security rules.

The **Department of Labor** (DOL), through the **Employee Benefits Security Administration** (EBSA), enforces the ERISA and COBRA provisions applicable to group health plans. The EBSA also has responsibility for the group health plan requirements contained in other federal laws such as HIPAA and the ACA.

The **Treasury Department** is responsible for developing federal tax policy as it relates to health coverage. Within the Department, the **Internal Revenue Service** (IRS) has primary enforcement responsibility of federal tax laws, including the application of excise tax penalties that may be applied to MCOs and other health insurers and employers that violate provisions of federal health coverage laws such as ERISA, HIPAA, and COBRA.

The **Department of Justice** (DOJ) enforces criminal penalties against health care entities that violate certain federal statutes such as HIPAA privacy provisions. The DOJ is also responsible for oversight with respect to federal fraud and abuse laws that protect government health care programs such as Medicare and Medicaid and for jointly enforcing federal antitrust requirements with the Federal Trade Commission (FTC).

The **Equal Employment Opportunity Commission** (EEOC) is responsible for oversight and enforcement activities with respect to the Americans with Disabilities Act.

The **Federal Trade Commission**, along with the DOJ, enforces federal antitrust provisions involving health care providers. In addition, the FTC has assumed responsibility for oversight with respect to federal laws that safeguard certain types of information, including health data.

■ INTERACTION OF STATE AND FEDERAL REQUIREMENTS

A major challenge for HMOs, health insurers, and health plans is determining when federal law applies, and situations when state requirements should be followed. In many cases, both Congress and the states have chosen to provide oversight with respect to the same set of issues. For example, in addition to the federal HIPAA privacy standards, many states passed laws about health information safeguards applicable to insurers. In other cases, such as the HIPAA Title I insurance market provisions, many states have directly incorporated the federal standards into state law.

A key part of this analysis is the concept of preemption—in other words, determining when the federal provisions are intended by Congress to take precedence over any conflicting state provisions. An example of this was seen back in Chapter 1 in the discussion about how the HMO Act of 1973 preempted state anti-HMO laws and regulations. As a general rule, Congress may choose to exercise "field preemption" (the federal law completely preempts any state laws on a subject) or "conflict preemption" (the federal law controls if it is impossible to comply with both the state and federal requirements). In practice, the preemptive effect of federal laws on managed care is more nuanced and depends on the particular set of laws.

ERISA Preemption Standards

The extent to which ERISA preempts state laws raises a number of key issues for payers that must balance the requirements imposed by states, which traditionally regulate insurance products including policies sold to group health plans, and the federal government, which regulates health benefits provided by group plans. ERISA includes two preemption standards that directly affect payers and health plans.

Section 502 of ERISA establishes civil enforcement standards for violations of the statute.[107] For example, participants and beneficiaries may file a legal action in federal court to recover the amount of a benefit due under the terms of the plan or to enforce the duties of a plan fiduciary.[108] Accordingly, federal courts "have exclusive jurisdiction of civil actions" brought to enforce a plan provision.[109] As a result, courts have generally held that participants and beneficiaries of a group health plan cannot litigate an issue involving their rights to receive health benefits from a group health plan in state court. As noted by the U.S. Supreme Court, a lawsuit challenging a decision by a payer to not cover services under a group health plan is subject to the "exclusive jurisdiction" of ERISA and the enrollee is not permitted to challenge the decision in state court.[110]

Section 514 of ERISA addresses state laws that are intended to regulate health insurance provided to group health plans and sets out three important principles with respect to preemption:

- ERISA preempts "any and all State laws insofar as they may now or hereafter relate to any employee benefit plan . . . ."[111]
- The ERISA "savings clause" permits states to enforce "any law . . . which regulates insurance, banking, or securities."[112]
- The ERISA "deemer clause" further provides that an employee benefits plan shall not "be deemed to be an insurance company or other insurer, bank, trust, or investment company or to be engaged in the business of insurance or banking, for purpose of any law of any state purporting to regulate insurance companies, insurance contracts, banks, trust companies, or investment companies."[113]

The issues related to Section 514 involve a complicated analysis of whether the state law affects health insurance and is therefore permissible, or the law affects the group health plan's provision of benefits and is therefore preempted by ERISA. This analysis is highlighted by three examples:

- In a 1995 case involving a New York law that imposed surcharges on hospital bills, the ruling was that the law was not preempted by ERISA; although the surcharges undoubtedly had an impact on a self-insured plan by increasing the cost of the benefits provided by the plan, the New York surcharge system did not relate to ERISA plans and therefore was not preempted.[114]
- In a case challenging a state law requiring independent review of decisions by an HMO to deny coverage based on medical necessity when the enrollee was in a fully insured group benefits plan, the Supreme Court held in 2002 that the state law was not preempted by ERISA because the statute regulated insurance and not the provision of health benefits.[115]
- As noted in Chapter 28, the Supreme Court ruled in 2003 that state "any willing provider" laws are not preempted under ERISA because it qualified as law regulating insurance.[116]

HIPAA Preemption Standards

Similar to ERISA, HIPAA establishes different preemption standards depending on the specific statutory requirements. In general, the health insurance reform provisions in Title I (with certain limited exceptions) preempt state laws that "prevent the application" of the federal requirements.[117] As a practical matter, this means that a health insurance issuer is required to follow both state and federal requirements unless it is impossible to do so.

The HIPAA requirements with respect to electronic transaction standards in Title II provides that the federal provisions "shall supersede any contrary provision of State law, including a provision of State law that requires medical or health plan records (including billing information) to be maintained or transmitted in written rather than electronic form." However, a state law is not preempted if the Secretary of HHS determines the state law is necessary to prevent fraud and abuse, to ensure appropriate state regulation of insurance, for state reporting on health care delivery, or to address controlled substances.[118]

The HIPAA health information privacy provisions do not preempt a contrary state law provision that imposes "more stringent" requirements. In general, this standard means that stricter state laws that are viewed as more consumer-friendly are not preempted (e.g., laws that require the consent of a minor child for disclosure of their health information to a parent or that place limits on the use and disclosure of patient records related to treatment for substance use disorders).[119]

■ CONCLUSION

As discussed in this chapter, there are an increasing number of federal laws that regulate the operations of MCOs. These laws directly govern payers or regulate the employers that contract with payers to administer their benefits plan and the health care providers that provide services to the organization. The federal requirements affect almost all aspects of managed care and payer operations including standards for how insurance coverage must be provided to individuals and employers, provisions affecting health benefits and group health plans, tax preferences for individual and group health coverage, and protections for health information. As discussed in Chapter 30, these protections and the federal oversight of payers has been greatly strengthened by the ACA.

Endnotes

1   P.L. 93-222, 42 U.S.C. §300e et seq.
2   P.L. 93-406, 29 U.S.C. §1001 et seq.
3   P.L. 104-191.
4   P.L. 111-148.

5   42 U.S.C. §300g-1.

6   P.L. 99-272, 42 U.S.C. §1395dd.

7   42 U.S.C. §§300e and 300e-4.

8   42 U.S.C. §300e-1.

9   42 U.S.C. §300e.

10 42 U.S.C. §300e-9.

11 29 U.S.C. §1001 et seq.

12 P.L. 99-272.

13 29 U.S.C. §1161. Some states have enacted "mini-COBRA" laws with similar continuation coverage standards for employers with under 20 employees.

14 42 U.S.C. §1395dd.

15 P.L. 101-336, 42 U.S.C. §12101 et seq.

16 42 U.S.C. §12112.

17 42 U.S.C. §12201(c).

18 See EEOC Enforcement Guidance on Disability-Related Inquiries and Medical Examinations of Employees, July 27, 2000.

19 P.L. 103-3, 29 U.S.C. §2601 et seq.

20 29 U.S.C. §2614.

21 P.L. 103-353, 38 U.S.C. §4301 et seq.

22 38 U.S.C. §4317, 20 C.F.R. Part 1002.

23 P.L. 104-191.

24 P.L. 104-204, Title VI.

25 P.L. 104-204, Title VII.

26 P.L. 105-277, Title IX.

27 P.L. 110-233.

28 42 U.S.C. §300gg-1.

29 P.L. 110-343, Division C, Title V, Subtitle B.

30 P.L. 110-381.

31 P.L. 111-5, Title XIII.

32 Ibid.

33 Ibid.

34 P.L. 111-148 as amended by the Health Care and Education Reconciliation Act, P.L. 111-152.

35 29 U.S.C. §1001(b).

36 29 U.S.C. §1003.

37 P.L. 80-101, 29 U.S.C. §141 et seq.

38 29 U.S.C. §1003.

39 Ibid.

40 29 U.S.C. §1102.

41 29 U.S.C. §1104.

42 29 U.S.C. §1106.

43 29 U.S.C. §§1105 and 1109.

44 29 U.S.C. §1022.

45 29 C.F.R. §2520.102-3.

46 29 C.F.R. §2520.102-2(c).

47 29 U.S.C. §1024(b).

48 29 C.F.R. Part 2520.

49 Ibid.

50 29 C.F.R. §2560.503-1.

51 29 U.S.C. §1161 et seq.

52 29 U.S.C. §1181.

53 29 U.S.C. §1169.

54 29 C.F.R. §2590.712.

55 29 U.S.C. 1185(d).

56 42 C.F.R. §164.522.

57 29 U.S.C. §1185b(b).

58 29 C.F.R. §§2520.104-1.

59 29 C.F.R. 2560.503-1.

60 Ibid.

61 29 U.S.C. §1161 et seq.

62 29 U.S.C. §1161.

63 29 U.S.C. §1163.

64 29 U.S.C. §1162.

65 29 U.S.C. §1164.

66 29 U.S.C. §1181, 42 U.S.C. §300gg.

67 Ibid.

68 Ibid.

69 29 U.S.C. §1182, 42 U.S.C. §300gg-1.

70 Ibid.

71 42 U.S.C. §§300gg-11.

72 42 U.S.C. §300gg-91.

73 42 U.S.C. §300gg-12.

74 29 U.S.C.§1181(f), 42 U.S.C. §300gg(f).

75 42 U.S.C. § 300gg-300gg-41.

76 42 U.S.C. §300gg-44.

77 42 U.S.C. §300gg-42.

78 45 C.F.R. §160.103.

79 Ibid.

80 45 C.F.R. §164.506.

81 45 C.F.R. §§164.510, 164,512, and 164-514.

82 45 C.F.R. §§164.524 and 164.526.

83 45 C.F.R. §164.522.

84 45 C.F.R. §160.400.

85 45 C.F.R. §164.520.

86 42 U.S.C. §1320d-2.

87 42 U.S.C. §1320d-1.

88 42 U.S.C. §1320d-2.

89 45 C.F.R. §164.306.

90 See: 42 C.F.R. §164.302 et seq.

91 Ibid.

92 P. L. 110-233, 29 U.S.C. §1182, 42 U.S.C. §300gg-1, and 42 U.S.C. §300gg-53.

93 Ibid.

94 P.L. 104-204, Title VII.

95 P.L. 110-343, Division C, Title V, Subtitle B.

96 45 C.F.R. §146.136(c).

97 Ibid.

98 Ibid.

99 Title XIII of P.L. 111-5, 42 U.S.C. §§17921 and 17931 et seq.

100 42 U.S.C. §17932.

101 42 C.F.R. §164.406.

102 26 U.S.C. §106.

103 26 U.S.C. §213.

104 26 U.S.C. §106 and 224.

105 26 U.S.C. § 223(c)(2)(A).

106 www.treasury.gov/resource-center/faqs/Taxes/Pages/
HSA-2011-indexed-amounts.aspx. Accessed August 26,
2011.

107 29 U.S.C. §1132.

108 29 U.S.C. §1132(a).

109 29 U.S.C. §1132(c).

110 Aetna Health Inc. v. Davila, 542 U.S. 200 (2004).

111 29 U.S.C. §1144(a).

112 29 U.S.C. §1144(b)(2)(A).

113 29 U.S.C. §1144(b)(2)(B).

114 De Buono v. NYSA-ILA Med. & Clinical Servs. Fund, 520
U.S. 806 (1997); N.Y. State Conference of Blue Cross
& Blue Shield Plans v. Travelers Ins. Co., 514 U.S. 645
(1995).

115 Rush Prudential HMO, Inc. v. Moran, 536 U.S. 355
(2002).

116 Kentucky Ass'n of Health Plans v. Miller, 538 U.S. 329
(2003).

117 42 U.S.C. §300gg-23(a).

118 42 U.S.C. §1320d-7(a)(1).

119 42 U.S.C. §1320d-2.

CHAPTER 30

The Patient Protection and Affordable Care Act

Tom Wilder

STUDY OBJECTIVES

- Understand the overall scope and impact of the Patient Protection and Affordable Care Act (ACA) on the health insurance and managed health care industry
- Understand the specific elements of the ACA affecting payers that went into immediate effect or into effect prior to 2014
- Understand the specific elements of the ACA affecting payers that go into effect beginning in 2014
- Understand the interaction of state and federal laws, regulations, and oversight of the payer industry
- Understand the potential impact on the ACA of judicial and political forces

DISCUSSION TOPICS

1. What are the primary goals of the ACA in regard to the health insurance and managed health care sector?
2. Discuss whether you think the ACA will achieve those goals, and why or why not.
3. Discuss what the impact of the ACA will be on payers and managed health care organizations, both positive and negative.
4. Discuss how states might implement elements of the ACA, identifying elements that can differ from state to state, and what might be the impact of differing implementation approaches.
5. Discuss the concept of guaranteed issue and its associated benefits and risks, and how those risks might be mitigated.

■ INTRODUCTION

The Patient Protection and Affordable Care Act (ACA) was signed into law by President Barack Obama on March 23, 2010.[1] The ACA has a significant impact on the provision of health coverage to Americans, and is the most far-reaching law affecting managed care since Medicare and Medicaid were enacted in 1965.

This chapter reviews the provisions of the ACA applicable to payers in the commercial market such as health insurers, health maintenance organizations (HMOs), and self-funded employer-sponsored group health benefits plans. The ACA provisions applicable to government health care programs such as Medicare and Medicaid are not included in this discussion, but are included in Chapters 24 and 25. Likewise, major sections of the ACA are applicable to providers, long-term care, and so forth, and they too are not addressed in this chapter.

As discussed at the end of the chapter, there have been and are legal challenges to the ACA, and the U.S. Supreme Court addresses the new law in its 2012 term. Because the outcome of their deliberations is not known at the time of publication, this chapter addresses the ACA as it exists at the close of 2011, meaning it is possible that some of the ACA's provisions may either change or no longer apply after that date.

As discussed in more detail below, the ACA amends four federal laws that relate to managed care:

- The Public Health Service Act (PHSA), which is a wide-ranging law (including amendments) that affects health care and health coverage in multiple places;
- The Employee Retirement Income Security Act (ERISA), which applies to group health plans sponsored by employers and employee organizations;
- The Internal Revenue Code (IRC) provisions dealing with the taxation of health insurance and group health plan benefits, and the application of certain excise and income taxes to individuals, employers, and health insurers; and
- The Health Insurance Portability and Affordability Act (HIPAA), which deals with administrative simplification, including electronic transactions and code sets, and privacy and security of protected health information (PHI).*

Managed care organizations are primarily affected by new requirements imposed on health insurers, including HMOs, that offer coverage in the individual and group markets. In addition, many of the ACA provisions apply to group health plans sponsored by employers and employee organizations. These group health plans either purchase health insurance from an insurer or HMO, or choose to "self-fund" the coverage and contract with a payer or a third-party administrator (TPA) to provide administrative services, as described in Chapters 2 and 29.

As discussed in this chapter, the ACA imposes the following changes to managed care:

- Reforms to the individual and group health insurance markets and to group health plans that were implemented within a short time period after enactment, referred to as the "immediate market reforms";
- Expansion of access to health coverage beginning in 2014 through the creation of state health insurance exchanges and additional health insurance market changes;

- Modification of the requirements for electronic health care transactions addressed in the "administrative simplification" provisions of HIPAA; and
- Provisions affecting the federal tax code.

The ACA combines very specific requirements with broad ones, but in all cases implementation requires that the federal regulatory agencies responsible for enforcing the ACA provisions—the Departments of Health and Human Services, Labor, and the Treasury (HHS, DOL and Treasury, respectively)—create interim and then final regulations. The ACA also calls for these departments, and HHS in particular, to consult with various designated organizations, most often the National Association of Insurance Commissioners (NAIC), that represent state insurance departments.

In addition, this chapter reviews the role of the states and federal government in carrying out the ACA provisions and of the political and legal challenges to implementation.

■ LEGISLATIVE HISTORY

Although various committees of the U.S. House of Representatives and Senate began consideration of health care reform legislation in early 2009, formal Congressional action on the ACA began on September 17, 2009, with the introduction of H.R. 3590, "the Service Members Home Ownership Tax Act of 2009." This bill, which provided a first-time homebuyer credit to members of the Armed Forces, was approved by the House on October 8, 2009. The Senate deleted the house provisions in H.R. 3590 and substituted a new version of legislative language addressing health care reform (including a new title, "the Patient Protection and Affordable Care Act"), which they approved on December 23, 2009. The House acceded to the Senate amendments to the bill on March 23, 2010. The ACA was signed into law by President Obama on March 23, 2010 (P.L. 111-148).[2]

Additional amendments to the ACA contained in the Health Care and Education Reconciliation Act (H.R. 4872) were approved by the House on March 21, 2010, and by the Senate on March 24, 2010. The Reconciliation Act was signed into law on March 30, 2010 (P.L. 111-132). Together, these two laws are referred to in this chapter as the ACA.

In some respects, the ACA is patterned after health care reform legislation approved by the Massachusetts Legislature in 2006. The bill, "An Act Providing Access to Affordable, Quality, Accountable Health Care," included many of the elements that make up the ACA:

- Subsidies to assist low-income individuals and families with the purchase of health insurance coverage;
- Expansion of Medicaid;
- A mandate, meaning a financial penalty, for all adults to have health coverage unless they have a financial hardship exemption; and

---

*Technically, HIPAA is an amendment to the PHSA, but for clarity's sake it is included with the others.

- The establishment of a state insurance "connector" that helps pair individuals and businesses with health insurance coverage options.[3]

■ IMMEDIATE REFORMS

A number of the ACA changes involving the health insurance market and group health plans were intended to go into effect within the first 12 months of enactment. These immediate reform provisions include restrictions on the use of annual and lifetime benefit limits, expansion of coverage to dependent children, access to emergency and preventive services, and creation of new mechanisms to provide health insurance information to consumers.

Unless otherwise indicated, the following immediate reform provisions were effective for health insurance policy or group health plan "years" that began on or after September 23, 2010 (6 months after enactment). A policy or plan "year" begins at the start of new coverage or the renewal of existing coverage under a health insurance policy or group health plan. As a result, most health insurance offered in the group market and group health plans needed to implement the changes as of January 1, 2011, because most health coverage offered through an employer is provided on a calendar-year basis.

"Grandfathered" Health Coverage

A key concept embodied in the immediate market reforms is the preservation of the right of individuals and employers to maintain their existing health insurance coverage. As discussed in more detail below, this so-called "grandfathered coverage" is not subject to some of the initial ACA changes. To qualify as grandfathered coverage, an individual or employer had to be enrolled in the health insurance or group health plan coverage as of the date of enactment of the ACA (March 23, 2010).[4] Employers are permitted to add new employees to a group health plan and individuals may add family members to existing coverage without losing grandfathered status.

Health insurers and group health plans must inform enrollees that they have grandfathered coverage and that, as a result, some of the consumer protections of the ACA may not apply. In addition, there are modifications to the existing health insurance or group health plan, such as increasing the enrollee's cost-sharing (premiums, deductibles, copayments, and coinsurance) above a certain amount, changing the annual or lifetime benefit limits, or dropping coverage for benefits.[5] For example, an MCO that provided mental health benefits through prescription drugs and counseling prior to March 23, 2010 that subsequently drops coverage for counseling will cease to be a grandfathered plan and will have to comply with all of the ACA provisions applicable to "nongrandfathered" plans.[6] A simplified list of events or conditions under which a grandfathered plan would lose that status may be seen in Table 16-3 in Chapter 16.

Table 30-1 outlines the ACA immediate reform provisions that apply or do not apply to grandfathered coverage.

TABLE 30-1	Impact of Reforms in Immediate Effect upon "Grandfathered Plans"

ACA provision	Grandfathered coverage	Nongrandfathered coverage
Restrictions on lifetime benefit limits	Yes	Yes
Restrictions on annual benefit limits	No – individual insurance market Yes – all other coverage	Yes
Prohibition against rescissions	Yes	Yes
Coverage of preventive services	No	Yes
Coverage of emergency services	No	Yes
Access to pediatricians and ob/gyns	No	Yes
Extending coverage for dependent children to age 26	Yes *	Yes
Uniform evidence of coverage documents	Yes	Yes
Medical loss ratio reporting and rebates for health insurers	Yes	Yes
Standards for internal appeals and external review	No	Yes
Prohibition on preexisting condition limitations	No – individual insurance market Yes – all other grandfathered coverage*	Yes
Medical loss ratio reporting and rebates†	Yes	Yes
Reporting of "unreasonable" premium increases	Yes	Yes

* Prior to January 1, 2014, a grandfathered group health plan does not have to extend dependent coverage if the individual has coverage available through another group health plan (such as through their employer).

†This provision only applies to health insurers and is not applicable to self-funded group health plans.

Restrictions on Annual and Lifetime Benefit Limits

The ACA prohibits health insurers and group health plans from imposing lifetime limits on the dollar value of benefits. This provision applies to all coverage offered by an insurer or group health plan, regardless of whether or not it is grandfathered.[7] In addition, prior to January 1, 2014, a health insurance issuer in the group market and a group health plan may only impose "restricted" annual limits on "essential health benefits" (grandfathered individual market insurance policies may continue to place annual limits on the dollar value of essential benefits).

As discussed later in this chapter, essential health benefits make up a standard coverage package that will be determined by the Secretary of HHS. Essential benefits are defined under the ACA to include very broad categories of coverage such as emergency care, hospitalization, ambulatory patient services, and prescription drugs.[8] Starting in 2014, all health coverage offered through the state insurance exchanges and any health insurance sold in the individual and small group markets (employers with up to 100 employees) must offer essential benefits.[9]

The term "restricted annual limits" is not defined by the ACA. The federal regulatory agencies responsible for enforcing the ACA provisions (HHS, DOL, and Treasury) determined the minimum restricted annual limits that health insurers and group health plans were permitted to apply until plan or policy years on or after January 1, 2014.[10] After that date annual limits may not be applied by an insurer or group health plan with respect to essential health benefits except for grandfathered coverage in the individual insurance market. Those limits are:

- For policy or plan years beginning on or after September 23, 2010, but before September 23, 2011—annual limits must be set at $750,000 or above.
- For policy or plan years beginning on or after September 23, 2011, but before September 23, 2012—annual limits must be set at $1.25 million or above.
- For policy or plan years beginning on or after September 23, 2012, but before January 1, 2014—annual limits must be set at $2 million or above.

The regulatory agencies also established a process for certain health insurers in the group market and group health plans to apply for a waiver from the application of the restrictions on the use of annual limits on the dollar value of benefits. The waivers are intended to provide relief in situations where the application of the annual limit restrictions "would result in a significant decrease in access to benefits under the plan or health insurance coverage or would significantly increase premiums for the plan or health insurance coverage."[11] The purpose of the waiver is to protect health insurance and group health plan coverage commonly known as "mini-med" or "limited benefit" plans that provided fewer health benefits, often with higher deductibles or lower annual lifetime benefit limits. These types of policies, which have significantly lower premiums, are frequently offered to individuals with lower incomes such as part-time workers or those in certain industries such as retail or food-service jobs.[12]

Coverage of Preventive and Emergency Services

Health insurers and group health plans that are not grandfathered are required to provide coverage for certain designated preventive care services.[13] These services must be provided without the imposition of any cost-sharing requirements (deductibles, copayments, or co-insurance). The following preventive services are included in the ACA coverage requirements:

- Services with a rating of "A" or "B" as recommended by the U.S. Preventive Services Task Force (USPSTF);
- Immunizations recommended by the Advisory Committee on Immunization Practices of the Centers for Disease Control and Prevention;
- Preventive care and screenings for infants, children, and adolescents supported by guidelines from the Health Resources and Services Administration (HRSA);
- Preventive care and screenings for women supported by HRSA guidelines; and
- Recommendations of the USPSTF regarding breast cancer screening, mammography, and prevention.

If new recommended preventive services are added by any of the designated organizations such as the USPSTF, the health insurer or group health plan must provide coverage no later than policy or plan years beginning 12 months after the service is added.[14]

In addition, nongrandfathered health insurance policies and group health plans must cover medical services for individuals with emergency medical conditions without requiring prior authorization for coverage or imposing cost-sharing requirements.[15] This prohibition applies regardless of whether the emergency services are provided at in-network or out-of-network care settings and whether or not the treating health care provider is a member of the insurer or plan network (for health insurers and group health plans that use networks of physicians and hospitals). An "emergency medical service" is defined as a medical screening examination and treatment to stabilize a patient.[16]

Access to Health Care Providers

Health insurance issuers and group health plans that are not grandfathered and that require enrollees to designate a primary care health care provider must allow enrollees to pick any primary care provider participating in the insurer or plan network who is available to accept new patients.[17] If the enrollee is a child, a nongrandfathered health insurer or group health plan must permit a covered parent to designate a provider who specializes in pediatrics as the child's primary care physician (if the health insurer or group health plan requires the designation of a health care provider for a child).[18]

In addition, nongrandfathered health insurers and group health plans are required to permit enrollees to access health care providers specializing in obstetrical and gynecological care without requiring the individual to obtain prior authorization for such services.[19] The health insurer or group health plan must provide enrollees a notice of their right to designate any primary care health care provider, to designate a pediatrician as the primary care provider for a child, and to obtain access to obstetrical or gynecological care without prior authorization.[20]

Limits on Preexisting Conditions for Children

As discussed in Chapter 29, HIPAA restricts the ability of health insurers and group health plans to impose limits on coverage for preexisting medical conditions, meaning a medical condition for which medical advice, diagnosis, care, or treatment was received prior to enrollment.[21] The ACA prohibits the use of all preexisting condition limitations as applied to children up to age 19 for all health insurers and group health plans, with the exception of grandfathered health insurance coverage in the individual market. As discussed later in this chapter, the use of preexisting condition limits will be prohibited with respect to all health insurance or group health plan coverage, except for grandfathered individual insurance market coverage, starting in 2014.[22]

Coverage for Children up to Age 26

With one exception, the ACA requires all health insurers and group health plans that offer family coverage to allow a dependent child to stay on the policy until he or she reaches age 26. However, in the case of a grandfathered group health plan for plan years prior to January 1, 2014, the plan does not have to cover the child if he or she is eligible for another employer-sponsored group health plan, for example, the child is employed and offered coverage through his or her work.[23]

The federal regulatory agencies provided additional requirements in the case of (1) children who had previously been covered by a parent's health insurance policy or through a group health plan, but had lost coverage because they "aged-out," meaning they no longer met the age-limit restrictions for coverage of a child under a family policy or plan; or (2) children who were not previously covered under the parent's policy or plan. In such cases, the health insurer or group health plan was required to offer parents a one-time opportunity to enroll the child.[24]

The agencies also made clear that the coverage must be offered to the dependent child without the imposition of any preexisting condition limits and on a guaranteed issue basis (i.e., the health insurer or group health plan must accept the child for coverage regardless of their health status). Health insurers were allowed (if permitted by applicable state law) to restrict the new enrollment of a dependent child to an annual open-enrollment period and to charge separate rates for children based on age.[25]

Prohibition on Rescissions

The ACA prohibits all health insurers and group health plans from rescinding coverage unless the individual has engaged in fraud or misrepresented a material fact prohibited by the terms of the coverage.[26] This provision is intended to address decisions by health insurers in the individual market to void the insurance policy because of a misrepresentation or other act by the individual applying for the insurance coverage (i.e., a valid contract between the insurer and the individual was never in effect). A rescission is different from a cancellation where the coverage is ended effective with the date of cancellation.[27]

The federal regulatory agencies provided two examples where a rescission is not permissible. The first example is a health insurer that requires applicants to complete a questionnaire that asks about prior medical history (which affects setting premium rates). The application includes the question, "Is there anything else relevant to your health that we should know?" The applicant inadvertently fails to list a visit to a psychologist on two occasions, 6 years previously. The individual is provided health coverage and is later diagnosed with breast cancer. The health insurer cannot rescind the coverage because the failure to disclose the visits to the psychologists was inadvertent.

The second example is a group health plan that provides coverage to employees who work at least 30 hours per week. The enrollee works at least 30 hours per week and is provided coverage as a full-time employee. The enrollee later switches to part-time status but the plan mistakenly continues to provide coverage, collect premiums, and pay claims. The group health plan cannot rescind coverage because there was no fraud or an intentional misrepresentation of a material fact.[28]

Health insurers and group health plans must provide enrollees with at least 30 days advance written notice that they are intending to rescind the coverage. A decision to rescind may be appealed by the enrollee, as discussed later, and coverage must be continued during the appeal.[29]

Disclosures of Information to Consumers

The ACA has several requirements for disclosures of information to consumers. Two major ones are below.

Summary of Benefits Coverage

The ACA requires the Department of Health and Human Services within 12 months of enactment of the legislation to develop standards for a uniform "explanation of coverage"

(EOC)* document, also referred to as a summary of coverage (SOC) and a summary of benefits (unsurprisingly, no acronym).[30]

In the ACA, the SOC is to be limited to four pages, but the NAIC recommendations contain language allowing two sections to be expanded by a page each under certain circumstances.[31] The SOC is supposed to describe the coverage provided under the insurance policy or plan, including the following information:[†]

- Description of the coverage including any cost-sharing for "essential health benefits" and other benefits as designated by HHS;
- Any exceptions, reductions, or limitations on coverage;
- Renewability and continuation of coverage provisions;
- A "coverage facts label" that includes examples of common benefits scenarios including pregnancy and serious or chronic medical conditions and applicable cost-sharing;
- A statement if the coverage includes minimum essential coverage (discussed later in this chapter and refers to the types of coverage that meet the requirements of the individual mandate provisions of the ACA); and
- A contact telephone number for consumers to call with questions and an Internet address where a copy of the entire health insurance policy or group health plan certificate of coverage may be obtained.

The SOC must be provided to individuals when they apply for coverage and at the time of enrollment or re-enrollment in health insurance coverage or a group health plan. HHS is also required to create uniform definitions of insurance and medical terms to be used in the SOC.[32]

As discussed in Chapters 28 and 29, ERISA as well as most states require that enrollees in health insurance coverage and group health plans be notified of any changes to the terms of their insurance policy or health plan. The ACA requires that individuals be notified of any "material modifications" to coverage no later than 60 days prior to the effective date of any changes.[33]

Internet Web Portal for Consumers and Businesses

HHS was required by the ACA no later than July 1, 2010, to create an internet web portal to provide consumers and businesses with information about the availability of health insurance choices in their states.[34] The portal must provide information on the following coverage options:

- Health insurance coverage available in the state (other than insurance covering a single disease or condition or

covering an "unreasonably limited set" of diseases or conditions);
- Medicaid coverage;
- Coverage under a state Children's Health Insurance Program (CHIP);
- Coverage under the state's high-risk pool (as discussed in Chapter 30, a high-risk pool provides coverage for individuals who are unable to obtain insurance on the private market due to a serious health condition); and
- Coverage within the state's small group insurance market.

HHS was also required by the ACA to create a standard format for the presentation of information allowing individuals and employers to compare the coverage offered through the private market listed on the web portal.[35]

Internal Appeals and External Review

All nongrandfathered health insurers and group health plans are required by the ACA to meet certain minimum standards for resolving an appeal of an adverse benefit decision, for example, a decision that a particular medical service is not covered because it is not medically necessary.[36] An adverse benefit determination subject to the appeal process is "a denial, reduction, or termination of, or a failure to provide or make payment (in whole or in part) for, a benefit . . ." and includes a decision by a health insurer or group health plan to rescind coverage (discussed earlier).[37]

The ACA requires that the internal appeals process conducted by health insurers and group health plans include the following protections:

- The procedures required for group health plans by ERISA (discussed in Chapter 29). As a practical matter most states already meet the ERISA standards with respect to their laws applicable to health insurers.
- Enrollees must be provided notices in a "culturally and linguistically appropriate manner" of the available appeals processes and contact information for any state office of insurance consumer assistance.[38]
- Individuals must be permitted to review their file and to present evidence and testimony during the appeals process.
- Enrollees must continue to receive coverage from the health insurer or group health plan during the appeals process.

In addition, health insurers and group health plans must ensure that the claimants receive a "full and fair" review of their appeal. The individuals must be provided, free of charge, with any new evidence that develops during the course of the appeal.[39] Health insurers and plans also must ensure the person reviewing the internal appeal is free from any conflicts of interest. As a result, any decisions regarding the hiring, termination, or promotion of, or compensation

---

*Not to be confused with the evidence of coverage—also referred to as an EOC—that is a far more detailed document described in Chapter 20.

[†]See Table 20-1 in Chapter 20 for a more detailed listing.

paid to, the individual handling the internal appeal must not be based on the likelihood they will deny an appeal.[40]

In addition, insurers and group health plans are required to implement external review requirements that allow certain disputes to be submitted to an external review process. The ACA provides that the external review process shall, at a minimum, include "the consumer protections set forth in the Uniform External Review Model Act promulgated by the National Association of Insurance Commissioners. . . ."[41] Many states have adopted the NAIC Model Act as the basis for external review laws applicable to health insurers.

The federal regulatory agencies have established additional requirements for the external review process divided into a "state process" (for health insurers in states that have established an external review process consistent with the consumer protections in the NAIC Model Act) and a "federal process" (for self-funded group health plans and health insurers in states that have not established an external review process that meets the consumer protection standards in the NAIC Model Act).[42] With one exception, discussed below, the state and federal process includes the same elements with respect to external review of adverse benefit decisions:

- Claimants must be provided a notice of the rights in connection with the external review.
- If the health insurer or group health plan fails to comply with any of the internal appeals requirements, the claimant has the right to immediately proceed to the external review process (in other words, the claimant is not required to first "exhaust their remedies" with the insurer or plan).
- Claimants on group health plans are not required to pay the cost of the external review, other than a nominal filing fee (not to exceed $25), which is refunded if the claimant is successful in his or her external review request.
- A restriction on the minimum dollar amount of a claim that is eligible for external review is not allowed.
- Claimants must be given a minimum of 4 months to submit a request for external review after they have received the notice of the final determination of their internal appeal.
- The appeal must be submitted to an independent review organization (IRO). The IRO is required to use medical or legal experts to review the appeal (e.g., an appeal involving an adverse benefit determination based on medical necessity criteria is reviewed by a health care provider with training and experience in the field of medicine that is the subject of the claim for benefits).
- The IRO must meet standards to ensure that it does not have a conflict of interest. For example, the IRO may not be owned or controlled by a health insurance issuer, group health plan, or plan sponsor.
- The claimant must be given at least 5 business days to submit in writing additional information to the IRO for consideration during the review.
- The decision by the IRO is binding on the health insurer or group health plan and on the claimant, "except to the extent other remedies are available under State or Federal law."
- The IRO must make its decision no more than 45 days after receiving a request for external review.
- If the review concerns an urgent care situation, the decision must be made as expeditiously as possible but no more than 72 hours after submission (e.g., a claim involving a medical condition for which the standard review timeframe would seriously jeopardize the life or health of the claimant).
- The external review process must be described in the Summary Plan Description, insurance policy, or other evidence of coverage provided to health insurer or group health plan enrollees.
- The IRO must maintain written records of reviews and make them available to regulatory agencies.

One critical difference between the state and federal process is the scope of adverse benefit determinations that may be submitted for external review. The state process applies to any adverse benefit determination "based on the issuer's [or plan's] requirements for medical necessity, appropriateness, health care setting, level of care, or effectiveness of a covered benefit."[43] The federal external review process applies to all benefit denials including both medically necessary decisions and a denial based on a decision that a service is not covered by the insurer or plan.[44] As a result, the federal external review process applies to a significantly larger number of issues.

Medical Loss Ratios

Health insurers in the individual and group markets, including grandfathered coverage, are required by the ACA to report to HHS the "medical loss ratio" (MLR) for each line of business (i.e., individual and group markets) in every state where they do business.[45] The MLR measures the percentage of premium revenue used to pay clinical services and activities that improve health care quality compared to the amounts spent on administrative costs and overhead. In making the MLR determination, certain state and federal licensing fees and taxes are excluded. The specifics of the MLR calculation are provided in Chapter 21.

Health insurers in the individual or small group markets (the ACA defines "small group" as employers with up to 100 employees[46]) must maintain an MLR of 80%. Health insurers selling coverage in the large group market are required to meet an 85% MLR standard. Insurers that fail to maintain a minimum loss ratio in a particular market, as measured on a state-by-state basis, are expected to refund the excess premium amount back to policyholders.[47] For example, an MCO selling coverage in the individual market that has a 75% loss ratio during the year in a state must refund 5% of the premium amount on a pro rata basis back to consumers who purchased coverage. Insurers also have the option of reducing future premiums.*

The HHS Secretary is authorized to adjust the 80% MLR standard for the individual health insurance market in a state if it is determined it will "destabilize" the market.[48] An adjustment may be needed if the health insurance issuers in a state will be required to pay rebates because they have MLRs below 80% and the payment of rebates would threaten the solvency of the insurers (in some states, insurers selling coverage in the individual market have higher administrative costs because of factors such as the cost to pay insurance agents who sell the policies and the volatility of the market).[49] As of the date this chapter went to press, several states had applied for a waiver with respect to the MLR standards for insurers selling coverage in the individual market.

Premium Review Process

The ACA directs HHS to establish a process, starting with the 2010 plan year, for health insurers in the individual and group markets to report "unreasonable" increases in premiums to the Department of Health and Human Services.[50] This provision applies to both grandfathered and nongrandfathered coverage. The request and supporting information (e.g., historical and projected claims experience, trend projections, and the allocation of the overall rate increase to claims and nonclaim costs) must be displayed on the insurer's website and also publically available through HHS.[51] In general, rate increases that are 10% or more for the first review period (increases that are effective between July 1, 2011, and December 31, 2011) must be submitted for review. Starting in 2012, there will be state-specific thresholds for the percentage rate increases that must be reported as determined by HHS.[52]

The ACA also established grants to states to help them review requests for premium increases.[53] Although most states require health insurers to submit some types of premium increases for review, not all states have the authority to deny premium increases that they believe are unreasonable.

---

*The reason is that a rebate is a one-time event, but a rate rollback goes on for 12 months. If the insurer rolled back rates but medical costs rose higher than predicted, it would have no way of recovering the shortfall.

Quality Care Payment Programs

The ACA directs the HHS Secretary, no later than 2 years after enactment, to develop reporting requirements for health insurers and group health plans regarding payment structures for payments to health care providers that:

- Improve health outcomes;
- Prevent hospital readmissions;
- Improve patient safety and reduce medical errors; and
- Implement wellness and health promotion activities such as smoking cessation or weight management.[54]

Health insurers and group health plans must report this information annually to HHS, and the reports will be publically available through an Internet website. HHS is authorized to impose fines on health insurers and group health plans that fail to provide the health quality program reports.[55]

Immediate Actions to Preserve and Expand Coverage

In addition to the web portal described previously that is intended to help consumers and businesses comparison-shop for coverage, the ACA included three near-term initiatives to help Americans obtain access to or maintain health coverage prior to the overall market changes that will take place in 2014.

Preexisting Condition Insurance Plan (PCIP)

The ACA established a temporary high-risk pool for individuals that are unable to find other insurance coverage. The PCIP will sunset on January 1, 2014.[56] Coverage is available to individuals who:

1. Are U.S. citizens or legal residents who reside in one of the 50 states or the District of Columbia;
2. Have not been covered under "creditable coverage," meaning other health insurance coverage, for a continuous 6-month period prior to applying; and
3. Have a preexisting medical condition.[57]

The ACA directed HHS to enter into contracts with states or private nonprofit entities to administer pools that meet the following requirements:[58]

- The pool may not impose any preexisting condition exclusions;
- The premiums cannot exceed 100% of the "standard risk" rate for coverage sold in the state's individual market;
- Specified limits are placed on cost-sharing amounts, meaning deductibles, coinsurance, and co-payments;
- Premiums charged to enrollees may not vary on the basis of age by a factor of more than 4 to 1; and
- The pool must cover required benefits including preventive care, professional services, hospital, home health, durable medical equipment, emergency services, and prescription drugs.

Early Retiree Reinsurance Program (ERRP)

The ACA provided funding to pay the health care claim costs for "early retirees," defined as individuals between age 55 and Medicare eligibility, who were covered by an employer-sponsored group health plan.[59] The program pays 80% of the annual claim costs between $15,000 and $90,000 incurred by early retirees and their qualified family members. HHS established a process for employers to apply for participation in the ERRP and submit claims to HHS for payment. The ACA appropriated $5 billion to pay for ERRP claims. HHS stopped accepting applications for the program as of May 5, 2011, because all of the anticipated funding was allocated.[60]

Small Business Tax Credit

The ACA established a tax credit program for small employers to help fund the cost of providing health coverage.[61] An eligible employer: (1) must have fewer than 25 full-time equivalent employees for the taxable year and (2) average annual wages for its employees of less than $50,000 per employee. To qualify for the credit, the employer must pay at least half of the cost of coverage. The tax credit amount is based on the average cost of coverage in the small group market in the state where the employee enrolls for coverage. Starting in 2014, the credit may only be used for coverage purchased through a state insurance exchange.[62]

■ 2014 REFORMS

Starting in 2014, a number of ACA provisions intended to expand access to health insurance coverage become effective. These include new state health insurance exchanges for individuals, creation of new insurance cooperative arrangements and small businesses to purchase coverage, and rules eliminating restrictions on premium rating and underwriting. Unless otherwise stated, the changes are effective for health insurance policy or group health plan years that begin on or after January 1, 2014.

Preexisting Condition Limits

As explained earlier in this chapter in the discussion on immediate market reforms, the ACA eliminated the use of preexisting condition restrictions as applied to dependent children under age 19. Starting January 1, 2014, the use of preexisting condition limits is not permitted for all individuals, regardless of age.[63] This prohibition applies to all health insurers (except "grandfathered" policies in the individual market) and group health plans.

Restrictions on Premium Rates

The ACA applies limits on premiums that may be charged by a health insurer in the individual and small group (meaning employers with up to 100 employees) markets starting in 2014. These new restrictions are described further in Chapter 22, but are summarized here. Health insurance rates may only be based on the following factors:

- The number of people covered under the policy;*
- The age of the enrollee, except rates may not vary by more than a ratio of 3 to 1 for all individuals; and
- Tobacco use, except rates may not vary by more than a ratio of 1.5 to 1.

In addition, the insurer may vary rates within a state based on specific rating areas, for example, a city or region. States are required to designate rating area or areas provided the Department of Health and Human Services has approved the rating areas within a state.[64]

Another restriction on premium rating affects the use of "health status factors" such as medical claims history in setting the cost of coverage paid by an individual. As discussed in Chapter 29, HIPAA prohibited health insurers in the group market and group health plans from denying coverage to an individual or from setting premiums paid by an individual based on a health status factor such as claims experience, the receipt of health care, medical history, genetic information, or the evidence of insurability. This prohibition on using a health status factor to deny coverage or set rates will be extended to health insurance in the individual market starting in 2014. In addition, the ACA gives the HHS Secretary the authority to designate other health status-related factors for both the group and individual insurance markets.[65]

Guaranteed Availability of Coverage

HIPAA also requires health insurers in the group market and group health plans to make coverage available to any individual who wants to be covered, assuming the applicant meets the group health plan's eligibility requirements, and to any employer that wishes to purchase an insurance policy. The ACA extends the guaranteed availability requirements to the individual insurance market starting in 2014.[66] As a result, a health insurer selling coverage in the individual market is not permitted to deny coverage to anyone that applies for coverage.

However, the ACA does not require payers to sell guaranteed coverage on a continuous basis, but allows them to restrict enrollment to open- or special-enrollment periods.[67] Open-enrollment periods are to be defined by the states; the minimum is 1 month per year, and the maximum is continuous open enrollment, meaning individuals and groups could opt in and out at will. Special events are generally the same as the "qualified life events" described in Chapters 17 and 29, for example, losing coverage associated with one's job or the birth of a child.

---

*Examples of different ways of looking at the number of people covered under one policy are described in Chapter 22.

Wellness Programs

As discussed above, HIPAA (in the group insurance market and for group health plans) and amendments made by the ACA (for all insurance markets and group health plans) prohibit the use of a health status factor to determine the premium rate paid by any enrollee. HIPAA recognized an exception that allows premiums to vary based on the participation by an enrollee in a "bona fide" wellness program.[68] The ACA adopted these regulations with a few modifications and extended them to health insurance coverage sold in the individual market.

The wellness program requirements apply where a premium discount or rebate or other reward is based on an individual satisfying a health status factor. For example, a wellness program that lowers the enrollee's monthly premium if they lose a certain amount of weight or meet a body mass index (BMI) target. Other types of wellness programs that are not based on a requirement to meet a health status factor target (such as a program that pays fitness center memberships) are permissible.[69] To qualify, a wellness program that is based on a health status factor must meet the following requirements:[70]

- The reward for the wellness program, together with rewards for other programs under the insurance or plan, cannot exceed 30% of the total cost of coverage; for example, if the employee and employer pay $1,000 per year in premiums, the wellness program incentive cannot exceed $300. The HHS Secretary is authorized to increase this percentage by up to 50% by regulation.
- The program must be reasonably designed to promote health or prevent disease.
- The wellness program must not be a subterfuge for discrimination against enrollees based on a health status factor.
- Individuals participating in the program must be given the opportunity to qualify for a reward at least once each year.
- The full reward must be made available to all individuals who qualify for participation in the program.
- Individuals must be given an alternative incentive target to satisfy if they are unable to meet the criteria based on a determination by their physician that the health status factor makes it unreasonably difficult to qualify. For example, a program that offers a reward based on the enrollee walking at least 1 mile per day must be given an alternative target such as weight loss, if their physician indicates it is medically inadvisable for them to walk any significant distances.
- All wellness program materials must describe the terms of the wellness program and the availability of a reasonable alternative standard.

Coverage for Approved Clinical Trials

Starting in 2014, all health insurers and group health plans must provide coverage to pay routine patient costs for items and services furnished in connection with participation in a clinical trial for the prevention, detection, or treatment of a life-threatening disease such as cancer. If a health insurer or group health plan requires enrollees to be treated through a network provider, they may require the qualified individual to use a network provider who is taking part in the clinical trial.[71]

Essential Health Benefits

Starting in 2014, health insurance coverage that is offered in the individual and small group markets[72] and qualified health insurance plans offered through the new state health insurance exchanges (discussed in more detail later)[73] must meet standards for "essential health benefits" and limitations on the amount of cost-sharing (deductibles, copayments, and co-insurance). The Secretary of Health and Human Services is required by the ACA to define essential health benefits, which must include the following categories of coverage:[74]

- Ambulatory patient services;
- Emergency services;
- Hospitalization;
- Maternity and newborn care;
- Mental health and substance use disorder services;
- Prescription drugs;
- Rehabilitative and habilitative services and devices;
- Laboratory services;
- Preventive and wellness services;
- Pediatric services; and
- Chronic disease management.

The HHS Secretary is required to ensure that the essential health benefits package "is equal to the scope of benefits provided under a typical employer plan. . . ."[75] In addition, the HHS Secretary must periodically review and update the essential benefits package as necessary to address any gaps in coverage. To facilitate this, the Secretary has requested the Institute of Medicine to formulate recommendations for the criteria and methods for determining and updating the essential health benefits package.[76]

The essential benefits coverage also must meet standards for "actuarial value." Actuarial value is determined based on the level of coverage expected to be provided to a standard population as a percentage of the cost paid for coverage.[77]

There are four actuarial value categories:

- Bronze level—60% actuarial value.
- Silver level—70% actuarial value.
- Gold level—80% actuarial value.
- Platinum level—90% actuarial value.

These levels do not refer to coinsurance, but to cost-sharing in aggregate. For example, an actuarial value of 70% means that a standard population enrolled in the Silver level coverage would be expected to have claims for health care services paid in an amount that is at least 70% of the in-network cost, net of deductibles, co-insurance, and copayments. The actuarial value specifically does not include premiums, balance billing amounts for non-network providers, or spending for noncovered services.[78]

Existing consumer-directed health plans (CDHPs; see Chapter 2) fit comfortably within a Bronze level of coverage. Even so, Congress recognized that individuals who are young and healthy are the least likely to purchase health insurance, and will be even less likely to do so when they can no longer buy it at the very low premium rates available before 2014 when new rating requirements go into effect. The ACA addresses this by permitting health insurers to offer a catastrophic coverage "young adult" plan in the individual or small group markets or through a state exchange if they are under 30 years of age. The catastrophic coverage plan may also be available to individuals if they are unable to afford other coverage, either by qualifying for a hardship exemption from the individual mandate as determined by HHS, or the cost of available coverage exceeds 8% of the individual's income. The catastrophic plan must cover essential benefits but may impose deductibles equal to the out-of-pocket cost limits required for high-deductible health plans (HDHPs) associated with tax-advantaged health savings accounts (HSAs); the annual out-of-pocket cost limits for HDHPs in 2011 is $5,950 for self-only coverage, and $11,900 for family coverage.[79] However, the plan must not impose any cost-sharing for preventive services or for three physician office visits before the deductible is met.[80]

State Health Insurance Exchanges

A key mechanism created by the ACA for expanding access to coverage for individuals and small businesses are the state health insurance exchanges that are scheduled to go into operation in 2014.[81] States may choose to have a single exchange or operate separate exchanges for individuals and for small employers (the Small Business Health Options Program or SHOP Exchange). In addition, a state may choose to operate regional exchanges within a state. If a state does not create an exchange mechanism by 2014, HHS is authorized to contract with one or more entities to establish an exchange in the state.[82] (Exchanges are also addressed in Chapter 16.)

All individuals and small employers (employers with up to 100 workers) in a state are permitted to obtain coverage through an exchange. States have the option to define the small group market as employers with up to 50 employees until 2016.[83] States may also allow large groups (employers

with over 100 employees) to purchase coverage through an exchange starting in 2017.[84]

Health insurers will be allowed, but not required, to sell qualified health plans (QHPs) through the exchange that meet the essential benefit and actuarial value standards discussed above. Health insurers offering qualified health plans through the exchange must agree to offer at least one plan at the Silver level and one plan at the Gold level in each state where they participate.[85] The HHS Secretary is required to develop rating systems based on quality and price for qualified health plans in each of the four benefit levels.[86]

The HHS Secretary is required to develop standards for QHPs that cover, at a minimum, the following requirements:

- Marketing standards; for example, plans are prohibited from marketing practices or benefit designs that discourage enrollment by individuals with significant health needs;
- Requirements to ensure that there are sufficient choice of health care providers to meet the needs of enrollees;
- Inclusion of essential community providers to serve low-income, medically underserved individuals;
- Requirements to meet clinical quality measures and standards for consumer access, utilization management, provider credentialing, network adequacy and access, complaints and appeals, and patient information programs;
- Provisions to implement a quality improvement strategy;
- Utilization of uniform enrollment forms and standard formats for presenting health benefits plan options;
- Provision of information to enrollees and prospective enrollees on quality measures for health plan performance; and
- Annual reporting to HHS on pediatric quality reporting measures.

Exchanges must require qualified health plans to make information available to the public on the following:

- Claims payment policies and practices;
- Periodic financial disclosures;
- Data on enrollment and disenrollment;
- Information on the number of claims that are denied;
- Data on rating practices;
- Information on cost-sharing and out-of-network payments; and
- Information on enrollee rights.

In addition, QHPs shall make information available to individuals on the amount of cost-sharing (deductibles, copayments, and insurance) under the individual's plan. All disclosures shall be in plain language that can be readily understood by the intended audience, including individuals with limited English proficiency.[87]

Multistate Plans

The Office of Personnel Management (OPM), the government agency responsible for personnel matters involving federal employees, is required by the ACA to contract with health insurers to offer at least two QHPs in each state exchange on a multistate basis. At least one of the insurers must be nonprofit.[88] The contract must address the multistate plan's medical loss ratio, profit margin, premiums, and other terms and conditions that are similar to provisions in the Federal Employees Health Benefits (FEHB) program. The plan must meet the state exchange requirements and provisions applicable to qualified health plans.

Consumer Operated and Oriented Plans

The ACA provides that the Department of Health and Human Services shall create a program to encourage the formation of consumer-operated and -oriented plans (CO-OPs) as nonprofit entities to offer insurance coverage in the individual and small group markets and state insurance exchanges. The Act included funding for loans and grants for CO-OP startup costs.[89] (CO-OPs are discussed in more detail in Chapter 4.) In general, the CO-OP must comply with the following standards:

- Health insurers in existence prior to July 16, 2009, and governmental organizations may not participate in the program;
- Governance must rest with the members of the CO-OP;
- CO-OPs must comply with all applicable state insurance laws regarding solvency, licensure, network adequacy, filing of premium rates and forms, and premium assessments;
- The organization must follow restrictions on lobbying activities;
- All CO-OP profits must inure to the benefit of its members through lower premiums, improved benefits, or other programs to improve the delivery of health care quality; and
- The entity must meet requirements applicable to nonprofit organizations under Section 501(c) of the Federal Tax Code.[90]

■ ADMINISTRATIVE SIMPLIFICATION

As discussed in Chapters 23 and 29, HIPAA established standards for electronic health care transactions between covered entities such as health insurers (including HMOs), TPAs, health care providers, and health care clearinghouses such as claims, payments, and eligibility inquiries. These standards provide a uniform system of data exchange to streamline the administrative process and to eliminate the exchange of paper documents.[91]

The ACA added a number of additional requirements intended to further encourage the use of electronic data transactions in health care and health care financing.[92]

The Department of Health and Human Services was directed to add an additional transaction for electronic funds transfers and to develop a series of "operating rules" for each transaction. These operating rules define the business rules for how transactions are conducted between health plans, providers, and clearinghouses.[93] The primary focus of the operating rules requirement is on the implementation of standardized transactions, as well as the means of electronic connectivity, although they may be developed for other covered operations as well. The ACA also requires health plans to certify that they are complying with the electronic transaction standards or pay penalties. These provisions are required to be implemented over the new few years. The new administrative simplification requirements are addressed further in Chapter 23.

■ REVENUE AND TAX PROVISIONS

The ACA included a number of tax and revenue provisions affecting individuals, employers, health insurers, and health care providers, including new taxes, a subsidy to assist low-income individuals with the purchase of health coverage through state insurance exchanges, and requirements for individuals and employers to maintain coverage or pay a penalty.

Subsidies for Purchase of Exchange Coverage

Starting in 2014, the ACA provides subsidies to assist low-income individuals with the purchase of coverage through the exchange. The subsidy is in the form of either a "refundable" or "advancable" tax credit. The subsidy is available for individuals with household incomes between 100% and 400% of the federal poverty level (FPL).[94] Household income is the taxpayer's modified adjusted income together with the modified adjusted gross income (AGI) of all other individuals in the taxpayer's family size for purposes of the credit. Modified AGI is the taxpayer's adjusted gross income plus any interest received or accrued during the tax year.[95]

The amount of the subsidies is based on the premium cost of the second lowest-cost silver plan offered in the exchange in the area where the individual resides (for self-only or family coverage). The subsidy amount is based on the percentage of income the premium represents. The subsidies are provided on a sliding scale, shown in **Table 30-2**.

In general, an individual is eligible to obtain a subsidy for the purchase of coverage through the exchange if they meet the household income requirements and if they do not have access to affordable coverage through an employer. Employer coverage is "unaffordable" if either: (1) the actuarial value of the coverage is less than 60% or (2) the premium they are required to pay is 9.5% or more of their household income.[96]

In addition, a cost-sharing subsidy is provided to reduce the individual's annual cost-sharing responsibilities for the plan purchased through the exchange.[97] The amount of the

TABLE 30-2 Premium Subsidies		
Household AGI (as a percentage of FPL)	**Initial premium**	**Final premium**
100–133%	2.0%	3.0%
133–150%	3.0%	4.0%
150–200%	4.0%	6.3%
200–250%	6.3%	8.05%
250–300%	8.05%	9.5%
300–400%	9.5%	9.5%

TABLE 30-3 Individual Responsibility Fines		
Year	**Penalty dollar amount**	**Penalty percentage of income amount**
2014	$95	1.0%
2015	$325	2.0%
2016	$695	2.5%

reduction is tied to the statutory out-of-pocket limits for HSA-qualified HDHPs as described earlier. For individuals with household income greater than 100% of FPL but not more than 200% of FPL, the out-of-pocket limit on the plan will be reduced by two-thirds. For individuals with household income between 201%o of FPL and 300% of FPL, the limits are reduced by one-half. In the case of individuals with household income between 301% of FPL and 400% of FPL, the out-of-pocket limits are reduced by one-third.

Individual Responsibility Mandate

Starting in 2014, all U.S. citizens and legal residents will be required to maintain qualified coverage or pay a penalty, unless they are exempted. Qualified coverage is defined to include:

- Government-sponsored health programs such as Medicare, Medicaid, Indian Health Service, or TRICARE;
- An eligible employer-sponsored plan, including a self-funded or insured group health plan, church plan, or government employee plan;
- Health insurance offered in the individual market; and
- Coverage purchased through a state insurance exchange.[98]

An individual can be exempted if:

- They meet a religious conscience standard;
- Are below the income threshold for filing federal income taxes;
- Are without insurance coverage for 3 months or less during the year;
- Are in prison, or
- Whose coverage options are "unaffordable," meaning the cost of the lowest-cost Bronze plan in the exchange in their state exceeds 8% of their household income.[99]

The penalty is determined based on the number of months during the year a taxpayer and any dependents do not have qualified coverage. The penalty is the greater of (a) $695 per year per each family member up to a maximum

of three family members ($2,085) or (b) 2.5% of the household income. However, these penalty amounts will be phased in as shown in **Table 30-3**.

Employer Responsibility Mandate

Also starting in 2014, employers with 50 or more full-time employees will be required to offer health coverage.[100] The penalty is applied as follows:

- Employers that do not offer health coverage and have at least one FTE receiving a subsidy for coverage purchased through a state insurance exchange will pay a penalty of $2,000 multiplied by the total number of full-time employees at the business (however, the first 30 FTEs are deducted for purposes of the penalty calculation).
- Employers that offer health coverage and that have at least one FTE receiving a subsidy for coverage purchased through the exchange must pay a penalty of $3,000 for each full-time employee covered through the exchange. As discussed above, an individual who purchases coverage through an exchange is not eligible for the subsidy if they have an "affordable" employer coverage option (i.e., the employer plan is at least the 60% actuarial value level or the employee's share of the premium cost does not exceed 9.5% of their household income).

Health Insurance Taxes

The ACA imposes two new taxes on health insurers that will result in increased health care costs for purchasers. They are described as follows.

Comparative Effectiveness Fee

The ACA establishes a new fee that will be assessed against health insurers in the individual and group markets and self-funded group health plans to help fund the cost of the Patient-Centered Outcomes Research Trust Fund. The fee will help fund research on the clinical effectiveness of health care treatments, procedures, therapies, medical devices, and pharmaceuticals.[101] The amount of the fee is as follows:

- For policy or plan years ending during fiscal year 2013 (i.e., October 1, 2012, through September 30, 2013), $1.00 for each covered life;

- For policy or plan years ending during fiscal year 2014 (i.e., October 1, 2013, through September 30, 2014), $2.00 for each covered life; and
- For policy or plan years ending in fiscal years after September 30, 2014, the fee is equal to the dollar amount for the preceding fiscal year multiplied by the percentage increase in the projected per capita amount of National Health Expenditures as most recently published before the beginning of the fiscal year.

Fee on Health Insurance Providers

Starting in 2014 an annual fee will be imposed on any health insurer providing coverage in connection with any United States health risk, for example, major medical, dental, and vision insurance. Self-funded group health plans are not required to pay the fee.[102] The aggregate annual fee is divided among all covered health insurers based on the net premiums written. The aggregate annual fee is as follows:

- 2014—$8.0 billion,
- 2015—$11.3 billion,
- 2016—$11.3 billion,
- 2017—$13.9 billion,
- 2018—$14.3 billion, and
- 2019 and thereafter—indexed to medical inflation.

■ LEGAL AND POLITICAL CHALLENGES

The ACA was controversial when it was enacted and that controversy has not stopped. At the time of publication, some polls showed that over half of Americans view the legislation unfavorably.[103] This view has translated into legal and political challenges to the law. It is a difficult topic to address in the chapter of a book since, by its nature, politics is volatile and how the political process will affect the law is simply not known at the time of publication. The political process may result in certain elements being changed in significant ways, or even eliminated.

Many in Congress remain opposed to the ACA and are attempting to repeal the law or "defund" the regulatory agencies charged with implementation. In the states, some governors and legislatures have refused to take action on specific ACA requirements such as establishment of insurance exchanges. The public opposition and attempts by Congress and state legislatures and governors to subvert the ACA requirements raises challenges to federal regulatory agencies attempting to implement the legislation, and to health insurers that are required to comply with its provisions.

In addition, at the time of publication, a number of legal actions had been filed arguing that the law is unconstitutional. In particular, the requirement that individuals maintain health coverage or pay a fine has been challenged on the basis that Congress lacks authority to penalize individuals for failure to take an action, referring to the purchase of

health insurance coverage. As of the writing of this chapter, the decisions handed down by the federal courts are mixed, with some courts dismissing the lawsuits outright, others denying the challenges to the law, and still other courts finding the law unconstitutional in whole or in part. The U.S. Supreme Court has agreed to address the ACA during its 2012 term, and it will decide whether, and to what extent, the provisions of the ACA will be carried out before the end of that term.

Since the Supreme Court ruling takes place after the publication date of this book, the reader will need to discover what elements, if any, described in this chapter or throughout the book have been changed in some substantial way. As noted elsewhere in the book, an excellent and unbiased source for this is the Kaiser Family Foundation, whose main website address is www.kff.org.

■ CONCLUSION

As discussed in this chapter, the ACA, if upheld by the courts and relatively unchanged by the political process, will have a significant effect on all segments of the health care system. The immediate reform provisions are already resulting in changes to the health benefits offered by health insurers and group health plans. Increasing regulation and oversight of health insurers and new processes to provide access to health coverage will ultimately add to the cost and complexity of health care financing. While it is still too early to gauge the impact of the cost of, and access to, health coverage, it is clear that how managed care is provided to Americans will be different after 2014, at least for some. How stakeholders, including health insurers and HMOs respond to these changes will determine the future of managed care systems.

Endnotes

1   The Patient Protection and Affordable Care Act (P.L. 111-148) as amended by the Health Care and Education Reconciliation Act of 2010 (P.L. 111-152), which was signed into law on March 30, 2010. For purposes of this chapter, the ACA includes both laws.

2   The full legislative history can be viewed at the U.S. Congress website, www.thomas.gov.

3   Dorn S, Hill I, Hogan S. "The Secrets of Massachusetts' Success: Why 97 Percent of State Residents Have Health Coverage," the Urban Institute and Robert Wood Johnson Foundation (November 2009).

4   ACA Section 1251, 42 U.S.C. §18011.

5   29 C.F.R. §2590.715-1251, 45 C.F.R. §147.140.

6   29 C.F.R. §2590.715-1251(g)(4) [Example 2], 45 C.F.R. §147.140(g)(4) [Example 2].

7   ACA Section 1001, 42 U.S.C. §300gg-11.

8   ACA Section 1302, 42 U.S.C. §18022.
9   ACA Section 1311, 42 U.S.C. §1303 and ACA Section 1201, 42 U.S.C. 300gg-61.
10 26 C.F.R. §54.9815-2711T(d), 29 C.F.R. §2590.715-2711(d), 45 C.F.R. §147.126(d).
11 Ibid.
12 See Department of Health and Human Services, OCIIO Sub-Regulatory Guidance (OCIIO 2010–1): Process for Obtaining Waivers of the Annual Limits Requirements of PHS Act Section 2711 (September 3, 2010).
13 ACA Section 1001, 42 U.S.C. §300gg-13.
14 29 C.F.R. §2590.715-2713(b), 45 C.F.R. §147.130(b).
15 ACA Section 1001, 42 U.S.C. §300gg-19a(b).
16 Ibid.
17 ACA Section 1001, 42 U.S.C. §300gg-19a(a).
18 ACA Section 1001, 42 U.S.C. §300gg-19a(c).
19 ACA Section 1001, 42 U.S.C. §300gg-19a(d).
20 29 C.F.R. §2590.715-2719A(a)(4), 45 C.F.R. §147.138(a)(4).
21 29 U.S.C. §1181, 42 U.S.C. §300gg.
22 ACA Section 1201, 42 U.S.C. §300gg-3 and ACA Section 1255 (effective date of the prohibition on applying preexisting limits to health coverage for children up to age 19).
23 ACA Section 1001, 42 U.S.C. §300gg-14 and ACA Section 1251 (provision regarding grandfathered group health plans).
24 29 C.F.R. §2590.715-2714(f), 45 C.F.R. §147.120(f).
25 See Department of Health and Human Services, "Questions and Answers on Enrollment of Children Under 19 Under the New Policy That Prohibits Pre-Existing Condition Exclusions" (October 13, 2010).
26 ACA Section 1001, 42 U.S.C. §300gg-12.
27 29 C.F.R. §2590.715-2712(a)(2), 45 C.F.R. §147.128(a)(2).
28 29 C.F.R. §2590.715-2712(a)(3), 45 C.F.R. §147.128(a)(3).
29 29 C.F.R. §2590.715-2712(a)(1), 45 C.F.R. §147.128(a)(1).
30 ACA Section 1001, 42 U.S.C. §300gg-15.
31 http://naic.org/documents/committees_b_consumer_information_ppaca_instructions_group_insurers.pdf. Accessed August 27, 2011.
32 Ibid.
33 Ibid.
34 ACA Section 1103, 42 U.S.C. §18003.
35 Ibid.
36 ACA Section 1001, 42 U.S.C. §300gg-19.
37 29 C.F.R. 2590.715-2719(a)(2), 45 C.F.R. §147.136(a)(2). The regulations cross-reference the definition of an adverse benefit determination included in the ERISA claims rule (29 C.F.R. §2560.503-1).
38 "Culturally and linguistically appropriate" notices are required to meet requirements for communications to individuals with limited English proficiency. See 29 C.F.R. §2590.715-2719(e) and 45 C.F.R. §147.136(e).
39 29 C.F.R. §2590.715-2719(b)(3), 45 C.F.R. §147.136(b)(3).
40 Ibid.
41 ACA Section 1001, 42 U.S.C. §300gg-19.
42 The "state process" is described at 29 C.F.R. §2590.715-2719(c), 45 C.F.R. §147.136(c), and guidance from the Department of Health and Human Services released on August 26, 2010 ("Technical Guidance for Interim Procedures for Federal External Review Relating to Internal Claims and Appeals and External Review for Health Insurance Issuers in the Group and Individual Markets under the Patient Protection and Affordable Care Act"). The "federal process" is described at 29 C.F.R. §2590.715-2719(d), 45 C.F.R. §147.136(d), and Technical Release 2010-01 issued by the Department of Labor on August 23, 2010.
43 29 C.F.R. §2590.715-2719(c)(2), 45 C.F.R. §147.136 (c)(2).
44 29 C.F.R. §2590.715-2719(d)(1), 45 C.F.R. §147.136(d)(1).
45 ACA Section 1001, 42 U.S.C. §300gg-18.
46 45 C.F.R. §158.103 (prior to 2016, states may choose to limit the small group market to businesses with up to 50 employees).
47 45 C.F.R. §158.210 et seq.
48 45 C.F.R. §158.301 et seq.
49 For a discussion of the waiver process and the factors impacting health insurer MLRs in the individual market, see the Preamble to the Interim Final Rule on the Medical Loss Ratio Requirements, 75 Fed. Reg. 74886 et seq. (December 1, 2010).
50 ACA Section 1003, 42 U.S.C. §300gg-94.
51 45 C.F.R. §§154.215 and 154.230.
52 45 C.F.R. §154.200.
53 ACA Section 1002, 42 U.S.C. §300gg-94.
54 ACA Section 1001, 42 U.S.C. §300gg-17.
55 Ibid.
56 ACA Section 1101, 42 U.S.C. §18001.
57 45 C.F.R. §152.14(a).
58 45 C.F.R. §152.1 et seq.
59 ACA Section 1102, 42 U.S.C. §18002.
60 Centers for Medicare and Medicaid Services Notice (CMS 9996-N), published in the *Federal Register* on April 5, 2010 (76 Fed. Reg. 18766).
61 ACA Section 1421, 26 U.S.C. §45R.
62 IRS Notice 2010-82 (December 2, 2010).
63 ACA Section 1201, 42 U.S.C. §300gg-3.
64 ACA Section 1201, 42 U.S.C. §300gg.
65 ACA Section 1201, 42 U.S.C. §300gg-4.
66 ACA Section 1201, 42 U.S.C. §300gg-1.
67 ACA Section 1201, 42 U.S.C. §300gg–1.
68 29 C.F.R. §2590.702, 45 C.F.R. §146.121.
69 ACA Section 1201, 42 U.S.C. §300gg-4.
70 Ibid.
71 ACA Section 1201, 42 U.S.C. §300gg-8.
72 ACA Section 1201, 42 U.S.C. §300gg-6.
73 ACA Section 1301, 42 U.S.C. §1804.
74 ACA Section 1302, 42 U.S.C. §18022.
75 Ibid.

76 www8.nationalacademies.org/cp/projectview. aspx?key = IOM-HCS-10-04. Accessed August 27, 2011.

77 McDevitt R. "Actuarial Value: A Method for Comparing Health Plan Benefits," California HealthCare Foundation (October 2008).

78 ACA Section 1302, 42 U.S.C. §18022(c)(3)(B).

79 www.treasury.gov/resource-center/faqs/Taxes/ Pages/HSA-2011-indexed-amounts.aspx. Accessed August 26, 2011.

80 ACA Section 1302, 42 U.S.C. §18022(e).

81 ACA Section 1311, 42 U.S.C. §3031.

82 ACA Section 1311, 42 U.S.C. §13031.

83 ACA Section 1304, 42 U.S.C. §18024.

84 ACA Section 1311, 42 U.S.C. §13031.

85 ACA Section 1301, 42 U.S.C. §18021.

86 Ibid.

87 ACA Section 1311, 42 U.S.C. §13031(e).

88 ACA Section 1334, 42 U.S.C. §18054.

89 ACA Section 1322, 42 U.S.C. §1322.

90 IRS Notice 2011-23 (March 11, 2011).

91 42 U.S.C. §1301 et seq.

92 ACA Section 1104, 42 U.S.C. §1320d et seq.

93 Ibid.

94 ACA Sections 1401, 1411 and 1422, 26 U.S.C. §36B.

95 Ibid.

96 Ibid.

97 ACA Section 1402, 42 U.S.C. §18071.

98 ACA Section 1501, 26 U.S.C. §5000A, 42 U.S.C. §18091.

99 Ibid.

100 ACA Section 1513, 26 U.S.C. §4980H.

101 ACA Section 6301, 42 U.S.C. §1320e-2.

102 ACA Section 9010.

103 A Kaiser Health Tracking Poll taken in March 2011 shows 46% of respondents view the ACA unfavorably while 42% had a favorable view of the legislation. "Kaiser Health Tracking Poll," Kaiser Family Foundation (March 2011).

Glossary of Terms and Acronyms*

24/7: Slang that means something is available 24 hours per day, 7 days per week. For example, the nurse advice line is available 24/7.

AAAHC: See Accreditation Association for Ambulatory Health Care.

AAC: See Actual Acquisition Cost.

AAHC: See American Accreditation HealthCare Commission.

Abandon Rate: The percentage of calls where the caller hangs up before reaching a live CSR due to lengthy average speed to answer times.

ABN: See Advanced Beneficiary Notice of Noncoverage.

Abuse or Health Care Abuse: A term that is not as well defined as fraud, abuse typically occurs if an activity abuses the health care system but does not meet the legal definition of fraud or is not medically necessary; for example, using billing codes that are related to, but pay higher than, the service actually provided, or charging outrageous fees.

ACA: Abbreviation commonly used for the Patient Protection and Affordable Care Act. See the latter for further definition.

Access Fee: A fee charged by a PPO or HMO for access to its provider network, including its payment terms, by an employer or another payer. See also Rental PPO.

Accountable Care Organization (ACO): The term coined by CMS and MedPAC, and now used in the ACA, to describe an organized group of physicians, possibly including a hospital, that are supposed to coordinate the care for beneficiaries in traditional FFS Medicare with high medical costs. Those beneficiaries are not locked in or required to use the ACO. CMS assigns or attributes them to the ACO through statistical means. An overall target cost is calculated, and the ACO shares in savings if costs are less than the target,

but pays back a portion of what they were paid if costs exceed the target. Despite being specifically addressed in the ACA, it is not known yet whether or not they will work.

Accreditation: Certification by a qualified neutral agency that an organization meets defined criteria for participation in a program. For payers, this means accreditation by NCQA, URAC, or (less commonly) AAAHC. For health care facilities, it most commonly means accreditation by JCI or, for ambulatory facilities, JCI or AAAHC. Other agencies exist for different types of facilities such as rehabilitation, osteopathy, and so forth. See also Deeming.

Accreditation Association for Ambulatory Health Care (AAAHC): An accreditation agency that focuses on ambulatory facilities such as ASCs, endoscopy centers, dialysis centers, and so forth. It is also one of three accreditation agencies certified by CMS to accredit MA plans, along with NCQA and URAC.

Accrete: The term used by CMS for the process of adding new Medicare enrollees to a plan. See also Delete.

Accrual: The amount of money that is set aside to cover expenses. The accrual is the plan's best estimate of what those expenses are and (for medical expenses) is based on a combination of data from the authorization system, the claims system, the lag studies, and the plan's prior history.

ACD: See Automated Call Distributor.

ACGs: See Ambulatory Care Groups.

ACO: See Accountable Care Organization.

ACR: See Adjusted Community Rate.

Actual Acquisition Cost (AAC): The actual cost a pharmacy paid to acquire a drug, as opposed to a published average. Usually applicable to generics and devices.

---

*These are working definitions of common terms and acronyms in the managed health care industry and related health care sectors. In an industry this dynamic, it is not possible to list every term or acronym in use since new ones come into use faster than any publication can keep up with. Other terms will become obsolete or fall out of use while this book is still in print, especially in the case of governmental agencies and programs. Some definitions in this glossary may also be disputed by others in the industry, and the editor is open to receiving such communication from any such nitpickers.

Actuarial Assumptions: The assumptions that an actuary uses in calculating the expected costs and revenues of the plan. Examples include utilization rates, age and sex mix of enrollees, and cost for medical services.

Actuarial Equivalent: The term is used in two similar but separate ways. In the ACA, it refers to an aggregate level of cost-sharing; for example, a Silver Plan has the actuarial equivalent of 30% cost-sharing, meaning the total of all deductibles, copayments, and coinsurance for an average member adds up to 30%. Under Medicare Advantage, it's a health benefit plan that offers similar coverage to a standard benefit plan. Actuarially equivalent plans will not necessarily have the same premiums, cost-sharing requirements, or even benefits; however, the *expected* spending by insurers for the different plans will be the same.

ADGs: See Ambulatory Diagnostic Groups.

Adjudication: The management and processing of claims by a payer or health insurance company.

Adjusted Average Per Capita Cost (AAPCC): CMS's estimate of the amount of money it costs to care for Medicare recipients under FFS Medicare in a given area. The AAPCC is made up of 142 different rate cells; 140 of them are factored for age, sex, Medicaid eligibility, institutional status, working age, and whether a person has both Part A and Part B of Medicare. The two remaining cells are for individuals with end-stage renal disease. Once used to set payments to private Medicare plans, it has been replaced with a payment model that factors in a beneficiary's level of illness.

Adjusted Community Rate (ACR): Used in the past by Medicare managed care plans. It is being phased out and replaced with an acuity-based methodology.

Administrative Contract Services (ACS) Contract: See Administrative Services Only.

Administrative Services Only (ASO): An ASO contract is between an insurance company or health plan administrator and a self-funded plan where the insurance company or administrator performs administrative services only and does not assume any risk. Services usually include claims processing and member services, but may include other services such as actuarial analysis, utilization review, and so forth. See also ERISA.

Admitted Asset: A financial asset of a health plan that can be converted to cash on short notice. See also Nonadmitted Asset, Net Worth, and Risk-Based Capital.

Advanced Beneficiary Notice of Noncoverage (ABN): A form designated by CMS for use by providers and suppliers for all situations where Medicare payment is expected to be denied.

Adverse Selection: The problem of attracting members who are sicker than the general population (specifically, members who are sicker than was anticipated when the budget for medical costs was developed).

Affordable Care Act (ACA): See Patient Protection and Affordable Care Act.

Age Band or Age-Banding: Applicable primarily to the individual insurance market, age-banding means putting individuals into different age groups for purposes of premium rate adjustments, with younger individuals paying lower premiums than older ones. Under the ACA, the maximum difference between the lowest and highest age-banded premiums is 3:1 as of 2014.

Agency for Healthcare Research and Quality (AHRQ): A federal agency charged with addressing a wide array of quality-related issues and evidence-based standards of care. An excellent resource for the most current thinking on these topics.

Agent: A person who is authorized by an HMO or an insurer to act on its behalf to negotiate, sell, and service coverage contracts. May be self-employed, employed by an agency, or employed by a broker.

AHIP: See America's Health Insurance Plans.

AHP: See Association Health Plan.

AHRQ: See Agency for Healthcare Research and Quality.

All Payer: A term that refers to the government, state or federal, setting payment rates for defined health services, which all payers, public and private, must follow. Potentially applies to hospitals and/or physicians. Used in many European nations but not (so far) in the United States with some exceptions at the state level. Also referred to as all payer rates or all payer fee schedule.

Allowed Charge: The maximum charge that a payer (such as Medicare or Medicaid) will pay for a specific service, even if the amount billed is greater than the allowed charge. This does not mean that it will be paid, however; cost-sharing by the member or beneficiary may still apply (e.g., a deductible or coinsurance).

ALOS: See LOS.

Alternative Medicine: See Complementary and Alternative Medicine.

Ambulatory Care Groups (ACGs): A method of categorizing outpatient episodes. There are 51 mutually exclusive ACGs, which are based on resource use over time, and modified by principle diagnosis, age, and sex. See also ADGs, APGs, and APCs.

Ambulatory Diagnostic Groups (ADGs): A method of categorizing outpatient episodes. There are 34 possible ADGs. See also ACGs and APGs.

Ambulatory Patient Classification (APC): A payment methodology used by CMS for payment to facilities for ambulatory services. Like DRGs, APCs bundle various charges into a single payment. Unlike DRGs, they are based primarily on procedures, not diagnoses. They also differ from DRGs in that they can be added together, while DRGs are used in a hierarchy for purposes of calculating payment. APCs are an outgrowth of APGs.

Ambulatory Patient Group (APG): A payment methodology developed by 3M Health Information Systems for CMS, but also used by some commercial health plans and by many state Medicaid agencies. APGs are to outpatient procedures what DRGs are to inpatient days. APGs provide for a fixed payment to an institution for outpatient procedures or visits, but unlike DRGS, they are based primarily on the procedure or procedures performed instead of the diagnosis. APGs prevent unbundling of ancillary services. Also see ACGs, ADGs, and APCs.

Ambulatory Surgical Category (ASC): The term also used by Medicare in its Hospital Outpatient Prospective Payment System (HOPPS) program. This use is specifically referring to a payment term using CMS's methodology.

Ambulatory Surgical Center (ASC): A facility for ambulatory procedures. The term is generally applied to several different types of outpatient facilities, not all of which are actually surgical such as dialysis facilities, endoscopy facilities, and so forth. This use is specifically referring to a facility.

American Accreditation HealthCare Commission (AAHC): A name once used by URAC, but not anymore. See URAC.

American National Standards Institute (ANSI): ANSI develops and maintains standards for electronic data interchange. HIPAA mandates the use of ANSI X 12N standards for electronic transactions in the health care system.

America's Health Insurance Plans (AHIP): The primary trade organization of managed care organizations. Their areas of focus include legislative and lobbying efforts, education, certification of training in managed health care operations, and representation of the health insurance industry to the public. Initially there were three groups: the Group Health Association of America (GHAA), the American Managed Care and Review Association (AMCRA), and the Health Insurance Association of America (HIAA). These predecessor organizations represented different types of health plan constituencies. GHAA and AMCRA merged to form the American Association of Health Plans (AAHP), which in turn merged with HIAA to form AHIP.

Ancillary Services: Health care services that are ordered by a physician, but provided by some other type of provider, for example, diagnostic testing or physician therapy. Does not apply to inpatient care, ambulatory procedures, or pharmacy.

Annual Limit: The maximum amount of coverage that a health plan will provide in a year. This may apply to either the aggregate of all costs in a year (e.g., coverage stops when costs exceed $1 million in a year), or it may apply to a specific service (e.g., no more than 20 behavioral health visits are covered in a year). Does not carry over into the next year. Some HMOs do not have annual limits on charges in the aggregate. Under the ACA, annual limits must be phased out for all benefits plans as of 2014.

ANSI: See American National Standards Institute.

Any Willing Provider (AWP): This is a form of state law that requires a payer to accept any provider willing to meet the terms and conditions in the payer's contract, whether the payer wants or needs that provider or not. Considered to be an expensive form of antimanaged care legislation.

APC: See Ambulatory Patient Classification.

APG: See Ambulatory Patient Group.

Appeal: A formal appeal by a member of a denial of coverage. It requires a response within a fixed timeframe. Under the ACA, a member can appeal at least twice—once for an internal review and once for an external review. It is not the same as a grievance.

ASA: See Average Speed to Answer (not to be confused with acetylsalicylic acid, aspirin).

ASC: See Ambulatory Surgical Center (facility term) or Ambulatory Surgical Category (payment term).

ASO: See Administrative Services Only.

ASP: See Average Sales Price.

Assignment of Benefits: A form signed by a patient directing their insurer to pay a nonparticipating provider directly, not paying the member. The member is still liable for whatever a nonparticipating provider bills versus what the plan pays. Health plans, especially Blue Cross and Blue Shield plans, long refused to directly pay nonparticipating providers since direct payment is a valuable reason to participate due to difficulties collecting from patients, even ones who receive a check from the insurer. Therefore, providers successfully lobbied state legislatures in several states to require it.

Association Health Plan: An association made up of smaller businesses that group together for purposes of providing health benefits to employees. This may be done by purchasing group health insurance in which all of the businesses in the association participate equally, or it may be done by creating a pool of employees sufficiently large so as to self-insure, thereby avoiding benefits mandates and premium taxes. See also MEWA and MET.

Attachment Point: A term used in reinsurance contracts, the attachment point is the size that a claim must be before any reinsurance coverage applies. For example, an 80/20 reinsurance contract with an attachment point of $100,000 means that if any individual incurred claims adding up to more than $100,000 in the contract period (usually a year), reinsurance would pay 80% of any amount in excess of $100,000.

Authorization: In the context of managed care, authorization refers to the need to obtain authorization before certain types of health care services are covered. Most commonly used in "gatekeeper"-type HMOs in which a PCP must authorize a referral to a specialist, or the HMO will not pay for the specialist visit. Sometimes referred to as preauthorization or preauth. Sometimes used synonymously with precertification (see Precertification); though no clear distinction is actually made, by convention authorization is applied more often to specialty referral services, while precertification is applied more often to facility-based services.

Auto-Adjudication: The complete processing of a claim without any manual intervention. May also be applied to claims processing following claims data entry, which is called claims capture. Claims capture is not a trivial cost, so comparing auto-adjudication rates between payers must use a consistent definition.

Automated Call Distributor (ACD): A computerized system to automatically route calls or contacts coming into a call center based on programmed distribution instructions.

Average Handle Time: The length of time it takes a CSR to resolve or complete a call or contact from a member.

Average Sales Price (ASP): A method to determine the amount that Medicare or a payer will pay for drugs, particularly biological or injectable drugs. It is based on the average price the manufacturers sells it for, not what is charged by whoever is administering it. Payment for giving the drug is usually the ASP plus 6%.

Average Speed to Answer (ASA): The average time it takes to answer a call, typically measured in seconds; it is commonly used in measuring the performance of a CSR.

Average Wholesale Price (AWP): Commonly used in pharmacy contracting, the AWP is generally determined through reference to a common source of information.

Avoidable Readmission: The unplanned readmission of a patient to a hospital within 30 or 60 days of discharge for the same medical problem or one related to the first admission, and that could have been prevented through intervention. For example, a patient with a chronic condition that does not receive office-based follow-up care from his or her doctor, or does not comply with his or her medications.

AWP: See Average Wholesale Price or Any Willing Provider.

BAA: See Business Associate Agreement.

Back Office: An informal term describing the administrative processes of a health plan; for example, claims processing or contract management.

Balance Billing: The practice of a provider billing a patient for all charges not paid for by the insurance plan, even if those charges are above the plan's UCR or are considered medically unnecessary. Managed care plans and service plans generally prohibit providers from balance billing except for allowed copays, coinsurance, and deductibles. Such prohibition against balance billing may even extend to the plan's failure to pay at all (e.g., because of bankruptcy).

Balanced Budget Act of 1997 (BBA '97): A sweeping piece of legislation, part of BBA '97, created the Medicare + Choice program (since replaced by Medicare Advantage) as well as demonstration MSAs.

BCBS: Blue Cross Blue Shield.

BD/K: See Bed Days per Thousand.

Bed Days per Thousand (BD/K): Also called Bed Days per Thousand per Year; a standard method of measuring inpatient utilization on an annualized basis. It is the number of hospital days that are used in a year for each thousand covered lives. It may be applied to differing time periods such as a single day, month-to-date, and year-to-date.

Behavioral Shift: A change in the behavior of an individual with health insurance or managed care coverage based on the design of the benefits. For example, higher cost-sharing may reduce unnecessary visits to the emergency department for nonurgent care.

Benefit Buy Down: Another term for increasing employee cost-sharing in order to reduce an employer's benefits costs. It's most often used by actuaries, underwriters, and benefits consultants.

Benefit Design: The exercise of designing a benefits package to effectively compete in the market by balancing the level of benefits and the costs.

Benefit Waiver: A part of most case management programs, benefit waiver means the case manager can authorize coverage for something that isn't normally a covered benefit in order to keep a member out of the hospital. For example, a plan may pay for a hospital bed in the home even though it does not cover durable medical equipment if it allows a member to receive home care rather than inpatient care.

Best Practices: If you do not know what those are, it is suggested that you turn to page 1, begin reading, and work your way back to this point.

Biologics: Refers to a type of specialty pharmacy drug that is biologic in nature. Usually created by recombinant DNA and administered via injection. Biologics exist for cancer, rheumatoid arthritis, anti-inflammatory diseases, and a host of other conditions. Usually extremely expensive, and often the focus of specialized utilization management by specialty pharmacy companies.

Biosimilar: A generic biologic drug, or a biologic drug that is similar enough to another one that it may be used in its place.

Book Rate: A premium rate developed using the experience of all individuals or groups in a specific block or pool. It may also be called a manual rate or a base rate. The book rate is used as the basis for calculating various market rates such as family rates, single rates, and so forth. See also Community Rating.

BPO: See Business Process Outsourcing.

Bridge: See Doughnut Hole.

Bronze Level of Benefits or Bronze Plan: As defined in the ACA, a qualified health benefits plan with the actuarial equivalent or average of 40% cost-sharing, when accounting for deductibles, copayments, and coinsurance as applied to in-network services.

Bundled Payment: An all-inclusive payment for all facility and professional services associated with an episode of care.

Business Associate: Under the privacy provisions of HIPAA, a business associate is a person or organization that, on behalf of a covered entity (health plan, health care clearinghouse, or health care provider) or organized health care arrangement, performs or assists in the performance of activities involving the use or disclosure of individually identifiable health information. A business associate is not an employee of the covered entity.

Business Associate Agreement (BAA): A contract between a covered entity under HIPAA and one of its business associates, requiring the business associate to comply with the privacy and security requirements placed upon covered entities.

Business Process Outsourcing (BPO): A form of outsourcing to a third party that focuses on one or more administrative processes of a payer such as claims or enrollment.

Buy Down: See Benefits Buy Down.

Cafeteria Plan: An informal term for a Flexible Benefits Plan; see Flexible Benefits Plan.

CAHPS®: See Consumer Assessment of Healthcare Providers and Systems.

Call Center: See Contact Center.

CAM: See Complementary and Alternative Medicine.

Capitated Risk Pool: See Risk Pool (Capitation).

Capitation: A set amount of money received or paid out; it is based on membership rather than on services delivered and usually is expressed in units of PMPM. May be varied by such factors as age and sex of the enrolled member.

Captive or Captive Insurer: The initial meaning was a restricted insurance company that provided coverage only for subsidiaries of its parent company or companies, not to the marketplace at large; for example, a national employer with a subsidiary providing long-term care insurance benefits to its employees. Captives are not subject to the same degree of regulation as regular insurers, and are often based offshore and regulated even less. Captives typically do not have reserves that are anywhere close to what commercial insurers do, putting them at more risk of failure; however, this is typically offset by having reinsurance from a commercial reinsurer. See also Fronting Insurer.

CAQH: See Council for Affordable Quality Healthcare.

Care Continuum Alliance: The organization for disease management, formerly called the Disease Management Association of America (DMAA).

Care Management: A broad term that is sometimes used in place of utilization management, or may be used as an umbrella-like term to refer to the combination of utilization management, disease management, case management, condition management, and so forth.

Career Limiting Move (CLM): A boneheaded mistake by a manager. What this book is designed to try to prevent.

Carve-Out: This term can be used in several different ways, depending on to what it is being applied. One common application is to payment terms, where it means that something is carved out of the basic payment methodology; for example, the cost of implantable devices might be carved out of hospital or ambulatory case rates and charged for separately. Applied to plan benefits, a carve-out typically refers to a set of benefits that are carved out and contracted for separately; for example, mental health/substance abuse services may be separated from basic medical/surgical.

Case Management: A method of managing the provision of health care to members with high-cost medical conditions. The goal is to coordinate the care so as to both improve continuity and quality of care as well as lower costs. This generally is a dedicated function in the utilization management department. The official definition according to the Certification of Insurance Rehabilitation Specialists Commission (CIRSC) is: "Case management is a collaborative process which assesses, plans, implements, coordinates, monitors, and evaluates the options and services required to meet an individual's health needs, using communication and available resources to promote quality, cost-effective outcomes" and "occurs across a continuum of care, addressing ongoing individual needs" rather than being restricted to a single practice setting. When focused solely on high-cost inpatient cases, may be referred to as large case management or catastrophic case management.

Case Mix: Refers to the mix of illness and severity of cases for a provider. The mix of cases in an inpatient setting, accounting for differences in potential or real cost and outcomes. Case mix adjustment refers to a methodology of using case mix to evaluate performance of a provider or project potential costs.

Cat Claim: Catastrophic Claim. See Shock Claim.

CCIIO: See Center for Consumer Information and Insurance Oversight.

CCIP: See Chronic Care Improvement Program.

CCO: Corporate Compliance Officer. See Corporate Compliance.

CCP: See Coordinated Care Plan.

CDH/CDHP: See Consumer Directed Health Plan.

Census: In the context of managed health care, it is the term used by hospitals themselves to refer to the number of filled inpatient beds, in whole numbers or a percentage of capacity. Payers may use it the same way to refer to the number of members who are inpatients at one hospital, or sometimes use it to refer to the number of hospitalized members overall.

Center for Consumer Information and Insurance Oversight (CCIIO): An agency within CMS, responsible for ensuring compliance with the ACA's market rules and medical loss ratio rules; assists states in reviewing insurance rates; provides guidance and oversight for state-based insurance exchanges; and compiles and maintains data on insurance.

Center for Medicare and Medicaid Innovation (CMMI): A branch of CMS created under the ACA to focus on identifying, testing, and ultimately spreading new ways of delivering and paying for care in Medicare and Medicaid.

Centers for Medicare and Medicaid (CMS): The federal agency within the Department of Health and Human Services (DHHS) responsible for Medicare and (with the states) Medicaid and implementation of the ACA.

CER: See Comparative Effective Research.

Certificate of Authority: The license required by an HMO that is issued by a state after the HMO meets regulatory requirements. A form of state licensure.

Certificate of Coverage: See EOC.

Certificate of Need (CON): The requirement that a health care organization obtain permission from an oversight agency before making changes. Generally applies only to facilities or facility-based services. Varies on a state-to-state basis.

CHAMPUS: Civilian Health and Medical Program of the Uniformed Services; see TRICARE.

Chase and Pay: A term used in COB that means determining which carrier is primary and which is secondary before paying anything. See also Pay and Chase and Coordination of Benefits.

Chargemaster: The list of charges a hospital has for each and every thing it can charge for on a pure, FFS basis. What a hospital is actually paid by a payer, Medicare, or Medicaid is rarely even close to what is listed on the chargemaster. However, the chargemaster is what is typically used to define when a case is classified as an outlier, and payment past that point is usually a discount on the chargemaster. Note: the word chargemaster is sometimes spelled as two words instead of a single word.

Chest Pain Unit: The term used to describe a specialized unit, usually either in or associated with the emergency department. The purpose of the chest pain unit is to rapidly identify an evolving cardiac event and initiate treatment as early as possible in order to decrease morbidity and mortality. The other (lesser) primary value of the unit is to rapidly identify chest pain that is noncardiac in origin, so as to avoid unnecessary hospitalization. Other terms that may be used include chest pain emergency room, chest pain evaluation unit, short-stay ED CCU, and ED-monitored observation beds.

CHIP: See State Children's Health Insurance Program (SCHIP).

Chronic Care Improvement Program (CCIP): A requirement of the MMA, the CCIP of a MA plan identifies enrollees with multiple or sufficiently severe chronic conditions who meet the criteria for participation in the program and have a mechanism for monitoring enrollees' participation. A form of a disease management program under MA. Plans must monitor enrollee participation in the program.

Churning: The practice of a provider seeing a patient more often than is medically necessary, primarily to increase revenue through an increased number of services. Churning may also apply to any performance-based payment system where there is a heavy emphasis on productivity (in other words, rewarding a provider for seeing a high volume of patients whether through FFS or through an appraisal system that pays a bonus for productivity).

Civilian Health and Medical Program of the Uniformed Services (CHAMPUS): The old term for the federal program providing health care coverage to families of military personnel, military retirees, certain spouses and dependents of such personnel, and certain others. Now called TRICARE. See also TRICARE and Military Health System.

Claims: The term used to describe a bill for services from a health care provider to the organization or person responsible for payment. Claims can be paper or electronic.

Claims Capture: The process of entering claims data into a claims processing system. Electronic claims without errors and containing all required data are captured quickly and at very little cost. Standardized paper claims such as the CMS-1450 and the CMS-1500 are usually scanned in using optical character recognition programs, which are manually reviewed and corrected as needed. Member-submitted claims may also be scanned in or may require manual key entry, all of which are very expensive.

Claims Clearing House: A company that accepts claims or other transactions from providers, formats them into HIPAA compliant standards, and electronically transmits them to the payer.

Claims Made Reinsurance or Insurance: A common type of reinsurance, and one of two primary types of professional liability insurance, applies to professional malpractice insurance for physicians, but is applicable to directors' and officers' liability policies as well. Claims Made means that the insurer has liability only when the event occurred and the insurer was informed of the potential for liability while the insurance is in force. If informed after the policy has lapsed, the insurer has no liability. See also Claims Paid and Occurrence.

Claims Paid Reinsurance: A reinsurance policy that applies to claims paid in a specific time period (e.g., 1 year). The coverage is for any claims paid during the contract period, regardless of when the costs were actually incurred. After the period of coverage has ended, there is no further coverage for costs even if they were incurred during the period when the reinsurance was in force if no claims were paid by the benefits plan. Not to be confused with Claims Made in which notification of the potential for liability, not necessarily the payment of a claim, is sufficient to activate coverage.

Claims Repricing: An activity in which a rental PPO (see Rental PPO) receives claims submitted by the participating providers, reprices them using the PPO fee schedule, and then transmits the repriced claim to the payer or insurance company for final processing.

Clean Claim: A claim that has no errors and contains all required data. The term can apply to either paper or electronic, but is increasingly being used only for electronic claims.

CLM: See Career Limiting Move.

Closed Panel: A managed care plan that contracts with physicians on an exclusive basis for services and does not allow those physicians to see patients for another managed care organization. Examples include staff and group model HMOs. Could apply to a large private medical group that contracts with an HMO.

CMMI: See Center for Medicare and Medicaid Innovation.

CMP: See Competitive Medical Plan.

CMS: See Centers for Medicare and Medicaid Services. Also stands for Contract Management System when used in the context of network management systems support.

CMS-1450: A paper claim form used by hospitals and facilities, standardized by CMS. It replaced the UB-92. Does not apply to electronic claims. CMS discourages paper claims, but if an institution submits one to any type of payer, this is what it uses. Also called the UB-04.

CMS-1500: A paper claims form used by professionals to bill for services. Developed for Medicare, but also used in the commercial sector. Does not apply to electronic claims. CMS no longer accepts paper claims, though most commercial health plans do.

CMS-Hierarchical Condition Categories System (CMS-HCC): A system that is based on diagnosis codes used in inpatient and outpatient settings as well as physician settings of care. The codes are assigned to groups of diagnoses called condition categories. The condition categories are ranked in a hierarchy, in which a higher category trumps a lower category for a patient whose diagnoses map to both categories. Each category is assigned a value (risk adjustment factor, or RAF) based on the statistical relationship between that category and the following year's claim costs, and is used to adjust payments to MA plans.

COA: See Certificate of Authority.

COB: See Coordination of Benefits.

COBRA: See Consolidated Omnibus Reconciliation Act.

Code Sets: Sets of codes used by providers to bill for services. As a practical matter, it is used when discussing the official codes that must be used for any electronic transaction covered under HIPAA. These code sets are ICD-9-CM (until October 1, 2012) or ICD-10 (after October 1, 2012),

CPT-4, NDC, HCPCS, and the Code on Dental Procedures and Nomenclature. Official code sets change over time.

Coinsurance: A provision in a member's coverage that limits the amount of coverage by the plan to a certain percentage, commonly 80%. Coinsurance may also vary depending on whether or not a service was received from an in-network versus out-of-network provider (e.g., 80% for in-network care, 60% for out-of-network care). Any additional costs are paid by the member out of pocket.

Commercial Health Insurance: Health insurance or HMO coverage for subscribers who are not covered by virtue of a governmental program such as Medicare, Medicaid, or SCHIP. May be group or direct-pay.

Commission: The money paid to a sales representative, broker, or other type of sales agent for selling the health plan. May be a flat amount of money or a percentage of the premium.

Community Rating: The rating methodology required of HMOs under the laws of many states, and occasionally PPOs and indemnity plans under certain circumstances. When required, it usually applies only to the small group market. The HMO must obtain the same amount of money per member for all members in the plan. Community rating may allow for variability by allowing the HMO to factor in differences for age, sex, mix (average contract size), and industry factors; not all factors are necessarily allowed under state laws, however. Such techniques are referred to a community rating by class and adjusted community rating. See also Experience Rating.

Comparative Effective Research (CER): The use of scientific studies to determine how effective one type of treatment or procedure is compared to another.

Competitive Medical Plan (CMP): A now archaic federal designation that allowed a health plan to obtain eligibility to receive a Medicare risk contract without having to obtain qualification as an HMO. Requirements for eligibility were somewhat less restrictive than for an HMO. Replaced by certain types of Medicare Advantage plans.

Complementary and Alternative Medicine (CAM): This is a general term that covers treatment modalities other than traditional allopathic medicine. Examples include acupuncture, chiropractic medicine, homeopathy, and various forms of "natural healing."

Compliance: See Corporate Compliance.

Computer Telephony Integration (CTI): A term used in a payer's call center or contact center. It means using information input by a member at the beginning of a call to access relevant data in the transaction system, route the call to the most appropriate CSR, and provide decision support to the CSR.

Computerized Physician Order Entry (CPOE): A system in which a physician enters medical orders into an electronic medical record or transactional system such as a drug dispensing program. This lowers the error rate caused by illegible handwriting. CPOE systems may also be partially or completely automated for certain things, such as routine or standing orders for a patient admitted to the ICU.

CON: See Certificate of Need.

Concurrent Review: Refers to utilization management that takes place during the provision of services. Almost exclusively applied to inpatient hospital stays, but also applicable to certain extended types of treatment such as long-term rehabilitation.

Condition Management: A term that may be used interchangeably with disease management, or may be used to refer to the management of those patients with multiple chronic conditions, a sort of multidisease management. See also Disease Management.

Consolidated Omnibus Reconciliation Act (COBRA): A portion of this Act requires employers to offer the opportunity for terminated employees to purchase continuation of health care coverage under the group's medical plan. See also Conversion.

Consumer Assessment of Healthcare Providers and Systems (CAHPS®): Begun by the federal government for use in Medicare and Medicaid managed care plans, it is now also used by commercial health plans. Maintained by the AHRQ and required as part of the NCQA accreditation process, its initial focus was on managed health care plans, but is being expanded to ambulatory providers, hospitals, and the Medicare prescription drug program. The hospital version in use is the Hospital Consumer Assessment of Healthcare Providers and Systems survey (HCAHPS).

Consumer Directed Health Plan (CDH/CDHP): A type of health plan that combines a qualified HDHP with a pretax fund such as an HRA or an HSA. The HRA or HSA is used to pay for qualified services on a first dollar basis, but are not large enough to cover the entire deductible, the so-called "doughnut hole." CDHPs also provide information such as cost data and decision-support tools to consumers to promote greater involvement on the part of the consumer in making health care choices.

Consumer Operated and Oriented Plan (CO-OP) Program: Defined in the ACA as a new type of consumer-operated, not-for-profit payer organization offering coverage through a state Health Insurance Exchange.

Consumer Portal: See Portal.

Contact Center: The place within a payer that supports inbound inquiries across a broad array of media (though most frequently, inbound telephone calls), blended with outbound contact and outreach transactions.

Contract Management System (CMS): A computer program or database management system used to keep track of the various provider contracts and their terms. The term may also sometimes be used to track employer group master contracts and benefits terms, but that is usually separate from the provider system. The acronym CMS may be used in context when it won't be confused for the federal Center for Medicare and Medicaid Services (also CMS).

Contract Year: The 12-month period that a contract for services is in force. Not necessarily tied to a calendar year.

Contributory Plan: A group health plan in which the employees must contribute a certain amount toward the premium cost, with the employer paying the rest.

Convenient Care Clinic (CCC): Another term used for a Retail Clinic. See Retail Clinic.

Conversion: The conversion of a member covered under a group master contract to coverage under an individual contract. This is offered to subscribers who lose their group coverage (e.g., through job loss, death of a working spouse) and who are ineligible for coverage under another group contract. See COBRA and HIPAA.

CO-OP: Prior to the ACA, a co-op was shorthand for cooperative or health care cooperative, and was (and still is) used by certain group model HMOs such as Group Health of Puget Sound. Under the ACA, it now also refers to Consumer Operated and Oriented Plan program (see also that term in the Glossary).

Co-op: See Healthcare Cooperative.

Coordinated Care Plan (CCP): Medicare Advantage plans that include HMOs, PPOs (both regional and local), provider-sponsored organizations that operate like HMOs, and HMOs with point-of-service products. CCPs can require enrollees to use a network of providers for coverage of Medicare services. Other than in an emergency, a CCP has no obligation to cover the cost of care if a non-network provider is used, even if the care would have been covered in FFS Medicare.

Coordination of Benefits (COB): An agreement that uses language developed by the NAIC to prevent double payment for services when a subscriber has coverage from two or more sources. For example, a husband may have Blue Cross Blue Shield through work, and the wife may have elected an HMO through her place of employment. The agreement gives the order for what organization has primary responsibility for payment and what organization has secondary responsibility for payment. The respective primary and secondary payment obligations of the two carriers are determined by the Order of Benefits Determination (OOBD) Rules contained in the NAIC Model COB Regulation, as interpreted and adopted by the various states. COB is not exactly the same as OPL. See also Other Party Liability.

Copayment: That portion of a claim or medical expense that a member must pay out of pocket. Usually a fixed amount, such as $20 in many HMOs.

Corporate Compliance: The function in a health plan or provider charged with ensuring compliance with federal rules and regulations. There are many compliance areas for Medicare; specific compliance requirements exist for privacy and security under HIPAA and financial requirements under Sarbanes-Oxley. Regulations for Medicare and HIPAA also require the existence of a corporate compliance officer (CCO).

Corporate Practice of Medicine Acts or Statutes: State laws that prohibit a physician from working for a corporation; in other words, a physician can only work for him- or herself or another physician. Put another way, a corporation cannot practice medicine. Often created through the effort on the part of certain members of the medical community to prevent physicians from working directly for managed care plans or hospitals.

Cost-Sharing: Any form of coverage in which the member pays some portion of the cost of providing services. Usual forms of cost-sharing include deductibles, coinsurance, and copayments.

Cost-Shifting: When a provider cannot cover the cost of providing services under the payment received, the provider raises the prices to other payers to cover that portion of the cost.

Council for Affordable Quality Healthcare (CAHQ): A not-for-profit alliance of health plans, networks, and trade associations, to foster industry collaboration on initiatives that simplify health care administration, including credentialing of providers.

Countercyclical: This term applies to Medicaid, which is countercyclical in that it expands to meet increasing need when the economy is in decline. During an economic downturn, more people become eligible for and enroll in the Medicaid program when they lose their jobs and their access to health insurance. As enrollment grows, program costs also rise.

CPOE: See Computerized Physician Order Entry.

CPT-4: See Current Procedural Terminology, 4th edition.

Credentialing: The most common use of the term refers to obtaining and reviewing the documentation of professional providers. Such documentation includes licensure, certifications, insurance, evidence of malpractice insurance, malpractice history, and so forth. Generally includes both reviewing information provided by the provider as well as verification that the information is correct and complete. A much less frequent use of the term applies to closed panels and medical groups and refers to obtaining hospital privileges and other privileges to practice medicine.

Credentialing Verification Organization (CVO): This is an independent organization that performs primary verification of a professional provider's credentials. The managed care organization may then rely on that verification rather than subjecting the provider to provide credentials independently. This lowers the cost and "hassle" for credentialing. NCQA (see NCQA) has issued certification standards for CVOs.

Credibility: The measure of credence or belief that is attached to a particular body of statistical experience for rate-making purposes, frequently defined in terms of specific mathematical formulas. Generally, as the body of experience increases in volume, the corresponding credibility also increases.

Credit: The pass-through to a payer or Medicare of a refund received by a hospital or ambulatory facility from a device manufacturer for a device that failed or needed to be removed while still under warranty. Credit applies when implantable devices are carved out of the payment methodology and charged for separately.

Critical Paths: Defined pathways of clinical care that provide for the greatest efficiency of care at the greatest quality. Critical paths are also an ever-changing activity as science and medicine evolve. This term is being replaced through common usage with the term "clinical guidelines."

CRM: See Customer Relationship Management.

CSR: See Customer Service Representative.

CTI: See Computer Telephony Integration.

Current Procedural Terminology, 4th edition (CPT-4): A set of five-digit codes that apply to medical services delivered. Frequently used for billing by professionals. See also HCPCS.

Custodial Care: Care provided to an individual that consists primarily of assistance with the basic activities of living. May be medical or nonmedical, but the care is not meant to be curative or as a form of medical treatment, and is often lifelong. Custodial care is not a covered benefit in any form of group health insurance, HMO, or Medicare. Only LTC insurance policies (which are property/casualty policies, not health) or, for the indigent, Medicaid, provide any coverage for custodial care.

Customer Relationship Management (CRM): Originally the term was used to describe all of the processes and information systems used by an organization in regard to its interactions with its customers, such as telephone calling systems and customer databases. It is now used more broadly to include the use of the same processes and technology in regard to any external constituency, such as a payer's nonroutine interactions with its providers.

Customer Service Representative (CSR): An individual in the member services function that has direct communications with members. There are usually different levels of CSRs consistent with different levels of experience, training, and authority. The Glossary can offer no good reason why the term "customer" is used for the acronym, while the term "member" is used for the department other than a guess: providing services to enrolled members has been around since the beginning, while the term CSR came along with software first developed for other industries—but that is no more than pure speculation.

Customer Services: See Member Services.

CVO: See Credentialing Verification Organization.

CWW: Clinic Without Walls. See Group Practice Without Walls.

Data Transparency: Refers to a payer or governmental agency making data about health care cost and quality available to consumers, usually via the Internet.

Date of Service: Refers to the date that medical services were rendered. Usually different from the date a claim is submitted.

DAW: See Dispense as Written.

Days per Thousand: See Bed Days per Thousand.

DCG: See Diagnostic Care Group.

Death Spiral: An insurance term that refers to a vicious spiral of high premium rates and adverse selection, generally in a free-choice environment (typically, an insurance company or health plan in an account with multiple other plans, or a plan offering coverage to potential members who have alternative choices, such as through an association). One plan ends up having continually higher premium rates such that the only members who stay with the plan are those whose medical costs are so high that they far exceed any possible premium revenue. Called the death spiral because the losses from underwriting mount faster than the premiums can ever recover, and the account eventually terminates coverage, leaving the carrier in a permanent loss position.

Deductible: That portion of a subscriber's (or member's) health care expenses that must be paid out of pocket before any insurance coverage applies, commonly $100–300. May apply only to the out-of-network portion of a point-of-service plan. May also apply only to one portion of the plan coverage (e.g., there may be a deductible for pharmacy services or hospital care, but not for anything else).

Deeming: If an organization is accredited by the appropriate accreditation agency as meeting defined requirements, it will be deemed as being in compliance with requirements of a governmental agency as well. For payers, accreditation by NCQA, URAC, or (less commonly) AAAHC is deemed by CMS as meeting at least some requirements for participation in Medicare Advantage. Many states also deem plans as being in compliance with certain requirements of licensure. For facilities, accreditation by JCI, or ambulatory facilities, AAAHC is usually deemed as being in compliance with certain state and Medicare requirements.

Defined Benefit: A term of insurance that refers to an employer (or governmental agency that provides benefits to employees) providing a benefit that is the same regardless of the cost (though cost-sharing with employees is not a part of the definition of defined benefit). In other words, an employee knows what type(s) of insurance or managed health care plans are offered and what the benefits are under each, and the employer's contribution to the cost of that coverage is a function of how expensive that coverage is. This is the most common form of employee health insurance benefit as of early 2000.

Defined Contribution: A term of insurance that refers to an employer designating a fixed amount of money for use in purchasing insurance or for funding a retirement account.

Delete: The term used by CMS for the process of removing Medicare enrollees from a plan. See also Accrete.

Demand Management: Services or support that a payer provides members in order to lower the demand for acute care services. Includes self-help tools, nurse advice lines, and preventive services.

Dental Content Committee of the American Dental Association: A DSMO under HIPAA that focuses on coding standards for dental procedures.

Dental Health Maintenance Organization (DHMO): An HMO organized strictly to provide dental benefits.

Department of Health and Human Services (DHHS or HHS): This is the cabinet-level federal agency that oversees many programs, including the CMS, which is responsible for Medicare and Medicaid (in conjunction with individual states), as well as oversight of HIPAA and other related federal legislation.

Department of Labor (DOL): Regulates coverage offered to employees when employers retain the insurance risk through self-funding pursuant to ERISA, either on a stand-alone basis or through a multiple employer welfare arrangement.

Certain ERISA requirements are also applicable to insured plans, and thus are regulated by the DOL as well.

Dependent: A member who is covered by virtue of a family relationship with the member who has the health plan coverage. For example, one person has health insurance or an HMO through work, and that individual's spouse and children, the dependents, also have coverage under that contract.

Designated Standards Maintenance Organizations (DSMOs): Organizations designated in HIPAA that are charged with making recommendations to DHHS regarding updates to existing standards as well as the addition of new standards to the transactions and code sets.

DFRR: See Disclosure of Financial Relationships Report.

DHHS: See the Department of Health and Human Services.

DHMO: See Dental Health Maintenance Organization.

Diagnosis-Related Groups (DRGs): A statistical system of classifying any inpatient stay into groups for purposes of payment. DRGs may be primary or secondary, and an outlier classification also exists. This is the form of payment that the CMS uses to pay hospitals for Medicare recipients. Also used by a few states for all payers and by many private health plans for contracting purposes. DRGs were replaced by MS-DRGs during 2008–2009. See also MS-DRG.

Diagnostic Care Group (DCG): A methodology commissioned by the CMS to look at how to adjust prospective payments to health plans based on retrospective severity. Replaced by the CMS-Hierarchical Condition Categories.

Direct Access: See Open Access.

Direct Contract Model: A managed care health plan that contracts directly with private practice physicians in the community, rather than through an intermediary such as an IPA or a medical group. A common type of model in open-panel HMOs.

Direct Contracting: A term describing a provider or integrated health care delivery system contracting directly with employers rather than through an insurance company or managed care organization. A superficially attractive option that occasionally works when the employer is large enough. Not to be confused with direct contract model (see preceding entry). Rarely used for long since it is almost always more costly than working through an existing health plan.

Direct-Pay Subscriber: An individual subscriber to a health plan who is not covered under a group policy, but rather pays the health plan directly. May be a commercial member that has passed underwriting screening, or may be a conversion plan holder (see Conversion). Is not used to describe Medicare or Medicaid subscribers by convention;

even though such subscribers are enrolled individually, part or all of their premiums are paid via a governmental agency.

Discharge Planning: That part of utilization management that is concerned with arranging for care or medical needs to facilitate discharge from the hospital.

Disclosure of Financial Relationships Report (DFRR): A mandatory hospital disclosure form applicable to Medicare. It was created by CMS to report any financial relationships between hospitals and physicians, and to measure compliance with the physician self-referral statute and regulations. Applicable to Medicare.

Disease Management: The process of intensively managing a particular disease. This differs from large case management in that it goes well beyond a given case in a hospital, or an acute exacerbation of a condition. Disease management encompasses all settings of care, and places a heavy emphasis on prevention and maintenance. Similar to case management, but more focused on a defined set of diseases. See also Condition Management.

Disenrollment: The process of termination of coverage. Voluntary termination would include a member quitting because he or she simply wants out. Involuntary termination would include leaving the plan because of changing jobs. A rare and serious form of involuntary disenrollment is when the plan terminates a member's coverage against the member's will. This is usually only allowed (under state and federal laws) for gross offenses such as fraud, abuse, nonpayment of premium or copayments, or a demonstrated inability to comply with recommended treatment plans.

Dispense as Written (DAW): The instruction from a physician to a pharmacist to dispense a brand-name pharmaceutical rather than a generic substitution.

Dispensing Fee: The fee paid to a pharmacy for that part of the cost of a prescription that is not the ingredient cost. Usually a flat dollar amount, not tied to the cost of the drug.

Disproportionate Share Hospital (DSH) Payment: An amount added to payments by Medicare to help defray the cost of uncompensated care. Different for each hospital and state depending on the actual documented amount of charity care, but going away in any event by 2014 under the terms of the ACA.

Distribution Channel or Distribution: An informal term used to describe the various ways that a payer sells its products, for example, brokers, consultants, employed sales force, electronic sales portals, and so forth.

DME: See Durable Medical Equipment.

DOL: See Department of Labor.

Doughnut Hole: The term applied to the difference between when first dollar coverage stops and then insurance begins.

Also referred to as a bridge. May be applied in a CDHP plan to the gap between the HRA or HSA, and when the high-deductible insurance plan starts to cover costs. Also existed in the basic Medicare Part D drug benefit passed under the MMA, but under the ACA it is being partially phased out by 2020. A term that may not necessarily have great persistency.

Dread Disease Policy: A peculiar type of health insurance that only covers a specific and frightening type of illness, such as cancer. Uncommon.

DRG: See Diagnosis-Related Groups.

Drive Time: The average amount of time it takes for a member to get to a provider. It is often used as a measure of network accessibility.

Drug Utilization Review: UM applied to the pharmaceutical benefit. It relies more on prospective review than does medical/surgical UM.

DSH: See Disproportionate Share Hospital Payments.

DSM-IV: *Diagnostic and Statistical Manual of Mental Disorders, 4th Edition.* The manual used to provide a diagnostic coding system for mental and substance abuse disorders. Far different from ICD-9-CM. See ICD-9-CM.

DSMO: See Designated Standards Maintenance Organization.

Dual Choice: An archaic term, sometimes also referred to as Section 1310 or mandating. That portion of the original HMO Act that required any employer with 25 or more employees that reside in an HMO's service area, pays minimum wage, and offers health coverage to offer a federally qualified HMO as well. The HMO had to request it. This provision of the HMO Act "sunseted" in 1995.

Dual Eligibles: Individuals who are entitled to both Medicare and Medicaid coverage. Sometimes referred to as "Medi-Medi's."

Dual Option: This once referred only to offering of both an HMO and a traditional insurance plan by one carrier. It now refers to offering two different health plans, regardless of type.

Duplicate Claims: When the same claim is submitted more than once, usually because payment hasn't been received quickly. Can lead to duplicate payments and incorrect data in the claims file.

DUR: See Drug Utilization Review.

Durable Medical Equipment (DME): Medical equipment that is not disposable (i.e., is used repeatedly) and is only related to care for a medical condition. Examples would include wheelchairs, home hospital beds, and so forth. An area of increasing expense, particularly in conjunction with case management.

EAP: See Employee Assistance Program.

Early and Periodic Screening, Diagnostic, and Testing: Usually referred to by its acronym EPSDT, these are a defined set of screening benefits provided to children covered under Medicaid.

Earned Premium: That portion of the premium paid to a payer for coverage for a time period that has already passed. Premium that is paid in advance is considered unearned premium until the entire time period that the premium is meant to cover has passed, on a proportionate basis.

eBusiness: See eCommerce.

eCommerce: A term that refers to the use of electronic communications to conduct business. Also called eBusiness. By convention, ecommerce applies to the use of the Internet for such transactions. Also by convention, the "e" is almost always in lowercase (and who knows why?). ee cummings would approve.

ED: See Emergency Department.

EDI: See Electronic Data Interchange.

Edit: A term used in claims processing. See Suspend.

Effective Date: The day that health plan coverage goes into effect or is modified.

EFT: See Electronic Funds Transfer.

EHR: See Electronic Health Record.

Electronic Data Interchange (EDI): A term that refers to the exchange of data through electronic means rather than by using paper or the telephone. Prior to the rise of the Internet, EDI was applied primarily to direct electronic communications via proprietary means. EDI now encompasses electronic data exchange via both proprietary channels as well as the Internet.

Electronic Funds Transfer (EFT): Getting paid by electronic transfer of funds directly to one's bank instead of receiving a paper check.

Electronic Health Record (EHR): A more expansive type of electronic record encompassing more than the care provided by a single provider or entity to a single patient.

Electronic Medical Record (EMR): An electronic version of the type of health record that a physician or a hospital keeps on a single patient.

Eligibility: When an individual is eligible for coverage under a plan. Also used to determine when an individual is no longer eligible for coverage (e.g., a dependent child reaches a certain age and is no longer eligible for coverage under his or her parent's health plan).

Emergency or Emergency Medical Condition: Specific language in EMTALA states "An emergency medical condition means a medical condition manifested by acute symptoms of sufficient severity (including severe pain) that the absence of immediate medical attention could reasonably be expected to result in: a) placing the patient's health in serious jeopardy; b) serious impairment to bodily functions; or c) serious dysfunction of any bodily organ or part."

Emergency Department (ED): The location or department in a hospital or other institutional facility that is focused on caring for acutely ill or injured patients. In earlier times, this was often a room or set of rooms, hence the older designation emergency room or ER. These days, at least in busy urban and suburban hospitals, volume is high, physicians are specially trained and certified in emergency care, and it has grown to be an entire department.

Emergency Medical Treatment and Active Labor Act (EMTALA) 1986. 42 USC 1395 dd (1986), Pub. L. No. 99-272, 9121: "Antidumping" legislation dictates that all patients presenting to any hospital emergency department must have a medical screening exam performed by qualified personnel, usually the emergency physician. The medical screening exam cannot be delayed for insurance reasons, either to obtain insurance information or to obtain preauthorization for examination.

Employee Assistance Program (EAP): A program that a company puts into effect for its employees to provide them with help in dealing with personal problems such as alcohol or drug abuse, mental health or stress issues, and so forth.

Employee Retirement Income Security Act (ERISA): One provision of this Act allows self-funded plans to avoid paying premium taxes, complying with state-mandated benefits, or otherwise complying with most state laws and regulations that apply to health insurance. Another provision requires that plans and insurance companies provide an explanation of benefits (EOB) statement to a member or covered insured in the event of a denial of a claim, explaining why the claim was denied and informing the individual of his or her rights of appeal; this aspect was significantly strengthened under the ACA. Numerous other provisions in ERISA are very important for a managed care organization to know.

EMR: See Electronic Medical Record.

EMTALA: See Emergency Medical Treatment and Active Labor Act.

Encounter: An outpatient or ambulatory visit by a member to a provider. Applies primarily to physician office visits, but may encompass other types of encounters as well. In FFS plans, an encounter also generates a claim. In capitated plans, the encounter is still the visit, but no claim is generated.

End-Stage Renal Disease (ESRD): While no other particular clinical definitions are found in this glossary, this one is only because Medicare treats beneficiaries with ESRD differently than other types for purposes of enrollment in MA plans.

Enrollee: An individual enrolled in a managed health care plan. Usually applies to the subscriber or person who has the coverage in the first place rather than to their dependents, but the term is not always used that precisely.

Enrollment Period: Defined in the ACA and applicable to the mandated open enrollment requirements that begin in 2014. See Open Enrollment Period.

Entitlement Program: Federal programs, such as Medicare and Medicaid, for which people who meet eligibility criteria have a right to benefits, and in which changes to eligibility criteria and benefits require legislation. The federal government is required to spend the funds necessary to provide benefits for individuals in these programs, unlike discretionary programs for which spending is set by Congress through the appropriations process. Enrollment in entitlement programs cannot be capped and neither states nor the federal government may establish waiting lists.

EOB: See Explanation of Benefits.

EOC: See Evidence of Coverage.

EPO: See Exclusive Provider Organization.

ePrescribing: When a physician uses electronic means to prescribe drugs.

EPSDT: See Early and Periodic Screening, Diagnostic, and Testing.

Equity Model: A term applied to a form of for-profit, vertically integrated health care delivery system in which the physicians are owners.

ER: Emergency Room; see ED.

ERISA: See Employee Retirement Income Security Act.

ESRD: See End-Stage Renal Disease.

Essential Health Benefits: A benefits design under the ACA that includes ambulatory patient services, pediatric services, including oral and vision care emergency services, hospitalization, maternity and newborn care, mental health and substance use disorder services, prescription drugs, rehabilitative and habilitative services and devices, laboratory services, preventive and wellness services, and chronic disease management. The specific definitions of each category are to be determined by each individual state using HHS guidelines. Up to four different levels of cost-sharing may be applied depending on the level of coverage.

Ethics in Patient Referrals Act: A law prohibiting physicians from referring patients to diagnostic, therapeutic, or supply services in which the physician has a financial interest. Also known as the Stark Laws after Fortney "Pete"

Stark, a congressional representative from California. The so-called Stark regulations are actually two sets of regulations: Stark I and Stark II. These regulations are not for amateurs to handle, and competent legal counsel is required for any provider system doing business with federal or state governments.

Evergreen Contract: A contract that continues in force unless one or both parties give notice of cancellation. Some evergreen contracts require a year's notice, while others use shorter terms.

Evidence-Based Medicine or Guidelines: Clinical practices or guidelines that are based on scientific studies, not habits or hope. Some would extend this definition to consensus-driven professional standards, but this book does not.

Evidence of Coverage (EOC): Also known as a certificate of benefits. The EOC is a document that describes in detail the health care benefits covered by the health plan, what is excluded, and how benefits are affected by UM requirements, medical necessity definitions, and so forth.

Evidence of Insurability: The form that documents whether or not an individual is eligible for health plan coverage when the individual does not enroll through an open enrollment period, or when applying for an extension of coverage under COBRA.

eVisit: Electronic visit, referring to an interaction between a provider (usually a physician) and a patient using a secure electronic communications channel rather than face-to-face or via telephone.

Exchange: See Health Insurance Exchange.

Exclusion: As used in managed care and health insurance, exclusions refer to those services or conditions for which there will be no (or very limited) coverage. The most common is an exclusion in an individual direct-pay policy for pre-existing conditions, in which there will be no coverage for conditions that existed at the time the policy was issued; there is also usually a time limit for this type of exclusion (e.g., after 2 years). An exclusion may also be a complete one, such as no coverage for experimental or scientifically unproven care.

Exclusive Provider Organization (EPO): An EPO is similar to an HMO in that it often uses primary physicians as gatekeepers, often capitates providers, has a limited provider panel, and uses an authorization system, and so on. It is referred to as exclusive because the member must remain within the network to receive benefits. The main difference is that EPOs are generally regulated under insurance statutes rather than HMO regulations. Not allowed in many states that maintain that EPOs are really HMOs. Now uncommon.

Experience Rating: The method of setting premium rates based on the actual health care costs of a group or groups.

Experimental and Investigational Treatment: The term used by payers and insurance companies to refer to medical care that is not yet proven, or that may be the subject of clinical investigation. Most plans will not cover costs for this unless the patient is enrolled in a qualified investigational trial.

Explanation of Benefits (EOB): A statement mailed to a member or covered insured explaining how and why a claim was or was not paid; the Medicare version is called an EOMB. See also ERISA.

External Review: The second part of an appeal of a denial of coverage, it refers to a panel of physicians who do not work for the payer organization reviewing the appeal, and whose decision is binding on the payer. Often required by states and addressed in ERISA, it is required for all plans under the ACA.

Extra-Contractual Benefits: Health care benefits beyond what the member's actual policy covers. These benefits are provided by a plan in order to reduce utilization. For example, a plan may not provide coverage for a hospital bed at home, but it is more cost-effective for the plan to provide such a bed than to keep admitting a member to the hospital.

Facility Fee: A fee added on to a physician office visit by a hospital or facility owner. Adding a facility fee to a charge is generally prohibited if the physician owns or leases the office, but if an independent entity owns or leases it, the extra charge is not prohibited. Facility fees have been increasing over the years as physicians become employees of hospitals. May or may not be covered by health insurance.

Faculty Practice Plan (FPP): A form of group practice organized around a teaching program. It may be a single group encompassing all the physicians providing services to patients at the teaching hospital and clinics, or it may be multiple groups drawn along specialty lines (e.g., psychiatry, cardiology, or surgery).

FAR: See Federal Acquisition Regulations.

Fast Track ED: A pathway in the ED allowing minor ailments to be managed quickly, at lower cost, often by non-physician practitioners.

Favored Nation Clause: See Most Favored Nation Clause.

Federal Acquisition Regulations (FAR): The regulations applied to the federal government's acquisition of services, including health care services, excluding Medicare. See also FEHBARs.

Federal Employee Health Benefit Acquisition Regulations (FEHBARs): The regulations applied to OPM's purchase of health care benefits programs for federal employees.

Federal Employee Health Benefits Program (FEHBP): The program that provides health benefits to federal employees. See OPM.

Federal Qualification: A term once applied to HMOs and CMPs that met federal standards regarding benefits, financial solvency, rating methods, marketing, member services, health care delivery systems, and other standards. Not used since 1995.

Federally Qualified Health Center: Health centers approved by the government to provide low-cost health care.

Fee-for-Service (FFS): A patient sees a provider, the provider bills the health plan or patient, and gets paid based on that bill. In the case of a contracted provider, the maximum payment may be limited to the fee schedule.

Fee Schedule: May also be referred to as fee maximums or as a fee allowance schedule. A listing of the maximum fee that a health plan will pay for a certain service, based on CPT billing codes.

FEHBARs: See Federal Employee Health Benefit Acquisition Regulations.

FFS: See Fee-for-Service.

File-and-Use Rating Laws: State-based laws that permit insurers to adopt new rates without the prior approval of the insurance department. Usually insurers submit their new rates with supporting statistical data.

Financial Services Modernization Act of 1999: Also called the Gramm-Leach-Bliley Act, it repealed the Glass-Steagall Act of 1933 that had been passed in the aftermath of the crash of 1929. Glass-Steagall prohibited most U.S. commercial banks from performing investment banking activities such as bringing new debt and equity issues to market, or other such underwriting, and from functioning as insurance companies. In addition to the repeal of Glass-Steagall, the Act also allows affiliations between securities firms, banks, and insurance companies.

First-Call Resolution: The percentage of contacts resolved on the first call. Typically used in call centers by member services.

First Pass Rate: The percentage of claims auto-adjudicated to completion the first time they go through the claims processing system.

Fiscal Intermediary: A company that processes the administrative transactions on behalf of Medicare, though the term may also be used by similar types of companies providing services to state Medicaid programs. May be limited to adjudication and payment of claims or may encompass other activities as well.

Flexible Benefits Plan: A benefits plan at a company that allows an employee to select from different options up to a set amount of money, and always includes an FSA. Also called a Cafeteria Plan or a Section 125 Plan.

Flexible Spending Account (FSA): A financial account funded with pretax dollars via payroll deduction by an employer. Funds may be used to reimburse the employee for qualified expenses not covered under insurance. FSAs exist for health care and, separately, for child care services. Unused FSA funds do not roll into following years; they are "use it or lose it" except that in some cases, unused FSA funds can roll over into an HSA account.

Formulary: A listing of drugs that a health plan provides coverage for, but almost always at differing levels. For example, drugs considered Tier 1 in the formulary may be covered with a $5 copay, Tier 2 at a $20 copay, Tier 3 at a $50 copay. May also list drugs that require precertification for coverage, or that are subject to other coverage limitations.

Foundation: A not-for-profit form of integrated health care delivery system. The foundation model is usually formed in response to tax laws that affect not-for-profit hospitals, or in response to states with laws prohibiting the corporate practice of medicine (see Corporate Practice Acts). The foundation purchases both the tangible and intangible assets of a physician's practice; the physicians then form a medical group that contracts with the foundation on an exclusive basis for services to patients seen through the foundation.

FPP: See Faculty Practice Plan.

Fraud and Abuse: A term with its roots in a description applied to fraud and/or abuse by health care providers or intermediaries in the provision of services to Medicare and Medicaid beneficiaries. Since that time nobody, and I mean nobody, uses either term separately, and it has taken on a generic meaning applied to any form of perceived skullduggery on the part of a provider or health plan doing business with the government. See also Fraud, Waste, and Abuse. See the individual definitions of Fraud and of Abuse

Fraud or Health Care Fraud: Actual fraud occurs when someone misrepresents a fact related to health care services to receive—or increase—payment from a health plan or the government. Fraud also occurs when someone misrepresents details in delivery of health care services or supplies.

Fraud, Waste, and Abuse (FWA): Not the name of a law firm or a rock band, this troika is used to cover fraud, abusive practices, and wasteful practices by either providers or health plans. It's also a handy catch-all for casting general blame at an industry sector. See also Fraud and Abuse and the individual definitions of Fraud and of Abuse.

Fronting or Fronting Insurer: A commercial insurer that has a market rating and meets state insurance requirements, and that "rents" its name to another nonrated insurer or captive insurer (see also Captive Insurer) and typically takes only 10–20% of the risk. A fronting company may be free-standing, but is often a subsidiary of a nonrated or captive insurer's reinsurer.

FSA: See Flexible Spending Account.

FTE: See Full-Time Equivalent.

Full Professional Risk Capitation: A loose term used to refer to a physician group or organization receiving capitation for all professional expenses, not just for the services they provide themselves; does not include capitation for institutional services (see Global Capitation). The group is then responsible for subcapitating or otherwise reimbursing other physicians for services to their members.

Full-Time Equivalent (FTE): The equivalent of one full-time employee. For example, two part-time employees are 0.5 FTE each, for a total of 1 FTE.

FWA: See Fraud, Waste, and Abuse.

Gag Clause: A clause in a provider contract that prevents a physician from telling a patient about available clinical treatment options (i.e., a "gag"). This clause was much like the Sasquatch—big, hairy and scary, but hard to actually find. The federal government conducted a review of managed care physician contracts and was unable to find any examples. Gag clauses have been banned by many states. Most or all contracts between payers and physicians do contain clauses that prohibit the physician from revealing business secrets such as payment schedules, but this is a different matter. In some cases in the past, contracts also required a physician to contact the payer before initiating a treatment option, which may have been interpreted or treated as such a clause, but the majority of contracts actually require the physician to actively discuss options with the patient.

Gatekeeper: An informal, though widely used term that refers to a primary care case management model health plan. In this model, all care from providers other than the primary care physician, except for true emergencies, must be authorized by the primary care physician before care is rendered. This is a predominant feature of most (but not all) HMOs.

Generic Drug: A drug that is equivalent to a brand name drug, but usually less expensive. Most managed care organizations that provide drug benefits cover generic drugs, but may require a member to pay a higher copay for a brand name drug.

Genetic Information Nondiscrimination Act (GINA): The Genetic Information Nondiscrimination Act of 2008 prohibits discrimination in health coverage and employment based on genetic information. GINA, plus certain provisions of HIPAA generally prohibit health insurers or health plan administrators from requesting or requiring genetic information of an individual or the individual's family members. It also prohibits using genetic information for decisions regarding coverage, rates, or preexisting conditions.

GINA: See Genetic Information Nondiscrimination Act.

Glass-Steagall Act: See the Gramm-Leach-Bliley Act of 1999.

GLB: Gramm-Leach-Bliley Act. See the Financial Services Modernization Act.

Global Capitation: The term used when an organization receives capitation for all medical services, including institutional and professional.

Global Payment: A single fixed payment for an episode of care. Most commonly used for well-defined types of care such as maternity or surgery. When combined with facility payment, it is referred to as a bundled payment. See Bundled Payment.

Gold Level of Benefits or Gold Plan: As defined in the ACA, a qualified health benefits plan with the actuarial equivalent or average of 20% cost-sharing, when accounting for deductibles, copayments, and coinsurance as applied to in-network services.

Grace Period: The amount of time that a payer or insurance company must allow a group or individual that hasn't paid their premium to make good on the payment before the plan can cancel the policy. If the delinquent company or individual pays up during the grace period, the policy is said to be reinstated and coverage is considered unbroken.

Gramm-Leach-Bliley Act (GLB): See Financial Services Modernization Act.

Grandfathered Plan: A health benefits plan meeting certain criteria is exempt from some, but not all, of the new requirements under the ACA. A grandfathered plan loses that exemption if it changes in any substantial way.

Grievance: A formal complaint by a member about a payer, requiring a response within fixed timelines. It does not apply to appeals, also a formal process.

Group: The members that are covered by virtue of receiving health plan coverage at a single company.

Group Health Insurance: A commercial health insurance policy (or HMO coverage policy) that is sold to an employer to provide coverage to employees. Does not apply to a conversion policy or a direct-pay policy, nor to Medicare or Medicaid plans.

Group Model HMO: An HMO that contracts with a medical group for the provision of health care services. The relationship between the HMO and the medical group is generally very close, although there are wide variations in the relative independence of the group from the HMO. A form of closed-panel health plan.

Group Practice: The American Medical Association defines group practice as three or more physicians who deliver patient care, make joint use of equipment and personnel, and divide income by a prearranged formula.

Group Practice Without Walls (GPWW): A group practice in which the members of the group come together legally, but continue to practice in private offices scattered throughout the service area. Sometimes called a Clinic Without Walls (CWW).

Guaranteed Issue or Renewal: A law that requires insurers to offer and renew coverage, without regard to health status, use of services, or preexisting conditions. The ACA will require both for all individuals and employer groups beginning in 2014.

HBP: See Hospital-Based Physician.

HCAHPS®: Hospital Consumer Assessment of Healthcare Providers and Systems Survey. See Consumer Assessment of Healthcare Providers and Systems (CAHPS®).

HCFA: See Health Care Financing Administration.

HCFA-1500: See CMS-1500.

HCPCS: See Healthcare (previously HCFA) Common Procedural Coding System.

HDHP: High-Deductible Health Plan; see High-Deductible Health Insurance.

Health Care: A term generally used to refer to the services that a health care professional or institution provides you (services from a physician, at a hospital, from a physical therapist, etc.); it is this use of the term that is universally used when discussing care management. There is a broader definition, however, that encompasses services from nontraditional providers and, more importantly, the health care that individuals self-administer, which is actually the majority of health care most people receive. When individuals use the broad sense of the term health care, they frequently use medical care to refer to what is considered the narrow meaning noted above. Broad or narrow—it is your choice depending on the context.

Health Care Anti-Fraud Association: A public-private partnership founded in 1985 to combat fraud in health care.

Health Care Financing Administration (HCFA): The older name of CMS; no longer used.

Health Information Exchange (HIE): An entity to facilitate the electronic exchange of health information between physicians, hospitals, laboratories, payers, and so on, that is sponsored by a state or the federal government. When so sponsored, they typically represent the only option.

Health Insurance: Technically, this term should be reserved for indemnity type of insurance as described later in this glossary. Its use, however, is much broader now, describing pretty much any type of health plan, though usually not an HMO. It is even used to describe self-funded benefits plans in which the employer is at risk for expenses, not an insurance company, but that is a legal distinction and not one made by most individuals who have such coverage.

Health Insurance Exchange (HIE or "Exchange"): The ACA requires states to set up and operate state-level Health Insurance Exchanges where individuals and small group employers may purchase qualified health plans. That part of the exchange used by small businesses is referred to as the Small Business Health Options Program (SHOP). States have some latitude in their approach. If a state does not create them, the federal government may come in and do so. Provisions in the ACA also allow for multistate Health Insurance Exchanges.

Health Insurance Portability and Accountability Act (HIPAA): Enacted in 1997, HIPAA provides for the ability of new employees to be covered in an employer's health plan as long as they were covered under some other plan, guaranteed issue of all health insurance products to small groups (but only if they have met requirements for prior continuous coverage), mental health parity, and the ability to purchase individual coverage when all other options run out (but only if a person meets "creditable coverage" requirements). More importantly, HIPAA's administrative simplification provisions mandate the use of certain standardized electronic transactions by covered entities, meet privacy and security requirements, and use standardized identifiers (except for members).

Health Insuring Organization (HIO): An organization that contracts with a state Medicaid agency as both a fiscal intermediary and to manage the beneficiaries covered by the HIO.

Health Level 7 (HL7): A DSMO under HIPAA, HL7 focuses on electronic connectivity standards for clinical information.

Health Maintenance Organization (HMO): The definition of an HMO has changed substantially, at least in common use. Originally, an HMO was defined as a prepaid organization that provided health care to voluntarily enrolled members in return for a preset amount of money on a PMPM basis. With the increase in self-insured business, or with financial arrangements that do not rely on prepayment, that definition is no longer accurate. Furthermore, only closed-panel HMOs actually provide care; most HMOs contract with independent providers of all types to provide the care. Enrollment in a Medicaid HMO is often mandatory, not voluntary. A working definition of an HMO in the current environment would include the following: it is licensed by the state under a COA; it is one of the few types of payers that may enter into risk-sharing payment arrangements with providers (though the shared savings program the ACA requires CMS to institute in the traditional FFS Medicare program includes risk, so this aspect of the definition is now a little shaky); it must meet network access needs that are more stringent than any other type of payer; it must have strong "hold harmless" language in its provider contracts; it usually (but not always) requires members to go through their PCP to access specialty services; it allows direct access to all types of PCPs and OB/Gyns, however; and it has policies and procedures for UM and QM that exceed any other type of payer. For a while, individuals involved in managed health care used the looser term managed care organization since it avoided having to make difficult definitions like this one, but its use is in decline.

Health Outcomes Survey (HOS): The HOS is a survey that health plans with a Medicare Advantage risk contract must conduct to look at clinical outcomes of covered Medicare beneficiaries. CMS arranges and pays for administration of the CAHPS survey, while Medicare Advantage health plans are responsible for administering the HOS survey.

Health Plan: A term loosely applied to any type of payer. However, technically it is the benefits plan, including its sponsor, not necessarily the administrator of the plan.

Health Reimbursement Account/Arrangement (HRA): A financial account associate with a CDHP and used to pay for first dollar qualified health care expenses up to a preset limit using pretax funds provided by an employer. Unused HRA funds may roll into the next year, but they do not follow an individual when they change employment. Always associated with an HDHP.

Health Risk Appraisal (HRA): Instrument designed to elicit or compile information about the health risk of any given individual. Initially these tools were fairly uniform, but they have now become quite specialized and targeted toward particular populations with distinctive risk profiles (e.g., Medicare, Medicaid, underserved, commercial population).

Health Savings Account (HSA): Created under the MMA, an HSA is a financial account of pretax dollars for current or future qualified medical expenses, retirement, or long-term care premium expenses. Unused funds roll into following years. This is the type of CDHP used by individuals. Always associated with a qualified HDHP, and regulated under tax law.

Healthcare (previously HCFA) Common Procedural Coding System (HCPCS): A set of codes used by Medicare that describes services and procedures. HCPCS includes CPT codes, but also has codes for services not included in CPT such as DME and ambulance. While HCPCS is nationally defined, there is provision for local use of certain codes. Many HCPCS codes will be replaced by special codes in ICD-10, but not HCPCS codes used by physicians.

Healthcare Cooperative: One of the earliest forms of what we now call managed care, a health care cooperative is a nonprofit organization operated by its members for providing care to its members. Generally look like prepaid group health plans. Once more common, the most well-known existing co-ops include Group Health Cooperative of Puget Sound, and Group Health Cooperative of Southern Wisconsin. See also CO-OP for its use as defined in the ACA.

Healthcare Effectiveness Data and Information (HEDIS®): Developed by NCQA with considerable input from the employer community and the managed care community, HEDIS is an ever-evolving set of data reporting standards. HEDIS is designed to provide some standardization in performance reporting for financial, utilization, membership, clinical data, and more. Employers and consumers then can compare performance between plans, if the plan reports HEDIS data. Originally called the Health Plan Employer Data Information Set, the initial focus was on HMOs, but it has become much more varied and different versions exist for commercial, Medicare Advantage, and managed Medicaid plans.

Healthcare Integrity and Protection Data Bank: An electronic data bank established under HIPAA that records information about providers around fraud and abuse, criminal convictions, civil judgments, injunctions, licensure restrictions, and exclusion from participation in any governmental programs.

HEDIS: See Healthcare Effectiveness Data and Information Set.

HHS: See Department of Health and Human Services.

HIE: See Health Information Exchange or Health Insurance Exchange, whichever fits the reason you had for looking up this acronym.

High-Deductible Health Insurance/High-Deductible Health Plan (HDHP): Just what it sounds like, a health insurance policy with a very high annual deductible, such as $1,100 for singles or $2,300 for families. The specific deductible amounts are determined each year by the Treasury Department for HDHPs associated with CDHP pretax savings options such as MSAs, HRAs, and HSAs.

High-Risk Pool: Programs in some, but not all, states designed to provide health insurance to residents who are considered medically uninsurable and are unable to buy coverage in the individual market. High-risk pools vary from state to state by who is eligible, cost-sharing requirements, availability of premium subsidies, and funding sources. The ACA provided extra funding for states to use to expand eligibility for uninsurable individuals. Beginning in 2014, guaranteed issue requirements under the ACA will make such pools unnecessary.

HIO: See Health Insuring Organization.

HIPAA: See Health Insurance Portability and Accountability Act.

HL7: See Health Level 7.

HMO: See Health Maintenance Organization.

HMO Act of 1973 (42 U.S.C. § 300e): A law passed by Congress in 1973 to promote the expansion of HMOs by putting aside state anti-HMO laws and requiring large employers to offer at least one closed-panel and one open-panel HMO. It also required HMOs to offer then-rare comprehensive benefits and abide by community rating. Many elements of the HMO Act are no longer in effect, though the law itself is.

Hold Harmless Clause: A contractual clause between a provider and a payer that prohibits the provider from balance billing a member even in the event the payer fails to pay the provider (i.e., the provider holds the member harmless).

HOPPS: See Hospital Outpatient Prospective Payment System.

HOS: See Health Outcomes Survey.

Hospice: A program or facility dedicated to palliative care at the end of life. May be a combination of a home-care program, an outpatient facility, and/or an inpatient facility.

Hospital Outpatient Prospective Payment System (HOPPS): The overall term used by CMS for its different methods of prospective payment to facilities for outpatient care such as surgery, dialysis, drug administration, and so forth.

Hospital-Based Physician (HBP): A specialty physician who practices primarily within a hospital or ambulatory surgical center in one of five clinical areas: anesthesia, radiology, pathology, emergency department, or as a hospitalist. Traditionally, this term is not applied to hospital-employed physicians except if they fit into one of these categories.

Hospital-Employed Physician: The direct employment of a physician by a hospital or health system. The term could be applied to an HBP, but the more common usage is for other specialties such as primary care, cardiology, and so forth.

Hospitalist: A physician who concentrates solely on hospitalized patients. In a payer or medical group, this physician may specialize in hospital care, or the duties may be undertaken on a rotating basis. More often, hospitalists are employed by the hospital.

HRA: See Health Risk Appraisal or Health Reimbursement Account, depending on the context.

HSA: See Health Savings Account.

IBNR: See Incurred But Not Reported.

ICD-9-CM: International Classification of Diseases, 9th Revision, Clinical Modification. ICD-9-CM classifies diseases by diagnosis using six-digit numbers. It will be replaced by ICD-10 by October 1, 2013.

ICD-10: International Classification of Diseases, 10th Revision. ICD-10 will replace ICD-9-CM and several other codes sets on October 1, 2013. It has up to seven alpha-numeric characters, allowing coding of up to 16,000 different diseases, procedures, patient complaints, and other clinical data.

IDN: See Integrated Delivery System.

IDS: See Integrated Delivery System.

Impaired Insurer: An insurer that is in financial difficulty to the point where its ability to meet financial obligations or regulatory requirements is in question.

Imputed Premium: Applies to self-funded plans where no actual premium is paid (other than reinsurance premium). Since the self-funded plan pays costs via a system of electronic lock-boxes, there is no pool of premium dollars that is regularly replenished. However, even a self-funded plan must budget for expected costs and must also determine the amount that should be deducted from an employee's paycheck for their portion of the cost of the plan; therefore, an imputed premium is calculated for these purposes.

In-Office Ancillary Services Exception (IOASE): A loophole that allows physicians to bill Medicare for ancillary services they provide as long as they're provided in the physician's office. Given how certain physicians who own costly diagnostic devices define their office, it's a loophole you can drive a truck through. Provisions in the ACA at least now require physicians who own and order such services to disclose it to Medicare, and to provide their patients with a disclosure form that also lists alternative providers.

In-Sourcing: Bringing back into the payer a process or activity that was once outsourced.

Incurred But Not Reported (IBNR): The amount of money that the plan had better accrue for medical expenses that it knows nothing about yet. These are medical expenses that the authorization system has not captured and for which claims have not yet hit the door. Unexpected IBNRs have torpedoed more managed care plans than any other cause.

Indemnity Insurance: Insurance that "indemnifies" the policyholder from losses. In health insurance, this applies to providing financial coverage for health care costs, with little or no attempt to manage that cost (other than, perhaps, a precertification program); most importantly, it is not based on a contracted network of providers, unlike a service plan that may otherwise appear the same. Indemnity insurance plans do limit the amount they will pay for a professional service, however, based on some form of fee scale; such limits are rarely in place for institutional costs, however. Once common, indemnity plans are quite rare now due to high cost.

Independent Practice Association (IPA): An organization that has a contract with a managed care plan to deliver services in return for a single capitation rate. The IPA in turn contracts with individual providers to provide the services either on a capitation basis or on a FFS basis. The typical IPA encompasses all specialties, but an IPA can be solely for primary care, or may be single specialty. An IPA may also be the "PO" part of a PHO.

Independent Review Organization: An independent group that a payer contracts with to provide a secondary external review of coverage denials based on medical reasons. The use of an IRO for external review is required in most states, and is required for all payers and health plans under the ACA.

Individual Mandate: A requirement that all individuals obtain health insurance. A mandate could apply to the entire population, just to children, and/or could exempt specified individuals. Massachusetts was the first state to impose an individual mandate that all adults have health insurance, and many health reform proposals include it. The individual mandate is the other side of the guaranteed issue requirement, thus ensuring that all individuals, not just the sick ones, will contribute funds to the overall risk pool.

Individual Policy: See Direct Pay.

Informatics: A loosely defined term that refers to collecting, classifying, storing and retrieving, and using data mining to create usable reports. It is intended to imply a more sophisticated approach to obtaining and using data than is used for routine operations. The term is preferentially used by many payers for the function and/or department that analyze medical data. Sometimes spelled as Infomatics.

Information Technology (IT): A blanket term referring to all of the computer hardware and software systems that support the operations of a health plan. Virtually all operational functions of a health plan are supported by IT in one way or another.

Integrated Delivery System (IDS): Also referred to as an integrated health care delivery system. Another acronym that means the same thing is IDN (integrated delivery network). An IDS is an organized system of health care providers spanning a broad range of health care services. Although there is no clear definition of an IDS, in its full flower an IDS should be able to access the market on a broad basis, optimize cost and clinical outcomes, accept and manage a full range of financial arrangements to provide a set of defined benefits to a defined population, align financial incentives of the participants (including physicians), and operate under a cohesive management structure. See also ACO, IHO, IPA, PHO, MSO, Equity Model, Staff Model, and Foundation Model.

Intelligent Call Routing or Skill-Based Routing: A computer system in a call center or contact center that sends the contact to the CSR group best prepared to handle the contact. Criteria for routing may include the issue type, severity of the issue, past history of interaction with a specific CSR or set of CSRs, employer group, or other business rules into which have been programmed.

Intensivist: A type of hospitalist (physician) that focuses solely on care provided in the intensive (or critical) care unit.

Intermediary: See Fiscal Intermediary.

Investigational Treatment: See Experimental and Investigational Treatment.

IOASE: See In-Office Ancillary Services Exception.

IPA: See Independent Practice Association.

IRO: See Independent Review Organization.

IS: Information Systems; see Information Technology.

IT: See Information Technology.

JCAHO: See Joint Commission.

J-Codes: A subset of the HCPCS codes used by Medicare, Medicaid, and commercial payers to identify injectable drugs and oral immunosuppressive drugs. May be created on the fly by CMS when a new drug first appears.

Joint Commission (JC): A not-for-profit organization that performs accreditation reviews primarily on hospitals, other institutional facilities, and outpatient facilities. Most managed care plans require any hospital under contract to be accredited by the Joint Commission. The old name was the Joint Commission for the Accreditation of Healthcare Organizations (JCAHO).

Lag Study: A report that tells managers how old the claims are being processed and how much is paid out each month (both for that month and for any earlier months) and compares

these to the amount of money that was accrued for expenses each month. A powerful tool used to determine whether the plan's reserves are adequate to meet all expenses. Plans that fail to perform lag studies properly may find themselves staring into the abyss.

Lag Table: The tool used by finance to manage the lag study.

Lapse: To drop coverage. This may refer to an individual who stops paying premiums, thereby allowing his or her policy to lapse, subject to a grace period (see Grace Period). When used as a ratio, it is the opposite of a persistency ratio (i.e., the percentage of commercially enrolled groups that drop the health plan).

Laser or Lasering: An actuarial and underwriting slang term referring to reducing or eliminating a very specific benefit (i.e., a benefit reduction that is focused like a laser). The more formal term used by reinsurers is a "Special Limitations" clause. Lasering is used only in self-funded employee benefits plans, and usually only small plans at that, because it is usually prohibited in state-regulated *health* insurance (reinsurance is not technically health insurance). An example of a laser might be placing a very high deductible for any claims incurred by a single individual with a history of high claims such as a disabled infant. A laser does not mean that the self-funded employee benefits plan can also reduce benefits for that individual, which would be considered discriminatory under ERISA. Only the reinsurer can apply the laser, while the employer remains liable for benefit costs.

Legend Drug: A drug that can only be provided with a prescription from a licensed provider.

Length of Stay (LOS): The total number of days spent in the hospital for an inpatient admission.

Levels of Coverage: Cost-sharing levels defined in the ACA as falling into four categories: Platinum (90% coverage), Gold (80%), Silver (70%), and Bronze (60%). Cost-sharing includes all out-of-pocket expenses, not just coinsurance. Applies to services provided by in-network providers.

Lifetime Maximum: Now prohibited under the ACA, a lifetime maximum referred to the maximum benefit available under a benefits plan, and once that maximum was reached, there was no additional coverage. A common example would be a $2 million lifetime maximum, so that if an individual with extremely high health care costs reached a point where that much coverage had been spent, that individual had no more coverage. See also Annual Limit.

Limited Benefits Plan: Very low cost health "insurance" plans that offer significant limits on benefits, most commonly through low annual and lifetime maximum coverage. For example, an LBP may cap coverage at only $10,000 or

$20,000 per year, and may cover outpatient care only up to a set amount of dollars per visit regardless of charges. LBPs do not provide adequate coverage for any serious illness or injury. Also called a "Mini-Med" plan.

Line of Business (LOB): A health plan such as an HMO, EPO, or PPO that is set up as a line of business within another, larger organization, usually an insurance company. This legally differentiates it from a free-standing company or a company set up as a subsidiary. It may also refer to a unique product type (e.g., Medicaid) within a health plan.

LIS: See Low-Income Subsidy.

LOB: See Line of Business.

Lock-In Period: Applicable to Medicare Advantage plans, it is the period of time during which a member cannot switch to another plan. MA annual open enrollment begins in the Fall and coverage begins on January 1, but beneficiaries can change plans until April 1 when the lock-in period begins.

Long-Term Care: Services needed by people to live independently in the community, such as home health and personal care, as well as institutional care such as nursing homes. Long-term care is paid either through special long-term care insurance policies, out of pocket, or (most commonly) by Medicaid. Most long-term care services are not covered by Medicare or private health insurance or managed care plans (aside from Medicaid managed care).

LOS/ELOS/ALOS: Length of stay/estimated length of stay/average length of stay. See Length of Stay.

Loss Ratio: See Medical Loss Ratio.

Low-Income Subsidy (LIS): A subsidy provided for dual eligible (Medicare–Medicaid) individuals for the Part D drug benefit.

MA Local Plan: A Medicare Advantage managed care plan that does not provide services throughout an entire region as designated by CMS.

MA Regional Plan: A Medicare Advantage PPO-type plan that provides services throughout an entire region as designated by CMS.

MAC: See Maximum Allowable Charge (or Cost).

MACPAC: See Medicaid and CHIP Payment and Access Commission.

Major Medical: An archaic but still used term to refer to health insurance that includes coverage of physician services. It can be traced back to the 1940s through the early 1960s when employer-sponsored group health coverage was usually "hospitalization," meaning hospital costs only. Commercial insurers of the time were essentially mimicking Blue Cross and Blue Shield plans with their historical

roots in hospitals and physicians, respectively. The term was never applicable to self-funded plans or HMOs, and will finally become a relic in 2014 when the ACA's qualified health benefit plans go into effect.

Managed Behavioral Health Care Organization (MBHO): A third party that manages the behavioral health services benefits for a payer. It may also contract directly with an employer. An MBHO may be at financial risk, or it may manage the services under an administrative contract only. A form of clinical outsourcing.

Managed Care Organization (MCO): A generic term applied to a managed care plan. In the past two decades, some payers used the term "payer" to refer to an HMO simply because they thought that there was less negative connotation. It then broadened out to encompass plans that do not conform exactly to the strict definition of an HMO (although that definition has itself loosened considerably) such as a PPO, EPO, CDHP, IDS, or even an OWA. Its use is in decline.

Managed Health Care: A regrettably nebulous term. At the very least, it is a system of health care delivery that tries to manage the cost of health care, the quality of that health care, and access to that care. Common denominators include a panel of contracted providers that is less than the entire universe of available providers, some type of limitations on benefits to subscribers who use noncontracted providers (unless authorized to do so), and some type of authorization or precertification system. Managed health care is actually a spectrum of systems, ranging from so-called managed indemnity, through CDHPs, POSs, PPOs, open-panel HMOs, and closed-panel HMOs. For a better definition, the reader is urged to read this book and formulate his or her own.

Management Information System (MIS): An older term for the computer hardware and software that provides the support for managing a plan. See also the more commonly used term, Information Technology.

Management Service Organization (MSO): A form of integrated health delivery system. Sometimes similar to a service bureau (see Service Bureau), the MSO often actually purchases certain hard assets of a physician's practice, and then provides services to that physician at fair market rates. MSOs are usually formed as a means to contract more effectively with managed care organizations, although their simple creation does not guarantee success.

Mandated Benefits: Benefits that a health plan are required to provide by law. This is generally used to refer to benefits above and beyond routine insurance-type benefits, and it generally applies at the state level where there is high variability from state to state. Common examples include in-vitro fertilization, defined days of inpatient mental health or substance abuse treatment, and other special-condition treatments. Self-funded plans are exempt from most mandated benefits under ERISA, but even the federal government gets into the act with a mandatory two-day length of stay for childbirth and mental health parity provisions under HIPAA that apply to both insured and self-funded plans. The ACA mandates benefits to a significant degree; some went into immediate effect, such as prevention, others go into effect beginning in 2014, such as "essential health benefits."

Manual Rate: See Book Rate.

MAO: See Medicare Advantage Organization (not to be confused with the pharmaceutical acronym MAO or MAOI: monoamine oxidase inhibitor, a type of antidepressant).

Margin: The amount of money left over, or lost, after costs are subtracted from revenues. There are two different types: operating margin and underwriting margin. See those definitions.

Master Group Contract: The actual contract between a health plan and a group that purchases coverage. The master group contract provides specific terms of coverage, rights, and responsibilities of both parties.

Master Member Index (MMI): The MMI is used in physician practice profiling to identify in a reliable manner each patient receiving care from a particular physician. Subject to the privacy and security provisions under HIPAA.

Maximum Allowable Charge of Cost (MAC): The maximum, although not the minimum, that a vendor may charge for something. This term is often used in pharmacy contracting; a related term, used in conjunction with professional fees, is fee maximum.

Maximum Out-of-Pocket Cost: The most amount of money a member will ever need to pay for covered services during a contract year. The maximum out of pocket includes deductibles and coinsurance. Once this limit is reached, the health plan pays for all services up to the maximum level of coverage. The level is determined by states for insured products, and the maximum is determined by the Department of the Treasury for all plans under the ACA.

MBHO: See Managed Behavioral Health Care Organization.

McCarran-Ferguson Act of 1945: The Act established that states had the authority and responsibility to regulate the business of insurance without federal government interference, and allows states to establish mandatory licensing requirements. It also contained a limited antitrust exemption allowing insurers to share certain underwriting information for purposes of rate development, but that aspect was not relevant to health insurers or payers.

MCE: See Medical Care Evaluation.

MCO: See Managed Care Organization.

Medicaid: Enacted in 1965 at the same time as Medicare, Medicaid is a federal entitlement program that provides health and long-term care coverage to certain categories of low-income Americans. States also contribute funding for Medicaid and design their own programs within broad federal guidelines.

Medicaid and CHIP Payment and Access Commission (MACPAC): A new commission created by the ACA to focus on Medicaid payment policy. MACPAC is similar to MedPAC, which focuses on Medicare payment policy.

Medicaid Management Information System (MMIS): The mechanized claims processing and information retrieval system that states are required to have, unless this requirement is waived by the Secretary of HHS.

Medicaid Waivers: Also known as a Section 1115 Waiver, it is a section of federal law allowing a state to opt out of the standard Medicaid FFS program and adopt a managed care approach to financing and providing health care services to Medicaid-eligible recipients. Usually requires that some of the savings be applied to broaden coverage of who is eligible for Medicaid.

Medical Care Evaluation (MCE): A component of a quality assurance program that looks at the process of medical care. The term is now archaic, but was used specifically when HMOs were federally qualified.

Medical Home: See Patient Centered Medical Home (PCMH).

Medical Informatics: See Informatics.

Medical Loss Ratio: The ratio between the claims or provider payment cost of medical care and the amount of money that was taken through premium payments. It only applies to fully insured or at-risk business. The ACA sets limits on the MLR of 80% for individual and small group coverage, and 85% for large groups; if the MLR is below those levels, the plan must rebate the difference. The medical loss ratio is dependent on the amount of money brought in as well as the cost of delivering care; thus, if the rates are too low, the ratio may be high, even though the actual cost of delivering care is not really out of line.

Medical Policy: From an operational point of view, medical policies are the internal rules about what will be paid for as medical benefits. Routine medical policy is linked to routine claims processing, and is typically automated. For example, the plan may only pay 50% of the fee of a second surgeon, or may not pay for two surgical procedures done during one episode of anesthesia. This also refers to how a plan approaches payment policy for experimental or investigational care, and payment for noncovered services in lieu of more expensive covered services. Health policy is also the term for public policy as applied to the overall health care sector.

Medical Savings Account (MSA): Created as a demonstration under BBA '97 and updated in the MMA, MSAs are specialized savings accounts into which a consumer can put pretax dollars for use in paying medical expenses in lieu of purchasing a comprehensive health insurance or managed care product. MSAs require a catastrophic health insurance policy as a "safety net" to protect against very high costs. They still exist, in both commercial form and for Medicare, but have been supplanted by CDHPs that are similar in approach but have additional features that make them more attractive to the market.

Medically Necessary: The term used to refer to whether or not a clinical service or supply such as a drug or a device is actually necessary to protect or preserve the health of an individual, based on evidence-based medical knowledge or practices. It is defined in the EOC of all benefits plans, and although those definitions are generally similar, they are typically not exactly the same.

Medicare: The entitlement health insurance provided by the federal government for citizens over the age of 65 as well as some others, such as individuals with end-stage renal disease. Regular Medicare is a FFS type of insurance; *Part A* covers hospital care and *Part B* covers professional services. *Part C* authorizes private plans such as Medicare Advantage. *Part D*, passed under the MMA, provides a drug benefit. Traditional FFS Medicare is administered by intermediaries on behalf of CMS, while Parts C and D come through various forms of private plans.

Medicare Advantage (MA): Created as part of the MMA, MA replaced and expanded other forms of Medicare managed care. MA plans may be HMOs, PPOs, or PFFS plans; they may also be local or regional. Special needs plans (SNPs) were also created to focus on specific types of beneficiaries. MA MSAs are also overseen under MA.

Medicare Advantage MSA Plan (MA MSA): See also MSAs. MSA plans are not network plans in the sense of being able to limit coverage to a network. Enrollees of such plans have the right to expect the plan to cover the cost of care at any provider willing to accept the individual as a patient, consistent with the rules of the plan regarding coverage (e.g., an MSA plan has no coverage before a deductible is met).

Medicare Advantage Organization (MAO): CMS's overall term used to refer to the various types of MA plans.

Medicare + Choice: The old name for Medicare private insurance options, created under BBA '97; most often applied to Medicare HMOs. The name has been replaced by various forms of Medicare Advantage plans under the MMA.

Medicare Improvements for Patients and Providers Act of 2008 (MIPPA): A law that reduced overpayments to the MA plan, required MA PFFS plans to establish networks, changed Part D marketing practices, and added preventive benefits (pre-ACA), among other things.

Medicare Modernization Act of 2003 (MMA): The federal act originally titled the *Medicare Prescription Drug Improvement and Modernization Act of 2003*. The MMA is the basis for both the Medicare Part D drug benefit and for the variety of Medicare Advantage (MA) plans described elsewhere, including MA Local, MA Regional, and MA PFFS.

Medicare Payment Advisory Commission (MedPAC): An independent congressional agency established by the Balanced Budget Act of 1997 to advise Congress on issues affecting the Medicare program. The Commission's statutory mandate is to advise the Congress on payments to providers in Medicare's traditional FFS program; private health plans participating in Medicare; and to analyze access to care, quality of care, and other issues affecting Medicare. See also MACPAC.

Medicare Recovery Audit Contractors (RAC): Auditors under contract to review the appropriateness of data supporting payment.

Medicare Severity Diagnosis-Related Groups (MS-DRGs): Implemented by Medicare to replace traditional DRGs. MS-DRGs are based not only on the diagnosis and procedures performed, but also take into account other chronic conditions and comorbidities, including those that are major. The intent was to reduce the number of cases classified as outliers, but chargemaster inflation has resulted in continued high numbers of outlier cases.

Medication Therapy Management (MTM): Required under the MMA for Part D sponsors, MTM is a program to ensure optimum therapeutic outcomes and reduced adverse events for targeted beneficiaries through improved medication use.

Medigap Insurance: A form of state-licensed health insurance that covers whatever Medicare doesn't. Medigap policies are subject to minimum standards under federal law and are restricted to 12 different benefits plans, labeled A through L, sold and administered by private companies. Medigap has been further restricted under the MMA.

MedPAC: See Medicare Payment Advisory Commission.

Member Months: The total of all months that each member was covered. For example, if a plan had 10,000 members in January and 12,000 members in February, the total member months for the year to date as of March 1 would be 22,000.

Member: An individual covered under a managed care plan. May be either the subscriber or a dependent.

Member Services: The department, as well as the actual services, that support a member's needs, not including the actual provision of health care. Examples of such member services include resolving problems, managing disputes by members about coverage issues, managing the grievance and appeals processes, and so forth. Member services also function in a proactive manner, reaching out to members with educational programs, self-service capabilities, and the like. Also known as customer services.

Mental Health Parity Act of 1996: This Act requires that annual or lifetime dollar limits on mental health benefits be no lower than any such dollar limits for medical and surgical benefits offered by a group health plan. It does not apply to benefits for substance abuse or chemical dependency, however. See Mental Health Parity and Addiction Equity Act of 2008.

Mental Health Parity and Addiction Equity Act of 2008: This acts requires group health plans and health insurance issuers to ensure that financial requirements (such as co-pays and deductibles) and treatment limitations (such as visit limits) for mental health or substance use benefits are no more restrictive than those used for medical/surgical benefits.

Messenger Model: A type of IDS that simply acts as a messenger between a payer and the providers participating in the IDS in regard to contracting terms. Does not have the power to collectively bargain, thus avoiding antitrust violations.

MET: Multiple Employer Trust; see Multiple Employer Welfare Association.

MEWA: See Multiple Employer Welfare Association.

MFN: See Most Favored Nation.

MHS: See Military Health System.

Midlevel Practitioner (MLP): Physician's assistants, clinical nurse practitioners, nurse midwives, and the like. Nonphysicians who deliver medical care, generally under the supervision of a physician but for less cost.

Military Health System (MHS): A large and complex health care system designed to provide, and to maintain readiness to provide, medical services and support to the armed forces during military operations and to provide medical services and support to members of the armed forces, their dependents, and others entitled to Department of Defense (DoD) medical care. See also TRICARE.

Mini-Med: See Limited Benefits Plan.

Minimum Creditable Coverage: The minimum level of health benefits coverage in order for an individual to be considered insured.

Minimum Premium Plan: A type of insurance plan that closely resembles self-funding in which the employer is responsible for claims costs up to a certain level, which is usually very high. After that, the insurer is at risk, similar to reinsurance. With the advent of ERISA, minimum premium plans have largely been replaced with self-funded plans and reinsurance.

MIPPA: See Medicare Improvements for Patients and Providers Act of 2008.

MIS: See Management Information System.

Mixed Model: A managed care plan that mixes two or more types of delivery systems. This has traditionally been used to describe an HMO that has both closed-panel and open-panel delivery systems.

MLP: See Midlevel Practitioner.

MMA: See Medicare Modernization Act.

MMI: See Master Member Index.

MMIS: See Medicaid Management Information System.

Moral Hazard: An old term of insurance that remains applicable today. Loosely defined for purposes of this glossary, moral hazard refers to changes in the behavior of an insured individual (or organization) caused by the existence of insurance itself, and for that behavior change to increase costs to the insurer. It can occur if the insured knows something the insurer doesn't, and which would have an impact on premiums or even providing insurance at all, for example, not buying health insurance until you discover a lump (i.e., a preexisting condition that insurers can refuse to cover until the ACA prohibits that beginning in 2014). It can occur if the insured engages in risky behavior only because they're insured, for example, insuring a cargo ship to shorten time at sea by sailing through pirate-infested waters. It can occur if having insurance encourages its use, even in the absence of risky behavior, for example, people with health insurance use it regularly, whereas people with life insurance use it once (and hope to never use it). Finally, it can occur if the insurer's agent (i.e., a person or organization that is able to save or spend the insurer's money) is not financially aligned with the insurer, for example, an auto body shop that overestimates damages to get the insurer to pay for a customer's new paint job, or in the case of health care, all providers who are paid via fee for services.

Most Favored Nation (MFN) Clause: A clause in a contract between a payer and a health system that requires the health system to give the payer the best rate; in other words, it prohibits the health system from giving any nongovernmental payer a more favorable rate than it gives the payer. Once commonly used by large hegemonic payers such as Blue Cross and Blue Shield plans that had most of the business in a state, it is illegal in many states, although it is not actually considered anticompetitive.

MSA: See Medical Savings Account. Not to be confused with Metropolitan Statistical Area.

MS-DRG: See Medicare Severity Diagnosis-Related Groups.

MSO: See Management Service Organization.

MTM: See Medication Therapy Management.

Multiple Employer Welfare Association (MEWA) or Multiple Employer Trust (MET): A group of employers who band together for purposes of creating a self-funded health benefits plan to avoid state mandates and insurance regulation. By virtue of ERISA, such entities are regulated little, if at all. However, they are subject to the ACA. Many MEWAs have enabled small employers to obtain cost-effective health coverage, but some have not had the financial resources to withstand the risk of medical costs and have failed, leaving the members without insurance or recourse. MEWAs and METs are also more susceptible to fraud than traditional insurance or a single employer self-funded benefits plan. See also Association Health Plan.

Mutual Insurance Company or Mutual Insurer or Mutual: Companies with no capital stock, and owned by policyholders. The earnings of the company—over and above the payments of the losses, operating expenses, and reserves—are the property of the policyholders.

NADDI: See National Association of Drug Diversion Investigators.

NAIC: See National Association of Insurance Commissioners.

National Association of Drug Diversion Investigators (NADDI): A nonprofit organization that facilitates cooperation between law enforcement, health care professionals, state regulatory agencies, and pharmaceutical manufacturers in the prevention and investigation of prescription drug diversion.

National Association of Insurance Commissioners (NAIC): An organization that represents all of the state insurance departments and that formulates model insurance laws and regulations. Provisions of the ACA require the HHS Secretary to seek the recommendations of the NAIC for many elements.

National Committee on Quality Assurance (NCQA): A not-for-profit organization that performs quality-oriented accreditation reviews on HMOs and similar types of managed care plans. NCQA also now accredits CVOs, PPOs, certain types of DM programs, and so forth. NCQA developed and maintains the HEDIS® standards.

National Council for Prescription Drug Programs (NCPDP): The NCPDP developed and maintains accepted electronic data interchange standards for pharmacy claims transmission and adjudication accelerated adoption of pharmacy e-commerce. This standard permits the submission of pharmacy claims and the adjudication of those claims in a real-time interactive mode. Recognized by ANSI, and addressed under HIPAA.

National Drug Code (NDC): The national classification system for identifying prescription drugs.

National Health Plan Identifier: An identifier mandated under HIPAA. These will be the identifiers used by health plans (broadly defined) when conducting all transactions, regardless of the type of customer (commercial health plan, Medicare plan, etc.) or provider. At the time of publication, neither the standards for the National Health Plan Identifier nor an implementation date have been announced. The actual name for this identifier may change when it is finally defined, which accounts for the distressing lack of an acronym.

National Practitioner Data Bank (NPDB): A databank established under the federal Health Care Improvement and Quality Act of 1986, it electronically stores information about physician malpractice suits successfully litigated or settled and disciplinary actions upon physicians. Accessible by hospitals and health plans under controlled circumstances as part of the credentialing process. Hospitals and health plans must likewise report disciplinary actions to the data bank.

National Provider Identifier (NPI): The NPI is mandated under HIPAA, and replaced almost all other types of provider (broadly defined) identifiers regardless of customer (commercial health plan, Medicare, Medicaid, TRICARE, etc.). The NPI is a 10-digit number, with the 10th digit being a checksum that can help detect keying errors. It contains no embedded intelligence; that is, it contains no information about the health care provider such as the type of health care provider or state where the health care provider is located. The NPI does not replace the DEA number or the Tax ID number of a provider, however.

National Quality Forum (NQF): A not-for-profit, public-private organization created to develop and implement a national strategy for health care quality measurement and reporting. It is a voluntary consensus standards-setting organization addressing quality measurements in patient care, electronic health records, patient safety, and so forth. Found at www.qualityforum.org on the Web.

Navigator: Aside from the usual meaning as an individual who keeps a ship on course, the ACA defines a navigator as a qualified entity that helps consumers and employers understand their options and select coverage through a state health insurance exchange.

NCPDP: See National Council for Prescription Drug Programs.

NCQA: See National Committee on Quality Assurance.

NDC: See National Drug Code.

NDP: See Notice of Denial of Payment.

Net Worth: See Statutory Net Worth.

Network Model HMO: A health plan that contracts with multiple physician groups to deliver health care to members. Generally limited to large single or multispecialty groups. Distinguished from group model plans that contract with a single medical group, IPAs that contract through an intermediary, and direct contract model plans that contract with individual physicians in the community.

Never Event: A medical error that occurs in a facility (hospital or ambulatory surgical center) that should never happen. An example of a never event is amputation of the wrong limb. Definitions exist for 27 such never events. Medicare as well as most payers will not pay for care required as a result of a never event.

NHCAA: See Health Care Anti-Fraud Association.

NIO: See Noninvestor Owned.

Nocturnist: A type of hospitalist that covers inpatients at night.

Nonadmitted Asset: An asset owned by an insurer or HMO that does not count toward its statutory net worth under SAP rules. It may vary from state to state, but usually is applied to assets that cannot be readily converted into cash in the event of a health plan failure. It may also apply to only a portion of such an asset; for example, no more than 5% of a plan's statutory net worth can consist of such assets as computers, real estate, and so forth.

Noninvestor Owned (NIO): An insurer that is not a for-profit company, but is not technically a nonprofit charitable organization either. It is most often a type of mutual insurer or mutual reserve company, and is taxed like a for-profit.

Nonpar: Short for nonparticipating. Refers to a provider that does not have a contract with the health plan.

Notice of Denial of Payment (NDP): A form CMS requires MA plans to use when notifying a beneficiary that a payment for a service is being denied, why it's being denied, and what appeal rights the beneficiary has.

NPI: See National Provider Identifier.

Observation Unit: A treatment room usually adjacent to the ED where rapid evaluation and stabilization of a medical problem can be managed, resulting either in admission or in discharge of the patient within 23 hours. A common example is a chest pain unit.

Occurrence Insurance or Reinsurance: One of two primary types of professional liability insurance, it applies to professional malpractice insurance for physicians, but is applicable to directors and officers liability policies and to reinsurance as well. Occurrence means that the insurer has liability if the policy was in force when the event occurred, regardless of whether or not the professional has notified the insurer. This differs substantially from the other common form of professional liability known as claims made, and from a third type of reinsurance called claims paid. See Claims Made and Claims Paid.

OCR: See Office for Civil Rights or Optical Character Recognition, depending on the context.

Office for Civil Rights: A department within the U.S. Department of Health and Human Services charged with enforcing HIPAA privacy and security standards, among other things.

Office of the Inspector General (OIG): The federal agency responsible for conducting investigations and audits of federal contractors or any system that receives funds or payment from the federal government. There are actually several OIG departments in different federal programs; examples pertinent to managed health care would include TRICARE, CMS, and the FEHBP.

Office of Personnel Management (OPM): The federal agency that administers the FEHBP. This is the agency with which a managed care plan contracts to provide coverage for federal employees.

OIG: See Office of the Inspector General.

Open Access: A term that refers to an HMO that does not use a primary care physician "gatekeeper" model for access to specialty physicians. In other words, a member may self-refer to a specialty physician rather than seeking an authorization from the PCP. HMOs that use an open-access model typically have a significant copayment differential between care received. May also be called direct access.

Open Enrollment Period: The period when an employee may change health plans; usually occurs once per year. A general rule is that most managed care plans will have around half their membership up for open enrollment in the Fall for an effective date of January 1. In some states there is an annual open enrollment period in which HMOs and not-for-profit payers must accept any individual applicant (i.e., one not coming in through an employer group) for coverage, regardless of health status. Under the ACA, beginning in 2014 open enrollment will become mandatory for all insurers and HMOs. The minimum requirement is for a month per year, but the ACA leaves it to the state to define when that will happen each year, including the possibility of continuous open enrollment.

Open-Panel HMO: A managed care plan that contracts (either directly or indirectly) with private physicians to deliver care in their own offices. Examples would include a direct contract HMO and an IPA model HMO.

Operating Margin: The amount of money left over, or lost, after subtracting the cost of care and the cost of operations from revenues. Generally does not include the cost of taxes, does include the revenue from investments, but may or may not include margin contribution from subsidiaries.

OPL: See Other Party Liability. See also Coordination of Benefits.

OPM: See Office of Personnel Management.

Opt Out: A managed care benefits design in which a member can opt out of using the plan's network and still receive some coverage for medical services; for example, a POS plan may be considered an HMO with an opt-out benefit.

Optical Character Recognition: A system of hardware and software that is able to recognize written characters scanned in from a paper source and convert those characters into standard data. Used in any processing systems in which paper forms may be submitted; claims and enrollment forms are the most common. Data scanned in via OCR is usually checked by clerks for accuracy and to correct errors; however, it is still more efficient than keying the data in manually.

Organization Provider: The term used by NCQA and some other organizations to describe facilities as providers, for example, hospitals, ambulatory care centers, dialysis centers, and so forth.

Out-of-Pocket: Any amount of money spent by a member on benefits. Usually synonymous with cost-sharing, but some include payroll deductions in the category as well.

Other Party Liability (OPL): A term that means another party is completely responsible to pay for the costs. The most common examples are workers' compensation and automobile liability policies. It is not exactly the same as COB. See also COB.

Other Weird Arrangement (OWA): Refers to some type of benefits plan, product design, or network contract that some bright person or consultant has created but for which there is no precedent, no track record, and no easy means of implementing.

Outlier: Something that is outside of a range. Most often applied to hospital payment under which inpatient cases that exceed a certain cost, based on chargemaster fees, receive additional payments based on a discount to chargemaster fees. May also be used to refer to a provider who is using medical resources at a much higher rate than their peers, or to a case in a hospital that is far more expensive than anticipated, or in fact to anything at all that is significantly more or less than expected.

Outsourcing: Having a process or activity that a payer provides done by a contracted third party. For example, contracting with an off-shore company to manually enter data from images of paper claims.

OWA: See Other Weird Arrangement.

P4P: See Pay for Performance.

PACE: See Programs for All Inclusive Care for the Elderly.

Package Pricing: An older term for bundled payment. See Bundled Payment.

Par Provider: Shorthand term for participating provider (i.e., one who has signed an agreement with a plan to provide services). May apply to professional or institutional providers.

Part D: The drug benefit created under the MMA. May be provided by a private, free-standing prescription drug plan, or included in an MA plan as an MA-PDP.

Partial Hospitalization: A hospital stay that lasts between 4 and 23 hours.

Patient-Centered Medical Home (PCMH): The term used by CMS and others to refer to a form of coordinated care through the use of designated primary care physicians and a clinical team. The medical home concept put forth by a joint statement by the AAFP, ACP, AAP, and AOA is to emphasize four key primary care elements: accessibility, continuity, coordination, and comprehensiveness, which research shows positively affect health outcomes, satisfaction, and costs. Also something that most well-run group model HMOs have been doing for decades. Sans substantial organizational changes, its long-term utility, durability, and replicability is unknown. Sometimes called a primary care medical home or simply medical home.

Patient Protection and Affordable Care Act (ACA or PPACA; Public Law 111-148): An Act signed into federal law by President Barack Obama in 2010. The ACA provides for a sweeping overhaul of the rules under which health insurance may operate, regardless of whether or not it is fully insured or self-funded. The ACA also contains many provisions beyond those that directly affect health coverage, including changes in funding for primary care, how hospitals are paid, changes to Medicare Advantage, and so forth. Provisions are addressed as appropriate throughout this text.

Patient Safety and Quality Improvement Act of 2005 (PSQIA): A law providing federal privilege and confidentiality protections for patient safety information (called a patient safety work product) that includes information collected and created during the reporting and analysis of patient safety events. Created in response to the difficulty in collecting information about patient safety problems due to the threat of such information being used as the basis for a lawsuit.

Patient Safety Organization (PSO): A new type of organization described by federal rules in which clinicians and health care providers can work to collect, aggregate, and analyze data within a legally secure environment of privilege and confidentiality protections to identify and reduce patient care risks and hazards. AHRQ administers provisions governing PSO operations, and HHS's Office for Civil Rights enforces confidentiality provisions. The same acronym was used for the now archaic term provider-sponsored organization.

Patient's Bill of Rights (PBR): A law or policy describing what rights a patient has regarding his or her health care and how he or she should be treated, and may be applied to either a provider or a payer. A voluntary PBR is often posted by hospitals. Some states also have PBR legislation regarding health insurers. In the 1990s, Congress made several attempts to pass a PBR, but never succeeded. With the passage of the ACA in 2010, however, various provisions falling under the broad category of consumer protections are now called a Patient's Bill of Rights.

Pay and Chase: The antonym is pursue and pay, or "chase" and pay. A term commonly used in COB, it refers to the health plan paying for the claim and then trying to recover all or some of the costs from the other insurance company. See also Chase and Pay and Coordination of Benefits..

Pay and Pursue: See Pay and Chase.

Pay for Performance: Term applied to providing financial incentives to providers (hospitals and/or physicians) to improve compliance with standards of care and to improve outcomes and patient safety. Usually referred to as P4P when in print.

Payer: Generic term applicable to any commercial health insurer or benefits administrator that pays medical claims. It is sometimes spelled "payor," as it was by your humble editor in earlier editions of this very book, but that once commonly used spelling has been slowly disappearing.

PCCM: See Primary Care Case Manager.

PCMH: See Patient-Centered Medical Home.

PCP: See Primary Care Physician.

PDP: See Prescription Drug Plan.

Peer Review Organization (PRO): The old name for organizations charged with reviewing quality and cost for Medicare. Since replaced by QIOs.

PEL: See Provider Excess Loss.

Pend or Pended: See Suspend, a term used in claims processing.

PEPM: See Per Employee per Month.

Per Diem Payment: Payment of an institution, usually a hospital, based on a set rate per day rather than on charges. Per diem payment can be varied by service (e.g., medical/surgical, obstetrics, mental health, and intensive care) or can be uniform regardless of intensity of services.

Per Employee per Month (PEPM): Like PMPM, but rolls the unit up to the level of the employee or subscriber, rather than measuring based on all members (subscriber plus dependents).

Per Member per Month (PMPM): The total revenue, cost, or unit of utilization during a time period, averaged across all enrolled members (both subscribers and dependents) as though on a monthly basis. To use a simple example, if an HMO has 100 members and during the course of the year one member has $70,000 in hospital expenses, one has $50,000 in hospital expenses, and one has $45,000 in hospital expenses, the HMO's hospital costs would be $137.50 PMPM [(($70,000 + $50,000 + $45,000) ÷ 12) ÷ 100].

Per Member per Year (PMPY): The same as PMPM, but based on a year (leave out the 12 in the above example).

Per Thousand Members per Year (PTMPY): A common way of reporting utilization. The most common example is hospital utilization, expressed as days per thousand members per year.

Persistency: Also called a persistency ratio. The term refers to a commercial group staying with a payer organization from year to year. A persistency ratio of 90 would mean that 90% of groups enrolled do not change health plans.

Personal Health Record: A record, usually created by a health plan, of an individual's health-related data. The sources of that data include claims from providers, prescription drugs the plan paid for, demographic data, and so forth. Clinical data such as results of diagnostic lab or imaging may be provided if the plan has access to it, and the member can add additional data such as drug allergies or the results of a health risk appraisal. The purpose is to provide at least a usable subset of important health-related information in an electronically portable or transmittable format to improve continuity of care and emergency care.

PFFS: See Private FFS Plan.

PHI: See Protected Health Information.

PHO: See Physician-Hospital Organization.

PHR: See Personal Health Record.

Physician Incentive Program: A generic term referring to a payment methodology under which a physician's income from a payer (or an IDS) is affected by the physician's performance or the overall performance of the plan (e.g., utilization, medical cost, quality measurements, member satisfaction). This term has a very specific usage by the CMS, which limits the degree of incentive or risk allowed under a Medicare HMO (refer to PIP regulations at 42 CFR 422.208/210 of the June 26, 1998, regulations that implement Medicare Part C). CMS essentially bans "gainsharing" via a PIP altogether in an IDS receiving payment under Medicare. Some states also now have laws and regulations regarding limits on PIPs and requirements for disclosure of incentives to members enrolled in payers. See also SFR.

Physician Practice Management Company (PPMC): An organization that manages physicians' practices, and in most cases either owns the practices outright or has rights to purchase them in the future. PPMs concentrate only on physicians and not on hospitals, although some PPMs have also branched into joint ventures with hospitals and insurers. Most PPMs failed spectacularly, but some still exist, particularly for single specialties.

Physician Quality Reporting System (PQRS): A program under Medicare in which physicians report data on selected measures of quality and receive an incentive payment. The potential value of the incentive in 2011 was up to 1% of a physician's total annual payments by Medicare. Most likely the amount of payment reductions and/or incentives will change periodically. Started out as a pilot called the Physician Quality Reporting Initiative (PQRI), and was changed to PQRS in 2011.

Physician-Hospital Organization (PHO): These are organizations that bond hospitals and the attending medical staff, developed for the purpose of contracting with managed care plans. A PHO may be open to any members of the staff who apply, or they may be closed to staff members who fail to qualify or who are part of an already overrepresented specialty.

Platinum Level of Benefits or Platinum Plan: As defined in the ACA, a qualified health benefits plan with the actuarial equivalent or average of 10% cost-sharing, when accounting for deductibles, copayments, and coinsurance as applied to in-network services.

PMPM: See Per Member per Month.

PMPY: See Per Member per Year.

POD: See Pool of Doctors.

Point of Service (POS): A plan where members do not have to choose how to receive services until they need them. The most common use of the term applies to a plan that enrolls each member in both an HMO (or HMO-like) system and a PPO or an indemnity plan. These plans provide a difference in benefits (e.g., 100% coverage rather than 70%) depending on whether the member chooses to use the plan (including

its providers and in compliance with the authorization system) or go outside the plan for services.

Pool of Doctors (POD): This refers to the plan grouping physicians into units smaller than the entire panel, but larger than individual practices. Typical PODs have between 10 and 30 physicians. Often used for performance measurement and compensation. The POD is typically not a legal entity, but rather a grouping. Not to be confused with the pod people from *Invasion of the Body Snatchers*.

Pooling: See Risk Pool.

Portability: Refers to the ability of people to obtain coverage as they move from job to job or in and out of employment. Individuals changing jobs are guaranteed coverage with the new employer without a waiting period. In addition, insurers must waive any preexisting condition exclusions for individuals who were previously covered within a specified time period. Portable coverage can also be health coverage that is not connected to an employer, allowing individuals to keep their coverage when they have a change in employment. Portability is provided under HIPAA, but is very expensive.

Portal: Also called an Internet portal. Refers to a single Internet website providing access to multiple other sites and/or functionalities. For example, payers in a region may jointly offer a single sign-on portal for providers to use for checking a patient's coverage eligibility. The ACA also required HHS to create a consumer portal for health insurance, and state health insurance exchanges will also have to create consumer portals.

POS: See Point of Service.

PPACA: Also called the ACA; see the Patient Protection and Affordable Care Act.

PPMC: See Physician Practice Management Company.

PPO: See Preferred Provider Organization.

PPS: See Prospective Payment System.

PQRI: Physician Quality Reporting Initiative, the pilot program replaced by the PQRS. See Physician Quality Reporting System.

PQRS: See Physician Quality Reporting System.

Preauthorization: See Authorization. See also Precertification.

Precertification: Also known as preadmission certification, preadmission review, and pre-cert. The process of obtaining certification or authorization from the health plan for routine hospital admissions or for ambulatory procedures. Often involves appropriateness review against criteria and assignment of length of stay. Failure to obtain precertification often results in a financial penalty to either the provider or the subscriber.

Preexisting Condition: A medical condition for which a member has received treatment during a specified period of time prior to becoming covered under a health plan. May have an effect on whether or not treatments for that condition will be covered under certain types of health plans.

Preferred Provider Organization (PPO): A plan that contracts with independent providers at a discount for services. The panel is limited in size and usually has some type of utilization review system associated with it. A PPO may be risk-bearing, like an insurance company, or may be non-risk-bearing, like a physician-sponsored PPO that markets itself to insurance companies or self-insured companies via an access fee. See also Rental PPO.

Premium: The money paid to a health plan for coverage. The term may be applied on an individual basis or a group basis. Recognized by the health plan as premium revenue; see earned Premium Revenue and Unearned Premium Revenue. See also Imputed Premium.

Premium Compression: The result of a law or regulation placing limits on how much difference is allowable between the highest and lowest premiums; for example, a community rated premium in which the most expensive rate can be no more than four times higher than the least expensive rate. Compressing the range of allowable rates results in more subsidization of costlier groups by healthier groups.

Premium Insufficiency: A term that means an insurer is not charging enough in premiums to cover medical and administrative costs. Out-of-control administrative costs can cause it, but it typically occurs when benefits costs rise higher than what was expected when the premium rates were originally calculated. It is particularly dangerous because an insurer must live with an insufficient premium for the entire year that policy is in place, so losses mount each month and the insurer cannot collect more money from the insured.

Premium Tax: A tax levied by a state on health insurance premiums for policies sold in that state. Employers that self-fund their health benefits plan, as well as Medicare Advantage plans, are not subject to premium taxes.

Premium-Cost Compression: The reduction in the difference between what a health plan is able to charge and what it costs to pay for care. May be a result of regulatory or competitive market forces. It not only reduces the plan's ability to generate a positive underwriting margin, but also reduces the ability to withstand errors or cost overruns.

Prepaid or Prepayment: Payment for services before they are incurred. Capitation is a form of prepayment since the provider is paid before the month that services will be provided. HMOs were once called prepaid health plans since premiums were paid in advance of the HMO providing the service. Can also be applied to the prepayment of any type of insurance premium, though health plans sometimes prefer to call it unearned premium revenue. Never applies to self-funding except when self-funded plans fund capitation to providers.

Prescription Drug Plan (PDP): A private, free-standing plan providing drug coverage to Medicare beneficiaries under MA. Does not provide coverage for other services.

Preventive Care: Health care that is aimed at preventing complications of existing diseases or preventing the occurrence of a disease. Often misspelled as "preventative."

Primary Care Case Manager (PCCM): Used in Medicaid managed care programs, it refers to the state designating PCPs as case managers to function as "gatekeepers," but paying those PCPs using traditional Medicaid FFS, as well as paying the PCP a nominal management fee such as $5 or $10 PMPM.

Primary Care Physician (PCP): Generally applies to internists, pediatricians, family physicians, and general practitioners and occasionally to obstetrician/gynecologists.

Private Fee-for-Service Plan (PFFS): A type of Medicare Advantage plan in which a private insurance company accepts risk for enrolled beneficiaries, but pays providers on a FFS basis that does not have any risk component to the provider. PFFS plans were originally not network plans in the sense of being able to limit coverage to a network, but are now required to have networks of contracted providers, consistent with the rules of the plan regarding coverage. Because of new network requirements and reductions in payment from CMS, PFFS plans have sharply declined in numbers.

Private Inurement: What happens when a not-for-profit business operates in such a way as to provide more than incidental financial gain to a private individual; for example, if a not-for-profit hospital pays too much money for a physician's practice, or fails to charge fair market rates for services provided to a physician. Prohibited by the Internal Revenue Service.

PRO: See Peer Review Organization.

Producer: In health insurance and managed care it refers to the brokers and agents who sell the plan's policies to businesses and individuals.

Professional Services Agreement (PSA): A contract between a physician or medical group and an IDS or payer for the provision of medical services.

Profiling: Measuring a provider's performance on selected measures and comparing that performance to similar providers. Usually applied to physicians. May be used for purposes of network selection or tiering, feedback reports, and/or P4P programs. Very complicated to perform properly.

Programs for All-Inclusive Care for the Elderly (PACE): A federally funded program for seniors who are state-certified as needing nursing home care, but who can live safely in their communities. PACE facilitates community resources to help those individuals continue to live in the community.

Prospective Payment System (PPS): Medicare's terminology for determining fixed pricing for payment of hospitals and facilities for care. The most well-known examples of PPS are DRGs, APCs, and now MS-DRGs. Prospective payment may be used by commercial plans as it applies to payment of facilities using the same methodologies.

Prospective Review: Reviewing whether or not a medical service will be covered before the care is rendered. See also Precertification.

Protected Health Information (PHI): That information that reveals medical information or data about an individual. PHI is addressed specifically by HIPAA in the Privacy and Security sections.

Provider: The generic term used to refer to anyone providing medical services. In fact, it may even be used to refer to any*thing* that provides medical services, such as a hospital. Most often, however, it is used to refer to physicians. How physicians migrated from being called physicians to being called providers is not very clear-cut, and certainly not embraced by physicians, but it is a term in general use, including in this book.

Provider Excess Loss (PEL): Refers to a stop-loss insurance policy purchased by risk-bearing provider organizations, full-risk-bearing medical groups, or IDSs in order to limit exposure to catastrophic claims costs.

Provider-Sponsored Organization (PSO): An archaic term referring to an entity allowed under the BBA '97. A PSO was a risk-bearing managed care organization that contracted directly with CMS (HCFA at the time) to cover Medicare enrollees. Unlike a typical HMO, the PSO was made up of the providers themselves, and they had to bear substantial risk for expenses; unlike an HMO owned by a large organized medical group, the providers were all independent. PSOs were the result of a belief by providers and legislators that there were fat profits to be had through "cutting out the middle man" by removing the HMO from the equation. With a few small exceptions, they failed utterly and lost considerable amounts of money. The federal waiver authority for PSOs expired quietly in 2002. CMS, being a green agency, recycled the acronym and it now stands for Patient Safety Organization.

Prudent Layperson: See Reasonable Layperson Standard.

PSA: See Professional Services Agreement.

PSO: See Patient Safety Organization (first definition) or Provider-Sponsored Organization (second and older definition); see those definitions.

PTMPY: See Per Thousand Members per Year.

Pursue and Pay: See Pay and Pursue.

QA or QM: Quality assurance (older term) or quality management (newer term).

QIO: See Quality Improvement Organization.

QIP: See Quality Improvement Program.

QISMC: See Quality Improvement System for Managed Care.

Qualified Health Plan: Defined in the ACA as a health plan that is certified or recognized by a state health insurance exchange, provides the ACA-defined essential health benefits, is licensed by the state, and offers at least one Gold- and one Silver-level benefits plans through the Exchange. See also Essential Health Benefits and Health Insurance Exchange.

Quality Improvement Expenses: Under the ACA, health plan costs associated with improving quality may be considered as a medical cost instead of an administrative cost, for purposes of calculating the MLR.

Quality Improvement Organization (QIO): An organization under contract to CMS to conduct quality reviews of providers, respond to beneficiary complaints about care, measure and report performance of providers, ensure that payment is made only for medically necessary services, and other functions. It applies to all types of plans and services, not just managed care.

Quality Improvement Program (QIP): The program put in place by CMS for Medicare Advantage plans of all types. The QIP uses data from HEDIS, HOS, and CAHPS, as well as financial and member disenrollment data. Accreditation by NCQA is also considered under the QIP.

Quality Improvement System for Managed Care (QISMC): The now discontinued CMS program regarding quality of care and member satisfaction for Medicare risk plans, it was replaced by the QIP.

Qui Tam Sui: A provision in tort law that allows a citizen to file suit on behalf of the (federal) government, and to collect one-third of the proceeds of that lawsuit. Such suits are usually also subject to treble damages, making success a lucrative endeavor. The point of this is to encourage citizens with knowledge of deliberate wrongdoing to blow the whistle on the transgressor, since the government cannot always know when fraud is occurring. In the context of this book, qui tam sui applies to health insurance programs paid with federal funds (i.e., Medicare, Medicaid, TRICARE, and the FEHBP).

RAC: See Medicare Recovery Audit Contractors.

Rate: Synonymous with premium rate. The amount of money that a group or individual must pay to the health plan for coverage.

Rate Band: Premium rates charged to all individuals within a specific age group, such as all individuals between the ages of 41 and 50. Rate banding was designed to provide low rates to the young and healthy and thereby entice them to buy coverage, and then progressively rise consistent with higher costs incurred by older people. The ACA does not prohibit rate banding, but restricts the rate spread to a maximum of 3:1 as of 2014.

Rate Spread: The difference between the highest and lowest premium rates within a risk pool, for example, all individual subscribers or small employer groups. The ACA prohibits a rate spread above 3:1 as of 2014, and even then based only on age.

Rating: Rating refers to the health plan developing premium rates. Not to be confused with various rating indicators such as the MA Stars program.

RBC: See Risk-Based Capital.

RBRVS: See Resource-Based Relative Value Scale.

Reasonable Layperson Standard: This means that the judgment of a reasonable nonclinician should be applied in determining if a service is warranted or not. This standard is almost always focused on the use of emergency or urgent care, when a layperson has good reason to believe that a medical problem must be addressed immediately, even if a trained provider may not feel that it was urgent. The specific language most often used, and addressed directly in the Balanced Budget Act of 1997 as pertaining to Medicare and Medicaid recipients, is: *"Health plans should provide payment when a consumer presents to an emergency department with acute symptoms of sufficient severity— including severe pain—such that a "prudent layperson" could reasonably expect the absence of medical attention to result in placing health in serious jeopardy, serious impairment to bodily functions, or serious dysfunction of any bodily organ or part."*

Rebate: In general usage, a rebate is simply returning some money to a purchaser. Under the ACA, it also means that a health insurer must return to consumers or employers the difference in their actual medical costs and the medical loss ratio (MLR). For large employer groups, the minimum MLR is 85%, and for individuals and small employer groups it is 80%.

Rebundlers: Software programs that roll up and reprice fragmented bills as well as apply industry-standard claims adjudication conventions.

Reference Pricing: A term that means benefits coverage is based on the lowest available market price, not necessarily what was charged. It's usually applied to biologics and other pharmaceuticals, as well as devices.

Regional Health Information Organization (RHIO): A nongovernmental entity that facilitates electronic health information to flow between different organizations such as physicians, hospitals, and payers. At the time of publication and for the last 18 + years, most RHIOs have consisted primarily of committee meetings. See Health Information Exchanges.

Reimbursement: A term commonly but incorrectly used to refer to payment of health care providers. Reimbursement is more applicable to something like an employer reimbursing an employee's out-of-pocket travel costs. The relationship of what it actually costs to provide care and how much a provider is paid is approximate at best, and payers (e.g., Medicare, Medicaid, HMOs, and PPOs) do not all pay the same amount for the same provider billing code. The accurate term is therefore payment, not reimbursement.

Reinstatement: When an insurance or managed care policy is reinstated after payment for delinquent premiums during a defined grace period. See Grace Period.

Reinsurance: Insurance purchased by a health plan to protect it against extremely high cost cases. See also Stop Loss.

Relative Value Units (RVUs): Numeric values used as multipliers in order to calculate the payment to a provider. It may be used for time units such as for anesthesia, but its most common use is the Resource-Based Relative Value Scale.

Relative Value Update Committee (RUC): A committee of the American Medical Association that reviews the weights placed on the relative value units in the Medicare RBRVS every 5 years, and CMS uses its recommendations to adjust payment rates.

Rental PPO: A PPO network owned and managed by a third party that rents access (and often services such as claims repricing) to a payer or health insurance company. Not the same as a risk-bearing PPO that combines a network with the insurance function.

Rescission: The retroactive rejection of an issued insurance policy "for cause." A common example is a policy issued to an individual who then incurs claims that the insurer believes to be related to a preexisting condition that the individual failed to disclose during the application process. The ACA places severe restrictions on this activity as a response to health insurers rescinding policies for failure to disclose a medical condition or past treatment that was irrelevant to the individual's current (and costly) medical condition.

Reserves: The amount of money that a health plan puts aside to cover health care costs. May apply to anticipated costs such as IBNRs, or may apply to money that the plan does not expect to have to use to pay for current medical claims, but keeps as a cushion against future adverse health care costs. Reserves can only be made up of admitted assets. They're also called statutory reserves because the accounting is done per Statutory Accounting Principles (SAP), not Generally Accepted Accounting Principles (GAAP). See also Admitted Assets, Non-Admitted Assets, and Risk-Based Capital.

Resource-Based Relative Value Scale (RBRVS): This is a relative value scale developed for the CMS for use by Medicare. The RBRVS assigns RVUs to each CPT code based on the level of skill and complexity required for that procedure, including office visits. Smaller RVUs are also assigned based on costs associated for the setting in which the care was provided, and for the cost of malpractice insurance. The RVUs are then added together and multiplied by a dollar amount conversion factor to calculate the actual payment. Commercial versions exist as well to cover procedures not typically used by Medicare.

Retail Clinic: A type of urgent care clinic, usually located in a drug store or grocery store, often staffed by nonphysician primary care providers who provide care for routine illnesses (sore throats, etc.), but are limited in what they can do. Often less expensive than a physician office visit, which also reduces primary care income. Also called a Convenient Care Clinic (CCC).

Retention: A term with two meanings depending on context. Retention is used to describe that portion of a health insurance premium that is for administrative costs, not medical claims costs. Retention may also be less commonly used as a synonym for persistency; see Persistency.

Retrospective Review: Reviewing health care costs after the care has been rendered. There are several forms of retrospective review. One form looks at individual claims for medical necessity, billing errors, or fraud. The other form looks at patterns of costs rather than individual cases.

RHIO: See Regional Health Information Organization.

Rider: An add-on to the core insurance or HMO policy; for example, coverage for dental or optometry services. Surprisingly, most regular drug benefits are provided via a rider and are not part of the main medical-surgical policy, while coverage for injectable drugs (including specialty pharmacy drugs) may be part of the main policy.

Risk Adjustment: A methodology to account for the health status of patients when predicting or explaining costs of health care for defined populations or for evaluating retrospectively the performance of providers who care for them. Also known as severity adjustment and acuity adjustment. Used by CMS in the payment of MA plans as well. Case mix is a related term.

Risk Contract: Also known as a Medicare risk contract; an informal term once common but now rarely used. A contract between a health plan and the CMS under Medicare Advantage under which the health plan is at risk for the cost of medical services to voluntary Medicare beneficiaries, and receives a monthly payment in return.

Risk Corridor: The upper and lower limits of financial risk for a health plan or provider that is at risk for medical costs. Both limits must exist to be considered a risk corridor. A risk corridor of 20%, for example, would mean that the plan or provider can have financial losses or gains of no more than 10% of the baseline payment.

Risk Management: A term that has at least two different but related meanings. As applied to the management of a health plan's operations, it refers to taking steps to reduce the risk of litigation or regulatory sanctions, for example, working with a member who has experienced a negative event in which the health plan may have had a role. The other use of the term applies to managing the overall risk of health care costs (i.e., managing the insurance risk).

Risk Pool (Capitation): In the case of capitation, it refers to a pool of funds that may be drawn against to cover medical costs, with any unused funds being paid to a provider or providers under capitation. See also Rule of Small Numbers.

Risk Pool (Premiums): In the case of premiums, a risk pool means a group of individuals (e.g., all individual subscribers, employees in a group, or Medicare enrollees) who all put in the same amount of money, thereby spreading out the risk even though some are healthier and some are sicker. Also called Pooling. Risk pools for premiums are also addressed specifically in the ACA.

Risk-Based Capital (RBC): A formula embodied in the Risk-Based Capital for Health Organizations Model Act, created under the auspices of the NAIC. RBC takes into account the fluctuating value of plan assets; the financial condition of plan affiliates; the risk that providers may not be able to provide contracted services; the risk that amounts due may not be recovered from reinsurance carriers; and general business risks (i.e., expenses may exceed income). The RBC formula gives credit for provider payment arrangements that reduce underwriting risk, including capitation as well as provider withholds, bonuses, contracted fee schedules, and aggregate cost arrangements. While not required in all states, RBC is the agreed-upon standard for an insurance department to determine whether or not a health plan meets minimum financial solvency requirements.

RUC: See Relative Value Update Committee.

Rule of Small Numbers: The notion that predictions that are based on large numbers are usually accurate, but as the numbers get smaller, chance plays a far more important role; eventually, chance completely outweighs predictability.

RVU: See Relative Value Unit.

Safe Harbor: The circumstances under which a hospital or other health care entity can provide something to a physician or other health entity and not violate the antikickback portion of the Stark laws and regulations. See Ethics in Patient Referrals Act.

Schedule of Benefits: The listing in the EOC of what is and what is not covered by a health plan, and under what circumstances.

SCHIP: See State Children's Health Insurance Program.

SCP: See Specialty Care Physician.

Second Opinion: An opinion obtained from another physician regarding the necessity for a treatment that has been recommended by another physician. May be required by some health plans for certain high-cost procedures. Once commonly used, now uncommon.

Section 1115 Waiver: See Medicaid Waiver.

Section 125 Plan: A section 125 plan allows employees to receive specified benefits, including health benefits, on a pretax basis. Section 125 plans enable employees to pay for health insurance premiums on a pretax basis, whether the insurance is provided by the employer or purchased directly in the individual market. See also Flexible Benefits Plan.

Self-Care: The series of steps "lay" individuals take to assess and treat an illness or injury, typically without the benefit of higher levels of training in the theory or science of medicine and with little or no consultation with a medical professional.

Self-Insured or Self-Funded Plan: A health plan where the risk for medical cost is assumed by the company rather than an insurance company or managed care plan. Self-funding makes up the majority of employer-sponsored coverage. Under ERISA, self-funded plans are exempt from most state laws and regulations such as premium taxes and mandatory benefits. They are also exempt from some, but not all, of the requirements created under the ACA. Self-funded plans typically contract with insurance companies or third-party administrators to administer the benefits. See also ASO.

Self-Referral: Self-referral means a physician refers a patient for a costly service or procedure that uses a facility or equipment in which the physician has a financial interest, thereby profiting by increasing its utilization above levels seen when a physician has no financial interest. In the earliest days of HMOs, self-referral meant a member saw a specialist without getting a PCP authorization, but that use of the term is archaic.

Sentinel Effect: The phenomenon that when it is known that behavior is being observed, that behavior changes, often in the direction the observer is looking for. Applies to the fact that utilization management systems and profiling systems often lead to reductions in utilization before much intervention even takes place, simply because the providers know that someone is watching.

Service Area: The geographic area that an HMO provides access to primary care. The service area is usually specifically designated by the regulators (state or federal), and the HMO is prohibited from marketing outside of the service area. It may be defined by county or by zip code. It is possible for an HMO to have more than one service area, and the service areas to either be contiguous (i.e., they actually border each other) or noncontiguous (i.e., there is a geographic gap between them).

Service Bureau: One definition refers to a weak form of IDS in which a hospital or other organization provides services to a physician's practice in return for a fair market price; it may also try to negotiate with managed care plans, but generally not considered to be an effective negotiating mechanism. The other definition is actually an older term used for Service Plans; see Service Plan.

Service-Level Agreement (SLA): The part of a contract specifying performance standards such as average speed to answer telephone calls, or percentage of claims processed within 14 days. A common part of an administrative services-only contract between a large self-funded employer group and a payer. It is also a common part of a contract between a payer and a company providing outsourced services.

Service-Level Percentage: A measurement in a call center of the specific percentage of calls to be answered within a given timeliness goal.

Service Plan: A health insurer that has direct contracts with providers but is not necessarily a managed care plan. The archetypal service plans are traditional (i.e., nonmanaged care) Blue Cross and Blue Shield plans, although a few non-Blue service plans do exist. The contract applies to direct billing of the plan by providers (rather than billing of the member), a provision for direct payment of the provider (rather than reimbursement of the member), a requirement that the provider accept the plan's determination of UCR and not balance bill the member in excess of that amount, and a range of other terms. The term has its roots in the formation as a prepaid service bureau created by the providers themselves, but providers no longer have any control over service plans. It is virtually indistinguishable from a health insurance company.

SFR: See Significant Financial Risk.

Shadow Pricing: The practice of setting premium rates at a level just below the competition's rates whether or not those rates can be justified. In other words, the premium rates could actually be lower, but to maximize profit the rates are raised to a level that will remain attractive but result in greater revenue. This practice is generally considered unethical and, in the case of community rating, possibly illegal.

Shared Savings: A payment methodology in traditional FFS Medicare in which an ACO is paid as usual, but an overall cost target is calculated for a cohort of individuals with high medical costs who are "assigned" to the ACO, and the ACO shares in a portion of any savings compared to that target. It also shares risk in that it must repay a portion of any costs in excess of the target. Unlike an HMO, there is no lock in, meaning those individuals are not required to use the ACO for care. Unlike other new payment models addressed in the ACA, CMS is specifically required to implement shared savings.

SHMO: See Social Health Maintenance Organization.

Shock Claim: Also referred to as a catastrophic claim. A shock claim is an extraordinarily expensive total cost of health care for an individual patient. Shock claims are taken into account by actuaries when they determine the trends for medical costs because shock claims have a certain amount of randomness to them, being they are infrequent and costly, unlike routine care that is predictable.

Shoe Box Effect: Refers to beneficiaries who save up their receipts of self-paid claims to file for reimbursement at a later time (i.e., saves them in a shoe box). Those receipts are sometimes lost, or the beneficiary never sends them in, in which case the insurance company doesn't have to reimburse the member.

SHOP: See Small Business Health Options Program.

Significant Financial Risk (SFR): A term used by the CMS that refers to the total amount of a physician's income at risk in a Medicare HMO. Such financial risk is considered "significant" when it exceeds a certain percentage of the total potential income that physician could receive under the payment program. SFR most commonly is defined as any physician incentive payment program that allows for a variation of more than 25% between the minimum and the maximum amount of potential payment.

Silent PPO: A term that is now rarely used since it is considered either unethical or illegal. A silent PPO was a form of rental PPO that a payer did not clearly identify by having the PPO's logo on the ID card somewhere, for example. A provider without a contract with the payer would bill full charges, but the rental PPO's payment terms would be applied to pay the claim, resulting in unanticipated reductions in booked revenue. See Rental PPO.

Silver Level of Benefits or Silver Plan: As defined in the ACA, a qualified health benefits plan with the actuarial equivalent or average of 30% cost-sharing, when accounting for deductibles, copayments, and coinsurance as applied to in-network services.

Single-Payer System: A health care system in which a single entity, usually the government, pays for health care services. This entity collects taxes and/or health care premiums, and pays for all health care costs, but is not involved in the delivery of health care. Canada uses a single payer system.

Single-Specialty Hospital: A hospital that provides services focusing on a single specialty such as cardiac procedures or orthopedics. Physicians often have an equity interest in them.

Skill-Based Routing: See Intelligent Call Routing.

SLA: See Service-Level Agreement.

Slice Business: A term referring to a large employer group offering more than one insurer or HMO to their employees.

Small Business Health Options Program (SHOP): That part of a state health insurance exchange that provides access to health insurance for small businesses as defined in the ACA.

SNP: See Special Needs Plan.

SOC: See Summary of Coverage.

Social Health Maintenance Organization (SHMO): A type of demonstration Medicare HMO that went beyond the medical care needs of its membership, to include their social and custodial needs as well. Authorized as demonstration projects under Medicare, SHMOs were always rare and Congress ended the Medicare demonstration project in 2008; however, four legacy SHMOs remain. See also Programs for All Inclusive Care for the Elderly.

Socialized Medicine: The government not only pays for health care as a single payer system, but also owns and operates significant portions of the health care provider system as well, for example, owning and operating the hospitals and paying the physicians based on a fixed schedule.

Solvency: Having sufficient assets to be eligible to transact insurance business and meet liabilities. For insurers and HMOs, solvency is based on Statutory Net Worth.

Special Limitations Clause: See Laser.

Special Needs Plan (SNP): A type of MA plan that may exclusively enroll, or enroll a disproportionate percentage of, special needs Medicare beneficiaries. Individuals with special needs include beneficiaries entitled to both Medicare and Medicaid ("dual eligibles"), institutionalized beneficiaries, and individuals with severe or disabling chronic conditions.

Specialty Care Physician (SCP): A physician who is not a PCP. SCP is not used as an acronym nearly as often as PCP.

Specialty Network Manager: A term used to describe a single specialist (or perhaps a specialist organization) that accepts capitation to manage a single specialty. Specialty services are supplied by many different specialty physicians, but the network manager has the responsibility for managing access and cost, and is at economic risk. A relatively uncommon model.

Specialty Pharmacy: This usually refers to biologics, which are injectable drugs, usually proteins created through recombinant DNA. May also apply more broadly to combine both biologics and special medical devices, either diagnostic or therapeutic.

Specialty Pharmacy Benefits Manager: Similar to a PBM, a specialty pharmacy benefits manager focuses on addressing costs in specialty pharmacy benefits. May be part of a PBM or a separate company.

Specialty Pharmacy Distributor (SPD): A company that distributes specialty pharmacy, from the manufacturer to the provider and/or directly to the patient, in order to address the unique distribution, storage, and utilization issues around these types of injectable drugs. May be part of a PBM or a separate company.

Staff Model HMO: A closed-panel HMO that employs providers directly and those providers see members in the HMO's own facilities.

Stark Laws or Stark Regulations: See Ethics in Patient Referrals Act.

Stars Program: A program developed by CMS for use in rating MA plans and that is also tied to a financial bonus program. At the time of publication, it is based on a combination of five categories that include 36 measures overall. That number will likely increase. The highest rating is five stars. An MA plan with fewer than 3 stars for 3 years in a row may not have its contract renewed.

State Children's Health Insurance Program (SCHIP or CHIP): A program created by the federal government to provide a "safety net" and preventive-care level of health coverage for children, funded through a combination of federal and state funds, and administered by the states in conformance with federal requirements.

State Insurance Exchange: A means for individuals and small employer groups to access coverage from a qualified health plan. An integral part of the ACA, a qualified health plan must offer at least one Silver and one Gold level of benefits if it participates in the exchange.

State Licensure: The license or certificate of authority issued by a state to a health plan that allows the plan to write business in the state. May be based on having a license in a different state; see State of Domicile.

State of Domicile: The state that an insurance company or payer is licensed in as its primary location. For example, a payer may have its state of domicile in Virginia, but also be licensed and doing business in Maryland and the District of Columbia. In many states, the insurance commissioner will defer primary regulation to the insurance department in the state of domicile as long as all minimum standards of the state are met.

Statutory Net Worth or Statutory Reserves: The total net worth of an insurer or HMO as defined under Statutory Accounting Principles (SAP) rules. For purposes of health insurance and managed care, net worth is what a health plan has in assets that can readily be converted into cash in the event of plan failure, such as unrestricted cash or investments, or other equally liquid and unencumbered assets. States have net worth minimum requirements for licensed health plans that vary with the size of the potential liability. States define the minimum statutory net worth an insurer or HMO must have before it's considered to be financially impaired. See also Non-Admitted Asset and Risk-Based Capital.

Stop Loss: A form of reinsurance that provides protection for medical expenses above a certain limit, generally on a year-by-year basis. This may apply to an entire health plan or to any single component. For example, the health plan may have stop-loss reinsurance for cases that exceed $100,000. After a case hits $100,000, the plan receives 80% of expenses in excess of $100,000 back from the reinsurance company for the rest of the year. Another example would be the plan providing a stop loss to participating physicians for referral expenses over $2,500. When a case exceeds that amount in a single year, the plan no longer deducts those costs from the physician's referral pool for the remainder of the year. Specific coverage refers to individual cases, while aggregate coverage refers to the total costs rather than a specific case.

Subacute Care Facility: A health facility that is a step down from an acute-care hospital. May be a nursing home or a facility that provides medical care but not surgical or emergency care. Some confine use of the term to services that are a step up from conventional skilled nursing facility intensity of services, adding RNs around the clock and intravenous medications.

Subordinated Note: Essentially a promise from a lender that a health plan can borrow money up to the limit of the note if it needs to in order to pay claims, and that the holder of the note will not be repaid before all claims costs are settled. This subordination allows the plan to claim it for purposes of net worth since it may be so used. A note or loan for which the plan must pay the note holder regardless of the plan's inability to pay claims is not subordinated and cannot be counted as part of its net worth.

Subrogation: The contractual right of a health plan to recover payments made to a member for health care costs after that member has received such payment for damages in a legal action. Subrogation is illegal in some states but required in others.

Subscriber: The individual or member who has the health plan coverage by virtue of being eligible on their own behalf, rather than as a dependent.

Summary of Coverage (SOC): A requirement under the ACA, the SOC is a brief and easily understandable standardized four- to six-page document summarizing benefits, requirements, and rights. Payers are required to provide before enrollment, each time a policy is renewed, and whenever there is a substantial change.

Surplus: The amount of money in a nonprofit insurer or HMO that equates to the margin or profit in a for-profit plan. Surplus may be used to boost reserves, to keep rate increases down, or to invest in operational improvements. Surplus may not be distributed like profits or dividends to shareholders or executives.

Suspend: When a claim is being processed but cannot be completed due to missing or inconsistent information, it is suspended until manual intervention allows it to be completed. Claims suspensions may also be called edits or pends. Although the terms *pend* and *suspend* are often used synonymously, some payers differentiate between claims that examiners place on hold (pends) and those that are placed on hold automatically by one or more systems edits (suspends).

Sutton's Law: "Go where the money is!" Attributed to the Depression-era bank robber Willy Sutton, who, when asked why he robbed banks, replied, "That's where the money is." Sutton denied ever saying it in a book he coauthored, *Where the Money Was* (Viking Press, 1976), but that if he'd been asked he probably would have said it. In any event, it is a good law to use when determining what needs attention in a managed care plan.

Switch or The Switch: The term applied to the computer that handles the telephone calling system. It's a charming holdover from the days when calls were routed by using a mechanical switchboard.

Taft-Hartley Plan: A type of association health plan under ERISA that is provided by a union to its members, usually using funds contributed by more than one employer or company. It is also eligible to be a type of MA plan.

TANF: See Temporary Assistance to Needy Families.

TAT: See Turnaround Time.

Tax Equity and Fiscal Responsibility Act of 1982 (TEFRA): One key provision of this Act prohibits employers and health plans from requiring full-time employees between the ages of 65 and 69 to use Medicare rather than the group health

plan. TEFRA also first enabled federally qualified HMOs to offer plans to Medicare beneficiaries if they met certain other requirements as well.

TCM: See Transitional Case Management.

TEFRA: See Tax Equity and Fiscal Responsibility Act of 1982.

Temporary Assistance to Needy Families (TANF): Administered by DHHS, TANF provides assistance and work opportunities to needy families by granting states the federal funds and wide flexibility to develop and implement their own welfare programs. TANF replaced the older term AFDC.

Termination Date: The day that health plan coverage is no longer in effect.

Third-Party Administrator (TPA): A firm that performs administrative functions such as claims processing, membership, and the like for a self-funded plan or a start-up managed care plan. See also Administrative Services Only.

Tiering: A term that applies to categorizing coverage into different tiers, or differential benefits. When used in pharmacy, Tier 1 drugs require lower copays than to Tier 2, Tier 3, and so forth. When applied to providers, members accessing Tier 1 providers likewise have less (or even no) cost-sharing than if they use a Tier 2 provider.

Time Loss Management: The application of managed care techniques to workers' compensation treatments for injuries or illnesses in order to reduce the amount of time lost on the job by the affected employee.

Total Capitation: See Global Capitation.

TPA: See Third-Party Administrator.

Transitional Case Management (TCM): Also called Transitional Care Management; a program to facilitate the discharge of a patient with complex medical problems or who is otherwise at risk for post-discharge complications and/or readmission. TCM programs function much like traditional case management, but focus on the immediate post-discharge period.

Transparency: Refers to making data available to the public. Also called pricing transparency when such data is the price for services from different providers of care.

Treaty: A reinsurance agreement between the reinsured company and the reinsurer, usually for 1 year or longer, which stipulates the technical particulars applicable to the reinsurance of some class or classes of business.

Triage: In health plans, this refers to the process of sorting out requests for services by members into those who need to be seen right away, those who can wait a little while, and those whose problems can be handled with advice over the phone. The origins of this term are grizzly: The process of sorting out wounded soldiers into those who need treatment immediately, those who can wait, and those who are too severely injured to even try and save.

TRICARE: The Department of Defense's worldwide managed health care program. TRICARE was initiated in 1995, integrating health care services provided in the direct care system of military hospitals and clinics with services purchased from civilian providers for anybody eligible for coverage (e.g., retirees and dependents). There are various different TRICARE benefits programs. See also Military Health System. The non-MTF portion of TRICARE is administered by private managed care companies in three regions in the United States.

Triple Option: The offering of an HMO, a PPO, and a traditional insurance plan by one carrier.

TrOOP: See below.

True-Out-of-Pocket Cost (TrOOP): The full amount of out-of-pocket costs paid by an individual before any annual limits on out-of-pocket costs apply. It is a term used for MA plans by regulation, and may be used for commercial plans.

Turnaround Time (TAT): The amount of time it takes a health plan to process and pay a claim from the time it arrives.

UB-04: See Universal Billing Form 04.

UB-92: No longer in use. See CMS-1450 and Universal Billing Form 04 (UB-04).

UCR: See Usual, Customary, or Reasonable.

UM: See Utilization Management.

Unbundling: The practice of a provider billing for multiple components of service that were previously included in a single fee. For example, if dressings and instruments were included in a fee for a minor procedure, the fee for the procedure remains the same, but there are now additional charges for the dressings and instruments.

Uncompensated Care: Health care services that are provided but not paid for by the patient or by insurance. These uncompensated costs are partly shifted to higher prices to private insurers, absorbed in part by health care providers, and partly to the federal government by calculating payments under Medicare, which will diminish greatly in 2014 under provisions of the ACA.

Underwriting: In one definition, this refers to bearing the risk for something (i.e., a policy is underwritten by an insurance company). In another definition, this refers to the analysis of a group that is done to determine rates and benefits, or to determine whether the group should be offered coverage at all. A related definition refers to health screening of each individual applicant for insurance and refusing to provide coverage for preexisting conditions.

Underwriting Margin: The amount of money left over, or lost, after medical costs are subtracted from premium income. It does not include the cost of operations such as administrative costs and sales and marketing, which makes up the operating margin. See also Operating Margin.

Universal Billing Form 04 (UB-04): The paper form that institutions must use if they submit a paper claim to Medicare. Its use is also required by commercial payers for paper claims. The UB-04 replaced the paper UB-92 from prior years. The more commonly used and interchangeable name is the CMS-1450.

Universal Provider Identification Number (UPIN): An identification number once issued by CMS for use in billing Medicare. The UPIN was replaced by the NPI in 2007 and is no longer in use. See NPI.

Upcoding: The practice of a provider billing for a procedure that pays better than the service actually performed. For example, an office visit that would normally be paid at $45 is coded as one that is paid at $75.

UPIN: See Universal Provider Identification Number.

UR: See Utilization Review.

URAC: A not-for-profit organization that performs reviews on external utilization review agencies (free-standing companies, utilization management departments of insurance companies, or utilization management departments of managed care plans). Its primary focus is payers, though they have expanded their accreditation activities; for example, accrediting health-related websites. States often require certification by URAC or another accreditation organization to operate. URAC once stood for the Utilization Review Accreditation Commission, but now is known only as URAC. URAC was also once known as the American Accreditation HealthCare Commission (AAHC), but that name is no longer used either.

URO: See Utilization Review Organization.

Usual, Customary, or Reasonable (UCR): A method of profiling prevailing fees in an area and reimbursing providers on the basis of that profile. One archaic method is to average all fees and choose the 80th or 90th percentile. Payers typically use another method to determine what is reasonable. Sometimes this term is used synonymously with a fee allowance schedule when that schedule is set relatively high.

Utilization Management (UM): The combined activities of a payer or IDS to reduce the cost of medical utilization by decreasing the amount of unnecessary utilization and by managing the cost of utilization. It encompasses the three types of utilization review: prospective review, concurrent review, and retrospective review. It also includes other activities such as case management.

Utilization Review (UR): An older term for UM, and somewhat less encompassing of all UM activities. See Utilization Management.

Utilization Review Organization (URO): A free-standing organization that does nothing but UR, usually on a remote basis, using the telephone and paper correspondence. It may be independent, or may be part of another company such as an insurance company that sells UR services on a stand-alone basis.

Value-Based Insurance Benefits Design (VBID, VBBD, or VBD): A benefits design that allows for improved coverage under certain conditions. For example, a member with congestive heart failure would be able to obtain certain drugs without having to pay a copay or coinsurance. Unlike benefits waiver, value-based benefits design is applied to all members of the group that has such a design, not on a case-by-case basis.

Value-Based Payment (VBP): Required under the ACA, VBP refers to modifications of payments to hospitals by CMS based on several factors such as Never Events (see that term), efficiency, consumer satisfaction, and other metrics.

VBID, VBD or VBBD: See above.

Waste, Fraud, and Abuse: See Fraud, Waste, and Abuse. Seriously, the order of these terms has changed at the federal level. Why it changed is a mystery.

Workgroup for Electronic Data Interchange (WEDI): A group that provides input on electronic transaction standards under HIPAA.

Workers' Compensation: A form of social insurance provided through property-casualty insurers. Workers' compensation provides medical benefits and replacement of lost wages that result from injuries or illnesses that arise from the workplace; in turn, the employee cannot normally sue the employer unless true negligence exists. Workers' compensation has undergone dramatic increases in cost as group health has shifted into managed care, resulting in carriers adopting managed care approaches. Workers' compensation is often heavily regulated under state laws that are significantly different than those used for group health insurance, and is often the subject of intense negotiation between management and organized labor. See also Time Loss Management.

Wraparound Plan: Commonly used to refer to insurance or health plan coverage for copays and deductibles that are not covered under a member's base plan. MediGap is a form of wraparound, and they exist for commercial plans as well.

Zero Down: The practice of a medical group or provider system distributing the entire capital surplus in a health plan (except for surplus required for statutory reserves) or the group to the members of the group, rather than retaining any capital or reinvesting it in the group or plan.

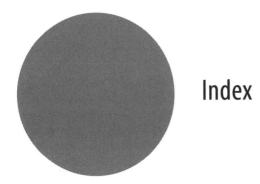

Index

Page numbers followed by *f* and *t* indicate figures and tables.

D